Critical Care
NURSING

A Holistic Approach

Carolyn M. Hudak, RN, PHD
Nurse Practitioner
Denver, Colorado

Barbara M. Gallo, RN, MS, CNAA
Assistant Professor
University of Hartford
School of Education, Nursing
   and Health Professions
Division of Nursing
Hartford, Connecticut

Special Editor
Julie J. Benz, RN, MS
Critical Care Clinical Nurse Specialist
Lutheran Medical Center
Denver, Colorado

Sixth Edition

Critical Care
NURSING

A Holistic Approach

J. B. Lippincott Company
Philadelphia

Coordinating Editorial Assistant: Patty L. Shear
Project Editor: Amy P. Jirsa
Indexer: Betty Herr Hallinger
Design Coordinator: Kathy Kelley-Luedtke
Interior Design: Anne O'Donnell
Production Manager: Helen Ewan
Production Coordinator: Maura C. Murphy
Compositor: Circle Graphics
Printer/Binder: Courier Book Company/Westford

6th Edition

6 5 4 3 2 1

Library of Congress Cataloging in Publications Data

Critical care nursing : a holistic approach / [edited by] Carolyn M.
   Hudak, Barbara M. Gallo ; special editor, Julie J. Benz. —6th ed.
       p.   cm.
   Includes bibliographical references and index.
   ISBN 0-397-54985-7
   1. Intensive care nursing.   2. Holistic medicine.   I. Hudak,
Carolyn M.   II. Gallo, Barbara M.   III. Benz, Julie J.
   [DNLM: 1. Critical Care—nurses' instruction.   2. Holistic Health—
nurses' instruction.   WY 154 C9328   1994]
RT120.I5C744   1994
610.73'61—dc20
DNLM/DLC
for Library of Congress   93-11419
                                                            CIP

To Thelma "Skip" Lohr, my mentor, my friend, and one of the most influential role models in my life.

Carolyn

To my sister Carole "Sammie" Jaehn, friend, supporter, and companion through tears and laughter.

Bobbie

CONTRIBUTING AUTHORS

Patricia Barry, RN, PHD, CS
Psychotherapist and Consultant in Private Practice
Clinical Faculty, University of Connecticut School of Nursing
and Yale University School of Nursing
Hartford, Connecticut
    Effects of the Critical Care Unit on the Nurse

Julie J. Benz, RN, MS
Critical Care Clinical Nurse Specialist
Lutheran Medical Center
Denver, Colorado
    Heart Failure
    Acute Myocardial Infarction
    Anatomy and Physiology of the Respiratory System
    Assessment: Respiratory System
    Pharmacologic Agents
    Common Pulmonary Disorders
    Adult Respiratory Distress Syndrome

Helen C. Busby, RN, BSN, CCRN
Critical Care Practitioner
Scripps Memorial Hospital
Chula Vista, California
    Assessment: Gastrointestinal System
    Management Modalities: Gastrointestinal System
    Acute Gastrointestinal Bleeding
    Hepatic Disorders

Karen D. Busch, RN, PHD
Assistant Professor
Intercollegiate Center for Nursing Education
Spokane, Washington
    Psychosocial Concepts and the Patient's Experience with
      Critical Illness
    Caring for the Patient's Family
    Patient and Family Teaching

Jacquelyn M. Clement, RN, PHD
Associate Professor, School of Nursing
Southern Illinois University at Edwardsville
Edwardsville, Illinois
    The Dynamics of Touch in Patient Care
    The Critically Ill Elderly Patient
    Assessment: Renal System
    Acute Renal Failure
    Diabetic Emergencies

Sarah Dillian Cohn, MSN, JD
Associate Counsel
Yale-New Haven Hospital
New Haven, Connecticut
    Applied Legal Principles

Lane D. Craddock, MD, FACP, FACC
Clinical Professor of Medicine
University of Colorado Health Sciences Center
Attending Physician, Cardiology
Rose Medical Center
Denver, Colorado
    Cardiopulmonary Resuscitation

Crystal A. Cranor, RN, BSN, CCRN
Staff Nurse, Coronary Intensive Care Unit
Loma Linda University Medical Center
Loma Linda, California
    Bioethical Issues in Critical Care

Anda Craven, RN, MS, CCRN
Assistant Professor of Nursing
Oregon Institute of Technology
Klamath Falls, Oregon
    Trauma

A. Gail Curry-Kane, RN, BS, ICP
Nurse Epidemiologist, Infection Control Specialist
Consultant to Hospital Shared Services of Denver, Colorado
Consultant to Department of Corrections, Colorado Prison
Systems
Immune System-Compromising Conditions

Mary de Meneses, RN, EDD
Associate Professor of Nursing
Southern Illinois University at Edwardsville
Edwardsville, Illinois
The Critically Ill Elderly Patient
Assessment: Renal System
Acute Renal Failure
Diabetic Emergencies

Martha M. Foley, RN, BSN, CSPI
Staff Nurse
Rocky Mountain Poison Center
Denver, Colorado
Drug Overdose and Poisoning

Marsha D. M. Fowler, PHD, MDIV, MS, RN
Professor, School of Nursing and Graduate School
of Theology
Director, Parish Nursing Clinical Specialization
Azuza Pacific University
Intern, Westminster Presbyterian
Church, Temple City, California
Fellow, W. K. Kellogg Foundation
Bioethical Issues in Critical Care

Barbara F. Fuller, RN, PHD
Professor of Nursing
School of Nursing
University of Colorado
Denver, Colorado
Anatomy and Physiology of Renal System
Anatomy and Physiology of Gastrointestinal System
Anatomy and Physiology of Endocrine System

Teresa Heise Halloran, RN, MSN, CCRN
Manager, Neonatal ICU
St. John's Mercy Medical Center and Critical Care Consultant
for Clinical Specialists in Critical Care, Inc.
St. Louis, Missouri
Common Endocrine Emergencies

Linda F. Hellstedt, RN, MSN, CCRN
Clinical Nurse Specialist
Department of Cardiac Nursing
Northwestern Memorial Hospital
Chicago, Illinois
Electrocardiographic Monitoring
Dysrhythmias and Conduction Disturbances
Effects of Serum Electrolytes on the Electrocardiogram

Eileen Brent Hemman, RN, MSN, CCRN
Director of Nursing Education
Fairbanks, Alaska
Bronchial Hygiene
Artificial Airways
Chest Tubes
Ventilatory Support

Elisa J. Ignatius
Freelance Writer and Editor
Mill Valley, California
Percutaneous Transluminal Coronary Angioplasty and
Percutaneous Balloon Valvuloplasty

Diane Korte-Schwind, RN, MSN
Instructor, Southern Illinois University at Edwardsville
and Staff Nurse, Barnes Hospital
St. Louis, Missouri
Assessment: Renal System

Barbara Krumbach, RN, MS, CCRN
Clinical Educator, Surgical ICU and Burn Unit
University Hospital
University of Colorado Health Sciences Center
Denver, Colorado
Commonly Used Antiarrhythmic Agents and Cardioversion
Cardiopulmonary Resuscitation

Joanne M. Krumberger, RN, MSN, CCRN
Critical Care Clinical Nurse Specialist
Veterans Affairs Medical Center
Milwaukee, Wisconsin
Assessment: Gastrointestinal System
Management Modalities: Gastrointestinal System
Acute Gastrointestinal Bleeding
Hepatic Disorders
Acute Pancreatitis

Mary Kay Knight Macheca, RN, MSN(R), CDE
Diabetes Clinical Nurse Specialist
Barnes Hospital at Washington University Medical Center
St. Louis, Missouri
Diabetic Emergencies

Margaret Marcinek, RN, MSN, EDD
Professor and Chair
California University of Pennsylvania
California, Pennsylvania
Burns

Barbara C. Martin, RNC, EDD
Assistant Professor of Nursing
Southern Illinois University at Edwardsville
Edwardsville, Illinois
The Critically Ill Elderly Patient

Joan D. Mersch, RN, MS
Nurse Manager, CCU/CSU
Stanford University Hospital
Stanford, California
Auscultation of the Heart
Hemodynamic Monitoring

Marilynn Mitchell, RN, MSN, CNRN
Assistant Professor
Clarkson College
Omaha, Nebraska
Anatomy and Physiology of the Nervous System
Common Neurological Disorders
Spinal Cord Injury

Kathleen S. Oman, RN, MS
Clinical Nurse Specialist
Surgery/Trauma Service
Denver General Hospital
Denver, Colorado
Septic Shock

Linda K. Ottoboni, RN, MS, CCRN
Clinical Nurse Specialist
Cardiac Electrophysiology & Arrhythmia Service
Stanford University Hospital
Stanford, California
Cardiac Pacing

Michele A. Parker, RN
Clinical Research Coordinator, Medical Intensive Care Area
Division of Nursing
Northwestern Memorial Hospital
Chicago, Illinois
Cardiac Enzyme Studies
Cardiovascular Diagnostic Procedures

Suzanne M. Provenzano, RN, BSN, CCRN, CNRN
Staff Nurse, Critical Care
St. Joseph Hospital
Tacoma, Washington
Assessment: Nervous System
Head Injury

Karen Robbins, RN, MS, CNN
Nephrology Nurse Consultant
West Hartford, Connecticut
Renal Transplantation

Carlena Robison
Clinical Consultant
Advanced Cardiovascular Systems
Pottstown, Pennsylvania
Percutaneous Transluminal Coronary Angioplasty and
Percutaneous Balloon Valvuloplasty

Lois Schick, RN, MBA, MNA, CPAN
Clinical Director SurgiCare One
Saint Joseph Hospital
Denver, Colorado
Recovery From Anesthesia

William A. Seiffert, MD
Internal Medicine
West Nebraska General Hospital
Scottsbluff, Nebraska
Assessment: Gastrointestinal System
Management Modalities: Gastrointestinal System
Acute Gastrointestinal Bleeding
Hepatic Disorders

Julie A. Shinn, RN, MA, FAAN, CCRN
Cardiovascular Clinical Nurse Specialist
Stanford University Hospital
Stanford, California
Intraaortic Balloon Pump Counterpulsation and Other
Ventricular Assist Devices
Disseminated Intravascular Coagulation

Janice S. Smith, RN, MS
Professor of Nursing
Front Range Community College and University of Phoenix,
Colorado Campus
Denver, Colorado
Psychosocial Impact of the Critical Care Environment

Rae Nadine Smith, RN, MS
Clinical Specialist
Medical Communicators & Associates
Salt Lake City, Utah
Autologous Blood Transfusion
Management Modalities: Nervous System

Marianne Stewart, RN, MSN, CCRN
Associate Degree Nursing Instructor
Antelope Valley College
Staff Nurse ICU/CCU
Antelope Valley Hospital Medical Center
Lancaster, California
Bioethical Issues in Critical Care

Mary Swanson, RN, MBA, CNN, CPTC, CCTC
Supervisor of Organ Procurement and Preservation
Hartford Transplant Center
Hartford, Connecticut
Renal Transplantation

Roslyn Sykes, RN, PHD
Associate Professor
School of Nursing Southern Illinois
University at Edwardsville
Edwardsville, Illinois
The Critically Ill Elderly Patient
The Dynamics of Touch in Patient Care

Barbara L. Weber, RN, MS, CVNS, CCRN
Critical Care Educator
Porter Memorial Hospital
Denver, Colorado
    Cardiac Surgery and Heart Transplantation

Kathleen M. Wruk, RN, MHS
Managing Director
Rocky Mountain Poison Center
Denver, Colorado
    Drug Overdose and Poisoning

Mary Zorzanello, RN, MSN, CNN
Clinical Nurse Specialist
Hemodialysis Unit
Yale-New Haven Hospital
New Haven, Connecticut
    Management Modalities: Renal System
    Acute Renal Failure

Sally Zouras-Meyerhofer, RN, BSN
Clinical Marketing Manager
Peripheral Systems Group, A Division of Advanced
Cardiovascular Systems, Inc.
Sacramento, California
    Percutaneous Transluminal Coronary Angioplasty
        and Percutaneous Balloon Valvuloplasty

PREFACE

This sixth edition of CRITICAL CARE NURSING: A HOLISTIC APPROACH continues to maintain its primary emphasis on the patient and the nurse within a framework that embraces the philosophy of holism. Our commitment to that philosophy however, did not preclude a major reorganization with this edition.

The section on Professional Practice Issues in the Critical Care Unit has been moved to the front of the book at the suggestion of instructors who tell us they prefer to teach content on ethical issues and legal principles at the beginning of a critical care course.

Chapters having to do with Assessment, Management Modalities, and Specific Disorders have been organized around similar outlines to increase ease of use and readability. In particular, the units on Cardiovascular, Respiratory, Renal, and Nervous Systems have been heavily reorganized. We have worked to eliminate repetition of content except in those areas where, although some general information is common, the specifics of drug use and practice protocols may differ, such as in the case of heart transplantation versus renal transplantation. We chose to tolerate some degree of information overlap for the sake of presenting the chapter as a complete package rather than requiring the student or practitioner to thumb back and forth between related chapters.

Three new chapters have been added to this edition: Septic Shock, Acute Pancreatitis, and Common Endocrine Emergencies. Nursing care plans accompany this new content and have been added to some of the existing content for a total of 51 care plans. Also new to this edition is the incorporation of case studies to provide the student with a foundation from which to apply the nursing care plan, synthesize the data, and make the nursing care plan more meaningful to the practice setting. Boxed displays pertaining to clinical research that impacts nursing practice and nursing decision making have been added to the chapters dealing with specific disease conditions. Also in this edition, references have been incorporated into the text and provide another source of learning for the student or practitioner.

The Self Study Guide that has accompanied this text for the past five editions has been dropped in favor of adding study questions at the end of each chapter to facilitate student learning and provide immediate feedback on knowledge of chapter content. A separate INSTRUCTOR's MANUAL has been developed for use with this sixth edition of the text.

Also new to this edition of the textbook is a companion book, HANDBOOK OF CRITICAL CARE NURSING, by Carolyn Hudak and Barbara Gallo, intended to serve as a quick and useful reference in the clinical setting. Drug information, troubleshooting guidelines, summary tables, symptomatology, patient teaching guides, laboratory values, assessment criteria, and nursing care plans are included in the HANDBOOK.

We are grateful that this text has withstood the challenges of time and the phenomenal advances that have occurred in the critical care field and in nursing practice over the past 20 years. We are also grateful for the comments and suggestions from those who have used the book. It has been our intent in this edition to provide you with a text geared to the level of sophistication of today's nurse, encompassing the depth and breadth of information that the patient of the 90s requires.

Carolyn M. Hudak, PHD, RN
Barbara M. Gallo, MS, RN

ACKNOWLEDGMENTS

From the first edition of this book back in the early 70s to this sixth edition, we have had the privilege of working with some very special people at the J. B. Lippincott Company.

Diana Intenzo edited several previous editions of our book and has since assumed the position of Vice President/Publisher of Nursing Books for Lippincott. She helped get this latest edition off the ground and her quick wit and wonderful sense of humor made the toughest situations seem manageable.

Patty L. Shear, Editorial Assistant, Nursing Division has been of immeasurable help in all those big and little things that crop up during the course of manuscript preparation. She always had the answer or got the job done.

Doris Wray, Administrative Assistant, Nursing Division also was involved in a past edition of this book and remains a friend and valuable resource.

Many of our difficult research questions were answered through the skillful work of Joyce L. Fedeczko, MALS, Medical Librarian for Midwestern University in Downers Grove, Illinois. We are grateful for her assistance and expertise. Also, thank you to Celia Conrad, Librarian at the Burgdorf Health Library Consortium, Hartford, Connecticut, for her assistance and support.

In Chapter 46, "Drug Overdose and Poisoning," Dr. Barry Rumack from the Rocky Mountain Poison Center in Denver, Colorado provided continual updating of information on the poisoned patient and we are grateful for his involvement.

We would also like to acknowledge the work of Julie J. Benz, RN, MS, Critical Care Clinical Nurse Specialist, Lutheran Medical Center, Denver, Colorado, who coordinated much of the rewriting of the unit on the Respiratory System and also reviewed every Nursing Care Plan to assure accuracy, consistency, and relevance to critical care nursing practice.

CONTENTS

PART I

The Concept of Holism Applied to Critical Care Nursing Practice

BEHAVIORAL OBJECTIVES

Based on the content in this chapter, the reader should be able to:

1. List four issues influencing current critical care nursing practice.
2. Define nursing diagnoses.
3. Outline the steps of the nursing process in critical care nursing practice.
4. Briefly describe how the principles inherent in Maslow's hierarchy of human needs can serve as a holistic framework for critical care nursing.
5. Describe the concept of adaptation.
6. Describe three specific nursing actions that foster adaptive functioning in the critically ill patient.

CHAPTER 1

Integrating Nursing Process and Nursing Diagnoses Within a Holistic Framework

Hudak: Critical Care Nursing:
A Holistic Approach, 6th ed. © 1994
J. B. Lippincott Company.

Description

Today more than ever the critical care nurse must have a base of knowledge that facilitates the ability to look at a wide range of issues as well as highly defined and specific pieces of information. Today's practitioner must also be as self-actualized as possible—physically, emotionally, and spiritually—in order to meet the challenges of caring for those who are critically ill. Increasingly ill patients, increasingly complex technology, an increasingly older population, ethical dilemmas, cost containment pressures, and changes in service delivery systems including nursing are some of the current issues facing critical care nurses.

Critical care nursing requires an ability to deal with crucial situations with a rapidity and precision not usually necessary in other health care settings. It requires adeptness at integrating information, making judgments, and establishing priorities, because when illness strikes one body system, other systems become involved in the effort to cope with disequilibrium. The essence of critical care nursing lies not in special environments nor amid special equipment but in a decision-making process based on a sound understanding of physiological and psychological entities.

Integrating Nursing Process and Nursing Diagnoses in Critical Care

Nursing Diagnoses

Nursing diagnoses are defined by the North American Nursing Diagnosis Association (NANDA) as clinical judgments "reflecting individual, family or community responses to actual or potential health problems/life processes."[1] They address physiological, psychological, and sociological alterations in health and involve interventions that the nurse can initiate independently to prevent, reduce, or resolve the problem. Nursing diagnoses serve as a classification system that organizes the nursing care plan. They are identified by using the nursing process.

Steps of the Nursing Process

The nursing process serves as a systematic framework within which the nurse seeks information, responds to clinical cues, and identifies and responds to issues affecting the patient's health. It begins with the collection of two types of information: subjective data (including all information obtained by history and interview) and objective data (including physical examination, laboratory values, and diagnostic tests). Clinical judgments are made after analysis of all available information. These judgments serve as the basis for formulating nursing diagnoses. The next steps in the process are to determine expected outcomes and nursing interventions. Interventions should be specific enough to guide care, and outcomes should clearly describe the patient behavior that will indicate that the goal has been achieved.

Expected outcomes are used to evaluate the effectiveness of the interventions. If the interventions are effective and restore equilibrium, the problem is resolved and the process is complete. If not, the process is repeated, beginning with data collection and continuing with analyzing data, formulating nursing diagnoses, further planning, implementing the plan, and reevaluating it based on patient outcomes (Table 1–1).

Steps in the Nursing Process:

- Collect information.
- Determine actual or potential nursing diagnoses.
- Identify outcomes which are measureable and reflect the patient's response.
- Develop individualized interventions aimed at achieving outcomes.
- Evaluate progress toward meeting outcomes.
- Adjust care plan based on evaluation by using the nursing process.

For example, the initial assessment of a patient with acute pancreatitis indicates that he has been experiencing pain. The nurse performs a pain assessment, noting onset, duration, intensity, location, and what relieves or worsens the pain. The nurse asks the patient to rate the pain using a pain rating scale. Additional assessment includes taking the blood pressure, heart rate, and respiratory rate, and observing for other signs that may accompany pain, such as restlessness, anxiety, and guarding. After analyzing these findings, the nurse formulates the following **nursing diagnosis**:

Pain: related to interruption of blood supply to the pancreas; edema and distention of the pancreas; peritoneal irritation from activated pancreatic exocrine enzymes.

The **expected outcome** is that the patient reports that the pain is within tolerable limits. **Interventions** include working with the patient to determine how to help reduce the pain. In this situation it involves administering analgesia (with physician orders), establishing a medication schedule, positioning the patient in a side lying position with knees flexed, and later giving mouth care. The nurse **evaluates** the effectiveness of these interventions by reassessing the patient's pain. If the outcome has not been

TABLE 1–1
Steps of the Nursing Process

Assessment:	Data are collected.
Diagnosis:	Data are analyzed to identify patient problems/nursing diagnoses.
Planning:	A plan of action is developed.
Implementation:	The plan is put into action.
Evaluation:	The results of implementation are evaluated.

met, the process of reassessment, further planning, intervention, and reevaluation continues until the outcome is met.

Holistic Framework

Hierarchy of Human Needs

The patient admitted to a critical care unit needs excellent care directed not only at the pathophysiological problems but also at the psychosocial, environmental, and family issues that become intimately intertwined with the physical illness. Within the framework of the nursing process, the concepts of the hierarchy of human needs, adaptation, and patient advocacy assume special relevance to critical care nursing.

Human beings seek to preserve their lives by directing all their energies toward the most basic unmet needs. For example, all the compensatory mechanisms of a person with inadequate cardiac output work to maintain the circulation of oxygen, thus meeting the most basic requirement for life. In this situation, energy is directed away from subsystems such as the gastrointestinal, skin, and kidney functions. This phenomenon can be described as *physiological amputation*. Energy is directed away from less critical functions in order to help the organism through the physiological crisis. If the crisis is not stabilized, the subsystems eventually move from a compensatory state (physiological amputation) to a decompensatory state.

Fundamental needs, although closely interrelated, are arranged in order of dominance. The most basic needs are physiological, aimed at self-preservation. Upper-level needs are security, belonging, self-esteem, and self-actualization.

The need for a sense of security to allay anxiety is always present, but it is not the most basic need at, for example, the time of inadequate cardiac output. Later, when needs for air, cellular nutrition, and elimination are met, the efforts of the patient are directed toward seeking security, a sense of belonging, and self-esteem (Fig. 1–1).

Although each of us has physiological and psychological mechanisms that compensate for disequilibrium, there are situations in which we cannot adapt without outside

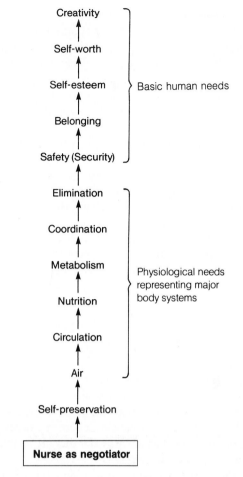

FIGURE 1–1
Hierarchy of human needs for critical care nursing, based on Maslow's theory.

intervention. It is in these situations that the critical care nurse becomes the patient's advocate and fosters adaptation.

Promoting Adaptation

The patient's attempts to cope with the environment include *avoidance*, in which one flees from the situation; *counteraction*, in which body defenses try to destroy the stressor, often at the expense of other systems; and *adaptation*, in which one seeks to establish a compatible response to the stress and still retain a steady state.

Although all mechanisms foster self-preservation, nursing intervention is aimed at adaptation. By fostering responses that encourage both physiologically and emotionally useful functioning, nurses enhance adaptation and aid the patient in reducing stress and conserving energy. Conversely, when nursing intervention or lack of it does not foster adaptation, the patient's energy is wasted, and a state of increased tension exists; that is, the patient has a diminished capacity to deal with a changing situation.

Thus, stress is increased when a patient's energy is devoted to maladaptive functioning that perpetuates the disequilibrium, and stress is minimized when the patient expends energy that fosters adaptation to the disequilibrium (see Figure 2–1).

An example of maladaptation versus adaptation is seen in a patient with restrictive lung disease who develops a lung infection resulting in $\uparrow$ Pco_2 and $\downarrow$ Po_2. This patient cannot compensate because of his restrictive lung disease; thus, his established pattern of breathing is maladaptive, perpetuating the problem of gas exchange. Adaptive nursing intervention involves helping the patient breathe more deeply and fostering the drainage of secretion either by having him do breathing exercises or by using mechanical aids. Although the energy is still expended, it is spent usefully. This concept of minimizing tension and stress is consistent with the ultimate goal of health care: to restore the person to a steady state with minimal stress to the rest of the body.

The Critical Care Nurse As Advocate

Fostering adaptive functioning means that the nurse negotiates for the patient. Because critically ill patients often cannot effectively cope with both the physiological problem and the rest of the environment, it becomes necessary for the nurse to do for the patients what they are unable to do for themselves so that energy is conserved. As patient advocate, the nurse must refrain from adding burdens that increase the patient's need to interact when such interaction does not foster adaptation. For example, patient energy spent in fearful suspense about the equipment nearby is not as helpful as energy spent in asking about it and then listening to a reply. Likewise, energy expended in persistently requesting a loved one to be present may not be as helpful as energy spent interacting with that person.

Fostering security in the critically ill patient involves decreasing both physiological and emotional vulnerability. The feeling of security is lost or at least significantly decreased whenever there is a decrease in control of body functions. Loss of control may vary from fatigue and weakness to paralysis. It may result from pathology, the environment (eg, restraint by IV tubing or machinery), or both; from fatigue and sleeplessness caused by physical discomfort; or from physiological fatigue (eg, dyspnea and sensory overload). Regardless of the decrease or loss of control, the nurse intervenes to increase the patient's feeling of safety. This is accomplished by using technical skill, tools, medication, and interaction; by providing assisted breathing with a respirator; by encouraging breathing exercises; or by staying with the patient during a time of anxiety or loneliness. Recognizing a patient's safety needs is an important element in the holistic approach to patient care. In addition, it is this very consideration of the "whole" patient that allows nurses to establish priorities as patient negotiators.

Negotiating for the patient is not without its hazards. This kind of caring and giving requires our energies in place of those that the patient is temporarily lacking. Therefore, to maintain our own emotional reserves, we also need to support one another as colleagues in the critical care unit and to enhance one another's feelings of belonging and self-esteem. Other hazards involve speaking on behalf of the patient, often as a minority voice and in the face of administrative, physician, or peer pressure. Acting as patient advocate means experiencing the joy of patients who recover as well as the sadness and anger of those who do not.

REFERENCES

1. Carroll-Johnson RM: Reflections on the ninth biennial conference. Nurs Diagn 1(2):50, 1990

BIBLIOGRAPHY

Carpenito LJ: Nursing Diagnosis Application to Clinical Practice. Philadelphia, JB Lippincott, 1992
Weber G: Making nursing diagnosis work for you and your client. Nurs Health Care 12(8):424–430, 1991

STUDY QUESTIONS

1. Mrs. N requests her pain medication. The nurse acknowledges this request and administers the medication. Which steps of the nursing process are *not* included in this scenario?

   1. nursing diagnosis identified
   2. information collected
   3. action taken
   4. outcome evaluated

   a. 1 & 3   b. 3 & 4   c. 2 & 3   d. 1, 2, & 4

2. Which of the following actions describe nursing efforts aimed at fostering patient/family adaptation?

    1. two family members may visit for five minutes every hour
    2. a plan is made in which the nurse will call the family with patient progress at 10:30
    3. the unit is short-staffed and has had several crises resulting in a temporary hold on visiting
    4. a family is asked to withhold visiting because the patient is sound asleep

        a. all of the above b. 1 & 2 c. 3 & 4 d. 2 & 4

3. Mrs. N is in the process of being weaned from the respirator. Which of the following actions are probably most in keeping with the principles of Maslow's hierarchy of human needs?

    1. remove indwelling catheter
    2. introduce new primary nurse
    3. focus on increasing respiratory reserves
    4. have consistent staff present during time off respirator

        a. 1 & 2 b. 2 & 4 c. 2 & 3 d. 3 & 4

CHAPTER 2

Psychosocial Concepts and the Patient's Experience With Critical Illness

BEHAVIORAL OBJECTIVES

Based on the content in this chapter, the reader should be able to:

1. Describe the relationship between stress and anxiety.
2. List the behavioral and physiological symptoms of anxiety.
3. Identify and describe methods to increase patients' sense of control and reduce their sense of helplessness.
4. Describe three methods to help patients cope with anxiety.
5. Identify and describe the stages of grieving and describe nursing interventions for each stage.
6. Discuss a nursing intervention that fosters the ability of patients to draw strength from their personal spirituality.
7. Describe the phenomena of transference and countertransference as they occur in critical care nursing.
8. Describe appropriate interventions for transference and countertransference.
9. Discuss the emotional implications of transferring a patient from the critical unit and describe interventions that help the patient cope with changes.

Hudak: Critical Care Nursing:
A Holistic Approach, 6th ed. © 1994
J. B. Lippincott Company.

Mind, Body, Spirit, and the Stress of Illness

This chapter is directed toward specific measures that nurses use to support their patients through the stress of crisis and adaptation to illness, health, or death. An understanding and appreciation of the intricate relationship among mind, body, spirit, and the healing process will help the critical care nurse provide emotional support to the patient. It is the caring and emotional support from the nurse that the patient will remember and value, regardless of the level of technical expertise the nurse may demonstrate.

Stress and Illness. Admission to the critical care unit signals a threat to life and well-being to all who are admitted. On the one hand, critical care nurses perceive the unit as a place where fragile lives are vigilantly scrutinized, cared for, and preserved. On the other hand, patients and their families frequently perceive admission to critical care as a sign of impending death because of their own or others' previous experiences. Because of these distinct differences in perception of the meaning of critical care between patients and nurses, communication breakdowns must be anticipated.

Communication breakdowns also are likely to be heightened by the stress of admission and introduction to the "sick role." In many cultures, sick role behaviors are associated with the often helpless role of the child. Anxiety associated with helplessness contributes to regression in the adult. Therefore, former modes of coping with anxiety and helplessness recur. Conflicts with the nurse concerning autonomy and dependency reveal this regression. Coping behaviors such as denial, anger, passivity, or aggression are commonly employed by patients.

These attempts at coping may be effective or ineffective in handling the stress and its resultant anxiety. If the coping behaviors are effective, energy is freed and may be directed toward healing. If coping attempts fail or are ineffective, however, the tension state is increased; accordingly, there is an increased demand for energy. Thus, the original stress of illness looms larger (Figure 2–1).

The relationships among stress, anxiety, and coping are complex and manifest themselves continuously in any critical care setting. Stress has been defined as any stimulus that results in a disequilibrium of psychological and physiological functioning. All hormone levels can be altered by stress. Extreme levels of stress damage human tissue and may interfere with adaptive responses to tissue pathology. If coping is ineffective, disequilibrium occurs, and the mind and body respond with increased efforts to restore balance.

Coping Behaviors

Anxiety

Anxiety can be viewed as a state of disequilibrium or tension that prompts attempts at coping. Coping can then be viewed as a transaction between the person and the environment. Successful transactions reduce tension and promote a sense of well-being.

Any stress that threatens one's sense of wholeness, containment, security, and control will cause anxiety. Illness is one such stress. The physiological responses of rapid pulse rate, increased blood pressure, increased respirations, dilated pupils, dry mouth, and peripheral vasoconstriction may go undetected in a seemingly cool, calm, self-contained patient. These autonomic responses to anxiety are frequently the most reliable index of the degree of anxiety when behavioral and verbal responses are not congruent with the circumstances.

Behavioral responses indicative of anxiety are often family-based and culturally learned. They vary from quiet composure in the face of disaster to panic in the presence of an innocuous insect. Such extremes of control and panic use valuable energy. If this energy is not directed toward eliminating the stressor, it serves only to perpetuate the discomfort of the tension state. The goal of nursing care is always to promote physiological and emotional equilibrium.

Whenever possible, the threat of stress must be reduced or eliminated. If this can be accomplished, the problem is quickly resolved and the patient is returned to a state of equilibrium. Usually, however, the stress is not

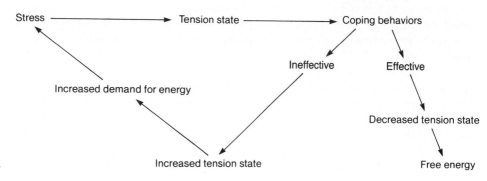

FIGURE 2–1
Stress and coping behaviors.

eliminated so easily, because many other stresses (secondary stresses) are introduced by attempts to remedy the original problem. For most people, hospitalization is an example of secondary stress. If coping defenses are effective, anxiety is reduced and energy is directed toward rest and healing.

For most patients, the fear that life is being threatened is justified, as is the feeling of being an alien in a foreign environment whose life is in the hands of strangers. A sense of inadequacy or inferiority results if patients are unable to understand what is happening physically and whether the personnel and surrounding machinery will return them to health. It is essential that the critical care nurse be knowledgeable about psychosocial dynamics so that appropriate assessment and intervention take place.

Nursing Assessment and Management

Helping the Patient Cope

It often is not possible for the nurse simply to remove the noxious stimulus that evokes anxiety. In these circumstances, the nurse must assess the effectiveness of the patient's coping behaviors and either support them, help the patient modify them, or teach new coping behaviors. Frequently, levels of anxiety are so high that the anxious state becomes the stimulus that demands additional coping responses.

> Assess coping behaviors for effectiveness and either
>
> • support them
> • help patient modify them
> • teach new ones

Coping behaviors may be directed toward eliminating the stress either of illness or of the anxiety state itself. The nurse must evaluate each behavior as to whether it functions to restore a steady state. Those behaviors that are consistent with movement toward a steady state can then be supported and encouraged. More likely, the nurse may need to help the patient modify or find substitutes for those coping devices that are disruptive or threatening to homeostasis. At times, it may be necessary for the nurse to teach or introduce new coping behaviors to facilitate movement toward the overall primary goal of homeostatic equilibrium.

The critical care arena is filled with anxiety-provoking stimuli. Intrusive procedures are among the most serious. At times, patients may be more capable of experiencing concern and worry over the variety of equipment that engulfs them than of focusing on the threat to life. This activity may allow some necessary **denial** of the reality of the crisis, but the worry itself may drain needed resources of energy. Information and explanation of the machinery

may reduce secondary anxiety, and expert nursing care may reassure the patients nonverbally of their security without stripping away the defense of denial.

> Anxiety occurs when there is
>
> • a threat of helplessness
> • a loss of control
> • a sense of loss of function and self-esteem
> • a failure of former defenses
> • a sense of isolation
> • a fear of dying

Anxiety is experienced whenever there is a threat of helplessness or lack of control. Nursing measures that reinforce a sense of control help increase the patient's sense of autonomy and reduce the overpowering sense of loss of control. Providing order and predictability allows the patient to anticipate and prepare for what is to follow. Perhaps it creates only a mirage of control, but anticipatory guidance keeps the patient from being caught off-guard and allows the mustering of those coping mechanisms that can be brought to bear.

Allowing small choices when the patient is willing and ready decreases the patient's feeling that there is no control over the environment. Would he prefer to lie on his right or left side? In which arm would he like his IV? How high does he want the head of his bed? Does he want to cough now or in 20 minutes after pain medication? Any decisions which permit the patient to participate in ways that allow a certain amount of control and predictability are important. These small choices also may help the patient accept lack of control of procedures that involve little choice. Minute decisions allow the patient to exercise some self-governance in a way designed to help reduce the anxiety-provoking sense of helplessness.

> Help increase patient's sense of control by
>
> • providing order and predictability
> • using anticipatory guidance
> • allowing choice whenever possible
> • including the patient in decisions
> • providing information and explanation

A second common cause of anxiety is a sense of isolation. Rarely is one lonelier than when in the midst of a socializing crowd of strangers. In such a situation, people attempt to either include themselves, remove themselves, or emotionally distance themselves. The sick person surrounded by active and busy persons is in a similar situation but with few resources available to reduce the sense of isolation. Hospital staff who ignore the presence of a patient, regardless of the patient's alertness, contribute to the patient's sense of isolation. This sense of isolation can be reduced by including the patient in conversations about treatment and by reassuring touching at frightening moments.

Serious illness and the fear of dying also separate the patient from his family. The immediate development of dependent and intimate relationships with strangers is required. The reassuring cliché, "You'll be all right," often offered by comforting nurses, only serves to reinforce the sense of distance that the patient is experiencing. It shuts off expression of fears and questions about what is to come next. The efficiency and activity that surround the patient increase the sense of separateness.

A third category of anxiety-provoking stimuli includes those that threaten the individual's security. Admittance to the critical care unit dramatically confirms for the family and patient that their security on all levels is being severely threatened.

After the patient is admitted to the unit, the initial insecurity undoubtedly concerns life itself. Later, questions regarding such issues as length of hospitalization, return to work, financial implications, well-being of the family, and permanent limitations arise. So, the patient's insecurity continues and needs to be sensitively considered.

Cognitive Techniques That Deal With Anxiety

Techniques that have evolved from cognitive theories of learning may help anxious patients and their families. These techniques are promising because they can be initiated by the patient and do not depend on complex insight or understanding of one's own psychological makeup. They can also be used to reduce anxiety in a way that avoids probing into the patient's personal life. Furthermore, the patient's friends and family members can be taught these techniques to help them and the patient reduce tension.

Internal Dialogue. Highly anxious people are most likely giving themselves messages that increase or perpetuate their anxiety. These messages are conveyed in one's continuously running "self-talk," or internal dialogue. The patient in the critical care unit may be silently saying things such as, "I can't stand it in here. I've got to get out." Another unexpressed thought might be, "I can't handle this pain." By asking the patient to share aloud what is going on in this internal dialogue, the nurse can bring to awareness those messages that are distracting the patient from rest and relaxation. Substitute messages should be suggested to the patient. It is important to ask the patient to substitute rather than delete messages because the internal dialogue is continuously operating and will not turn off, even if the patient wills it to do so. Therefore, asking the patient to substitute constructive, assuring comments is more likely to help him significantly

reduce the tension level. Comments such as, "I'll handle this pain just one minute at a time" or "I've been in tough spots before, and I am capable of making it through this one!" will automatically reduce anxiety and help the patient shape coping behaviors accordingly. Any message that enhances the patient's confidence, sense of control, and hope, and that puts him or her in a positive, active role rather than in the passive role of a victim, will increase the patient's sense of coping and well-being.

Help patient develop self-dialogue messages that increase

- confidence
- sense of control
- ability to cope
- optimism
- hope

External Dialogue. A similar method can be applied to the patient's external conversation with other people. By simply requiring patients to speak accurately about themselves to others, the same goals can be accomplished. For example, patients who exclaim, "I can't do anything for myself!" should be asked to identify the things that they are able to do, such as lifting their own bodies, turning to one side, making a nurse feel good with a rewarding smile, or helping the family understand what is happening. Even the smallest movement in the weakest of patients should be acknowledged and claimed by the patient. This technique is useful in helping patients correct their own misconceptions of themselves and the way others see them. This reduces patients' sense of helplessness and therefore their anxiety.

Mental Imagery and Relaxation. These are two other useful techniques that can be taught to the patient to help reduce tension. The nurse can encourage the patient to imagine either being in a very pleasant place or taking part in a very pleasant experience. The patient should be instructed to focus and linger on the sensations that are experienced. For example, asking the patient, "What colors do you see?" "What sounds are present?" "How does the air smell?" "How does your skin feel?" "Is there a breeze in the air?" helps increase the intensity of the fantasy and thereby promote relaxation through mental escape.

Guided mental imagery also can be used to help reduce unpleasant feelings of depression, anxiety, and hostility. Patients who must relearn life-sustaining tasks such as walking and feeding themselves can use imagery to prepare themselves mentally to meet the challenge successfully. In these instances, patients should be taught to visualize themselves moving through the task and successfully completing it. If this method seems trivial or silly to the patients, they can be reminded that this method demands concentration and skill and is commonly used by athletes to improve their performance and to prepare themselves mentally before an important event.

Techniques that induce deep muscle relaxation also can be used by the nurse to help the patient decrease anxiety. Deep muscle relaxation may reduce or eliminate the use of tranquilizing and sedating drugs. In *progressive relaxation*, the patient is first directed to find as comfortable a position as possible and then to take several deep breaths and let them out slowly. Next, the patient is asked to clench a fist or curl toes as tightly as possible, to hold the position for a few seconds, and then to let go while focusing on the sensations of the releasing muscles. The patient should practice this technique, beginning with the toes and moving upward through other parts of the body—the feet, calves, thighs, abdomen, chest, and so on. This procedure is done slowly while the patient gives nonverbal signals (eg, lifting a finger) to indicate when each new muscle mass has reached a state of relaxation. Extra time and attention should be given to the back, shoulders, neck, scalp, and forehead, because these are the areas in which many people experience physical tension.

Once a state of relaxation is achieved, the nurse can suggest that the patient fantasize or sleep as deeply as the patient chooses. The patient must be allowed to select and control the depth of relaxation and sleep, especially if the fear of death is prominent in the patient's mind. A moderately dark room and a soft voice will facilitate relaxation. Asking the patient to relax is frequently nonproductive compared with directing him to actively release a muscle mass, to let go of tension, or to imagine tension draining through the body and sinking deeply into the mattress. Again the patient is assisted to an active rather than passive role by the nurse's careful use of language.

Dependency

Critical care patients commonly demonstrate unresolved dependency conflicts typically found in healthy adults. Adults tend to reveal unresolved dependency issues when they take on a sick role by either craving or denying the need for nursing attention. Those who crave dependence will more readily adjust to the protective environment of an intensive care unit. They also are more likely to have difficulty in withdrawing from it. These patients may attempt to develop overly dependent relationships with nurses and may make many demands on their time and attention. Some nurses may view them to be somewhat hypochondriacal. The convalescence of these patients tends to be drawn out, characterized by frequent requests for pain-relieving and tranquilizing medications.

Patients who crave dependency can be especially frustrating for busy nurses. These patients seem to wait for the nurse to leave and then request or demand a service that could have been provided earlier. The manipulation to keep the nurse present is obvious and annoying, especially if the nurse has sicker patients waiting for care. The nurse senses the ever-present bind: If one is brisk, the patient's feelings are hurt; if one is yielding, other patients are neglected.

In the patient's view, however, being dependent is equivalent to being cared about and perhaps even prescribed by the patient role. Moreover, the patient must find congruent role behaviors with a variety of personalities. Some nurses reinforce dependency in patients by their own behavior, whereas others are intolerant of patients who they believe are demanding services that they could accomplish themselves.

Patients who deny their dependency needs demonstrate more difficulty in assuming the patient role. Although they also long for their dependency needs to be satisfied, their unresolved childhood conflict between being an adult and being a dependent, cared-for child arouses a good deal of anxiety. They make demands on themselves instead of others, and are less likely to ask for help when needed. These patients are both afraid and ashamed of dependency. Like their counterparts who crave dependency, they also are likely to have a more protracted convalescence than those who have learned to balance their need for dependency with their need for independence.

Overly independent patients will not wait for a nurse's help. They attempt to get out of bed by themselves, they hesitate to request pain medication when needed, or they fear that they will be viewed as helpless or childish by others. These patients are likely to lack confidence in themselves and ultimately resent their dependence on others. They may carry the nursing diagnosis of ineffective coping related to dependency needs.

Nursing Assessment and Management

For most nurses, coping with and providing optimal care to the overly dependent or overly independent patient are challenging both emotionally and physically. The reaction of nurses to these frustrating patients can be as much a problem as the patients' behavior. A first approach is for the nurse to determine which type of patient is easier to accept and like. It is this personality type with which the nurse is most likely to identify. The nurse will probably avoid the patient of whom she feels less accepting. Because both overly dependent and overly independent patients are dealing with conflicts of dependence, the nurse's avoidance of either type of patient is likely to *increase* the undesirable behavior. Dependency issues are fraught with anxiety for nurses and patients.

The nursing goal is to lower the level of anxiety around unresolved dependency. Order and predictability are likely to help the patient control anxiety that is associated with the dependency. The nurse should inform the patient of how much time is available and then let the patient know when there are only 5 or 6 minutes left for the visit. The nurse should also tell the patient when the next visit will be and then make every effort to return as scheduled. Each patient should have a clock, because knowing the time can help provide a sense of control and predictability.

Allowing the patient to impose order on the routine of care and to establish priorities of how to use the nurse's time may help reduce less important requests. By encouraging the patient to identify and talk about feelings of weakness, disability, and helplessness, the nurse helps the patient begin to distinguish feelings and fears from what is potential and what is real. Patients often have so little understanding about what is occurring within their bodies and what events in the environment mean that they can only guess and therefore frequently distort what is happening to them. Their behavior is likely to reveal their misunderstandings. It is important to clarify in as simple a way as possible what is occurring and why.

If nurse–patient encounters are short by necessity, they also must be frequent. Touching the patient physically in a gentle, warm way can help compensate for unspent time and unspoken conversations. Touch often can convey feelings that some nurses are unable to verbalize and some patients are unable to hear when verbally expressed.

Although it is not likely that the nurse will alter dependency conflicts in patients, anxiety can be alleviated and physical and emotional health promoted by offering constructive dependency experiences.

Responses to Loss

The threat of illness precipitates coping behaviors associated with loss. Dying patients must adapt to the loss of life; other patients must adjust to the loss of health or loss of a limb, a blow to self-concept, or a necessary change in lifestyle. All these events require a change—a loss of the familiar self-image and its replacement with an altered one. All losses include at least a temporary phase of lowered self-esteem. Regardless of the nature of loss, the dynamics of grief present themselves in some form.

The response to loss can be described in the following four phases:

1. Shock and disbelief
2. Development of awareness
3. Restitution
4. Resolution

Each phase involves characteristic and predictable behaviors that fluctuate among the various phases in an unpredictable way. Through recognition and assessment of the behaviors and an understanding of their underlying dynamics, the nurse can plan interventions to support the healing process.

Shock and Disbelief

In the first stage of response to loss, patients demonstrate the behaviors characteristic of denial. They fail to comprehend and experience the rational meaning and emotional impact of the diagnosis. Because the diagnosis has no emotional meaning, patients often fail to cooperate with precautionary measures. For example, patients may attempt to get out of bed against the physician's advice, deviate from the prescribed diet, and assert, "I am here for a rest!" Denial may go so far as to allow patients to project difficulties onto what is perceived as ill-functioning equipment, mistaken laboratory reports, or—more likely—the sheer incompetence of physicians and nurses.

When such blatant denial occurs, it is apparent that the problem is so anxiety-provoking to the patient that it cannot be handled by the more sophisticated mental mechanisms of rational problem solving. The stressor is temporarily obliterated. This phase of denial also may serve as the period during which the patient's resources, briefly blocked by the shock, can be regrouped for the battle ahead. Therefore, stripping away denial may render the patient helpless. Furthermore, although denial has its obvious hazards, denial has been associated with higher rates of survival after myocardial infarctions.

Nursing Management

The principle of intervention consists not in stripping away the defense of denial but in supporting the patient and acknowledging the situation through nursing care.

The nurse recognizes and accepts the patient's illness by watching the monitor or changing the dressings. In these ways, the nurse communicates acceptance of the patient through tone of voice, facial expression, and touch. The nurse must be able to reflect statements of denial back to the patient in a way that allows the patient to hear them—and eventually to examine their incongruity and apply reality—by saying something such as, "In some ways you believe that having a heart attack will be helpful to you?" The nurse can also acknowledge the patient's difficulty in accepting restrictions by making comments such as, "It seems hard for you to stay in bed." By verbalizing what the patient is expressing, the nurse gently confronts behavior but does not cause anxiety and anger by reprimanding and judging. In this phase the nurse supports denial by allowing for it, but does not perpetuate it. Instead, the nurse acknowledges, accepts, and reflects the patient's new circumstance.

Development of Awareness

In this stage second of grief, the patient's behavior is characteristically associated with anger and guilt. The anger may be expressed overtly and may be directed at the

When the patient is denying, the nurse demonstrates acceptance by:

- tone of voice
- congruent facial expression
- use of touch
- use of reflection of inaccurate statements
- avoiding joking with patient about serious issues

staff for oversights, tardiness, and minor insensitivities. In this phase, the ugliness of reality has made its impact. Displacement of the anger onto others helps soften the impact of reality on the patient. The expression of anger itself gives the patient a sense of power in a seemingly helpless state. A demanding manner and a whining tone often characterize this stage and represent the patient's primitive attempts to regain the control that appears to have been lost. However, such behavior often alienates the nurse and other personnel. The patient who does not demand or whine has probably withdrawn into depression because of anger directed toward self rather than toward others. This patient will demonstrate verbal and motor retardation, will likely have difficulty sleeping, and may prefer to be left alone.

During this phase, the nurse is likely to hear irrational expressions of guilt. Patients seek to answer the question, "Why me?" They attempt to isolate their human imperfections and attribute the cause of the malady to themselves or their past behavior. Both patients and their families may look for a person or object to blame.

Guilt feelings concerning one's own illness are difficult to understand unless one examines the basic dynamic of guilt. Guilt arises when there is a decrease in the feeling of self-worth or when the self-concept has been violated. In this light, the nurse can understand that what is behind an expression of guilt is a negatively altered self-concept. Blame thus becomes nothing more than projection of the unbearable feeling of guilt.

Nursing Management

During the patient's development of awareness, nursing intervention must be directed toward supporting the patient's basic sense of self-worth and allowing and encouraging the direct expression of anger. Nursing measures that support a patient's sense of self-worth are numerous and include calling the patient by name; introducing strangers, particularly if they are to examine the patient; talking to, rather than about, the patient; and, most importantly, providing and respecting the patient's need for privacy and modesty. The nurse needs to guard against verbal and nonverbal expressions of pity. It is more constructive and productive to empathize with the patient's

specific and temporary feelings of anger, sadness, and guilt rather than with a condition.

The nurse can create outlets for anger by listening and by *refraining from defending* the physician, the hospital, or his or her own actions. A nondefensive, accepting attitude will decrease the patient's sense of guilt, and the expression of anger will avert some of the depression. Later, when the patient apologizes for an irrational outburst, the nurse can interpret the patient's need to make this kind of verbalization as a necessary step toward rehabilitation and health.

Restitution

In this stage, the griever puts aside anger and resistance and begins to cope constructively with the loss. The patient tries new behaviors that are consistent with the new limitations. The emotional level is one of sadness, and time spent crying is useful. As the patient adapts to a new image, considerable time is spent going over and over significant memories relevant to the loss. Behaviors in this stage include the verbalization of fears regarding the future. Often these go unexpressed and undetected because they are unbearable for the family to hear. Furthermore, after severe trauma, which may have resulted in scarring or removal of a body part or loss of sensation, patients may question their sexual adequacy. They worry about the future response of their mates to their changed bodies. The patient probably also questions a new role in the family. Most likely, the patient has a variety of concerns that are specific to his or her individual lifestyle. Thus, in the mourning process such manifestations as reminiscing, crying, questioning, expressing fears, and trying out new behaviors help the patient modify the old self-concept and begin working with and experiencing a revised concept.

Nursing Management

During restitution, nursing care should again be supportive so that adaptation can occur. Listening to the patient for lengthy periods of time is necessary. If the patient is able to verbalize fears and questions about the future, he or she will be better able to define the anxiety and solve new problems. Furthermore, hearing oneself talk about fears helps put them into a more rational perspective. The patient may require privacy, acceptance, and encouragement to cry so that respite from sadness can be found.

During this stage, the nurse may have the patient consider meeting someone who has successfully adapted to similar trauma. This measure provides the patient with a role model as a new identity is assumed, which often occurs after the crisis period. There are many support groups made up of recovering people with all types of illnesses and injuries who will send someone to support and be a role model for patients and families.

The patient, with appropriate support from the nurse,

begins to identify and acknowledge changes that are arising from adaptation to illness. Relationships can and do change. Because friends may respond differently to the patient who has suffered a permanent disability than to a healthy person, the patient may not feel or believe that attitudes toward and feelings for him or her are the same as before the injury or illness.

During this time the family have also been going through a similar process. They too have experienced shock, disbelief, anger, and sadness. After they are ready to try to solve their problems, their energies are directed toward wondering how the changes in the patient will affect their mutual relationship and their lifestyle. They, too, experience the pain of turmoil and uncertainty. Nurses must also help the family. By allowing the family to ventilate their repulsion and fear and by showing acceptance of these feelings, the nurse can help the family be more useful to, and accepting of, the patient. Through intensive listening, the nurse provides a sounding board and then redirects the members of the family back to each other so that they can give and receive each other's support. Asserting the normality of untoward feelings also assists with future acceptance, while decreasing guilt and blame.

Resolution

Resolution is the stage of identity change. At first patients may *over*identify themselves as invalids. They may discriminate against themselves and make derogatory remarks about their bodies. Another method patients may use is to detach themselves emotionally from the source of trauma (eg, a stoma, prosthesis, scar, or paralyzed limb) by naming it and referring to it in a simultaneously alienated and affectionate way. Patients are sensitive to the ways in which health care workers respond to their bodies. A patient may make negative remarks to test the acceptance of the nurse. Chiding or telling the patient that many others share the problem will be less helpful than acknowledging feelings and indicating acceptance by continuing to care for, and talk with, the patient.

As time passes and the patient adapts, the sting of the endured hurt abates, and the patient moves toward an identification as an person who has certain limitations due to illness rather than as a "cripple" or an "invalid." The patient no longer uses a defect as the basis of identity. As the resolution is reached, patients are able to depend on others if necessary and should not need to push beyond their endurance or to overcompensate for an inadequacy or limitation. Often, the patient reflects on the crisis as a time of growth or maturation. Such a patient achieves a sense of pride at accomplishing the difficult adaptation and is able to look back realistically on successes and disappointments without discomfort. At this time, the patient may find it useful and gratifying to help others by

serving as a role model for those people in the stage of restitution who are experiencing their own identity crises.

Unfortunately, the critical care nurse is rarely in a position to observe the successful outcome of resolution. It is useful to know the process in order to work with and communicate an attitude of hope, especially when the patient is most self-disparaging.

Nursing Management

The goal of nursing care during the resolution stage is to help the patient attach a sense of self-esteem to a rectified identity. Nursing intervention centers on helping the patient find the degree of dependence that is needed and can be accepted. The nurse must accept and recognize with the patient that periods of vacillation between independence and dependence will occur. The nurse should encourage a positive emotional response to a new state of modified dependence. Certainly, the nurse can support and reinforce the patient's growing sense of pride in rehabilitation. For those nurses who have had the experience of successfully working through the process with one person, the problem is to stand back and allow the patient to move away from them (see Nursing Care Plan 2–1: Grieving and Loss).

Spirituality and Healing

The influence of spirituality on healing, the management of illness, anxiety, and acceptance of death is being given increasing attention by nurses. Nursing care includes recognition and support of the spiritual nature of human beings. Spirituality in nursing care refers to the recognition that a realm of invisible and intangible factors influences thought and behavior. This recognition includes religious beliefs and goes beyond. When people sense power and influence outside of time and physical existence, they are said to be experiencing the metaphysical aspects of spirituality.

Spirituality includes one's system of beliefs and values. Intuition and knowledge from unknown sources, and origins of unconditional love and belonging, typically are viewed as spiritual power. A sense of universal connection, personal empowerment, and reverence for life also pertain to the existence of spirituality. These elements also may be viewed as benefits of spirituality.

Critical care patients and their families frequently pray for miraculous healing. Miracles of healing, when they are experienced by believers, can be viewed as normal healing events occurring in collapsed time. Nursing goals related to spirituality or the nursing diagnosis spiritual distress include the recognition and promotion of patients' spiritual sources of strength. Allowing and supporting patients to share their beliefs about the universe without disagreement help them recognize and draw on their own sources of spiritual courage. Recognition of the unique spiritual nature of each patient is thought to assist personal empowerment and healing.

Spirituality includes

- religion
- beliefs and values
- intuition
- knowledge from the unknown
- unconditional love
- a sense of belonging
- a sense of connection with the universe
- reverence for life
- personal empowerment

Nurses who find their own spiritual values in religion must acknowledge and respect that non-religious people may also be spiritual and experience spirituality as a life force. Regardless of personal views, the nurse is obligated to assess patients' spiritual belief system and assist them to recognize and draw on the values and beliefs already in existence for them.

Furthermore, critical illness may also deepen or challenge existing spirituality. During these times it may be useful for the nurse or family to call on spiritual or religious leaders or teachers to help the patient make meaningful use of the critical illness experience.

Adaptation to Illness

Another method of understanding the characteristic problems of adapting to limitations enforced by illness is to understand the relationship between emotional regression and physical disability or illness. There is an observable lag between the physical onset of illness and its emotional acknowledgement; that is, the patient experiences illness and disability physically before they can be acknowledged fully on an emotional level. Denial is an example of this lag. Likewise, after physical health has been reestablished or stabilized, the patient still experiences concerns and fears related to acute illness. At this point,

the patient is likely to resist independence and be reluctant to cooperate with increased expectations for activity and self-care. Preparation for return to health, acknowledgment of concerns about increased activity, and the reassurance of watchful eyes will help alleviate anxiety as the patient progresses.

Figure 2–2 demonstrates one pattern of adapting to various stages of illness. The shaded area represents transition into illness and shows the disparity between a person's actual health and his perception of his health. In this situation there is denial. The acceptance phase demonstrates that physical well-being and mental well-being are congruent, whereas the convalescent phase shows that an emotional lag exists between physical and emotional well-being.

One principle that greatly affects understanding the patient's response is that during stress the patient regresses in an attempt to conserve energy. During times of acute exacerbation or heightened expectations, or during any significant change, the initial response is regression to an earlier emotional position of safety. Weaning from a respirator, removal of monitor leads, increased activity, and reduction in medication often trigger anxiety and regression. This regression may even include a retreat into increased dependency, depression, and anger. At such times, the patient may find comfort in regressing to a state that has already been coped with or mastered. The regression is usually temporary and brief and can be used to identify the cause of anxiety. Nurses may become disappointed, anxious, or angry with the patient's regression and may wish to retreat. It is more helpful, however, to acknowledge that regression is inevitable and to support the patient with intervention appropriate to earlier stages. Help the patient understand what is happening by explaining the emotional lag phenomenon. Diagramming the emotional lag response may also increase the patient's understanding of the relationship between what is experienced emotionally and what is occurring physiologically.

If different patients' responses to illness could be plotted on a graph, they would show both common and unique points, just as electrocardiograms from different people show common characteristics as well as individual differences. There will be variations in time and in the congruence between physical and sociopsychological responses, but the stages will occur predictably. Like the electrical events of the heart, responses to illness, both

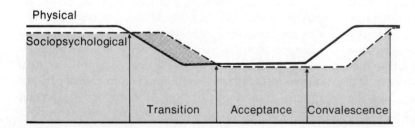

FIGURE 2–2
The solid line represents a normal level of physical well-being, the broken line a corresponding degree of sociopsychological integration.

adaptive and maladaptive, can be anticipated. The nurse's responsibility is to:

- anticipate, assess, and monitor the response to illness;
- recognize and support effective behaviors; and
- minimize and redirect ineffective behaviors.

Transference and Countertransference

There are some types of irrational behavior directed toward nurses that cannot be explained by adaptation or grieving. The phenomenon of *transference* may be used to explain some reactions patients have toward nurses that are inappropriate in intensity and, sometimes, in attitude. *Transference* can be thought of as an unconscious response that represents feelings and attitudes that originated in early childhood. Transference reduces the patient's anxiety by allowing him or her to experience current anxiety-provoking situations in terms of previous situations. Transference reactions are usually marked by an expression of intense feelings that seem inappropriate to the event that has triggered them. Exhibitionism, extreme dependency, and irrational demands are some behaviors that can often be accounted for by transference.

It may be that in times of crisis and regression, reality testing is impaired, and the patient is more likely to act and react to the irrational fears and feelings that originated when he or she was a helpless child. In such instances, the patient must be treated and addressed as an adult and helped to test reality in the current environment. For example, if a patient fears that the nurses do not care, the patient can be encouraged to ask specific nurses how they feel, or can be helped to identify what it is about the nurses that suggests they do not care. At that time, specific explanations can be given about nurses' behavior. This type of intervention satisfies the patient's need to be cared about far better than global reassurance that the nurses do care.

Critical care nurses must be ready to be subjected to powerful positive and negative feelings. An understanding of the regressive nature of these inappropriate and intense expressions and the dynamics involved can help the nurse retain composure and respond constructively rather than react impulsively with rejection or withdrawal.

Countertransference is the same phenomenon as transference when it occurs in the helper or nurse. Intensity of positive or negative feelings directed toward the patient should suggest to the nurse that this reaction is a product of countertransference rather than objective observation of, and response to, patient behavior. Clues that suggest countertransference include an inability to empathize with the patient, spending unusually short or long periods with certain patients, feelings of anger and discourage-

ment at the patient for not responding to care, personal and social involvement, and daydreaming about and preoccupation with the patient. The desire to argue with a patient or extreme protectiveness of a particular patient are common ways that nurses display countertransference. Strong negative transference from a patient may elicit an equally negative countertransference in the nurse.

Countertransference is viewed as destructive to patient care and the nurse–patient relationship because it is likely to interfere with accurate appraisals of the patient's condition. Countertransference does occur in nurses and other personnel; nurses need to be supportive of each other in confronting and dealing with these reactions. If countertransference occurs, it is helpful for nurses to recognize the dynamics of transference and countertransference and work together to achieve an accurate appraisal of nurses' and patients' responses, with the objective of providing nursing care that will potentiate reality testing and constructive interactions. If nurses observe the clues of countertransference in themselves and others, the most practical and useful intervention is to talk about the nurse's feelings and reactions toward the patient in the context of the countertransference phenomenon. If the nurse cannot work through the countertransference and react to patient behavior in a neutral and objective way, the nurse should be given a different patient assignment.

Transfer from the Critical Care Unit

Regression is often elicited when the patient is told it is time to be transferred to the general unit. The stage of illness greatly influences the patient's response to transfer. If the patient is transferred at the denial stage, the move can be accomplished with ease because it further fortifies the feeling that one isn't very sick. On the other hand, if the patient is transferred at the stage in which he or she is improving physically more than can be acknowledged emotionally, anxiety will be heightened. The patient is saying, "I'm sick, and being transferred means you think I'm improving when I'm not." While trying to cope with the anxiety generated by the move, the patient regresses and becomes more dependent. Transferring at the time when the patient first acknowledges the severity of illness may create discomfort for nurses because the patient is likely to be frightened, angry, uncooperative, and demanding.

Preparing for the Transfer. Regardless of the timing, in preparing for transfer both the nurse and the patient need to accept the fact that their relationship with each other is ending. They may accomplish this by reminiscing about an initial meeting or a special moment and by talking about the move.

If the patient is feeling dependent, more time may be needed to talk about what it will be like to leave. Often, because of discomfort associated with saying goodbye, nurses withdraw under the guise that it is easier for the patient if the nurse ignores the termination process. This unexplained withdrawal may be interpreted by the patient as a lack of interest or as anger over earlier unresolved outbursts made during a time when a change in body image and lowered self-esteem were being experienced.

The news of transfer often comes without warning or preparation. Even though patients may be pleased with their progress, they are at the same time concerned about losing the reassurance of special equipment, close surveillance, and the presence of familiar faces. It has long been advocated that continuity of care be provided by thoughtful preparation. Introduction to the new nurses who will take over care of the patient, and follow-up visits by the critical care nurses, increase familiarity, enhance security, and let the patient feel important. Disconnecting equipment and monitors before the time of transfer will lessen the strain of having to give up the room, equipment, and the nursing vigilance all at the same time.

Family members can provide valuable support during the transfer process if they know what will happen and have had their questions answered and their concerns addressed. Family members who either accompany patients during the transfer or meet them at the new room and then stay with them during the remainder of the day can lessen the stress associated with the change.

The process of preparing for and carrying out the transfer of a patient is an important aspect of nursing care. Even if the patient is prepared for transfer, regression and anxiety may occur; however, if the nurse acknowledges these concerns and offers support, the patient will again mobilize the needed energy. Because these processes have proved predictable, they give the nurse a basis for care and provide rationale for appropriate intervention. Despite the predictability of these responses in human behavior, their impact on a particular patient will be unique. By the time they are modified by personality and by sociocultural and economic variables, they have become a significant part of life and are indeed made unique as they become an historical and living part of one's identity.

NURSING CARE PLAN 2–1:
Grieving and Loss

Mr. James Saunders, age 41, was admitted to the critical care unit conscious but unresponsive to verbal questioning. According to the accident report, a large truck had swerved out of control on an icy road, killing Mr. Saunders' fiancée and injuring him. He had been hospitalized for observation and treatment of chest wounds and blood loss. Mr. Saunders' leg was amputated above the left knee as a result of an injury incurred in Vietnam 25 years ago.

While trying to reach Mr. Saunders' family, the nurse learned that his mother had died of cancer about 1 year ago and that 3 months later his father, suffering from depression, had killed himself. He had one sister who was flying to see him.

The primary nursing problems were maintenance of ventilation and vital signs, pain control, and immobility. Mr. Saunders remained uncommunicative though he was tearful. When he did talk, he expressed hopelessness and said he wanted to die. He asked, "Why me, God? What have I done to deserve this?"

The following care plan focuses on nursing diagnoses related to Mr. Saunders' psychosocial problems.

NURSING DIAGNOSIS	OUTCOME CRITERIA/ PATIENT GOALS	NURSING INTERVENTIONS
Ineffective coping: related to depression over multiple serious losses.	• Patient will be able to verbally and nonverbally express frustration, anger, and rage at events.	1. Express possible feelings that nurse might have if in similar situation. 2. Ask patient to agree or disagree regarding accuracy of nurse reflection of feelings. 3. Use gentle touch and sit quietly with patient, so that he does not experience physical pain in addition to emotional pain.

(continued)

NURSING CARE PLAN 2–1: (Continued)
Grieving and Loss

NURSING DIAGNOSIS	OUTCOME CRITERIA/ PATIENT GOALS	NURSING INTERVENTIONS
		4. Acknowledge the magnitude of the losses.
		5. Acknowledge the patient's reaction as a normal, expected human response to multiple and severe loss.
Powerlessness: related to losses, physical injuries, and incapacitation.	• Patient will demonstrate a sense of control over his own life by making sound decisions.	1. Allow patient as many choices as possible. Acknowledge soundness of choices.
		2. Question poor choices in a sensitive way (eg, "You believe that giving up will somehow help you feel better about what has happened?").
	• Patient will experience a decrease in feelings of guilt regarding the collision.	1. Allow expression of irrational thoughts (eg, "I must have done something very bad to deserve all this.").
		2. Reflect back statements emphasizing faulty logic (eg, "You believe that if you had been a better person, you could have controlled someone else's driving and the weather?").
		3. Teach patient about the stages of grieving and emphasize its necessity for health.
		4. Refer patient for mental health follow-up care and support.
Spiritual distress: related to questions such as "Why me, God?"	• Patient will share spiritual belief system with nurse.	1. Ask patient to share religious/ spiritual beliefs.
	• Patient will reenlist former spiritual sources of empowerment (eg, prayer, rosary, icons, etc.).	2. Contact appropriate religious or spiritual teacher (eg, priest, chaplain, etc.).
	• Patient will decrease expressions of hopelessness and the wish to die.	3. Ask patient to share other times of spiritual distress and their outcomes.
		4. Place meaningful spiritual/religious items near patient.
		5. Use readings of scripture, verse, or stories with patient as he desires.
		6. Assess patient for suicide ideation and impulse control. Observe frequently.

(continued)

NURSING CARE PLAN 2–1: (Continued)
Grieving and Loss

NURSING DIAGNOSIS	OUTCOME CRITERIA/ PATIENT GOALS	NURSING INTERVENTIONS
Grieving: related to actual loss.	• Patient will begin to grieve loss of fiancée and begin or continue to grieve loss of parents and loss of leg.	1. Provide honest information in simple terms, when requested. 2. Acknowledge own feelings to self regarding loss and identify separateness from patient in order not to over-identify with patient and lose objectivity. 3. Enlist other staff to act as resources for nurse and patient. 4. Assess stage of grief related to death of parents, loss of leg, and Vietnam experience. 5. Assess patient's stage of grief in relationship to ability to make sound decisions (ie, post discharge psychiatric followup). 6. Support denial, as needed, to let patient move at own pace in perceiving degrees of loss. 7. Consult psychosocial liaison nurse and spiritual counselor to assist in coping and facilitating appropriate grieving. 8. Avoid the temptation to reduce pain with false reassurance. 9. Acknowledge depth and breadth of loss. 10. Offer hope by letting patient know that time will ease the degree of pain. 11. Acknowledge that the patient has already demonstrated enormous personal strength by surviving the accident and his other losses. 12. Provide hope that he will recover by talking about the future. 13. Provide positive reinforcement for crying and grieving behaviors. ("Don't apologize for your tears; it's very important that you cry as much as you need to express your grief."). 14. Reframe the catastrophic event from a tragedy to the challenge of a lifetime.

The Meaning of Critical Care to the Patient

Former patients speak for years about their critical care experience. What happens to a patient in a critical care unit holds lasting meaning for the patient and the family members. Although actual painful memories are blurred by drugs and the mind's need to forget, attitudes that are highly charged with feelings about the nature of the experience survive. These attitudes shape the person's beliefs about nurses, physicians, health care, and about the vulnerability of life itself. Their attitudes and conversations with others contribute to the shaping of future patients' expectations and attitudes toward critical care nurses. Therefore, it is important that the patient and family have as positive an experience as possible, regardless of the outcome.

BIBLIOGRAPHY

Barr W: Teaching patients with life-threatening illnesses: Cardiovascular disease, transplantation, organ donation. Nurs Clin North Am 24(3):639–644, 1989

Barry PD: Mental Health and Mental Illness. Philadelphia, JB Lippincott, 1990

Burgess AW: Psychiatric Nursing in the Hospital and Community. Norwalk, CT, Appleton & Lange, 1990

Compton P: Critical illness and intensive care: What it means to the client. Crit Care Nurse 11(1):50–56, 1991

Cook JS: Essentials of Mental Health Nursing. Redwood City, CA, Addison-Wesley Nursing, 1990

Groër M: Psychoneuroimmunology. Am J Nurs 91(8):33, 1991

Haber J: Comprehensive Psychiatric Nursing. St. Louis, Mosby Year Book, 1992

Shaffer JL: Spiritual distress and critical illness. Crit Care Nurse 11(1):42–45, 1991

STUDY QUESTIONS

1. Denial is a response that

   a. is viewed as normal in the early phase of grieving
   b. helps the patient gather emotional resources to deal with problems ahead
   c. is a defense that should not be stripped away by the nurse
   d. all of the above

2. The best way to help the patients handle anxiety is to

   a. reassure them that they will receive the best possible care
   b. assist them to talk about their fears and concerns
   c. be direct and honest with them
   d. limit visitors' time with them

3. The nurse can help provide a sense of control in patients by

   a. providing order and predictability
   b. offering as many choices as possible
   c. including them in decision making
   d. all of the above

4. Anxiety occurs when patients

   a. are occupied with internal dialogue
   b. are overly dependent on the nurse
   c. have a long term recovery ahead
   d. perceive a threat to their well-being

5. If patients deny their illness, the nurse should

   a. confront their denial and talk about their illness
   b. ignore their denial and avoid talking about their illness
   c. be accepting of their denial and talk about other topics
   d. be accepting of their denial and talk about their illness

6. Countertransference relates to

   a. the nurses's feelings about a patient
   b. significant early relationships of the nurse
   c. positive and negative feelings of the nurse for the patient
   d. all of the above

7. If the patient is transferred to another unit, the nurse should

   a. expect some regression by the patient
   b. continue to monitor the patient electronically until transferred
   c. help the patient prepare by decreasing the length of time spent in the room
   d. all of the above

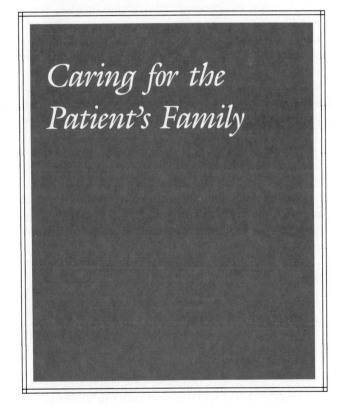

CHAPTER 3

Caring for the Patient's Family

BEHAVIORAL OBJECTIVES

Based on the content in this chapter, the reader should be able to:

1. Identify and describe the characteristics of a crisis event.
2. Identify variables that determine the meaning of crisis events for patients and family members.
3. Identify goals that assist families in coping with crises.
4. Describe the nurse's role in a helping relationship during times of crisis.
5. Identify and describe nursing behaviors that help families cope with crises.
6. Identify and describe nursing goals and behaviors associated with caring for dying patients and their families.

Hudak: Critical Care Nursing:
A Holistic Approach, 6th ed. © 1994
J. B. Lippincott Company.

Description

A holistic approach to critical care nursing must include the patient's family. For the purposes of this chapter, *family* means any persons who share intimate and routine day-to-day living with the critical care patient—in other words, those persons whose social homeostasis is altered by the patient's entrance into the arena of critical illness or injury. Anyone who is a significant part of the patient's normal lifestyle is considered a family member.

Stress and Family Adaptation

The patient's entrance into a life–death sick role threatens and alters the family's homeostasis for many reasons. Beyond realistic fears about loss of life, the contributions of the hospitalized member are lost to the family. The patient's responsibilities must now be added to the responsibilities of others. This alters their schedules and activities. When these responsibilities are left undone, family members experience various degrees of discomfort and annoyance. Financial concerns are usually major, and daily activities that previously were of little consequence now become important and often difficult to manage. Such activities as packing school lunches for children, keeping the family car filled with gasoline, taking out the garbage, and balancing the checkbook can, when unfulfilled, become critically significant.

In addition to the responsibilities the patient normally carries, the social role that the patient plays in the family is missing. Disciplinarian, provider of affection, lover, humorist, timekeeper, motivator, comforter, and so on, are all important roles in family life. If these roles are unfulfilled, considerable havoc and even grief in the family may ensue.

The family enters into a crisis under several conditions:

- A stressful event occurs and threatens lasting changes for the family.
- Usual problem-solving activities are inadequate or unemployed and therefore do not lead rapidly to the previous state of balance.
- The present state of family disequilibrium cannot be maintained and will lead either to improved family health and adaptation or to decreased family adaptability and increased proneness to crisis events.

By using these conditions to identify and define families in crisis, one can appreciate the stress of normal maturational events of family life, such as marriage, pregnancy, enrollment in school, and retirement, in a different light. Scales have been developed that score these stressful life events. These scales help predict who is at risk for developing illness. Significant life events all require readjustment and may include such things as marital reconciliation, change in finances, and trouble with in-laws or the boss. Not only situations of disease and injury propel families into crisis. A family that has been coping adequately with unemployment may not be able to deal with the added stress of a critically ill family member. What appears to be a family's overreaction to a small stress may be explained as having a "last straw" effect added onto formerly manageable stress.

Some families experience many more crises than others. Often challenges and demands that face these families are similar to the ones that present themselves to all families. An additional factor of *cognitive appraisal* must be considered. Some persons or families assign catastrophic meaning to some events that others would not. If family members appraise a situation by giving it the proportions and labels of a crisis event, the emotions, stress, and anxiety associated with a crisis, as well as attempts to cope, will follow. This phenomenon implies that crises based on cognitive appraisal are individual and unique—that is, a crisis for one family is not necessarily a crisis for another. The wide range of family behaviors and reactions observed by critical care nurses can in large part be explained by this concept. Cultural and age variables can also be accounted for in this way.

There are four important generalizations about crises that form a basis for nursing care of families:

1. Whether people emerge stronger or weaker as a result of a crisis is not based so much on their character as on the quality of help they receive during a crisis state.
2. People are more amenable to suggestions and open to help during actual crises.
3. With the onset of a crisis, old memories of past crises may be evoked. If maladaptive behavior was used to deal with previous situations, the same type of behavior may be repeated in the face of a new crisis.
4. The only way to survive a crisis is to be aware of it.

Families typically maintain a steady state. When a family member is in a critical care unit, other family members may try to maintain their equilibrium at first by either minimizing the significance of the illness or being overprotective.

The family member in the critical care unit is primarily in a biological crisis, whereas the rest of the family is experiencing an emotional crisis. At first, coping mechanisms may seem to work, and the family system may appear to improve despite increasing stress. However, as stress continues, the family system is likely to disintegrate unless there is intervention based on the reality of the situation.

Reactions to crises are difficult to categorize because they depend on individual responses to stress, and, within a family, several mechanisms for handling stress and anxiety may be used. In general, the nurse may observe behaviors signifying feelings of helplessness and urgency. An inability to make decisions and mobilize resources may be noted. A sense of fear and panic pervades. Irrational acts, demanding behavior, withdrawal, perseveration, and fainting all have been observed by critical care nurses. Just as the patient is experiencing shock and disbelief about the illness, so too is the family. A nurse must be able to perceive the feeling that a crisis victim is experiencing, particularly when that person cannot identify the problem or feeling to himself or others.

Assessment

Aside from the patient, the critical care nurse deals with many other people in crisis. Almost all patients and their families who populate the waiting room experience some degree of discomfort associated with crises. The problem is to assess the immediate events causing the disruption and then to help the families assign priorities to their needs so that they can act accordingly.

The nurse needs to identify current methods of coping and to evaluate them in terms of adaptation (see Chapter 2). The nurse will need to determine, and *sometimes* point out to the patients, chronic problems resulting from the threatening crisis. When the situational crisis seems inconsequential or obscure, the nurse should try to understand the meaning that the patients have attributed to the event. Furthermore, the meaning ascribed to the crisis will help the nurse evaluate current maturational problems with which the family is already coping. Understanding the parameters of the crisis may give the direction for action.

Management

Nursing intervention must be designed to help families

- reach a higher level of adaptation by learning from the crisis experience
- regain a state of equilibrium
- experience the feelings involved in the crisis to avoid delayed depressions and allow for future emotional growth.

The Use of the Relationship

Establishing an emotionally meaningful relationship with people in crisis tends to be easier than at any other time. Persons in crisis are highly receptive to an interested and empathetic helper. When first meeting the patient's family, the *nurse must demonstrate an ability to help*.

The family must be prepared for their experience in the critical care unit. The patient's condition, alertness, and appearance should be described in terms suitable to the family's level of understanding. Any equipment should be explained before the family views the patient. At the bedside, further explanation can be made.

Other specific help can be given at this time to demonstrate the nurse's interest. Looking up telephone numbers can be extremely difficult for the highly anxious family member. Even deciding who is to be notified of the patient's status can be an overwhelming decision. Assisting the family to determine immediate priorities is essential in the early phase of crisis work.

With this kind of timely intervention, the family will begin to trust and depend on the nurse's judgment. This process then allows family members to believe the nurse when she convey feelings of hope and confidence in their ability to deal with whatever is ahead of them. It is important to avoid giving false reassurance; rather, the reality of the situation can be expressed in statements such as, "This is a complicated problem; together we can work on it."

Problem Definition

As the relationship develops from one interaction to another, the nurse can formulate the dynamics of the problem. Formulations include items such as the following:

- the meaning the family has attached to the event
- other crises with which the family may be already coping
- the coping mechanisms previously used in times of stress, with an idea of why these behaviors are or are not working at this time
- the normal resources of the family, which may include friends, neighbors, relations, colleagues, and so forth. The nurse, having identified these areas, will best use them with the family to help them deal with their predicament.

A vital part of the problem-solving process is to help the family clearly state what the immediate problem is. Often people feel overwhelmed and immobilized by the free-floating anxiety or panic caused by acute stress. Stating the problem in words helps the patient achieve a degree of *cognitive mastery*. Regardless of the difficulty or threat the problem implies, being able to state it as such reduces anxiety by helping the family realize that they have achieved some sort of understanding of what is happening. Defining the problem is a way of delimiting its parameters.

Defining and redefining problems must occur many times before the crisis is resolved. Stating the problem clearly automatically helps the family assign priorities and direct the needed actions. For example, in the event of a tragic injury, finding a babysitter may become the number one priority, superseding notification of close relatives. Goal-directed activity will help decrease anxiety and irrational acts that sometimes go with it.

In high levels of stress, some people expect themselves to react differently. Rather than turning to the resources they use daily, they become reluctant to involve them. Simply asking people to identify who it is that they usually turn to when they are upset and finding out what has gotten in the way of turning to these people now helps direct the patient back to the normal mechanisms used to maintain homeostasis. When the patient or family is reluctant to call on a friend, the nurse can help resolve the indecision by asking, "Wouldn't you want to help her if she were in your place?" Most families are truly not without resources; they only have failed to recognize and call on them.

Defining and redefining the problem may also help put the problem in a different light. It is possible in time to view a tragedy as a challenge and the unknown as an adventure. The process of helping the family view a problem from a different perspective is called reframing.

The nurse can also help the family call on their own strengths. How have they handled stress before? Have they used humor, escape, exercise, or friendship? Do they telephone close friends and relatives who are far away? Even though the family may be threatened financially at this time, some expenditures of this sort may be well worth the money.

Problem Solving

A problem-solving technique that emphasizes choices and alternatives helps the family achieve a sense of control over part of their lives. It also reminds them, and clarifies for them, that they are ultimately responsible for dealing with the event and that it is they who must live with the consequences of their decisions.

Helping the family focus on feelings is extremely important to avoid delayed grief reactions and protracted depressions later on. The nurse can give direction to the family to help each other cry and to share their fear and sadness. Reflection of feelings or active listening is necessary throughout the crisis. If the nurse can starts a statement by saying, "You feel . . . ," he or she is reflecting a feeling. If the nurse says, "You feel *that* . . . ," he or she is reflecting a judgment instead of a feeling. Describing and recognizing one's feelings decreases the need to blame others. Valuing the expression of feelings can help the patients avoid the use of tranquilizers, sedatives, and excessive sleep to escape painful feelings. In sad and depressing times, the nurse can authentically promise the family that they will feel better with time. Adaptation takes time.

During the difficult days that a person is critically ill, the family may become very dependent on the judgment of professionals. It can be difficult for them to identify the appropriate areas in which to accept others' judgments. The nurse can best handle inappropriate expectations such as, "Tell me what I should do?" by acknowledging the feelings involved in an accepting manner and stating the reality of the situation; for example, "You wish I could make that difficult decision for you, but I can't, because you are the ones who will have to live with the consequences." This type of statement acknowledges the family's feelings and recognizes the complexity of the problem while emphasizing each person's responsibility for his or her own feelings, actions, and decisions.

Once the problem has been defined and the family begins goal-directed activity, the nurse may help further by asking them to identify the steps they must take. This anticipatory guidance helps reduce anxiety and make things go more smoothly.

Crisis victims should always be left with a specific plan of action. This plan may be as simple as, "Call me tomorrow at 2:00 PM"; regardless of its simplicity, it implies hope, responsibility, and a reason to get through the night.

The critical care nurse's time with families is often limited because of the nature of the work, so it is important to make every interaction as useful to the family as possible. The nurse must take responsibility for directing the conversation and focusing on the *here and now*. He or she must avoid the temptation to give useless advice in favor of emphasizing a problem-solving approach. However, the nurse must use judgment and recognize those moments when direction is vital to health and safety. It is often necessary to direct families to return home to rest. This can be explained by telling family members that by maintaining their own health they will be more helpful to the patient at a later time. To make each interaction meaningful, the nurse must focus on the crisis situation and avoid involvement in long-term chronic problems and complaints. For example, a nurse should help the family of the overdose patient deal with the events immediately preceding the suicide attempt rather than with long-standing family problems (see Nursing Care Plan 3–1: Caring for the Patient's Family).

Referral

Regardless of the nurse's ability in this area, some families will profit most by referral to a mental health nurse clini-

When working with family members

- provide choices
- help them identify and focus on feelings
- encourage respite from the crisis
- give direction in a way which confers responsibility and hope

NURSING CARE PLAN 3-1:
Caring for the Patient's Family

NURSING DIAGNOSIS	OUTCOME CRITERIA/ PATIENT GOALS	NURSING INTERVENTIONS
Altered family process: related to impact of critically ill members on family system.	• Family members will verbalize feelings to nurse. • Family members will participate in care of ill family member. • Family members will facilitate return of ill family member from sick role to well role.	1. Assess ability of family to meet outcome criteria. 2. Assist in verbalizing feelings by asking about them and showing interest and concern. Follow-up on previous discussions. 3. Provide opportunities for family members to participate in care. Encourage family members to use touch and talk with unconscious and conscious patients. 4. Assist family in identifying changes taking place in regard to role. 5. Assist family member in allowing patient to function in a modified role, as needed.
	• Family members will maintain functional system of mutual support for all.	1. Assist family in seeking respite and recreation during crisis periods. 2. Reassure family that they may call unit, or that a nurse will call them if things change for the worse.
	• Family members will seek appropriate resources when needed.	1. Have family members identify their typical pattern for coping with stress. Encourage them to call on old resources and refer them to new ones, *e.g.,* psychosocial nurse, social worker, chaplain. 2. Assist family members in identifying rational priorities, *e.g.,* find sitter or transportation.

cian, a social worker, a psychologist, or a psychiatrist. A nurse can best encourage the patient to accept help from others by emphatically acknowledging the difficulty and complexity of the problem and providing a choice of names *and* phone numbers. At times, it even can be appropriate for the nurse to set up the first meeting; however, the chances of follow-through are greater if the patient or family makes the arrangements. Many hospitals have skilled mental health nurses and social workers who, with very short notice, can help the nurse intervene.

When the Patient is Dying
Assessment and Management

For the most part, the goals of the critical care nurse are to preserve life and facilitate healing. Too often nurses experience a sense of disappointment and failure when a patient dies. Nurses naturally experience sadness when their patients die. Nurses and colleagues may interpret the signs of compassion and healthy involvement as indications of

---

Clinical Research

Freichels TA: Needs of family members of patients in the intensive care unit over time. Crit Care Nur Q 14(3):16–29, 1991

The purpose of this study was to compare the importance family members placed on particular needs when they had a relative in the intensive care unit. Forty-one family members completed the Critical Care Family Needs Inventory (CCFNI) at two time intervals: within 72 hours of admission to the CCU and one week after admission. Family members ranked their needs from most important to least important.

Results showed that seven of the ten most important needs identified by families in the first 72 hours were related to relieving anxiety. The ten needs ranked as least important were related to family support and comfort. Family needs identified as most and least important one week after admission were about the same as during the first time period. Measures related to assurance and information ranked high, while support and comfort remained low. The greatest need during both time periods was to have questions answered honestly. Being informed of patient progress and being assured that the patient was receiving the best possible care ranked high during both time periods. Recommendations based on study findings included use of a family assessment protocol, policies for more flexible visiting hours, and continued focus on providing family centered nursing care.

---

overinvolvement. A nurse whose eyes become filled with tears at a sensitive moment conveys a sense of empathy to patients, not loss of control. The major goal for many nurses is to learn to *demonstrate comfortably* the concern and compassion that are already an integral part of their emotional makeup.

Comfort

The aggressive pursuit of comfort is the primary nursing goal for the dying patient. This is especially important when a decision has been made to discontinue treatments and the goal changes from curing to supporting and comforting.

Pain relief is an important part of providing comfort for many critical care patients. The nurse must communicate closely with the patient and the physician to create a regimen in which the patient's integrity and peace of mind are not reduced by pain or the need to beg for medication. If a patient is in continuous pain, it is more appropriate to give medication on a predetermined schedule (eg, q3h) rather than as needed (eg, PRN). Furthermore, few patients who are given narcotics for pain develop a serious problem of addiction. In the terminally ill patient, concern for comfort supersedes concern for the problems of addiction. Knowing the patient's concern and desires about the pain experience is of utmost importance. For example, some patients elect not to trade alertness for pain reduction. Many nurses want to medicate these patients because working with people in excruciating pain is trying and frustrating. It also increases the nurse's feelings of helplessness and, therefore, the nurse's anxiety.

In addition, nurses should be made aware that staff attitudes appear to have much to do with the ordering and giving of analgesic medication. In general, patients who are young and female tend to receive more powerful analgesics than others. Age, rather than physical condition, degree of pain, or other variables, may be the determining factor relating to the nurses' implementation of PRN medication orders for patients with pain. This phenomenon points out that nurses must be careful to assess the patient's need and capacity for pain medication and separate this assessment from other irrelevant factors.

Finally, *every possible comfort measure* that can be used without greatly increasing discomfort should automatically be taken. Mouth care can be easily overlooked in a patient who is not eating. Dryness, drooling, odor, and poor nutrition may cause pain and discomfort. The family can be involved in applying lip balm to the patient's lips and washing saliva from the skin. Positioning, skin care, and massage are all useful measures in promoting comfort. Some family members may choose to participate in this type of care, whereas others may be uncomfortable or fear that they will hurt the patient. Usually, the family's participation means more work for the nurse; however, this participation in care can be a highly significant and useful experience for the grieving family.

Promoting comfort for the dying requires constant and judicious decision-making. Should a febrile patient be covered when cold? Should someone with depressed respirations be sedated when restless and anxious? Comfort measures that break the usual protocol of the critical care unit may be required. Honest and direct communication with the patient and the family help guide the actions of nurses and physicians on complicated matters.

Communication

Listening, and listening well, is the cornerstone of effective communication. Some patients do not wish to talk about dying. To do so strips them of whatever hope they are holding. Others deal with death in a symbolic way. They speak of autumns and winters and other subjects that symbolize endings. This is an effective way of terminating one's life; no interpretation is necessary, and to do so would be inappropriate.

Family members may elect to use the time to go over special memories, reconcile past misunderstandings, and forgive each other for past transgressions. It is hoped that they will have the time and atmosphere to say the things they need to say.

The nurse's responsibility is to establish an atmosphere in which this type of communication can occur. What does the family need to be comfortable on the unit—a cup of coffee, a pillow, a place to sit, permission to leave? Does the family wish to be present at the time of death? How can they be reached? All these questions require sensitive timing and a straightforward approach on the part of the nurse. If words escape the nurse, as they often may in difficult moments, or if words seem inadequate, much can be conveyed by touching a shoulder or an arm.

Children

Allowing children to visit a critical care unit may require special arrangements on the part of the staff. If the patient wishes to see a child or grandchild and if the child wishes to see the patient in a critical care unit, the child should be offered short, simple explanations concerning the patient's condition. Answering the child's questions in terms that the child can understand helps reduce possible fears. The person who is taking care of the child should be made aware that invasive procedures and equipment such as nasogastric tubes are likely to upset the youngster. If a visit from the child is not possible, arrangements for a telephone visit should be made.

Family Cohesion and Integration

The family in crisis is vulnerable to all types of other stresses. Helping family members provide support for one another is of paramount importance. Often they wish to have a family members stay with the patient. Family members can support one another by providing meal and rest breaks. Being together and being available to one another is sufficient for many families. The nurse may choose to say to some family members that even though it seems that they are not doing anything for the patient, their presence seems to relax or comfort the patient or the patient's spouse.

Cheerfulness

Not even dying people like a sad and grumpy nurse. Keeping one's sense of humor and expressing it appropriately offer relief in a difficult situation. Generous smiles and a sense of humor also help the family relax and share themselves in their usual ways. A good joke can also be appreciated by a dying patient.

Sensitivity to the patient's mood and a sense of timing are useful in assessing a patient's receptivity to light-heartedness. Talking to the patient in one's typical fashion helps the family relax and communicate more easily with one another and with the patient. In turn, the patient feels less isolated and alone in this final crisis.

Consistency and Perseverance

During times of crisis, complaints and criticisms are frequently directed toward the nurse. A nondefensive, tolerant attitude and a willingness to continue working with the patient and family are the most effective ways of conveying compassion and understanding. Continued interest in a patient and family demonstrates a sense of worth and respect to those involved.

As patients get closer to death, nurses are likely to spend less time with them. This decreased contact may evoke feelings of abandonment, sadness, and hopelessness in both patients and family. Moreover, changes in staff shifts increase their sense of isolation and cause them to use up energy adjusting to new people. Providing consistent staff who do not withdraw helps the patient and family develop trust and a sense of belonging that can become a rewarding experience for everyone involved.

Equanimity

Equanimity can be described as the ability to be comfortable with the dying patient. For many nurses, being comfortable about death depends on the ability to modify goals that are aimed at preserving life with goals that are designed to preserve personal integrity and family stability when a patient is dying. Rather than considering death as a symbol of failure, nurses can view it as a life-enriching and professionally gratifying experience.

Near Death Experiences

Description

Advances in medical and nursing technology have increased the number of people who have survived moments of death or a state of near death. Patients who are seriously ill or injured, who move alarmingly close to death, and then recover, have provided health care professionals with a growing understanding of the near death experiences (NDEs). Through the descriptions of memories of NDEs, remarkable patterns of the experiences have emerged.

There are commonalities in the descriptions of NDEs even though each experience is also unique and individualized. The typical pattern of NDEs nearly always begins with an out-of-body experience. Patients describe floating above their bodies and even moving out of the room. After, or concurrent with, the out-of-body experience are reports of visitors unseen by staff or family. These visitors are usually dead family members or other people who have significant meaning to the patient. Patients sometimes talk out loud to these visitors and tell others who the visitors are.

The next phase of the experience includes movement through a long dark enclosure, like a tunnel. Some report a bright, yet comfortable, light at the end of the enclosure. Most report an extraordinary sense of peacefulness. The environment beyond the enclosure is described as inviting and difficult to leave. Feelings of joy, euphoria, and an overwhelming sense of peace pervade the experience.

Assessment and Management

Some patients recover from the near death event. When the patient "returns" to life and eventually shares the experience with others, the responses of families and staff vary. Whatever the cause or interpretation placed on the experience, the NDE is likely to have a powerful effect on the individual. Attitudes toward life and death can be dramatically altered. Life becomes more meaningful and appreciated and death becomes less frightening.

Nurses can assist patients and family members by acknowledging the importance and meaning of the experience to them. Nurses should never attempt to denigrate the reality of the experience by explaining it away as a biochemically induced hallucination which occurs when the brain nears the point of death. Whether the experience is biologically or divinely caused should not detract from its importance for the individual and family. Family members can be told that many have survived years beyond the NDE, and that having this experience does not mean that the patient will die. Instead, the nurse genuinely can emphasize the choice to return to life as an important indicator of a positive prognosis. Even so, a positive prognosis should not be promised. Because reports of NDEs seem to emotionally touch all who hear them, the nurse must be careful to protect the patient's need for time and privacy to process the meaning and significance of the experience.

Although the NDE can end at any point, many who continue with the experience describe being given a choice to return to life, while others are not given a choice but are directed to return to life. Somehow they are told that it is not time for them to enter this new realm. At this point patients recount returning to their bodies.

There are several compelling explanations of this interesting phenomenon. The biologic explanation argues the NDE is nothing more than an hallucination of an anoxic, dying brain, while others interpret the episodes as a close encounter with God and a spiritual domain. In fact, NDEs typically are reported in the context of the culture and faith of the patient.

Only out-of-body experiences and encounters with others not physically present tend to be described by patients who experience NDE and who eventually die. Dying patients sometimes tell family members that dead relatives are present. Nurses can help teach the family about NDEs, should this happen. If the patient has been suffering and waiting for death, the family is probably ready to let go. The nurse may tell the family that the patient might need their permission to leave this world with those who have come for him or her.

Family members who are unaware of NDEs can become very disturbed when they see the patient talking to someone who is not there. The nurse can support the family through role modelling. The nurse may ask the patient about the visitors and about why he or she believes they are present.

Summary

The nature of critical care nursing is such that the nurse is exposed to repeated losses. When the nurse has experienced this type of loss as a result of death in her personal life, dealing with dying patients may at times reactivate feelings and memories associated with these personal losses. Therefore, it is essential that the nursing staff support one another, especially by listening in a tolerant way when a colleague is expressing what is generally considered to be unacceptable feelings.

Few nurses come to the critical care unit with these abilities. It is necessary for most nurses to request specific educational experiences, consultation, and supervision from appropriate resources. The intensity of emotion and involvement demanded by a nursing role in critical care makes these nurses particularly vulnerable to the "burnout" syndrome (see Chapter 10).

Crisis intervention for families undergoing acute stress is an important preventive mental health function that nurses can provide. Their knowledge of and proximity to the problem allow them to be first-line resource professionals. As patient advocates, their role is to realize and point out that dealing with a psychological crisis in the family greatly affects the recovery and well-being of the patient and decreases the chances for further disequilibrium in the family unit (see Nursing Care Plan 3–1).

BIBLIOGRAPHY

Freichel TA: Needs of family members of patients in the intensive care unit over time. Crit Care Nurs Q 14(3):16–29, 1991

Fremit MR: Near death experiences: A new understanding. Physician Assist 8:42–50, 1989

Kleinpell R: Needs of families of critically ill patients: a literature review. Crit Care Nurse 11(8):34–40, 1991

Kleinpell R, Powers M: Needs of family members of intensive care unit patients. Appl Nurs Res 5(1):2–8, 1992

Koller PA: Family needs and coping strategies during illness crisis. AACN Clin Issues Crit Care Nurs 2(2):338–345, 1991

Leske JS: Overview of family needs after critical illness: from assessment to intervention. AACN Clin Issues Crit Care Nurs 2(2):220–228, 1991

Moody R: Life After Life. A Bantam book (New York, NY) published by arrangement with Mockingbird Books, Covington, GA, 1975

Murphy PA, Forrester DA, Price DM, Monaghan JF: Empathy of intensive care nurses and critical care family needs assessment. Heart Lung 21(1):25–30, 1992

Nyamathi A, Jacoby A, Constancia P, Ruvevich S: Coping and adjustment of spouses of critically ill patients with cardiac disease. Heart Lung 21(2):160–166, 1992

Rukhorm E, Bailey P, Coutu-Wakulczyk G, Bailey WB: Needs and anxiety levels in relatives of intensive care units patients. J Adv Nurs 16(8):920–928, 1991

STUDY QUESTIONS

1. To help the family develop a sense of control the nurse may
   a. offer reassurance that the patient is receiving the best possible care
   b. refer family members to a grief counselor or clergy
   c. offer choices to family members whenever possible
   d. all of the above

2. During an immediate crisis, the family members will
   a. easily form a relationship with a helpful nurse
   b. have greater than usual problems forming a relationship with a helpful nurse
   c. follow the family's previous pattern of forming a relationship
   d. avoid forming a relationship because of a fear of loss

3. Assisting the family members to define or state a problem associated with a crisis is useful because it
   a. increases their sense of understanding of the problem
   b. implies parameters or limits of the problem
   c. helps family members achieve a sense of cognitive mastery
   d. all of the above

4. The family enters a crisis under several conditions. Identify the conditions most likely to increase the probability that a family will enter a crisis:
   a. an event has lasting consequences for a family
   b. a family's ability to problem-solve is inadequate
   c. the equilibrium of the family is thrown off
   d. all of the above

5. After a crisis has subsided the nurse can expect that the family
   1. has returned to its pre-crisis state of equilibrium
   2. has grown in its ability to adapt
   3. has decreased its ability to adapt
      a. 1 only
      b. 2 only
      c. 2 or 3
      d. 1, 2, and 3

6. If family members' expectations of the nurse are unreasonable, the nurse should first
   a. honestly tell the family that their requests or expectations are unreasonable
   b. offer alternative assistance related to their requests or expectation
   c. reflect back to the family the feeling beneath the demands
   d. all of the above

CHAPTER 4

Psychosocial Impact of the Critical Care Environment

BEHAVIORAL OBJECTIVES

Based on the content in this chapter, the reader should be able to:

1. List five factors that can adversely affect patients in the critical care unit.
2. Identify five nursing interventions that can minimize the effects of sensory deprivation and sensory overload.
3. Explain how periodicity affects the patient in the critical care environment.
4. Discuss potential problems caused by sleep deprivation.
5. List ten possible causes of acute confusion.
6. Identify five nursing interventions that encourage reality orientation.
7. Identify actions that acknowledge the patient's need for personal space and privacy.

Hudak: Critical Care Nursing:
A Holistic Approach, 6th ed. © 1994
J. B. Lippincott Company.

Introduction

Many factors affect patients in critical care environments in addition to the illness or injury for which they are admitted. This chapter discusses ways in which nurses can avoid or minimize the negative effects of the following factors:

- sensory input (deprivation, overload, the hospital phenomenon)
- periodicity
- sleep
- acute confusion

Patients in today's critical care units are surrounded by advanced technology that, although essential to save lives, may create an alien and even life-threatening environment for them. Critical care nurses must possess expertise in the use of this technology yet remain aware that a patient's fear of the equipment can create serious stress reactions. The nurse must be aware of care beyond the patient's physical needs and the mechanical workings of the ever-increasing array of equipment that medical technology produces.

The psychosocial support needed by the patient in the critical care unit includes assistance in dealing with the effects of the hospitalization as well as with a critical illness. The sounds and activities of the unit bombard the patient 24 hours a day; in addition, the patient must cope with fears concerning illness. Normal coping defense mechanisms are diminished in all patients and probably absent in the unresponsive patient. The unresponsive person has lost the ability to run from a frightening or painful stimulus and the ability to analyze a situation objectively and take action to control it.

To appreciate how devastating confinement to a critical care unit can be, think of how it would feel to reverse roles with a patient. When asked if they would volunteer to spend 24 hours in the patient role in the crisis care unit, nurses respond readily with a definite "No!" Because of awareness of the environmental threats of such units, the nurse, as primary caretaker, can function as the negotiator for the patient. The following concepts can help nurses be effective negotiators.

Sensory Input

Description

The broad concept of sensory input deals with stimulation of all of the five senses: visual, auditory, olfactory, tactile, and gustatory. Stimuli to all the senses may be perceived in a qualitative manner as pleasant or unpleasant, acceptable or unacceptable, desirable or undesirable, soothing or painful. Individual perceptions of stimuli vary drastically. Some persons may consider the sounds and smells of a metropolitan business section to be pleasant, acceptable, and desirable, whereas others may find them undesirable.

Everyday activities, including the choice of food or drink, are based on a person's likes and dislikes. Thus, people tend to choose, whenever possible, the environment or stimuli from the environment most acceptable to them. Patients in the critical care unit, however, have no control over the choice of their environment or most of its stimuli.

In addition to the *quality* of a stimulus, the nurse must also consider the *quantity*. Too much of a desirable stimulus can become as unacceptable as too little stimulation. For example, gorging oneself with a favorite food to the point of revulsion is "too much of a good thing." In the critical care unit, too many undesirable stimuli, such as excessive and constant noise, bright light, and hyperactivity, can be as distorting and bothersome as too few stimuli, such as gloom, silence, and inactivity.

In trying to control environmental stimuli in a critical care unit, the nurse must be aware of both the type and the amount of sensory input. If sensory stimuli are diminished too drastically, the patient is exposed to *sensory deprivation*, which can cause severe disorganization of normal psychological defenses. If sensory stimuli occur in excessive quantity, the phenomenon of *sensory overload* creates an equally undesirable response to the environment, including confusion and withdrawal.

Sensory Deprivation

Sensory deprivation is a term used to identify a variety of symptoms that occur after a reduction in the quantity or quality of sensory input. Other terms used to denote sensory deprivation or some form of it include *isolation, confinement, informational underload, perceptual deprivation,* and *sensory restriction*. A variety of symptoms has been observed in normal adults after exposure to sensory deprivation for varying periods. These include:

- loss of sense of time
- boredom
- presence of delusions, illusions, and hallucinations
- anxiety and fear
- restlessness
- depression
- any type of behavior or symptom present in psychoses

Sensory deprivation need not be present for a period of days or weeks for psychopathological reactions to occur. For example, it is well documented that normal young adults undergoing an 8-hour period of sensory deprivation may experience an acute psychotic reaction followed by continuation of delusions for several days and severe depression and anxiety for a period of several weeks.[1]

The degree of sensory deprivation possible in a laboratory setting is greater than that likely to occur in a critical care unit. However, laboratory subjects are aware of the time involved in the experiment and have the ability to stop whenever they wish. They also possess clinically normal defense mechanisms and total control of the situation. Hospitalized patients do not have these advantages.

Sensory Overload

The area of sensory overload has not received as much attention as that of sensory deprivation, but some of its effects on humans are known. Decreased hearing after long-term exposure to high noise levels has been well documented. It is also recognized that tension and anxiety increase when a person is exposed to continuous noise without quiet periods. Edgar Allan Poe capitalized on such knowledge in "The Pit and the Pendulum" and other horror stories that deal with the effect of continuous rhythmic sounds such as the dripping of water or the whirring of machinery. Continuous noise has also been used as a means of torturing prisoners of war. Florence Nightingale, in her "Notes on Nursing," warned nurses that "unnecessary noise is the most cruel absence of care which can be inflicted on either sick or well."[2] Therefore, consider sensory overload from the environment to be a possible cause of a patient's anxious or restless behavior.

Excessive stimuli in the environment are significant causes of psychological problems in patients in critical care units. In addition, the quantity and quality of noise can be a significant factor in a patient's recovery. For example, high noise levels can increase the need for pain medication, and loud laughter among personnel can cause resentment in patients. The normal egocentricity of critically ill persons may cause them to interpret all surrounding conversation and action as pertaining to them. Therefore, all talking and laughing not intended to be heard by the patients should occur outside the patient area.

If environmental stimuli exceed the limits to which the human organism can comfortably adapt, the coping system fails. If this occurs, behaviors such as anxiety, panic, confusion, delusions, illusions, or hallucinations may result.

DISPLAY BOX 4–1
Symptoms Related to High Noise Levels

- Increased need for pain medication
- Inability to sleep
- Feelings of fear, helplessness, forgetfulness, withdrawal
- Reaction that talk, laughter, and so forth is aimed at patient
- Confusion, delusions, illusions, or hallucinations

DISPLAY BOX 4–2
Information Overload Responses

- No processing of information
- Incorrect processing of information
- Selective processing of information
- Escape from the flow of information

The Hospital Phenomenon

The hospital environment often deprives patients of normal sensory stimuli while bombarding them with continuous strange sensory stimuli not found in the average home environment. This situation, a combination of sensory deprivation and sensory overload, is referred to as *the hospital phenomenon*.

Normal sounds at home include voices of loved ones and friends; barking of neighborhood dogs; automobile, bus, and train traffic and horns; the television or radio on a familiar station; children at play; the washing machine or dishwasher; daytime telephone calls; and many other sounds and sights that diminish when night comes. Sounds in critical care units, however, include voices of strangers in large numbers; movement of bed rails; beeping of cardiac monitors; paging systems calling strange names; suctioning of tracheostomies; telephones ringing at all hours; whispers, laughter, and muffled voices. These are accompanied by continuous lighting, strange views of equipment, fear, and pain. Such abnormal sounds and sights cause additional stress on patients in critical care environments. Therefore, the patient's surroundings must be controlled as much as possible so that environmentally induced stress can be minimized.

It is possible that nurses in critical care units like the noisy, hectic environment and inadvertently encourage rather than control it. Whether or not that is so, more than 25 years of evidence suggests that psychotic behavior can result when sensory deprivation or sensory overload occurs.

The combination of the loss of familiar stimuli and continuous exposure to strange stimuli elicits different types of defensive responses from patients. Withdrawal is a common coping mechanism and can cause a patient to be labeled erroneously as confused or disoriented unless a complete assessment is done. Some degree of withdrawal from the frightening reality of the situation is common.

Nursing Assessment and Management

Both sensory deprivation and sensory overload can adversely affect patients. Therefore, *assess* the environment for sensory stimuli (sounds, lights, touches, interruptions) throughout the entire day and night. *Note* each type of stimulus and its source, location, duration, and frequency. *Evaluate* the quality and quantity of stimuli and how they affect the patient.

Using the Nursing History to Plan Sensory Stimulation

A nursing history taken in the initial phase of planning can provide information to help tailor nursing interventions. Such a history requires that individualized questions be asked of both patient and family members. A brief outline of a normal 24-hour period of activity for the patient and his or her sleep habits gives the nurse a good starting point in compiling data. A simple rule to use in collecting a nursing history is to determine what is significant or familiar and expose the patient to it, if possible.

Additional information included in the nursing history can be anything from food likes and dislikes to favorite type of music or TV programs. It may be desirable to provide exposure to familiar stimuli by playing a favorite record from home, finding the right radio station to listen to, or requesting a taped message from a loved one who cannot visit. Such actions offer meaningful sensory stimulation to the patient in an otherwise unfamiliar environment. Family and friends should be involved in planning and providing such sensory input, especially for unresponsive patients. The potential value of a familiar voice in giving information or encouragement to a patient is made clear in the following patient situation.

CASE STUDY

A young woman was admitted to a critical care unit shortly after Christmas. She had a diagnosis of viral encephalopathy and a guarded prognosis. She became unresponsive within a few hours, and her husband was told that she was not expected to live. In spite of this, she held on to life for 2 months, during which the hopeless prognosis remained. Twice more, the husband was told that death was imminent.

Finally, after another message from the hospital, the young husband told his 2½-year-old son that his mother was dying. The child repeatedly told his father not to worry because his mommy wouldn't die. The father took the boy to the critical care unit to see his mother for the last time.

While there the boy said, "I love you, Mommy." To the shock of all except the boy, his mother opened her eyes for the first time. The young woman later told everyone, "I had forgotten everything until I heard his voice say 'I love you, Mommy.'" She is well on the road to recovery now.

Reality Testing

For reality testing to occur, there must be continuous input of familiar, meaningful information from the person's outside world. If this information is lacking, the person's internal mental events can be mistaken for exter-

nal ones. This may explain why some critical care patients appear to have illusions or hallucinations.

As human beings we take our physical environment for granted. But if we suddenly awoke in a world without grass or sunlight or the sounds of traffic or human speech, we would not have the necessary stimuli to keep our minds in contact with reality. We would try to interpret unknown stimuli on the basis of that with which we have always been familiar. In reality, however, our interpretations might be wrong. This is especially true of patients who suffer temporary loss of any of the senses, particularly vision or hearing, because people normally use a combination of senses to interpret their environment.

Absence of reality testing may offer at least partial explanation for the high incidence of psychosis in patients assigned to critical care units for long-term care because of altered levels of consciousness. The fact that no physical reason has ever been identified to explain posttraumatic psychosis offers additional support for the theory that it is caused by a lack of meaningful sensory input.

The following example of sensory deprivation in the critical care unit describes an unresponsive patient assumed to be unconscious by both the medical and nursing team members.

CASE STUDY

Carol was a 20-year-old college student with severe basal skull trauma and multiple injuries. She was unresponsive throughout the 8-day period she spent in a critical care unit.

When Carol began responding verbally, her first words to her mother were, "Am I free now? I was in the hands of the Soviet Union!" An immediate interpretation of such a statement could be that she was totally out of contact with reality because of the injury and had dreamed such an episode. It is just as reasonable to assume that she could have perceived that the actions in the unit and the treatments she received were related to torture and that she was the victim for some unknown reason.

Carol had no noticeable motor control of her facial muscles, so she was "blind." She had a tracheostomy that required frequent suctioning. She was almost immobile because of fractures and spasticity necessitating plaster casts or cloth restraints on all extremities. Because she had no means of interpreting her experience realistically from meaningful cues in the environment, such a situation could have caused her to believe that she was being tortured.

Providing Sensory Input for the Unresponsive Patient

Although all patients are susceptible to sensory deprivation and overload, those who are at highest risk and most likely to be seriously affected include the very young, the very old, those recovering from anesthesia, those with sensory deficits, and those who are unconscious (unresponsive).

The patient who can communicate is likely to seek out relevant and meaningful information by questioning visitors and those involved in his care. However, the nurse in the critical care unit serves as the eyes, ears, and voice for those at risk, specifically the unresponsive patient.

Because unresponsive patients may suffer the greatest psychological trauma related to the effects of the environment, their psychosocial needs require the greatest attention. One barrier to providing this attention is the attitude of hopelessness fostered by the patient's being referred to as "unconscious" rather than "unresponsive." "Unconscious" denotes a lack of sensory awareness, which cannot currently be measured in the absence of concurrent motor response, whereas "unresponsive" means that motor- and sensory-coordinated responses cannot be elicited.

Replacing the label "unconscious" with the term "unresponsive" helps remove the connotation of lack of awareness. This attitude paves the way for providing therapeutic sensory input to unresponsive patients.

In order to provide intentional, meaningful sensory stimulation, the nurse must collect data from any person who knows the patient and who is available to give information. For example, the nurse can ask about the patient's musical tastes, favorite radio station, hobbies, and activities during a typical week. Answers to the last question make it possible for the nurse to provide familiar activities that can help keep the patient oriented to time. The nurse must always be on the lookout for clues and information to make it easier for the patient to keep in contact with the familiar world. Other ways of creating a structured and familiar environment include having care given, as much as possible, by the same person on each shift. Encouraging family and friends to visit and to communicate results in further meaningful sensory stimulation.

Family and friends need instruction and encouragement about approaching the unresponsive patient. The nurse should let them know that they may speak to and then touch the patient. The nurse should communicate to them that it is not only all right but also very desirable for them to touch the patient's hand, arm, or face or to kiss the patient if it is part of their usual relationship (and does not interfere with any equipment attached to the patient). Do not assume that loved ones standing at the bedside know that they may touch the unresponsive person. Most visitors must be given permission as well as instruction.

One of the most agonizing feelings is that of uselessness on the part of a family member or friend at the bedside of an unresponsive loved one. The scene of a mother, father, husband, wife, or other close relative standing at the bedside and staring with a variety of emotions at the unresponsive patient is an opportunity for intervention. A simple direction or, in some cases, encouragement to touch the patient's hand and talk may bring a look of relief and gratitude to their faces. With further assistance concerning what to say to the patient, visitors can be very effective in diminishing sensory deprivation by discussing familiar people or subjects normally of interest to the patient.

The value of simple conversation about everyday activities is underestimated in the care of the unresponsive patient in critical care units. This is pointed out vividly in the following case study.

CASE STUDY

While caring for a patient in her late 50s who was comatose as a result of metastatic carcinoma of the brain, I carried on a one-sided conversation about many things, including a daily introduction of myself, explanations of care to be given, and discussion of the day and the weather. There was no perceptible response from the patient. Her condition appeared to be slowly deteriorating. I lost contact with her after 4 days because of an assignment change.

While boarding a train about 2 months later, I was approached by a woman on crutches who called me by name and asked if I were a nurse. I answered yes and eventually recognized her. Our discussion revealed much about our initial relationship. The patient expressed how she had felt during the days she lay in the hospital bed, totally defenseless and at the mercy of those on the nursing team. She said it was very important to her that I had identified myself and talked to her each day.

Of particular interest to the patient was information about when I would leave and when I would return. When I said I would be leaving for another assignment she cried, she said, because she anticipated receiving no further information about the outside world. The patient recalled much more about the interaction than I did.

Providing Security Information

Security information helps prevent unnecessary anxiety and disorientation, particularly for people with altered levels of consciousness or memory. It includes information

---

DISPLAY BOX 4–3
Providing Familiar, Meaningful Sensory Input

- Collect data from any person who knows the patient. Include such areas as musical tastes, favorite radio stations, hobbies.
- Have as much care given, as much as possible, by the same people.
- Encourage family and friends to visit and communicate.
- Provide instruction and encouragement to family and friends about approaching the unresponsive patient.
- Use simple conversation about everyday activities during your care.
- Provide security information (time and place orientation, explanation of treatment and procedures).

about the month, date, year, time of day, and place. It also includes explanation of treatments and procedures. This is particularly important for patients with altered levels of consciousness due to trauma, drugs, or toxicity. Encourage orientation to date and time not only by including the information in conversation but also by providing large-faced clocks that are readily visible to the patient and calendars that display the day, month, and year in large figures. These simple items increase the patient's comfort by providing information that we take for granted. In addition, it is necessary to provide this information because an assessment of the patient's state of orientation is often based on answers to questions concerning time and place.

Because many patients cope by withdrawing, anticipate a delayed response after calling the patient's name, and provide repetition to orient the patient to time, date, and place. In addition to the voices of the nursing staff, a familiar person's voice can be very helpful in providing such information.

Controlling Noise

A study of psychosocial parameters in critical care units revealed that a major patient concern was noise. The specific noises patients reported were those from personnel and the sound of chairs squeaking on the floor. The noisiest time was night. Suggestions to reduce noise included increasing staff awareness of the sources of noise, posting signs, and using drapes and carpeting to muffle sounds.[3]

Hospital personnel can reduce the amount of noise they create and nursing staff can control the general environmental stimuli, with the exception of some equipment essential to life-support systems. Nurses may be able to control various sounds on monitors that have light alarms instead of sound alarms. Machines that make continuous noise (eg, beeping cardiac monitors, cycling respirators) should not be kept in areas in which patients can hear the noise. However, methods have not yet been devised for protecting a patient from such machines' noises. If individual soundproofed patient units are not provided, at least one unit should be available for use by all patients who are on noisy life-support systems.

Sleep and Periodicity

Description

Sleep is an essential part of the 24-hour cycle within which human organisms must function. There is a 24-hour periodicity in which the typical major sleep period recurs once a day.[4] We spend about one-third of our lives sleeping, and sleep is essential to physical and mental well-being. The purpose of sleep is to prevent physiological and psychological exhaustion and/or illness; lack of sleep extends the time needed to recover from illness. There are four stages of sleep:

Stage I   Sleep Latency
Stage II   Slow Wave Sleep (SWS) or Delta Sleep
Stage III   Rapid Eye Movement (REM) Latency
Stage IV   REM Sleep

The first stage covers the time between trying to go to sleep and actually falling asleep. Stages I and II together compose Non-REM (NREM) Sleep; Stages III and IV are REM phases. A person normally experiences at least four to six cycles of sleep each 24 hours. The average time for a normal sleep cycle is 90 minutes, but it varies from 70 to 120 minutes.[5]

REM sleep is essential for mental restoration. REM stages become longer and more intense in later sleep cycles, occurring primarily in the last cycles of an uninterrupted night of sleep. Because of REM sleep's importance, it is likely that sleep deprivation is most significant when it occurs during the REM stage. In the critical care unit, sleep deprivation in the REM stage probably results most often from disruption of the continuity of sleep cycles. This is one more threat to the psychological well-being of the patient in critical care.

There are numerous adverse effects in people who are deprived of SWS and REM sleep for even a few days. Such effects include irritability and anxiety, physical exhaustion and fatigue, and disruption of metabolic functions including adrenal hormone production. Even respiratory distress is associated with disrupted sleep, with periods of apnea and hypopnea occurring. Increasing age and certain acute illnesses may further increase sleep apnea or hypopnea.[6]

The broad concept of **periodicity** is another area of knowledge necessary for the nurse in the critical care unit. Other related terms are *circadian rhythm, biological clock, internal clock,* and *physiological clock*. It has been recognized for many years that all living creatures have not only an identifiable life cycle but also short-term cycles that are rhythmic in nature. Disruption of those rhythms can cause deviations from the norm or cessation of life.

The human organism possesses a 24-hour cycle that is resistant to change, and long-term disruption can be fatal. Many of the biochemical and biophysical processes of the human body have rhythms, with peaks of function or activity that occur in consistent patterns within the daily cycle.

Physiological Variations

Knowing when physiological functions are at their lowest level helps the nurse evaluate the significance of fluctuations. For example, normal variations in the quantity of urine output should be expected, because the kidneys possess their own unique rhythm as demanded by sleep and activity patterns. This accounts for a normal decrease in the quantity of urine produced during the night.

Clinical Research

Topf M: Effects of personal control over hospital noise on sleep. Res Nurs Health 15:19–28, 1992

This study sought to determine whether a link exists between simulated CCU noise, subjective stress levels, and the quality of sleep. Research subjects were 105 women who volunteered and were paid to sleep overnight in a simulated hospital environment. They were randomly assigned to one of three groups: (1) instruction in personal control over noise by use of a sound conditioner, (2) no instruction in personal control over noise, or (3) quiet conditions. An audiotape of nighttime CCU sounds provided the noise for the first two groups.

The results provided support for the hypothesis that poorer sleep would be linked to an objective sound level and greater subjective stress. Subjects in the groups with noise had more difficulty in both falling and staying asleep and in progressing from one stage of sleep to another. They also woke up more times during their sleep, spent less time in the later REM sleep stage than the group without noise, and reported poorer sleep. Instruction in personal control over the sound conditioner (in an effort to mask CCU noises) did not result in better sleep. Sleep was measured by polysomnograph equipment and by self-report. Even though subjects were paid volunteers who were in a simulated CCU setting, results show strong support for the premise that CCU sounds cause poorer sleep.

Health care personnel may schedule drug dosage, sleep periods, and stressful procedures such as surgery on the basis of their knowledge of individual circadian rhythms, thus avoiding further stress on the most vulnerable parts of the cycle and capitalizing on the strongest parts of the cycle.

Nursing Assessment and Management

When assessing the patient's condition, consider whether there have been adequate uninterrupted time periods for all stages of sleep to occur. The plan must provide such periods as soon as possible after the patient's admission to the unit. The necessity of taking vital signs every 1 or 2 hours during the night must be weighed against the damage caused to the human organism when it is deprived of sleep. Because a cycle of sleep measured from REM stage to REM stage requires from 70 to 120 minutes, it is important to provide periods of a minimum of 2 hours of uninterrupted sleep during the night.

Physiological functions reach their lowest levels in the middle of the night, whereas in the later morning hours functions are beginning to reach a maximum level. Therefore, normal fluctuations in vital signs should be expected and patients should not be subjected to activity or stressful procedures in the early morning hours. Only life-preserving activities should be allowed to disturb the patient at night. For example, critically ill patients should not be bathed between 2:00 and 5:00 AM because at this time physiological functions are usually at their lowest levels.

Visiting hours should be adjusted to allow for longer periods of rest. For example, allowing visitors a few min-

utes with the patient every hour makes it impossible to have 70 to 120 uninterrupted minutes to complete a sleep cycle. Instead, longer periods of visiting time can be provided during the nonsleeping hours. Families usually acknowledge the need for their ill member to sleep and can work out an acceptable arrangement for sharing time with the patient.

Recent studies do not support the validity of the usual rationales for restricting visiting in critical care units (eg, visits are upsetting to the patient; there is an increased risk for infection to the patient; visits disrupt the unit, causing staff problems with time and energy; visits are physiologically damaging to patients).[7]

Nursing care measures should not always take priority over time for relatives or significant others. Including the family in planning the schedule for some nursing care may decrease their sense of helplessness.

Rest periods for the patient should be provided with the same emphasis as that given to assessing cardiac status and other aggressive physical measures of care. Some patients are receptive to wearing darkened eye shades (or eye masks) and ear plugs to shut out light and sound and promote rest.

Acute Confusion (Delirium)

Description

Patients admitted to a critical care unit have either a serious trauma or a sudden illness that automatically places them at risk for developing acute confusion. Acute confusion is a common condition seen in all ages but one to which elderly persons are especially prone. It has a rapid onset and is generally reversible, differentiating it from dementias, which develop slowly and are irreversible. An acute confusional state affects cognitive functions, attention, and the sleep–wake cycle. The following symptoms may occur:

- fluctuation in the level of awareness
- visual hallucinations
- misidentification of persons (usually in the form of thinking a nurse is some close relative)
- severe restlessness
- memory impairment

Table 4–1 lists other symptoms of acute confusion.

Nursing Assessment

In addition to assessing the patient's current status, obtain as much information as possible about recent functioning. Talk to people who had close contact with the patient before the hospital admission. If the patient's functioning was adequate for self-care before admission to the critical care unit, it should be assumed that any confusion or mental malfunctioning is potentially reversible.

The environmental stresses of the unit coupled with

TABLE 4–1
Symptoms of Acute Confusion

Disorders of Cognition

Impairment in perception, memory, and thinking
Behavior includes
    disorientation for location and time
    confusion of unknown persons with familiar ones
    memory impairment
    delusions that food is poisoned

Abnormal Sleep–Wake Cycle

Disorders of attention, vigilance, and sleep dysfunction
Behavior includes
    insomnia
    vivid night dreams
    agitation as darkness occurs ("sundown syndrome")
    reduced attention time
    under-alertness or over-alertness
    fluctuating awareness from drowsiness to lucidity

Disorders of Psychomotor Behavior

Generally nonspecific
Behavior includes
    wandering
    fluctuation from intense agitation to somnolence
    combative behavior, usually due to fear

the physical and psychosocial impact of illness can precipitate mental impairment that may be labeled acute confusion. Other causes also need to be considered, and they are described in Table 4–2.

A sudden change in a person's life, such as removal from familiar surroundings, a traumatic situation, or administration of certain sedative or tranquilizing drugs, can precipitate symptoms of acute confusion. The following situation illustrates these points.

CASE STUDY

Mrs. Marlow, a 70-year-old retiree, was among several passengers injured when their bus veered off the road and down an embankment. Although apparently not physically injured, Mrs. Marlow had a rapid heart rate, low blood pressure, weakness, and pallor. She was taken to the emergency room, where she described the accident coherently and expressed anxiety and concern over the condition of her injured friend and the loss of her purse and eyeglasses. A physical examination was done, and no injury was evident. Her blood pressure and pulse returned to normal ranges and her ECG was normal. During the latter part of the examination, however, she displayed increasing confusion and soon became disoriented, not knowing where she was or how she got there. Because of the escalating confusion, she was admitted for further observation and evaluation. She was taken to a four-bed room. Bed rails were raised, and she was instructed to use the call light if she needed to use the bathroom. Over the next few evening hours, she was first restless, then agitated; she thought she was home and was frightened by the presence of others in her home. She kept trying to get out of bed and finally climbed over the bed rails. After staff members gently assisted her return to bed, she began screaming and became resistive. She was given 1 mg Haldol intramuscularly and put into a vest restraint in bed.

The shock of these events and the changes that they created for this woman were further aggravated by:

- decreased sensory input (due to loss of her glasses)
- misinterpreted sensory input
- use of restraint
- use of drugs

It is easy to see how situations like this can escalate. One can even imagine that these events could lead to institutionalization in an extended care facility if thoughtful assessment, planning, and care did not short-circuit or eventually help reverse the symptoms.

Nursing Management

Although a comprehensive evaluation is made to determine possible causative factors that can be corrected, the nurse must use all knowledge available to make the environment a therapeutic tool rather than a stressor for the

TABLE 4–2
Possible Reversible Causes of Acute Confusion

Pharmacological factors:	Narcotics, sedatives, digitalis, tranquilizers, steroids, antihypertensives, antidepressants, diuretics, chemotherapeutic agents, bronchodilators, anticholinergics
Environmental factors:	Abrupt change in environment, sensory deprivation, sensory overload, isolation
Psychosocial factors:	Depression, loss, grief
Nutritional imbalances:	Vitamin deficiencies (B_{12}, folic acid, niacin), starvation
Elimination imbalances:	Fecal impaction, urinary retention
Trauma:	Fractures, surgery, concussion/contusion, subdural hematoma, cerebral hemorrhage
Alcohol abuse:	Alcohol withdrawal when hospitalized may be overlooked
Pain:	Due to trauma of external or internal origin
Fluid and/or electrolyte imbalances:	Sodium excess of depletion, dehydration, acid–base imbalance
Metabolic factors:	Hypo- or hyperthyroidism, renal impairment, liver malfunction
Cardiovascular factors:	Congestive heart failure, hypotension, myocardial infarction, dysrhythmias
Bacteriological factors:	Infection (eg, pneumonia)
Body temperature:	Hyperthermia, hypothermia

patient (see Nursing Care Plan 4–1: The Patient With Acute Confusion).

Need for Reality Orientation

Reality orientation requires a rigid, repetitive regimen of giving security information at predetermined times around the clock. A concerted effort by the nurses to help the patient achieve reality orientation must be started immediately as a primary treatment, regardless of the cause of symptoms. The monotony of the procedure may make nurses want to give up the regimen when there is no positive response after a few days. However, the regimen should continue until the patient can repeat the information on request. After a few days, repetition is more comfortable if the nurse prefaces the information with a statement to the patient that she knows the information has been stated many times but that it is important to repeat it until the patient is able to repeat it. In addition, the nurse should:

- answer questions in short simple sentences;
- demonstrate things concretely and nonverbally;
- tell the patient if the nurse does not understand him or her;
- avoid encouraging the disorientation;
- orient using visual props such as clocks and calendars.

Other nursing actions that may foster orientation include spending time with the patient, encouraging socialization with family and friends, positioning the bed so the patient can see outside, and, possibly, turning on the radio or television. Therapeutic touch can also be helpful in conveying concern and providing comfort (see Chapter 5).

Need for Personal Space (Territoriality)

All people have an unconsciously marked territory around them that is known as personal space. The actual size of this space is generally thought to be flexible and to provide a margin of safety and security. Factors that influence the size of the space include the social situation, the physical area, the person's cultural background, and the person's relationship to others who are present.

Invasion of one's personal space may cause discomfort, anger, and anxiety. It is normal to defend against such threats in order to maintain control of the space. In a hospital setting, personal space is severely limited and is often invaded by the nursing staff.

Nurses can provide the patients with some control over their personal space by practicing some common courtesies, such as knocking on the door before entering, asking permission to perform a procedure or inspect a dressing, and using covers and curtains to provide some privacy.

At a time in life when adapting to change becomes increasingly difficult and painful, the elderly patient is confronted with an extreme limitation of territory. Even the patient coming from a long-term care facility has had more space to claim and greater freedom to organize it in the manner desired. The historically diminishing size of the territory possessed and controlled by the elderly patient creates psychological pain and a decrease in self-esteem. The nurse in a critical care unit can show sensitivity to this situation by avoiding unnecessary intrusion into the patient's diminished territory.

A visit to the home or room of an elderly person characteristically reveals the presence of multiple treasures on walls, tables, and shelves, including pictures, books,

NURSING CARE PLAN 4–1:
The Patient With Acute Confusion

NURSING DIAGNOSIS	OUTCOME CRITERIA/ PATIENT GOALS	NURSING INTERVENTIONS
Thought Processes Altered: related to inability to evaluate reality.	• Patient will demonstrate the ability to differentiate between reality and fantasy.	1. Provide reality orientation. 2. Give security information at predetermined times around the clock. 3. Repeat this information until patient is able to say it to you.
Sensory-Perceptual Alterations, tactile: related to altered sensory integration and/or sensory overload.	• Patient will verbalize awareness of sensory needs.	1. Use therapeutic touch (eg, gently touch patient's hand or arm often). 2. Speak before touching those with impaired sight. 3. Instruct family and friends to touch patient while with them (hold hands or kiss patient if appropriate). 4. Assess the environment for sensory stimuli (sounds, light, touch, interruptions) throughout the entire day and night. 5. Evaluate the quality and quantity of stimuli and how they affect the patient. 6. Provide meaningful sensory stimulation. 7. Provide care that prevents unnecessary environmental overload, such as reducing excessive light and noise, explaining sounds of the unfamiliar environment (monitors, respirators), and promoting reorientation.
Powerlessness: related to hospitalization (loss of privacy and critical illness).	• Patient's privacy and personal space will be respected.	1. Ask permission to look at dressing or to perform any procedure. 2. Knock before entering the patient's room. 3. Use covers and curtains to provide some privacy. 4. Preface entry into the patient's personal space with an explanation.
Sleep Pattern Disturbance: Related to environmental changes.	• A healthy balance of rest and sleep will be maintained.	1. Plan and provide periods of a minimum of 2 h uninterrupted sleep during the night (at least three 2-h periods per night). 2. Plan nursing care so activity and stressful procedures are not undertaken in the early morning hours. 3. If possible, provide sleep time during patient's sleeping hours as determined from history.

glass items, and so forth. No matter how poverty-stricken the person is, there are usually some highly prized items. These objects develop increased value for the elderly person as the years pass, and the nurse must protect such possessions brought to the unit and allow the patients to position them wherever they wish within the small territory allotted to them.

Intrusions also occur in the form of impersonal equipment kept at the bedside (eg, suction machines, monitors, oxygen equipment, and IV equipment). This creates a situation in which territory is limited to the confines of the bed and, possibly, a bedside stand. For this reason, the patient usually clusters all personal possessions on the small stand.

There are also ways in which we all extend the boundaries of our personal space. Radio, television, and telephones are examples which can be used in some critical care unit settings. The availability of small television sets or radios with earplugs for sound control and of telephones with wall jacks makes it more feasible to use these items in a critical care unit. A telephone call from a special person may do more than any medication to help a patient relax. Certainly the judicious use of earphones to enjoy a favorite program helps counteract the adverse effects of the strange sounds of the critical care unit. Nursing assessment can determine the patient's ability to benefit from these territorial extensions, and the nurse who recognizes this therapeutic effect should incorporate them into a humanistic care plan.

REFERENCES

1. Curtis GC, Zuckerman M: A psychopathological reaction precipitated by sensory deprivation. Am J Psychiatry 125: 255–260, 1968
2. Nightingale F: Notes on nursing: What it is, what it is not, page 27. Philadelphia: JB Lippincott, 1992 (commemorative edition)
3. Williams M, Murphy JD: Noise in critical care units: A quality assurance approach. J Nurs Care Qual 6:53–59, 1991
4. Broughton RJ: Chronobiological aspects and models of sleep and napping. In Dinges D, Broughton R: Sleep and Alertness, pp 72–73. New York, Raven Press, 1989
5. Davis-Sharts J: The elder and critical care: Sleep and mobility issues. Nurs Clin North Am 24:755–767, 1989
6. Davis-Sharts J: The elder and critical care: Sleep and mobility issues. Nurs Clin North Am 24:755–767, 1989
7. Tughan L: Visiting in the PICU: A study of the perceptions of patients, parents, and staff members. Crit Care Nurs Q 15:57–68, 1992
8. Topf M: Effects of personal control over hospital noise on sleep. Res Nurs Health 15:19–28, 1992

BIBLIOGRAPHY

Espinoza H: Sleep fragmentation and ventilatory responsiveness to hypercapnia. Am Rev Respir Dis 144:1121–1124, 1991

Fairman J: Watchful vigilance: Nursing care, technology, and the development of intensive care units. Nurs Res 41:56–58, 1992

Fontaine DK: Measurement of nocturnal sleep patterns in trauma patients. Heart Lung 18:402–410, 1989

Grant JS, Kinney M: Altered level of consciousness: Validity of a nursing diagnosis. Res Nurs Health 13:403–410, 1990

Hopping BL, Sickbert S, Ruth J: A study of factors associated with CCU visiting policies. Crit Care Nurse 12(2):8–15, 1992

Hunt L: Eye risks for ventilated or unconscious patients. Insight 16:7, 1991

Johnson JC, Kerse NM, Chen MB, Gottlieb G, Wanich C, Sullivan E et al.: Prospective versus retrospective methods of identifying patients with delirium. J Am Geriatr Soc 40:316–319, 1992

Lloyd F: Eye care for ventilated or unconscious patients. Nurs Times 86:36–37, 1990

McQuillen MP: Can people who are unconscious perceive pain? Issues Law Med 6:373–383, 1991

Monk TH: Sleep and circadian rhythms. Exp Gerontol 26:233–243, 1991

Moore T: Making sense of sensory deprivation. Nurs Times 87:36–38, 1991

Reynolds CF: Rapid eye movement sleep deprivation as a problem in elderly subjects. Arch Gen Psychiatry 47:1128–1136, 1990

Rockwood K: Acute confusion in elderly medical patients. J Am Geriatr Soc 37:150–154, 1989

Salto T, Yoshikawa T: Sleep apnea in patients with acute myocardial infarction. Crit Care Med 19:938–941, 1991

Sullivan J: Neurological assessment. Nurs Clin North Am 25:795–809, 1990

STUDY QUESTIONS

1. Sensory deprivation
   a. will not be a problem for a patient for at least 24 hours
   b. is a term used to identify symptoms that occur related to a reduction in the quantity or quality of sensory input
   c. does not occur in a patient with normal defense mechanisms
   d. is not likely to be a problem in a critical care unit because there is activity and sound most of the time

2. The hospital phenomenon is best described as

   a. an ideal environment for anyone who is ill because it is conducive to rest and recuperation
   b. a situation in which stress is limited for patients because of the structure of the environment
   c. a combination of sensory deprivation and sensory overload related to the environment
   d. the desirable control of aspects of patient care by the health care team

3. The patient likely to suffer the *greatest* psychological trauma related to the effects of the environment is the

   a. unresponsive patient
   b. patient with sensory deficits
   c. very old patient
   d. patient recovering from anesthesia

4. Based on knowledge of the sleep cycle, it is likely that the most significant sleep deprivation occurs in the stage of

   a. SWS
   b. NREM
   c. Delta sleep
   d. REM

5. Symptoms of acute confusion include

   a. unconsciousness
   b. disorganized thinking which has worsened over years
   c. visual hallucinations, restlessness, and fluctuations in the level of awareness
   d. impaired remote memory

CHAPTER 5

The Dynamics of Touch in Patient Care

BEHAVIORAL OBJECTIVES

Based on the content in this chapter, the reader should be able to:

1. Discuss the concept of caring and how it is expressed through touch behaviors in nursing.
2. Identify messages sent and responses to touch as described in nursing literature.
3. Delineate situations/factors that put patients at high risk for touch deficit.
4. List nursing assessment guidelines for evaluating touch needs of patients and families.
5. Apply the nursing process, including nursing diagnosis, to address touch needs of patients.
6. Formulate a nursing care plan for patients threatened by touch deficit.

Hudak: Critical Care Nursing:
A Holistic Approach, 6th ed. © 1994
J. B. Lippincott Company.

Description

Since the 1960s, there has been a prolific growth of critical care units in general hospital settings. Along with this growth and progress have come previously unimagined developments in technology, highly modern facilities, and increasingly available invasive and noninvasive devices for measuring, monitoring, and regulating body systems.

Being a patient in a critical care setting is potentially more frightening, more lonely, more confusing, and, in many ways, more dehumanizing than ever before. The dimensions of the nursing role in this setting have similarly changed. The role is more technological, more physiologically oriented, more intense, and more intellectually demanding than in previous years. Because of these changes, the aspect of caring as the major dimension of nursing has become more important and increasingly threatened.

The nurse can express care for a patient in a many ways. There are descriptions in the nursing literature of mechanisms for providing emotional, social, spiritual, and physical support in the care setting. One behavior that permeates all these endeavors is that of touch. By using touch in a meaningful, genuine, sincere way, nurses can clearly convey caring and support to patients and families. By understanding the power of touch in interactions, nurses can successfully plan it into their care and develop their own skills by including it in communication processes.

Caring and Touch: A Review of the Literature

Caring

There is little dispute among nursing authorities that caring is the central focus of nursing. Leininger expresses a firm belief in the importance of caring behaviors in nursing. She describes a strong link between curing (the major focus of health care) and caring by health care practitioners. "I hold [that] it [caring] is the central concept and essence of nursing. Moreover, care is a vital factor for human growth, health maintenance, and survival. . . . Human caring and human relationships are closely interrelated. Human caring remains an essential dimension of professional work, especially in dealing with life crises, health maintenance problems, and changes in health practices."[1]

Watson[2] portrays the "science of caring" as a balance of science and humanism: "Preservation of human care is a critical agenda for nursing and the health care system of today. . . . [N]ursing must achieve a delicate balance between scientific knowledge and humanistic practice behaviors" (pp. xx, 3). Watson also addresses the close relationship between curing and caring. "Whereas curative factors aim at curing the patient of disease, carative factors aim at

the caring process that helps the person attain (or maintain) health or die a peaceful death" (p. 7). The philosophical foundation for the science of caring is composed of "(1) the formation of a humanistic–altruistic system of values, (2) the instillation of faith–hope, and (3) the cultivation of sensitivity to one's self and to others" (p. 9).

Other authors address the notion of caring from a slightly different perspective. Noddings states, "As human beings, we want to care and be cared for. Caring is important in itself. . . . [It] involves stepping out of one's own personal frame of reference into the other's. When we care, we consider the other's point of view, his objective needs, and what he expects of us."[3]

Benfield examines the concept of caring as it has evolved in the modern world of health care. He describes two distinct philosophies of care: (1) disease-oriented care, and (2) person-oriented care. In disease-oriented care, the focus and attention are on the pathology and illness, not necessarily within the context of the person. In person-oriented care, the focus is on the quality of life of the person and the family.[4] The complexity of health care today calls for the inclusion of both of these philosophies of care. If nurses provide the major person-oriented care and physicians the major disease-oriented care, the ultimate challenge rests in making both of these caring foci coexist to the enhancement of each other.

For this to become a reality, several barriers must be overcome:

- nurses and physicians must develop more effective communication and teamwork;
- the time required to provide patient-oriented care by nurses must be valued by the institutions in which the nurses practice;
- nurses must break out of, or expand, the technician-focused stereotype in critical care in order to include the role and skills of person-oriented care providers.

For many years, nursing literature has discussed the activities that reflect caring. Cohn describes these behaviors as humanistic attributes of patient care that cannot be replaced by technology: listening, caring, humor, involvement, and sharing.[5] Cowper-Smith suggests the preservation of courtesy, compassion, respect, dignity, and genuineness as essentials in caring for patients.[6] Kalisch describes high-level empathy as the major ingredient in the caring process.[7]

Jourard vividly describes his feelings about the nurse–patient relationship, caring, and the influence that they have on patient recovery. According to Jourard, the recovery of the patient depends, to a great extent, on the understanding that someone cares. Caring by the nurse increases patient comfort, identity, and integrity. Lack of caring can actually cause detrimental effects on the health and recovery of a patient. Human warmth, love, and responsive care are among the essentials in any recovery. The nurse is the professional who is most likely and able to provide these humane aspects of care.[8]

Communicating Caring Through Touch

Meaningful communication is a vehicle for the caring process used in meeting psychosocial needs of the patient. One important form of communication in any health care setting is touch. The need for tactile contact is present in everyone at birth and continues throughout life. It is a need that, if met, adds richness and growth to human potential and is basic to the healthy development of the person. The need for touch is thought to intensify during episodes of high stress and cannot be totally met by other forms of communication. Nurses, when using touch, are usually trying to convey understanding, support, warmth, concern, and closeness to the patient. This communication is an activation of the caring process. Touching not only improves the sense of well-being of the patient but also promotes physical recovery from disease.

The role of touch in nursing care can be viewed from many perspectives. It serves a multitude of purposes within nurse–patient interactions. Communication with touch is simple, straightforward, and direct. Touch is a positive behavior that produces a satisfying effect on the patient and is among the elementary needs for healthy mental and physical development. It is one of the most important senses. Touch confirms the reality perceived through other senses and is a central part of human communication processes. It has a positive effect on perceptual and cognitive abilities and can influence physiological parameters such as respiration and blood flow. In summary, touch represents a positive, therapeutic element of human interaction.

The act of touching or being touched involves the stimulation of receptors in the skin that transmit messages to the brain that are then interpreted by the person. A large segment of the brain is devoted to touch. Undoubtedly, touch contributes greatly to many aspects of communication, learning, and understanding.

Touch alone is a frequently used form of interpersonal communication carried out with little space or distance between persons. Intimate space is considered to be the area of approximately 6 to 18 inches from a person's body. The fact that touching invades this intimate space is of great significance to the message being sent.

There is an increased need for touch in the critical care unit, where machines and technology contribute strongly to depersonalization of the patient. Before this modern technology developed, the greatest things that a nurse could offer a patient were the comfort and caring of his or her presence and touch, and these accomplished much. Nurses may be tempted to think that touching is too simple to be effective. However, few medical advances can supersede the benefits of warm and caring touch.

Touch that is non-task related (*affective touch*) is a powerful therapeutic intervention that communicates caring. Nursing authorities generally believe that an increase in meaningful affective touch in conjunction with treatment-related touch can significantly improve the nurse–patient communication process.

Other Effects of Nursing Touch

The effects of touch in the clinical environment are far-reaching. Touch has played a major part in promoting and maintaining reality orientation in patients prone to confusion about time, place, and personal identification.[9] Nursing touch may be most helpful in situations in which people are experiencing fear, anxiety, or depression. It may also be beneficial for patients who have a need for encouragement or nurturing, who have difficulty verbalizing needs, or who are disoriented, unresponsive, or terminally ill.

The age of the patient greatly affects the perception of touch. In Day's study, younger patients felt that touch should be used as an everyday positive component of nursing care, whereas elderly patients felt that it should be used for therapeutic purposes in episodes of pain, loneliness, and depression. Patients also felt that the desire for touch increased with the seriousness of the illness and decreased with increased closeness of the family.[10]

Hollinger[11] suggests that nurses be aware that, for older patients, the need to communicate is paramount. Communicative strategies should include both verbal and nonverbal means, "with touch being an important form of nonverbal interaction between the nurse and the patient." Touch gains its importance because of the need to optimally stimulate the remaining sensorium owing to impairments in more than one sensory modality, or in neurological or psychosocial processes. In addition to a decrease in the use of the senses, older persons may also experience greater need for affective communication because of their increased likelihood for isolation and loneliness. It is believed that these factors greatly influence the physical and mental health of the older person.

In another study, the use of touch by nurses in critical care units did not vary according to the age or sex of the patient.[12] Unfortunately, the most ill patients—those who probably needed and desired touch the most—were touched the least. A study of touching habits and behaviors of nurses in a geriatric home found that people with little or no evidence of physical impairment were touched the most. Men and those who were physically impaired received little touching.[13]

Patients with hearing or vision loss demonstrate particularly high needs for effective, creative communication from nurses. The use of deliberate, planned touch seems to give these patients a greater sense of control over the unfamiliar setting of the hospital.[14] Using touch as a planned part of care (eg, in preoperative teaching) can be

Clinical Research

Mulaik J, Megenity J, Cannon R, Chance K, Cannella K, Garland L, Gilead M: Patients' perceptions of nurses' use of touch. West J Nurs Res 13(3):306–323, 1986

This exploratory study set out to gather data concerning patients' beliefs and attitudes about touch; their experiences, preferences, and responses to touch; their perceptions of the amount and kind of touch provided by nurses; and factors that might influence their perceptions of touch.

Two instruments were used in this study: the Patient Touch Questionnaire (PTQ) developed by the author and the Interpersonal Behavior Survey (IBS) developed by Mauger and Adkinson (1980).

Results indicated that patients perceived most touch by nurses to be "instrumental," in that touching was used for conducting treatments, examining the patient, and giving medications. Except for patting the patients' hands, very little "optional" touch was used.

The only patient characteristic which correlated significantly with differences in touch practices by nurses was patient sex. Male patients perceived receiving more "optional" touch then did women patients.

While most patients agreed that touch by nurses conveyed caring and affection, a moderate number of patients believed that touch also conveyed control. Of the patients preferring nurse touch, 72% expressed a desire for more touch during care. The patients who preferred that nurses limit touch were patients who received a greater amount of essential treatment-related touch in their required care. The researcher suspected that their touch may have been tiring or painful.

A large proportion of patients responded that the touch felt comfortable. One-fourth of the patients indicated that they would respond to touch by moving closer, although a small number would move away. Overall, patients' responses to touch by nurses were very positive.

an extremely effective nursing intervention.[15] These findings point to the need to include touch as a specific intervention in the nursing care plan. If efforts are coordinated by nurses, the use of touch can be more relaxing to a patient than sedatives or tranquilizers. More importantly, there is growing evidence that the nature of patient–nurse interaction influences physical and psychological outcomes of illness.[16] "The reason that touch is such an emotional word is that people so often experience it as a lack or deficit."[17]

Nurses convey a wide variety of messages through the use of touch in nursing care, including security, understanding, sincerity, respect, support, warmth, concern, reassurance, interest, empathy, comfort, closeness, encouragement, acceptance, willingness to help, and willingness to become involved. Despite the convictions of nurses concerning these messages, approximately one-third of them consciously use touch in their practice only in conjunction with verbal communication because of possible misinterpretation by patients.

The Messages of Touch

Touch can be interpreted in a variety of ways depending on the following characteristics: duration, location, frequency, action, intensity, and sensation.

Duration of touch is the total time over which the touch episode occurs. Generally, longer duration of touch allows increased opportunity for the patient to identify and integrate the touch. Longer duration also allows for more realization of body parts and boundaries and higher self-esteem.[18]

Location of touch pertains to the areas and parts of the body being touched. The location of touch gives messages concerning specific body parts and the integration of these parts into the whole. Touching the trunk more than the limbs (referred to as *centripetality*) often conveys a message of closeness and intimacy with the toucher. The number of locations touched in relation to those available to be touched can transmit a positive message of self-evaluation to the person who is being touched.

Frequency of touch, or the total amount of touching experienced, has the most potential for affecting self-esteem, closeness with others, cognitive and emotive ability, and sexual identity.

Action of touch refers to "the rate of approach to a body surface" and the energy used in the initiation of touch.[19] A rapid-approach action of touch increases the self-perception of the person who is being touched, allowing the patient to see himself or herself as an independent sexual being.

Intensity of touch refers to the pressure used on the body surface during touch. Intensity is measured by degree of skin indentation. Moderate intensity of touch has been reported to produce the least therapeutic effects, whereas a variation of strong and weak intensity has the highest potential for positive effects.

Sensation is the body interpretation of touch as being either pleasurable or painful. Painful sensations distort the body image by impairing normal use of the body's perceptual abilities. Pleasurable touch is more apt to provide a feeling that one's body is worthwhile and valuable.

Although these symbols of touch provide measurable components to look for in our behaviors, the messages sent and received and the contexts in which they occur will vary. It is helpful to remember that touching is a "language" that can be a powerful part of nurse–patient interaction.

Taxonomy of Touching

Taxonomies of touching have been developed and proposed with the major emphasis on categorization as determined by the roles and relationships of the persons involved. Heslin developed a very graphic taxonomy based on research findings on touch as a widely used nonverbal form of communication. The taxonomy illustrates an informal set of relationships that exist to regulate the kinds of touch allowed by society. Within the context of this taxonomy, the intensity of the relationship between the toucher and the recipient increases as they progress through the levels.[20–22]

Level I: Functional/Professional

In this level of relationship, touching is done in order to accomplish a professional task. Often the touching is intimate; however, it remains appropriate within the functional/professional relationship. Examples of this level of relationship are nurse–patient, nurse–patient's family, respiratory therapist–patient, and physician–patient.

Level II: Social/Polite

This level of relationship is typical of touching behaviors that are indicative of cultural restraints and prescriptions. The handshake is an example of a touch behavior at this level; it functions as a neutralizing act between two people.

Level III: Friendship/Warmth

This level of relationship is often thought of with uneasiness. Because it is less formal than the social/polite level, it is often misinterpreted as representing a higher level of love or sexual attraction. It carries with it a message of

caring and affection but often is misunderstood for more intense feelings. The messages that some people sense concerning sexuality with people of the same sex or opposite sex may make them wary of touch at this level. A very common touch behavior at this level is the hug.

Level IV: Love/Intimacy

This level of touching conveys the message of deep caring and commitment. Discomfort with gestures on this level often reflects ambivalence in the commitment to a relationship. People are more comfortable with touch gestures if the level of the relationship is appropriate for the message that is being sent.

Level V: Sexual Arousal

This is the level of intensity in relationships in which touch conveys sexual meaning and stimulation. This message may include or exclude love and commitment.

Heslin[23] hypothesizes that there are two possible ways in which this taxonomy provides a score of intensity for personalizing and humanizing another person. One model predicts that the level of humanizing and individualizing increases in correlation with the level of the taxonomy, from levels I to V. In this situation, an individual becomes less of an object and more of a person as the level of the relationship increases.

Heslin's alternate model is one in which the most appreciation of another individual occurs at the friendship/warmth level. Within this level of a relationship, there is more open acceptance of another person and greater tolerance of individual idiosyncrasies. It would be ideal if this same acceptance always occurred at levels IV and V in this taxonomy.

Nurse–Patient Bond

From Heslin's work the question arises, "Where does the nurse–patient relationship fit within this taxonomy?" It is certainly appropriate that many of our task-related interactions correlate with the functional/professional level, which allows for numerous care activities requiring touch (eg, physical assessment, repositioning the patient, bathing, changing a dressing, or attaching cardiac monitor electrodes). But what about "affective touch?" The acceptance, concern, caring, and support transmitted by these behaviors are more indicative of interaction at the friendship/warmth level. It is possible that the nurse has the capacity for moving between those two levels in a way that maintains the professional role while also relating on a very human level with genuine caring for each patient as an individual. It is this combination that makes the nurse–patient relationship unique and powerful.

The caring, trust, and support that develop between

the nurse and the patient constitute the foundation of the nurse–patient bond. No other health care professional has the consistent and frequent opportunities to interact with the patient within this same framework. No other framework of interaction can offer the patient a more powerful source of support: a professional, knowledgeable foundation and a caring, human acceptance as a person of worth and dignity.

"Hypohugganemia"

The concept of "hypohugganemia" signifies a state of touch deficiency in a patient. Because touch is a basic need from birth through adulthood, every person strives to meet this need as it varies with life experiences. Being ill or hospitalized, losing a loved one, or experiencing a crisis can increase a person's need or desire for touch. If such events occur and the need is not sufficiently met, the person is in a state of "hypohugganemia." Even though other forms of stimuli may reduce the immediacy of this need, only human touch can satisfy it.

High Risk Patients and Families

Although any patient admitted to an intensive care unit (ICU) is likely to experience some threat of touch deficiency, particular situations signal the high risk patient or family. Conscious, well planned touch can be an effective strategy for alleviating the state of touch deficiency that can occur in these situations.

Sensory Deprivation

Because of impaired use of the senses or inadequate quality and quantity of sensory input, an ICU patient may be less able to relate to the environment meaningfully. Such a patient may benefit from planned, individualized touch by the nurse. Tactile stimulation can be used to convey meaningful messages to the patient about himself or herself, body boundary perception, self-esteem, wholeness, and contact with reality. Touching can be very effective if used alone or in conjunction with other forms of verbal or nonverbal communication.

Body Boundary Threats

The critical care setting offers a particular challenge to patients to maintain a clear understanding of the boundaries of their own bodies. The increasing use of machinery and technology at the bedside as well as invasive monitoring and treatment techniques can frighten and confuse critically ill patients. Tubes, catheters, and wires extend beyond the body surface to connect with intravenous feeding equipment, monitoring equipment, and mechanical devices to support life. It can become difficult for a patient to know where the body ends and the machinery begins. This difficulty can increase if the nurse spends much time at the bedside touching and manipulating the equipment. In this situation, the nurse may find it helpful to make the effort to touch the patient while at the bedside. It is believed that touching a large number of the body areas available encourages the patient's ability to perceive the body's form and shape accurately and to integrate information about body parts and the body as a whole.

Fear, Anxiety, and Loss of Control

The critical care setting is an environment that makes it difficult for even the strongest and bravest patient to feel fearless, calm, and content. The nurse must give attention to the patient's psychological processes if optimal progress is to be made in the care regimen. One goal for care must always be that the patient be allowed to participate as much as possible. Participation depends to a great extent on the communication and support processes used to build trust, decrease fear, reduce anxiety, and maintain dignity. These processes can be greatly enhanced by the nurse's conveyance of genuine caring, warmth, support, and understanding through the use of touch. The messages transmitted through touch can be vivid and profound, even during a crisis. If used in conjunction with a calm and clear verbal message, eye contact, or effective listening, the communication of caring is enhanced.

Separation From Family

Even the most liberal visiting policies in a critical care unit cannot assure that family and other loved ones will be nearby when a patient is in crisis. A crisis need not be an abrupt physiological change or life-threatening event. It may be a sudden episode of feeling alone, awakening in an unfamiliar environment, the fear of dying, or simply a lack of physical contact with loved ones. The nurse has the opportunity to assist a patient through episodes like these by being with the patient and touching in therapeutic ways to give contact with the environment, the feeling of closeness with another person, and the belief that someone nearby cares.

Communication Barriers

Patients need to experience communication with their caregivers to maintain perceptions of themselves as worthwhile individuals who have contact with reality and can interact with other people. The challenge of communicating increases if patients are deaf, are unable to speak or understand the language of the nurse, or are unable to communicate verbally owing to intubation or a physical disorder or illness. The patient who is unable to move his or her hands, arms, or facial muscles has even more restricted options for communication. Using touch to enhance verbal communication, to get a patient's attention, or to convey a message can be very effective. Allowing the patient to touch the nurse may also be an acceptable way to promote communication with the caregiver. Patients can convey many emotions and messages using touch. Fear, pain, understanding, calmness, and joy are among the messages that may be transmitted by a patient who can hold the hand of the nurse, touch the nurse's face, or grasp his or her arm. This can be a very productive and useful vehicle for patients who offer unusual challenges with regard to communication.

The Family of a Critical Care Patient

The family is an extension of the patient, and caring for a patient also requires caring for loved ones. In numerous ways, families experience many of the same crises as patients in critical care. They are often anxious and fearful and feel very helpless in their abilities to intervene and help the patient. Like the patient, they have to some extent surrendered control to the health care team. They find themselves separated from their loved ones and become victims of visitation policies, a strange and fearful environment, and the unknown. Aside from the time actually spent with the patient, the most meaningful and supportive communication for the family often comes from the nursing staff. Nurses can decrease "communication barriers" for families by using clear, understandable terminology, taking the time to listen to questions and concerns, and using touch with the family members. By touching an arm or shoulder or holding hands, the nurse can enhance genuine listening and give support while sharing information with the family. Frequently, nurses encounter situations in which they feel unable to offer verbal support or understanding. Touching alone can be a very powerful silent transmission of support during these episodes.

Family's Fear of Touching the Patient

The family often feels helpless and fearful at the bedside of a critically ill patient. The tubes, dressings, wires, and machinery to which the nurse is so accustomed are frightening to family members. They see this equipment attached to their loved one and may be reluctant to reach out and touch for fear of causing harm to the patient or the equipment. They are often startled and shocked at the sight of someone they love who now appears so ill.

The nurse has the opportunity at this time to offer support to the family and patient in a unique way. By explaining and describing the equipment and the patient's appearance to the family before they go to the bedside, the nurse can prepare them for this often difficult experience. During this explanation, the nurse can use touch to develop a feeling of trust and support with the family. Again, touching an arm or shoulder or putting an arm around a family member while he or she is approaching the bedside can convey understanding, caring, and support. At the bedside, the nurse can touch the patient while talking with the patient and a family member to demonstrate that tactile contact is safe. By taking a family member's hand and touching the arm, face, shoulder, or hand of the patient, the nurse can help initiate touching behavior and assist in alleviating the fear of harming the patient or the equipment. The process of acting as a role model for the family is an excellent way of decreasing the anxiety of the family and patient and helping them feel more comfortable in a strange environment.

Nursing Assessment of Patient and Family Need for Touch

Individual assessment of touching needs is a very important step for the nurse. Because so many factors affect desire for touch, the nurse must keep in mind that people's needs and reactions to touch are individualized. There is no absolute formula for quantifying and qualifying these aspects of each person because of the complexity of factors that contribute to one's beliefs and feelings about touch. Individual family practice, cultural practices, and coping styles are other powerful influences on desire for—and interpretation of—touch by another person. Nurses must use information available in the care setting as well as their subjective instincts and interpretations of family interaction patterns to determine their strategies for meeting the touch needs of their patients and families.

There are some key questions that the nurse must consider when assessing the touch needs of the patient and family (Figure 5–1). Some of the *major signals of increased need for touch* are the following:

T Total amount of touching is low by family and health team members. The patient may require little physical care, may be in isolation, or may be using a kinetic bed. This could also be a patient who is relatively stable and situated in an area in the unit in which there is little traffic. Thus, few people go near the bedside unless it becomes necessary to implement a procedure or treatment. Often, this patient has few or no visitors, or the family members are very hesitant to touch the patient. When with the patient, they remain distant

Assessment Guide

T Total amount of touching is now by family and health team members.

O Older patient.
Orientation problems.

U Unusual threats to body image or body boundary.

C Consciousness level?
Communication problems? Intubated? Tracheostomy?
Crisis situation?

H High technology at bedside?
High stress period?
Helplessness and Hopelessness? Signs of depression?

I ICU psychosis? Confused: Restless?
Initiation of touch by patient?

N Normal use of senses?

G Giving behavior cues? Verbally? Nonverbally?

FIGURE 5–1
Assessment guide.

from the bed and appear fearful or uncomfortable with touching or displays of affection and caring.

O Older patients often have an increased need for meaningful touch during episodes of crisis. The aging process may also make them more prone to sensory deprivation, confusion, and communication difficulties that can sometimes be decreased by the meaningful use of touch in care. Having few visitors and little verbal interaction may intensify their touching needs.

U Unusual threats to body image and body boundary occur when patients experience discomfort and confusion about their body parts and the integration of those parts into the whole body. They also may experience difficulty with differentiating their bodies from the mechanical equipment used in their care. Patients who have undergone surgery or other invasive procedures or who have experienced side effects from medications, weight loss or gain from the illness or treatments, or dependency on life support equipment all are likely to have body perception problems. Patients who have received organ transplants may also experience some confusion about their body perceptions. Transplantation of other people's organs into one's body may create mixed feelings about wholeness, self-identity, and self-image.

C Consciousness level of the patient may render clues about touching needs. There may be less tendency to touch alert patients if they are stable and able to participate in their own care. This tendency, if prolonged, may actually contribute to an unmet need for touch. Patients who are less alert, lethargic, stuporous, semicomatose, or comatose may need more touching by the nurse. Because their modes of communication are limited by altered levels of consciousness, touching may be an avenue of communication that is very therapeutic. Using touch with these patients conveys all the messages of caring and support and provides them with some meaningful contact with the environment. The comfort and security transmitted through touch can be extremely meaningful to these patients.

Communication difficulties are common challenges to the ICU nurse. Patients who are intubated, who have tracheostomies, or who are physically unable to communicate verbally because of their illness or disability have always posed a communication challenge for the ICU nurse. Patients who cannot speak or understand the language of the nurse are equally disabled in an ICU setting. All these patients experience an increased need for meaningful communication. The importance of effective touch may be increased with these patients.

Crisis can trigger an increased need for support, closeness with others, and clear communication. Often, there is little opportunity for the nurse to provide prolonged verbal support during a crisis situation, even though the need for support and caring may be intense. Patients experiencing a crisis episode may have an increased need for supportive touch.

H High technology has contributed greatly to the intensive care regimen. It may also, however, contribute to the dehumanization process that can occur in the ICU setting. Attention to machinery and equipment can make ICU patients feel very insignificant and invisible among the tubes, wires, computers, and so forth. These patients may need human touch as a reassurance of their humanness, dignity, and self-worth in a setting that is frightening, awesome, and highly technological.

High stress episodes in the ICU need not always be physiological crises. Whenever a patient experiences feelings of fear, increased anxiety, or loss of control there may be a need for increased communication of support and caring. Some routine care activities, such as repositioning, feeding, or even moving a pillow, may remind patients of their inability to do these things themselves. The nurse who recognizes that these "routine" interventions may be psychologically threatening to the patient's self-esteem can use touch to convey understanding, closeness, and caring.

Some recent research[24] reminds us of the complexities of communicating effective support during an episode of high stress. Henneman conducted a study in which 26 patients were randomly assigned to either a control or an experimental group during attempts to wean them from mechanical ventilators. The experimental group received touch and verbal interaction during the weaning process, although the control group did not. Heart rates, mean arterial pressures and respiratory rates five minutes after ventilators were discontinued were recorded for both groups. These measures represented patient stress responses to the weaning process. No significant differences were found in any measures between the two groups. Henneman reminds readers that the messages conveyed by touch depend on the situation and the meaning to the persons involved. More research is needed on touch that is specific to particular patient experiences.

Helplessness and Hopelessness are feelings that patients may experience if they perceive that they are unable to improve their situations to an acceptable level. These feelings can leave them devastated and depressed. They may exhibit these feelings by appearing apathetic about their conditions or care, by being withdrawn and uncommunicative, or by weeping and looking hurt. Feelings of being alone in their crises only make them feel more hopeless. These patients may be very open to supportive and caring touch by the nurse as a sign that someone cares and is with them.

I ICU psychosis, confusion, and restlessness are possible side effects of the critical care environment in combination with the patient's stress level. Lack of restful sleep, altered nutritional status, and use of medications also contribute to the psychological disequilibrium that the patient experiences. Careful and planned touch can assist the patient through such episodes.

Initiation of touch by the patient may be a cue to his or her need for tactile contact by another person. Patients who reach out to the nurse or who cling tightly to the nurse's hand or arm may be signaling their need for closeness and contact with another human being.

N Normal use of the five senses and a normal amount and quality of sensory input enhance a person's ability to cope with anxiety, a strange environment, and crisis. Unfortunately, critical illness, aging, and the critical care setting often distort sensory input and its use. The nurse can at-tempt to increase the patient's use of sensory input by evaluating each person in an attempt to identify behaviors of touch that can reinforce a balanced sensory process. Giving sensitive attention to a patient's behavior is the first step in achieving this balance. The second step involves using meaningful touch in an attempt to communicate caring and the patient's connection with reality, dignity, and esteem. The third step requires the nurse to watch for the patient's response in order to evaluate the intervention on an individual level.

G Giving behavior cues about touching needs may be a subconscious phenomenon for a patient. Facial expression, eye contact, verbalization, initiation of touch, and frequent calling for the nurse may signal that the patient needs to have someone near. Sometimes, the desire for touch is transmitted so subtly that it is difficult to identify the exact characteristics of the message. Whether the message is overt or subtle and whether the nursing assessment is objective or intuitive make no difference. The nurse who is sensitive to the touch needs of the patient can identify the messages and cues much of the time. The nurse who spontaneously and genuinely uses touch with patients to convey caring may already be processing patients' subtle cues.

It is equally important to be alert to patient cues to avoid touch. Keep in mind the individuality of patients, changes in mood, cultural influences, and physiological changes which may cause fluctuations in a patient's need or readiness for physical contact. Openness to touch at one time does not assure that the patient will feel comfortable with touch under other conditions. It is important to understand that the patient's needs and responses to touch may change from hour to hour or day to day.

Moving From "Knowing" to "Doing"

It is always interesting to be enlightened by new information or to gain a new perspective on a frequently observed phenomenon. However, new insight does not always give a person the practical means by which new awareness can be transformed into useful strategies. It is with this in mind that the following case study is presented. This is one example of how a critical care nursing staff made some relatively simple but very meaningful and effective changes in their care on the basis of their increased awareness of patient–nurse interactions using touch.

CASE STUDY

Mrs. Bello was admitted to a large medical center critical care unit approximately 10 days ago. She is a 79-year-old married woman who was transferred from a small community hospital approximately 100 miles away after having undergone a bowel resection for cancer. After her difficult surgery, Mrs. Bello exhibited signs of acute renal failure and congestive heart failure. She suffered from severe fluid and electrolyte imbalance and was found to have toxic levels of gentamycin in her blood. Her major treatment since transfer has been hemodialysis.

Mrs. Bello's condition has remained stable throughout the week, yet she has shown signs of continued confusion and disorientation. It is suspected at this point that she has suffered a severe hearing loss as a result of her toxic drug levels. She has a very anxious facial expression and appears very restless. She has been using her nurse call light every 10 to 15 minutes and has great difficulty communicating her needs when the nurse arrives.

Nancy Smith, RN, has been taking care of Mrs. Bello for several days. She suspected that, along with other necessary aspects of care, Mrs. Bello could benefit from some planned touch interaction by the nurses. She scheduled a nursing care conference for the purpose of assessing Mrs. Bello's touch needs and developing some strategies for care in which all the nursing staff would participate.

The conference was productive and thought-provoking. The staff rapidly identified the high risk factors for touch deficiency and the symptoms that might be associated with decreased tactile stimulation. They include the following:

- Mrs. Bello is elderly and may have less effective use of available sensory stimuli because of the effects of the aging process.
- This is a crisis experience for the patient.
- There is increased use of highly technical equipment at the bedside that may be frightening and awesome.
- The patient is experiencing increased separation from family and loved ones because of the increased distance from home and limited visiting times available in the critical care unit.
- Because she has suffered some hearing loss, Mrs. Bello is having extreme difficulty interpreting her new surroundings and communicating effectively with other people.
- The sensory stimuli available to Mrs. Bello are strange to her and add to her confusion about her surroundings. Her bed is located on the end of the unit, where there is no window and little traffic flow. The head of her bed has been in low Fowler's position much of the time, limiting her visual access to her immediate surroundings.
- Mrs. Bello has experienced a variety of threats to her body image. She has a long incision on her abdomen, intravenous needles and tubes in her arms, an oxygen mask on her face, and an unfamiliar hospital gown covering her body. Her heart rhythm is on display on a cardiac monitor next to her bed.
- Lastly, the body that for so long was strong and agile is now weak and helpless. She cannot turn from side to side by herself, comb her own hair, or use the toilet. These all represent significant alterations in how she now sees herself.

Based on the assessment phase of the nursing care conference, the staff developed a care plan (see Nursing Care Plan 5–1). At the conclusion of the conference, the nurses agreed to document the implementation of their touch behaviors and evaluate the responses by the patient. They planned to have a follow-up conference in 2 days to evaluate the results.

Two days later, the nursing staff met to discuss the progress with Mrs. Bello and reevaluate their strategies. They identified the following changes in the patient and family status that they felt were associated with their planned uses of touch:

- Mrs. Bello appeared to communicate more effectively using the chalk board to read the messages from the nurse. She still seemed to have difficulty speaking clearly because her hearing was diminished, but she was noticeably improved. She occasionally reached for the nurse and touched her during the verbal and written exchanges.
- Mrs. Bello exhibited symptoms of confusion only rarely. She began to address one nurse by her name and asked about her family. Mrs. Bello frequently reached for the nurse at the bedside.
- Mrs. Bello appeared less restless and anxious. She rarely used the call light, and when she did, she was calmer and could communicate her needs more clearly. The nurses observed that her sleep habits were more clearly delineated. She slept more soundly at night and seemed to be more alert during the day.
- Mrs. Bello's family visited regularly at times that best met their schedules. They seemed more comfortable at the bedside, hugged and kissed Mrs. Bello on arriving and leaving, and used a lot of touching and handholding while there. They also approached the nurses more freely, asked questions, talked about Mrs. Bello's condition, and seemed more relaxed.

Interestingly, the nurses in the conference described feeling closer to Mrs. Bello and her family than to some other patients. They agreed that their feelings and the changes that they had identified in the patient were difficult to measure objectively. However, they did feel that their plans had had a positive effect on progress. They agreed to continue to give attention to their strategies with the goal of refining their abilities in using more effective touch in patient care.

Summary

The dynamics of patient–nurse interaction are rapidly changing along with the evolution of health care in general. Patients are not the same as they were many years ago. Likewise, the health care environment has undergone massive changes, with technology and science guiding the way. It is important that nurses respond to patients' needs, which have evolved with, and as a result of, modern health care. It is vital that the patient remain the central focus of care and that nurses develop new insights and skills to assure individualized care. Perhaps a revitalization of the basic caring acts, such as the use of touch, can bring new life and humanization into care as nurses face the challenges of the future.

(*Text continues on page 56*)

NURSING CARE PLAN 5–1:
Caring and Touch

NURSING DIAGNOSIS	OUTCOME CRITERIA/ PATIENT GOALS	NURSING INTERVENTIONS
Sensory-Perceptual Alterations, auditory, visual, kinesthetic and tactile: related to altered state of wellness.	• Patient will develop effective communication.	1. Plan frequent visits to patient's bedside. Use a combination of communication techniques: talk while using touch and eye contact; use a chalkboard to write messages; use a variation of moderately firm and gentle touch while communicating. 2. Monitor mental status for signs and symptoms of sensory deprivation.
Social Isolation: related to inadequate personal resources secondary to hospitalization.	• Patient will maintain frequent meaningful interaction with nurses and family.	1. Relocate patient in ICU to provide her clear view of the main nursing area and frequent, easy access by nurse. Go to bedside frequently; use touch and eye contact while communicating.
Alteration in thought processes: related to hearing changes and hospitalization.	• Patient orientation to time, place, person will be maintained.	1. Arrange regular visiting times with family. 2. Keep clock and calendar within patient's view.
Anxiety: related to fear of illness/death and critical care environment.	• Patient will demonstrate effective coping mechanisms.	1. Approach bed using verbal greeting and touch hand and arm immediately for a long duration. 2. Use touch to arm and shoulders when talking; continue touch while listening. 3. Stay with patient/during treatments or procedures to provide support and reassurance through touch. 4. Use eye contact and verbal interaction with touch to reinforce the message of support and caring. 5. Allow patient to verbalize feelings about illness and environment. 6. Instruct patient on relaxation techniques.
Powerlessness: related to feelings of helplessness and ineffective communication patterns.	• Patient–nurse communication will be maintained.	1. Be alert to patient cues for more or less touch. 2. Observe facial expression, body movements, visible responses to touch, or any attempts to initiate touch; encourage patient to initiate touch.

(continued)

NURSING CARE PLAN 5–1: *(Continued)*
Caring and Touch

NURSING DIAGNOSIS	OUTCOME CRITERIA/ PATIENT GOALS	NURSING INTERVENTIONS
		3. Observe for changes in behavior, restlessness, anxiety reduction, heart rate changes, and any other responses to touch.
		4. Encourage patient to verbalize needs; use eye contact while listening.
		5. Use moderate to long duration of touch to limbs and trunk and good eye contact.
		6. Visit bedside for purpose of touching and communicating.
Disturbance in self-concept, body image, self-esteem, role performance, and personal identity: related to altered state of wellness and decreased strength and activity.	• Patient will maintain self-esteem and verbalize self-worth and feelings of support and caring.	1. Incorporate planned meaningful touch into care activities. During physical assessment, use reasonably long periods of touch to extremities to clarify perceptions of body boundaries. Touch trunk when possible; touch shoulder while auscultating heart or lungs; massage back when assessing sacral edema.
		2. Use eye contact generously to reinforce communication process that occurs during touch.
		3. Plan progressive strengthening activities with patient and nurse or patient and family.
		4. Provide frequent verbal and nonverbal positive feedback about performance.
		5. Assist with personal hygiene and grooming.
		6. Touch legs, feet, arms, shoulders, back, head in assessment procedure. Provide adequate duration of touch.
Alteration in family process: related to decreased communication and social interaction secondary to hospitalization.	• Maintenance of effective family–patient communication.	1. Assist in planning family visiting; allow for flexibility in visiting policies to increase time with patient.
		2. Plan nursing care to not interfere with visits.
		3. Be a role model of touch for family members. Use touch in interactions with them to build trust. Greet family with a handshake; accompany them to bedside.

(continued)

NURSING CARE PLAN 5–1: (Continued)
Caring and Touch

NURSING DIAGNOSIS	OUTCOME CRITERIA/ PATIENT GOALS	NURSING INTERVENTIONS
		4. Demonstrate touch with patient to show family that they will not harm her or equipment.
		5. Encourage family to use touch alone or with verbal interaction with the patient. Tell them areas to avoid touching.
		6. Provide family and patient with uninterrupted visiting periods. Lower side rails; provide chair at bedside.
	• Patient will demonstrate effective coping mechanisms.	7. Encourage patient to identify situations that interfere with the ability to cope (eg, fear of loss of health and independence).
		8. Meet regularly with family to monitor effectiveness of coping. Instruct on effective coping strategies. Encourage use of touch with patient.
		9. Offer to contact clergy, social worker, or other means of support.

REFERENCES

1. Leininger M: Forward. In Watson J: Nursing: The Philosophy and Science of Caring, pp xii–xiii. Boulder, Colorado Associated University Press, 1985
2. Watson J: Nursing: The Philosophy and Science of Caring, Boulder, Colorado Associated University Press, 1985
3. Noddings N: Why care about caring. In Wright RA: Human Values in Health Care: The Practice of Ethics, pp 253, 267. New York, McGraw-Hill, 1987
4. Benfield DB: Two philosophies of caring. In Wright, RA: Human Values in Health Care: The Practice of Ethics, pp 246–252. New York, McGraw-Hill, 1987
5. Cohn L: Barriers and values in the nurse/client relationship. J Assoc Rehabil Nurs III:3–8, 1978
6. Cowper-Smith F: Nurse could you care more? Nurs Times 74:1882–1883, 1978
7. Kalisch BJ: An experiment in the development of empathy in nursing students. Nurs Res 20:202–211, 1971
8. Jourard S: The Transparent Self: Self-Disclosure and Well-Being. Princeton, D Van Nostrand, 1964
9. Cashar L, Dixson B: The therapeutic use of touch. J Psychiatr Nurs 5:442–451, 1967
10. Day F: The patient's perception of touch. In Anderson E et al (eds): Current Concepts in Clinical Nursing, pp 00–00. St. Louis, CV Mosby, 1973
11. Holinger LM: Communicating with the elderly. J Gerontol Nurs 12:8–13, 1986
12. Clement JM: A Descriptive Study of the Use of Touch by Nurses with Patients in Critical Care. Doctoral dissertation, The University of Texas, Austin, Texas, 1983
13. Watson W: The meaning of touch: Geriatric nursing. J Communication 25:104–111, 1975
14. Steffee DR, Suty KA, Delcalzo PV: More than a touch: Communicating with a blind and deaf patient. Nursing 15:36–39, 1985
15. Clement JM: Touch: Research findings and implications for preoperative teaching. AORN J 45:1429–1439, 1987
16. Fenton MV: Development of the scale of humanistic nursing behaviors. Nurs Res 36:82–87, 1987
17. Smoyak SA: High tech high touch. Nurs Success Today 3:13, 1986
18. Weiss SJ: Psychophysiologic effects of care-giver touch in incidence of cardiac dysrhythmia. Heart Lung 15:495–504, 1986
19. Weiss S: The language of touch. Nurs Res 28:76–80, 1979

20. Heslin R: Steps toward a taxonomy of touching. Paper presented to the Midwestern Psychological Association, May 1974

21. Heslin R, Alper T: Touch: A bonding gesture. In Wiemann JM, Harrison RP (eds): Nonverbal Communication, pp 47–75. Beverly Hills, Sage, 1982

22. Thayer S: Touch. In Barnouw E (ed): International Encyclopedia of Communications. New York, Oxford University Press, 1989

23. Heslin R: Steps toward a taxonomy of touching. Paper presented to the Midwestern Psychological Association, May 1974

24. Henneman E: Effect of nursing contact on the stress response of patients being weaned from mechanical ventilation. Heart Lung 18(5):483–489, 1989

BIBLIOGRAPHY

Mulaik J, Megenity J, Cannon R, Chance K, Cannella K, Garland L, Gilead M: Patients' perceptions of nurses' use of touch. West J Nurs Res 13(3):306–323, 1991

Oliver S, Redfern S: Interpersonal communication between nurses and elderly patients: refinement of an observation schedule. J Adv Nurs 16:30–38, 1991

Walleck A: Controversies in the management of the head-injured patient. Crit Care Nurs Clin North Am 1(1):67:74, 1989

STUDY QUESTIONS

1. Location of touch in patient care is an important factor. Of the following, all are true except

    a. touching of the body trunk is referred to as centrapetality
    b. patients receive messages about self-esteem from the toucher according to the number of body locations touched
    c. location refers to the "rate of approach to the body surface"
    d. location of touch gives messages about body parts and the integration of these parts into a whole being

2. Literature supports the following to be true in the use of touch with patients:

    a. patient touch needs can easily be assessed by nurses
    b. during a crisis, all patients need more touch
    c. patients who are not used to touch will never be comfortable with it
    d. patient touch needs may change rapidly and nurses should be alert to cues

3. The following are examples of patients at high risk for touch deficiency:

    a. a 70-year-old man who is brought in with chest pain by his daughter, two sons, and wife
    b. an elderly widow who is almost deaf and has no family in the city
    c. a 40-year-old married man with two teenage children
    d. a young mother of twins who is admitted with acute appendicitis

4. Ways to include touch in care include all of the following, except:

    a. hold the patient's hand while listening to complaints of pain
    b. massage the patient's back when repositioning the patient on his or her side
    c. touch the patient's arm and shoulder while preparing to measure the blood pressure
    d. stand at the foot of the bed while talking to the patient

CHAPTER 6

Patient and Family Teaching

BEHAVIORAL OBJECTIVES

Based on the content in this chapter, the reader should be able to:

1. Assess, carry out, and evaluate a patient education plan.
2. Identify and describe a seven-step process for planning and carrying out a patient education plan.
3. Identify specific cognitive and psychomotor knowledge deficits and related patient goals and outcome criteria.

Description

Patient teaching has always been considered an important part of holistic nursing care. However, in the past it often occurred in the last 5 minutes of hospitalization. Three societal trends—litigious action, a tightening economy, and a sense of personal responsibility for one's own health—have underscored the importance of extending nursing care through patient education. Americans have become more litigious as a tightening economy has increased the cost of medical care and insurance. The high cost of lawsuits has increased the cost of malpractice insurance, which in turn has added to the cost of care. Furthermore, adults now make concerted efforts to exercise and eat a balanced diet, in response to expanded knowledge regarding health promotion. Because of the impact of these trends, there is renewed interest in the need for nurses to plan, carry out, and *document* patient teaching as part of routine nursing care. Audits of records for reimbursement, accreditation, and quality control have reinforced the nurse's historical role in patient education by requiring documentation that education has been provided. In many health care institutions, patients are required to sign forms acknowledging that patient education has taken place and that the patient *understands* what has been taught.

Teaching and Learning

Recognizing the patient's response to illness helps the nurse predict when teaching will be best absorbed and most useful to the patient. The adaptation to illness model can be applied (see Figure 2–1). Learning is most likely to occur during quiet stages, when the patient's emotional outlook corresponds to physical condition. This means that the patient feels just about as sick or as well as he or she actually is. Providing information during this phase of illness helps the patient move on to the next phase of recovery. When there is less congruence between the patient's physical condition and emotional acknowledgement of it, motivation for learning is impaired and teaching is less effective.

Nursing Assessment and Management

To enhance teaching effectiveness, the nurse can use the following seven-step plan for assessment and management (Fig. 6–1).

Motivation

Motivation for learning should be assessed in two areas. Intrinsic motivation includes the learner's attitudes, values, personality, and lifestyle. The teaching method and what is taught must be adjusted for these aspects of the patient's

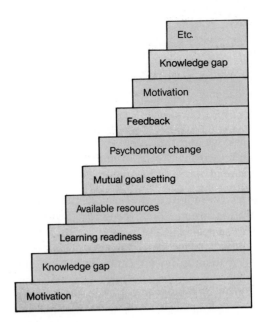

FIGURE 6–1
Staircase of patient teaching and learning.

life. Extrinsic motivation includes the learning climate, physical environment, time of teaching, possible reinforcers, interpersonal relationship with the teacher, and skill of the instructor. The nurse has far more control over the extrinsic sources of motivation. Does the patient respond best alone or with others? Does he or she prefer the solarium to the bedroom? Do touching, smiling, and encouraging enhance learning? Does the patient like to spend time with the nurse? Has the nurse developed teaching skills and methods for this particular type of learner? Trial-and-error attempts at teaching each patient can be shared with other nurses to increase extrinsic motivation skills.

Knowledge Gap

Assessing the knowledge gap includes recognizing what needs to be taught and learned to effect behavior change. A knowledge gap can also be assessed in terms of "what is" compared with "what could be." An honest, accurate appraisal leads to realistic, achievable goals rather than unrealistic ones that, if attempted, would result in the patient's experiencing failure. In this phase of the plan, it is important for patients and their families to recognize the advantages inherent in learning the new knowledge, skills, and attitudes. As this phase is completed, patients should become aware that they have a better basis for choice concerning whether they will learn and change. The patient's right to make this choice should be acknowledged and accepted by the nurse. However, the nurse has the responsibility to make certain that the patient is making a knowledgeable choice.

Learning Readiness

The step of learning readiness deals with:

- the patient's level of adaptation to illness
- the patient's anxiety level
- the patient's developmental level
- the opportunities for immediate application of new knowledge and skill
- an interpersonally safe learning environment that allows trial and error without recrimination

As patients adjust to the sick role, they become more receptive to learning about the illness. Because progress heightens anxiety, teaching is usually more effective during the period of emotional acceptance than during times when the patient is moving either into or out of the sick role. Whenever there is movement forward or backward on the health–illness continuum, there is likely to be an emotional response of anxiety, worry, or depression that can interfere with concentration and learning. Therefore, admission, transfer, readmission to the critical care unit, and *hospital discharge* are poor times for learning to occur. During periods of anxiety it is useful for the nurse to ascertain the patient's perceptions of what is happening so that misunderstandings that may cause unnecessary worry can be corrected.

Informal teaching and the provision of information that enhances equilibrium are best woven into the other nursing procedures occurring throughout the patient's stay in the critical care unit. For effective learning to take place, the high levels of anxiety commonly found in critical care units must be decreased to no more than mild anxiety states in which the patient demonstrates alertness without fear, motivation to learn, and interest. The more facts there are to absorb and the more behavior change is implied by the information, the more likely the patient is to respond with increased levels of anxiety. Therefore, there is a need to teach during times of decreased or mild anxiety.

Anxiety levels, physiological function, and the patient's own priorities must be assessed during the evaluation of learning readiness. Worry, pain, and some medications also interfere with the patient's ability to learn.

The patient's developmental stage must also be considered in the plan. For example, young adolescents do not deal as well with philosophical issues regarding their care and life choices as do older adolescents and adults. Their level of abstract thinking is not nearly as well developed as in the older adolescent or adult.

Because of anxiety associated with serious illness, patients are likely to have trouble remembering details. It is especially important that they be provided with written material so that they can review what they need to learn. Pamphlets, booklets, and customized lists and directions are useful to everyone. These educational items can be personalized by adding handwritten notes and explanations at the bedside. These notes should also address the patient's questions and concerns.

It is also important to have immediate opportunities for the learner to try new skills and behaviors. Early successful application of new knowledge is a reinforcer that cannot be replaced effectively by anything else. Often, anticipation of hospital discharge and return to home can be a powerful motivator and increase readiness for learning and carrying out new skills.

Because of the trend toward early hospital discharge, specialized teaching in the home is usually necessary to complete instruction that was begun in the hospital. At the home, in the patient's own surroundings and with his or her own routines, home health nurses can evaluate patient and family in terms of their knowledge and their ability to apply it. Appropriate records about nurse teaching and patient response should be forwarded to the proper agency. Areas not addressed should be identified so that other nurses do not assume that the teaching is complete.

Informal teaching and rehabilitation programs that involve structure and extended periods of time should occur after the crisis, when the patient has reached a fairly stable period of adjustment. Often, this stage of readiness does not occur until after discharge. To provide this type of essential health teaching, hospital-based personnel can conduct programs for patients to attend after discharge. In addition, community-based classes can be conducted, and teaching can be done in the home. Follow-up learning sessions are necessary, regardless of where they take place.

Most of the learning required of a patient who is recovering from critical illness involves changes in behavior that will alter his or her lifestyle. Dietary changes that restrict calories, sodium, cholesterol, or carbohydrates are common. A change in activity level may be imposed, exercise may be prescribed, and a decrease in smoking may be imperative. None of these changes is easy to make. Providing information is rarely sufficient to alter behavior.

Group teaching is a technique that is well-suited to learning that involves lifestyle changes. Group members can provide support, offer encouragement and motivation, and reinforce information and accomplishments.

An effective approach to learning includes a combination of informal teaching, group instruction, and specialized learning and evaluation at home. Teaching may be begun in the hospital, but it can rarely be completed there. Referral is now part of a complete nursing care plan.

Providing a safe environment conducive to learning is included in this phase. Learning occurs more easily if security, a sense of belonging, and self-esteem are high. Often, learning about illness means that the patient and family not only must learn facts and techniques but also must apply and adapt to their own lives what is taught. This is difficult if there are high degrees of anxiety, depression, or acute physical dysfunction. It is impossible for patients to respond creatively if they are struggling to maintain basic physiological stability. Therefore, much of the teaching is directed toward the family. A key concept to teach family members is how to support and encourage one another during a change process.

When the teachable moment appears, the following reminders will help keep communication open:

- find out about the learner's concerns before teaching
- ask for the learner's ideas and perceptions of what is happening
- avoid judgmental statements
- ask yourself, "Is what the patient or family wants to learn what I want to teach?"

The nursing process helps the nurse answer the last question. This process can be used to determine the teaching plan in the same way that it is used to determine any other nursing action.

Available Resources

A careful assessment of the availability of resources has an important effect on the outcome of patient learning. Without a realistic appraisal of resources, the nurse may spend valuable time teaching the patient activities impossible to implement once he or she is discharged. Equipment, adequate finances, values and cultural influences, family involvements, and community support all are resources that are likely to need careful appraisal to ensure a successfully implemented teaching plan. For example, if the nurse is teaching the patient how to reduce carbohydrate or sodium intake, the nurse should find out the types of foods eaten (a sample meal plan) and the ways they are prepared. This information can then be used to help the patient and family tailor the diet regimen to their meals.

The appropriate teaching media for the patient's learning style are evaluated in this phase. Audio and video tapes are increasingly available to nurses for teaching. These media are especially valuable because they can be repeated continually without embarrassing the patient or frustrating the nurse. Despite the availability of new media, nothing can replace a warm, encouraging, supportive relationship between the patient and a skilled and knowledgeable nurse. Even if mechanical media are frequently used, it is important to offer time for questions, support, and encouragement.

Mutual Goal Setting

During the phase of mutual goal setting, the nurse and patient formulate a contract about what is to be learned and how they will know that the specified material has been learned. An understanding is developed about what the nurse will do to help the patient learn and what the patient must do to meet the established goal. The actual goals or objectives to be accomplished provide direction about the content to be taught and prescribe behaviors for teacher and learner.

Words that define or specify behaviors are more useful and less ambiguous than words that make vague statements about what the patient is to accomplish. For example, "The patient will list 10 common foods that are high in sodium (or salt)" is better than "The patient will develop an understanding regarding high-sodium foods to be avoided." Furthermore, stating the goal in a positive "can do" statement is more likely to lead to success than the negatively stated list of "foods to be avoided." Return demonstrations of how to care for equipment and appliances or of how to perform exercises also are specific objectives likely to lead to success. For example, "After 1 week of practice, the patient will be able to make three bed-to-chair or chair-to-bed transfers within 2 hours" is a useful goal-oriented objective. It tells the nurse and patient how much time is available for learning, the exact behavior expected, and how many times it should be accomplished within a specified period of time.

Goals can and should be renegotiated as the situation or circumstances change, but, more importantly, they should be formulated so that success is achievable. Therefore, goals should be written in increments of complexity and for short periods of time. After one goal is achieved, it can be increased or modified. If it does not appear to be attainable, it should be modified downward so that the patient who makes a reasonable effort does not fail and give up, but rather is reinforced to go on by the feeling of success.

Psychomotor Change (Compliance)

Achieving actual psychomotor change or compliance in patients is one of the most difficult aspects of patient teaching and learning. In seriously ill patients, compliance typically demands a difficult long-term lifestyle change. For example, a nurse who is trying to lose 6 pounds gained on a vacation may feel frustrated, but the situation is in no way comparable to that of a patient who, having experienced the threat of severe illness, must lose and keep off 50 pounds. The patient's physical and emotional energies have probably been compromised by the illness and hospitalization. Now, medical personnel are demanding extensive lifestyle changes that seem necessary and logical to them for restoring the patient's health. The patient, after the emotional and physical depletion caused by illness, is more likely to experience the demand for change as deprivation.

Giving up smoking, eliminating salt from the diet, and losing weight are difficult objectives, even for the most knowledgeable and motivated health professional. Finding ways to help patients comply with lifestyle changes is a nursing problem that deserves intensive attention and extensive research. Appropriate teaching plans, reinforcement, support, and encouragement, even when there is regression, constitute a beginning. Involving the patient and the family in mutual goal setting and connecting them with community support systems are likely to enhance and sustain the necessary lifestyle changes.

Sometimes, serendipitous changes occur that can be used to encourage behavior modification. For example, a patient who loses 20 of a prescribed 50 pounds may be more reinforced by his or her improved self-image than by health improvement. This kind of change in self-image motivates the patient to lose more weight. Nurses can observe changes that improve attitude and use them to increase reinforcement and enhance motivation.

Feedback

Feedback is useful for evaluation of gains and modification of goals. It must be descriptive rather than judgmental and specific rather than general. Thus, "You've lost 3 pounds!" is more constructive than "You're doing well!" Timely feedback is more reinforcing than delayed feedback and is more useful in helping the patient resist temptations to transgress.

Helpful negative feedback promotes choices rather than guilt. The observation, "You've smoked more cigarettes today than yesterday" provides the patient with more support to modify or control behavior than the statement, "You're ruining your health," a judgment of self-destruction that fills the patient with guilt.

Positive feedback reinforces successes and extends the previously established motivation. As the teaching plan continues, undiscovered knowledge gaps are recognized and a new plan can be established according to the alterations that have been experienced.

Family Participation

Although most of the preceding discussion has focused on the patient, each of these learning steps and concepts should also be applied to the instruction of family members or others who are involved with the patient in daily activities. Most of the time, it is necessary and valuable for these people to acquire the same knowledge and skills as the patient, especially if they are involved in the patient's lifestyle changes. Examples of such involvement include performing a procedure (eg, injection, irrigation, dressing), shopping or cooking for a special diet, offering support, and sometimes even participating with the patient in certain activities (eg, accompanying the patient on a walking regimen).

Writing the Patient Education Plan

There are three domains to consider in the patient education plan:

- the cognitive domain
- the affective domain
- the psychomotor domain

Nursing Diagnosis

It may be helpful for the nurse to identify the precise domain in order to sharpen teaching interventions. For example, a cognitive deficit exists when the patient gives an incorrect explanation for the cause of current illness. A psychomotor deficit exists when the patient contaminates sterile equipment. The knowledge deficit diagnosis and patient goals should be listed on the plan in order of their importance, but they should be carried out according to a logical learning sequence and the patient's receptiveness to learning emotionally threatening content. Careful notes are needed to track what has been learned and what still must be taught and evaluated.

Outcome Criteria/Patient Goals

Defining the type of knowledge deficit assists the nurse in identifying the appropriate content to teach and the outcome criteria to evaluate the effectiveness of the teaching (eg, "The patient will be able to state the main action of digoxin," or "The patient will be able to *demonstrate* drawing up and administering insulin without contamination"). The affective domain objectives deal with clarification of the patient's values, attitudes, and feelings about what is happening to his or her life or lifestyle. A nurse cannot expect to make a patient change his or her feelings. However, by assisting the patient to understand and clarify the feelings associated with illness and disability, the nurse can better ascertain learning readiness. The patient is likely to be more accepting of negative feelings if they are understood in the context of an adaptation process (see Chapter 2).

Nursing Interventions

In this section of the plan, the nurse should identify the content to be taught, the method and media of teaching, and the special and personalized patient needs that can be met to promote learning (eg, privacy, reinforcement, hearing aids). In the critical care setting, the patient may be too ill or debilitated to cope with essential learning. In these cases, the teaching part of the plan should be written and customized for responsible family members or friends. The same points apply, especially in regard to feelings and attitudes, because they affect readiness for learning and motivation to follow through (see Chapter 3). A verbal, or perhaps written, contract among the responsible friend or relative, the patient, and the nurse helps motivate each partner to carry out his or her responsibilities. In designing such a contract, apply the content related to mutual goal setting (see Patient Education Plan 6–1).

PATIENT EDUCATION PLAN 6-1:

Mr. Chang was admitted to the emergency room with a severe myocardial infarction. Within hours after admission, bypass surgery was completed. Mr. Chang is 50 years old, 30 pounds overweight, and rarely exercises. As an engineer, he maintains a sedentary lifestyle with his wife. He enjoys high sodium oriental food at least three times a week. Now recovering from surgery, he expresses interest in losing weight and improving his general health.

NURSING DIAGNOSIS	OUTCOME CRITERIA/ PATIENT GOALS	NURSING INTERVENTIONS
Knowledge deficit: related to weight loss strategies, food choices, caloric intake, exercise.	• Patient will be able to state content presented.	1. Time teaching sessions during minimal interruption for care needs. 2. Include wife in content presentation. 3. Provide written materials to reinforce verbal information. 4. Modify weight reduction program to meet patient needs. 5. Refer patient to full service cardiac rehabilitation program that includes exercise and nutrition. 6. Include dietician in meal planning. 7. Continue education after transfer from ICU. 8. Use in-hospital menu selection to validate patient understanding of food choices. 9. If available, give list of cookbooks that prepare foods low in calories, fat, and cholesterol. 10. Gradually increase exercise (ambulation) while assessing physiologic tolerance (eg, heart rate, rhythm, angina).
Health-seeking behavior: related to desire for weight loss.	• Patient will participate in goal setting for weight loss.	1. Plan and set goals with patient for methods of weight loss. 2. Have patient identify favorite moderate exercises. 3. Have patient identify ways to lose weight. 4. Provide chart with caloric values. 5. Refer patient to weight loss group. Provide information about cost and location.

(continued)

PATIENT EDUCATION PLAN 6–1: (Continued)

NURSING DIAGNOSIS	OUTCOME CRITERIA/ PATIENT GOALS	NURSING INTERVENTIONS
High risk for anxiety: related to fear of failure, lifestyle changes, impact of diet on heart disease.	• Patient can begin to demonstrate effective coping mechanisms.	1. Have patient discuss feelings about changing diet. 2. Discuss with patient his feeling about his weight loss program. 3. Mobilize patient's resources (family or others) for support. 4. Help patient design chart which will graphically demonstrate weight loss achievement. 5. Acknowledge all questions and responses as meaningful and important (eg, "That's a great idea").

Summary

Patient education occurs throughout hospitalization. A formal written plan regarding specific content to be taught, documentation of nurse teaching, and patient response is now required for most patients. The areas of assessment and intervention include motivation, knowledge gap, learner readiness, available resources, mutual goal setting, psychomotor change, and feedback. Referral for follow-up after hospital discharge is usually essential to determine how well the patient is adhering to the plan of care.

BIBLIOGRAPHY

Anderson C: Patient Teaching and Communicating in an Information Age. New York: Delmar Publishing Co., 1990

Barr W: Teaching patients with life threatening illnesses: Cardiovascular disease, transplantation, organ donation. Nurs Clin North Am 24(3):639–644, 1989

Brannon PHB, Johnson R: The internal cardioverter defibrillator: Patient–family teaching. Focus Crit Care 19(1): 44–46, 1992

Duryee R: The efficacy of inpatient education after myocardial infarction. Heart Lung 21(3):217–227, 1992

Fornet K: The challenge of teaching the elderly cardiac patient. ACCN Clin Issues Crit Care Nurs 3(1):143–162, 1992

Kerner-Slemons S, Berron K, Oteham A: Bypass supported angioplasty: What your patient needs to know at discharge. Crit Care Nurse 12(2):55–57, 1992

Mullen PD, Mains DA, Velez R: A meta-analysis of controlled trial of cardiac patient education. Patient Educ Couns 19(2):143–162, 1992

Rankin SH: Patient Education: Issues, Principles, and Practices. Philadelphia, JB Lippincott, 1990

Rakel B: Interventions related to patient teaching. Nurs Clin North Am 27(2):397–405, 1992

STUDY QUESTIONS

1. Learning is most likely to occur under the following conditions:

   a. anxiety is mild and acceptance is congruent with the illness
   b. anxiety is moderate and the patient is motivated
   c. anxiety is high and the patient is highly motivated
   d. anxiety is low and the patient can deny the severity of the illness

2. The term "intrinsic learning" deals with the patient's

   a. motivation to learn
   b. lighting and noise within the environment
   c. ability to abstract meaning from inner resource
   d. values, attitudes, personality, and lifestyle

3. The nurse can expect the patient's anxiety to increase

   a. when the family is present
   b. as the expectations for change increase
   c. in a group environment
   d. when teaching plans are not individualized

4. To maintain open communication, the nurse should

   a. identify the learner's concerns before teaching
   b. ask the learner to share perceptions and ideas about what is happening
   c. avoid judgmental statements
   d. all of the above

5. The affective domain of learning refers to

   a. the learner's thinking
   b. the learner's psychomotor behavior
   c. the learner's feelings
   d. all of the above

CHAPTER 7

The Critically Ill Elderly Patient

BEHAVIORAL OBJECTIVES

Based on the content in this chapter, the reader should be able to:

1. Identify ten physical changes occurring as a result of the normal aging process.
2. Identify the development tasks of the elderly.
3. Describe prevalent conditions which affect the major body systems of the elderly.
4. Discuss age-adjusted parameters for the elderly.

Hudak: Critical Care Nursing:
A Holistic Approach, 6th ed. © 1994
J. B. Lippincott Company.

5. Describe why the principle *start low, go slow* is important for the elderly in regard to the absorption, distribution, metabolism, and excretion of medications.
6. Formulate a nursing care plan, using the nursing diagnosis format, for the gerontologic patient.

Description

Critical care nurses are caring for increasing numbers of older patients. As a result there is a need to understand the age-related physiological changes that occur with normal aging. All physiological processes are altered as a function of aging. Although these alterations are progressive, they are usually not apparent or pathological. Nevertheless, because of these age-related changes, the elderly critically ill patient requires more intense observation.

The leading causes of death among older patients are heart disease, malignant neoplasms, cerebrovascular accident, influenza, and chronic obstructive pulmonary disease. Chronic conditions are also prevalent among elderly persons (eg, arthritis, hearing and visual deficits). These conditions become more common with advancing age and result in increased hospitalizations. The longer life span has been the single most important cause of the increased numbers of elderly patients with multiple chronic and acute illnesses.

General Psychobiological Characteristics of Aging

Biologic Issues

It is important to distinguish changes due to the aging process from those due to a particular disease process. Conditions that occur as a result of aging and include the following:

- reduced resistance to stress
- poor tolerance of extremes of heat and cold because of hypothalamic changes
- reduced reaction to sounds and other external stimuli
- greater fluctuation in blood pH

The process of aging differs between men and women; the differences are more distinctive in middle life than in later years. Aging (in one organ or the entire body) may be premature or delayed in relation to actual chronological age. The effect of aging on cellular tissues is asymmetrical. For example, the changes resulting from aging in relation to the brain, bone, cardiovascular, and lung tissues may be fairly obvious, whereas changes affecting the liver, pancreas, gastrointestinal tract, and muscle tissues are less obvious. Several organic changes that result from aging are listed in Display Box 7–1.

DISPLAY BOX 7–1
Organic Changes With Aging

Increased amounts of connective and collagen tissue
Disappearance of cellular elements in the nervous system, muscles, and other vital organs
Reduction in the number of normally functioning cells
Increased amount of fat
Decreased oxygen utilization
Decreased blood pumped during rest
Less air expired by the lungs
Decreased muscle strength
Decreased excretion of hormones
Reduced sensory and perceptual activity
Alterations in blood pressure
Decreased absorption of lipids, proteins, and carbohydrates
Presbyesophagus
Thickening of the arterial lumen

Psychosocial Issues

In addition to physical signs of aging, nurses caring for acutely ill elderly patients must be aware of the general *developmental tasks* of the elderly as well as the specific dreams or wishes of an particular senior. Developmental tasks of the elderly are listed in Table 7–1.

TABLE 7–1
Developmental Tasks of the Elderly

Decision of where and how to live for their remaining years
Preservation of supportive, intimate, and satisfying relationships with spouse, family, and friends
Maintenance of adequate and satisfying home environment relative to health and economic status
Provision of sufficient income
Maintenance of maximum level of health
Attainment of comprehensive health and dental care
Maintenance of personal hygiene
Maintenance of communication and adequate contact with family and friends
Maintenance of social, civic, and political involvement
Initiation of new interests (in addition to former activities) that increase status
Recognition and feeling of being needed
Discovery of meaning in life after retirement and when confronted with illness of self/spouse and death of spouse and other loved ones; adjustment to death of loved ones
Development of a significant philosophy of life, and discovery of comfort in a philosophy/religion

The need for *support* and meaningful relationships continues throughout life. Support can be described as a feeling of belonging or as a belief that one is an active participant in the surrounding world. The feeling of mutuality with others in the environment lends strength and helps decrease the sense of isolation. Support by family, friends, and the community can provide an elderly patient with a greater sense of stability and security.

Self-worth and perceived well-being are feelings that usually coincide in elderly persons. The perception of well-being arises from the satisfaction of meeting an acceptable proportion of one's life goals. It can be described as an inner contentment one has in one's life as a whole. Related to this, a feeling of self-worth is derived not only from a sense of well-being but also from satisfaction with one's image or acceptance by others. Self-worth also reflects the quality of interactions with family and friends.

The *family environment* for the gerontologic patient includes, among others, dimensions of interpersonal relationships, personal growth, integrity of the family unit, and adaptation to stress. As family members age, all of these areas of concern intensify because of changes in roles of family members, alterations in the family power structure, and changes in financial and decision-making dynamics. Acute illness increases the urgency for effective cooperation among all family members as the traditional family structure is suddenly challenged.

When elderly patients are admitted to critical care, issues of *family cohesion and adaptability* often surface. Frequently, families face immediate changes in roles, with adult children and grandchildren assuming the roles of caretakers and nurturers for the elderly family members. The family must suddenly adjust to dramatically different demands. Frequent visits to the hospital; dialogues with nurses, physicians, and social workers; and efforts to support and communicate with the patient become primary tasks. Amid these activities, families often find themselves being pressed for decisions about immediate and long-term care. At this time, the issue of patient involvement in decision making may arise. Effective communication and a willingness to listen to and respect the wishes of the elderly patient become foremost. If this is achieved, the stress on families is reduced because of increased acceptance of the plan of care by all family members. These issues are addressed in Nursing Care Plan 7–1.

Physical Assessment

During the physical assessment process, keep in mind that changes in one organ system do not predict changes in other systems. For example, decreased renal function does not necessarily mean that the cardiovascular, hepatic, or neurologic systems are also impaired. In addition, although physiological changes can be expected with normal aging, the manifestations of the changes cannot be chronologically predicted. It is important to consider a wide variability and evaluate each person on the age-related changes actually present rather than on those that are "normal" for a particular age.

It is equally important to distinguish age-related changes from those associated with a chronic disease or acute illness and to avoid prematurely attributing some findings to age if they may be caused by illness. A discussion of the effects of aging on various body systems follows.

Auditory Loss

There is a gradual loss of hearing with age. One source estimates that 7 million persons older than 65 years of age have significant hearing loss, and continuation of current trends suggests that by the year 2000 there will be more than 11 million people with the problem.[1] The same source suggests that the aging process affects hearing in two critical ways: reduction in threshold sensitivity and reduction in the ability to understand speech.

Threshold elevations that occur between 8,000 and 20,000 Hz are not detectable with a routine hearing test; therefore, hearing loss because of aging or other factors is not documented clinically until frequencies are at or below 8,000 Hz.

Conductive hearing loss and sensorineural (perceptive) hearing loss are the two major types of hearing problems in older persons. Treatment may vary dramatically from simple removal of impacted ear wax to surgical removal of an auditory nerve tumor.

Blockage of sound transmission from the external ear through the tympanic membrane and small bones in the middle ear may cause a conductive hearing loss. Sensorineural hearing loss is by far the most common type of hearing problem in elderly people. The loss of cochlear hair cells occurs during the aging process and initially involves the high-frequency range loss commonly known as presbycusis. Presbycusis is defined as a hearing loss associated with normal physiological aging. There are varying degrees of presbycusis, which becomes severe if the lower frequencies in the speech range (2,000 Hz and below) are involved. Thirteen percent of persons 65 years of age and older, if tested, would show signs of presbycusis.[2]

The older patient may retain the ability to hear pure tones, but if these pure tones are grouped to form words, the ability to understand and perceive these sounds as intelligible speech may be lost. This is known as impairment of discrimination ability. The patient has increased difficulty hearing high-frequency, stimuli-sibilant sounds (-f-, -s-, -th-, -ch-, and -sh-). Noisy environments further hamper the ability to hear certain sounds. Selected nursing interventions for hearing-impaired patients are listed in Table 7–2.

TABLE 7–2
*Nursing Interventions for
Hearing-Impaired Patients*

Stand close and face patient.
Touch patient to get attention before communicating (personal space should be protected).
Speak slightly louder and slowly. (Do not shout.)
Pause more often than usual.
Avoid exaggerated lip movement.
Use facial expressions and gestures.
Use short phrases.
Repeat misinterpreted communication using different words.
Don't turn and walk away while talking.
Help family/support system with communication techniques.
Discourage social withdrawal (a problem associated with hearing loss).
Make sure hearing device works properly.

Impaired Vision

Like all other body systems, the eye is affected by aging. Structural and functional changes occur slowly and gradually. Visual perception depends on the integration of various neurosensory systems and structures that age at different rates.

The eyelids lose elasticity and become wrinkled. Ptosis (upper eyelid drooping) may be observed. Changes in tissues beneath the eyelid skin may allow fatty tissue formation and accumulation that result in "pouches."

The conjunctiva may develop a yellowish or discolored membrane or become thickened as a result of environmental hazards such as dust and exposure to drying and irritating pollutants. Arcus senilis, which is a white or gray ring around the limbus (junction of the cornea and sclera), may be related to a high blood level of fatty substances accumulated with advancing age.

The iris loses its ability to accommodate rapidly to light and dark and develops an increased need for light. The pupil becomes smaller and fixed. The lens becomes inflexible with less complete accommodation for near and far vision; it is also the site of cataract formation. The vitreous humor behind the lens may pull on the retina to produce holes or tears, risking detachment. The ciliary muscle becomes stiff, which contributes to the problems of accommodating to distances. By age 60, presbyopia may develop. This is the inability to shift focus from far to near. A possible rationale for this loss is that the older, aging lens is less flexible and cannot easily change shape from the action of the focusing muscle to which it is attached. Dark–light adaptation slows as the pupillary response slows and rods degenerate. Peripheral vision may decline because of decreased extraocular muscle strength, and depth perception may decline because of a thickening

lens. Therefore, allow time for the person to adapt when moving between dark and light environments and when getting out of bed. In addition to normal changes in vision, there is an increased incidence of many of the pathologies of the visual system with advancing age—cataracts, glaucoma, senile macular degeneration, and diabetic retinopathy. These pathologies must be studied in relation to normal aging of the eye structure and must consider the cognitive factors (orienting and attentional selectivity) affecting the visual function.

Cataracts

A cataract is a clouding of the normally clear and transparent lens of the eye. This condition of the lens makes it less able to send a focused picture to the retina. Assessing vision is especially important because almost 50% of those 75 to 85 years old have cataracts.

Glaucoma

With glaucoma an elevation of pressure within the eye causes damage to the nerve cells in the retina. Continued pressure can lead to blindness. Age-related changes in the canal of Schlemm, infection, injury, swollen cataracts, and tumors are etiologic factors for glaucoma.

Retinal Degeneration

Retinal degeneration is also known as senile macular degeneration. Central vision is either so dark or so distorted that the patient cannot see straight ahead.

Diabetic Retinopathy

Diabetic retinopathy is caused by the deterioration of the blood vessels nourishing the retina at the back of the eye. Microaneurysms and small hemorrhages in the eye may leak fluid or blood and cause swelling of the retina. If this leaking blood or fluid damages or scars the retina, the image sent to the brain becomes blurred. This can progress to blindness.

Selected nursing interventions for vision-impaired patients are listed in Table 7–3.

Other Sensory Changes

Although hearing and vision are the most researched sensory changes occurring in the elderly, these patients may also show declines in the other three senses.

Taste buds are reported to decrease with age, in conjunction with a decline in the ability to taste substances. Sweet and salty substances are less detectable as one ages. Hence, many elderly persons complain that food tastes

TABLE 7–3
Nursing Interventions for Visually-Impaired Patients

Identify yourself on approach.

Approach blind patients from the front.

Assess impact of failing vision and patient's ability to adapt both during hospitalization and after discharge.

Instill all prescribed medications.

Assess stress level because increased stress can necessitate higher dosages of eye medication for patients with glaucoma.

Be alert to side effects that other medications may have on the eyes (ie, medications containing antihistamines, caffeine, and atropinelike substances).

Provide eye lubrications when eyes are dry.

DISPLAY BOX 7–2
Changes in Sleep With Aging

Time falling asleep is lengthened.
Total sleep time usually decreases.
Lighter sleep occurs in stages III and IV.
Sleep is interrupted by increased number awakenings.

---

bitter or sour. There is very little data on smell sensation, but it is thought that a decrease in the sense of smell can result from atrophy of the olfactory organ and increased hair in the nostrils. The loss of taste and smell affect the elderly person's ability to identify food and make odor discriminations.

The threshold of touch varies with the part of the body stimulated. There is a loss of tactile sensation as one ages. Elderly persons may not feel the effects of lying too long in one position. A key nursing intervention is to vary the positions of the immobile elderly patient.

Sleep Changes

It is estimated that sleep disturbances occur in more than one-half of those older than 65 years of age.[3] An important aspect of the critical care nurse's assessment is to determine whether sleep problems are the result of normal aging, sleep disorders, or sleep disturbances due to the acute care environment.

Although some age-related changes in sleep patterns are the normal consequences of aging, the prevalence and potential for severe sleep disorders call for increased clinical awareness and evaluation. Such complaints as habitual snoring, frequent awakening, nocturnal sweating, and awakening with anxiety may be signs of a genuine sleep disorder.

The daily total number of sleeping hours decreases with age, as does the amount of time in stage IV and rapid eye movement (REM) sleep. Sleep changes accompanying normal aging include increased fragmentation of nighttime sleep due to intrusions of wakefulness and less time spent in the deeper stages of sleep (stages III and IV) where slow wave sleep takes place. Common abnormal complaints such as anxiety, waking up choking, headaches, sweating at night, nocturia, and snoring are a few of the symptoms the nurse should assess more thoroughly.

The most prevalent and most serious age-related sleep disorder is sleep apnea. There is evidence of an association between sleep apnea and circulatory disorders, including hypertension, stroke, and angina pectoris, and also between sleep apnea and reduced life expectancy. In addition, there may be a link between habitual snoring, stroke, and angina pectoris in older men.[4]

The prevalence of disordered breathing in the elderly is high; therefore, care should be taken in dispensing sedative hypnotics for persons with risk factors for sleep apnea. Nursing intervention includes encouraging elderly patients with disordered breathing to sleep on their sides and to lose weight if weight affects breathing. Other interventions include giving supplemental oxygen if hypoxemia, caused by chronic lung disease or hypoventilation, is present (see Chapter 4).

Normal aging, chronic illness, and drug therapy increase the elderly person's susceptibility to insomnia. Treatment depends on the problem. Behavior modification has been used successfully for many sleep problems; however, the conservative use of medications may be indicated in more problematic sleep disorders, periodic movements of sleep, and dementing illness.[5]

Skin Changes

As the skin ages, the decrease of subcutaneous fat resulting in the loss of skin elasticity and support allows for sagging and wrinkling of the skin. The stratum corneum (outer layer) of the epidermis thins and flattens, increasing permeability. In addition, sweat glands are decreased in number, and decreased sweating results.

The skin changes create many considerations for nursing care. Increased permeability allows increased penetration of chemical substances. Therefore, care must be taken to avoid overdose of transdermal medications. The thinning of the epidermis and loss of support tissue can result in easy bruising and avulsion. As the skin becomes looser, shearing forces can cause more damage.

Given these conditions, care must be taken when moving the older patient. Nursing interventions should be

Clinical Research

Cullum N, Clark M: Intrinsic factors associated with pressure sores in elderly people. J Adv Nurs 17:427–431, 1992

This prospective study examined the intrinsic factors associated with pressure sore development in a population of elderly patients with intact skin who were admitted to acute care units. The results of biochemical and hematological tests taken on admission, together with details of nursing care obtained from medical and nursing notes, were analysed in relation to the condition of the pressure areas of each patient. The same person observed and documented patient pressure areas throughout the study. The relations between intrinsic factors (eg, serum protein concentration, systolic blood pressure) and the presence of (or tendency to develop) pressure sores were examined and discussed in the light of a need for more specific and sensitive risk assessment tools.

No relation was found between diastolic blood pressure, serum urea, sodium, potassium, and bicarbonate concentrations, peripheral cell volume, or red and white blood cell counts and the development of pressure sores in this study.

planned to reduce shearing forces when turning or changing the patient's position. Incidental injury that can cause bruising or avulsion must be prevented. Even padded soft restraints can cause damage and should be avoided. Padding of the side rails may be indicated if the patient thrashes in bed. Although always important, keeping the bed free from foreign objects and the sheets free from wrinkles becomes essential with the older patient. Early recognition of pressure areas, frequent turning, and use of a pressure relief mattress are prime considerations.

Keep the patient appropriately covered to assist with temperature regulation. This is necessary because the loss of subcutaneous fat and impaired sweating mechanism diminish the patient's thermoregulating capabilities. Decreased lubrication of the skin increases the need for attention to skin care. Soap use should be minimal, and moisturizing lotions should be applied.

Cardiovascular Changes

The aging heart does not manifest anatomic change; there is, however, a gradual decrease in function. Stroke volume decreases, and the resting heart rate may increase slightly. In response to exercise, the rate increase is less, and the return to base line requires more time. Stroke volume during exercise increases to compensate for the lower pulse rate.

Arteries tend to lose their elasticity and become less compliant with increased output (arteriosclerosis). This may result in a higher systolic pressure with minimal, if any, changes of diastolic pressure.

In the absence of vascular disease, these changes should not interfere with normal tissue perfusion. In the older patient, the likelihood of atherosclerosis is increased. The narrowing of vessels, coupled with their decrease in

compliance, may produce tissue ischemia. This, along with bed rest, contributes to tissue injury and decubitus formation.

The decrease in vessel compliance affects large and small arteries. As a result, even a small increase in intravascular volume can be accompanied by a substantial rise in aortic pressure (and, in turn, systolic blood pressure) which may lead to pressure produced ventricular hypertrophy.[6]

The older patient may also have a greater amount of pooling in the lower extremities because of decreased muscle mass and poor venous return. If the patient is placed on bed rest this fluid pool is redistributed and may cause an overload in the cardiovascular system. The nurse must be alert for vascular overload and congestive heart failure.

Another factor to consider is the shifting of fluids when a patient arises after having been on bed rest. The sudden shift in fluid to the lower extremities and the lowered fluid volume that results from bed rest can produce extreme lightheadedness. A slow progression of head elevation and dangling before moving the patient to sitting or standing is necessary to prevent syncope and possible injury from falling.

Respiratory Changes

Decreased expansion and flexibility of the pulmonary structure results in a decreased volume exchange. In addition, cilia are lost and surfactant diminishes in the alveolar sacs; mucus production may increase. The number of alveoli is thought to remain constant except in respiratory disease. The older adult with a healthy respiratory system should experience only minimal respiratory difficulty during daily activities. There may be some respiratory compromise with exercise related to decreased exchange.

In many older patients changes related to disease arise

from damage to the lungs from smoking, environmental pollutants, or previous infections. Bony abnormalities such as kyphosis may also cause further restriction of respiratory excursion.

The decreased expansion of the thorax, increased secretions, and decreased number of cilia render the older patient susceptible to respiratory infections. In addition, a decreased immune response in older persons may contribute to the increased incidence of respiratory infection.

Careful attention to nutrition, especially to sufficient calories, protein, and fluid intake, is needed to reduce the risk of infection. Frequent position changes also assist in the clearance of secretions and aid ventilation and perfusion of the lungs.

Renal Changes

A loss of renal glomeruli accompanies the aging process. This loss in conjunction with decreased kidney perfusion results in a decreased glomerular filtration rate (GFR). The decrease in filtration may result in decreased clearance of substances normally excreted. An increase in blood urea nitrogen (BUN) or creatinine may indicate the extent to which the GFR is diminished. However, creatinine from muscle breakdown may be less than in younger patients and could mask an elevated creatinine. Creatinine clearance is a more accurate measure of renal function for the older patient. Evaluation of renal function is extremely important if the patient is receiving drugs normally excreted by the kidney.

There may also be a lessened response to antidiuretic hormones that can result in a decreased ability to concentrate urine. This may lead to problems of fluid and electrolyte balance as excess sodium, potassium, and water are lost. Loss of hydrogen ions may also make the acid–base balance more difficult to maintain.

Older persons tend to drink less fluid. This leaves them vulnerable to dehydration if fluids are further restricted or if medications with diuretic actions are administered. The older patient may also have decreased thirst. Care must be taken to ensure that the hospitalized older patient has adequate fluid intake by oral, enteral, or parenteral routes. Fluid balance may also be precarious because the elderly patient is taking more than one drug with diuretic action; diuretics and digoxin are a frequently prescribed combination, and disease states such as diabetes can also produce diuresis. Further, potassium and sodium levels may already be low when the patient arrives in the unit. Care must be taken to ensure that electrolyte balance remains stable or is restored. Confusion, dysrhythmias, coma, and death can occur quickly in the older patient with a precarious electrolyte balance.

As bladder muscle tone is lost, incomplete emptying with retention can foster the development of urinary tract infections that can ascend and become renal infections. Hypertrophy of the prostate gland also places older men at risk for urinary tract infection.

Loss of muscle tone, retention with overdistention, and loss of sphincter control lead to incontinence in the elderly. For the alert patient, this loss of control is embarrassing and disconcerting. Bladder training, observation for distention, and appropriate medications are nursing measures to assist the patient with maintaining continence. If incontinence does occur, rapid linen changes and proper skin care diminish physical and mental discomfort.

If an elderly patient develops any type of incontinence or retention during the stay in the critical care unit, evaluate the medication regime to see if any drugs affect bladder contractility or tone. If an indwelling (Foley) catheter is necessary during acute illness, it should be removed as soon as the primary reason for inserting it (eg, hourly urine measurements) has passed. Early removal may prevent deterioration of bladder function and urinary tract infection.

Gastrointestinal Changes

The gastrointestinal system experiences many age-related changes. The mechanical and chemical processes of digestion that begin in the mouth may be impaired because of loss of teeth and decrease in salivary secretions. Many old persons experience diminished senses of taste and smell, which may lead to decreased food intake.

Slowing of peristalsis may interfere with swallowing, gastric emptying, and passage through the bowel. The decrease in hydrochloric acid, digestive enzymes, and bile may contribute to incomplete digestion of nutrients. Diminished intrinsic factor in some persons as the result of decreased vitamin B_{12} synthesis may produce pernicious anemia.

Data are insufficient to make assumptions regarding changes in absorption in the large and small bowel. Some evidence indicates that absorption is somewhat impaired. Given that the eating patterns of older persons may not include all food groups, deficiencies may arise from lack of intake rather than malabsorption.

The decreased motility of the large bowel is probably not sufficient to produce constipation in the active adult. However, while on bed rest and with decreased intake of food and fluids, patients may experience constipation and fecal impaction. Dependence on or misuse of laxatives must be assessed when the history is taken.

Nursing intervention for gastrointestinal changes begins with a careful history. Eating habits, including time and frequency of food intake, food preferences, usual intake, food intolerances, and intactness of taste and smell, must be assessed. Use of laxatives, enemas, and vitamin supplementation should be explored. Evaluation of the teeth and gums helps to establish how well food can be handled mechanically.

In planning care, the nurse must consider that bed rest slows peristalsis and aggravates any preexisting condition related to motility. Adequate fluid intake, bulk in the diet, use of natural laxatives (eg, prune juice, warm liquids), and as much active or passive exercise as the condition of the patient allows may help maintain a normal pattern of bowel movements. Stool softness and mild laxatives are often included in the regimen.

Hospitalized patients of any age can become rapidly malnourished secondary to the stress of acute illness, an increased demand for energy, and lack of nourishment. Therefore, it is important to look for indicators of nutritional risk. They include a history of recent weight loss, a diet lacking in protein and calories, an albumin level < 3.5 g/dl, and a lymphocyte count < 1,500. The elderly patient who enters the hospital already mildly to moderately malnourished and with a poor intake of protein and calories may quickly become severely malnourished. This state can markedly compromise the immune response and increase the incidence and severity of infection. Therefore, it is crucial to see that critically ill elderly patients maintain adequate nutritional intake.

Musculoskeletal Changes

Mobility limitations of the elderly patient may be related to loss of muscle strength. Muscle mass may be lost because of a reduction in the number and size of muscle fibers or, possibly, an increase in connective tissues. This results in less muscle tension and decreased strength of the contraction. The decrease of lean muscle mass and the loss of elasticity contribute to lost flexibility and increased stiffness.

There may be a loss of bone mass with aging that, in the presence of osteoporosis, increases the risk of fracture. Lack of exercise, poor nutrition, and calcium malabsorption contribute to the loss of bone mass. The bedfast patient may rapidly lose bone mineral concentration. The calcaneus (heel) and spine are most susceptible, with a loss of approximately 1% per week. This loss is related to lack of weight-bearing. Having the patient stand quietly as soon as the condition allows acts to slow the loss of bone mineral concentration.

Forced fasting of the critically ill hospitalized patient may further accelerate muscle loss through catabolism and gluconeogenesis. The added burden of bed rest leads to a rapid loss of mobility, strength, and energy in the older patient. Maintaining nutrition, changing position frequently, active and passive exercise, and getting out of bed as much as permitted by condition are essential to preserving strength, energy, and bone mass. If the patient is comatose or has suffered loss of function, proper positioning and splinting can help prevent permanent deformity.

Endocrine Changes

No significant changes occur in hormone production during the aging process except for the female reproductive hormones. Therefore, with this exception, changes in the circulating hormones may reflect a disease process or a drug-altered response.

Glucose tolerance decreases with age. In fact, an increase in blood glucose of 200 mg/dl occurs in about 50% of persons older than 70 years of age.[7] Interpretation of this glucose intolerance requires the use of age-adjusted parameters to avoid the inappropriate diagnosis and treatment of diabetes mellitus. Evaluating glycosylated hemoglobin (HbA_{1c}) or glycosylated albumin may help establish the presence or absence of diabetes mellitus in the older patient with elevated glucose.

Diabetes mellitus is frequently seen in conjunction with acute illness, trauma, or surgery. The end-organ damage of diabetes mellitus is a factor in stroke, myocardial infarction, decreased renal function, and peripheral vascular disease. In fact, long-standing non–insulin-dependent diabetes may only be diagnosed when the patient presents with a stroke or acute myocardial infarction. Therefore, it is important to distinguish among the impaired glucose tolerance of aging, a transient rise in glucose related to acute illness, and the disease process of diabetes.

Recognition of the underlying diabetes and possible end-organ damage may alter the course of the acute illness. For example, knowing that the incidence of congestive heart failure after myocardial infarction is higher in diabetics than in nondiabetics, the nurse can be alert for early signs of fluid retention.

Older diabetics are, for the most part, non–insulin-dependent. Even if they develop extremely high blood sugars they are rarely ketoacidotic. In fact, the coma of this age group is usually hyperglycemic, hyperosmolar, and nonketotic (HHNK). Managing this state requires a delicate balance of hydration and rapid reduction of blood sugar without massive brain edema and death. The critical care nurse must be aware that HHNK coma can be triggered by acute illness or surgery.

Nursing interventions for patients with diabetes include the following:

- observe for skin problems related to decreased peripheral circulation and neuropathy
- select a diet to help correct elevated glucose levels
- watch for dehydration, which increases the risk of hyperosmotic coma
- assess for end-organ damage such as renal impairment and absorption problems that may determine medication therapy

Although diabetes mellitus is probably the most common disease process encountered in the older critically ill patient, thyroid conditions are frequent. The symptoms of thyroid disease in the older patient may not be as pronounced as in younger persons. In elders, symptoms such as apathy, weakness, and weight loss may be attributed to old age rather than to hyper- or hypothyroidism. The elderly patient with hyperthyroidism is more likely to be anorexic than hyperphagic and may not suffer from heat intolerance. The most prominent sign of hyperthyroidism may be atrial tachycardia. The hypothyroid patient may be more susceptible to hypothermia if exposed to cold. Accelerated aging, fatigue, or dizziness and a tendency to fall may signal hypothyroidism. However, dizziness with a tendency to fall may be the only symptom of hypothyroidism in the older person.

Thyroid conditions may be difficult to diagnose because they mimic other disease states. However, once diagnosed, thyroid disease in the older patient is usually readily corrected with medication.

Being aware of the atypical presentation of thyroid disease in elderly persons leads the critical care nurse to recognize that untoward medication responses may be caused by endocrine imbalance. Depression, agitation, and weight loss may also be identified as symptoms of thyroid dysfunction. Correcting the thyroid hormone imbalance can help the patient return to the base line health status. Early recognition of symptoms that may be related to endocrine dysfunction and interventions leading to accurate diagnosis enable the nurse to anticipate and plan care to prevent complications.

Psychological Assessment

Cognitive Changes

Cognition refers to the process of obtaining, storing, retrieving and using information. Some observable and studied changes in cognition occur with aging. They include some decline in perceptual motor skills, concept formation, complex memory tasks and quick-decision tasks. However, age itself is not the criterion for making decisions about a patient's cognitive functions. Each person's abilities must be judged individually rather than against a norm.

Cognitive function should be assessed and described on admission and then monitored routinely over time and whenever the patient's condition changes. While assessing cognitive functions during the patient's stay in critical care, it is important to remember that physiological deficits, some medications, and internal and external stress, including environmental stressors, affect cognitive skills.

A mental status questionnaire can be used to assess cognitive function systematically. One example is the Folstein Mini Mental Status Examination. It has 11 questions that provide information about orientation, attention, memory, perception, and thought process. It takes 5 to 10 minutes to complete, and the patient must be able to give oral and written responses.[8] Use of a consistent assessment

tool helps the nurse compare responses and monitor results over time. The main drawback to the use of a questionnaire is that some critically ill patients may not be able to hear, see, talk, or write well enough to respond to the questions. Longer, more sensitive tools may also be more fatiguing for critically ill elders.

Learning

Older adults may take longer to respond to and assimilate new material. They may also be hesitant to take on new tasks. Motivation continues to be an important aspect of learning new material. If the material is irrelevant or meaningless, motivation is decreased—which is often interpreted as inability to learn. In teaching elderly patients, it is important to consider sensory abilities along with cognition. It may be necessary to present information using small segments and varied stimuli, including touching, seeing, hearing, and (if vision permits), writing. If movements are slowed, allow time for the completion of motor tasks such as manipulating equipment or carrying out exercises.

Memory

The older person's memory decline occurs with short-term memory rather than long-term and remote memory. Recall of memory from the past is least impaired by age. Remote memory recall (items learned many years ago) can be a positive therapeutic strategy for elderly patients. Reminiscence is an adaptive mechanism that helps the nurse learn about the patient and contributes to feelings of increased self-worth and competence for the patient.

A summary of cognitive changes in the elderly patient is found in Table 7–4.

Depression

Depression disorders are among the most common complaints of older adults and the leading cause of suicide in

TABLE 7–4
Summary of Cognitive Changes With Aging

Intelligence

Remains stable
More hesitant with new tasks

Learning

Takes longer to respond
Needs motivation to learn new material

Memory

Decline in short-term memory
Remote memory remains intact

DISPLAY BOX 7-3
Some Drugs that May Cause Depression in the Elderly

Analgesics/anti-inflammatory agents
Anticonvulsants
Antihistamines
Antihypertensive agents
Antimicrobials
Antiparkinsonian agents
Cytoxic agents
Hormones
Immunosuppressive agents
Tranquilizers

---

later life. Depression evidenced in clinical behaviors and symptoms in later life can be masked by the exaggeration of changes commonly associated with normal aging. For example, difficulty sleeping, early morning awakening, and lethargy are the cardinal symptoms of major depression and are also common physical complaints of the normal aging person. Therefore, it is important to use an assessment tool, such as the Geriatric Depression Scale, that is age specific.[9]

Other common complaints of the elderly depressed patient are fatigue, pain, gastrointestinal disturbances, and sleep disorders. In some patients, the dominant emotional mood may not be sadness but anger, anxiety, or irritability. Depression can also mimic other diseases to which the elderly are especially susceptible, such as occult carcinoma, thyroid disease, collagen disease, substance abuse, and Alzheimer's disease. Some medications, such as the major and minor tranquilizers, barbiturates, cardiotonics, and steroids, can potentiate or enhance depression. Others, such as digitalis, beta blockers, and diuretics, can produce symptoms and complications that either suggest depression or in fact produce a true depression.

The nurse must also be aware of cardiovascular side effects of antidepressive drugs. On the electrocardiograph, ST segment and T wave changes may become evident but are not necessarily indicative of myocardial damage. Ventricular dysrhythmias and disturbances in cardiac conduction are considered serious side effects of antidepressive drugs, which may result in the drug being reduced or discontinued. The elderly may also experience changes related to sleep, appetite, and blood pressure with antidepressive drugs. Anticholinergic effects, especially in Alzheimer's disease, benign prostatic hypertrophy, or coronary artery disease, may also be seen.

Specific agents with a high incidence of causing depression are methyldopa, reserpine, corticosteroids, barbiturates, minor tranquilizers, alcohol, and Inderal.

Suicide is a serious problem among the elderly. Of all suicides committed in this country annually, 25% are persons older than 65 years of age. White men older than 85 years of age are at particular risk. Multiple changes and losses over a short period, isolation, and decreased independence diminish the self-esteem and coping abilities of the aging person. Because of their many losses and changes, suicide may for some older persons fulfill a fantasy of "reunion" with their dead spouse or significant other.

The nurse should help the depressed elderly patient regain feelings of self-worth, be watchful of suicide attempts or warnings, and be aware of drugs that may cause depression.

Abuse of the Elderly

Rough estimates indicate that one of ten elderly persons living with family members is subject to abuse. Abuse of the elderly occurs in both homes and institutions, and it takes many forms. It may be blatant or subtle; physical, psychological, or material (eg, financial). It may involve neglect (by others or by self), exploitation, or abandonment. The abused elderly are often physically or mentally frail and unable to report the abusive situation. Abuse can also happen to emotionally and intellectually stable older people, who may feel unable to stop the abuse and also unable to report it because of their financial or emotional dependence on the abuser. They may also be afraid of being abandoned.

The abuse can be by people who do not live with the elderly person. It can occur because of a lack of knowledge about the elderly person's basic needs and lack of resources to help. Sometimes it occurs because adult children don't want to subject their parents to tests perceived as harmful, or when they are limiting their parents' spending to protect an inheritance. The abuse can be by caretakers who are extremely stressed. And, of course, the abused

---

DISPLAY BOX 7-4
Indicators of Potential Abuse or Neglect

Unexplained:
- injuries, burns, bruises
- sores, excoriations, decubiti
- malnutrition, dehydration
- poor care: unclean hair, nails, body
- fear, anxiety, or withdrawal from caretaker
- highly stressed caretaker
- too much or too little medication

person may be the caretaker (and not the patient). Frequently self neglect occurs if the elderly person either is not able or chooses not to take adequate care of his or her basic needs.

The nurse should be alert to any indications of abuse (eg, bruises, burns, broken bones) and any failure to thrive (eg, underhydration, underweight, and poor hygiene). Any suggestion by the patient or family that things aren't well at home or that they are worried about someone should be pursued. A statement such as, "My son hasn't been here yet. He sometimes forgets his commitments," should open the door for further conversation. It might uncover a mother who is worried about her son's drinking . . . and perhaps about the way he treats her when he's drinking. Ask elderly patients how they were managing before they became ill. Also ask the caretaker and family members. Is the history given by the patient different from that given by the family? Ask the caretakers if they were able to give the care they felt was needed. Indications that the patient was "getting to be a handful" may be a clue to mismanaged care or a caretaker in need of support and assistance. In either situation, the nurse can provide information and support and possible referral to a social worker or mental health nurse for further assistance. In addition, health care workers, including nurses, should know their responsibility under state law for reporting abuse of the elderly.

Alcohol Abuse

Alcohol abuse occurs in the aging population although there is little documentation about its prevalence. Problem drinking in the elderly occurs for the same reasons as during the adult years. However, smaller amounts of alcohol create larger problems for the elderly, and they may be more susceptible to alcohol-induced pathology. In the past, it was thought that the many stresses of advancing age and difficulty in managing them contributed to increased alcohol abuse. This may remain true for a small percentage of elderly persons. Recently, it has been recognized that differences in metabolism of alcohol in the elderly, the smaller volume of body water, and the decrease in lean body tissue may increase the propensity to alcoholism or alcohol problems. In addition, elderly persons are high consumers of psychotropic drugs and are at risk for drug–alcohol interaction.

Nursing interventions include assessing the reasons for drinking and assessing for physical deterioration resulting from alcohol consumption. The immediate goal is to stabilize physiological and psychological response to alcohol withdrawal and determine its impact on whatever other diagnoses have resulted in the need for critical care. As soon as possible, the nurse should refer the patient to a social worker, psychiatric liaison nurse, or alcohol counselor.

Medication Assessment

Start low, go slow, and *be patient* is the rule for giving therapeutic medications to the older patient. Changes related to aging can have a great impact on drug response. Changes in renal function, gastrointestinal secretions and mobility, and cell receptor sites as well as concurrent disease states can alter the absorption, distribution, and excretion of drugs.

Before admission to the critical care area, older patients may have been taking a multitude of drugs, including over-the-counter (OTC) medications such as vitamins, tonics, laxatives, antacids, and pain relievers. They may also have a history of heavy alcohol intake. Any of these drugs can cause problems if combined with medications administered in the hospital.

The nurse needs to elicit a careful history of drug usage from the patient and family. As part of collecting this information, the family can be asked to bring in all medications the patient has been using including OTC drugs. Although alcohol use may be a sensitive topic, establishing the pattern of use can be essential in preventing untoward drug interactions and anticipating problems with liver damage or withdrawal.

Special considerations concerning administration of drugs to the older patient include knowing the drugs the patient has been taking, assessing renal, hepatic, endocrine, and digestive systems, and evaluating lean body mass. Impairment within the body systems may affect the absorption, metabolism, and excretion of drugs. A decrease in lean body mass and an increase in total body fat may alter the distribution of the drug within the body.

Drug Absorption

The increased pH of gastric secretions and delayed stomach emptying time can alter the degradation, and thus the absorption, of drugs. Drugs that are not stable in an acid medium can be severely reduced in bioavailability if they remain in the stomach for long periods. Drugs that are designed to be acted on in the small intestine may be affected by the higher pH of the aging stomach. A coated, pH-sensitive medication such as erythromycin may lose its coating in the stomach and be degraded before reaching the absorption sites in the small intestine. Coated gastric irritants may lose their coatings and cause bleeding or nausea and vomiting.

Drug Distribution

Distribution of drugs in the body can be affected by a decrease of lean body mass, an increase in total body fat, or a decrease in total body fluid, all of which may accompany

(*Text continues on page 84*)

NURSING CARE PLAN 7–1:
The Aging Patient

Mrs. Jamison, an 82-year-old woman who lived on a fixed income, was admitted to the intensive care unit with a diagnosis of septicemia and impending septic shock (BP 92/60 mm Hg) resulting from a gram-negative infection of her postoperative incision. Initial assessment revealed that the patient lived alone and had a history of hypertension, neck pain, and difficulty sleeping. Her daughter reported that she had had no appetite and had lost 20 pounds in the last year. She had become increasingly weak and was barely able to take care of herself. She had taken prescribed hypnotic agents for the past 20 years. The daughter stated that her mother had been highly anxious for the past 3 days.

On admission, the patient complained of malaise, fever, shaking chills, headache, nausea and vomiting, and mental cloudiness. She appeared restless, fearful, and apprehensive; her skin was warm, dry, flushed, and pink; respirations were tachypneic with decreased respiratory depth; her urine output was decreased and dark amber in color. Her temperature was 101° F (38.4° C).

DIAGNOSTIC STUDIES

Serum electrolytes: Showed acidosis, fluid shifts, and altered renal function.

Blood: Hematocrit was elevated because of hemoconcentration. White blood cells (WBC) were decreased because of early septicemia (hyperdynamic stage).

Clotting studies: Platelets were decreased because of platelet aggregation. Prothrombin time/partial thromboplastin time (PT/PTT) was slightly prolonged, indicating beginning coagulopathy associated with circulating toxins and impending shock state.

Serum lactate: Increased level consistent with metabolic acidosis and shock.

Serum glucose: Hyperglycemia reflecting gluconeogenesis and glycogenolysis in response to cellular starvation (caused by inability of cells to use glucose, then use of fat and finally protein as energy sources).

BUN/creatinine: Increased levels associated with dehydration, renal impairment.

ABGs: Metabolic acidosis caused by failure of compensatory mechanisms.

Urine: Increase WBCs/bacteria suggestive of infection.

Wound culture: Gram-negative organisms causing sepsis. Intravenous fluids and antibiotics were started immediately. When her vital signs were stable, Mrs. Jamison was bathed, assisted with oral hygiene, and given oral fluids as tolerated. The nurses developed the following care plan.

Initial Plan of Care

NURSING DIAGNOSIS	OUTCOME CRITERIA/ PATIENT GOALS	NURSING INTERVENTIONS
Decreased cardiac output: related to gram-negative sepsis, renal dysfunction, dehydration, and metabolic acidosis.	• Maintain cardiac output to ensure adequate tissue perfusion.	1. Assess BP, heart rate and rhythm, and respiratory rate q15–60 min, as indicated. 2. Provide bed rest and minimal activity. 3. Supplemental oxygen, as ordered. 4. Administer IV fluids and antibiotics, as ordered. 5. Assess volume status (eg, auscultate lungs, assess skin turgor and edema, measure urine output, weigh patient, evaluate jugular vein distention) q2–4 h, as indicated. 6. Evaluate all laboratory data, as available.

(continued)

NURSING CARE PLAN 7–1: (Continued)
Initial Plan of Care

NURSING DIAGNOSIS	OUTCOME CRITERIA/ PATIENT GOALS	NURSING INTERVENTIONS
		7. Control fever with antipyretics or cooling blanket, as ordered.
		8. Obtain and evaluate available hemodynamic parameters (PAP, PCWP, PAS, PAD, and CO) q1 h.
Ineffective breathing pattern: related to pain, hypoxemia, loss of muscle strength, and poor nutrition.	• Maintain normal breathing patterns and adequate gas exchange.	1. Administer oxygen as ordered.
		2. Plan activities to include periods of comfort and rest.
		3. Assist patient into comfortable positions for eating, sleeping, reading.
		4. Ambulate or sit patient in chair for frequent limited periods of time. Do not overfatigue.
		5. Monitor oxygen saturation with oximetry.
Fluid volume deficit: related to abnormal fluid loss, decreased fluid intake, and hyperglycemia.	• Maintain fluid balance and correct electrolyte imbalances.	1. Note signs/symptoms of dehydration (eg, dry mucous membranes, thirst, dulled sensorium, peripheral vasoconstriction).
		2. Measure intake and output.
		3. Weigh daily; monitor changes.
		4. Calculate insensible fluid losses.
		5. Monitor vital signs and hemodynamic pressures if available.
		6. Monitor laboratory reports (eg, serum K, serum and urine Na).
		7. Administer IV fluids per order; correct fluid deficit gradually.
		8. Provide scheduled oral fluids throughout the 24-hr period.
Altered nutrition, less than body requirements: related to alterations in taste, loss of appetite, nausea and vomiting, decreased strength, and medications.	• Promote adequate nutrition to meet body requirements.	1. Weigh daily, record.
		2. Observe, record liquid, solid food intake.
		3. Provide a pleasant environment at mealtime.
		4. Monitor laboratory reports (eg, transferrin, albumin, electrolytes).
		5. Maintain accurate intake, output.
		6. Record amount, color, consistency of vomitus. Keep a record of all stools.
		7. Administer medications; observe effect and record.

(continued)

NURSING CARE PLAN 7–1: (Continued)
Initial Plan of Care

NURSING DIAGNOSIS	OUTCOME CRITERIA/ PATIENT GOALS	NURSING INTERVENTIONS
Anxiety: related to fear and social isolation, secondary to emergency admission to the hospital.	• Patient will verbalize decreased feelings of anxiety.	1. Assess level of anxiety. 2. Maintain calm, unhurried manner when assisting patient. 3. Listen to patient with respect and interest. 4. Provide clear, simple explanations to patient.
	• Patient's participation in health-care decisions will increase.	1. Assist patient to develop communication skills. 2. Encourage participation in diversional activities. 3. Encourage development of new coping methods.
	• Patient will increase expressions of security, safety, well-being.	1. Assist patient to label feelings. 2. Encourage patient to engage in activities using large muscle groups. 3. Establish and maintain familiar routines in self-care. 4. Assist and teach patient to use relaxation techniques.
Fear: related to feeling of powerlessness, real or imagined threat to well-being secondary to disease process and hospitalization.	• Patient involvement in care and decisions about care will be maintained.	1. Involve patient and family in planning care and setting goals. 2. Administer antianxiety medication as ordered. 3. Instruct in relaxation techniques (eg, guided imagery, progressive muscle relaxation).
	• Patient will verbalize trust and understanding of disease process and treatment.	1. Assist patient and family in identifying source(s) of fear; determine understanding of the situation. 2. Spend uninterrupted time with patient and family. 3. Instruct patient and family on disease process and necessary treatments; evaluate understanding of same. 4. Orient to surroundings; make adaptations to compensate for sensory deficits.
Sleep pattern disturbance: related to noxious stimuli, stress, pain, undesirable side effects of medications, and critical care environment.	• Normal sleep patterns will be established.	1. Assist patient in identifying potential underlying causes of sleep disturbances (eg, fear, unresolved problems, conflicts).

(continued)

NURSING CARE PLAN 7–1: (Continued)
Initial Plan of Care

NURSING DIAGNOSIS	OUTCOME CRITERIA/ PATIENT GOALS	NURSING INTERVENTIONS
		2. Provide comfort measures during sleep and rest periods.
		3. Provide quiet, peaceful environment, minimize interruptions.
		4. Consult with physician regarding need to revise medication regimen where nonhypnotic medications interfere with sleep pattern.
High risk for self-care deficit: related to inability/limitations in feeding, bathing/hygiene, grooming, toileting, and ambulating.	• Functional independence will improve.	1. Assist patient in planning care activities to increase patient participation.
		2. Schedule care and hygiene activities as desired by patient.
		3. Provide privacy for personal care that patient can manage.
		4. Listen to patient's expression of desires, fears, and other feelings.
		5. Provide assistive devices for care activities (eg, bedside commode, walker, special silverware for meals).
High risk for powerlessness: related to lack of control over hospital environment and dependence on others.	• Increased decision-making ability and independence will be promoted.	1. Allow patient to share in the decision-making process concerning care activities.
		2. Provide as many situations as possible where patient takes control (eg, positioning self, visiting).
		3. Encourage patient to express feelings about present situation.
Knowledge deficit: related to limited understanding of disease process, limited understanding of prescribed treatment, and impaired communication.	• Patient will demonstrate increased knowledge about illness and treatment. • Patient will comply with medical and pharmacological therapy.	1. Assess and record patient's level of understanding of disease process and prescribed treatment.
		2. Evaluate patient's readiness to learn about disease process and treatment plan.
		3. Involve patient's support system in the teaching process.
		4. Provide written information specific to the patient's learning needs.
		5. Reassess patient's understanding of all teaching material and content.

(continued)

NURSING CARE PLAN 7–1: *(Continued)*
Initial Plan of Care

NURSING DIAGNOSIS	OUTCOME CRITERIA/ PATIENT GOALS	NURSING INTERVENTIONS
Altered family process: related to lack of respite from care of elderly family member and change in family roles.	• Positive patient–family interaction will be promoted.	1. Identify who will assume the role of head of the family. 2. Provide emotional support to head of family in regard to added responsibilities. 3. Recognize and provide support to all family members. 4. Facilitate communication among family members so they can express their feelings about their present situation.
	• Family members will demonstrate increased tolerance related to the demands of the caregiver role.	1. Assess coping ability of family members for purposes of referral to social services and community agencies. 2. Assist family to plan family conferences. 3. Instruct family members on relaxation techniques. 4. Include social worker and discharge planning nurse in family conferences. 5. Include patient in decisions. 6. Identify community resources for assistance in home care.
High risk for impaired home maintenance management: related to limited financial resources, home environment obstacles, inadequate support system, and insufficient family resources or planning.	• Patient's ability to manage the home environment with assistance of family, friends, and community resources will increase.	1. Assist patient and family to examine resources necessary to ease the transition from hospital to home. 2. Instruct patient and family on matters that will require independent decision-making. 3. Involve patient and family in decision-making concerning care before discharge.

Mrs. Jamison continued to gain strength over the next 2 days. The social worker and clergy were involved in planning long-term care after hospitalization. She was transferred from critical care to a medical unit where the focus of care became efforts to increase her lost strength and to resolve her diarrhea, which had started on the third day of hospitalization, probably as a result of antibiotic therapy.

Mrs. Jamison began to express her feelings openly to the nurses. She complained of feeling that her life was over and that her weakness could prevent her from being independent again.

On Day 6 the nurses met with the family members and Mrs. Jamison to confirm plans for discharge to a convalescent center. She was to go there for 4 to 6 weeks to regain her strength before moving back home. Her 19-year-old granddaughter planned to live with her at least 6 months to assist her and monitor her progress and ability to live alone.

(continued)

NURSING CARE PLAN 7–1: (Continued)
Expanded Assessment

On the next day, treatment IV antibiotics and fluid therapy continued. Mrs. Jamison began a full liquid diet. Her temperature returned to near normal (99° F) and urine output averaged 30 to 40 cc per hour. Her BP was 100 to 130/180 to 90 mm Hg. Her daughter spent most of the day visiting, frequently expressing her own exhaustion to the nurses. She explained to the staff that her mother lived alone by her own insistence and was not really able to care for herself adequately. She reported that her mother frequently stopped taking her heart medications because they "made her feel weak." She also suffered frequent episodes of depression. The nursing staff conducted a nursing care conference and developed the following expanded plan of care.

Expanded Plan of Care

NURSING DIAGNOSIS	OUTCOME CRITERIA/ PATIENT GOALS	NURSING INTERVENTIONS
Noncompliance: related to undesirable side effects of treatment regimen.	• Patient will comply with prescribed regimen and report side effects to primary health care provider.	1. Allow patient to verbalize reasons for noncompliant behavior. 2. Identify areas of patient's noncompliant behavior. 3. Acknowledge patient's right to choose not to carry out the prescribed treatment regimen.
Bowel incontinence: related to dietary changes, medication, and stress.	• Previous elimination pattern will be restored.	1. Auscultate, record bowel sounds. 2. Monitor frequency, characteristics of stools. 3. Administer antidiarrheal medications as ordered. Monitor, report effectiveness. 4. Observe skin condition daily and report excoriation, irritation, ulceration. 5. Weigh daily. 6. Maintain accurate intake and output. 7. Provide fluid and electrolyte replacement per physician's order. 8. Oversee collection of stool specimens.
Grieving: related to loss of function/ health/life role.	• Patient will maintain effective coping mechanisms during the illness process.	1. Encourage patient to use expressions of feelings that are comfortable (ie, crying vs. talking). 2. Encourage patient to assist in self-care activities. 3. Instruct patient and family about existing support groups and community agencies.

(continued)

NURSING CARE PLAN 7–1: (*Continued*)
Expanded Plan of Care

NURSING DIAGNOSIS	OUTCOME CRITERIA/ PATIENT GOALS	NURSING INTERVENTIONS
Self-esteem disturbance: related to body image, personal identity, role, performance, self-esteem, or diminished power.	• Patient will verbalize positive feelings of self-worth.	1. Assess and record evidence of disturbance in self-concept (eg, "Why me?", expressed concern about ability to continue role performance). 2. Allow patient to verbalize consequences of physical and emotional changes that influence self-concept. 3. Offer listing of community resources to patient and family. 4. Assist patient and family in identifying coping mechanisms related to body usage disturbance, personal identity disturbance, and role performance disturbance.
Impaired physical mobility: related to decreased strength and endurance, musculoskeletal impairment, neuromuscular impairment, lack of transportation, enforced bed rest, and depression.	• Patient will maintain muscle tone and muscle mass.	1. Evaluate the degree to which patient's mobility is impaired. 2. Assess patient's needs regarding safety precautions. 3. Perform passive, and instruct on active, range-of-motion exercises to maintain/develop muscle strength and endurance. 4. Encourage patient to verbalize limitations in strength and endurance. 5. Get patient up on feet and walking as soon as possible. 6. Note and record any increase or decrease in strength and endurance. 7. Provide adequate nutrition and fluid intake.
High risk for impaired skin integrity: related to altered sensation, immobility, and incontinence of stool/urine.	• Skin breakdown and infection will be absent.	1. Assess and record condition of skin (especially over bony prominences for breakdown). 2. Observe for presence/absence of redness, excoriation, pain, itching, tenderness. 3. Use protective measures (eg, skin protector products, pressure relief mattress, foam protectors). 4. Provide foods high in proteins, minerals, vitamins.

(*continued*)

NURSING CARE PLAN 7–1: *(Continued)*
Expanded Plan of Care

NURSING DIAGNOSIS	OUTCOME CRITERIA/ PATIENT GOALS	NURSING INTERVENTIONS
		5. Cleanse perinanal area with water and nondrying soap after incontinence.
High risk for ineffective individual coping: related to anger, anxiety, denial, dependent behavior, depression, and lack of information/communication.	• Patient will demonstrate effective coping strategies.	1. Identify and reduce unnecessary environmental stimuli.
		2. Spend uninterrupted periods with patient to encourage expression of feelings.
		3. Ask the psychiatric clinical nurse specialist to visit patient and assist with plan of care.
		4. Assist patient and family to establish visiting routine without taxing resources of patient or family.
		5. Provide patient and family with clear, concise information about patient's condition.
		6. Allow patient to identify short-term and long-term goals for care.
		7. Assist family to support patient's independence.

aging. Drugs that bind to muscle (eg, digoxin) become more bioavailable as lean body mass diminishes, increasing the risk of toxicity. Fat-soluble drugs (eg, Dalmane, Thorazine, phenobarbital) can be deposited in fat and result in cumulative effects of oversedation. In the presence of a volume deficit, drugs that are water soluble (eg, Garamycin) may have a higher concentration and may reach toxic levels rapidly.

Drug Metabolism

The liver is the major organ for biotransformation and detoxification of medications. In the older patient, there may be some decrease in the metabolism of drugs requiring hepatic enzymes for transformation. This results in an increased plasma level and prolonged half-life of the drug. The benzodiazepines (eg, Valium, Dalmane) may have a half-life increase from 20 to 90 hours in the older patient. Hepatic oxidation of these drugs can further be affected by alcohol-induced changes in the liver. There may be a decrease in drug metabolism with occasional

alcohol use. However, in chronic alcohol use drug metabolism is increased and excretion is accelerated.

Drug Excretion

The kidney is the primary excretory organ for clearing drugs. Drugs that are excreted unchanged (eg, digoxin, cimetidine, antibiotics) may have a decreased renal clearance. Given the decreased renal function of the older adult, the dosage of these drugs may need to be reduced. Serum creatinine alone is not a good determinant of renal function in the elderly. A creatinine clearance study reflects a more accurate estimation for drug clearance.

In summary, it is important to remember the following points if giving medication to the older patient:

1. Drug dosage guidelines are usually based on studies in younger persons, and recommended adult dosage guidelines may not be appropriate for older patients.

2. Elderly persons may be taking numerous prescrip-

DISPLAY BOX 7–5
Factors That can Affect Drug Absorption, Metabolism, or Excretion

> pH of gastric secretions
< lean body mass
< total body fat
< total body fluid
< metabolism of drugs needing hepatic enzymes
< glomeruli filtration rate
< creatinine clearance

tion drugs and may also self-medicate with borrowed, old prescription and OTC drugs.

3. The effects of alcohol use must be considered.
4. The potential for drug interactions and adverse reactions is increased because of the effects of aging on drug absorption, distribution, metabolism, and excretion. See Nursing Care Plan 7–1: The Aging Patient.

REFERENCES

1. Rees TS, Duckert LG, Auditory and vestibular dysfunction in aging. In Hazzard WR, Andres R, Bierman EL, Blass JP (eds): Principles of Geriatric Medicine and Gerontology, 2 ed, pp 432–444. New York, McGraw Hill, 1990
2. Robert JC: Clinical Issues. In Maddox GL (ed): The Encyclopedia of Aging, p 426. New York, Springer-Verlag, 1988
3. Treatment of Sleep Disorders of Older People. NIH Consensus Development Conference Statement Mar 8(3): 26–28, 1990
4. Koskenvuo M, Taprio J, Partinen M: Snoring as a risk factor for hypertension and angina pectoris. Lancet 11:893–896, 1985
5. Becker PM, Jamieson AO: Common sleep disorders in the elderly: Diagnosis and treatment. Geriatrics 47(3):41–52, 1992
6. Rebenson-Piano M: The physiologic changes that occur with aging. Crit Care Nurs Q 12(1):1–14, 1989
7. Halter JB: Endrocrinology and aging. In Kent B, Butler RN (eds): Human Aging Research: Concepts and Techniques, p 185. New York, Raven Press, 1988
8. Foreman MD, Gillies DA, Wagner D: Impaired cognition in the critically ill elderly patient: Clinical implications. Crit Care Nurs Q 12(1):61–73, 1989
9. Yesavage JA, Bunk TL, Rose TL, Lum O, Huang V, Adey M et al: Development and validation of a Geriatric Screening Scale: A preliminary report. Journal of Psychiatric Research 17(1):37–49, 1982–1983

BIBLIOGRAPHY

Andresen G: How to assess the older mind. RN 55(1):34–41, 1992
Fournet K: The challenge of teaching the elderly cardiac patient. Clin Iss in Crit Care Nurs 3(1)79–88, 1992
Gawlenski A, Jensen G: The complications of cardiovascular aging. Am J Nurs 91(11):26–30, 1991
Hoffman NB: Dehydration in the elderly: insidious and manageable. Geriatrics 46(6):35–38, 1991
Holm K, Hedricks C: Immobility and bone loss in the aging adult. Crit Care Nurs Q, 12(1):46–51, 1989
Kee CC: Age-related changes in the renal system: causes, consequences and nursing implications. Geriatric Nursing 13(2): 80–83, 1992
Maas M, Buckwalter KC, Hardy M: Nursing Diagnosis and Interventions for the Elder. Redding, MA, Addison-Wesley Publishing Co. Inc., 1991
Prinz PN, Vitiello NV, Raskind MA, Thorpy MJ: Geriatrics: sleep disorders and aging. N Engl J Med 323(8):520–526, 1990
Schwertz DW, Buschmann MBT: Pharmacogeriatrics. Crit Care Nurs Q 12(1):26–37, 1989
Stanley M: Elderly patients in critical care: an overview. Clin Iss in Crit Care Nurs 3(1):120–126, 1992

STUDY QUESTIONS

1. Physical changes that occur as a result of the normal aging process include which of the following?

   a. reduced sensory and perceptual activity
   b. extremes of heat and cold are tolerated well
   c. decreased amounts of connective and collagen tissue
   d. increased excretion of hormones

2. Major concerns in administration of drugs to elderly patients include all of the following except

   a. status of renal function
   b. assessment of hydration
   c. assessment of muscle strength
   d. medications taken before admission

3. Frequent turning and early ambulation are essential with the elderly patient for all of the following reasons *except*:

   a. to slow bone loss
   b. to maximize loss of strength
   c. to prevent respiratory complications
   d. to prevent skin breakdown

4. Types of elderly abuse are

   a. physical, social, biological
   b. social, psychological, biological
   c. material, emotional, social
   d. physical, psychological, and material

5. Visual pathologies of aging include

   a. glaucoma, diabetic retinopathy, cataracts, retinal generation
   b. diabetic retinopathy, cataracts, presbyopia, stria vascularis
   c. cataracts, glaucoma, arcus senilis, retinal degeneration
   d. presbyopia, stria vascularis, diabetic retinopathy, arcus senilis, retinal degenerations

6. Age-related factors that can put elderly persons at greater risk for alcohol-related problems are all of the following except

   a. a smaller volume of body water
   b. poor dentition
   c. decreased lean body tissue
   d. alcohol–drug reactions

PART II

Professional Practice
Issues in the
Critical Care Unit

CHAPTER 8

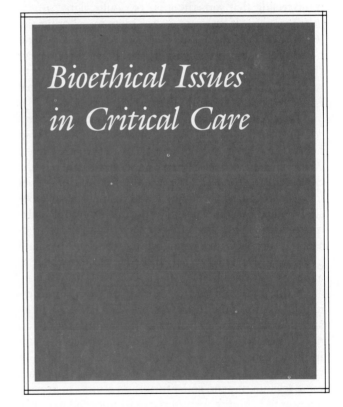

*Bioethical Issues
in Critical Care*

BEHAVIORAL OBJECTIVES

Based on the content in this chapter, the reader should
be able to:

1. Briefly explain the way in which ethics assists in
   reaching answers to moral dilemmas.
2. Name the ethical principles most relevant to the
   withholding or withdrawing of life-sustaining
   treatment and to the Patient Self-Determination
   Act.
3. Explain the basic difference between the two major
   ethical systems: consequentialism and nonconse-
   quentialism.
4. Discuss the terms moral uncertainty, moral distress, and moral dilemma.
5. Name the two guidelines that provide the nurse
   with basic directions needed to address ethical
   issues.

Hudak: Critical Care Nursing:
A Holistic Approach, 6th ed. © 1994
J. B. Lippincott Company.

Description

Hemodialysis is in some measure representative of the advances in contemporary health care. To mechanically replace the function of kidneys was once a dream of science fiction, yet now we can not only mechanically replace the function of the kidneys but also control the functions of the lungs, stomach, and heart. In the future, perhaps even the function of the uterus will be replaced by total *in vitro* gestation. The once simple questions of life and death have become frighteningly complex. Moral conflicts give rise to feelings of moral uncertainty, dilemma, and distress. The function of ethics is to clarify and illuminate moral issues and to help relieve these feelings.

But how does ethics accomplish this? How does ethics illuminate moral conflict? Identifying a problem as a source of moral uncertainty, distress, or dilemma begins the process of reasoning through the complexity. *Moral uncertainty* exists if one is unable to identify clearly a moral conflict within a situation, but experiences the troublesome feeling that something is "not quite right." *Moral dilemmas* occur if there are two or more moral principles involved in a situation, but to honor one principle would be to violate another. *Moral distress* is caused if one can clearly identify a moral conflict and the right action to resolve it, but institutional protocol or rules of professional etiquette prevent morally appropriate action.

Ethics education, consultation with institutional ethics committees, and the use of institutional ethics policies can help nurses reason through moral conflicts in the clinical environment. The major purpose of ethical analysis in the clinical area is to clarify the moral issues and principles involved in a particular situation, to examine one's responsibilities and obligations, and to provide an ethically adequate rationale for the decision made. This chapter presents an overview of nursing ethics, the principles and guidelines of nursing ethics, and a process by which to apply them clinically.

Critical care nurses are not immune to moral uncertainty, dilemma, and distress, particularly about such issues as withholding or withdrawing treatment and "do not resuscitate" (DNR) orders, two issues discussed later in this chapter. The unnerving and unending stream of technological advances in critical care makes ethical issues more relevant, urgent, and difficult; yet ethics can provide a means to help specify nurses' moral duties and to clarify these issues.

Ethics

Before applying the tools of ethics to moral conflicts in critical care, some basic definitions need to be discussed. The concept of ethics itself is difficult. What exactly is ethics? Are morals and ethics the same? Where do our personal values and feelings fit into such discussions? Does the nursing profession have its own realm of ethics differ-

ent from that of the medical profession? And on what do we base the tenets of nursing ethics?

Definitions

The original meanings of the terms *morals* and *ethics* are quite similar. The word *moral*, derived from the Latin *mores*, meant customs and habits; the word *ethics*, derived from the Greek *ethos*, meant customs, habitual usages, conduct, and character. Even in current discussion, the terms are used interchangeably, although their definitions are somewhat different.

Morals are personal or codified standards of conduct derived from societal expectations of behavior. They are the standards of behavior and values to which we are committed as members of society. *Ethics*, a more formal term, refers to the systematic study of those standards and values. Ethical inquiry, which is a form of philosophical or theological inquiry, allows us to think reasonably about, question, critique, and ultimately understand the dimensions of moral conduct.

The term ethics is sometimes used to refer to the formal beliefs or practices of a particular group of people, such as "Jewish ethics" or "business ethics." It is also used to denote the formal codes of conduct for professional groups. Within the profession of nursing, conduct is guided by the American Nurses' Association's (ANA's) *Code for Nurses With Interpretive Statements*. Further guidance can be found in the ANA's *Social Policy Statement* and other documents that communicate the values of the profession. We use the term ethics specifically to mean a method of inquiry that helps us answer questions about what is right or good and what ought to be done in specific situations.

Divisions of Ethics

Ethical inquiry, falling under the broad umbrella of philosophy or theology, can be subdivided into three categories: descriptive ethics, normative ethics, and metaethics. Descriptive ethics focuses on moral judgments made and carried out, and it is often studied within the fields of sociology, psychology, and anthropology; in other words, descriptive ethics *describes behavior*. Normative ethics, on the other hand, *applies standards of behavior* and value to specific situations. Normative ethics involves moral recommendations, judgments, and evaluations; its focus is what we *ought* to do, be, or cherish. It is normative ethics that most concerns us here. The third category, metaethics, is concerned with the nature of ethical inquiry. Metaethics researches the connections between human conduct and morality, between beliefs and reality, and between ethical theories, conduct, principles, and rules; it is generally the province of professional ethicists. Metaethics is the study of the *theoretical* basis of ethics.

Bioethics in Medicine and Nursing

Bioethics, a form of applied normative ethics, is the study of ethical issues in health care. In the past, nursing ethics was considered a branch of medical ethics, with medical ethics falling under the rubric of biomedical ethics. However, nursing ethics today is acknowledged as a discipline distinct from medical ethics.

The field of medical ethics involves ethical norms for the practice of medicine. It involves applying general moral principles to problems encountered in medicine. Medical ethics has a long tradition of focusing on influential codes of professional and research ethics, with very specific rules that apply to practicing physicians. Many physicians continue to equate medical ethics with specific, authoritative rules of conduct, rather than understanding medical ethics as a means for reasoning through moral conflicts.

Bioethics in nursing, or nursing ethics, asks specifically what our obligations are as nurses, what makes a good nurse, and what are the ends that nursing ought to seek. The *Code for Nurses* and the *Social Policy Statement* provide nurses with basic guidelines for addressing those questions. They are general guidelines for professional conduct that must be applied to specific clinical situations, rather than specific rules to be imposed on the nurse.

Values and Feelings

In addition to the ANA guidelines and general moral principles, personal values and emotions help determine the action the nurse takes in a particular situation. In Plato's *Crito*, Socrates directs us to allow reason rather than emotion to guide our decisions. By definition, ethics involves systematic study, in which reason must play some part.

How we feel about an issue, however, is a manifestation of our moral convictions that we cannot and should not ignore. To reach an ethical decision allowing reason to temper emotions and emotions to tutor reason would be ideal. Although nursing is a moral endeavor based on the idea of service, the nurse must be allowed to practice in a manner that maintains the practitioner's sense of self-respect while also maintaining the dignity of the patient.

Nursing practice takes place within a team of health care professionals reflecting a multiplicity of values, often in conflict. Differing personal, professional, and institutional values compound moral conflict—all must be considered. In the end, these competing values must be weighed and assigned priority in light of the ethical norms that guide us.

The Tools of Ethics

To one involved in moral conflict, resolution may seem impossible. Systematically applying the tools of ethics, basic moral principles, and nursing's professional guide-lines, however, helps us identify our ethical obligations and decide which "right" actions can help us meet them. A systematic decision-making process is another tool that can help us identify and meet ethical obligations.

Ethical decision-making does not promise absolute answers, however. Ethical dilemmas are dilemmas because compelling reasons exist for taking each of two or more opposing actions. Decisions about which action to take should be analyzed and eventually justified on the grounds of the basic moral principles discussed below.

Systems of Ethical Thought

Within normative ethics, there are two major ethical systems by which we determine what is right or wrong. The first category includes theories that determine an action to be right or wrong on the basis of its consequences. These theories are termed *consequentialistic* theories. Utilitarianism is, today, chief among the consequentialistic theories. The second category includes theories that judge an action right or wrong on the basis of features other than consequences, usually on the basis of the conformity of the action to a moral rule. These theories are called *deontological* or *nonconsequentialistic* theories. Both utilitarian and deontological theories use principles and rules, although for different reasons.

As we apply the basic moral principles to specific situations, we are sometimes unaware of our own professional values and obligations that color our ethical reasoning. Awareness of differences in professional and personal obligations can provide insight into the sources of interprofessional or interpersonal ethical conflict.

Ethical Principles

The principles most pertinent to analyzing the moral conflicts faced by practicing nurses are *beneficence* ("doing good"), *nonmaleficence* ("not inflicting harm"), *autonomy* ("respecting self-determination"), and *fidelity* ("faithfulness in relationships"). These principles help us determine what our duties are, that is, what is right or wrong for us to do.

These principles are found in the *Code for Nurses*. The *Code* lists them in its Preamble and applies them throughout the Interpretive Statements.

Nonmaleficence and Beneficence

The principle of nonmaleficence says that we have an ethical duty not to inflict harm or evil. It is a duty foundational to our society. In fact, the duty not to harm others bears more weight than the duty to benefit others. Citing statements from the Hippocratic oath and the words of Nightingale, Jameton argues that "it is more important to avoid doing harm than it is to do good."[1]

DISPLAY BOX 8–1
Ethical Principles

These are the principles most pertinent to analyzing the moral conflicts faced by the critical care nurse.

BENEFICENCE	Doing good
NONMALEFICENCE	Not inflicting harm
AUTONOMY	Respecting self-determination
FIDELITY	Faithfulness in relationships

Beneficence involves taking deliberate steps to benefit another person. Beauchamp and Childress state that this duty compels us to provide benefits by preventing and removing harm and to balance benefits and harms by performing a risk–benefit analysis, such as weighing the side effects of a drug against its therapeutic actions.[2]

Beneficence and nonmaleficence, like all moral norms, specify what are called prima facie obligations. A prima facie obligation is binding on all occasions unless it is in conflict with another prima facie obligation of equal or stronger claim. Often beneficence and nonmaleficence conflict; the noninfliction of harm usually is given the greater weight. The following case study illustrates a type of conflict that can occur involving these two ethical principles.

CASE STUDY

George Edwards, a 59-year-old male, came into the emergency room complaining of dizziness and chest pain for the past week. A cardiac monitor showed ventricular tachycardia, and he was successfully cardioverted and placed on Tridil. After admittance to the coronary care unit, Mr. Edwards required multiple cardioversions for recurrent ventricular tachycardia. At one point he required cardiopulmonary resuscitation (CPR) for sustained symptomatic ventricular tachycardia. Lab work indicated a massive myocardial infarction, and an echocardiogram showed an ejection fraction of 25 percent. Mr. Edwards' cardiologist planned electrophysiology studies with a possible implantable defibrillator when the patient became stable.

On Day 14 of his hospital stay, Mr. Edwards went into congestive heart failure and sustained ventricular tachycardia, requiring CPR and multiple defibrillations. The cardiologist continued to show optimism that the electrophysiology studies and the automatic implantable cardiac defibrillator (AICD) would provide good results. Mr. Edwards was tired, confused at times, and began to seek frequent reassurance from the nurses that he would live long enough for the AICD insertion. He expressed fear about the frequent cardioversions and the discomfort they caused him. The nurses began to question what kind of long-term benefit such treatment would offer this severely compromised patient.

This case shows the dilemma of providing treatment that can give the benefit of defibrillation for recurrent ventricular tachycardia to a patient already suffering severe cardiac damage. Without this therapy, the patient will die, but do the benefits of avoiding sudden cardiac death outweigh the risks of the physical and emotional harm caused by repeated defibrillations and cardioversions while the patient awaits an AICD?

The desire to prevent harm by postponing death is one shaped by nonmaleficence. Perhaps a greater harm than death, however, is the frequent physical and psychological discomfort caused by aggressive treatment. The desire to act beneficently by providing comfort and less aggressive treatment may have a greater weight in the above case.

Respect for Autonomy and the Rule of Informed Consent

To respect autonomy is to treat another with respect and to respect the plan of action that the other person chooses. The principle of autonomy gives rise to the rule or doctrine of informed consent. The nurse's duty with regard to this principle is to see that the patient or patient surrogate is truly autonomous before a health care decision is made. A surrogate is someone who is able to make a "substituted judgment" for the patient; it is usually a spouse or adult child, because such a person is usually in the best position to express the patient's feelings and desires about treatment. For the patient or surrogate to be autonomous requires that he or she be fully informed and freely consenting.

To be fully informed, the patient or surrogate needs all the information a "reasonable person" would need to make a particular decision. If, because of who he or she is as a person (ie, because of age, physical condition, educational level, sex, position, etc.), the patient or surrogate needs any additional process to understand the information, that must also be supplied. The patient may give free consent with a waiver of informedness if he or she does not want the information.

Free consent refers to "voluntariness." The patient is not to be subject to coercion, fraud, or deceit. A fully informed, freely consenting patient has a right to make an autonomous decision, whether or not it corresponds with what others think he or she should do, with the exception that the decision may not harm others.

In most cases in which health care professionals and hospitals have wished to override patient or surrogate autonomy, the issue has involved forcing the patient to receive or to continue to receive medical care deemed necessary by the health care professionals or hospitals. In such cases, the patient's or surrogate's decision has been supported, both in the view of ethics and in the law. A recent case presented a reversal of the situation. The patient's surrogate wished continued treatment that physicians and the hospital went to court to have withdrawn.

Since a respiratory arrest in May 1990, 87-year-old Helga Wanglie had been in a persistent vegetative state in a hospital in Minneapolis. Her physicians believed that continuing to maintain her on a ventilator was futile treatment because she was severely brain damaged and had no hope of recovery. Her husband was emphatic, nevertheless, that his wife would want her life maintained at all costs and that nobody knew better than he what her wishes would be. The case was the first time that a hospital had gone to court to withdraw treatment against a family's wishes. In her ruling, the judge supported the husband's power to make medical decisions for his wife, saying that he was in the best position to know his wife's religious and moral beliefs.[3] Again, the finding was in support of patient autonomy.

The Wanglie case stimulated a great deal of discussion among ethicists, health care professionals, and patients' rights groups. Some believe that patients' wishes should be kept in the center of medical decisions; others believe that patients should not be allowed to ask for options that are not seen as viable. The Wanglie case is a current example of how the courts view the importance of patient autonomy even in light of physician opposition to continued treatment that is considered medically futile.

Fidelity

When a person becomes a nurse, he or she assumes the "promises" and obligations of the nursing profession. Making promises involves the principle of fidelity. Fidelity and faithfulness to patients are fundamental to the nurse–patient relationship. Ramsey calls fidelity the single, foundational moral principle, a moral covenant between people.[4]

When a person makes a promise, whether implicitly or explicitly, the party to whom the promise is made expects it to be fulfilled. The person who made the promise now has an obligation to fulfill it. In promising, there is an invitation to trust. Emphasizing a spirit of trust, the principle of fidelity obliges health care professionals to act in patients' best interests and to fulfill promises made to patients.

CASE STUDY

Jack Crawford was a 44-year-old male with protracted pain from metastatic cancer. After a slowly deteriorating stay in a university intensive care unit, Mr. Crawford, thin, jaundiced, and in respiratory distress, confided to his primary nurse, Mrs. B, that he was ready to die and did not want life-sustaining treatments of any kind. Mrs. B knew that Mr. Crawford's wife had not come to terms with her husband's prognosis and was ready to try any treatment to extend his life. Mrs. B dreaded the impending conflict between the unit's aggressive oncologist, the patient with no hope of life without pain, and the wife not ready to let her husband die.

As the primary nurse, Mrs. B had worked to develop a trusting relationship with Mr. Crawford and his wife and felt keenly her responsibility to act as her patient's advocate. She realized that the desires confided to her carried implicit expectations to relay his wishes to the physician. She thought that Mr. Crawford might even expect her to ensure that these wishes be carried out.

To avoid conflict if life-sustaining became necessary, Mrs. B decided to contact the physician and set up a family conference to discuss the plan of care with the Crawfords, the physician, and the nursing staff. Hopefully, the health care team and the Crawfords could discuss Mr. Crawford's grave prognosis and come to an agreement on what types of treatment would be of benefit.

A fiduciary relationship between the nurse and the patient is one of trust, expectation, and action. Such a relationship is exemplified in the above case study. Although it does not guarantee that expectations will be fulfilled, it does guarantee they they will be represented.

Ethical Decision Making Within a Nursing Process Model

The interests of the patient, professional and personal values of the health care professionals, institutional values, personal feelings, moral principles, and legal issues are all important aspects of a moral conflict. At first glance, it might seem impossible to integrate them into anything other than an incoherent mass of conflicting possible actions.

Ethical decision making models provide us with a process for systematically and thoughtfully examining a conflict, ensuring that participants consider all important aspects of a situation before taking action. The steps of ethical analysis and evaluation are much like the steps of the nursing process. Both ethical analysis and the nursing process provide an orderly approach to resolving dilemmas.

DISPLAY BOX 8–2
Ethical Decision Making

Examining an ethical problem in the clinical setting usually involves five steps:

- Identify the ethical problem.
- Gather the morally relevant facts.
- Analyze the situation using ethical principles and rules.
- Analyze action alternatives in the light of those principles or rules and act.
- Evaluate and reflect.

Identify the Problem

The first step is to clearly identify the problem. Is this truly a problem involving conflicting ethical principles or values, or is it primarily a legal issue or communication problem? Communication problems and legal restrictions are often a *part of* an ethical problem; some clinical problems, however, can be resolved solely through better communication or legal counsel, without ethical analysis.

Gather the Ethically Relevant Facts

The next step is to identify the information needed to fully understand the situation. Who are the principal agents involved? Are the values and goals for treatment of the patient clear? How do the values of the others involved affect the problem? Are cultural, religious, or other aspects relevant to the situation?

It is also important to understand the various contexts of the dilemma, including its physiological dimensions and its legal dimensions. What are the medical diagnoses, possible treatment modalities, and prognosis? Are there legal ramifications, institutional protocols, or economic factors to consider?

Analyze the Situation Using Ethical Principles and Rules

It is at this step that the person who is to make the final decision must be identified. Is the patient competent, fully informed, and free to choose (ie, the principle of respect for autonomy applies)? Is there a family member who is able to speak forthrightly for the comatose patient (principle of beneficence applies) or a durable power of attorney for health care designating a surrogate decision maker (principle of respect for autonomy applies)? Are there vested interests (principles of justice and nonmaleficence apply)?

Consider the ethical principles. Which are most applicable to the case? There can be several competing claims, all of which are reasonable and justifiable. Does honoring one of the principles lead to conflict with legal or institutional requirements?

Analyze Alternatives and Act

Identify all the possible and reasonable intervention options; then, evaluate those options on the basis of their conformity to ethical principles and rules:

1. Will the action respect patient autonomy?
2. Is the patient fully informed and freely consenting?
3. Is the family informed and consenting?
4. Will the action and its probable outcome harm or benefit any or all of those involved?
5. Will this action strengthen patient–professional bonds and reaffirm society's expectations of nurses?

In considering the alternatives, one must also determine which actions are realistically open to the nurse. What variables can the nurse influence or control? There are ethical problems about which the nurse can do very little, but usually there are variables on which the nurse can act readily, such as facilitating communication, pointing out pertinent facts to the participants, or ensuring that the participants are aware of all reasonable options. After careful reasoning, the nurse must choose and then act on the option that is consistent with sound ethical analysis and personal moral convictions.

Evaluate and Reflect

After the action has been taken, it is important to further analyze the ethical problem and its final outcome. Compare the outcome with what was hoped for or intended; how can a similar situation be handled with greater sensitivity or wisdom in the future? Evaluation is especially helpful if it is undertaken in a quiet, nonthreatening atmosphere conducive to reflection.

Ethical reasoning in the decision-making process can enable the nurse to move beyond initial feelings of helplessness. It points to areas that nurses must address to reach decisions and actions based on principled reasoning. Although the process directs us to a *range* of right actions, and sometimes indicates specific actions that would be wrong, it does not necessarily specify a single cut-and-dried answer, because applications of the principles must always be sensitive to the unique moral features of specific clinical situations.

Applied Ethics

Patients being cared for in the critical care unit today are older and more acutely ill than in years past. The technologies available to the physician to extend life are awesome, but their application is often the cause of ethical conflict. Does the 96-year-old woman with severe upper gastrointestinal bleeding truly want to be intubated after aspirating bloody vomitus? Should we resuscitate—without question—the 30-year-old, multiple trauma patient with adult respiratory distress syndrome (ARDS) who has remained unresponsive since a motor vehicle accident two weeks ago? The questions go on and on.

The major concern of the public in such matters has emerged as a fear of being forced to endure an existence supported by machines without hope of a meaningful life and without the ability to have a say in the decision making surrounding the care or treatment given. It is such concern that spurred development of legislation resulting in the Patient Self-Determination Act (PSDA) of 1990.

The PSDA, effective December 1, 1991, requires that all health care facilities receiving Medicare or Medicaid provide to all adults admitted written information about their rights under state law to make decisions about medical care, including the right to accept or to refuse such care. It also requires that information be given about their rights to formulate advance directives such as living wills or durable powers of attorney for health care. There is the assumption that such involvement by patients in decision making about their medical care will result in care more responsive to their values and needs.[5]

Most states have now enacted health care legislation regarding living wills and durable powers of attorney. The living will allows a person to specify in advance his or her wishes about health care should he or she lose the capacity to decide. The durable power of attorney for health care provides a procedure by which a person can designate a surrogate and indicate preferences for general levels of medical treatment in specific circumstances.

This legislation has come about as a result of the public's fears of losing control over personal medical care decisions and of being subjected to the physical and emotional indignity and suffering that can occur with inappropriate use of today's technology. The publicity surrounding the Nancy Cruzan case made the public even more aware of the advisability of an advance directive.

Cruzan v. Cruzan

Nancy Cruzan was a young woman rendered in a persistent vegetative state since being in an automobile accident in 1983. Her parents had petitioned the Missouri Supreme Court to have her gastrostomy feeding tube removed, contending that she would not have wanted to be maintained in such a manner if there were no hope for her recovery. The Missouri Court denied the request, based on the fact that there was no clear and convincing evidence that Miss Cruzan had ever stated her feelings with regard to artificial feeding. The case went to the United States Supreme Court, the first case to come before it regarding termination of medical care. On June 25, 1990, the Supreme Court upheld the Missouri decision, finding that it did not violate federal constitutional rights, but it did acknowledge that competent persons enjoy a constitutional right to refuse medical treatment. In the other 49 states, where the laws in this regard are more liberal and do not require specific expression of patient wishes with regard to types of treatment, the judgment reaffirmed the right of competent patients to request that medical treatment be withheld or withdrawn.[6]

The discussion here focuses on the withholding or withdrawing of life-sustaining treatment. Such treatment can include CPR, emergency medications, mechanical ventilation, intravenous fluids, artificial nutrition and hydration, antibiotics, and dialysis.

Withholding and Withdrawing Treatment

What does nursing ethics say about withholding or withdrawing treatment? The first provision of the *Code for Nurses* states that "clients have the moral right to determine what will be done with their own person . . . [and] to accept, refuse, or terminate treatment without coercion." The *Code* goes on to say that nurses "must protect and preserve human life when there is hope of recovery or reasonable hope of benefit from life-prolonging treatment."[7]

What is meant by the terms "withholding" and "withdrawing"? Withholding refers to never initiating a treatment, whereas withdrawing refers to actually stopping a treatment once started. Health care professionals often find it emotionally more difficult to withdraw a treatment than to withhold it in the first place. The difference between not starting a treatment and stopping it, however, is not one of moral or legal importance. Ending treatment for sound moral reasons does not violate professional obligations. A presidential commission has acknowledged that "the distinction between failing to initiate and stopping therapy is not itself of moral significance."[8] Because it is not a routine medical order, the presence of both the physician and the nurse at the bedside is encouraged when treatment is to be ended. This offers the opportunity for mutual support to all involved during a time that is often emotionally charged.[9]

The Hastings Center's *Guidelines on the Termination of Life-Sustaining Treatment and Care of the Dying* states that "there is strong reason to prefer stopping treatment over not starting it in some cases. . . . There is often uncertainty about the efficacy of a proposed treatment, or the burdens and benefits it will impose on the patient. It is better to start the treatment and later stop if it is ineffective than not to start treatment for fear that stopping will be impossible."[10]

When the patient or surrogate decides that a proposed treatment will impose undue burdens and refuses such treatment, it is morally correct for the health care professional to respect that decision. If the patient or surrogate decides that a treatment in progress and the life it provides have become too burdensome for the patient, then the treatment may permissibly be stopped. Imposing harmful or futile treatment against the patient's wishes violates the autonomous patient's right to self-determination and, where patient wishes cannot be known, it violates the nonautonomous patient's best interests. Stopping treatment acknowledges that a patient has a right to refuse treatment and to determine what constitutes "benefit" for him or her. It also acknowledges the principle of nonmaleficence, or not harming the patient's dignity and quality of life by forcing unwanted, painful, or futile treatment on the patient. The Nancy

Cruzan case involved a request for withdrawal of medical treatment.

An example of withholding of a treatment is a "do not resuscitate" (DNR) order, an order not to do CPR. The original intent of CPR was to resuscitate or revive patients suffering specific types of sudden cardiac or pulmonary arrest: victims of drowning, electric shock, untoward effects of drugs, anesthetic accidents, heart block, and acute myocardial infarction. In time, CPR became a routine medical intervention extended to almost all patients suffering cardiac or pulmonary arrest, no matter what the underlying disease process. Although CPR has proven dramatically effective for the patients mentioned above, it is of little, if any, benefit to many others.

The immediate, reflexive intervention to preserve life without the express consent of the patient is been supported by the principle of beneficence. Health care personnel assume that a "reasonable person" would wish to be resuscitated. We act on the assumption that death is undesirable to the patient. Yet, some patients can express or have expressed their wishes not to be resuscitated. In such cases, to presume to understand the needs of a patient and to act against the patient's expressed wishes (or to avoid ascertaining what those wishes might be) is paternalistic. Paternalism is the act of overriding another's actions or requests to bring about what is believed to be the most good for that person. From the medical perspective, which is protective, paternalistic interventions tend to be viewed as morally acceptable.

The perspective of nursing, however, as stated in the Preamble of the *Code for Nurses*, acknowledges respect for persons as the most fundamental principle in professional practice.[11] Respect for self-determination is essential to respect for persons and is undermined whenever intervention takes place without informed consent (if the patient can participate in decision making) or against the patient's wishes. Paternalistic interventions are usually contrary to the spirit and obligations of nursing ethics.

To ensure patient self-determination and the opportunity to refuse treatment, discussion must occur when the patient is alert and possessed of a reasonably clear sensorium. Before making a voluntary and informed decision to accept or to refuse CPR, the patient or surrogate must understand what CPR is and how it will most likely affect the disease process and future quality of life. This process applies to any life-sustaining treatment. Hence, the need for advance directives.

Decisions should be made jointly by the health care professional and the patient (or patient surrogate). The physician must supply the necessary information about realistic outcomes and possible interventions. The nurse must ensure that the patient or surrogate understands that information by clarifying technical terms and helping the patient to weigh treatment options. By providing the patient an opportunity to discuss personal choices about end-of-life care, the nurse assists the patient. It is the patient who then must consider his or her own values and wishes in the context of prognoses and realistic options. The final decision should reflect the patient's wishes.

It is morally permissible for a nurse to refuse to participate in withholding or withdrawing treatment on the grounds of personal moral conviction, or if he or she believes it is against the patient's best interests. In the former case, the nurse can remove himself or herself from the situation as long as there is another nurse available to care for the patient. In the latter case, under the principle of fidelity, the nurse must make his or her patient-based objections known and request reassignment, if necessary.

Summary

The courts have held nurses increasingly accountable for protecting the patients' well-being through the exercise of their professional judgment. Sound professional judgment requires both clinical excellence and a determined belief that one of nursing's primary responsibilities is to

---

Clinical Research

Tittle MB, Moody L, Becker MP: Nursing Care Requirements of Patients With DNR Orders in Intensive Care Units. Heart Lung 21(3):235–242.

Many family members and physicians worry that a "do not resuscitate" (DNR) order ultimately means that the patient will not receive the same attention and care that a non-DNR patient receives. But a recent study of hospital ICUs confirmed that patients with DNR orders actually receive more nursing care. Sixty-two patients with DNR orders were compared to 62 patients without such orders. Characteristics such as length of ICU stay and nursing care requirements, which were rated on an acuity scale, were examined. In the middle range of acuity, DNR patients received *more* nursing care than patients without DNRs who were equally ill.

This study confirmed what many critical care nurses have intuited all along, although the study did not investigate why these patients receive more care. The researchers speculated, "The nursing staff may have felt the needs of the family could be met by knowing that the patient continued to receive maximal nursing care."

ensure the patient's right to self-determination, or to assure that the patient's best interests are served if self-determination is not possible.

Knowledge of basic ethical principles and the ability to apply them systematically is essential to professional nursing practice. However, our responsibility does not end with knowledge and ability but lies in actively trying to understand our patients' values and beliefs. To fulfill such a responsibility we must become familiar with the ethical principles and rules that nursing espouses and incorporate them into professional practice as habits of thought. To maintain one's professional ethical integrity requires habitual, systematic examination of the autonomous patient's course of treatment and action to ensure that the patient receives the information and counseling necessary to make informed decisions without duress.

The role of the critical care nurse is to foster an environment in which informed decision making about treatment preferences is valued and considered an essential element of care.[12] We must help develop compassionate and ethically correct institutional and public policies, policies that create an ethical environment supportive of patient autonomy and that protect the free exercise of moral agency by nurses.

REFERENCES

1. Jameton A: Nursing Practice: The Ethical Issues, p 93. Englewood Cliffs, NJ, Prentice-Hall, 1984
2. Beauchamp T, Childress J: Principles of Biomedical Ethics, 2nd ed. New York, Oxford University Press, 1983
3. McCormick B: Can families require doctors to continue futile treatment? Amer Med News 34:1,32, 1991
4. Ramsey P: The Patient as a Person. New Haven, Yale University Press, 1970
5. Rouse F: Patients, providers, and the PSDA. Hastings Cent Rep 21:S2–S3, 1991
6. Wolf S: Honoring Broader Directives. Hast Cent Rep 21:S8–S9, 1991
7. American Nurses' Association: Code for Nurses With Interpretive Statements. Kansas City, MO, American Nurses' Association, 1985
8. President's Commission for the Study of Ethical Problems in Medicine and Biomedical and Behavioral Research: Deciding to Forego Life-Sustaining Treatment, p 61. Washington, DC, Government Printing Office, 1983
9. The Hastings Center: Guidelines on the Termination of Life-Sustaining Treatment and Care of the Dying. Briarcliff Manor, NY, The Hastings Center, 1987
10. The Hastings Center: Guidelines on the Termination of Life-Sustaining Treatment and Care of the Dying. Briarcliff Manor, NY, The Hastings Center, 1987
11. American Nurses' Association: Code for Nurses With Interpretive Statements. Kansas City, MO, American Nurses' Association, 1985
12. Reigle J: Preserving patient self-determination through advance directives. Heart Lung 21:196–198, 1992

BIBLIOGRAPHY

Bedell S, Pelle D, Maher P, Cleary P: Do-not-resuscitate orders for critically ill patients in the hospital: How are they used and what is their impact? JAMA 256:233–237, 1986
Callahan S: The role of emotion in ethical decision-making. Hastings Cent Rep, 18:9–14, 1988
Capron A: The burden of decision. Hastings Cent Rep 20:36, 1990
Fowler M, Levine-Ariff J: Ethics at the Bedside. Philadelphia, JB Lippincott, 1987
McCann J: Ethics in critical care nursing. Crit Care Nurs Clin North Am 2:1, 1990
Mitchell PH, Armstrong S, Simpson TF: American Association of Critical Care Nurses Demonstration Project: Profile of excellence in critical care nursing. Heart Lung 18:219, 1989
Shannon SE: Living your ethics: Strategies of experienced nurses. Paper presented at American Association of Critical Care Nurses National Teaching Institute, San Francisco, May 1990
Wlody G: Ethical issues in critical care: A nursing model. Dimens Crit Care 9:224, 1990

STUDY QUESTIONS

1. Choose the most correct answer to describe the primary purpose of the Patient Self-Determination Act:

   a. requires patients to complete an advance directive
   b. assures treatment preferences for the terminally ill patient
   c. gives the patient surrogate the power to make decisions for the patient
   d. makes patients aware of their rights to accept or to refuse medical treatments so that they can make choices while they are still capable

2. Ethics helps people reach answers to moral dilemmas by

   a. clarifying the moral issues and principles involved in a situation
   b. helping the person to examine his or her responsibilities and obligations
   c. providing an ethically adequate rationale for a decision
   d. all of the above

3. A nurse believes medical treatment being given her patient is ethically inappropriate and refuses to give the patient care, leaving the workplace that day in order to not be a part of the situation. This is an example of

   a. a nurse standing up for his or her right not to participate in morally objectionable care
   b. violation of the principle of fidelity through patient abandonment
   c. a nurse's support for the principle of nonmaleficence, noninfliction of harm
   d. the exercise of professional nurse judgment

4. All of the following are true except

   a. withholding life-sustaining treatment is ethically acceptable, but withdrawing such treatment is not
   b. to be truly autonomous, a patient must be fully informed and freely consenting
   c. DNR is a medical order to withhold CPR
   d. a nurse's duty always to act in the best interests of his or her patient is based on the principle of fidelity

5. Which of the following set of guidelines is most important in providing the nurse with basic directions needed to address ethical issues

   a. hospital policies
   b. ANA Social Policy Statement and the Code for Nurses With Interpretive Statements
   c. the Code for Nurses With Interpretive Statements and the state boards for registered nursing
   d. position statements of various nursing specialty organizations

CHAPTER 9

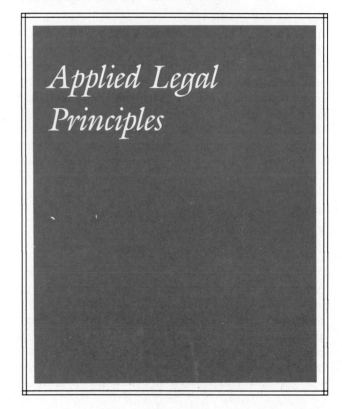

Applied Legal Principles

BEHAVIORAL OBJECTIVES

Based on the content in this chapter, the reader should be able to:

1. Define the four elements of a malpractice suit.
2. Describe the concept of negligence.
3. List three allegations commonly made against nurses.
4. Explain the concept *respondeat superior*.
5. List three possible actions to be taken if there is an unclear medical order, inadequate staffing, or defective equipment.
6. Identify the nurse's responsibilities if there is a do not resuscitate (DNR) order.
7. Summarize five principles that can guide nursing practice.

Description

Legal issues involving critical care have been highly publicized and are of increasing concern to health care providers, hospitals, and the public. Our society seems to be more litigious than ever, and the number of malpractice suits that name or involve nurses is increasing. Issues such as refusal and termination of treatment have been widely discussed and written about; even legislatures have acted—so-called living will statutes have been enacted in many jurisdictions.

This chapter begins with a discussion of principles of negligence as they apply to the critical care nurse (CCN). It then proceeds to identify and address certain current legal issues most applicable to the CCN.

Nursing Negligence in Critical Care

There are few reported cases of negligence by nurses in a critical care area. This does not mean that cases necessarily are rare; instead, the hospital may be the only named defendant (as the employer of the nurse), the case may be settled in advance of trial, or a judgment simply may not be appealed. The incidents in many reported nurse malpractice cases, however, could have taken place in a critical care area and can serve as examples of potential CCN negligence.

If a malpractice case is presented, the legal principles are the same as those applicable to non-critical care nurses. They are not difficult to understand, and an awareness of them can reinforce some of the fundamental requirements of competent nursing practice.

Duty and Dereliction of Duty

A nurse who cares for a patient has a duty to that patient to use reasonable care. Failure to do so is negligence, for which the patient may recover monetary damages. Generally, the law does not require a CCN or any other health care professional to have been perfect or always to have made the correct decision. Instead, the standard is what

a reasonably prudent CCN would have done under the same or similar circumstances. If a reasonable, prudent CCN would have avoided the problem, the defendant nurse will be held to be negligent. However, if the reasonable CCN would have acted as the defendant did, no negligence exists, and there will be no recovery of damages despite the plaintiff's very real and substantial injuries.[1] This standard permits variation among cases regarding the education and experience of the nurse and the equipment and personnel available at the time of the incident.

The plaintiff must prove the standard of care as it existed at the time of the incident, and this proof is often one of the most difficult parts of the case. The standard must be established by an expert witness. For example, the generalist nurse would be competent to explain injection technique and sites; however, if the case involves the reading of an electrocardiogram (ECG), the expert must be a nurse who is competent in that clinical area. Testimony is based on such items as written standards or position statements from relevant professional organizations, the current literature, job descriptions, and hospital policies and procedures. The defendant nurse can also use experts in an effort to show that the standard of care is different from the one that the plaintiff has demonstrated.

Once the duty is established, a breach of that duty is required—that is, the nurse must have been negligent. Negligence is found or refuted by a comparison of the nurse's conduct with the standard of care. Generally, negligence is either ordinary or gross. Ordinary negligence implies professional carelessness, whereas gross negligence suggests that the nurse willfully and consciously ignored a known risk of harm to the patient. Most cases involve ordinary negligence, but gross negligence can be present if a nurse harmed a patient while under the influence of drugs or alcohol.

Causation and Damage

There must be a causal relation between what the CCN did or failed to do and the damages suffered by the patient. A negligent medication error that occurred near the time of the patient's death could have had nothing to do with the death or could have caused it; expert testimony on the cause of death is critical in this case because the nurse, even if negligent, is not liable if his or her actions did not contribute to the patient's suffering or death. Generally, however, the law interprets damages broadly. Any physical injury is sufficient to award monetary damages. Small injuries merit small compensation, whereas larger injuries merit larger amounts. If there were physical injuries, compensation for emotional distress may also be required; in a few states, under some circumstances, compensation for emotional anguish may be awarded even in the absence of physical injury.

A merely undesirable event or outcome does not con-

DISPLAY BOX 9-1
Elements of a Malpractice Suit: The 4 Ds

Duty
Dereliction of duty
Direct causation
Damages

stitute negligence. Not every fall from a hospital bed is a result of some negligent act on the part of a health care provider. The facts surrounding the event must be examined in light of the applicable standard of care. Further, the plaintiff must prove all four elements of the action to the jury. In summary, the plaintiff (the patient) must prove "upon a preponderance of the evidence" that the nurse breached a duty and caused harm.

CCN Negligence and Case Law

The following cases illustrate the legal and professional principles that apply in malpractice cases. There are numerous allegations that are commonly made against members of the nursing staff. One is failure to *monitor the patient's condition* properly, as illustrated in the first case.

CASE 1

A 4-month-old boy was admitted for correction of a congenital trachea condition and underwent a tracheotomy. The surgery was uneventful, and he was last examined by the surgeon in the critical care unit (CCU) at 11:00 PM. The physician left orders and went home. At that time, the infant's condition was satisfactory, and he had no manifestations of postoperative complications. At 3:55 AM, he stopped breathing and suffered devastating and irreversible brain damage when the resuscitation team was unable quickly to restore respirations or a heartbeat. The cause of the arrest was a massive pneumothorax from the gradual accumulation of trapped air beneath the skin (subcutaneous emphysema), which had entered the body at the site of tracheotomy and had subsequently worked down until it broke through the surface of the lung. Expert testimony determined that the infant had exhibited signs and symptoms of the complication for almost 2 hours before the arrest occurred. The jury found the hospital liable for the negligence of the nurses and the resident.[2]

The infant in this case was a fresh postoperative patient, and the standard of care required diligence in observing his condition. This included the prompt recognition and treatment of complications. In essence, the court held that even though the complication itself might have been unavoidable, the failure to recognize it and treat it constituted negligence.

This principle also applies in other circumstances. A patient had surgery for acute gallbladder disease. He fell from his bed during his first postoperative night. Twenty-four hours after the fall, he went into shock, and the drug Levophed was ordered. He had infusions running into both arms, but they were discontinued when they infiltrated. An intravenous infusion was begun in the patient's leg, infiltrated, and caused a permanent partial disability. Evidence at the trial determined that the infusion containing the Levophed had been infusing into the tissues for 2 hours. The court found the evidence sufficient to warrant a finding of negligence for failing to detect the situation within a reasonable time.[3] Infiltration of intravenous fluids is fairly common, and tissue necrosis is an acknowledged and not unusual complication with the administration of Levophed. Generally, the courts have held that as long as the drug is indicated by the patient's condition and the patient has constant attention during the infusion, the occurrence of tissue necrosis is an unavoidable side effect, and damages will not be awarded.[4]

Failure to record observations can lead to the conclusion that the patient was improperly monitored, as illustrated in the following case.

CASE 2

A 6-year-old boy was admitted after he was struck by an automobile while riding his bicycle. In addition to sustaining several other injuries, the boy had a fractured left leg, which was placed in traction on the day of admission (May 7). That night, the nurse who was observing the patient wrote several entries in the nurse's notes suggesting that the circulation in the affected leg was good. The next day, the left leg circulation remained adequate at least until 11:00 PM, when the patient was last examined by a physician. By 6:00 AM, the circulation was seriously compromised. Nurse's notes for that night contained no information about circulation in the leg, although the nurse wrote that the boy was medicated for pain and that he was unable to sleep. Ultimately, it was necessary to amputate the patient's left leg. The court held that the failure by the nurse "who was on duty during the crucial period to make any entry of observations that she made concerning the circulation in [the patient's] foot . . . could very well have led the jury to infer than no such observations were made between 11:00 PM and 6:00 AM, when the nurse wrote that the left foot was cold, had no feeling, and was dusky." The case was remanded for trial on the hospital's liability (as the nurse's employer) in this case.[5]

Another common malpractice allegation is that the *nurse failed to notify the physician* of abnormalities in the patient's condition or history. This is illustrated in the next case.

CASE 3

The Ramsey family lived in a rural county in Maryland. In May 1974, the parents brought their infant sons (aged 1 and 2 years) to the emergency room of a hospital when each developed a rash and a high fever. While there, Mrs. Ramsey told the nurse on duty that she had removed two ticks from one of the boys; the nurse did not tell the examining physician of that history. The physician testified that he asked the parents about exposure to ticks and was told nothing. The children were treated as if they had measles for several days, and one boy died. The second boy was subsequently treated for, and recovered from, Rocky Mountain spotted fever; an autopsy on the younger child revealed that he had died of the same disease. Because of the rarity of the disease in Maryland and the atypical nature of the children's symptoms, the physicians involved were held not liable. However, the emergency room nurse was found negligent because she had not recorded or communicated significant medical data and because expert testimony indicated that this failure was a contributing cause of the death of one child and of serious illness in the other.[6]

Finally, *medication and transfusion errors* have frequently been the subject of malpractice actions. The next case is an example.

CASE 4

A 3-month-old infant had congenital heart disease and was admitted to the hospital. The physician ordered "elixir pediatric digoxin (Lanoxin) 2.5 ml (0.125 mg) q6h × 3 then once daily." In a later hospitalization, an order stated, "Give 3.0 ml Lanoxin today for 1 dose only." The route of administration was not indicated on either order. A nursing supervisor assisting on the unit that day administered 3 ml of Lanoxin in its injectable form, a lethal overdose. Medical testimony revealed that 3 ml of Lanoxin in its elixir form and administered orally would not have harmed the child. The infant died 75 minutes after receiving the intramuscular injection. The physician was found negligent in failing to specify the intended route of administration when the same dose would be fatal by one route and therapeutic by another. The nurse was also negligent because she was in doubt about the medication order and did not call the prescribing physician. Furthermore, the nurse was unfamiliar with the drug and did not know that it was available for administration in an oral form and an injectable form.[7]

Vicarious Liability

Potential liability exists for both the hospital and the health care provider. The hospital, as a corporation, can be liable for an equipment failure or for failure to provide a competent medical and nursing staff in a critical care unit (CCU). It is also liable as an employer for the negligence of its physician and nursing employees. These staff members are also independently liable for injuries that were directly and proximately caused by poor decision-making skills or for theory and skill incompetency.

The doctrine of *respondeat superior* ("let the master answer") is the major legal theory under which hospitals are responsible for the negligence of their employees. As long as the nurse acts within the scope of employment, the hospital is be liable as well; it is not liable if the nurse acts outside the scope of employment.

Because the hospital is also liable, hospitals carry professional liability insurance for the activities of their employees. Generally, a hospital will defend a nurse named in a malpractice case. However, some CCNs choose to carry their own personal malpractice insurance. Personal insurance is important if the CCN feels, for example, that the hospital liability coverage is inadequate.

Protocols

If the CCN is required to perform medical acts and is not under the direct and immediate supervision of a delegating physician, the activities must be based on established protocols. These protocols should be created by the medical and nursing departments and should be reviewed for compliance with state nurse practice acts. They must be frequently reviewed so that health care professionals can determine whether they reflect current medical and nursing standards of care. In the event of a malpractice suit, the critical care protocols and procedures can be introduced as evidence to help establish the applicable standard of care. Although it is important that protocols provide direction, excessive detail restricts the flexibility that a CCN needs to select a proper course of action.

The Questionable Medical Order

In addition to protocols, a policy statement should exist (in procedures or by directive) that indicates the manner of resolving the issue of the "questionable" medical order. This is important for all medical orders, but particularly for those given for critically ill patients because of the unusual doses of medication that are frequently ordered. The nurse who questions a particular order should express her specific reasons for concern to the physician who wrote the order. This initial approach frequently results in an explanation of the order and a medical justification for the order in the patient's medical record. If this approach is unsuccessful, many hospitals require that the attending physician or the nursing supervisor be notified; others have a policy that the chief of service must be consulted about questionable orders. If these options are unavailable or are unsuccessful, a CCN or any other nurse can refuse to give a medication.

It is important for the CCN to realize that an order that is patently wrong can harm the patient if it is followed; a secondary consequence can be liability for both the physician and the nurse (and the hospital, her employer) if the patient suffers harm as a direct result of the order.

Inadequate Staffing

One of the most important factors that sets the CCN apart from a generalist medical and surgical nurse is the CCN's knowledge of scientific theories and nursing skills unique to a critical care setting and necessary to meet the needs of critically ill patients. The nurse functioning in a CCU, for example, must be competent to make immediate nursing judgments and to act on those decisions. A nurse who does not possess the theory and skills required of a CCN should not be rendering critical care. If a generalist nurse is floated to a CCU, she should inform her nursing supervisor that she lacks the necessary critical care skills. The nurse should make it clear that she can carry out only nursing care activities in which she is competent. The CCU staff should also know of the skills of the generalist nurse and should delegate only those activities in which the floated nurse is competent. It is reasonable to expect any hospital that has a CCU or an emergency room to take precautionary measures to assure that it is adequately staffed. Increasingly, nurses are regarding the adequacy of staff as a professional practice issue and are bringing this issue to the attention of hospital administrators.

Nevertheless, a nurse must still make priority decisions that consider the patient's situation and available staff. The following case illustrates this point.

CASE 5

Mr. Horton was admitted to a private room with a fever of unknown origin (later diagnosed as pneumonitis). He was also confused at times. The room had a window opening onto a small balcony which was encircled by a railing 2 to 3 feet high. At about 3:30 PM, Mr. Horton was observed standing on the balcony and calling to nearby construction workers for a ladder. The workers notified hospital personnel, who then returned the patient to his room and placed him in restraints. The charge nurse called the attending physician, who instructed the nurses to "keep an eye on the patient." The charge nurse then called the patient's wife at work and asked her to come in and sit with Mr. Horton because no hospital staff were free to do so. Mrs. Horton responded by saying that she would call her mother, who lived within a few minutes of the hospital. She asked that a staff member sit with Mr. Horton until her mother arrived. She was told that the staff could not "possibly do that." Mrs. Horton called her mother, who hurried to the hospital. She arrived in time to observe construction workers surrounding something on the ground. The object of their attention was Mr. Horton, who had fallen from the second floor balcony. Mr. Horton survived the fall. In the lawsuit which followed, the evidence showed that the patient unit was at capacity. There were no emergencies; all the staff were engaged in routine duties that could have been postponed. Further, an aide assigned to the unit was sent to supper at the time the charge nurse indicated that there was not enough staff to assign a member to stay with Mr. Horton for 15 minutes, until the family member arrived. The staff did not place Mr. Horton in additional restraints either, something they had the power to do without an order. The trial court found the defendants negligent and awarded damages to the family; an appeals court affirmed the lower court judgment.[8]

Medical Equipment

A medical device, defined as virtually anything used in patient care that is not a drug, includes more complicated pieces of equipment (eg, intraaortic balloon pumps, endotracheal tubes, pacemakers, defibrillators) along with less obvious ones such as bedpans, suture materials, patient restraints, and tampons. Before 1976, medical devices were unregulated; since 1976, medical devices have been regulated by the Food and Drug Administration (FDA). Before November 1991, hospitals, their employees and staffs were permitted but not required to report device malfunctions to the device manufacturer or to the FDA.

On November 28, 1991, the Safe Medical Devices Act of 1990 became effective (PL 101-629), just after proposed regulations (called the Tentative Final Rule) were published for comment.[9] This act requires user facilities (which include hospitals and ambulatory surgery facilities but not physician offices) to report to the manufacturer medical device malfunctions that result in serious illness or injury to a patient, and to report to the FDA those that result in a patient's death. A serious illness or injury includes not only a life threatening injury or illness but also an injury that requires "immediate medical or surgical intervention to preclude permanent impairment of a body function or permanent damage to a body structure." Thus, the rupture of an intraaortic balloon pump that requires that the balloon-dependent patient immediately be transported to the operating room for removal and replacement of the device is a reportable event.

Nursing and other staff now must participate in reporting device malfunctions, even those associated with user error, to a designated hospital department. Personnel in that area are generally responsible for determining which malfunctions engender an obligation to report and to whom.

More recently, the FDA has proposed a new tracking system in which hospitals must participate. As of March 1, 1993, facilities that implant certain devices (eg, pacemakers, heart valves, silicone breast implants) must notify the manufacturer when the devices are implanted and maintain files from which the hospital can determine the identities and certain other information about patients in whom the devices have been implanted.[10]

There is a duty not to use equipment that is patently defective. If the equipment suddenly ceases to do what it was intended to do, makes unusual noises, or has a history of malfunction and has not been repaired, the hospital could be liable for damage caused by it, and nurses also could be liable if they know or should know of these problems and use the equipment anyway. The following cases involved liability for defective equipment.

CASE 6

A woman who had a complex pancreatic condition was being transferred from one hospital room to another. The new room was a short distance from her old room, and during the transfer she experienced severe respiratory distress. It was known that she had previously experienced respiratory difficulty. When the nurses reached the new room and attempted to attach the oxygen supply to the wall outlets, they discovered that the oxygen plugs did not fit into the outlets. The patient expired before emergency oxygen could be obtained. The court held that death was attributable to the negligence of the hospital as a corporation for its failure to standardize the outlets and the oxygen plugs. There was no liability on the part of the nurses. If the woman had been experiencing respiratory problems before the transfer began or if the rooms had been separated by a great distance, there might have been a duty to have the woman transferred with portable oxygen or to delay the transfer until her status improved.[11]

CASE 7

An infant suffered a cardiac arrest during surgery and was treated postoperatively with a hypothermia machine. Although the nurse knew that the continuous readout thermometer often malfunctioned, she did not check it with a glass thermometer. After the infant's temperature did not decrease, the nurse did not use other methods to lower body temperature, nor did she call the physician. The infant had a seizure and required mechanical ventilation. The nurse noticed poor air exchange but did not correct a kink in the ventilator tubing. The infant suffered permanent neurologic damage. The court held that the injury was proximately caused by the negligence of the hospital's employees and by the defective equipment used in the intensive care unit.[12]

Consent

Frequently, surgical and medical procedures are required by patients who are being cared for in critical care settings. In some institutions, consent forms are used, whereas in others the patient's consent is documented in the medical record notes. In general, it is the responsibility of the physician to obtain consent for treatment from the patient or the family, but a CCN may be asked to sign a consent form as a witness. Unless there is a statute stating otherwise, a witness who signs the form is simply able to testify that the signature is not a forgery. The witness is not required to state that legal consent was obtained.[13]

Issues That Involve Life-Support Measures

There are several basic issues regarding refusal and termination of treatment that can involve the CCN. Do not resuscitate (DNR) orders, living wills, and withdrawal of life-support measures are only three. As the following discussions indicate, these are complex topics for which only an overview can be provided.

Do Not Resuscitate Orders

It has been reported that cardiopulmonary resuscitation (CPR) takes place in 30% of patients who die at a major Boston hospital.[14] However, CPR is not appropriate for all patients who experience a cardiac arrest because it is highly invasive and may constitute a "positive violation of an individual's right to die with dignity."[15] Furthermore, CPR may not be indicated in cases in which the illness is terminal and irreversible and in which the patient can gain no benefit.

Prestigious authorities (eg, the President's Commission for the Study of Ethical Problems in Medicine and Biomedical and Behavioral Research) have recommended that hospitals have an explicit policy on the practice of writing and implementing DNR orders.[16] Several hospitals[17] and medical societies[18] have published DNR policies.

Whether to resuscitate any particular patient is a decision that is made by the attending physician, the patient, and the family, although CCNs and other nurses often have substantial input into the decision. Generally, however, the consent of a competent patient should be required when a DNR order is written. If the patient is incompetent, the physician and family members make the decision. Of course, the situation can be more complex, and the physician and the family or patient can disagree. The President's Commission has published advisory tables regarding the resuscitation of both competent and incompetent patients that take into account the patient's preference and the likelihood that CPR would benefit the patient.[19]

Once the DNR decision has been made, the order should be written, signed, and dated by the responsible physician. It should be reviewed periodically; hospital policies may require review every 24 to 72 hours.[20] More informal methods of designating those patients in whom CPR is not to be undertaken can lead to errors if an arrest occurs. For example, the wrong patient can be allowed to die.

If an arrest occurs in an emergency room or in another situation in which a formal DNR decision has not been made and written, the presumption of the medical and nursing staffs should be in favor of life, and a code should be called. A "slow code" (in which the nurse takes excessive time to call or the team takes its time responding) should never be permitted—either CPR is indicated or it is not.

Courts are beginning to be involved in DNR decisions. In 1978, a Massachusetts appellate court ruled that an attending physician may lawfully write a DNR order for an incompetent patient for whom there is no life-saving or life-prolonging treatment.[21] More recently, a New York grand jury investigated a hospital that indicated DNR decisions by using purple dots stuck to nursing cards that were discarded after the death of the patient. Nurses from the hospital complained that the decals could be stuck to the wrong patient's card; one card had two dots affixed to it. The grand jury found that the dot system "virtually eliminated professional accountability, invited clerical error and discouraged physicians from obtaining informed consent from the patient or his family."[22]

Advance Directives: Living Wills, Health Care Agents, and Powers of Attorney

A living will is a directive from a competent patient to family and medical personnel about the treatment he or she wishes to receive if in a terminal condition or permanently comatose. These directions are used if the person is incompetent and unable to make decisions.[23] In general, a living will is not needed if a patient is competent and can communicate, because under these circumstances treatment can be refused when it is offered.

At least 39 United States jurisdictions (Table 9–1) have so-called natural death statutes, or living will statutes, although provisions of these laws vary. Usually, a person who is 18 years of age or older may execute a living will. It must be written, signed, and witnessed. Because many statutes bar medical personnel who are attending the patient or who are employed by the facility in which the patient is hospitalized from being witnesses, a CCN should not witness a document for her patient. The directive should be reviewed and re-signed by the patient annually.

Even in states with living will statutes, the directive may not be binding on the physician. However, in a few

TABLE 9–1
Jurisdictions That Have Living Will Statutes*

Alabama	Missouri
Alaska	Montana
Arizona	Nevada
Arkansas	New Hampshire
California	New Jersey
Colorado	New Mexico
Connecticut	North Carolina
Delaware	North Dakota
District of Columbia	Ohio
Florida	Oklahoma
Georgia	Oregon
Hawaii	Rhode Island
Idaho	South Carolina
Illinois	South Dakota
Indiana	Tennessee
Iowa	Texas
Kansas	Utah
Kentucky	Vermont
Louisiana	Virginia
Maine	Washington
Maryland	West Virginia
Minnesota	Wisconsin
Mississippi	Wyoming

* As of November, 1991. To update this information, contact Concern for Dying at (212) 246-6973.

TABLE 9–2
Jurisdictions Authorizing Health Care Proxy/Agent Appointments*

Arkansas	Nevada
Connecticut	New Jersey
Delaware	New York
District of Columbia	South Carolina
Florida	Texas
Idaho	Utah
Massachusetts	Virginia
Minnesota	Wyoming
Montana	

* As of November 11, 1991.

states, it is unprofessional conduct for a physician to refuse to comply with the directive, although the physician may transfer the patient to the care of another. In all states with statutes, personnel and facilities that comply in good faith with the directive are immune from civil and criminal prosecution.

In states without statutes, it is likely that a recent living will would be taken as evidence of what the patient would have wanted had he or she been competent when the decision was presented. Although there have not been any cases concerning a written living will, there have been several involving patients who had expressed wishes orally about life-sustaining measures.

CASE 8

Brother Fox was an 83-year-old member of a religious order who became permanently comatose during hernia surgery. After hospital officials and physicians refused to cease respirator therapy, Brother Fox's order began court proceedings. New York's highest court, the Court of Appeals, ruled (after the death of the priest) that Brother Fox's oral, solemn statement of his wishes, made to members of his order after the Karen Ann Quinlan case had occurred, was sufficient to authorize termination of treatment.[24]

If a patient or family member reveals the existence of a written living will, a copy should be placed in the medical record, and the attending physician should be notified. If the patient is competent, attempts should be made to clarify the meaning of terminology in the directive; these discussions should be well documented in the medical record. This is necessary to enable nursing and medical personnel to understand exactly what treatment the patient wishes to avoid.[25]

Although living wills are the most commonly seen advance directive, legislatures have now created others that are increasing in popularity. As of early 1992, sixteen states had statutes in place that would permit a competent adult to appoint a decision maker either in addition to a living will or in lieu of that document (Table 9–2). Authority to appoint a health care agent or proxy usually is found within the state's living will statute. Execution formalities are generally the same as those for a living will.

Powers of a health care agent or proxy are effective if the patient cannot decide and are usually limited to making decisions about implementation or withdrawal of life-support treatment if the patient is in a terminal condition. In effect, these documents appoint a person with whom the health care team can discuss decisions that seem appropriate under a living will.

The third type of advance directive is a durable power of attorney. Most states have general statutes that permit the appointment of a proxy to act if a person becomes incompetent. Although these statutes were not originally intended to delegate health care decisions, some authorities feel that language contained in these acts is broad enough to authorize health care decision making.[26] California was the first state to pass a special act for durable power of attorney for health care. When reviewing its provisions, the CCN must remember that each durable power of attorney law is different and that it is important to understand the law in the jurisdiction in which it is applied.

The California statute permits a patient to designate another as his or her "attorney in fact" to make certain health care decisions on his or her behalf. The power to make health care decisions can include consent, refusal of consent, or withdrawal of consent to any care or treatment of a mental or physical condition. The document may limit the powers of the attorney in fact, and the statute does not permit consent to certain treatments (eg, sterilization, commitment to a mental health facility).

To be effective, a durable power of attorney in California must be executed as required by statute. Two witnesses are required. Generally, the power expires after 7 years, but it may be revoked at any time by oral or written notification of the attorney in fact or the health care provider. Treatment authorized by the attorney in fact may not be administered over the objection of the patient.[27]

Patient Self-Determination Act

On December 1, 1991, the Patient Self-Determination Act went into effect. This federal statute is applicable to facilities that receive Medicare reimbursement for patient care. As a condition of reimbursement, the law requires that hospitals, nursing facilities, home health care services, hospice programs, and certain health maintenance organizations provide information to adults about their rights concerning decision making in that state. For hospitals, this information must be provided to every adult on admission regardless of diagnosis and regardless of whether he or she is a Medicare patient. The material distributed must include information about the types of advance directives that are legal in that state. Documentation that the

patient has received this information must be placed in the medical record. If the patient is incapacitated on admission, the information must be provided to a family member, if available. This action, however, does not relieve the hospital of its duty to provide information to the patient once he or she is no longer incapacitated.[28]

Surrogate Decision Making

Most patients do not have guardians, and many do not have advance directives to guide decision making. If a patient can no longer make decisions for himself and no other guidance is available, hospitals and health care providers consult family members or, if there are none, then close friends, about what the patient would have wanted under the circumstances. More than 15 states and the District of Columbia now have statutes addressing this long-standing practice. These statutes usually establish a list of persons, in order of priority, who may make decisions for an incompetent patient who has not left a living will or other instructions. (See, for example, the District of Columbia Health-Care Decisions Act of 1988–1989.)[29]

Withdrawal of Life-Support Measures

What constitutes life support, when these measures must be used, and when they may be terminated have been issues raised in many court cases. However, the law in these areas is still developing and will continue to do so as each jurisdiction creates its own guidelines.

Given the regularity with which life-support decisions must be made in health care facilities, it is remarkable that it was not until 1976 that the first case, *In re Quinlan*, focused national attention on the "right to die" controversy. The cases have concerned minors and adults, competent patients and incompetent ones, afflicted with a disease or condition that would eventually be terminal. States have not been consistent in their decisions, even when the situations are arguably similar. For example, the New Jersey court in the case of Karen Ann Quinlan, a 21-year-old woman in a persistent vegetative state, held that the decision about treatment is in the hands of the patient's guardian in consultation with the hospital ethics committee.[30] Massachusetts, however, rejected the New Jersey approach in favor of judicial review of decisions made by physicians and family members.[31] The President's Commission for the Study of Ethical Problems in Medicine and Biomedical and Behavioral Research stated that judicial review of these decisions should be reserved for occasions when "adjudication is clearly required by state law or when concerned parties have disagreements that they cannot resolve over matters of substantial import."[32]

The Florida case of *Satz v. Perlmutter* involved a competent patient and his right to refuse treatment.

CASE 9

Abe Perlmutter was 73 years old, suffered from amyotrophic lateral sclerosis, and was dependent on respirator therapy. He was conscious, competent, and able to speak, although he found speech difficult and painful. He had expressed his suffering and had attempted to disconnect his respirator himself. State officials argued that anyone who helped him disconnect his respirator would be guilty of aiding suicide. The Florida Supreme Court ruled that disconnection of the respirator was not suicide because Mr. Perlmutter's condition was not self-inflicted.[33]

The following three cases concern whether it is necessary to provide patients with fluids and nutrition if they cannot feed themselves.

CASE 10

In re Conroy involves an 84-year-old nursing home patient who suffered from severe organic brain syndrome. Her guardian, a nephew, petitioned the court to permit removal of her nasogastric tube, on which she was dependent. The trial court held that the tube could be removed.[34] An appeals court held removal of the tube improper because the bodily invasion suffered by the patient as a result of the treatment was small, and death by dehydration and starvation would be painful.[35] Although the patient had died, the New Jersey Supreme Court held in 1985 that treatment (including artificial feeding and hydration) for nursing home residents may be terminated under certain circumstances and set forth the procedures to be followed. This decision was restricted to nursing home residents who were once competent and who would probably die within approximately 1 year, even with treatment.[36]

CASE 11

Mrs. McConnell was a 57-year-old woman who was in a chronic vegetative state for three years after an auto accident. Before the accident, she had been the head nurse in an emergency department and had expressed her views orally about the maintenance of life if useful recovery was hopeless. The patient was being fed by gastrostomy tube in the nursing home in which she was a resident. After considerable discussion, the husband (who was the conservator) and adult children asked that the tube be removed and the patient be allowed to die. The nursing home declined to comply without court authority. After considerable testimony about the patient's wishes, the lower court ruled that there was sufficient evidence of Mrs. McConnell's wishes and that the nursing home must comply with the conservator's request. The case was appealed and, in January 1989, the Connecticut Supreme Court affirmed the lower court decision.[37] Mrs. McConnell's feeding tube was disconnected; she died on February 28, 1989.

Another case involved the criminal liability of physicians who order termination of treatment.

CASE 12

Clarence Herbert was 55 years old when he had a cardiac arrest in the recovery room after elective surgery for closure of a colostomy. Three days later, he was deeply comatose and unlikely to recover; the respirator was removed with the consent of the family. Mr. Herbert then began to breathe on his own. Two days later, intravenous lines and the nasogastric tube were removed. Mr. Herbert died 7 days later from dehydration and pneumonia.[38] Two physicians were charged with murder for terminating intravenous feeding. Finding that the physicians did not have a legal duty to continue life-sustaining treatment that is futile or ineffective, a California appellate court ordered the criminal charges dropped.[39]

Only one case involving the termination of food and fluids has been decided by the U.S. Supreme Court.

CASE 13

The case concerned Nancy Cruzan, a young woman who suffered anoxic brain damage in an automobile accident. She remained in a persistent vegetative state in Missouri and was fed by gastrostomy. After rehabilitation was unsuccessful, Ms. Cruzan's parents (as co-guardians) requested withdrawal of the feeding tube. After the employees of the rehabilitation center where she was a patient declined, the Cruzans sought judicial review of their request. After testimony, the trial court approved the parents' request. On appeal, the Missouri Supreme Court reversed the lower court. First, it held that Missouri law does not permit surrogate decision making in decisions of this importance. In order for a person to exercise the right to terminate artificial feeding in Missouri, that person must have previously expressed his or her wishes, either orally or in writing. Evidence of those wishes had to meet a relatively high evidentiary standard, a standard that the court held had not been met in the lower court proceeding.

This case was appealed to the U.S. Supreme Court and, in 1990, it was affirmed on constitutional ground.[40] After the decision was issued, the Cruzans returned to the Missouri lower court and presented further evidence (through additional witnesses) about what their daughter had expressed while competent. The lower court found that they had presented clear and convincing evidence and affirmed the rights of the co-guardians to authorize withdrawal of the feeding tube. After withdrawal of the tube, Nancy Cruzan died on December 26, 1990.

Although this case received much publicity, it did not change the law in any state but Missouri. Most states continue to permit surrogate decision making by relatives and require a lower evidentiary standard than that required in Missouri.

In recent years, as health care providers have become more comfortable recommending termination of treatment in selected cases, they have met resistance from some families who wish to continue treatment no matter what its chance of success. Although no law or legal principle requires that extraordinary, but clearly futile, treatment be provided, it is probably also true that health care providers have no legal recourse against families who refuse to withdraw life support (unless the patient has left written indications of his or her wishes prior to incompetence). There has been one case addressing this complicated problem.

CASE 14

In December 1989, Helga Wanglie broke her hip. After a complicated course, Mrs. Wanglie, who was 86 years old, ventilator dependent and competent, had a cardiopulmonary arrest. After this event, she remained in a persistent vegetative state. Pursuant to the wishes of the family, she was nourished by feeding tube and treated aggressively for recurrent pneumonia. Hospital staff disagreed with the family in this case; intervention by the hospital ethics committee did not resolve the conflict. Therefore, the hospital filed an application for a non-family member guardian to decide for the patient. The Minnesota court instead appointed the husband as guardian, finding that he was in the best position to know his wife's wishes. The court found that the hospital had requested the appointment of a non-family member, not because Mr. Wanglie was incompetent to be guardian, but because he disagreed with hospital staff.[41]

So far, there have been no cases where hospital staff directly challenged a family's decision to continue life support. Most commentators believe that such a challenge to family authority would not prevail, at least where the family is available and interested in making decisions for the patient.

In most states, problems of terminating treatment need not be resolved in court. Decisions regarding treatment or nontreatment that meet accepted medical standards and with which the patient concurs are made virtually every day in health care settings. If the patient is incompetent to decide, generally family members may do so, although they may not refuse therapy that would benefit the patient. Finally, a distinction should be made between termination of treatment and termination of care: even patients who are not being treated for their terminal condition require competent and sensitive nursing and medical care so that their final days are as comfortable as possible. The families of these patients may also require information along with sensitive emotional support. The need for good nursing care does not end with the decision "not to treat."

Brain Death

In 1968, the Harvard criteria established standards for determining brain death. The criteria have been found quite reliable. In fact, no case has "yet been found that met these criteria and regained any brain functions despite continuation of respirator support."[42] Some states adopted the Harvard criteria by statute, whereas other states enacted legislation defining brain death in broader, less restrictive terms.

The President's Commission for the Study of Ethical Problems in Medicine and Biomedical and Behavioral Research published *Defining Death* in July 1981. The Commission recommended a uniform statute defining death; it recommended that the statute address "general physiological standards rather than medical criteria and tests, which will change with advances in biomedical knowledge and refinements in technique."[43]

A patient who is brain dead is legally dead, and there is no legal duty to continue to treat him or her. It is not necessary to obtain court approval to discontinue life support on a patient who is brain dead. Furthermore, although it can be desirable to obtain family permission to discontinue treatment of a brain dead patient, there is no legal requirement. However, before terminating life support, physicians and nurses should be sure that organs are not intended for transplant purposes.[44]

Organ Donation

Every state in the United States has a law based on the Uniform Anatomical Gift Act. The statutes establish the legality of organ donation by individuals and their families and set procedures for making and accepting the gift of an organ. Every state also has some provision to enable persons to consent to organ donation using a designated place on a driver's license. More recently, many states have enacted "required request" laws. These laws attempt to increase the supply of organs for transplant by requiring hospital personnel to ask patients' families about an organ gift at the time of the patient's death. New York was the second state to enact such a law; it became effective in 1986.[45] A recent Connecticut law goes much further; it requires that hospital personnel ask each patient (aged 18 years or older) whether he or she is an organ donor. The answer must be placed in the medical record.[46] Further proliferation of these statutes is to be expected. We hope that new legislation balances the needs of the patient and family and the needs of the organ recipient.

Summary

The legal responsibility of the registered nurse in the CCU does not differ from that of the registered nurse in any work setting. The registered nurse adheres to five principles for the protection of both patient and practitioner:

- A registered nurse performs only those functions for which he or she has been prepared by education and experience.
- A registered nurse performs those functions competently.

• A registered nurse delegates responsibility only to personnel whose competence has been evaluated and found acceptable.
• A registered nurse takes appropriate measures as indicated by observations of the patient.
• A registered nurse is familiar with policies of the employing agency.

REFERENCES

1. Holder AR: Medical Malpractice Law, 2d ed, p 43. New York, John Wiley & Sons, 1978
2. Variety Children's Hospital, Inc. v. Perkins et al: 382 So2d 331, Florida, 1980
3. North Shore Hospital v. Luzi: 194 So2d 63, Florida, 1967
4. Holder AR: Medical Malpractice Law, 2d ed, p 158. New York, John Wiley & Sons, 1978
5. Collins v. Westlake Community Hospital: 312 NE2d 614, Illinois, 1974
6. Ramsey v. Physicians Memorial Hospital, Inc et al: 373 A2d 26, Maryland, 1977
7. Norton V. Argonaut Insurance Company et al: 144 Ao2d 249, Louisiana, 1962
8. Horton v. Niagra Falls Memorial Medical Center: 380 NYS 2d 116 (NY App Div 1976)
9. Department of Health and Human Services, Food and Drug Administration: Medical devices: Medical device, user facility, distributor, and manufacturer reporting, certification and registration. Federal Register 56:64004–64182 (December 6, 1991)
10. Department of Health and Human Services, Food and Drug Administration: Medical devices: Device tracking. Federal Register 57:22971–22981 (May 29, 1992)
11. Bellaire General Hospital v. Campbell: 510 SW2d 94, Texas, 1974
12. Rose v. Hakim: 335 F. Supp. 1221 (DDC 1971), affirmed in part, reversed in part, 501 F. 2d 806 (DC Cir 1974)
13. Holder AR: What commitment is made by a witness to a consent form? IRB 1:7, 1979
14. Bedell SE, Delbanco TL, Cook EF, Epstein FH: Survival after cardiopulmonary resuscitation in the hospital. New Engl J Med 309:569, 1983
15. Matter of Dinnerstein: 380 NE2d 134, Massachusetts, 1978
16. President's Commission: Deciding to Forego Life-Sustaining Treatment. Washington DC, Government Printing Office, March, 1983
17. Doudera AE, Peters JD (eds): Legal and Ethical Aspects of Treating Critically and Terminally Ill Patients (Appendices B–E). Ann Arbor, MI, Health Administration Press, 1982
18. Parrella GS: No Code? Conn Med 47:49, 1983
19. President's Commission: Deciding to Forego Life-Sustaining Treatment, Washington DC, Government Printing Office, March, 1983
20. Greenlaw J: Orders not to resuscitate: Dilemma for acute care as well as long term care facilities. Law Med Health Care 10:30, 1982
21. Matter of Dinnerstein: 380 NE2d 134, Massachusetts, 1978
22. Panel accuses hospital of hiding denial of care. New York, New York Times, March 21, 1984
23. Cohn S: The living will from the nurse's perspective. Law Med Health Care 11:121, 1983
24. In re Eichner (Fox), 420 NE2d 64, New York, 1981
25. Eisendrath SJ, Jonsen A: The living will: Help or hindrance? JAMA 249:2054, 1983
26. President's Commission: Deciding to Forego Life-Sustaining Treatment, Washington DC, Government Printing Office, March, 1983
27. Cal Civil Code, sections 2430–2443
28. Department of Health and Human Services, Health Care Financing Administration: Medicare and Medicaid programs: Advance directives. Federal Register 57:8194–8204, 1992
29. District of Columbia Health-Care Decisions Act of 1988, DC Code Annotated Section 21-2210 (1989)
30. In re Quinlan, 70 NJ 10, 355 A2d 647, New Jersey, 1976
31. Superintendent of Belchertown State School v. Saikewicz: 373 Mass. 728, 370 NE2d 417, Massachusetts, 1977
32. President's Commission: Deciding to Forego Life-Sustaining Treatment, p 6, Washington DC, Government Printing Office, March, 1983
33. Satz v. Perlmutter: 379 So2d 359, Florida, 1980
34. In the matter of Claire C Conroy: 457 A2d 1232, New Jersey Superior Court, 1983
35. In re Conroy, 464 A2d, 303, New Jersey, 1983
36. In the matter of Claire C Conroy: Slip Opinion 98 NJ:321, A2d, 1985
37. McConnell v. Beverly Enterprises, 209 Conn. 692 (1989).
38. Steinbock B: The removal of Mr. Herbert's feeding tube. Hastings Cent Rep 13:13, 1983
39. Barber v. Superior Court of California for the County of Los Angeles: 195 Cal Rptr 484, California Appeals Court, 1983)
40. Cruzan v. Director, Missouri Department of Health et al, III L Ed2d 224, 110 SCt 2841 (1990)
41. In re the Conservatorship of Wanglie, No. PX-91-283 (Minn Dist Ct, Probate Ct Division, July 1991)
42. President's Commission for the Study of Ethical Problems in Medicine and Biomedical and Behavioral Research: Defining Death, p 25, July, 1981
43. President's Commission for the Study of Ethical Problems in Medicine and Biomedical and Behavioral Research: Defining Death, p 1, July, 1981
44. Robertson J: The Rights of the Critically Ill, p 121. New York, Bantam Books, 1983
45. New York Public Health Law Article 43-A
46. Connecticut Public Act 88-318 (effective 7/1/88)

STUDY QUESTIONS

1. In a professional liability action, the standard of care is an important part of the plaintiff's burden of proof and often of the defendant's case. The applicable standard of care is that which was in effect

   a. at the time of the incident
   b. at the time the claim is made or suit is brought
   c. at the time the expert witness is retained
   d. at the time the case is tried

2. The doctrine of respondeat superior is the legal theory under which

   a. a hospital is directly liable for its corporate hiring decisions
   b. a health care provider is personally liable for acts of negligence
   c. an employer is vicariously liable for the negligent acts of its employees as long as they act within the scope of employment
   d. a hospital is liable for injuries to its employees

3. The Patient Self-Determination Act went into effect in 1991. This federal law requires that hospitals, nursing homes, and certain other providers

   a. provide patients with information about advance directives and require them to execute at least one type of advance directive
   b. provide patients with information about living wills only
   c. provide patients with information about all types of advance directives applicable in that state
   d. provide patients with information about all types of advance directives whether or not applicable in that state

4. A living will is applicable under which of the following circumstances?

   a. if the patient is incapacitated and is terminally ill
   b. if the patient is incapacitated and has a life threatening but curable illness
   c. if the patient is competent to express his wishes and has expressed a desire to be treated and has subsequently become incapacitated

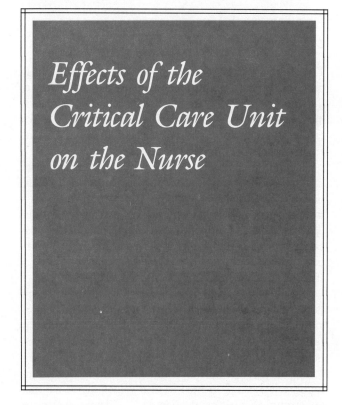

CHAPTER 10

*Effects of the
Critical Care Unit
on the Nurse*

BEHAVIORAL OBJECTIVES

Based on the content in this chapter, the reader should be able to:

1. Describe the change of focus from initial studies of stress in critical care nurses in the early 1970s to the studies currently being conducted.
2. Identify the self-expectations of critical care nurses that can contribute to burnout.
3. Name the different characteristics of assertive, passive, and aggressive behavior and the reactions of others to those characteristics.
4. Define "coping."

(*continued*)

Hudak: Critical Care Nursing:
A Holistic Approach, 6th ed. © 1994
J. B. Lippincott Company.

BEHAVIORAL OBJECTIVES (Continued)

5. Name the personality characteristics described under the coping style of "hardiness."
6. Describe the steps of the quieting reflex.
7. List five changes that can decrease nurses' stress levels in the critical care unit.

Introduction

Critical care nurses have been the focus of more study than perhaps any other population of nurses. There are many reasons why this is so. One of the main ones is that critical care units (CCUs) are places in which the forces of life and death are in constant battle. Nurses and physicians are the main defenders of the patient—but it is the nurses who are in constant attendance. Accordingly, they are continually charged with the responsibility of maintaining the patient's homeostasis.

Stress and its Effects on the Critical Care Nurse

The effects of stress on both psychological[1-3] and physical[4-5] health have been well documented. The delivery of nursing care in specialized CCUs became widespread in most hospitals by the early 1970s.[6] The advent of CCUs caused a strong interest in the effects of intensive working environments on nursing personnel.[7-12]

These initial studies explored the factors that caused job stress, job satisfaction, and job dissatisfaction in CCU nurses. They used many concepts and research findings from the general field of organizational psychology. Studies of workers in a variety of industries (eg, police work, day care) revealed certain traits that seemed related to burnout; others appeared to reduce the negative effects of stress.

Some of these characteristics apply to nurses and some do not. It appears likely that the values and general personality characteristics found in nursing differ from those in other fields that are primarily male-dominated or have a general mix of both male and female workers. Gilligan has found in her studies of men and women that women are highly relationship-oriented in their value judgments; men are strongly achievement oriented.[13-14] These differences could potentially affect a person's response to job-related decisions, valuing of one's work role, and response to patients. Because nursing is a woman-dominated profession, nurses can be more stressed by factors that affect their relationships, whether with supervisors, physicians, peers, patients, or patients' families. Certain aspects of these relationships have been reported as potential stressors in various studies of CCU nurses.

These studies were authored by a variety of mental health clinicians, including psychiatrists, psychologists, social workers, and nurses. The development of nursing research on CCU stressors was concomitant with the acquisition of research skills by increasing numbers of nurses with advanced degrees.

In the 1980s, research on the stressful effects of the CCU on the nurse clarified the particular CCU factors that cause stress. In addition, certain personality characteristics, and factors related to level of education and years of experience in the CCU, were found to have an effect on potential for burnout.[15-19] These are discussed later in the chapter.

The study of nursing stress by nurses is a positive trend in understanding the adverse effects of the CCU on nurses. A profession is more than the scientific body of knowledge that it utilizes: it also socializes its members so that they acquire qualities and dynamics that are unique to that profession. These factors can contribute to nurses' stress responses and can be best articulated by other nurses who understand their importance and effects. This chapter examines the different types of stressors experienced by CCU nurses. It also reviews the most recent trend in CCU nursing stress research—identifying personality factors that are helpful in coping with the CCU—as a way of better understanding the potentially adverse effects on the nurse and what can be done about them.

Socialization as a CCU Nurse

Nurses in CCUs often feel a special sense of pride in themselves. The level of work that they perform and the knowledge required to do their jobs well are known to be more complex than those of any other staff nursing position in the hospital. Accompanying this justified self-pride and positive professional self-image is another self-expectation that many critical care nurses experience: the ability to be calm and cool under pressure. This calmness has been commented on by several authors.[6,20-23]

It is frequently the nurses who impose this expectation on themselves. Physicians (who, it should be noted, have the opportunity to go into and out of the CCU, rather than remaining for assigned tours of duty) frequently remark on the nurses' apparent ability to tolerate the very high level of stress that exists there. Many doctors believe that the environment is difficult to tolerate for any period of time.[24] This implies that physicians would find it difficult to remain for several hours and still maintain an outward calm. Patients and families react well and are calmed by a cool, professional nurse's demeanor. Importantly, they are also comforted by nurses who are able to become emotionally involved with them and occasionally "let go" of the professional demeanor and demonstrate their caring.

If physicians, patients, and families are all willing to accept the need for the nurse to be human and occasionally slip out of the cool, professional role, why then do so many CCU nurses impose this rigid expectation on themselves?

Stressful Factors in the CCU

Unquestionably, the most important reasons that CCU nurses set such high expectations for themselves is that they view this as a way of maintaining emotional equilibrium. This is the greatest coping defense that most nurses use in dealing with the constant pressures of the CCU. Before explaining and discussing the need for coping abilities in nurses, it is important to accurately present the variety of stresses on the intensive care nurse.

Most nurses would immediately identify the unpredictability of the CCU environment as a leading stressor. Other stressors are the "incessant repetitive routine . . . ; every step must be charted . . . ; floating in nurses from elsewhere . . . ; frequent situations of acute crisis . . . ; physical dangers (inadequate protection from x-rays, needles, isolation patients, and those who are delirious) . . . ; lifting heavy, unresponsive patients . . . ; distraught relatives . . . ; (constant sounds of) moaning, crying, screaming, buzzing and beeping monitors, gurgling suction pumps, and whooshing respirators . . . "[6] Another very important stress on the nurse, and one that should not be underestimated, is that everywhere there are human bodies, many of them wasted, mutilated, or discolored. There are exposed genitalia and excretions of feces, blood, chest mucus, vomitus, and urine. Some patients' dressings are soaked with purulent discharge or serous or bloody drainage.[6]

STOP READING

Think back to your *honest* reaction as you read each of the stressors in the preceding section. Be honest with yourself.

TAKE A BIG BREATH
AND LET IT OUT SLOWLY

Now, pretend that you are on a beautiful, green hillside that slopes gently downward to a sandy beach. There are large, crashing waves that you can see and hear. The sun is shining. You are lying under a graceful old maple tree that protects you from the sun. A breeze is gently blowing your hair. Beautiful! Right? Now, slowly reread the list of stressors and let yourself *feel* a response. You may feel nothing as you read some of them. For others you may feel disgust, anxiety, or boredom. Are you able to detect a difference between your first set of responses and your second set? If not, is it possible that the coping strategies that you have unconsciously developed have resulted in an emotional detachment that is causing you to miss many of the good and positive aspects of life in and *out* of the CCU? It is very difficult to deaden one's response to negative emotional experiences without concurrently deadening it to pleasure and joy. What a high cost! What causes it to happen?

A common personality trait in many nurses is selflessness. This trait is nurtured and praised by nursing educators and administrators. If people are selfless, they deny their own physical or emotional needs in the service of others. Nurses who legitimately refuse to work a double shift, float to another unit, or take on extra assignments because of chronic understaffing usually are not as popular with supervisors as those who deny their own needs and acquiesce immediately.

Because in the past selflessness has been a desired trait in nurses and because the selfless nurse has received far more approval from peers and supervisors than the outspoken nurse who tries to assert various rights, many nurses have been socialized into denying their own needs, their own feelings—their own humanness!

Remember that nowhere on earth are people born knowing how to deny their own needs and feelings. Instead they have *learned* to deny them. The most important motivation in this process is the need for approval.

Traditional Personality Traits of Nurses

Think for a moment: if it is true that physicians, patients, and families are all able to recognize the nurse's humanness and accept that, on occasion, the professional, calm, cool exterior shell can safely slide away, revealing the real person who is underneath, why then is it necessary to hold on so tightly to the cover and try to stifle our own humanness?

If we are looking for approval, to whom are we looking? Nursing peers and supervisors are the obvious answer—the easy answer! The tough answer could be to admit that we do it ourselves. Sometimes nurses are their own severest critics. If they fail in their own, sometimes very difficult self-expectations, the result is guilt.

Many nurses were taught that it is not good to feel grief, fear, disgust, or love when working intimately with patients. Despite their own humanness they were taught that it was not "professional" to feel such emotions about patients. If a person feels something he or she was taught not to feel, the result is guilt. Because guilt is an unpleasant feeling, the mind (the ego, specifically) helps defend the person so that the guilt does not occur. Repression is a defense or coping mechanism that buries the original feelings of grief, fear, and so forth so that they are no longer felt. It is important to know, however, that the memories of the experiences that *normally* cause such feelings remain stored in our unconscious memories. The repression does not get rid of those memories.

The *constant* burying of these feelings is *not* healthy. Remember that the nursing educators and supervisors who have taught that it is "professional" to bury them have been socialized by other nurses. Theirs is not a helpful approach. It will not change until they themselves are socialized into a more humane approach and become kinder to themselves and to other nurses.

Burnout

The result of constant denial of self is probably one of the most important, yet underrecognized, dynamics of burnout. Critical care nurses, because of the stressful nature of their work, are at risk for burnout. Burnout can be the result of working in a stressful environment. The worker eventually feels resigned, ineffective, and hopeless about working in such an environment. The result of burnout is that the employee either leaves the job or remains in the position functioning ineffectively. Burnout is an energy-less state.

There are other important causes of burnout. Alvin Toffler, in *Future Shock*,[25] suggests that we live in a highly technological environment in which change is occurring at a faster and faster rate. The result is that the knowledge needed by critical care nurses and the complexity of the patients they care for are constantly increasing, imposing even greater stress in an already stressful milieu.

If nurse–patient ratios were improved to be proportionate to the increasing complexity of care, nurses would be able to adapt to the stress of the CCU more readily. Otherwise, chronic understaffing results. The effects of chronic understaffing are many. Frustration occurs if nurses are consistently under pressure and repeatedly feel that they are not giving the full kind of care that their patients need. This type of frustration can lead to burnout.

Burnout is causing many nurses to leave nursing. As a result, the problem of burnout is receiving more attention in both the professional and lay sectors. As nurses, it is important for us to understand the causes of burnout.[26] Certainly the aforementioned root problems have always been there. Until the 1970s, if nurses were victims of burnout because of overwork or because of repression of self, they frequently remained in their positions, but in a diminished state. Today, however, nurses are responding to a different current in society.

Another cause of burnout in the CCU can be attributed to dysfunctional communication. Management of the staff dynamics in the CCU can be a challenging role for the nursing manager. If important staff issues are consistently avoided or are dealt with in an autocratic rather than democratic manner, staff members often feel angry and unrecognized.[27]

The presence of co-dependent personality characteristics can also cause high self-expectations in nurses. Co-dependence is a phenomenon addressed by Beattie[28] in which a person sacrifices his or her own needs in service of another person who is perceived as dysfunctional. Schaef and Fassel[29] have applied this concept to organizational dynamics. A staff member with a manager or hospital cultural environment that does not respect the need for reasonable working conditions can become co-dependent with a dysfunctional organization.

Consciousness Raising in Nursing

The feminist movement, with its strong emphasis on selfhood, has made women increasingly aware of their right to experience their lives fully. The essential goal of this movement is improvement in the quality of life for all women. It attempts to make them aware of the traditional role that they have filled in society and to present alternatives that they can then choose or reject. Nursing is a predominately female profession. Its members, whether men or women, strongly represent the most traditional female qualities of caring, nurturing, and selflessness.

The women's movement has created more of an awareness in women that they are "givers." In her book, Jean Baker Miller[33] quoted a woman who said, "I can't give anymore, but I don't feel allowed to stop." Insightful women have begun to realize that the permission to stop has to come *first* from the giver—not from the takers. After all, why would anyone who is receiving good things tell the giver to stop?

This giving–taking relationship has been the traditional relationship between nurse and hospital. A new dynamic is being observed in nurses that is probably directly related to their raised consciousness as women. In the past they became burned out, resigned, and ineffective care givers as a result of difficult working conditions. Today, it is far more common for nurses to feel angry and frustrated by these conditions. They leave their positions rather than allowing their selfhood and their own needs to be diminished.

In many cases, their anger and frustration are justifiable, and they have few options other than leaving. Frequently, however, when they move to other positions, the cycle repeats itself. It is possible that after several of these moves the nurse still becomes burned out. After all, the resiliency of any human being eventually has a breaking point.

Hopeless? No! There are many alternatives. The important point is that the alternatives must be considered before the breaking point is in view. Baker says, "Clearly, women need to allow themselves to take, openly, as well as give."[30] The amount of energy necessary to create this change of thinking in nurses can be likened to pulling teeth—from a whale! Or stopping a 50-ton locomotive as it is hurtling down a hill! Nurses have always been givers. It is why they entered nursing. It is okay to give. It is beautiful to give. But it is also okay and beautiful to be a full human being and to value one's own worth. Judeo-Christian teaching has frequently been the basis of giving to others. It is important to note, however, that the most basic rule is "love thy neighbor as thyself." This rule assumes that we first love ourselves, and that we should love others as much as—not more than—we love ourselves!

Assertiveness: An Important Factor in Effective Coping

One of the catchwords of the feminist movement is "assertiveness." This movement has encouraged women to become more assertive. For many women who favor the traditional feminine characteristics, the word *assertiveness* has some negative implications. It is possible that this is due to a lack of distinction between the behavioral characteristics of assertiveness and those of aggressiveness. The differences between being aggressive, being assertive, and being passive, or nonassertive, are presented in Table 10–1.

The difference between the passive person and the assertive person is that the passive person is "done unto" by another who has no awareness of the passive person's needs or desires. Passive people seem more like nonpersons. Actually, they often put their faith in others to know what they need, usually with unexpressed expectations (also called a *hidden agenda*). If the others fail them in any way there can be two outcomes:

1. They further submerge their "selves" and needs. The implied meaning is "I have no worth."
2. They feel resentment. "Why did they do this to me?" Actually, the agency or other person had no idea of the unexpressed needs.

Assertive persons, however, are aware of their own needs and the treatment that they are entitled to as human beings. They express these needs when appropriate. If their rights are openly violated, they speak up and express their feelings. Assertive persons are not offensive and do not infringe on the rights of other people or institutions. They place value on their own thoughts and beliefs. They place value on themselves.

Aggressive persons are offensive people. They impose their beliefs on others, expecting them to agree, and become angry if the others do not acquiesce. They actually deny others the right to their own thoughts or opinions.

Which is in Control: Thinking or Feeling?

Learning to distinguish thoughts from feelings can help us change behavior from passive to assertive. For example, if a person feels guilty, he or she has a gut reaction inside. Guilt is a *feeling*. A person can't think guilt; he or she feels it. Accordingly, if he or she thinks that Bill Clinton was a good president, he cannot *feel* that Clinton was a good president. He can think that it is time to paint his house; he cannot *feel* that it is time to paint his house.

In the beginning of the chapter guilt was briefly discussed. Guilt is a strong feeling. It is not pleasant to feel guilty. Most people go to any lengths to avoid feeling guilty. As a result, guilt is a very strong motivator. For most nurses, it is a troublesome and frequent companion in the working place. There are so many things nurses *think* they have to do. If they are unable to accomplish all of them, even though the limitations are beyond their control, they *feel* guilty. To avoid feeling guilty, they frequently push themselves harder and harder.

Nurses' work is "never really done." It is impossible to make a finite list of things to be done within an 8-hour shift. For example, once the absolutely required tasks are

TABLE 10–1
Assertiveness, Passivity, and Aggressiveness

	Characteristics	Feelings in Self	Reactions of Others
Assertive	Open	At peace inside	Respect
	Honest	Good self-esteem	
	Does not impinge on others' beliefs	Respects others' rights	
Passive	Weak	Uncertain	Pity
	Yielding	Tries to please others	Uncertainty
	Self-denying	Resentful	Unconcern
	Hidden bargaining		Annoyance
	Deceptive about real feelings		
Aggressive	Quarrelsome	Anger	Indignation
	Bold	Contempt	Displeasure
	Degrades others	Extreme self-pride	Hurt
	Bulldozes over others' opinions, beliefs, and feelings	Anxious when aggressiveness is out of control	Disgust

accomplished and charted, you could still give Mrs. Jones, the woman with the cardiac bypass in isolation, some more time; she seemed depressed today. Or, you could update some nursing care plans; they've been neglected because the unit was so busy.

Even if nurses push themselves to do more and more, the end result can be continued feelings of guilt—and sometimes resentment. There is an important point to be remembered, however. No person can *make* another person feel guilty. Even though individuals or institutions may make unreasonable demands on a person, only that person can allow himself or herself to feel guilty. The intellect, the thinking side of a person, can be a strong ally in preventing unreasonable demands from creating guilty feelings. It can be consciously willed into action. A non-nursing example of this concept follows.

If a mother buys her youngster four electronic games for his birthday and the child demands to know why he did not receive five, the mother can either *think* to herself, "How ungrateful; I did far more than was necessary," or she can *feel* guilty. The child did not make her feel guilty. She allowed his statement to cause her guilt feelings. By not consciously guarding ourselves against guilt-inducing statements or expectations of others, we become victims of guilt.

In working with nurses the author has repeatedly found that feelings of guilt are the greatest cause of nurses' inability to break away from passivity. It is necessary to understand how to suppress unnecessary guilt before we can learn to be assertive, fully actualized persons.

Will the Real You Please Stand Up?

Another concept that is important in the process of being comfortable with assertiveness is one that is explained by Bowen as the *pseudo* self and the *solid* self.[31] The pseudo self is the side of ourselves we allow others to know. Some people are all pseudo self. They are to their family members, friends, patients, and physicians exactly what those people need them to be. Their own needs, desires, and so forth are submerged to meet the expectations of others.

The solid self is the real you. Many nurses have a difficult time identifying the real self. It has almost entirely been given away to meet the demands of others. The real self must be dug up and reinflated. It's still there. It can return and be bigger and better than it ever was. It requires hard work and concentration and a strong imposition of intellect to break the chains of passivity. It requires control over feelings that can quickly undermine the best intentions. The greatest challenge to your success will be the same family, friends, patients, and physicians who have previously been very successful at "pulling your strings." Being assertive means speaking up for what you need, what you think, and what you believe in. It means knowing your real self.

Coping: Keeping it all Together

Coping was a popular word used during the stress-conscious era of the 1980s. It appears frequently in articles about the responses of CCU nurses to their environment.[32–40] It could be helpful to review the concept of coping before proceeding. Coping is "a combination of conscious strategies that have worked successfully in the past that join with unconscious defense mechanisms in order to reduce the level of stress that a person is experiencing."[41]

It is very important to remember that coping includes the *automatic* use of defense mechanisms by the ego. These automatic mechanisms (eg, denial, avoidance, repression) are used whenever the ego senses a threat to the self. It is also important to remember that an event that is perceived as threatening to one person may not be to another. The following case study is an example.

CASE STUDY

Evelyn, Joan, and Carol were working nights in the coronary intensive care unit. Evelyn had worked there for 12 years. Joan and Carol had been hired as new graduates 6 months previously. Joan was an astute nurse who learned quickly but was not yet fully confident in all situations. Carol was currently on probation because her nurse manager had found her to be lacking in both assessment and problem-solving skills. During the night a patient developed a severe episode of tachycardia. Within 5 minutes another patient arrested. The perception and responses of the three nurses were as follows:

Evelyn was skilled in all aspects of emergency cardiac assessment and intervention. She was alert and fully monitoring the initial patient's condition. When the other patient arrested she rapidly assessed the condition of the two patients, gave orders to Joan to assume care of the first, and moved to call the code and resuscitate the second. Her ego had become so accustomed to these events that it automatically switched on the cognitive or thinking mode and switched off her emotional response. If her emotions had prevailed, she would have reacted with anxiety. Moderate to high levels of anxiety markedly lower a person's problem-solving abilities. Joan, when thinking in advance about emergency situations in the CCU, experienced many symptoms of anxiety (eg, increased heart and breathing rates, cold perspiration). During the critical situation just described, however, she maintained full control and awareness of herself and felt little anxiety. Her emotional response was repressed by her ego.

As the double emergencies began, Carol reacted to them by "freezing." Her ego shut out her initial anxiety about the situation by denial. With Evelyn and Joan pushing her to action, she quickly began to work with them but was highly anxious. Her ego was not repressing her anxiety. Accordingly, her problem-solving skills were decreased.

In the situation just described, each of the three nurses experienced the emergency in a different way. *No two human beings ever perceive the same event in the same way.* This is because every person is born with a basic temperament.[42] This inborn set of basic personality traits is then affected by the environment in which the child is raised.

The ego evolves as a response to the surroundings of the child. It determines what is good, bad, harmless, or threatening during the first several years of life.[43] It develops consistent patterns of defenses against situations that it decides are harmful. Depending on the types of experiences the child encounters and the capacity of the ego to defend against feelings of anxiety, the child perceives a situation as stressful or not stressful.[44]

Coping is actually a complex process that involves a usually consistent response in each person. For example, a person who copes well in one type of stressful situation usually copes well in all situations. The exceptions are if a person is profoundly fatigued; has had a previous similar experience in which coping failed, so that another similar event causes a burst of anxiety; or has experienced several stressful incidents over a brief period of time, so that the new stressor is like "the straw that can break the camel's back."

Coping Styles of CCU Nurses

The most recent research on CCU nursing stress has focused on the way that CCU nurses perceive their working environment(s) and the manner in which they adapt to it.

Because there has been so much emphasis on CCU nursing stress, turnover, and so on, the following question is being asked: are there particular coping abilities or certain personality styles that help CCU nurses adapt successfully to a stressful environment?

Maloney and Bartz[45] approached this question by studying the personality and coping characteristics of nurses in intensive care and non-intensive care settings. They examined several factors to determine whether there were differences between the two groups of nurses. Their findings showed that the intensive care nurses differed significantly in several ways.

Adventurousness and Challenge

These qualities were found to be present more often in CCU nurses than in non-CCU nurses and are believed to contribute toward their attraction to the CCU environment and their capacity to experience satisfaction in it.

Power

The CCU nurses generally felt less powerful and more controlled by the environment than the non-CCU staff. This is a realistic finding of adaptation in view of the emergency and unpredictable nature of the CCU setting.

Detachment

The CCU nurses were found to be more detached than their non-CCU counterparts. It was suggested by the authors that this quality helped the nurses cope with the perceptual bombardment present in the CCU. The capacity for detachment is based on use of the defense mechanisms of denial, repression, intellectualization, and similar defenses that reduce the level of anxiety that a person might normally feel in a threatening situation.

In an earlier study, Maloney[46] had compared the coping capacity of CCU nurses with that of non-CCU nurses by examining the ways that both groups experienced anxiety. It was found that CCU nurses experience less anxiety in both normal and new situations than do non-CCU nurses. This information can lead to speculation that CCU nurses have a stronger capacity to cope with anxiety. One can further wonder whether persons who are not attracted to CCU settings are motivated by the desire to avoid excessive anxiety.

Another finding of the study revealed that non-CCU nurses had higher scores on somatic complaints, personal and family problems, and work load dissatisfaction. The generalized conclusion is that CCU nurses have a stronger capacity for coping and adaptation than do nurses attracted to non-CCU settings.

Hardiness: A Deterrent to Burnout

Hardiness is a term applied to a particular set of personality characteristics described by Kobassa and Puscetti.[47] Their research revealed that people who perceived that their lives and choices were under their own control, felt committed to their current goals and lifestyle, and experienced the strains of life as challenges were less likely to become ill as the result of stressful life events. These characteristics were described by the authors as the way a person responds to stress with a sense of **control versus powerlessness, commitment versus alienation, and challenge versus threat**.

Based on this study and others, it appears that the use of conscious coping mechanisms, such as reframing one's perspective of a stressful situation, can be important to the CCU nurse. Shifting from a sense of powerlessness, lack of commitment, and threat to a positive perspective can restore hope and an increased feeling of well-being.

Nursing Stress Factors Identified in CCU Research

Research on the effects of the CCU environment on the nurse demonstrates many important stress-related factors. By understanding the underlying causes of burnout, the value of assertiveness in combating burnout, the importance of instituting personal change, and accepting one's authenticity, nurses can improve their working environments. By analyzing these factors, nursing administrators, managers, and staff members themselves can design interventions that can improve the quality of work life of critical care nurses.

The need for CCU nurses continues to increase. One current estimate of the annual increase in CCU beds per year in this country is approximately 2500.[48] It behooves nursing administrators to address the needs of their CCU staff members so that CCUs themselves do not experience crises as the number of their staff members decrease.[49]

Anderson et al[32] found that the three most significant stressors reported by CCU nurses were (1) interpersonal conflict with physicians; (2) the care of sicker patients; and (3) nursing administrator and manager issues. This third factor was also identified by Oehler et al[38] as lack of overall support from nursing managers and administrators. Hart et al[37] found that organization dynamics, such as (1) communication patterns; (2) staff utilization and planning; (3) interdisciplinary politics with division level nursing administrators and physicians; (4) reward, including salary, promotion, and educational opportunities; and (5) availability of support from nonnursing departments and other health care professionals, are the critical determinants of nurses' job satisfaction and turnover rates.

Rosenthal et al[39] found that ethical issues regarding dying patients were highly stressful to nursing staff.

The review of these factors indicates that the CCU environment continues to exert strong demands on nurses. Regardless of the type of stress, it appears that the nurses' perception of control of these factors may be the critical element in whether effective or ineffective coping occurs.

Effective coping prevents the development of mental or physical exhaustion.[41] Cavanagh[35] has described these forms of exhaustion as the cause of burnout. In order to cope with the CCU stressors described above, it can be helpful to classify them according to their controllability. Some of them are subject to changes in the environment, some not. Those that are not can then be addressed by a change in nurses' attitudes or expectations, or by modifying coping techniques. They can be classified as *environmental responses* and *personal responses*.

Environmental Responses

Interpersonal Conflict With Physicians

The use of a consultation/liaison psychiatry consultant can support problem solving and effective communication by nurses. Such problems can also be addressed within the medical administration by creating a joint committee of nurses and physicians to consider this specific problem. This problem also raises the need for more active education of and role-playing by student nurses to increase effective and assertive communication when they become nursing professionals.

The Care of Sicker Patients

The use and support of nursing staff as they care for acutely ill patients can be important to the coping responses of CCU staff members.

One of the most difficult stressors for CCU nurses is the death of patients.[36] If a patient's death involves an ethical conflict or conflict with a physician, the effects on the nurse can be severe. Two important interventions can assist with these factors. The first is the support of or development of an ethical review panel.[39] There should be active participation by nurses on such a panel. Difficult ethical considerations or conflicts can be brought forward, addressed, and, ideally, resolved in such a forum. If the decisions of such panels are physician-dominated, the needs of patients, families, and nurses are usually not well met.

If a conflict with a physician is not ethical in nature and seems unresolvable to the staff nurse, the nursing manager can negotiate with the physician director of the unit for review of the problem. In addition, psychiatric consultation/liaison services can be requested to work with the nursing and medical staff members to develop alternative solutions to the existing conflict. Ongoing, unresolved conflicts are active contributors to nurses' perceptions of lack of control and helplessness.

Even though the actual acuity level of the very sickest patients is be fully controllable by the environment, the support of the nurse can be directly related to (1) a supportive relationship with the nursing manager; (2) technical and equipment resources; (3) positive interpersonal relations with nursing and other health care disciplines; (4) good benefits and wages to balance heavy work demands; and (5) reasonable working hours with limited overtime expectations.

Nursing Administrator and Management Issues

The job satisfaction of a staff nurse can be directly proportional to the value system and attitudes of the Vice President for Nursing toward the quality of work life of each nurse in the department. His or her attitude drives the decision making in all hospital departments that interface with nursing. This person also sets the tone for the management styles of middle-level and nursing unit managers.

Oehler et al[38] found that the support of the CCU manager is critical to the job satisfaction of the CCU nurse. Volk and Lucas[50] described four different organizational management styles and their effects on nursing job performance, job satisfaction, and turnover rates. They are (1) Exploitative–Authoritative, (2) Benevolent–Authoritative, (3) Consultative, and (4) Participative. Each of these management styles was rated by the factors of leadership, motivation, communication, decision making, goals, and control. The Exploitative–Authoritative style was rated by CCU nurses as lowest in preference. The Benevolent–Authoritative and Consultative styles result in increased staff involvement. The Participative style is characterized by the confidence and trust of superiors in their staff members and a democratic decision-making and goal-setting pattern of staff participation.

Overall, CCU nurses ranked their managers' styles

midway between Benevolent–Authoritative and Consultative. The turnover rates of nurses increased in direct proportion to the presence of the management factors present in the Exploitative–Authoritative style.

Personal Responses

If environmental stressors in the intensive care unit are resistant to change or, by their nature, are an inherent factor of working in the CCU (eg, the death of patients), nurses are wise to address these demands by use of either an emotion/stress reduction or a problem-solving approach. The first involves reducing emotional distress, such as anxiety or emotional fatigue. The Quieting Reflex[51] reduces the emotional overload that nurses can experience while working in a stressful environment.

The Quieting Reflex

There is a very effective relaxation technique that requires only 6 seconds to do. It is called the Quieting Reflex. It was developed by Dr. Charles Stroebel, a research psychiatrist, who created it to reduce the stressful effects of our society on a person's normal mental and physical functioning.

If a person is stressed and feels helpless, the sympathetic nervous system arouses responses that can lead to physical and mental illness. The most common problems are gastrointestinal distress, skeletal and muscle tension, headaches, hormonal problems, and psychological strain. All of these problems range on a continuum beginning with occasional, momentary distress. They can proceed to moderate problems that are chronic, leading potentially to unyielding pain and ultimate death if the person's resistance is completely overwhelmed.

Stroebel's Quieting Reflex is a coping device that can break the cycle of stress. He recommends using it frequently during the day—as many as 75 or 100 times. It purpose is to alter the neurophysiology that causes wear and tear on the various body systems. In time, the body reflexively learns to take care of itself by programming the Quieting Reflex as an automatic response to any stressful event.[51]

The Quieting Reflex consists of five steps:

- Inhale an easy, natural breath.
- Think "Alert mind, calm body."
- Smile inwardly (with your internal facial muscles).
- As you exhale, allow your jaw, tongue, and shoulders to go loose.
- Allow a feeling of warmth and looseness to go down through your body and out through your toes.

The Problem-Solving Process

The second type of personal response that nurses can use if experiencing high levels of personal stress is a problem-solving process. It supports an intellectual approach to increase nurses' sense of control and decrease their feelings of helplessness. Feelings of loss of control and helplessness are primary factors in job burnout[47] and depression.[41] The problem-solving process is effective whether used as an individual written exercise or in a group problem-solving process with a facilitator.

The problem-solving process to reduce stress or create change as a desired outcome is based on the steps in standard problem solving, using the nursing process as a guideline for these steps. It includes the following stages:

Assessment
1. Identify the problem
2. Analyze the causes of it

Planning
3. Identify the primary cause
4. What are the possible solutions to it?
5. What are the possible outcomes of each of the solutions?
6. Choose the best solution
7. At this point determine how you will evaluate its effectiveness: What criteria will indicate the desired outcome? What type of evaluation process will you use?

Implementing
8. Implement your change

Evaluating
9. Evaluate the outcome using the criteria and process described in #7

Group Meetings

Mohl[18] speculated that factors other than the primary task of delivering specialized care to patients could contribute to the stress of CCU nurses. They studied the work attitudes and levels of stress reported by the staff members of two non-intensive care units and two intensive care units. The results of the study indicated that the nature of the work in the CCU does affect the nurses' level of stress. More importantly, this study also showed that factors within the unit and nursing organization social system have a significant effect on nurses' stress levels. These include:

- support and respect from nursing supervisors;
- acceptance by staff and supervisors that mutual support in the form of informed one-on-one and formal support groups are important stress reducers;
- staff nurse/unit cohesiveness that includes the head nurse.

A recommendation unanimously presented by authors who have addressed the problem of stress in the CCU nurse is to have the CCU nursing staff meet regularly with an objective outsider who is trained in individual and group dynamics.[52–57]

The ideal leader is one who is schooled in *liaison psychiatry*, which is based on the study of the effects of stress on the person and on the social systems to which he or she belongs: the family, working environment, hospital, and so on.

Other successful leaders reported in the literature have been psychiatrists and nurse clinicians from the field of general psychiatry, social workers, and hospital chaplains trained in group process.

These are professionals employed by the hospital who usually are willing to give an extra hour of their time to this type of group. The request for such a group should come from the nursing staff. Meetings should be held once a week, at a regularly scheduled time, when the largest number of staff members can attend. A quiet meeting place adjacent to or in the CCU should be used.

The discussion group is used to address any CCU-related issue. The time is nonstructured, with the nurses raising the issues to be discussed. In the beginning weeks of the group, these issues frequently are centered on the emotional management of problem patients or families. Once the staff members feel trusting of themselves and their leader, they frequently discuss some of their own psychological reactions to specific incidents, such as the hopelessness of weaning a specific patient from a respirator, grief about the death of a long-term CCU patient, anger about house staff who are not there when needed, frustration with an insensitive nursing administration, or helplessness in dealing with the spouse of a dying 30-year-old patient.

Critical care nurses invest large amounts of energy and time in the care of one or two patients a day. It is inevitable that they will lose these patients, either by discharge from the unit or by death. When patients die, their nurses are left with many emotions: grief, sadness, depression, guilt, and anger. Without a safe place to talk about these repetitive losses, nurses unconsciously repress or deny their feelings in order to survive emotionally. Two other coping mechanisms that they use are avoidance and withdrawal.

Although avoidance and withdrawal are two different coping mechanisms, they have the same result. They occur when nurses consciously or unconsciously become numb to their own feelings and the emotional needs of patients and families. Another name for this phenomenon is *professional distancing*.

As a result, nurses care for the physical needs of patients but hold back from an emotional commitment. This helps them avoid the intolerable grief that occurs when the people they care for are repeatedly lost to them.

In a liaison group meeting, these feelings of grief and loss can be talked about in a supportive setting. The nurses' needs for rigid defenses against these feelings are eventually decreased. If it feels safe for them to experience their own honest feelings once again, they usually become more aware of the emotional needs of patients and their families. Their care becomes humanistic rather than technical.

Another issue that can cause conflict in the staff and also be alleviated is intrastaff conflict. The CCU staff nurses are bright, ambitious, and highly motivated. If they are working in close contact with others like themselves in a stress-filled environment, competition, staff schisms, or conflicts can result. Ideally, they should be resolved quickly. Without an available forum this is not easily accomplished.

Another problem in the CCU is nurse–doctor relationships. Eisendrath and Dunkel suggest that this may be a masked male–female issue. "This is particularly so when, despite a broader base of experience with critically ill patients, the nurse has to defer to a junior house officer with less relevant background."[54]

In addition, a problem that causes much resentment in nurses is that some doctors consistently avoid family members who need to ask questions or need reassurance. If these concerns are discussed in a liaison group and the anger is vented, nurses can learn better ways of discussing these issues directly with the doctors rather than allowing resentment to grow.

Stress: Is There Any Way to Make it Better?

The final section of this chapter includes suggestions for reducing stress during off-duty hours and recommendations that can also alleviate stress during working hours in the CCU. It is important to understand that the body's normal physiological reaction to stress was designed to help cavemen fight or flee from danger. In today's CCU, the nurse's response to stress causes a strong increase in tension and an increase in physical activity to help with the increased workload. There is an excess of energy available, however. If a nurse finishes work and feels tense, it is frequently a result of this unexpended energy.

Because of the sedentary trend in our society, many people live with chronic tenseness. The proliferation of tranquilizer and alcohol usage attests to the uncomfortable levels of tenseness in people. The best way to reduce physical and mental tension is by physical exercise. One mile of jogging or brisk walking every day returns the body's equilibrium to normal. Many people are pleasantly surprised to discover that their emotional state also improves if they begin a regular exercise program. Their depression, anxiety, or fatigue is lessened and gradually disappears.

The relation between physical tension and emotional disequilibrium is not fully understood. It is known, however, that adrenaline and the other catecholamines, which are the biochemical stimulators of the stress response, are

DISPLAY BOX 10–1
Recommended Changes
for Reducing Stress

- Institute 4-d work weeks with 10-h shifts.
- Employ a full-time physician as permanent CCU director. He or she would be available, especially during emergencies, and could supervise and teach house staff as they rotate into the unit.
- Schedule automatic rotations out of the CCU every 3 mo for 2 wk. These should be to an adjacent clinical area, preferably the step-down unit to which CCU patients are routinely discharged.[50]
- Allow nurses time to visit their "special" patients who are discharged from the CCU to other hospital units.
- Schedule a senior staff nurse on the day shift with a light patient assignment; he or she can assist and teach the less experienced nursing staff.
- Pay CCU nurses an extra wage increment—especially when chronic understaffing occurs.
- Upgrade the nurse–patient ratio in direct proportion to increased technology.
- Allow 6 wk for a comprehensive orientation and training period for new CCU nurses.
- Require orderlies or other non-CCU personnel to prepare the body of a deceased patient for the morgue.

In construction of new CCUs hospitals should

- Allow larger space between patient beds.
- Ideally, build small rooms for one or two patients or install permanent partitions between patient units.
- Build nurses' lounge out of view of patients, in the center of the CCU.
- Install windows in the unit. Install clocks within sight of patient. These are important orienting cues for patients *and* nurses. If patients are less disoriented, the stress on the nurse is less.
- Seek advice from CCU nurses in the architectural design.
- Install extra amounts of sound-proofing material.

also an integral part of the limbic system—the anatomical part of the brain that is the center of emotions. If adrenaline and the other neurotransmitters return to normal levels as a result of physical exercise, it is possible that the response of the limbic system is to regain emotional equilibrium as well.

If there is mental stress about specific patients, sadness about losing a special patient, or discouragement about the working environment, the best solution is to become involved in an activity that causes you to mentally focus on something else. This could be an academic course or something like an arts and crafts class—anything that requires intense concentration. The mental stress-reducing should always be accompanied by physical stress-reduction activities, such as walking or jogging.

The stress that occurs as a result of working in a CCU can also, ideally, be alleviated by changes within the CCU. Recommended changes will not be instituted by nursing or hospital administrators unless there is the impetus of strong recommendations by the CCU nursing staff.

REFERENCES

1. Borysenko J: Minding the Body, Mending the Mind. Reading, MA, Addison-Wesley, 1987
2. Kasl SV: Stress and health. Annu Rev Public Health 5: 319–341, 1984
3. Kiecolt-Glaser JK, Glaser R: Psychological influences on immunity. Psychosomatics 27(9):621–624, 1986
4. Ader R, Felten D, Cohen N: Psychoneuroimmunology. New York, Academic Press, 1991
5. Megargee EI: The dynamics of aggression and their application to cardiovascular disorder. In Chesney MA, Rosenman RH (eds): Anger and Hostility in Cardiovascular and Behavioral Disorders, pp 31–57. New York, McGraw-Hill, 1985
6. Hay D, Oken D: The psychological stresses of intensive care nursing. Psychosom Med 34:109–118, 1972
7. Cassem N, Hackett T: Sources of tension for the CCU nurse. Am J Nurs 72:1426–1430, 1972
8. Gardam J: Nursing stresses in the intensive care unit. JAMA 208:2337–2338, 1969
9. Gardam J: Observations on intensive care units. Superv Nurse 3:27–28, 33–42, 44, 1972
10. Gentry W, Foster S, Froeling S: Psychologic response to situational stress in intensive and non-intensive care units. Heart Lung 1:793–796, 1972
11. Kornfield D: Psychiatric problems of an intensive care unit. Med Clin North Am 55:1353–1363, 1971
12. Koumans A: Psychiatric consultation in an intensive care unit. JAMA 194:633–637, 1965
13. Gilligan C: Mapping the Moral Domain: A Contribution of Women's Thinking to Psychological Theory and Education. Cambridge, MA, Harvard University Press, 1988
14. Gilligan C: Making Connections: The Relational Worlds of Adolescent Girls at Emma Willard School. Cambridge, MA, Harvard University Press, 1990
15. Esteban A, Ballestros P, Cabbalero J: Psychological evaluation of intensive care nurses. Crit Care Med 11:616–620, 1983
16. Jacobsen S: Stressful situations for neonatal intensive care nurses. MCN 3:144–150, 1978
17. Maloney J, Bartz C: Stress-tolerant people: Intensive care nurses compared with non-intensive care nurses. Heart Lung 12:389–394, 1983
18. Mohl P, Denny N, Mote T, Coldwater C: Hospital unit stressors that affect nurses: Primary task vs. social factors. Psychosomatics 23:366–374, 1982
19. Nichols K, Springford V, Searle J: An investigation of distress and discontent in various types of nursing. J Adv Nurs 6:311, 1981

20. Alberts M: Doctor–nurse communication. RN 39: ICCU-6, 1976
21. Gardner D, Parzen Z, Stewart N: The nurse's dilemma: Mediating stress in critical care units. Heart Lung 9: 103–106, 1980
22. Nadelson T: The psychiatrist in the surgical intensive care unit. Regist Nurse 39:ICCU/CCU-6, 7, 1976
23. Simon N, Whitely S: Psychiatric consultation with MICU Nurses: The consultation conference as a working group. Heart Lung 6:497–504, 1977
24. Gardner D, Parzen Z, Stewart N: The nurse's dilemma: Mediating stress in critical care units. Heart Lung 9: 103–106, 1980
25. Toffler A: Future Shock, pp 19–47. New York, Bantam Books, 1970
26. Nelson M, Fells R: What job attributes are important to nurses? Aust J Adv Nurs 7:350–355, 1989
27. Dodds A, Lawrence J, Wearing A: What makes nursing satisfying: A comparison of college students' and registered nurses' views. J Adv Nurs 16(6):741–753, 1991
28. Beattie, M: Codependent No More. San Francisco, Harper & Row, 1987
29. Schaef AW, Fassel D: The Addictive Organization. New York, Harper & Row, 1988
30. Miller J: Toward a New Psychology of Women. Boston, Beacon Press, 1986
31. Bowen M: Theory in the practice of psychotherapy. In Guerrin P (ed): Family Therapy: Theory and Practice, pp 42–90. New York, Gardner Press, 1976
32. Anderson M, Chiriboga D, Bailey J: Changes in management stressors on ICU nurses. DCCN 7(2):111–117, 1988
33. Bartz C, Maloney J: Burnout among intensive care nurses. Res Nurs Health 9:147–153, 1986
34. Brack G, La Clave L, Heumann K: Consultation on the medical frontier. Gen Hosp Psychiatry 11:174–181, 1989
35. Cavanagh S: Nursing turnover: Literature review and methodological critique. J Adv Nurs 14:587–596, 1989
36. Foxall M, Zimmerman L, Standley R, Captain BB: A comparison of frequency and sources of nursing job stress perceived by intensive care, hospice and medical-surgical nurses. J Adv Nurs 15:577–584, 1990
37. Hart SK, Moore M: The relationship among organizational climate variables and nurse stability in critical care units. J Prof Nurs 3:124–131, 1989
38. Oehler J, Davidson MG, Starr L, Lee D: Burnout, job stress, anxiety, and perceived social support in neonatal nurses. Heart Lung 5:500–505, 1991
39. Rosenthal S, Schmid K, Black M: Stress and coping in a NICU. Res Nurs Health 12:257–265, 1989
40. Sosnowitz B, Hriceniak J: Neonatal intensive care units can be hazardous to nurses' health. J Perinatol 3:253–257, 1988
41. Barry P: Psychosocial Nursing Assessment and Intervention, p 327. Philadelphia, JB Lippincott, 1989
42. Chess T, Chess S: Temperament and Development. New York, Brunner/Mazel, 1977
43. Blanck G, Blanck R: Ego Psychology II: Psychoanalytic Development Psychology. New York, Columbia University Press, 1979
44. Lazarus R: Cognitive and coping processes in emotion. In Monat A, Lazarus R (eds): Stress and Coping: An Anthology. New York, Columbia University Press, 1977

45. Maloney J, Bartz C: Stress-tolerant people: Intensive care nurses compared with non-intensive care nurses. Heart Lung 12:389–394, 1983
46. Maloney J: Job stress and its consequences on a group of intensive and non-intensive care nurses. ANS Adv Nurs Sci 4:31, 1982
47. Kobasa S, Puscetti M: Personality and social resources in stress resources in stress resistance. J Pers Soc Psychol 45:839–850, 1983
48. Hart SK, Moore M: The relationship among organizational climate variables and nurse stability in critical care units. J Prof Nurs 3:124–131, 1989
49. Coleman B: Advanced nursing apprenticeship program: A strategy for retention of experienced critical care nurses. Heart Lung 19(3):236–242, 1990
50. Volk M, Lucas M: Relationship of management style and anticipated turnover. DCCN 10(1):35–40, 1991
51. Stroebel C: QR: The Quieting Reflex. New York, Berkley Books, 1982
52. Baldwin A: Mental health consultation in the intensive care unit: Toward a greater balance and precision of attribution. J Psychiatr Nurs 2:17–21, 1978
53. Cassem N, Hackett T: The setting of intensive care. In Hackett T, Cassam N (eds): Massachusetts General Hospital Handbook of General Psychiatry, pp 319–341. St Louis, CV Mosby, 1978
54. Eisendrath S, Dundel J: Psychological issues in intensive care unit staff. Heart Lung 8:751–758, 1979
55. Gowan N: The perceptual world of the intensive care unit: An overview of some environmental considerations in the helping relationship. Heart Lung 8:340–344, 1979
56. Melia K: The intensive care unit: A stress situation? Nurs Times 73:17–20, 1977
57. West N: Stresses associated with ICUs affect patients, families, staff. Hospitals 49:62–63, 1975

BIBLIOGRAPHY

Allen D, Calkin J, Peterson M: Making shared governance work: a conceptual model. J Nurs Adm 18(1):37–43, 1988
Bailey JT, Steffen SM, Grout JW: The stress audit: Identifying the stressors of ICU nursing. J Nurs Educ 19:15–25, 1980
Bartz C: Re: Stress in ICU and non-ICU nurses (letter). Nurs Res 35:59, 1986
Blackburn S: The neonatal ICU: A high-risk environment. Am J Nurs 82:1708–1712, 1982
Bryson RW, Aderman M, Sampiere JM et al.: Intensive care nurse: Job tension and satisfaction as a function of experience level. Crit Care Med 13:767–769, 1985
Buscherdorf J: On my own terms: the redefinition of success in nursing. Image J Nurs Sch 22(2):84–88, 1990
Caldwell T, Weiner M: Stresses and coping in ICU nursing: A review. Gen Hosp Psychiatry 3:119, 1981
Caraway B: The day I "quit" nursing. Nursing '89 1:100, 1989
Dolan S: The relationship between burnout and job satisfaction in nurses. J Adv Nurs 12:3–12, 1987
Gentry W, Parks K: Psychologic stress in intensive care unit and non-intensive care unit nursing: A review of the past decade. Heart Lung 11:42–47, 1982
Gilligan C: In a Different Voice: Psychological Theory and

Women's Development. Cambridge, MA, Harvard University Press, 1982

Horowitz M: Stress Response Syndromes. New York, Jason Aronson, 1976

Huckaby L, Jagla B: Nurses' stress factors in the intensive care unit. J Nurs Adm 2:21–26, 1979

Keane A, Ducette J, Adler DC: Stress in ICU and non-ICU nurses. Nurs Res 34:231–236, 1985

Kelly JG, Cross DG: Stress, coping behaviors, and recommendations for intensive care and medical surgical ward registered nurses. Res Nurs Health 8:321–328, 1985

Kernoff P et al: The job context index: A guide for improving the 'fit' between nurses and their work environment. J Adv Nurs 14:501–508, 1989

Kiecolt-Glaser JK, Speicher CE, Holliday JE, Glaser R: Stress and the transformation of lymphocytes by Epstein-Barr virus. J Behav Med 7:1–12, 1984

Kobasa S, Maddi S, Kahn S: Hardiness and health: a prospective study. J Pers Soc Psychol 1:168–177, 1982

Kobasa SC, Maddi SR, Courington S: Personality and constitution as mediators in the stress illness relationship. J Health Soc Behav 22:368–378, 1981

Meyerholz S: Find a nurse. Nurs Manage 21:25–26, 1990

Mitchell BK: Re: Stress in ICU and non-ICU nurses (letter). Nurs Res 36:135, 1987

Paternak I: The effects of primary care nursing and feeling of isolation/depersonalization of the critical care nurse, Part I: Background for the study. Nurs Manage 19:112I–112P, 1988

Pilkington P: Reclaim the role: Definition and examination of the nursing role. Lamp 46:22–28, 1989

Seymour E, Buscherhof J: Sources and consequences of satisfaction and dissatisfaction in nursing: findings from a national sample. Int J Nurs Stud 2:109–124, 1991

Spragg J: CC and med/surg nurses: Another story. Nurs Manage 10:8–9, 1990

Stehle J: The findings revisited. Nurs Res 30:182–186, 1981

Summers S: Re: Stress in ICU and non-ICU nurses (letter). Nurs Res 36:135, 1987

Trobaugh M: Preceptorship: A quality issue in the PACU. J Post Anesth Nurs 5:321–322, 1989

Vincent P, Coleman WF: Comparison of major stressors perceived by ICU and non-ICU nurses. Crit Care Nurse 6:64–69, 1986

STUDY QUESTIONS

1. Effective coping in the intensive care unit is assisted by the following personality traits:
   a. boldness
   b. respect
   c. assertiveness
   d. aloofness

2. Which one of the following is *not* a normal response to acute anxiety?
   a. decrease in skin temperature
   b. increase in problem-solving ability
   c. increase in diastolic blood pressure
   d. increase in pulse

3. Research has shown that CCU nurses demonstrate higher scores on which one of the following traits if compared with non-ICU nurses?
   a. detachment
   b. personal problems
   c. maladaption
   d. somatic complaints

4. A significant cause of stress commonly identified by critical care nurses is
   a. conflict with the nursing manager
   b. poor CCU design
   c. high noise levels
   d. conflict with physicians

PART III

The Critical Care Nursing Process Applied to Alterations in Core Body Systems

UNIT 1

Cardiovascular System

CHAPTER 11

Anatomy and Physiology of the Cardiovascular System

BEHAVIORAL OBJECTIVES

Based on the content in this chapter, the reader should able to:

1. Briefly describe the characteristics of cardiac muscle cells.
2. Explain the difference between electrical events and mechanical events in the heart.
3. Define *depolarization*.
4. Describe the normal conduction system of the heart.
5. State the formula for calculating cardiac output.
6. Briefly explain the role of the parasympathetic and sympathetic nervous systems in the regulation of heart rate.
7. State the three factors involved in the regulation of stroke volume
8. Define *preload* and *afterload*.

Hudak: Critical Care Nursing:
A Holistic Approach, 6th ed. © 1994
J. B. Lippincott Company.

Description

During the 70 years in the life of the average person, the heart will pump approximately 5 quarts of blood a minute, 75 gallons an hour, 57 barrels a day, and 1.5 million barrels in a lifetime. Although the work accomplished by this organ is out of proportion to its size, for most people the heart functions normally throughout the life span. The pumping action of the heart moves blood, a vital substance, throughout the body, supplying oxygen and nutrients to cells and removing waste. Without this action, cells die. For those people in whom cardiac problems develop, the results may be dramatic and the outcome drastic. This chapter will discuss the following aspects of heart action:

- Cardiac microstructure
- Anatomic and physiological bases for contraction
- Physiological basis for events of the cardiac cycle
- Factors influencing cardiac output and perfusion
- Coronary circulation
- Peripheral circulation

Physiological Principles

Cardiac Microstructure

Microscopically, cardiac muscle contains visible stripes, or striations, similar to those found in skeletal muscle (Fig. 11–1). The ultrastructural pattern also resembles that of

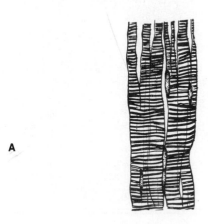

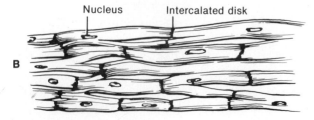

Nucleus   Intercalated disk

FIGURE 11–1
Histologic features of the two types of contractile tissue. (**A**) Striated muscle. (**B**) Cardiac tissue.

striated muscle. The cells branch and connect freely, and they form a three-dimensional, complex network. The elongated nuclei, like those of smooth muscle, are found deep in the interior of the cells and not next to the cell membrane as they are in striated muscle.

Cardiac muscle (myocardial) cells are endowed with extraordinary characteristics, most of which belong to the cell membrane or sarcolemma. To pump effectively, the heart muscle must begin contraction as a single unit. To contract myocardial cells simultaneously, cell membranes must depolarize at the same time. The heart does this, without using much neural tissue, by rapidly conducting impulses from cell to cell through intercalated disks. At each end of every myocardial cell, adjacent cell membranes are folded elaborately and attached strongly. These areas comprise the intercalated disks, where depolarization is conducted from one cell to the next extremely rapidly (see Fig. 11–1B).

Another extraordinary characteristic of myocardial cells, seen mainly in cell membranes, is automaticity. Selected groups of cardiac cells are capable of initiating rhythmic action potentials, and thus waves of contraction, without any outside humoral or nervous intervention.

Within each cardiac cell lie thousands of contractile elements, the overlapping actin and myosin filaments. Figure 11–2 illustrates these elements and the changes seen during diastole and systole. Not shown are the many cross-bridges that extend like rows of oars from the surface of the thicker myosin filaments. During diastole, these bridges are unattached to other filaments. The arrangement of actin and myosin filaments gives cardiac muscle its banded or striated appearance. One grouping of actin and myosin filaments, bounded by sarcoplasmic reticulum (SR), is called a sarcomere.

Mechanical Events of Contraction

Before mechanical contraction, an action potential travels quickly over each cell membrane and down into each cell's SR. When an action potential causes depolarization of the SR, calcium ions move from the SR into the myocardial cell cytoplasm and bind to troponin molecules on actin filaments. Calcium-bound troponin moves slightly to uncover binding sites on the actin, to which myosin filaments then attach. With a release of energy stored in adenosine triphosphate (ATP), these binding sites move so that actin and myosin slide past each other and new couplings between actin and myosin occur. Rapid, successive uncoupling of cross-bridges and their reattachment to new actin-binding sites lead to rapid and dramatic shortening of the sarcomere (see Fig. 11–2). This shortening is the essence of myocardial contraction (systole). Contraction ceases when the calcium ions return to their storage sites on the SR, thereby causing the binding sites on the actin filaments to be covered again. The separated actin and myosin

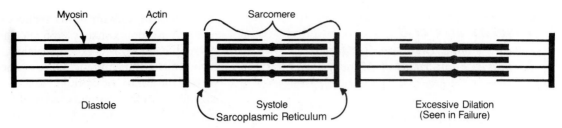

FIGURE 11–2
Contractile elements lying inside a single sarcomere of a myocardial cell.

filaments then slip past each other in the reverse direction, lengthening the sarcomere to its relaxed state.

Contraction requires both calcium and energy. The presence of adequate ATP stores and the movement of calcium provide the essential link between electrical events of depolarization and the mechanical events of contraction in the heart.

Electrical Events of Depolarization

Membranes of all the cells in the human body are charged, that is, they are polarized and therefore have electrical potentials. This means simply that there is a separation of charges at the membrane. In humans, all cell membranes, regardless of type, are positively charged at rest, with more positively charged particles at the outer surface of the cell membrane than at the inner surface.

Figure 11–3A illustrates this "resting stage." This does not mean that there is a lack of negatively charged particles at the outer surface, nor that there is a lack of positively charged particles at the inner surface. It merely means that there is a net difference in the number and kind of charged particles at the outer surface compared to the inner surface.

Cardiac muscle membranes are polarized, and the electrical potential can be measured, as it can in any of the cells in the human body. The potential results from the difference between intracellular and extracellular concentrations of electrolytes. When salt compounds of various elements are dissolved in aqueous solutions, they dissociate into their charged particles, called ions.

In the resting myocardial cell, there are more potassium ions inside than outside the cell, and more sodium and unbound calcium ions outside than inside the cell. All three of these positively charged ions (cations) may diffuse through pores, or channels, in the cell membrane. If each ion freely obeyed the law of diffusion, however, potassium would diffuse out of the cell, whereas sodium and calcium would diffuse into it. Very soon there would be equal concentrations of each ion between the intracellular and extracellular fluids, and no resting potential would exist. It is through the selective regulation of the concentrations of these ions on either side of the membrane that the resting membrane potential is maintained (see Display Box 11–1). Several factors contribute to this regulation. The first factor is the presence of sodium–potassium "pumps" within the cell membrane. These pumps move sodium out of the cell and potassium into the cell, with both movements occurring against the concentration gradients for each of these ions. The second factor is the active movement of calcium out of the cell against the concentration gradient in response to the passive diffusion of sodium into the cell. The third factor is the regulation of membrane channels whereby calcium ions can enter the resting myocardial cell. The fourth factor is the presence of intracellular anions (negatively charged particles) that are too large to exit from the cell. Keeping these factors in mind, let us now look at the physiological events underlying both the resting potential and the action potential.

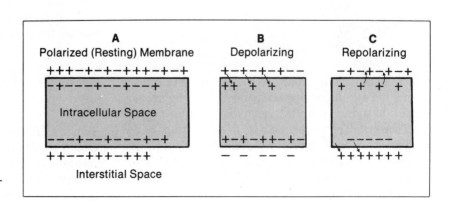

FIGURE 11–3
Electrical events at rest (diastole) and preceding contraction (systole).

Physiological Basis of the Resting Potential

The cardiac cell contains large anions that cannot exit the cell. These anions attract sodium and potassium cations, which diffuse through membrane channels into the cell. The anions would attract the calcium cation also, except that the membrane channels for the entry of this ion are closed when the cell is at rest. The potassium ions remain within the cell, but the sodium ions are pumped out of the cell almost as fast as they can enter by the sodium–potassium "pumps" located within the cell membrane. While forcing sodium out of the cell, these pumps actively transport potassium ions into the cell, against their concentration gradients. This increase in intracellular potassium still is insufficient to offset all the intracellular anions. Thus, the inside of the myocardial cell remains negative with respect to the outside—as long as the pumps are operative. This produces the resting potential, which is approximately -80 mV. For each molecule of an ion "pumped" from the cell, one molecule of ATP is required to provide the energy necessary to effect the chemical bond between ion and carrier. Maintaining a resting potential thus requires energy.

Physiological Basis of the Action Potential

When a stimulus is applied to the polarized cell membrane, the membrane that ordinarily is only slightly permeable to sodium permits sodium ions to diffuse rapidly into the cell. This occurs because of inactivation of the sodium active transport enzymes (pumps). The result is a reversal of net charges. The outer surface is now more negative than positive, and the membrane is said to be depolarized (see Fig. 11–3B).

When the sodium influx reduces the polarity from -80 mV to approximately -35 mV, the electrical change opens the previously closed "calcium channels" in the myocardial cell membrane. Once opened, these channels permit the influx of calcium. The entry of this cation, together with the continued entry of sodium, is responsible for the remainder of the depolarization, which continues until the polarity of the extracellular side equals approximately $+30$ mV. Such a maximal depolarization inactivates sodium–potassium pumps in nearby membranes. This can cause depolarization in these areas. When the original depolarization becomes self-propagating in this way, it is termed an action potential. In a myocardial cell, an action potential triggers the release of intracellular calcium from its storage sites on the SR. This plus the calcium influx across the sarcolemma elevates intracellular calcium levels, thereby initiating muscular contraction, as previously described.

If the depolarization remains below a certain critical (threshold) point, it will die out without having opened any calcium channel or inactivated any adjacent sodium–potassium pumps. Because it does not become self-propagating and remains localized, such a depolarization is termed a local depolarization.

During depolarization, the elevated intracellular sodium concentration frees potassium ions to diffuse out of the cell in accordance with their concentration gradient. Just as this potassium efflux gains some momentum, however, the sodium–potassium pumps automatically reactivate (they can be inactivated only temporarily). Once reactivated, they begin to restore the original resting potential. This is termed repolarization (see Fig. 11–3C). During the initial phase of repolarization, the efflux of both potassium and sodium ions exceeds their influx, but as the intracellular sodium ions are removed from the cell, potassium ions remain as the major cation to be electrostatically held within the cell by the intracellular anions. This halts the potassium efflux. The remainder of repolarization consists of pump activity that increases intracellular potassium and decreases intracellular sodium. Thus, the resting potential is reestablished. The electrical events at the start of repolarization also reclose the calcium entry channels, thereby halting calcium influx. Intracellular calcium levels are reduced when the diffusion of sodium into the cell causes a movement of calcium out of the cell against the latter's concentration gradient.

Cardiac Macrostructure and Conduction

To pump effectively, large portions of cardiac muscle must receive an action potential nearly simultaneously. Special cells that conduct action potentials extremely rapidly are arranged in pathways through the heart. All these cells have automaticity.

The heart chambers and specialized tissues are diagrammed in Figure 11–4. In the wall of the right atrium is the sinoatrial (SA) node. The cells of the SA node have the property of automaticity. Because the SA node normally discharges at a rate faster than any other heart cell with automaticity (60 to 100 beats/minute), this specialized tissue acts as a normal cardiac pacemaker. In the lower right portion of the interatrial septum is the atrioventricular (AV) node. This tissue acts to conduct, yet delay, the atrial action potential before it travels to the ventricles.

Atrial action potentials travel through atrial cells by intercalated disks, although some specialized conductive tissue in the atria has been discovered. Action potentials reach the AV node at different times, however. The AV node slows conduction of these action potentials until all potentials have exited the atria and entered the AV node. After this slight delay, the AV node passes the action potential all at once, to the ventricular conduction tissue, allowing for nearly simultaneous contraction of all ventricular cells. This AV node delay also allows time for the atria fully to eject their load of blood into the ventricles, in preparation for ventricular systole.

From the AV node, the impulse travels down the bundle of His in the interventricular septum into either a right or left bundle branch, and then through one of many Purkinje fibers to the ventricular myocardial tissue itself. An action potential can traverse this conducting tissue three to seven times more rapidly than it can travel through the ventricular myocardium. Thus, the bundle, branches, and Purkinje fibers enable a near-simultaneous contraction of all portions of the ventricle, thereby allowing the maximal unified pump action to occur.

Electrocardiograms

Conduction of an action potential through the heart can be shown by an electrocardiogram (ECG; Fig. 11–5). Because ECGs will be extensively covered in a later chapter, discussion here is brief. An ECG does not show mechanical events of the heart, but in the normal heart, coupling of electrical and mechanical events can be assumed (see Chapter 12).

In Figure 11–5, point 1 shows early ventricular diastole, when both the atria and the ventricles are at rest. Blood is passively filling both atria from the large veins and is spilling over into the ventricles. The AV valves are open.

At point 2, the beginning of late ventricular diastole, both ventricles remain relaxed and are about three-quarters full.

Due to automaticity, the SA node fires spontaneously and both atria depolarize, generating a P wave. Blood is moved actively from the atria into the ventricles.

At point 3, late in the PR interval (PR), the action potential begun in the SA node is being delayed and "collected" in the AV node, and travels to the bundle of His. Both the atria and ventricles are at rest.

At point 4, the action potential moves to the septum, which depolarizes and leads to the Q wave. Septal depolarization is rapidly followed by action potential movement down the right and left bundles into the Purkinje fibers, to all cardiac muscle cells. These electrical events are seen as the RS waves on the ECG, and are followed rapidly by mechanical contraction of both ventricles. The AV valves close, and the aortic and pulmonic valves open.

At point 5, the heart returns to early ventricular di-

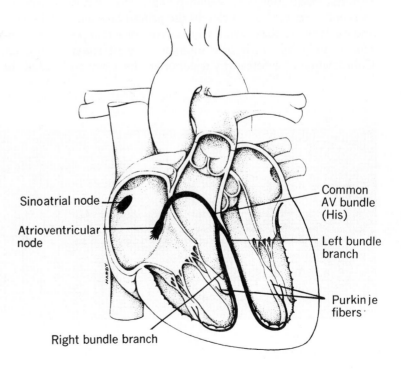

FIGURE 11–4

Distribution of the conductive tissue in the human heart.

Sinoatrial node

Atrioventricular node

Common AV bundle (His)

Left bundle branch

Purkinje fibers

Right bundle branch

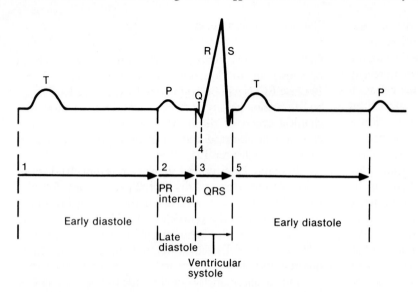

FIGURE 11-5

A comparison of electrical and mechanical events during one cardiac cycle, using a normal ECG tracing.

astole, and the ventricles repolarize. This repolarization shows as a large, wide T wave. The aortic and pulmonic valves close about midway through repolarization.

Because the QRS represents ventricular depolarization, shortly after a QRS is seen on the ECG, a single pulse will be felt in an artery. The number of QRSs seen, or the number of pulsations felt, in 1 minute, equals the heart rate. Figure 11-6 illustrates a normal ECG tracing. There is no Q wave in Figure 11-6, which can be a normal occurrence.

Rhythmicity and Pacing

Automaticity is an inherent property of myocardial conduction cells, and occurs as a result of a spontaneous and rhythmic inactivation of the sodium pumps. Under abnormal conditions, cardiac muscle cells also gain automaticity, and can produce their own rhythmic series of action potentials and, thus, their own stimulus for contraction. Coordination of automaticity is important for rhythmic cardiac contraction and is achieved through the varying rates of automaticity found in different cardiac tissues.

The SA node, located between the openings of the inferior and superior venae cavae in the right atrial wall, discharges at a resting rate of 60 to 100 times/minute. The remainder of the conduction system and ventricles have progressively slower rates of discharge. The AV node discharges at a rate of 40 to 60 times/minute. The conduction tissues in the ventricles discharge about 20 to 40 times/minute. The group of cells with the fastest rate of automaticity paces the heart. Normally, this is the SA node.

If conduction from the SA node to the AV node is disrupted, the fastest pacemaker tissue on both sides of this interruption will govern their respective areas, and the ECG may evidence two independent rhythms. Atrial systole is not needed for the ventricle to fill with blood because most ventricular filling is passive and occurs in early diastole. The clinically important rhythm is that of the ventricles; they are the chambers that supply the lungs and the rest of the body with blood. Their systolic rate

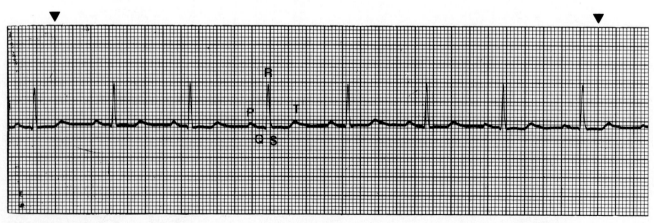

FIGURE 11-6
Normal ECG tracing.

helps determine true perfusion. The slower the rate, the less able are the ventricles to meet the perfusion needs of the body during exercise or activities of daily living. A very rapid ventricular rhythm also will compromise perfusion needs, because the shorter the diastole, the less time for filling of the chambers. Decreased ventricular filling will reduce cardiac output.

Cardiac Output

Cardiac output (CO) is a traditional measure of cardiac function. It is the amount of blood, in liters, ejected from the left ventricle each minute, and is the product of heart rate (HR) and the volume ejected per ventricular contraction or stroke volume (SV):

$$CO = HR \text{ (beats/min)} \times SV \text{ (liters/beat)}$$

Normal CO ranges from 4 to 8 liters/minute. The output can be altered to meet changing bodily demands for tissue perfusion, but the cardiac output equation does not account for differences in body size. An output of 5 may be adequate for a 50-kg man but insufficient for a 120-kg man. Because perfusion is a function of body size, a newer and more accurate measure of cardiac function is cardiac index (CI), which represents the amount of blood, in liters, ejected each minute from the left ventricle (or CO) per square meter of body surface area:

$$CI = \frac{CO \text{ (liters/min)}}{body \text{ surface area (m}^2)}$$

It typically averages 3.0 ± 0.2 liters/minute and ranges from 2.8 to 4.2 liters/minute/m^2.

Because of the relationship of stroke volume and heart rate with cardiac index, we will examine these further.

Regulation of Heart Rate

Although the heart has the ability to beat independently of any extrinsic influence, cardiac rate is under autonomic and adrenal catecholamine influence. Both parasympathetic and sympathetic fibers innervate the SA and AV nodes. In addition, some sympathetic fibers terminate in myocardial tissues.

Parasympathetic stimulation releases acetylcholine near the nodal cells. This decreases the rate of depolarization, thereby slowing cardiac rate. Stimulation of sympathetic fibers causes the release of norepinephrine. This chemical increases the rate of nodal depolarization. It also has ino-

---

DISPLAY BOX 11–2
α *and* β *Effects of Autonomic Nervous System on the Heart and Vascularity*

Effector Organ	Cholinergic Impulses Response	Noradrenergic Impulses Receptor Type	Response
Heart			
SA node	Decrease in heart rate; vagal arrest	β_1	Increase in heart rate
Atria	Decrease in contractility and (usually) increase in conduction velocity	β_1	Increase in contractility and conduction velocity
AV node and conduction system	Decrease in conduction velocity; AV block	β_1	Increase in conduction velocity
Ventricles	—	β_1	Increase in contractility and conduction velocity
Arterioles			
Coronary, skeletal muscle, pulmonary, abdominal viscera, renal	Dilation	α β_2	Constriction Dilation
Skin and mucosa, cerebral, salivary glands	—	α	Constriction
Systemic Veins	—	α β_2	Constriction Dilation

tropic effects on myocardial fibers, which will be discussed later. Thus, sympathetic stimulation increases heart rate (see Display Box 11–2). The adrenal medulla also releases norepinephrine and epinephrine into the bloodstream. These circulating catecholamines act on the heart in the same way as sympathetic stimulation.

There are two reflexes that adjust heart rate to blood pressure: the aortic reflex and the Bainbridge reflex. In the aortic reflex (Fig. 11–7A), a rise in arterial blood pressure stimulates aortic and carotid sinus baroreceptors to fire sensory impulses to the cardioregulatory center in the medulla. This causes an increase in parasympathetic stimulation or a decrease in sympathetic stimulation to the heart. Thus, a rise in arterial blood pressure reflexively causes a slowing of cardiac rate. That results in a decrease in output, which, in turn, can decrease arterial blood pressure. Conversely, a fall in arterial blood pressure, such as in shock, will reflexively increase heart rate. This aortic reflex is an ongoing regulatory mechanism for homeostasis of arterial blood pressure.

The Bainbridge reflex (see Fig. 11–7B) uses receptors in the venae cavae. An increase in venous return stimulates these receptors, which then fire sensory impulses that travel to the cardioregulatory center. These reflexively cause a decrease in parasympathetic cardiac stimulation and an increase in sympathetic cardiac stimulation, thereby increasing cardiac rate. A fall in venous return causes a decrease in heart rate. Thus, the Bainbridge reflex adjusts cardiac rate to handle venous return.

Regulation of Stroke Volume

Stroke volume is the amount of blood ejected by the left ventricle during systole. Normal values range from 60 to 100 ml/beat. Three factors are involved: 1) preload, 2) afterload (or wall tension), and 3) inherent inotropic myocardial contractility.

Preload

Preload is the amount of stretch placed on a cardiac muscle fiber just before systole. Usually, the amount of stretch in any chamber is proportional to the volume of blood the chamber contains at the end of diastole, before systole. Thus, many practitioners equate volume with preload.

The concept of preload is related to Starling's Law of the heart, which states that the force of myocardial contraction is determined by the length of the muscle cell fibers.

Within a certain range (0.05–2.2 μm), increasing myofibril stretch will increase the force of systole. Beyond optimal fibril length (about 2.2 μm), it is hypothesized that too few actin–myosin binding sites overlap to provide an adequate contraction. Below optimal shortening (about 0.05 μm), there is little room for filaments to slide, and cell walls limit further sliding. Also, actin filaments may have begun to overlap, decreasing the number of binding sites available to myosin fibers.

When the force of systole decreases, the chamber

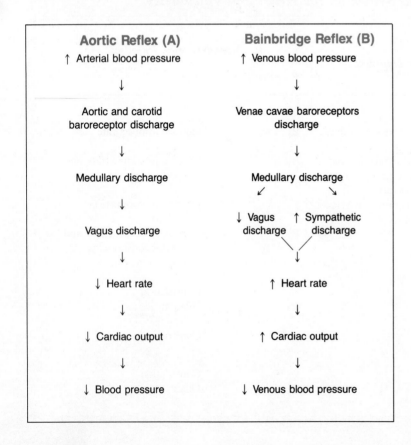

FIGURE 11–7
Effects of (**A**) aortic reflex and (**B**) Bainbridge reflex on heart rate.

pumps poorly, and does not empty properly. Excessive blood is left in the chamber at the end of systole. During diastole, when the chamber fills, this extra blood causes overfilling of the chamber and increases stretch. The next systole will be even weaker, as preload increases during every diastole.

Because preload is a measure of volume at the end of diastole, it often is equated with end-diastolic volume or pressure. Thus, left ventricular preload is represented by left ventricular end-diastolic pressure.

An example of rapid and normal adjustments to changes in preload occurs during the Valsalva maneuver. The first part of the Valsalva occurs when one holds one's breath and bears down, such as during defecation or heavy lifting. Bearing down increases intra-abdominal and intra-thoracic pressures, which decreases venous return to the right atrium and ventricle. Right heart preload decreases. Bearing down also stimulates the vagus nerve, and the heart rate slows.

On exhalation, during the second part of the Valsalva maneuver, intrathoracic pressures decrease rapidly, allowing a sudden increase in venous return. Right atrial and ventricular preloads increase dramatically, stretch increases, and the right ventricular stroke volume increases. Atrial stretch receptors also signal the medulla and lead to sympathetic nervous discharge. Heart rate increases.

Afterload

Afterload is the force or pressure against which a cardiac chamber must eject blood during systole. The most critical factor determining afterload is vascular resistance, in either the systemic or pulmonic vessels. Afterload often is equated with systemic vascular resistance or pulmonary vascular resistance.

Afterload affects stroke volume by increasing or decreasing the ease of emptying a ventricle during systole. A decrease in systemic vascular resistance, through vasodilation, presents the left ventricle with relatively large, open, relaxed arteries into which it can pump. Because it is easier to pump, the left ventricles will empty easily, which increases stroke volume.

If systemic vascular resistance increases, for example through catecholamine-induced constriction of arteries, it takes a great deal more force for the left ventricle to pump into such a tightened vasculature. Stroke volume will decrease.

Inotropic Action

Inotropic capabilities and cardiac workload refer to contractile forces. Cardiac muscle forces change in response to neural stimuli and to circulating levels of catecholamines. It is thought that, through cyclic adenosine monophosphate mechanisms, cardiac cells change intracellular levels of calcium and ATP. These changes lead to increased inotropic actions, although the mechanisms remain unknown.

It is known, however, that increased inotropic action increases the oxygen consumption of heart cells. This increased consumption also is called increased workload and increased oxygen demand.

Cardiac output depends on heart rate and stroke volume. Regardless of the initial cause of increased stroke volume (increased preload, increased afterload, or increased inotropic force), an increase in stroke volume increases workload. Similarly, an increased heart rate, no matter the cause, increases oxygen demand.

Coronary Circulation

Blood supply to the myocardium is derived from the two main coronary arteries that originate from the aorta, immediately above the aortic valve. The left coronary artery supplies the major portion of the left ventricle, and the right coronary artery supplies the major portion of the right ventricle.

Shortly after its origin, the left coronary vessel branches into the anterior descending artery, which traverses the groove between the two ventricles on the anterior surface of the heart, and the circumflex artery, which passes to the left and posteriorly in the groove between the left atrium and the left ventricle. The circumflex branch may terminate before reaching the posterior side of the heart, or it may continue into the posterior groove between the left and right ventricles. The coronary circulation is referred to as *dominant left* if this branch of the left coronary artery supplies the posterior aspect of the heart, including the septum.

Seventy-five percent of human hearts are *dominant right*. When this situation prevails, the right coronary artery passes posteriorly and is responsible for the blood supply to the posterior side of the heart and the posterior portion of the interventricular septum.

Because of their anatomic deviation from the aorta (above the aortic valve) and the fact that they lie between myocardial fibers, blood flow through the coronary arteries occurs during ventricular diastole, not systole. Therefore, anything that decreases the diastolic time (eg, tachycardia) will decrease coronary perfusion.

Peripheral Circulation

The biologic significance of the cardiovascular system is tissue perfusion. Such perfusion supplies the body's cells with oxygen and nutrients while carrying away metabolic wastes, including carbon dioxide. Tissue perfusion is directly proportional to the rate of blood flow, which, in turn, depends on several factors. One factor is the difference between the mean arterial blood pressure and right atrial pressure (usually represented by the central venous pressure). The greater this difference, the faster the flow rate (all else being unchanged). Conversely, if arterial pressure falls or venous pressure rises, flow rate and, thus, tissue perfusion will be decreased.

Another factor affecting flow rate is vascular resistance, already discussed. The relationship between vascular resistance and blood flow has two general applications. One is to describe the flow rate through vessels of differing diameters (eg, arteries, capillaries). The other application concerns the ongoing regulation of blood flow by means of adjustments in arteriole diameters (ie, constriction, dilation). Arteriole constriction reduces the radius, thereby increasing resistance and decreasing the flow rate. Conversely, arteriole dilation increases the flow rate.

The other two factors that can affect the flow rate normally are held constant. They are 1) the sum of all vessel lengths, and 2) blood viscosity. Because these factors do not normally change significantly, they usually are omitted from flow rate considerations. Their relationships are obvious, however. The greater the length of a vessel, the more resistance, and thus the slower the flow rate. Also, the more viscous the blood, the slower the rate of its flow. Blood viscosity is determined by the proportion of solvent (water) to solute and other particles, including blood cells and platelets. The less water and the more particles, the more viscous the blood. The complete equation that describes all four factors is as follows:

$$\text{flow rate} = \frac{\text{mean arterial pressure} - \text{central venous pressure}}{\substack{\text{resistance} \times \text{viscosity} \\ \times \text{ vessel length}}}$$

Because blood volume and pressure have such an important influence on tissue perfusion, we will examine the factors that alter and regulate them.

Blood Volume

Urinary output and fluid input are the major normal mechanisms for regulating volume. The greater the output or the less the fluid input, the less the volume—if all else is held constant. Factors that alter the volume of urine excreted every 24 hours include those that alter the glomerular filtration rate and the tubular reabsorption of water, with or without electrolytes. (For a more detailed explanation of these factors, see Chapter 31, specifically the discussion of normal endocrine physiology that considers the antidiuretic hormone.) Pathologic conditions that promote any type of fluid loss (eg, burns, severe diarrhea, osmotic diuresis) or a shift of water from the

vascular to the interstitial compartment have the potential for reducing blood volume.

Blood Pressure

Because the difference between arterial and venous pressures is the driving force for blood circulation and tissue perfusion, we will examine first those factors that influence central venous pressure, then the factors that regulate arterial blood pressure. Central venous pressure is, strictly speaking, the pressure of blood in the venae cavae just before its entry into the right atrium. It can be increased by either an increase in blood volume (eg, intravenous fluid overload) or a decrease in the pumping ability of the heart (eg, cardiac failure).

Because the pulsatile effects of the cardiac cycle are removed by capillary networks, venous pressure is recorded as an average, or mean, and reported in millimeters of mercury (mm Hg).

Arterial blood pressure is the pressure of blood in the arteries and arterioles. This is a pulsatile pressure, due to the cardiac cycle, and systolic (peak) and diastolic (trough) numbers are reported, in millimeters of mercury. Average or mean arterial blood pressure can be clinically useful as an indicator of average perfusion pressures.

Arterial blood pressure is regulated by the vasomotor tone of the arteries and arterioles, the amount of blood entering the arteries per systole (ie, cardiac output), and blood volume itself. The greater the volume or output, the greater would be the blood pressure, and *vice versa*—if vasomotor tone were held constant. The normal regulation of vasomotor tone involves both neural and hormonal mechanisms.

Neural regulation is mediated by the vasomotor center of the medulla oblongata. This center consists of vasopressor and depressor subdivisions. It receives neural input from 1) baroreceptors in the carotid sinuses and aorta, 2) atrial diastolic stretch receptors, 3) the limbic system and hypothalamus, 4) the midbrain, and 5) pulmonary stretch receptors. In addition, it is directly responsive to local hypoxia or hypercapnia. Neural outputs from the vasopressor center result in increased sympathetic stimulation to arterial smooth muscle cells. This results in arterial constriction and a rise in arterial blood pressure. Stimulation of the depressor area decreases such sympathetic stimulation.

Rapid adjustments in arterial blood pressure are effected primarily by the baroreceptor reflexes. Here, an increase in the pressure on these receptors (directly by elevated blood pressure or manual compression, and indirectly by increased blood volume) reflexively stimulates the depressor area. This results in decreased sympathetic stimulation to major arteries and the aorta, which causes a fall in arterial blood pressure. Decreased baroreceptor stimulation by a fall in arterial blood pressure reflexively stimulates the pressor area and results in increased sympathetic stimulation to arterial muscles, causing a rise in arterial blood pressure. Thus, homeostasis of arterial pressure is maintained.

In orthostatic hypotension, the baroreceptor reflex is sluggish. Arterial pressure is not elevated rapidly enough, so the postural change results in a temporary decrease in brain perfusion that leads, in extreme cases, to syncope.

Various other factors may alter arterial blood pressure reflexively by their influences on the vasomotor center. Nerve fibers from the limbic system and hypothalamus are believed to mediate emotionally produced alterations in blood pressure. An example of this is fainting, caused by neurally mediated vasodilation in response to the sight of blood or very bad news—or very good news! Neural inputs from the midbrain and possibly from ascending spinothalamic fibers in the medulla result in both the elevation in arterial pressure that initially accompanies severe pain and in the later fall in arterial pressure that occurs when severe pain is prolonged. Lung inflation stimulates pulmonary stretch receptors. Their input to the vasomotor center reflexively decreases arterial pressure. Hypercapnia, and, to a lesser extent, hypoxia of vasomotor neurons stimulate the pressor area, reflexively causing a rise in arterial pressure. Such stimuli obviously are not part of a normal daily regulatory mechanism but can operate as a normal compensatory mechanism in certain pathologic situations. Elevated intracranial pressure can promote medullary hypercapnia and hypoxia. This increase in arterial pressure reflexively produced by these stimuli (Cushing's reflex) increases medullary perfusion, which can ameliorate the medullary hypoxia or hypercapnia, or both. Hormonal regulation of arterial blood pressure is effected by adrenal medulla catecholamines and the renin–angiotensin system. In the former, adrenal medullary catecholamines mimic the action of sympathetic fibers innervating the muscle layer or arteries (tunica media), causing arterial constriction and elevating arterial pressure. The renin–angiotensin system is discussed in Chapter 22. Briefly, a decreased glomerular filtration rate, which can result, for example, from a fall in blood volume or renal perfusion, stimulates the secretion of renin from the juxtaglomerular apparatus. This leads to the production of angiotensin II, which acts directly on tunica media to promote vasoconstriction. Thus, renin elevates arterial pressure, which, in turn, increases renal perfusion and glomerular filtration.

Finally, arterial blood pressure can be influenced by alterations in the level of unbound calcium within tunica media cells. Such levels are, in turn, influenced by factors that open or close calcium channels in the membranes of these muscle cells. Drugs that block calcium channels ("calcium blockers") inhibit the entry of calcium into cells. Such decreased calcium influx can lower intracellular calcium levels sufficiently to decrease muscle contractility, including contractility of the heart, thereby promoting a degree of vasodilation and lowering the arterial pressure.

BIBLIOGRAPHY

Akesson EJ, Loeb JA, Wilson-Pauwels L: Thompson's Core Textbook of Anatomy, 2nd ed. Philadelphia, JB Lippincott, 1990

Chatterjee K, Cheitlin M, et al: Cardiology: An Illustrated Text Reference, vol. 1. Philadelphia, JB Lippincott, 1991

Ganong WF: Review of Medical Physiology, 15th ed. Norwalk, CT, Appleton & Lange Medical Publications, 1991

Guyton AC: Textbook of Medical Physiology, 8th ed. Philadelphia, WB Saunders, 1991

Hole JW Jr: Essentials of Human Anatomy and Physiology, 4th ed. Dubuque, IA, WC Brown, 1992

Memmler RL: Human Body in Health and Disease, 7th ed. Philadelphia, JB Lippincott, 1992

Porth CM: Pathophysiology: Concepts of Altered Health States. Philadelphia, JB Lippincott, 1990

STUDY QUESTIONS

1. Preload refers to

    a. the pressure against which the cardiac chamber must eject blood during systole
    b. cardiac workload
    c. the amount of stretch placed on the cardiac muscle fiber just before systole
    d. the amount of stretch placed on the cardiac muscle fiber just before diastole

2. Cardiac output is determined by

    a. heart rate times stroke volume
    b. heart rate times end-diastolic volume
    c. stroke volume plus end-diastolic volume
    d. afterload times preload

3. Sources of neural input that regulate the myocardium include

   a. atrial stretch receptors
   b. the limbic system
   c. baroreceptors in the carotid sinus and aorta
   d. all of the above

4. In the normal heart the impulse for cardiac contraction originates in the

   a. AV node
   b. SA node
   c. Bundle of His
   d. Purkinje fibers

Auscultation of the Heart

CHAPTER 12

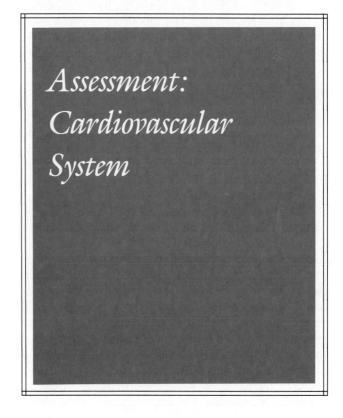

Assessment: Cardiovascular System

BEHAVIORAL OBJECTIVES

Based on the content of this section, the reader should be able to:

1. Discuss four important considerations in preparing a patient for a cardiac examination.
2. Locate the four areas of auscultation on the anterior chest wall.
3. Discuss the mechanisms responsible for the production of the first and second heart sounds and the phases of the cardiac cycle these sounds represent.
4. Discuss the clinical significance of the third and fourth heart sounds and their timing in the cardiac cycle.

(continued)

Hudak: Critical Care Nursing:
A Holistic Approach, 6th ed. © 1994
J. B. Lippincott Company.

BEHAVIORAL OBJECTIVES (Continued)

5. Describe each type of murmur, its timing in the cardiac cycle, and the area on the chest wall where it is most easily auscultated.

Description

Observation and auscultation are by far the most crucial components of the cardiac examination. For a clinician to become adept in the skill of cardiac auscultation, a basic understanding of normal cardiac anatomy and physiology must be mastered. This is only the first step, however. Perfection of the skill can be accomplished only by endless hours of listening. The data obtained by careful and thorough auscultation of the heart are essential in planning and evaluating care of the critically ill patient.

In this section the basic principles underlying examination of the patient, the factors responsible for the production of normal heart sounds, and the pathophysiological conditions responsible for the production of extra sounds, murmurs, and friction rubs will be discussed. This information must then be taken to the clinical area and applied.

Physical Examination

To facilitate accurate auscultation the patient should be relaxed and comfortable, in a quiet warm environment, with adequate lighting. The patient should be in a recumbent position with the trunk elevated 30° to 45°.

A good-quality stethoscope is essential. The earpieces should fit the ears snugly and comfortably, and follow the natural angle of the ear canals. Sound waves that travel a shorter distance are more intense and less distorted; therefore, the tubing of the stethoscope should be approximately 12 inches in length and somewhat rigid. It is best to have two tubes leading from the head of the stethoscope, one to each ear. The head of the stethoscope should be equipped with both a diaphragm and a bell on a valve system that allows the clinician to switch easily between the two components. The diaphragm is used to hear high-frequency sounds such as the first and second heart sounds (S_1, S_2), friction rubs, systolic murmurs, and diastolic insufficiency murmurs. The diaphragm should be placed firmly on the chest wall to create a tight seal. Low-frequency sounds like the third and fourth heart sounds (S_3, S_4) and the diastolic murmurs of mitral and tricuspid stenosis are best heard with the stethoscope bell, which should be placed lightly on the chest wall only to seal the edges.

Auscultation of the precordium should be done systematically (Fig. 12–1). The nurse should begin the examination listening with the stethoscope diaphragm at the

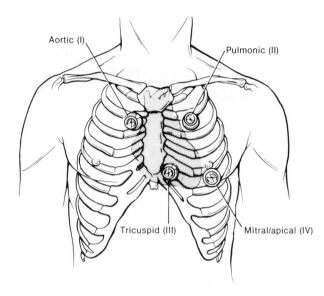

FIGURE 12–1
Areas of auscultation.
  I. Aortic area (second intercostal space to the right of the sternum).
 II. Pulmonic area (second intercostal space to the left of the sternum).
III. Tricuspid area (fifth intercostal space to the left of the sternum).
 IV. Mitral or apical area (fifth intercostal space midclavicular line).

aortic area where S_2 is loudest, then move to the pulmonic area, and from there inch the stethoscope down the left sternal border to the tricuspid area and out to the mitral area or apex of the heart, where S_2 is the loudest. This pattern should then be repeated with the stethoscope bell.

In each area auscultated, the clinician should identify S_1, noting the intensity of the sound, respiratory variation, and splitting. S_2 should then be identified and the same characteristics assessed. After S_1 and S_2 are identified, the presence of extra sounds is noted—first in systole, then in diastole. Finally, each area is auscultated for the presence of murmurs and friction rubs.

Heart Sounds

The First Heart Sound

S_1 (Fig. 12–2) is timed with the closure of the mitral and tricuspid valves at the beginning of ventricular systole. Because mitral valve closure is responsible for most of the sound produced, S_1 is heard best in the mitral or apical area. The upstroke of the carotid pulse correlates with S_1 and can be used to help distinguish S_1 from S_2.

The intensity (loudness) of S_1 varies with the position of the atrioventricular (AV) valve leaflets at the beginning of ventricular systole and the structure of the leaflets (thick-

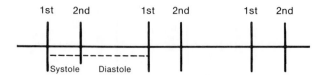

Normal: S₁ is produced by the closure of the AV valves and correlates with the beginning of ventricular systole. It is heard best in the apical or mitral area.

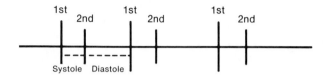

Loud First Sound: The intensity of the first heart sound may be increased when the PR interval is shortened, as in tachycardia, or when the valve leaflets are thickened, as in mitral stenosis.

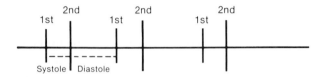

Soft First Sound: A soft S₁ is heard when the PR interval is prolonged.

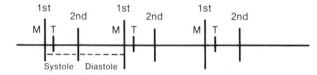

Split First Sound: A split S₁ is heard when right ventricular emptying is delayed. The mitral valve closes before the tricuspid valve and "splits" the sound into its two components.

FIGURE 12–2
Variations in the first heart sound.

ened or normal). A loud S₁ is produced when the valve leaflets are wide open at the onset of ventricular systole and corresponds to a short PR interval on the surface electrocardiogram (ECG) tracing. A lengthening of the PR interval will produce a soft S₁ because the leaflets have had time to float partially closed before ventricular systole. Mitral stenosis also will increase the intensity of S₁ due to a thickening of the valvular structures.

Generally, S₁ is heard as a single sound. If right ventricular systole is delayed, however, S₁ may be split into its two component sounds. The most common cause of this splitting is delay in the conduction of impulses through the right bundle branch; the splitting correlates with a right bundle branch block pattern on the ECG. Splitting of S₁ is heard best over the tricuspid area.

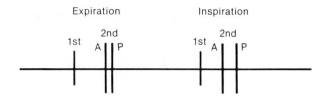

FIGURE 12–3
The second heart sound is produced by the closure of the semilunar valves (aortic and pulmonary). During inspiration there is an increase in venous return to the right heart, which causes a delay in the emptying of the right ventricle and the closure of the pulmonic valve. This allows the two components of the second heart sound to separate or split during inspiration.

The Second Heart Sound

S₂ (Fig. 12–3) is produced by the vibrations initiated by the closure of the aortic and pulmonic semilunar valves and is heard best at the base of the heart. This sound represents the beginning of ventricular diastole.

Like S₁, S₂ consists of two separate components. The first component of S₂ is aortic valve closure; the second component is pulmonic valve closure.

With inspiration, systole of the right ventricle is slightly prolonged owing to increased filling of the right ventricle. This causes the pulmonic valve to close later than the aortic valve and S₂ to become "split" into its two components. This normal finding is termed "physiological splitting." Physiological splitting is heard best on inspiration with the stethoscope placed in the second intercostal space to the left of the sternum.

The intensity of S₂ may be increased in the presence of aortic or pulmonic valvular stenosis or with an increase in the diastolic pressure forcing the semilunar valves to close, as occurs in pulmonary or systemic hypertension.

The Third Heart Sound

S₃ (Fig. 12–4) may be physiological or pathologic. A physiological S₃ is a normal finding in children and healthy young adults; it usually disappears after 25 to 35 years of

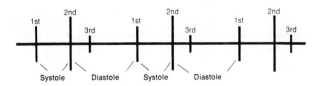

FIGURE 12–4
The third heart sound. An S₃ or ventricular gallop is heard in early diastole, shortly after the second heart sound. The presence of a pathologic S₃ can be indicative of heart failure.

age. An S_3 heard in an older adult with heart disease signifies ventricular failure. S_3 is a low-frequency sound that occurs during the early, rapid-filling phase of ventricular diastole. A noncompliant or failing ventricle cannot distend to accept this rapid inflow of blood. This causes turbulent flow, resulting in the vibration of the AV valvular structures or the ventricles themselves producing a low-frequency sound. An S_3 associated with left ventricular failure is heard best at the apex with the stethoscope bell. The sound may be accentuated by turning the patient slightly to the left side. A right ventricular S_3 is heard best at the xiphoid or lower left sternal border and varies in intensity with respiration, becoming louder on inspiration.

The Fourth Heart Sound

S_4 or atrial gallop (Fig. 12–5) is a low-frequency sound heard late in diastole just before S_1. It is rarely heard in healthy patients. The sound is produced by atrial contraction forcing blood into a noncompliant ventricle that, by virtue of its noncompliance, has an increased resistance to filling. Systemic hypertension, myocardial infarction, angina, cardiomyopathy, and aortic stenosis all may produce a decrease in left ventricular compliance and an S_4. A left ventricular S_4 is auscultated at the apex with the bell of the stethoscope. Conditions affecting right ventricular compliance, such as pulmonary hypertension or pulmonic stenosis, may produce a right ventricular S_4 heard best at the lower left sternal border; it increases in intensity during inspiration.

The Summation Gallop

With rapid heart rates, as ventricular diastole shortens, an S_3 and S_4, if both present, may fuse together and become audible as a single diastolic sound. This is called a summation gallop (Fig. 12–6). This sound is loudest at the apex and is heard best with the stethoscope bell while the patient lies turned slightly to the left side.

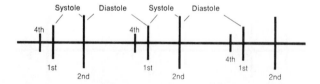

FIGURE 12–5
The fourth heart sound is a late diastolic sound that occurs just prior to S_1. It is a low-frequency sound heard best with the bell of the stethoscope.

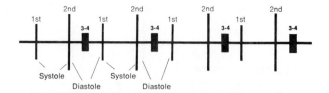

FIGURE 12–6
With rapid heart rates, S_3 and S_4 may become audible as a single, very loud sound that occurs in mid-diastole. This sound is called a summation gallop.

Heart Murmurs

Murmurs are sounds produced either by the forward flow of blood through a narrowed or constricted valve into a dilated vessel or chamber or by the backward flow of blood through an incompetent valve or septal defect. Murmur classification is based on timing in the cardiac cycle. Systolic murmurs occur between S_1 and S_2. Diastolic murmurs occur after S_2 and before the onset of the following S_1. Murmurs are described further according to the anatomic location on the anterior chest where the sound is heard the loudest. Any radiation of the sound also should be noted. The quality of the sound produced is described as blowing, harsh, rumbling, or musical in nature. The intensity or loudness of a murmur is described using a grading system. Grade I is faint and barely audible; grade II is soft; grade III is audible but not palpable; grade IV and V murmurs are associated with a palpable thrill; and a grade VI murmur is audible without a stethoscope.

Systolic Murmurs

As previously described, S_1 is produced by mitral and tricuspid valve closure and signifies the onset of ventricular systole. Murmurs occurring after S_1 and before S_2 are therefore classified as systolic murmurs.

During ventricular systole the aortic and pulmonic valves are open. If either of these is stenotic or narrowed, a sound classified as a midsystolic ejection murmur is heard. Because the AV valves close before blood is ejected through the aortic and pulmonic valves, there is a delay after S_1 and the beginning of the murmur. The murmurs associated with aortic stenosis and pulmonic stenosis are described as crescendo–decrescendo or diamond shaped (Fig. 12–7), meaning that the sound increases, then decreases in intensity. The quality of these murmurs is harsh, and they are of medium pitch. The murmur caused by aortic stenosis is heard best in the aortic area and may radiate up into the neck. The murmur of pulmonic stenosis is heard best over the pulmonic area.

Systolic regurgitant murmurs are caused by the back-

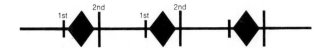

FIGURE 12–7
Blood flow through a stenotic aortic or pulmonic valve will produce a crescendo–decrescendo midsystolic ejection murmur.

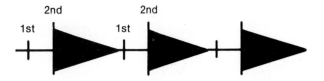

FIGURE 12–9
Murmur of aortic or pulmonic insufficiency. Regurgitant flow through an incompetent aortic or pulmonic valve produces a decrescendo diastolic murmur.

ward flow of blood from an area of higher pressure to an area of lower pressure. Mitral or tricuspid valvular insufficiency or a defect in the ventricular septum will produce systolic regurgitant murmurs, which are harsh and blowing in quality. The sound is described as holosystolic, meaning that the murmur begins immediately after S_1 and continues throughout systole up to S_2 (Fig. 12–8).

Mitral insufficiency produces this type of murmur, heard most easily in the apical area with radiation to the left axilla. This type of murmur, associated with tricuspid insufficiency, is heard loudest at the left sternal border and increases in intensity during inspiration. This murmur may radiate to the cardiac apex.

A ventricular septal defect also will produce a harsh, blowing holosystolic sound caused by blood flowing from the left to the right ventricle through a defect in the septal wall during systole. The associated murmur is heard best from the fourth to sixth intercostal spaces on both sides of the sternum, and is accompanied by a palpable thrill.

Diastolic Murmurs

Diastolic murmurs occur after S_2 and before the next S_1. During diastole the aortic and pulmonic valves are closed while the mitral and tricuspid valves are open to allow filling of the ventricles.

Aortic or pulmonic valvular insufficiency produces a blowing diastolic murmur that begins immediately after S_2 and decreases in intensity as regurgitant flow decreases

through diastole. These murmurs are described as early diastolic decrescendo murmurs (Fig. 12–9).

The aortic insufficiency murmur is heard best in the aortic area and may radiate along the right sternal border to the apex. Pulmonic valve insufficiency produces a murmur that is loudest in the pulmonic area.

Stenosis or narrowing of the mitral or tricuspid valve also will produce a diastolic murmur. The AV valves open in mid-diastole shortly after the aortic and pulmonic valves close, causing a delay between S_2 and the start of the murmur of mitral and tricuspid stenosis. This murmur decreases in intensity from its onset, then increases again as ventricular filling increases due to atrial contraction. This is termed decrescendo–crescendo (Fig. 12–10).

The murmur associated with mitral stenosis is heard best at the apex with the patient turned slightly to the left side. Tricuspid stenosis produces a murmur that increases in intensity with inspiration and is loudest in the fifth intercostal space along the left sternal border.

Friction Rubs

A pericardial friction rub can be heard when the pericardial surfaces are inflamed. This high-pitched, scratchy sound is produced by these inflamed layers rubbing together. A rub may be heard anywhere over the pericardium with the diaphragm of the stethoscope. The rub may be accentuated by having the patient lean forward and exhale. A pericardial friction rub, unlike a pleural friction rub, does not vary in intensity with respiration.

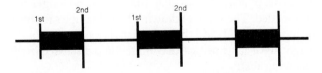

FIGURE 12–8
A holosystolic murmur is caused by the regurgitant flow of blood through an incompetent mitral or tricuspid valve. Flow of blood from the left ventricle to the right ventricle through a ventricular septal defect also will produce this type of murmur.

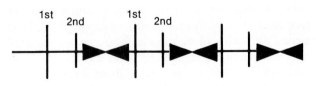

FIGURE 12–10
The murmur of mitral or tricuspid stenosis is a low-frequency murmur heard best with the bell of the stethoscope. It occurs after S_2 and has a decrescendo–crescendo configuration.

Cardiac Enzyme Studies

BEHAVIORAL OBJECTIVES

Based on the content in this section, the reader should be able to:

1. Describe the role of enzyme studies in diagnosing an acute myocardial infarction.
2. Compare and contrast the usefulness of creatine kinase (CK) and lactate dehydrogenase (LDH) isoenzyme studies.
3. List possible etiologies of serum CK and LDH elevations other than acute myocardial infarction–ischemia.
4. Interpret CK and LDH isoenzyme studies when providing patient care.

Description

Knowledge of the purpose and significance of laboratory values in relation to the diagnosis and prognosis of acute myocardial infarction can enhance the quality of nursing care available to patients. With a basic understanding of serum enzyme determinations, the nurse can exercise judgment in interpreting results relative to other information about the patient. The ability to use this kind of judgment may well affect the patient's clinical course or prognosis. It certainly is as important to the physical and mental well-being of these patients to rule out the presence of acute myocardial infarction as it is to confirm its existence. In addition, knowledge about serum enzymes can result in their more judicious use and cost savings to the patient.

Enzymes. Enzymes are found in all living cells and act as catalysts in biochemical reactions. They are present in low amounts in the serum of normal people, but when cells are injured, enzymes leak from the damaged cells, resulting in serum enzyme concentrations above the usual low levels. No single enzyme is specific to the cells of a single organ. Each organ contains a variety of enzymes and there is considerable overlap among organs in the enzymes they contain. The distribution of enzymes within the cells of organs is relatively organ specific, however. When organ damage occurs, the presence of abnormally high levels of enzymes in the serum, their distribution, and the time patterns for their serum appearance and disappearance make the clinical use of serum enzyme studies relevant.

Cardiac enzymes. Cardiac enzymes are those enzymes found in cardiac tissue. When cardiac injury occurs, as in acute myocardial infarction, these enzymes are released into the serum, and their concentrations can be measured (Fig. 12–11). Unfortunately, the cardiac tissue enzymes also are present in other organs so that elevation of one or more of these enzymes is not a specific indicator of cardiac injury. Because cardiac damage does result in above-normal serum concentrations of these enzymes, however, the quantification of cardiac enzyme levels, along with other diagnostic tests and the clinical presentation of the patient, is routinely used for diagnosing cardiac disease, particularly acute myocardial infarction.

Only three of the many enzymes present in cardiac tissue have widespread use in the diagnosis of acute myocardial infarction. Lactate dehydrogenase and serum glutamic-oxaloacetic transaminase (SGOT) were first used in the 1950s. Since the mid-1960s, CK has become the most important addition to the enzyme diagnosis of acute myocardial infarction. None of the three is specific to cardiac tissue; however, CK and LDH can be divided further into components, or isoenzymes. In each case, at least one of the isoenzymes is more specific for cardiac disease, and it is the increase in these more specific components of LDH or CK relative to their other isoenzymes that has resulted in their common use. Because of the nonspecificity of SGOT and the widespread availability of CK and LDH isoenzymes, the routine sampling of serum for SGOT for the diagnosis of acute myocardial infarction is no longer recommended. The value of drawing blood samples for measuring CK, LDH, and their associated isoenzymes for the diagnosis of acute myocardial infarction is discussed in the following text.

Creatine Kinase

The level of total CK in plasma usually becomes abnormal 6 to 8 hours after onset of infarction and peaks between 24 and 28 hours. When patients appear at the hospital soon

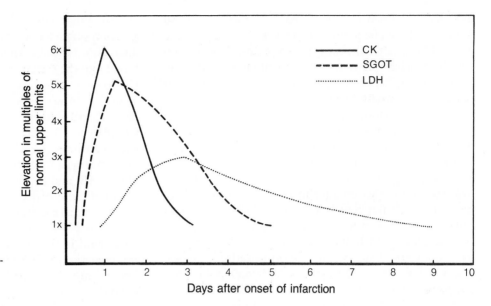

FIGURE 12–11
Peak elevation and duration of serum enzymes after acute myocardial infarction.

after the onset of symptoms, the initial CK frequently is within normal limits and, at the time of hospital admission, it is not possible to discriminate on the basis of CK those who are having an acute myocardial infarction from those who are not. For this reason, serial sampling of CK for the first 24 hours after the onset of symptoms usually is done every 4 to 6 hours. Within 2 to 4 days after myocardial infarction, serum concentration of total CK usually will have returned to normal. Therefore, abnormal total CK levels may be missed in patients who present more than 24 hours after the onset of infarction. The normal level of total CK typically is higher in men than women and in blacks compared to whites. The upper limit of normal may vary between laboratories, and nurses must be aware of the normal value used in their laboratory. In general, the amount of total CK correlates with the amount of myocardial damage and is of prognostic importance. With a small infarction, total CK may rise two to three times the initial levels but never reach the upper limit of normal; CK isoenzymes can be valuable in these situations.

Skeletal muscle contains more CK than the heart, whereas the cerebral cortex has slightly less CK. Conditions that result in damage or injury to the brain or skeletal muscle also may result in abnormal levels of CK in plasma. Skeletal muscle diseases such as polymyositis and muscular dystrophy as well as the effects of alcohol, strenuous exercise, convulsions, trauma, surgery, and intramuscular injections within skeletal muscle may give rise to abnormal CK levels. Cerebrovascular disease also may result in abnormal CK levels; however, the increase occurs later, lasts longer, and is not as high as the abnormal CK levels due to acute myocardial infarction. Although the clinical presentation of the patient, the ECG, and the amount and time course of abnormal CK levels are useful in determining whether or not the diagnosis of acute myocardial infarction is appropriate, it is not always possible to distinguish myocardial infarction from other clinical conditions. For this reason, CK isoenzymes, in addition to total CK, generally are obtained serially.

Creatine Kinase Isoenzymes

Electrophoresis, glass bead, and radioimmunoassay are techniques used to measure CK isoenzymes. The three CK isoenzymes routinely reported are CK-MM, CK-BB, and CK-MB, found to the greatest extent in skeletal muscle, brain, and heart muscle, respectively. Total CK usually consists entirely of CK-MM, and neither CK-BB nor CK-MB is present; in other words, the normal levels of CK found in healthy people are due entirely to skeletal muscle. Normal skeletal muscle may contain up to 2% CK-MB, and values of CK-MB of up to 5% are not necessarily considered diagnostic. The amount of CK-MB in cardiac muscle is 15% to 22%, with the remainder being CK-MM. When cardiac damage occurs, as in acute myocardial infarction, total CK rises, and the percentage due to CK-MB is greater than 5%. Although other organs, such as the tongue, small intestine, uterus, and prostate, contain CK-MB, the presence of CK-MB in amounts greater than 5% generally is considered diagnostic for myocardial damage in the presence of chest pain or other symptoms believed to represent myocardial ischemia.

CK-MB usually begins to appear in serum 4 to 6 hours after the onset of infarction and peaks at approximately 24 hours. The appearance time and peak, however, may be significantly earlier in patients who have a non-Q wave infarction, or who have undergone successful recannulation of the infarct-related coronary vessel by angioplasty or thrombolytic therapy. Those who present more than 24 hours after the onset of symptoms may not benefit from CK isoenzymes because the levels already may have returned to normal. As with total CK, serial sampling should be performed every 4 to 6 hours for the first 24 hours after the onset of symptoms. Patients who continue to have signs or symptoms of myocardial ischemia after hospital admission should continue to undergo serial CK isoenzyme sampling.

Most laboratories report the absolute amount of each CK isoenzyme present in the serum, although some also report the percentage. Normal values for absolute amounts of each of the CK isoenzymes vary by laboratory and by the measuring technique used. The amount of CK-MB released into the serum after an acute myocardial infarction offers a better correlation with infarction size than total CK because of its specificity to cardiac muscle.

Because total CK and CK isoenzymes are the cardiac enzymes whose levels become abnormal earliest after the onset of infarction, the routine serial sampling for other cardiac enzymes is unnecessary. Serial analysis of CK isoenzymes is the most specific, sensitive, and cost effective means of diagnosing acute myocardial infarction. Perhaps more important, CK isoenzymes also have made possible the ability to "rule out" an acute myocardial infarction more quickly and reliably. It no longer requires 2 to 3 days of CCU hospitalization to determine that SGOT or LDH enzyme levels remain normal; rather, patients can be "ruled out" in less than 24 hours if their CK isoenzyme levels do not become abnormal. Nurses and physicians not only are able to provide earlier reassurance to the patients who are found not to have acute infarction, but patients also can be discharged sooner to a less costly environment than the CCU.

Cardiac disorders other than acute myocardial infarction also may be associated with abnormal total CK and CK-MB levels. These include pericarditis, myocarditis, and trauma. In addition, CK-MB levels have been reported to be abnormal after cardiac surgery and cardioversion. The clinical presentation of the patient and the ECG usually are helpful in distinguishing patients with acute myocardial infarction.

Creatine Kinase Isoforms

Creatine kinase-MB and CK-MM isoenzymes may be divided further into isoform or subform components using electrophoretic or immunoassay techniques. The laboratory performance of these tests is time consuming and labor intensive; however, they are being used clinically in some hospitals. Because isoforms may offer earlier confirmation or exclusion of myocardial infarction than CK isoenzymes, efforts are underway to develop faster and less labor-intensive CK isoform measurements that will result in their widespread clinical use.

Two subforms of CK-MB and three subforms of CK-MM have been identified. Because CK-MB is more specific to cardiac muscle than is CK-MM, CK-MB isoforms are appropriate for the patient with suspected myocardial infarction. Creatine kinase-MB$_2$ (tissue CK-MB) is released into the serum and converted to CK-MB$_1$ (plasma CK-MB) by carboxypeptidase N, another enzyme present in serum. In normal patients, the amounts of CK-MB$_2$ and CK-MB$_1$ present in serum are small and the ratio of CK-MB$_2$ to CK-MB$_1$ is approximately one. In patients with acute myocardial infarction, CK-MB$_2$ is released into the serum in larger quantities than normal and the amount of CK-MB$_2$ and the ratio of CK-MB$_2$ to CK-MB$_1$ in the serum of these patients becomes elevated.

Abnormal elevations of CK-MB$_2$ have been reported as early as 2 hours after onset of symptoms of myocardial infarction.[1] In their study, in patients with acute myocardial infarction, 59% had diagnostic CK-MB isoforms on serum samples obtained within 2 to 4 hours of onset of symptoms, whereas only 23% were diagnostic by the conventional CK isoenzyme assay. In addition, CK-MB isoforms were positive in all patients in whom blood samples were obtained within 8 hours of onset of symptoms, compared to 71% for CK isoenzymes.

Because the ratio of CK-MB$_2$ to CK-MB$_1$ may remain elevated only for up to 12 hours after onset of infarction, CK-MB isoforms likely will not be as useful as CK isoenzymes in patients presenting to the hospital more than 12 hours after the onset of symptoms. Nevertheless, the importance of a reliable early laboratory marker of infarction cannot be underestimated. The period of early sensitivity of CK-MB isoforms is similar to the therapeutic window for the administration of thrombolytic therapy and may be useful in identifying additional patients who could benefit. Also, acute myocardial infarction can be excluded as a diagnosis within 8 hours of symptom onset using CK-MB isoform assay, compared to the 18 to 24 hours required for the conventional CK isoenzyme assay (see Display Box 12–1).

Lactate Dehydrogenase

Lactate dehydrogenase may be found in many organs besides the heart, including the liver, skeletal muscle, kidney, lung, fat, and red blood cells. Total LDH is less specific than CK for cardiac disease. It usually begins to appear in the serum within 24 hours after the onset of acute myocardial infarction and does not peak until 2 to 3 days; it may remain elevated for 7 to 10 days before returning to normal levels. The use of LDH in the diagnosis of acute myocardial infarction is unnecessary if the diagnosis can be confirmed by CK and CK-MB. Patients who present more than 24 hours after the onset of symptoms (CK and CK-MB levels already may have returned to normal) or those who have been having symptoms of myocardial ischemia for several days may be appropriate

DISPLAY BOX 12–1
Cardiac Enzymes After Acute Myocardial Infarction

	Increase	Peak	Return to Normal
CK	3–8 hr	10–30 hr	2–3 days
CK-MB	3–6 hr	10–24 hr	2–3 days
CK-MB$_2$	1–6 hr	4–8 hr	12–48 hr
LDH	14–24 hr	48–72 hr	7–14 days
LDH$_1$	14–24 hr	48–72 hr	7–14 days

for sampling for total LDH and LDH isoenzymes. Although LDH rises more slowly and remains elevated longer than CK, the time course of abnormal levels for both enzymes overlaps. A single sample for LDH may be obtained in patients presenting more than 24 hours after symptom onset, and, if abnormally elevated, be further analyzed for LDH isoenzymes. Routine serial sampling of LDH or LDH isoenzymes in these patients is not recommended because, in the face of nondiagnostic CK isoenzymes, there is no evidence that serial LDH or LDH isoenzyme sampling improves the diagnostic yield.[2]

Because LDH is present in many organs, it may be abnormally elevated in various conditions, including hemolytic anemia, pulmonary infarction, renal infarction, hepatic disorders such as hepatitis and hepatic congestion, and skeletal muscle disorders. Care must be taken when obtaining blood samples for LDH because hemolysis may result in LDH being released from red blood cells, causing falsely elevated levels.

The upper limit of normal for LDH, like CK, is higher in men than women and also varies by laboratory. Nurses must know the normal values for their laboratory.

Lactate Dehydrogenase Isoenzymes

Lactate dehydrogenase isoenzymes are measured by electrophoretic techniques. The isoenzyme that moves most quickly toward the positive pole of the electrical field, LDH$_1$, is found most abundantly in heart muscle. Somewhat lesser amounts of LDH$_1$ are present in kidney, brain, and red blood cells. Lactate dehydrogenase$_5$, the LDH isoenzyme that moves most slowly toward the positive electrode, is found most abundantly in liver and skeletal muscle. Lactate dehydrogenase$_2$, LDH$_3$, and LDH$_4$ are present in intermediate amounts in these organs between the extremes of LDH$_1$ and LDH$_5$. In normal healthy people, LDH$_1$ comprises between 17% and 27% of total LDH, whereas LDH$_2$ comprises 28% to 38%; LDH$_1$ is always present in a lesser percentage than is LDH$_2$. Because the heart contains relatively more LDH$_1$ than LDH$_2$, the ratio of the percentage of LDH$_1$ to LDH$_2$ usually becomes one or more whenever cardiac injury occurs. This "flip" in the ratio of the percentage of LDH$_1$ to LDH$_2$ occurs between 1 and 3 days after the onset of myocardial infarction. Although LDH isoenzymes are not as specific as CK isoenzymes in the diagnosis of acute myocardial infarction, they nevertheless are helpful in patients whose CK isoenzyme levels may have returned to normal.

Diagnostic Limitations

As yet, enzyme determinations can serve only as adjuncts to ECG and clinical diagnosis. To be of most value they should be used with discretion. Consideration must be given to the length of time since the onset of symptoms, because each enzyme rises and returns to normal at different intervals.

Enzyme determinations have been of greatest value to the patient whose ECG and clinical picture are equivocal for diagnosis of myocardial infarction. Enzyme elevation may well confirm a suspected diagnosis in this case. Sometimes it is difficult or impossible to interpret infarction on ECG because of previous infarction changes, the effects of certain drugs or electrolyte imbalances, conduction defects such as bundle branch block or Wolff–Parkinson–White syndrome, dysrhythmias, or a functioning pacemaker. Enzyme determination may be a distinct advantage here. If a definite diagnosis can be made by ECG, enzyme tests may not be needed, except for academic and prognostic interest.

Because serum enzyme elevations are nonspecific in the diagnosis of myocardial infarction, they must be considered in view of the total clinical picture. We are in a highly technical age of nursing, and must not forget to look at and listen to the patient before making judgments and decisions.

Cardiovascular Diagnostic Procedures

BEHAVIORAL OBJECTIVES

Based on the content in this section, the reader should be able to:

1. Describe four current techniques used for diagnostic purposes in cardiology.
2. Outline the patient and family teaching appropriate to prepare the patient for exercise ECG studies.
3. Explain the preparation necessary before cardiac catheterization.
4. Outline the nursing care to be delivered during and after exercise ECG and cardiac catheterization.
5. List potential complications of invasive cardiac studies such as cardiac catheterization.

Description

Cardiovascular diagnostic techniques have expanded dramatically in the past few years, especially in the area of noninvasive testing. This permits a more careful screening of the population for high-risk procedures, as well as low-risk methods for monitoring disease progression and response to treatment. In addition, many of the technologies are being combined so that a functional assessment of a patient's cardiac status can be made to select the best treatment option.

The critical care nurse often cares for patients who undergo one or more of these procedures. Understanding the principles on which the procedures are based enables the nurse to answer questions, incorporate diagnostic findings into the patient's plan of care, and provide high-level nursing care. The critical care nurse also can decrease the anxiety of patients and their families by providing them with an explanation of the procedure the patient is to experience.

Noninvasive Techniques

Standard 12-Lead Electrocardiogram

Purpose

The standard ECG records electrical impulses as they travel through the heart. In patients with normal conduction, the first electrical impulse for each cardiac cycle originates in the sinus node and is spread to the rest of the heart via the specialized conduction system—the intra-atrial tracts, AV node, Bundle of His, and right and left bundles. As the impulse traverses the conduction system, it penetrates the surrounding myocardium and provides the electrical stimuli for atrial and ventricular contraction. The change in electrical potential in cells of the specialized conduction system as the impulse proceeds is very small and cannot be measured from electrodes outside the body. The change in electrical potential of myocardial cells, however, produces an electrical signal that can be recorded from the surface of the body, as is done with an ECG.

Impulses that originate in sites other than the sinus node or impulses that are prevented from traversing the conduction system because of disease or drugs interrupt the normal order of electrical sequences in the myocardium. An ECG may be used to record these abnormal patterns of impulse formation or conduction. The clinician then has a visual record of the abnormal pattern from which to identify the arrhythmia.

In addition, an abnormal ECG tracing may result from diseased myocardial cells. For example, in patients with left ventricular hypertrophy, impulses traversing the enlarged muscle mass of the left ventricle produce a bigger electrical signal than normal. In contrast, impulses are unable to traverse myocardial cells that are irreversibly damaged, such as in myocardial infarction, and no electrical signal is present in the infarcted cells of the left ventricle.

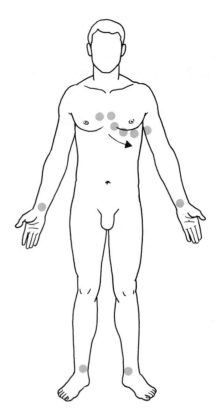

FIGURE 12–12
Standardized 12-lead ECG positions.

Procedure

The standard 12-lead ECG is so named because the usual electrode placement and recording device permit the electrical signal to be registered from 12 different views. The four limb and six precordial leads are attached to the patient as depicted in Figure 12–12. For the limb leads, the recording device alternates the combination of electrodes that are active during recording of electrical signals from the heart (Fig. 12–13). This results in six standard views or leads (I, II, III, aVR, aVL, and aVF) that are recorded in the heart's frontal plane. The six precordial leads (V1, V2, V3, V4, V5, and V6) are arranged across the chest to record electrical activity in the heart's horizontal plane (Fig. 12–14). Abnormal localized areas of myocardial conduction such as occur with ischemia or infarction may be identified in the leads that are nearest to that part of the heart. For example, an inferior myocardial infarction produces changes in the leads that view the inferior aspect of the heart, or leads II, III, and aVF.

Electrocardiograms are used routinely in CCU patients to assess arrhythmias and myocardial ischemia or infarction. The test is performed easily at the bedside with the patient ideally placed in the supine position and the electrodes arranged as previously described. In some patients, chest bandages may preclude placement of the pre-

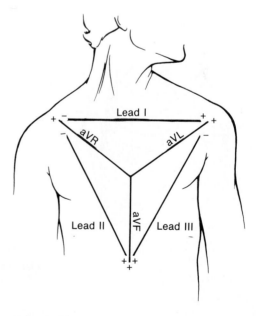

FIGURE 12–13
Frontal plane leads = standard limb leads, I, II, III, plus augmented leads aVR, aVL, and aVF. This allows an examination of electrical conduction across a variety of planes (eg, left arm to leg, right arm to left arm).

cordial leads. It is important that the patient remain still during the ECG recording so that skeletal muscle movement does not result in extraneous noise or artifact in the electrical signal. Additional horizontal plane leads may be recorded by placing electrodes on the right side of the chest to view right ventricular activity or the back of the chest to view left ventricular posterior wall activity.

Nursing Assessment and Management

Critical care nurses often record an ECG in the event of a change in patient status. This change in status includes the development of dysrhythmias. Often, an ECG is obtained during episodes of chest pain before the administration of sublingual nitroglycerin. The ECG provides documentation of ST changes associated with the pain.

Some patients fear they will receive an electrical shock from the ECG recorder, so preparatory instruction for the patient should include an explanation of the manner in which the electrical impulses of the heart are recorded.

Holter Monitoring

Purpose

Ambulatory monitoring of coronary care or telemetry patients provides a noninvasive method of assessing for

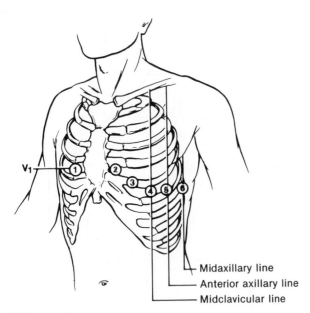

FIGURE 12–14
ECG chest lead placement.
V_1: fourth intercostal space at the right sternal border.
V_2: fourth intercostal space at the left sternal border.
V_3: midway between V_2 and V_4.
V_4: fifth intercostal space at the midclavicular line.
V_5: directly lateral to V_4 at the anterior axillary line.
V_6: directly lateral to V_4 at the midaxillary line.

dysrhythmias, response to dysrhythmia treatment, pacemaker failure, and ECG signs of myocardial ischemia. Patients who present to the hospital with syncope, near syncope, or palpitations may not have recurrence of symptoms while at rest; Holter monitoring permits the patient to be ambulatory while heart rhythm is recorded continuously to ascertain whether the etiology of the symptoms is due to dysrhythmia. Many patients with unstable angina have transient episodes of ST segment depression or elevation without associated angina pectoris; Holter monitoring enables the documentation and quantification of these episodes of "silent ischemia."

Procedure

The Holter monitor is a battery-powered tape recording device that may be worn on a belt around the patient's waist or carried on a shoulder strap. Commonly, two leads are recorded continuously on tape via four or five electrodes placed on the patient's anterior chest; the electrodes are arranged so that one lead reflects the inferior wall of the heart and the other lead reflects the anterior wall. Continuous recording of ECG leads usually is performed for 24 to 48 hours. The Holter monitor contains a clock so that time also is recorded on the tape. After completion of the test, the tape is removed and played back for identification and quantification of ST segment changes or dysrhythmias.

Nursing Assessment and Management

Patients who are scheduled to undergo Holter monitoring should be instructed to bathe before the test because the electrodes cannot be removed during the 24- to 48-hour recording. Skin preparation and electrode placement are crucial to obtaining high-quality ECG recordings. It may be necessary to wrap material or fishnet over the electrodes and cables on the patient's torso to reduce movement artifact. Often, the skin under and around the electrodes becomes irritated, and the patient must be cautioned to avoid pulling at the electrodes because loss of electrical contact can mimic sinus pauses or heart block, making the diagnostic interpretation of the test difficult.

Most Holter monitors have an "event" button that can be pushed whenever symptoms occur; this button sends a signal to mark the tape. Patients are asked to maintain a diary of symptoms and activities and the time they occurred, and should be instructed to record the time from the Holter monitor clock. Patients should be encouraged to maintain normal activities while wearing the monitor and told that it is desirable to record an entry in the diary at least every 2 hours. Hospitalized patients may need the assistance of nursing staff in maintaining their diaries.

Signal-Averaged Electrocardiography

Purpose

Signal-averaged ECG is a noninvasive method for assessing patients who are at high risk for sudden cardiac death due to ventricular arrhythmias. In recent years, it has been used primarily in patients who are recovering from or have a history of myocardial infarction to define the risk for development of ventricular tachycardia. In addition, patients who are admitted with unexplained syncope may benefit from signal-averaged ECG after other noncardiac causes have been excluded.[3]

The major mechanism of ventricular tachycardia in patients with a history of myocardial infarction relates to an area of slow conduction in the left ventricle. This area of slow conduction depolarizes late after most of the ventricle has depolarized, producing small-amplitude and late electrical potentials not visible on the normal 12-lead ECG. The signal-averaged ECG allows these late potentials to be identified by (1) repetitively mapping the patient's QRS complexes onto each other, (2) filtering out noise such as movement or electrical interference, (3) averaging the repetitively mapped QRS complexes, and, finally, (4) amplifying the averaged signal. There is some variation between laboratories in the definition of a positive signal-averaged ECG; however, in general, late potentials are considered to be present if the QRS duration is prolonged, the terminal low amplitude portion of the QRS complex is prolonged, or the root mean square voltage of the terminal portion of the QRS is less than 20 microvolts.

Procedure

In addition to a ground electrode, six other electrodes are placed on the patient's chest during the 20 minutes required for performing the signal-averaged ECG. The six electrodes constitute three paired leads that are at right angles to each other; one set of leads is placed horizontally on the mid-right and left anterior chest, a second set is placed vertically at the top and bottom of the sternum, and the third set is placed anteroposteriorly just to the left of the sternum and on the posterior thorax. The patient must rest quietly in a supine position for the duration of the study. Extraneous noise such as muscle movement interferes with interpretation of the test, and patients who are restless or agitated or have difficulty lying supine are not good subjects for signal-averaged ECG.

Nursing Assessment and Management

The critical care nurse may be responsible for explaining the general format of the test and for emphasizing the need to remain as motionless as possible during the study to achieve accurate data.

Chest Radiography

Purpose

Chest radiography is a routine diagnostic test used in assessing critically ill patients with cardiac disease. The test can be performed easily at the bedside in patients too ill to be transported to the radiology department. The image obtained on a radiograph that allows visualization of vascular and cardiac shapes is based on the premise that thoracic structures vary in density and permit different amounts of radiation to reach the film.

Chest radiography may be used for the evaluation of cardiac size, pulmonary congestion, pleural or pericardial effusions, and the position of intracardiac lines such as transvenous pacemaker electrodes or pulmonary artery catheters.

Procedure

Cardiac size is evaluated best in the radiology department, where the procedure can be standardized with the patient standing and the radiograph taken from a posterior view at a distance of 6 feet. Portable bedside chest radiographs usually are taken from an anterior view with the patient lying supine or sitting erect, and are not standardized.

Patients undergoing radiography of the chest should be instructed to not move while the radiograph is being taken. Proper positioning of the radiographic plate behind the patient is important to ensure that thoracic structures will be aligned on the film. Care should be taken to remove all metal objects, including fasteners on clothing, from the field of view because metal will block the x-ray beam. Patients usually are asked to take a deep breath and hold it when the radiograph is taken to displace the diaphragm downward; this may be uncomfortable for patients who have undergone recent thoracic surgery.

Nursing Assessment and Management

The critical care nurse's role in obtaining diagnostic thoracic radiographic films often is limited to the CCU, where portable radiographs are made. With unstable patients, the nurse must decide when the film can be taken. It is important that intravenous lines not become tangled or loosened while one is trying to place the radiographic plate in the proper position.

Female patients of childbearing potential should have a lead drape placed over the abdomen to protect the ovaries from any radiation scatter. For the same reason, caregivers and family members should leave the patient's room when the radiograph is taken. In those instances where caregivers cannot leave the patient's bedside, a lead apron should be worn.

Echocardiography

Purpose

The use of echocardiography in diagnosing and monitoring heart disease has increased dramatically since its introduction in the 1960s. It now refers to a group of tests that use ultrasound either alone or in combination with other technologies. For many patients, echocardiography has been an invaluable substitute for more invasive procedures in the management of their heart disease. The growth of echocardiography for clinical application is likely to continue. Because of miniaturization of the equipment, research is being conducted on intravascular ultrasound devices that would permit the identification of intraluminal defects.

Echocardiography is used clinically in many cardiac conditions. The type of echocardiogram that is to be performed depends on the condition being evaluated. In critical care patients, echocardiography is used most often to assess ejection fraction, segmental wall motion, systolic and diastolic ventricular volumes, and mitral valve regurgitation due to papillary muscle dysfunction, and to detect the presence of mural thrombi, valve vegetations, or pericardial fluid. It also may be used in the evaluation of function of all four cardiac valves, including calculation of gradients and orifice size, intracardiac tumors, and aortic dissection. In some centers, echocardiography has made it possible for young patients unlikely to have coronary artery disease to undergo valve replacement without requiring a preoperative cardiac catheterization. Although M-mode and two-dimensional echocardiography can be performed easily at the bedside, the reduced noise and light levels of the laboratory usually result in better recordings.

Procedure

The first and simplest use of ultrasound in cardiac patients is *M-mode echocardiography*. It requires a transducer that acts both as a sound transmitter and sound receiver. The transducer is placed on the anterior chest in an intercostal space or subcostal position to avoid bony structures. A single ultrasound beam is sent from the transducer and directed toward the heart. As the sound waves reach various structures in the path of the beam, some pass through and around the structures, and some are reflected back to the transducer by the interface between two structures of differing densities. The more distant the interface, the longer it takes for the reflected sound waves to reach the transducer. A recording device is connected to the transducer so that as the reflected sound waves are received, they are converted to an electrical signal. If only one ultrasound wave beam is emitted from the transducer, the recording will contain echoes from structures in the beam's path. For example, based on transducer position #1 in

Figure 12–15, the recording would contain sound waves reflected from the chest wall, the free right ventricular wall, a space representing the right ventricular cavity, the intraventricular septum, a space representing the left ventricular cavity, and the posterior wall of the left ventricle.

In M-mode echocardiography, ultrasound waves are transmitted intermittently; the remainder of the time, the transducer is receiving the reflected sound waves. Typically, an M-mode recording is made with the reflected sound waves on the vertical axis and time on the horizontal axis. As the heart moves during the cardiac cycle, the recording displays this movement. Because M-mode echocardiography is based on a single beam, the so-called "ice-pick" view, only a small region of the heart can be visualized at any one time. The four positions of the transducer depicted in Figure 12–15 are the typical views used during an M-mode echocardiogram.

Two-dimensional (2D) echocardiography is performed in a similar manner except for two major differences: the ultrasound waves are transmitted in a pie-shaped beam, resulting in a "plane" of reflected echoes, and the recording device is a video camera so that the two dimensions of the plane as well as movement over time are recorded. In addition to parasternal and subcostal transducer positions,

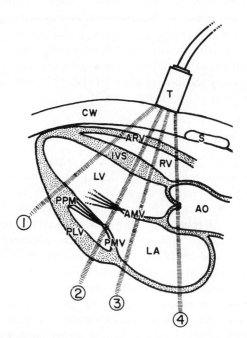

FIGURE 12–15
A cross-section of the heart showing the structures through which the ultrasonic beam passes as it is directed from the apex (1) toward the base (4) of the heart. CW = chest wall; T = transducer; S = sternum; ARV = anterior right ventricular wall; RV = right ventricular cavity; IVS = interventricular septum; LV = left ventricle; PPM = posterior papillary muscle; PLV = posterior left ventricular wall; AMV = anterior mitral valve; PMV = posterior mitral valve; AO = aorta; LA = left atrium. (Feigenbaum H: Clinical applications of echocardiography. Prog Cardiovasc Dis 14:535, 1972)

apical and suprasternal positions also may be used in 2D echocardiography. In recent years, exercise or pharmacologic stress testing has been used in conjunction with 2D echocardiography. A comparison of an image taken at rest is made with an image taken immediately after exercise. In patients with significant coronary artery disease, ventricular wall motion abnormalities will develop after exercise in the segments supplied by diseased arteries.

Doppler echocardiography superimposes Doppler techniques on either M-mode or 2D images. The direction of blood flow can be assessed by measuring echoes reflected from red blood cells as they move away or toward the transducer. This type of study is particularly useful in patients with valvular stenosis or regurgitation; blood flow is quite turbulent through a stenotic valve, and in the opposite direction with regurgitation. When the direction of flow is color encoded, the study is known as a color Doppler echocardiogram. Audio signals usually are recorded during Doppler studies. Contrast material also may be used in conjunction with M-mode or 2D echocardiography. Although many agents have been used as contrast material, almost any liquid injected intravenously contains microbubbles. As the microbubbles travel through the heart, they produce multiple echoes. This technique is especially useful in identifying right-to-left intracardiac shunts because of the early appearance of the microbubble echoes in the left atrium or ventricle.

The most recent type of ultrasound study to be used clinically is *transesophageal echocardiography*. This is made possible by placing a 2D transducer on the end of a flexible endoscope and positioning it at various locations in the esophagus. Doppler and color Doppler also can be added. Because the transducer is closer to cardiac structures, the images are usually superior to those obtained with transthoracic techniques. Transesophageal echocardiography is useful in situations where it is technically impossible to image structures of interest from the usual transthoracic position—in particular, the aorta, atria, and valves.

Nursing Assessment and Management

There are no specific prestudy restrictions for patients undergoing transthoracic echocardiography. During the study, the patient usually is placed in the supine position or turned slightly to the left side. Noise and light should be kept to a minimum during the test. There is no discomfort associated with transthoracic echocardiographic studies; however, the patient may experience chest wall discomfort after the study due to the positioning of the transducer. Suboptimal imaging may occur in patients who are obese or have obstructive lung disease.

Patients who are scheduled to undergo transesophageal echocardiography should take nothing orally (NPO) for 6 or more hours before the study. Mild to moderate sedation may be administered intravenously both before

and during the test. Emergency equipment should be readily available in case of oversedation. A local anesthetic spray usually is applied to the posterior oropharynx to block the gag reflex before the endoscope is inserted orally. After the procedure, the patient should remain NPO until return of the gag reflex.

Phonocardiography

In phonocardiography, heart sounds are recorded by a microphone and converted to electrical activity that is recorded. This procedure may be used to obtain precise measurements of the timing of cardiac cycle events, to determine the characteristics and timing of murmurs and abnormal heart sounds, to measure systolic time intervals, and to teach cardiac auscultation. There are no contraindications or risks associated with this procedure.

Procedure

For a phonocardiogram, the patient is brought to a quiet room and asked to lie on a comfortable table or bed. Microphones are applied to the chest wall over areas where the heart sounds and murmurs are auscultated best. The microphones pick up the sound of the heartbeat and convert it to an electrical impulse that is then amplified, filtered, and recorded. Some of the microphones are allowed to lie free on the chest; others are attached by straps or Ace bandages. A recording of sound waves is obtained, usually in conjunction with an ECG and a carotid pulse wave recording. These accessory recordings provide a reference point for the timing of cardiac events.

Special maneuvers or the use of pharmacologic agents may accentuate certain heart sounds and murmurs. These include the inhalation of amyl nitrate, injection of intravenous isoproterenol or vasopressors, changes in position (sitting or squatting), variations in breathing (deep inspiration and expiration), and the performance of a Valsalva maneuver.

Nursing Assessment and Management

Generally, phonocardiography takes 1 to 2 hours. Patients should be told beforehand that they may be asked to perform certain maneuvers or may be given certain agents to facilitate the diagnostic value of the test.

Exercise Electrocardiography

Purpose

Exercise ECG is used primarily in outpatients to assess patients at risk for the presence of coronary artery disease; however, its use in patients in coronary care and telemetry units is becoming more widespread. Patients who have presented to the hospital with chest pain but without associated ECG changes, have had the diagnosis of infarction excluded, and remained symptom free may undergo exercise ECG to evaluate the etiology of their presenting symptoms and whether continued hospitalization is warranted. It also may be used to evaluate patients with dysrhythmias whose symptoms are exacerbated by exercise. Low-level exercise ECG, a modification of the standard exercise test, is commonly performed predischarge in patients hospitalized with acute myocardial infarction.

Patients with significant coronary artery disease may have normal ECGs at rest when myocardial oxygen supply is sufficient to meet oxygen demands. With increased oxygen demands during exercise, however, coronary blood flow cannot increase adequately owing to coronary artery stenoses, and ECG changes may occur.

Exercise ECG should not be performed in patients who have left bundle branch block or preexcitation at rest because the baseline QRS abnormalities preclude interpreting the ST segment response to exercise. The test also is less specific in women, especially young or middle-aged, than in men. It is common practice to perform a low-level exercise test before hospital discharge after acute myocardial infarction to identify patients at risk for ischemic events as well as to determine exercise prescription. The low-level test exercise target is approximately 70% to 80% of the predicted age-adjusted maximum. In patients with uncomplicated myocardial infarction, the low-level exercise test has been performed safely as early as 3 days after infarction.[4]

Procedure

Although there are various exercise protocols, most are based on either walking on a treadmill or riding a stationary bicycle. The test usually begins at a low level of exercise and increases every 2 to 3 minutes until the patient reaches a target level of oxygen consumption or manifests signs or symptoms of coronary artery disease. Oxygen consumption, the amount of oxygen used in milliliters per minute per kilogram, usually is expressed in metabolic equivalents that take into account the age of the patient. If a treadmill is used to perform exercise, the speed or the uphill slope of the treadmill is increased at the beginning of each 2- to 3-minute stage; in cycling, the resistance of the pedals or braking mechanism is increased at the beginning of each stage.

Patients who have not previously undergone exercise testing should be allowed briefly to practice walking on the treadmill or riding the bicycle. Before starting the test, a resting ECG and blood pressure are obtained with the patient in sitting and standing positions. During the test, an ECG and blood pressure are obtained at the end of each stage of the protocol and immediately before termination. The test usually is terminated when signs or symptoms of

myocardial ischemia develop or the patient manifests other symptoms such as fatigue or dyspnea and cannot continue. In the absence of myocardial ischemia or serious arrhythmias, every effort should be made to reach the patient's predicted level of exercise to avoid a nondiagnostic test. During the recovery period, monitoring of the ECG and blood pressure continues until the patient has reached baseline values. It is mandatory that emergency resuscitation equipment and trained personnel be available in areas where exercise testing is performed.

Indications of myocardial ischemia during exercise testing are the development of: (1) ST segment depression of 1 mm or more; (2) angina pectoris; or (3) failure to increase systolic blood pressure to 120 mm Hg or more or a sustained decrease of 10 mm Hg or more with progressive stages of exercise. The ECG leads in which ST segment depression occurs during exercise are not specific to the coronary artery involved; however, the greater the number of leads with ST segment depression, the more likely it is that the patient has multivessel coronary artery disease. The development of ST segment elevation or T wave changes during exercise testing is not specific for myocardial ischemia, and their significance requires further assessment. Often, exercise ECG is performed in conjunction with echocardiography, radionuclide perfusion imaging, or radionuclide ventriculography to assess better the extent of coronary artery disease and its effect on ventricular function.

Nursing Assessment and Management

Patients who are scheduled to undergo exercise ECG should abstain from eating or drinking caffeine-containing beverages several hours before testing to prevent abdominal cramps or nausea from developing at maximal exercise. They also should have available comfortable shoes for walking on a treadmill or riding a bicycle. The ECG lead system is the same as used for the standard 12-lead cardiogram; however, the limb leads are moved to the torso so that arm or leg movement during exercise will not interfere with ECG recording. Extreme attention is paid to skin preparation and electrode attachment to permit interpretable recordings during maximal exercise. It may be necessary to wrap material or fishnet over the electrodes and cables on the patient's torso to reduce movement artifact.

The critical care nurse may be responsible for explaining the general format of an exercise test to the patient and family. It is important that patients understand why the test is indicated and what will be expected of them. It is reassuring for patients to know that someone will be observing them closely throughout the test and that they are encouraged to express all concerns before, during, and after the procedure. Patients also should understand that they may have to continue exercising after the development of angina but will not be expected to do more exercise than is safe.

Radionuclide Imaging

Purpose

The noninvasive assessment of cardiac structure and function using radiotracers has increased dramatically in the past few years. In particular, radionuclide perfusion studies are playing a bigger role in the diagnosis and treatment of patients with coronary artery disease. The ability of perfusion studies to separate ischemic, viable myocardium from infarcted, nonviable myocardium is used by clinicians to select noninvasive versus invasive strategies such as angioplasty or coronary bypass grafting for treating the underlying coronary artery disease.

Radionuclide perfusion studies provide information not only about the presence of coronary artery disease but also the location and quantity of ischemic and infarcted myocardium. In addition, they offer advantages over exercise ECG when ischemic changes cannot be assessed easily on the ECG, such as in patients with LBBB, paced rhythm, or those receiving digitalis.

New on the horizon and not discussed in detail here is positron emission tomography (PET). The equipment required for PET is expensive and currently is available in only a few centers. Because it offers the ability to image and quantify myocardial metabolism and blood flow, however, it will be useful in distinguishing viable myocardium and evaluating the response of the myocardium to treatment with pharmacologic agents.

Perfusion Imaging

Procedure

Cardiac radionuclide perfusion imaging is based on the fact that a radioactive tracer is taken up in abnormal myocardial cells in either increased or decreased amounts compared to normal myocardium. After injection of the tracer, a gamma camera is used to record an image of radioactive counts from the entire myocardium. An abnormal area with decreased uptake is commonly known as "cold spot" imaging and is the type of study used to assess myocardial perfusion. An abnormal area with increased myocardial uptake or "hot spot" imaging is the type of study used to assess myocardial necrosis.

Perfusion studies are performed most commonly in conjunction with exercise testing so that radionuclide scans obtained at rest and with exercise can be compared. Typically, during rest, the radiotracer is spread uniformly throughout the myocardium and the camera reads counts equally from throughout the myocardium. A similar scan is obtained during exercise in patients without significant coronary artery stenosis as blood flow increases uniformly to meet myocardial oxygen demands. In patients with significant coronary artery disease, however, the image during exercise is altered. The amount of coronary blood flow is limited in stenotic arteries and the quantity of tracer in myocardial segments supplied by stenotic arteries is diminished or absent in comparison to segments supplied by nonstenotic arteries. The presence of an area of decreased tracer uptake during exercise compared to rest is known as a *reversible perfusion defect*.

In patients with previous infarction, decreased uptake may be present on both the rest and exercise scans in the infarcted segments; this pattern is known as a *fixed perfusion defect* and usually signifies nonviable myocardium. It is possible for patients to have fixed perfusion defects in some myocardial segments, reversible defects in others, and normal perfusion in the remaining segments.

Because of the many patients who are physically unable to exercise, pharmacologic agents may be used to mimic the heart's response to exercise. Vasodilating agents such as dipyridamole, adenosine, and dobutamine administered intravenously mimic exercise conditions in the heart by dilating nonstenotic coronary arteries. Coronary blood flow is increased preferentially through normal, nonstenosed arteries; this results in relative hypoperfusion in myocardial segments supplied by stenosed coronary arteries. A radiotracer injected during the peak action of the pharmacologic agent produces images similar to those seen with exercise. As of this writing, only dipyridamole is approved by the Food and Drug Administration for use in perfusion imaging.

Two methods are used to record radioactive images—planar and tomographic. With the planar technique, images of the heart are obtained by the gamma camera from three views—anterior, left anterior oblique (45° to the left of the anterior view), and left lateral, as shown in Figure 12–16. Tomographic or single-photon emission computed tomographic (SPECT) images are obtained by rotating the head of the camera over a 180° arc from the left lateral to the anterior position while stopping to record 32 to 64 times for 20 to 40 seconds each. A computer uses the recorded images to reconstruct multiple slices of the heart along its short axis and both horizontal and vertical long axes.

Three radioactive tracers, thallium-201 (^{210}Tl), technetium-99m-sestamibi (^{99m}Tc-sestamibi) and technetium-99m-teboroxime (^{99m}Tc-teboroxime), are approved for perfusion imaging. Because thallium has been available since 1974, most experience in radionuclide perfusion studies has occurred with this agent. Characteristics of the three agents differ and are responsible for the varying imaging protocols used.

Thallium Protocol

The cardiac half-life of thallium is approximately 7.5 hours, meaning that 50% of the tracer still will be present in myocardial cells 7.5 hours after it is administered. It also redistributes readily, so that thallium in normally perfused areas will move to previously underperfused areas after the

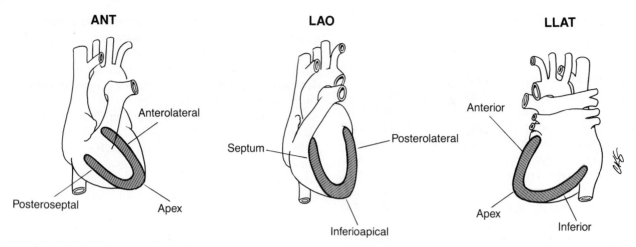

ANT　　　　**LAO**　　　　**LLAT**

FIGURE 12–16
Ventricular segments as projected on radionuclide planar views. ANT = anterior; LAO = left anterior oblique; LLAT = left lateral.

myocardial blood flow demands in that territory have decreased. The standard protocol for thallium perfusion studies begins first with the exercise portion; thallium is injected at the peak of exercise and imaging starts within 5 minutes of injection. The rest scan is obtained 2 to 4 hours later. Because of redistribution, no additional thallium is required. In some patients with perfusion defects on both the rest and exercise scans, however, significant redistribution may not occur, and it is recommended that an additional dose of thallium be administered.[5]

Sestamibi Protocol

Perfusion imaging with sestamibi typically begins with the rest scan first. Because significant uptake also occurs in the liver, imaging is delayed for approximately 60 minutes. This time delay allows sestamibi to be cleared from the liver but not the heart. In addition, a glass of milk or small fatty meal is taken shortly after radiotracer injection to enhance hepatic clearance. A second dose of sestamibi is administered during peak exercise and the exercise scan is obtained 60 minutes after injection, again allowing time for hepatic clearance. Because sestamibi redistributes very slowly, the image obtained 60 minutes after peak exercise reflects the perfusion conditions at the time of injection. Initially, perfusion studies with sestamibi were performed on two different days, but it now is customary to complete both portions of the study in one day.

Teboroxime Protocol

Because of the very short cardiac half-life of teboroxime, two injections of tracer are required. As with sestamibi, hepatic uptake also occurs. Redistribution is not an issue because of the short half-life. Imaging must begin within 2 to 5 minutes of injection and be completed within 15 minutes. The sequence of imaging, exercise versus rest,

is not of concern, and typically the two scans are obtained 60 to 90 minutes apart.

Planar imaging usually is performed with the patient in the supine position, although some laboratories place patients on their right side to obtain the left lateral image. When teboroxime is used as the radiotracer, scans may be obtained with the patient in a sitting or standing position to avoid hepatic interference. With tomographic studies, it is extremely important that the patient not move during image acquisition because computer reconstruction of the images requires the same reference points. If significant movement occurs, the entire tomographic scan may have to be repeated.

Nursing Assessment and Management

All of the directions and precautions that pertain to exercise ECG also apply to exercise radionuclide imaging. When pharmacologic agents are used in place of exercise, minor side effects such as flushing, headache, and nausea may occur; medications to counteract serious side effects should be readily available. Serious side effects due to the radiotracer are extremely rare. Some patients who receive sestamibi report a metallic taste several minutes after injection. Patients often are anxious about the radiation involved and the appearance of the equipment; the nurse plays an important role in allaying these anxieties.

Infarct Imaging
Procedure

Infarct or "hot-spot" imaging may be useful in patients who present to the hospital several days after myocardial infarction when serum cardiac enzymes have returned to normal. Accumulation of the radiotracer in the area of myocardial necrosis compared to the surrounding normal myocardium is responsible for the hot-spot image obtained.

^{99m}Tc-Sn-pyrophosphate is the only radiotracer currently approved by the Food and Drug Administration for infarct imaging and is sensitive for 1 to 5 days after onset of symptoms. Because aneurysm formation in the area of a previous infarction may result in a false-positive study, a second pyrophosphate scan may be performed 7 to 10 days after symptom onset. In patients with recent infarction, little or no radiotracer uptake will be seen on the repeat scan. The diagnostic sensitivity of pyrophosphate imaging in patients with small or nontransmural infarction is poor.

Indium-111 antimyosin is a monoclonal antibody that binds to damaged myocytes and is under investigation as an imaging agent for myocardial necrosis. Planar or tomographic images are obtained 24 to 48 hours after injection of the indium-labeled antibody. Although the study usually is performed within 1 week of a myocardial infarction, a positive scan may be obtained for up to 1 year after myocardial necrosis. Initial results suggest that antimyosin is more sensitive than pyrophosphate scans for the detection of infarction. In addition, antimyosin may be useful in other clinical conditions that result in myocardial necrosis, such as myocarditis and rejection after cardiac

transplantation. The pattern of radiotracer uptake is more diffuse and global in these conditions, compared to the localized pattern of uptake in infarction.

Nursing Assessment and Management

No special preparation is required for patients undergoing infarct imaging other than an explanation of procedure. Views usually are obtained with the patient in the supine position. If an antimyosin tomographic study is to be performed, the importance of not moving during image acquisition should be reinforced. No serious side effects have been reported with either pyrophosphate or antimyosin administration.

Table 12–1 outlines some of the tests that are used to detect the presence of myocardial ischemia.

Angiocardiography

Purpose

Radionuclide angiocardiography for the assessment of cardiac performance has been in clinical use since the 1970s. Such studies may include information about right and left ventricular ejection fractions, left ventricular regional wall motion abnormalities, ventricular volumes,

TABLE 12–1
Diagnostic Tests Used to Detect Myocardial Ischemia

Procedure	Abnormal Findings	Special Considerations
Standard 12-Lead ECG*	Transient ST segment and T wave changes in patients with chest pain at rest or of prolonged duration	
Holter monitoring	Transient ST segment and T wave changes occurring at rest or with activity	Only two ECG leads monitored
Stress echocardiogram	Segmental wall motion abnormality associated with echocardiogram obtained during exercise	May be used in patients with ventricular conduction defects Pharmacologic agents may be used in patients who cannot exercise
Exercise ECG	Transient ST segment and T wave changes occurring with exercise	Cannot be used in patients who are unable to exercise or who have left bundle or paced rhythm Does not provide good information on the location of the coronary artery disease
Radionuclide perfusion stress study	"Cold spot" image or perfusion defect associated with scan obtained during exercise	May be used in patients with ventricular conduction defects Pharmacologic agents may be used in patients who cannot exercise

* ECG, electrocardiogram.

and cardiac shunts. The measurement of left ventricular ejection fraction, the percentage of blood ejected with each contraction of the left ventricle, has been a key prognostic index for patients with myocardial infarction or cardiac arrest.

Two approaches are used for the evaluation of cardiac performance. The technique used most commonly is known as equilibrium angiocardiography. It is performed easily at the bedside in patients too critically ill to be transported to the laboratory. The other technique, first-pass angiocardiography, likely will enjoy wider use in the future because it can use technetium radiotracers such as teboroxime or sestamibi and can be performed at the same time as perfusion imaging.

Procedure

With *equilibrium radionuclide studies*, an aliquot of the patient's blood is drawn and the erythrocytes are tagged with ^{99m}Tc radiotracer. The blood sample is then returned intravenously to the patient. Imaging can begin within a few minutes after administration and performed serially over a period of 4 to 6 hours because the radiotracer-tagged erythrocytes remain within the vascular system. An ECG signal from the patient is used to separate radioactive counts acquired during systole from those during diastole; imaging continues over several hundred cardiac cycles; images are averaged for both systole and diastole to obtain a representative cardiac cycle.

At the end of diastole, when the left ventricle is maximally filled with blood containing tagged erythrocytes, the amount of radioactivity will be greatest. As the ventricle contracts during systole, blood is ejected into the aorta. The amount of blood and therefore radioactivity in the left ventricle is lowest at the end of systole. Because radioactive counts are proportional to the blood volume, the difference in counts obtained at the end of systole and the end of diastole permit the calculation of left ventricular ejection fraction. Left ventricular impairment due to previous infarction or cardiomyopathy usually results in a reduction in left ventricular ejection fraction from the normal values of 55% to 70%. Comparisons in ejection fractions at rest and with exercise also can be made. An inability to increase left ventricular ejection fraction by at least 5% with exercise is considered abnormal and may represent ischemic myocardium.

Left ventricular volumes and wall motion also can be assessed with equilibrium angiocardiography. By tracing the images obtained during the end of diastole and the end of systole, abnormalities in systolic or diastolic volumes can be ascertained. In addition, global versus regional impairment of ventricular function can be differentiated, including the identification of aneurysm formation after infarction. Baseline data may provide information about the etiology of the ventricular impairment and serial measurements often are used to assess response to treatment.

First-pass radioangiocardiography also use ^{99m}Tc tracers; however, they are not tagged to any blood components. An image is obtained immediately after intravenous injection of the radiotracer as it enters the central circulation. The appearance time of the tracer in the various cardiac chambers as well as right and left ventricular systolic and diastolic counts provide diagnostic information. Because the time required for the tracer to traverse the central circulation is only a few cardiac cycles, the image acquisition time is very short.

Intracardiac shunts may be diagnosed by first-pass techniques. For example, in a patient with a ventricular septal defect and right-to-left shunt, the tracer appears in the left ventricle at the same time or before its appearance in the left atrium. In addition, this technique allows the amount of shunting to be quantified.

Right ventricular ejection fraction and volumes are measured best by first-pass angiocardiography. Because the tracer is present in the right ventricle before it appears in the left ventricle, there is no contamination of counts from the overlapping left ventricle. The methods for measuring right ventricular volumes and ejection fraction are similar to those used for the left ventricle.

Nursing Assessment and Management

Three planar views similar to those used in perfusion imaging are obtained during equilibrium angiocardiography. If exercise angiocardiography is to be performed, the patient should be instructed to wear comfortable shoes for treadmill walking or bicycle riding. Emergency equipment should be readily available, as is required with other types of exercise testing. Although imaging usually is performed with the patient in the supine position, semierect or erect positioning may be used. It is important that the patient not move during image acquisition for either equilibrium or first-pass studies because of the effect on systolic and diastolic images.

Nurses caring for patients who have undergone radionuclide imaging should be aware of any precautions that need to be taken; this information is available through the Radiation Safety Department of their institution. The length of time that any precautions may be necessary is related to the half-life of the radiotracer used. In general, nurses who are pregnant should avoid caring for patients for 24 to 48 hours after the study, and all nurses should wear gloves when handling body fluids during the 24- to 48-hour period.

Invasive Techniques
Cardiac Catheterization

Cardiac catheterization is a generic term that refers to a variety of procedures that are performed in the catheterization laboratory. Such procedures include selective coronary, saphenous vein bypass graft or internal mammary angiography, ventriculography, and right or left heart catheterization. All of the procedures are performed using invasive techniques and require a sterile environment.

Procedure

Coronary angiography is used to evaluate the presence and location of coronary artery disease. A catheter is introduced via the arterial system under fluoroscopy retrograde to the ascending aorta. The right or left main coronary artery is then selectively cannulated and a radiopaque dye is injected directly into the artery via the catheter. As dye flows down the artery, the lumen of the artery can be visualized and the image recorded on film. Disease in the coronary artery or one of its branches will delay or obstruct the flow of dye and may be visualized on the film as a site of lumen narrowing and slow filling of the artery with dye. In patients who have undergone previous coronary bypass surgery, selective injections of saphenous vein bypass grafts or internal mammary arteries can be performed in a similar manner.

Ventriculography is accomplished by injecting dye directly into the left ventricle, and commonly is performed in conjunction with selective coronary angiography. A catheter is directed retrograde into the left ventricle via the arterial system under fluoroscopy. Dye is injected rapidly and an image of the left ventricular cavity is recorded on film as the ventricle contracts. Left ventricular ejection fraction, the percentage of blood present in the left ventricle during diastole that is ejected during systole, can be calculated from the film images. Outlines of the ventricle during diastole and systole are traced and the areas inside each outline are proportional to the amount of blood present. In addition, regional ventricular wall motion abnormalities due to myocardial infarction or severe ischemia can be visualized. The competence of the mitral valve also may be evaluated during ventriculography. In patients with mitral regurgitation, dye is observed being ejected not only into the aorta during systole but also into the left atrium through an incompetent mitral valve. In patients with suspected aortic regurgitation, dye may be injected into the aorta; if regurgitation is present, the dye will flow retrograde into the left ventricle during diastole.

A *left heart catheterization* is done to measure intracardiac or intravascular pressures in the structures of the left side of the heart. The chambers are accessed with a catheter introduced retrograde via the arterial system under fluoroscopy. If either the mitral or aortic valves are stenosed, the pressures required to eject blood forward will be higher than normal due to the small valve orifice. For example, with normal mitral valve function, the left atrial pressure and left ventricular pressure are nearly equal during ventricular diastole because blood flows rather easily from the left atrium through the mitral valve into the left ventricle. In contrast, mitral stenosis will result in a left atrial pressure that is significantly higher than the pressure in the left ventricle during ventricular diastole because the left atrium has to generate more pressure to force blood forward through the stenosed valve. This difference in pressure is known as a "gradient," and is related to the degree of stenosis present. Similar pressure comparisons are made in the left ventricle and aorta during systole to evaluate aortic stenosis. If a cardiac output measurement is available, the area of either the mitral or aortic valve opening may be calculated.

Mitral or aortic valve regurgitation also may be assessed by pressure measurements as well as with ventriculography, as previously described. The abnormal retrograde flow of blood into the left atrium during ventricular systole that occurs with mitral regurgitation produces higher-than-normal left atrial pressures. In patients with severe mitral regurgitation, the pressure in the left atrium may nearly equal the peak systolic pressure in the left ventricle. Similar pressure measurements are made in the left ventricle and aorta to evaluate aortic regurgitation.

A *right heart catheterization* procedure is performed to measure intracardiac and intravascular pressures in structures of the right side of the heart. A catheter is inserted antegrade via the venous system under fluoroscopy; the procedure is similar to the insertion of a pulmonary artery catheter. Pressures are recorded from the vena cava, right atrium, right ventricle, pulmonary artery, and pulmonary capillary wedge position. In addition, blood samples may be drawn from each chamber as the catheter is advanced, and the amount of oxygen present in each blood sample is measured. Because the right side of the heart normally contains venous blood, a significant increase in the amount of oxygen present in a blood sample may indicate a left-to-right intracardiac shunt.

Cardiac output, the amount of blood pumped by the heart in a minute, may be measured during a right heart catheterization using the thermodilution technique. Because cardiac output can be expected to vary with body size, the term "cardiac index," which takes height and weight into consideration, is used more often (see page 202 for a discussion of cardiac output measurement).

Arterial and venous accesses usually are achieved with percutaneous techniques from femoral sites. Typically, a needle is inserted into the artery or vein. A guidewire is then inserted through the needle and advanced to the appropriate position in or near the heart. After removing the needle, a catheter may be placed over the guidewire and advanced to the desired position. Changing catheters over guidewires allows specific preformed catheters to be used during the procedure. In some patients, percutaneous access cannot be accomplished from a femoral site and a cutdown at a brachial site may be required. A bolus of intravenous or intra-arterial heparin is administered to patients requiring arterial access to prevent clot formation on the guidewire or catheter.

Nursing Assessment and Management

Patients undergoing elective cardiac catheterization are NPO for at least 6 hours before the procedure. Because the dye may be nephrotoxic, hydration with intravenous fluids may be started before the procedure and continued afterward. Patients with low cardiac output or renal impairment are especially susceptible to dye nephrotoxicity, and their renal function should be monitored closely after the procedure. Patients may be prescribed a mild sedative before the procedure. When percutaneous access is used, pressure usually is applied over the site until bleeding has ceased. A pressure dressing and, in some laboratories, a sandbag is left in place for several hours after the procedure.

Patients typically are placed on bed rest for 6 hours after the procedure and instructed not to flex the affected extremity. After the procedure, the access site should be checked frequently for signs of bleeding, swelling, or hematoma formation. If a femoral arterial access site was used, peripheral pulses in the affected extremity should be monitored. In addition, bleeding may occur in the retroperitoneal space in patients who have undergone femoral arterial access; close monitoring of blood pressure and heart rate and an awareness that retroperitoneal bleeding frequently presents as low back pain are useful in preventing a significant bleed.

Before catheterization, patients should be informed about the procedures that will be performed and questioned about any possible dye allergies. They should be instructed that they will be placed on a table with rounded sides and that their body will be strapped down so that they will not move as the table rotates from side to side. If they are to undergo ventriculography, they should be instructed that they may experience a temporary hot flash or flushing when dye is injected into the left ventricle. Postcatheterization procedures also should be explained to the patient, including bed rest and monitoring of the access site and vital signs. If the patient is to be discharged after the procedure and a cutdown was used for access, the patient should be instructed to make a follow-up appointment with the physician for suture removal.

Electrophysiology Studies

Purpose

Electrophysiology studies are used both for diagnosing and evaluating interventions in the treatment of arrhythmias. The testing protocol may include the measurement of conduction and recovery times in the specialized conduction system of the heart, identification of abnormal or accessory conduction pathways, and stimulation of atrial or ventricular tissues to induce arrhythmias. All of the procedures are performed using invasive techniques and require a sterile environment.

Patients presenting with symptoms suggestive of supraventricular or ventricular tachycardias or syncope frequently are studied with electrophysiological testing. The intracardiac electrodes are used to stimulate atrial or ventricular tissue at various pacing rates and numbers of extra stimuli. The induction and subsequent recording of a supraventricular tachycardia provides information about the mechanism of the arrhythmia. If an accessory pathway is identified as the mechanism, radiofrequency or surgical ablation of the pathway may be successful in eliminating future episodes of the tachycardia.

The successful induction of ventricular tachycardia with electrophysiological testing is of both diagnostic and prognostic value for the risk of sudden cardiac death. Treatment with pharmacologic agents can be evaluated with subsequent studies. Antiarrhythmics that prevent induction or slow the rate of a ventricular tachycardia in a patient who was inducible in the control state may be used in the long-term management of the arrhythmia. Ventricular arrhythmias usually are not treated with ablation methods because the areas of ventricular tissue responsible for the tachycardia are not easily identified and are widespread.

Procedure

To measure electrical activity from the specialized conduction system of the heart, it is necessary to place electrodes at various intracardiac sites. Special catheters with multiple electrodes are inserted via arterial or venous access and advanced to locations within the heart; a separate access site is required for each electrode. In most studies, venous access is adequate for proper positioning of the electrodes; however, arterial access may be required for blood pressure monitoring. The high right atrium, bundle of His, and right ventricular apex sites typically are used for recording and stimulation. In addition, several body surface leads are recorded simultaneously.

Venous and arterial accesses usually are achieved with percutaneous techniques from femoral sites in a manner similar to that used during cardiac catheterization. A sheath may be left in place during the procedure, however, so that electrode catheters may be repositioned as necessary. In some patients, access cannot be accomplished from a femoral site and percutaneous access via the jugular vein or a cutdown at a brachial site may be required. A bolus of intravenous or intra-arterial heparin is administered to patients requiring arterial access to prevent clot formation on the electrode catheter.

Conduction times from the atria to the bundle of His and bundle of His to ventricles are measured. Sites of block—supra-His or infra-His—can be identified and provide information that is used to direct treatment. In addition, the atrium can be paced over a range of rates to identify the rate at which heart block develops. Sinus node function is evaluated by pacing the atrium at various rates, suddenly stopping pacing, and measuring the amount of time it takes for the sinus node to initiate an impulse. The development of heart block at slow heart rates or prolonged sinus node recovery times may indicate a causal factor in patients presenting with syncope or presyncope.

Nursing Assessment and Management

Patients undergoing electrophysiological testing are NPO for at least 6 hours before the procedure, although a sedative administered orally may be prescribed. When percutaneous access is used, pressure is applied over the site until bleeding has ceased. A pressure dressing usually is left in place for several hours after the procedure.

Patients typically are placed on bed rest for 6 hours after the procedure and instructed not to flex the affected extremity. The access site should be checked frequently for signs of bleeding, swelling, or hematoma formation. If a femoral arterial access site was used, peripheral pulses in the affected extremity should be monitored.

Before electrophysiological testing, patients should be instructed that they will be placed on a table with straps over their torso. They should be informed that they may experience palpitations or syncope if rapid tachyarrhythmias are induced. Post-study procedures also should be explained to the patient, including bed rest and monitoring of the access site and vital signs. If the patient is to be discharged after the procedure and a cutdown was used for access, the patient should be instructed to make a follow-up appointment with the physician for suture removal.

Patients with ventricular tachycardia who are being initiated on antiarrhythmic therapy are at risk for sudden cardiac death because some medications may have adverse proarrhythmic effects. These patients often are kept in a monitored setting for most of their hospital stay until appropriate therapies have been identified. Most of these patients are otherwise healthy and physically active, and it becomes a challenge for the nursing staff to care for these patients as well as the more severely ill patient population.

Electrocardiographic Monitoring

Behavioral Objectives

Description

Equipment Features

Hard-Wire Monitoring Systems

Telemetry Monitoring Systems

Monitoring Lead Systems
    Three-Electrode Systems
    Four- and Five-Electrode Systems
    Lead Selection

Procedure

Electrode Application

Monitor Observation

Troubleshooting ECG Monitor Problems

BEHAVIORAL OBJECTIVES

Based on the content in this section, the reader should be able to:

1. State the major features of an ECG monitoring system.
2. Discuss the rationale for using the various types of monitoring leads.
3. Describe a method for applying ECG electrodes to achieve an optimal tracing.
4. Identify approaches for troubleshooting ECG monitor problems.
5. List priorities in caring for the patient undergoing ECG monitoring.

Description

Cardiac monitoring is used in a variety of settings in health care today. Besides the traditional use in ICU and operating rooms, cardiac monitors are found in other inpatient units where it is necessary continuously to monitor a patient's heart rate and rhythm or the effects of a therapy. Cardiac monitors are used outside of the hospital in settings such as paramedic ambulances, outpatient rehabilitation programs, and transtelephonic monitoring.

Although the type of monitor may differ in each of these settings, all monitoring systems use three basic components: (1) an oscilloscope display system; (2) a monitoring cable; and (3) electrodes. Electrodes are placed on the patient's chest to receive the electrical current from the cardiac muscle tissue. The electrical signal is then carried by the monitoring cable to an oscilloscope, where it is magnified over 1,000 times and displayed. The display can be obtained both at the patient's bedside and at a central station, along with displays from other patients' monitors.

Equipment Features

Two types of cardiac monitoring equipment in use are continuous hard-wire monitoring systems and telemetry monitoring systems.

Hard-Wire Monitoring Systems

Hard-wire monitors, which are the standard type of monitors used in the ICU setting, require that the patient be linked directly to the cardiac monitor via the ECG cable. Information is displayed and recorded at the bedside along with simultaneous display and recording at a central station. Although this type of cardiac monitoring limits patient mobility, patients using this system usually are confined to bed rest or are allowed to be up at the bedside only. Hard-wire monitors operate on electricity but are well isolated so that water, blood, and other fluids do not pose an electrical hazard as long as the machine is maintained adequately.

Telemetry Monitoring Systems

In telemetry monitoring, no direct wire connection is needed between the patient and the ECG display device. Electrodes are connected by a short monitoring cable to a small battery-operated transmitter that the patient carries in a disposable pouch tied to his or her body. The ECG is then sent by radiofrequency signals to a receiver that picks up and displays the signal on an oscilloscope, either at the bedside or at a distant central recording station. Antennas are built into the receiver and may be mounted in the vicinity of the the receiver to widen the range of signal pickup. Batteries are the power source for the transmitter, thus making it possible to avoid electrical hazards by isolating the monitoring system from potential current leakage and accidental shock. Telemetry systems are used primarily for arrhythmia monitoring in areas where the patient is fairly mobile, such as an arrhythmia surveillance or "step-down" unit. Because the patient is mobile, stable ECG tracings often are more difficult to obtain. Some hard-wire systems have built-in telemetry capability so that patients may be switched easily from one system to another as monitoring needs change.

Modern electronics continues to make sophisticated advances in monitoring equipment, and current display systems incorporate such features as:

- Improved freeze/hold modes, which allow the ECG pattern to be held for more detailed examination
- Storage capability, either by tape loops or an electronic memory, which permits retrieval of dys-

rhythmias from 8 to 60 seconds after their occurrence
- Automatic chart documentation, in which the ECG recorder is activated by alarms or at preset intervals
- Heart rate indicators, which display the rate either by meter or by digital display (the alarm system is incorporated into the heart rate monitor with adjustments for both the high and low settings)
- Multilead ECG display, which facilitates complex dysrhythmia interpretation
- ST segment analysis, for monitoring ischemic events
- Multiparameter displays, which offer display of hemodynamic pressures, temperature, intracranial pressure, and respirations
- Computer systems that store, analyze, and trend ECG data; the information can then be retrieved at any time to aid in diagnosis and to note trends in the patient's status

Monitoring Lead Systems

All cardiac monitoring systems use leads to record the electrical activity generated by cardiac tissue. Each lead is composed of a positive or recording electrode, a negative electrode, and a third electrode used as a ground. As the heart depolarizes, the waves of electrical activity move inferiorly, because the normal route of depolarization moves from the sinoatrial (SA) node and atria, downward through the AV node, His–Purkinje system, and ventricles, and to the left as the left heart muscle mass predominates over the right heart. Each lead system looks at these waves of depolarization from a different location on the chest wall and thus produces P waves and QRS complexes of varying configuration.

Cardiac monitoring systems currently on the market vary from two- and three-electrode telemetry devices to three-, four-, and five-electrode hard-wire systems. These systems produce limited selections of the standard limb leads for single-channel recordings, to the possibility of any of the 12 standard ECG leads on multichannel recordings.

Three-Electrode Systems

Monitors that require three electrodes use positive, negative, and ground electrodes that are placed in the right arm (RA), left arm (LA), and left leg (LL) positions on the chest as designated by markings on the monitor cable. When the electrodes are placed appropriately, standard limb lead equivalents may be obtained by moving the lead selector on the bedside oscilloscope to the lead I, II, or III position (Fig. 12–17). The lead selector automatically adjusts which lead is positive, which lead is negative, and which lead is ground to obtain an appropriate tracing. These same limb leads can be obtained manually by using the LA lead as the positive electrode, the RA lead as the negative electrode, and the LL lead as ground and manu-

	LA	RA	LL
.... Lead I	+	−	G
- - - - - Lead II	G	−	+
———— Lead III	−	G	+

FIGURE 12–17

System for obtaining simulation of the standard limb leads. Three-electrode monitoring systems use a "floating ground," eliminating the right leg electrode. A four-electrode monitoring system includes the right leg electrode as a permanent ground electrode.

ally placing each electrode in the correct position while the lead selector is maintained in the lead I position.

A modified version of a standard chest lead also may be obtained when using a three-electrode monitoring system. By positioning the negative electrode (RA) below the left clavicle and the positive electrode (LA) in the appropriate "V" position on the chest and with the lead selector in the lead I position, a modified chest lead (MCL) can be created. The two most commonly used modified chest leads are an MCL_1, where the positive electrode is placed in the fourth intercostal space to the right of the sternum, and an MCL_6, where the positive electrode is placed in the midaxillary line, fifth intercostal space (Fig. 12–18).

Four- and Five-Electrode Systems

Four-electrode, as well as five-electrode, systems increase the monitor's capability beyond the three-electrode system. The four-electrode monitor requires a right leg (RL) electrode that is the ground for all leads described in the three-electrode system. The five-electrode monitor adds an exploring "chest" electrode that allows one to obtain any one of the six modified chest leads as well as the

standard limb leads. It is necessary to have this type of system when multilead recordings are desired.

Lead Selection

The optimal lead for ECG monitoring is the one that shows the best P waves and QRS complexes (and pacing spikes, if present). No single monitoring lead is ideal for every patient (Table 12–2). Lead II is used commonly because it records well formed upright complexes that are easy to identify and measure. MCL_1 is helpful in recognizing RBBBs and LBBBs, and in differentiating ventricular ectopy from supraventricular rhythms with aberrancy; MCL_6 also can be used for this purpose. In addition to lead II, leads III and AVF, as well as MCL_1, show well formed P waves and therefore are helpful in identifying atrial dysrhythmias. The Lewis lead also can be used to record atrial activity and is obtained by placing the positive electrode in the V_1 position and the negative electrode in the second intercostal space to the right of the sternum. Lead I may be tried with the respiratory patient who has much artifact on the tracing because there is less movement of the positive electrode in this lead than in a lead II or an MCL_1.

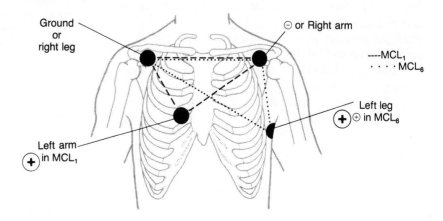

FIGURE 12–18

System for obtaining simulation of V_1 and V_6 chest leads. For an MCL tracing, use lead "1" selection.

TABLE 12–2
Suggested Monitoring Lead Selection

Lead	Rationale for Use
II	• Produces large, well formed P waves and QRS complexes for strip interpretation
	• Produces large ECG signal for easy monitoring
MCL₁	• Produces characteristic BBB configuration for differentiating RBBB from LBBB, VEA from aberrancy, and RV from LV ectopy
	• Produces well formed P waves for analyzing atrial dysrhythmias
III, AVF, Lewis Lead (& II, MCL₁)	• Produce well formed P waves, helpful in identifying atrial dysrhythmias
I	• Use with patients in respiratory distress to decrease motion artifact; affected less by chest movement than other leads

ECG, electrocardiogram; BBB, bundle branch block; R(L)BBB, right (left) bundle branch block; VEA, ventricular ectopic activity; RV, right ventricle; LV, left ventricle.

As mentioned, there is no one ideal monitoring lead for every patient, and, in several situations, a multilead recording is desirable. Multilead ECG systems offer multiple views of the heart because they reflect a tracing from each of the major heart surfaces. One of the major uses for this type of system is in the interpretation of complex cardiac dysrhythmias, especially when differentiating aberrancy from ventricular ectopy and in identifying complex atrial dysrhythmias, uncharacteristic-looking ventricular premature beats, and fascicular blocks. Another role for multilead monitoring is in assessing myocardial ischemia and infarction. By continuously viewing one lead from each area of the heart, episodes of anginal pain or silent ischemia can be documented. Later, these changes should be confirmed by a full 12-lead ECG because monitor leads are only simulations of comparable leads on the 12-lead ECG and cannot be relied on for diagnosis.

Procedure

Electrode Application

Proper skin preparation and application of electrodes are imperative for good ECG monitoring. An adequate tracing should reflect (1) a narrow, stable baseline; (2) absence of distortion or "noise"; (3) sufficient amplitude of the QRS complex to activate the rate meters and alarm systems properly; and (4) identification of P waves.

The type of electrode currently used for ECG monitoring is a disposable silver- or nickle-plated electrode centered in a circle of adhesive paper or foam rubber. Most electrodes are pregelled by the manufacturer. They may have disposable wires attached to the electrodes or nondisposable wires that snap onto the electrodes. They are comfortable for the patient, but if not properly applied, may result in undue artifact and false alarms.

When electrodes are applied, this procedure should be followed:

1. Select a stable site. Avoid bony protuberances, joints, and folds in the skin. Areas in which muscle attaches to bone have the least motion artifact.
2. Shave excessive body hair from the site.
3. Rub the site briskly with a dry gauze pad to remove oils and cellular debris. Skin preparation with alcohol may be necessary if the skin is greasy; allow the alcohol to dry completely before applying the electrode. Follow the the electrode manufacturer's directions because the chemical reaction between alcohol or other skin-preparation materials and the adhesives used in some electrodes may cause skin irritation or nonadhesion to the skin.
4. Remove the paper backing and apply each electrode firmly to the skin by smoothing with the finger in a circular motion. Attach each electrode to its corresponding ECG cable wire. Sometimes it is necessary to tape over the cable wire connection or make a stress loop with the cable wire for extra stability.
5. Change electrodes every 2 to 3 days and monitor for skin irritation.

While applying the electrodes to the patient, it is important to explain the purpose of the procedure. In addition, the patient should be reassured that every time the monitor alarm sounds, it does not indicate a problem with the patient's heartbeat—it often occurs when an electrode becomes loose or disconnected.

Monitor Observation

Cardiac monitors are useful only if the information they provide is "observed," either by computers with alarms for programmed parameters or by the human eye, and appropriately acted on by competent, responsible people. Some critical care units use monitor technicians whose sole responsibilities are to observe monitors, obtain chart samples, and give appropriate information to the nurse as to each patient's ECG status. Those observing the monitor should know the acceptable dysrhythmia parameters for each patient and should be notified of any interruptions in monitoring, such as those caused by changing electrodes or by changing the patient to a portable monitor. The observer also should be aware of the presence of artifact from chest physical therapy or hiccoughs so that it may be considered in dysrhythmia diagnosis.

Regardless of the system used for monitor observation, certain practices always should be followed. If the monitor alarm sounds, the nurse should evaluate the clinical status of the patient before *anything else* to see if the problem is an actual dysrhythmia or a malfunction of the monitoring system. Asystole should not be mistaken for an unattached ECG wire, nor should a patient inadvertently tapping on an electrode be misread as ventricular tachycardia. In addition, the monitor alarms always should be in the functioning mode. Only when direct physical care is being given to the patient can the alarm system safely be put on "standby." This ensures that no life-threatening dysrhythmia will go unnoticed.

Troubleshooting ECG Monitor Problems

Several problems may occur in monitoring ECG, including baseline but no ECG trace, intermittent traces, wandering or irregular baseline, low-amplitude complexes, 60-cycle interference, excessive triggering of heart rate alarms, and skin irritation. The steps to follow when such problems occur are outlined in Table 12–3.

TABLE 12–3
Electrocardiogram (ECG) Monitor Problem Solving

Excessive Triggering of Heart Rate Alarms

- Is high-low alarm set too close to patient's rate?
- Is monitor sensitivity level set too high or too low?
- Is patient cable securely inserted into monitor receptacle?
- Are the lead wires or connections damaged?
- Has the monitoring lead been properly selected?
- Were the electrodes applied properly?
- Are the R and T waves the same height, causing both waveforms to be sensed?
- Is the baseline unstable, or is there excessive cable or lead wire movement?

Baseline But No ECG Trace

- Is the size (gain or sensitivity) control properly adjusted?
- Is appropriate lead selector being used on monitor?
- Is the patient cable fully inserted into ECG receptacle?
- Are electrode wires fully inserted into patient cable?
- Are electrode wires firmly attached to electrodes?
- Are electrode wires damaged?
- Is the patient cable damaged?
- Call for service if trace is still absent.
- Is the battery dead (for telemetry system)?

Intermittent Trace

- Is patient cable fully inserted into monitor receptacle?
- Are electrode wires fully inserted into patient cable?
- Are electrode wires firmly attached to electrodes?

Intermittent Trace (continued)

- Are electrode wire connectors loose or worn?
- Have electrodes been applied properly?
- Are electrodes properly located and in firm skin contact?
- Is patient cable damaged?

Wandering or Irregular Baseline

- Is there excessive cable movement? This can be reduced by clipping to patient's clothing.
- Is the power cord on or near the monitor cable?
- Is there excessive movement by the patient? Muscle tremors from anxiety or shivering?
- Is site selection correct?
- Were proper skin preparation and application followed?
- Are the electrodes still moist?

Low-Amplitude Complexes

- Is size control adjusted properly?
- Were the electrodes applied properly?
- Is there dried gel on the electrodes?
- Change electrode sites. Check 12-lead ECG for lead with highest amplitude and attempt to simulate that lead.
- If none of the above steps remedies the problem, the weak signal may be the patient's normal complex.

Sixty-Cycle Interference

- Is the monitor size control set too high?
- Are there nearby electrical devices in use, especially poorly grounded ones?
- Were the electrodes applied properly?
- Is there dried gel on the electrodes?
- Are lead wires or connections damaged?

Dysrhythmias and Conduction Disturbances

Atrioventricular Blocks

First-Degree AV Block
    Definition
    Etiology
    Clinical Significance
    Treatment

Second-Degree AV Block—Mobitz I (Wenckebach)
    Definition
    Etiology
    Clinical Significance
    Treatment

Second-Degree AV Block—Mobitz II
    Definition
    Etiology
    Clinical Significance
    Treatment

Third-Degree (Complete) AV Block
    Definition
    Etiology
    Clinical Significance
    Treatment

Bundle Branch Block
    Definition
    Etiology
    Clinical Significance
    Treatment

BEHAVIORAL OBJECTIVES

Based on the content in this section, the reader should be able to:

1. Define the components used in the evaluation of an ECG tracing.
2. State the criteria for diagnosis of normal sinus rhythm.

3. Identify the ECG criteria used to interpret dysrhythmias commonly encountered in monitored patients.
4. Describe the etiologies, clinical significance, and treatment for each of the dysrhythmias discussed.
5. Discuss the nursing management for those patients exhibiting dysrhythmia disturbances.

Description

Dysrhythmias commonly encountered in monitored patients can be recognized with a little practice. The types that occur most frequently are discussed in this chapter. Before presenting the individual dysrhythmias, the method for evaluating a rhythm strip will be addressed. The approach to nursing management of the patient with a cardiac dysrhythmia is presented in a nursing care plan at the end of this chapter.

Understanding of dysrhythmias is helped by knowledge of the conduction system. Before beginning the study of this section, review the discussion of the cardiac conduction system in Chapter 11.

Evaluation of a Rhythm Strip

ECG Paper

An ECG tracing is a graphic recording of the heart's electrical activity. The paper consists of horizontal and vertical lines, each 1 mm apart. The horizontal lines denote time measurements. When the paper is run at a sweep speed of 25 mm/second, each small square is equal to 0.04 seconds, whereas a large square (five small squares) equals 0.20 seconds. Height or voltage is measured by counting the lines vertically (Fig. 12–19). Most ECG paper also is marked at 3-second intervals along the top or bottom for rate calculation.

FIGURE 12–19
Schematic representation of the electrical impulse as it traverses the conduction system, resulting in depolarization and repolarization of the myocardium.

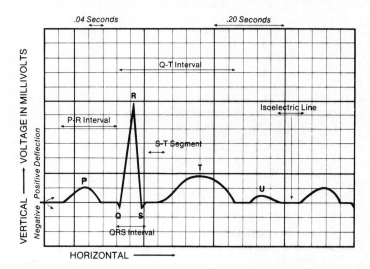

Waveforms and Intervals

During the cardiac cycle, the following waveforms and intervals are produced on the ECG surface tracing (see Figure 12–19):

P wave: A small deflection representing depolarization of the atria. It normally is seen before the QRS complex at a consistent interval.

PR interval: The interval representing conduction time through the atria, AV node, bundle of His, and bundle branches, up to the point of activation of the ventricular muscle tissue. The interval is measured from the beginning of the P wave to the beginning of the QRS. A normal PR interval is 0.12 to 0.20 second.

QRS complex: A large waveform representing ventricular depolarization. Each component of the waveform has a specific connotation. The initial negative deflection is a Q wave, the initial positive deflection is an R wave, and the negative deflection after the R wave is an S wave. Not all QRS complexes have all three components, even though the complex is commonly referred to as the QRS complex. A normal QRS complex is 0.06 to 0.11 second in width.

ST segment: The segment between the end of the QRS complex and the beginning of the T wave. Normally it is isoelectric at baseline but may be elevated or depressed in a variety of conditions.

T wave: A deflection that represents ventricular repolarization or recovery. It appears after the QRS complex. An atrial T wave reflects atrial repolarization but usually is not apparent because it occurs at the same time as the QRS.

U wave: A small, usually positive deflection after the T wave. Its significance is uncertain, but it typically is seen with hypokalemia.

QT interval: The interval representing total duration of ventricular electrical systole. The QT interval is measured from the beginning of the QRS complex to the end of the T wave. Because the QT varies with heart rate, it is necessary to use a table in which QT intervals for various heart rates are listed. Tables such as Table 12–4 are available in most arrhythmia texts for this purpose. If a table is not available, a corrected QT interval (QT_c) can be calculated for comparison to normal values. A normal QT_c usually does not exceed 0.42 second for men and 0.43 second for women. A quick method for obtaining a QT_c is to use half of the preceding RR interval.

Calculation of Heart Rate

Although monitors provide a continuous display of heart rate, it usually is necessary also to determine atrial and ventricular heart rates on the rhythm strip. To calculate heart rate using the 6-second strip method, find the number of complexes in a 6-second strip and then multiply the number of complexes by 10. This method can be used for regular as well as irregular rhythms and is accurate within ± 5 beats/minute. The reader is referred to a dysrhythmia text for description of other methods.

Steps in Assessing a Rhythm Strip

The following represents a systematic approach for analyzing a cardiac rhythm strip. Whether this method or another method is used, it is important to take the time to go through each step, because many dysrhythmias are not as they first appear.

1. Identify the QRS complexes.
2. Look for the P waves.
   If present, are they all the same configuration?
   Is there a P wave for every QRS complex?
3. Measure the PR interval.
   Is it normal?
   Is it the same throughout the strip or does it vary?

TABLE 12–4
Approximate Normal Limits for QT Intervals in Seconds*

Heart Rate per Minute	Men and Children	Women
40	0.45–0.49	0.46–0.50
46	0.43–0.47	0.44–0.48
50	0.41–0.45	0.43–0.46
55	0.40–0.44	0.41–0.45
60	0.39–0.42	0.40–0.43
67	0.37–0.40	0.38–0.41
71	0.36–0.40	0.37–0.41
75	0.35–0.38	0.36–0.39
80	0.34–0.37	0.35–0.38
86	0.33–0.36	0.34–0.37
93	0.32–0.35	0.33–0.36
100	0.31–0.34	0.32–0.35
109	0.30–0.33	0.31–0.33
120	0.28–0.31	0.29–0.32
133	0.27–0.29	0.28–0.30
150	0.25–0.28	0.26–0.28
172	0.23–0.26	0.24–0.26

* Adapted from Frye SJ, Lounsbury P: Cardiac Rhythm Disorders: An Introduction Using the Nursing Process, p 38. Baltimore, Williams & Wilkins, 1988.

4. Evaluate the QRS complex.
   Is it normal in width or is it wide?
   Are all complexes of the same configuration?
5. Determine the atrial and ventricular rates:
   Are they within normal limits?
   Is the atrial rate the same as the ventricular rate? If not, is there a relationship between the two (ie, is one a multiple of the other)?
6. Measure the PP and RR intervals:
   Are the intervals regular or irregular?
   Are the PP and RR intervals the same?
7. Identify the rhythm and determine its clinical significance:
   Is the patient symptomatic? (Check skin, neurologic status, renal function, coronary circulation, hemodynamic status/blood pressure.)
   Is the dysrhythmia life threatening?
   What is the clinical context?
   Is the dysrhythmia new or chronic?

Normal Sinus Rhythm

Definition

Normal sinus rhythm (Fig. 12–20) is the normal rhythm of the heart. The impulse is initiated at the sinus node in a regular rhythm at a rate of 60 to 100 beats/minute. A P wave appears before each QRS complex. The PR interval is within normal limits (0.12–0.20 second) and the QRS is narrow (<0.12 second) unless an intraventricular conduction defect is present.

Dysrhythmias Originating at the Sinus Node

Sinus Tachycardia

Definition

In sinus tachycardia, the sinus node accelerates and initiates an impulse at a rate of 100 times/minute or more (Fig. 12–21). The upper limits of sinus tachycardia extend to 160 to 180 beats/minute. All other ECG characteristics,

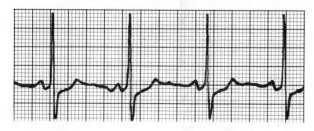

FIGURE 12–20
Normal sinus rhythm. (Rate = 60–100 beats/minute.)

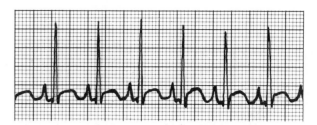

FIGURE 12–21
Sinus tachycardia. (Heart rate = 100–180 beats/minute.)

except for heart rate, are the same as in normal sinus rhythm.

Etiology

Sinus tachycardia usually is caused by factors relating to an increase in sympathetic tone. Stress, exercise, and stimulants such as caffeine and nicotine can produce this dysrhythmia. Sinus tachycardia also is associated with such clinical problems as fever, anemia, hyperthyroidism, hypoxemia, congestive heart failure (CHF), and shock. Drugs such as atropine (which blocks vagal tone) and the catecholamines (eg, isoproterenol, epinephrine, dopamine) also can produce this rhythm.

Clinical Significance

The cause of the sinus tachycardia and the underlying state of the myocardium determine its prognosis. Sinus tachycardia in and of itself is not a lethal dysrhythmia but often signals an underlying problem that should be pursued. In addition, the rapid rate of sinus tachycardia increases oxygen demands on the myocardium and decreases the filling time of the ventricles. In people who already have depleted cardiac reserve, ischemia, or CHF, the persistence of a fast rate may worsen the underlying condition.

Treatment

Treatment usually is directed toward eliminating the underlying cause. Specific measures may include sedation, oxygen administration, digitalis if heart failure is present, or propranolol if the tachycardia is due to thyrotoxicosis.

Sinus Bradycardia

Definition

Sinus bradycardia is defined as a rhythm with impulses originating at the sinus node at a rate of less than 60 beats/minute (Fig. 12–22). The rhythm (RR interval) may become less regular as a slower heart rate prevails; otherwise, all other parameters are normal.

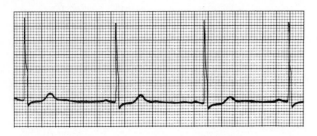

FIGURE 12-22
Sinus bradycardia. (Heart rate less than 60 beats/minute.)

Etiology

Sinus bradycardia is common among all age groups and is present in both normal and diseased hearts. It may occur during sleep and in highly trained athletes, as well as with severe pain, inferior wall myocardial infarction, acute spinal cord injury, and with certain drugs (eg, digitalis, β-blockers, verapamil, diltiazem).

Clinical Significance

Slow rates are tolerated well in people with healthy hearts. With severe heart disease, however, the heart may not be able to compensate for a slow rate by increasing the volume of blood ejected per beat. In this situation, sinus bradycardia will lead to a low cardiac output.

Treatment

No treatment is indicated unless symptoms are present. If the pulse is very slow and symptoms are present, appropriate measures include atropine (to block the vagal effect), isoproterenol, or cardiac pacing.

Sinus Arrhythmia

Definition

Sinus arrhythmia is a disorder of rhythm (Fig. 12–23). It is said to be present if the RR intervals on the ECG strip vary by more than 0.12 second, from the shortest RR

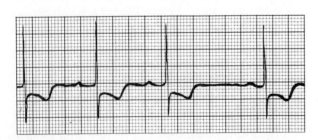

FIGURE 12-23
Sinus arrhythmia. (The difference between the shortest and longest PP interval is greater than 0.12 second.)

interval to the longest. This dysrhythmia is due to an irregularity in sinus node discharge, often in association with phases of the respiratory cycle. The sinus node gradually speeds up with inspiration and gradually slows with expiration. There also is a nonrespiratory form of this dysrhythmia.

Etiology

Sinus arrhythmia is a normal phenomenon, seen especially in young people in the setting of lower heart rates. It also occurs after enhancement of vagal tone (eg, digitalis, morphine).

Clinical Significance

Sinus arrhythmia is a normal finding and therefore does not imply the presence of underlying disease. Symptoms are uncommon unless there are excessively long pauses.

Treatment

Usually, no treatment is required.

Sinus Arrest and Sinoatrial Block

Definition

Sinus arrest is a disorder of impulse formation. The sinus node fails to discharge one or more impulses, producing pauses of varying lengths due to the absence of atrial depolarization. The P wave is absent and the resulting PP interval is not a multiple of the basic PP interval. The pause ends either when an escape pacemaker from the junction or ventricles takes over or sinus node function returns.

Sinoatrial block often is difficult to differentiate from sinus arrest on a surface ECG tracing. In SA block, the sinus node fires but the impulse is delayed or blocked from exiting the sinus node. If the block is complete, the duration of the pause is a multiple of the basic PP interval (Fig. 12–24).

Etiology

Both dysrhythmias may be due to involvement of the sinus node by infarction, degenerative fibrotic changes, drug effects (digitalis, β-blockers, calcium channel blockers), or excessive vagal stimulation.

Clinical Significance

These rhythms usually are transient and not significant unless a lower pacemaker fails to take over to pace the ventricles.

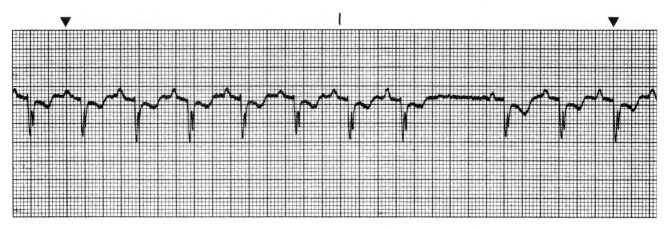

FIGURE 12–24
SA block. The pause is a multiple of the basic PP interval.

Treatment

Treatment is indicated if the patient is symptomatic. The goal is to increase the ventricular rate, which may require the use of atropine or, in the presence of serious hemodynamic compromise, the use of a pacemaker.

Sick Sinus Syndrome

Definition

Sick sinus syndrome refers to a chronic form of sinus node disease (Fig. 12–25). Patients exhibit severe degrees of sinus node depression, including marked sinus bradycardia, SA block, or sinus arrest. Often, rapid atrial dysrhythmias, such as atrial flutter or fibrillation (the "tachycardia–bradycardia syndrome") coexist and alternate with periods of sinus node depression.

Treatment

Management of this condition requires control of the rapid atrial dysrhythmias with drug therapy and, in selected cases, control of very slow heart rates, often requiring implantation of a permanent pacemaker.

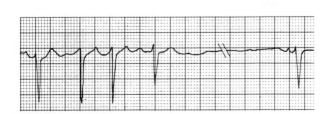

FIGURE 12–25
Sick sinus syndrome. Atrial fibrillation is followed by atrial standstill. A sinus escape beat is seen at the end of the strip.

Atrial Dysrhythmias

Premature Atrial Contraction

Definition

A premature atrial contraction (PAC) occurs when an ectopic atrial impulse discharges prematurely and, in most cases, is conducted in a normal fashion through the AV conducting system to the ventricles (Fig. 12–26). On the ECG tracing, the P wave is premature and may even be buried in the preceding T wave; it differs in configuration from the sinus P wave. The QRS complex usually is of normal configuration but, due to timing, may appear wide and bizarre if conducted with some degree of delay (aberrant PAC) or not at all if the atrial impulse is blocked from being conducted to the ventricles (blocked PAC). A short pause, usually less than "compensatory," is present (see later definition of ventricular premature beat).

Etiology

This is a common dysrhythmia seen in all groups. It may occur in normal people and in patients with rheumatic heart disease, ischemic heart disease, or hyperthyroidism. It often is seen in the setting of CHF.

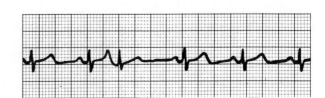

FIGURE 12–26
Premature atrial contraction.

Clinical Significance

Premature atrial contractions may be a precursor to an atrial tachycardia, indicating an increasing atrial irritability. They also may indicate an underlying condition (eg, CHF). Patients may have the sensation of a "pause" or "skip" in rhythm when PACs are present.

Treatment

In many cases, no treatment is necessary. The patient should be monitored and the frequency of the premature beats documented. In addition, the patient should be assessed for underlying conditions and treated. Specific drugs such as digitalis or quinidine may be in order.

Paroxysmal Supraventricular Tachycardia

Definition

Paroxysmal supraventricular tachycardia (PSVT) describes a rapid atrial rhythm occurring at a rate of 150 to 250 beats/minute (Fig. 12–27). The tachycardia begins abruptly, in most instances with a PAC, and it ends abruptly. P waves may be seen preceding the QRS but at faster rates may be hidden in the QRS or preceding T wave. (If some of the P waves are not followed by a QRS, this is referred to as PSVT with block, and usually is due to digitalis toxicity.) The P waves usually are negative in II, III, and AVF owing to retrograde conduction from the AV node to the atria. The QRS usually is normal unless there is an underlying intraventricular conduction problem. The rhythm is regu-

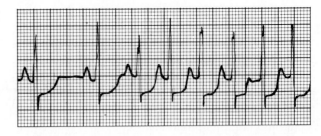

FIGURE 12–27
Paroxysmal supraventricular tachycardia (begins with a premature atrial contraction).

lar and the paroxysms may last from a few seconds to several hours or even days.

The term "PSVT" is used to identify rhythms previously referred to as paroxysmal atrial tachycardia (PAT) and paroxysmal nodal or junctional tachycardia (PNT or PJT), rhythms similar in all respects except in their sites of origin. PSVT also is known as *AV nodal reentrant tachycardia* because the mechanism most commonly responsible for this dysrhythmia is a reentrant circuit or chaotic movement at the level of the AV node.

Paroxysmal supraventricular tachycardia must be differentiated from other narrow QRS (supraventricular) tachycardias (Table 12–5). The following points favor the diagnosis of PSVT versus a sinus tachycardia:

An atrial premature beat often initiates the rhythm

It begins and terminates abruptly

The rate often is faster than a sinus tachycardia and tends to be more regular from minute to minute

In response to a vagal maneuver, such as carotid

TABLE 12–5
Differential Diagnosis of Narrow QRS Tachycardia

Type of SVT	Onset	Atrial Rate	Ventricular Rate	RR Interval	Response to Carotid Massage
Sinus tachycardia	Gradual	100–180 beats/min	Same as sinus rate	Regular	Gradual slowing
PSVT	Abrupt	150–250 beats/min	Usually same as atrial; block seen with digitalis toxicity and AV node disease	Regular, except at onset and termination	May convert to NSR
Atrial flutter	Abrupt	250–350 beats/min	Occurs with 2:1, 3:1, 4:1, or varied ventricular response	Regular or regularly irregular	Abrupt slowing of ventricular response, flutter waves remain
Atrial fibrillation	Abrupt	400–650 beats/min	Depends on ability of AVN to conduct atrial impulse; decreased with drug therapy	Irregularly irregular	Abrupt slowing of ventricular response, fibrillation waves remain

SVT, supraventricular tachycardia; paroxysmal supraventricular tachycardia; AV, atrioventricular; NSR, normal sinus rhythm; AVN, atrioventricular node.

sinus massage, the ectopic tachycardia either will be unaffected or will revert to a normal sinus rhythm; sinus tachycardia, however, will slow slightly in response to increased vagal tone

Etiology

Paroxysmal supraventricular tachycardia occurs often in adults with normal hearts, and for the same reasons as PACs. When heart disease is present, such abnormalities as rheumatic heart disease, acute myocardial infarction, and digitalis intoxication may serve as the background for this dysrhythmia.

Clinical Significance

Often the patient is without underlying heart disease and may experience only palpitations and some light-headedness, depending on the rate and duration of the PSVT. With underlying heart disease, dyspnea, angina pectoris, and CHF may occur as ventricular filling time, and thus cardiac output, is decreased.

Treatment

Vagal stimulation often will terminate the PSVT, either through carotid massage or the Valsalva maneuver. If vagal stimulation is unsuccessful, intravenous verapamil usually is the drug of choice. Diltiazem, β-blockers, or adenosine also are indicated in this setting. Cardioversion or overdrive pacing may be required if drug therapy is unsuccessful. Long-term prophylactic therapy may be indicated for some patients.

Atrial Flutter

Definition

Atrial flutter is a rapid atrial ectopic rhythm occurring at atrial rates of 250 to 350 beats/minute (Fig. 12–28). Unless an abnormal AV conduction path is present, the ventricles can respond only at half the atrial rate, initially producing a 2:1 flutter. With treatment, the degree of AV block increases and the ventricular rate slows further (3:1 flutter, 4:1 flutter, or flutter with a varying ventricular response).

The rapid and regular atrial rate produces a "saw-tooth" or "picket fence" appearance on the ECG. It is usual for a flutter wave to be partially concealed within the QRS complex or T wave. The QRS complex exhibits a normal configuration except when aberrant conduction is present.

When the ventricular rate is rapid, the diagnosis of atrial flutter may be difficult. Vagal maneuvers such as carotid sinus massage often will increase the degree of AV block and allow recognition of flutter waves (see Table 12–5).

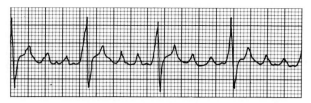

FIGURE 12–28
Atrial flutter. (Atrial rate = 250–350 beats/minute. P wave shows characteristic saw-toothed pattern.)

Etiology

Atrial flutter often is seen in the presence of underlying cardiac disease including coronary artery disease, cor pulmonale, and rheumatic heart disease.

Clinical Significance

If atrial flutter occurs with a rapid ventricular rate, the ventricular chambers cannot fill adequately, resulting in varying degrees of hemodynamic compromise.

Treatment

No immediate treatment is necessary if flutter is associated with a high degree of AV block so that the ventricular rate remains within normal limits. When the ventricular rate is rapid, prompt treatment to control the rate or revert the rhythm to a sinus mechanism is indicated. Drugs of choice include digitalis, diltiazem, or verapamil, which increase the degree of AV block and thus control the ventricular rate. Reversion to a sinus mechanism may follow. Quinidine may be helpful in converting the flutter to a normal sinus mechanism after the ventricular rate has been slowed. Atrial flutter is not desirable in the long term, because the ventricular response often is difficult to control; synchronized cardioversion may be necessary to convert the rhythm to sinus or a more stable atrial fibrillation.

Atrial Fibrillation

Definition

Atrial fibrillation is defined as a rapid atrial ectopic rhythm, occurring with atrial rates of 400 to 650 beats/minute (Fig. 12–29). It is characterized by chaotic atrial activity with the absence of definable P waves. The ventricular rate and rhythm depend on the ability of the AV junction to respond to the rapid stimuli from the atria. Initially, the ventricular response may be 140 to 170 beats/minute, but with treatment or disease of the AV conduction system, the ventricular response may be slower. The ventricular rhythm is characteristically irregularly irregular. Atrial fibrillation usually is preceded by PACs.

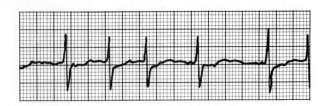

FIGURE 12–29
Atrial fibrillation. (Atrial rate = 400–600 beats/minute with a variable ventricular response. Characteristic atrial fibrillatory waves seen.)

Etiology

Although atrial fibrillation may occur as a transient dysrhythmia in healthy young people, the presence of permanent atrial fibrillation almost is always associated with underlying heart disease. One or both of the following are present in patients with permanent atrial fibrillation: atrial muscle disease or atrial distension together with disease of the sinus node. This rhythm commonly occurs in the setting of CHF, ischemic or rheumatic heart disease, pulmonary disease, and after open heart surgery. It also is seen in congenital heart disease.

Clinical Significance

Atrial fibrillation causes the cardiac output to fall because of (1) a rapid rate that allows less time for the ventricles to fill, and (2) loss of effective atrial contractions (atrial kick). Patients with borderline cardiac function may experience signs and symptoms of hemodynamic compromise while in this rhythm. A pulse deficit often will be seen in this setting. The radial pulse is slower than the apical pulse because some systolic contractions are weak and not palpable in the peripheral arteries.

In addition, patients with chronic atrial fibrillation are at high risk for an embolic event, including stroke. Because of the passive dilated state of the atria, thrombi can form on the atrial wall and dislodge, producing embolization. The incidence of embolization can be reduced by anticoagulation.

Treatment

If cardiac output remains sufficient and the patient is not hypotensive or in significant heart failure, drug therapy usually is tried first. Digitalis is specifically useful because it increases AV block and allows more time for diastolic filling of the ventricles. The rhythm also may convert with digitalis to a normal sinus mechanism. Diltiazem or verapamil also can be used for this purpose. Quinidine aids in maintenance of normal sinus rhythm. Cardioversion is indicated when drug therapy fails or in the setting of hemodynamic compromise.

Multifocal Atrial Tachycardia

Definition

Multifocal atrial tachycardia (MAT) is a rapid atrial rhythm with varying P wave morphology, due to the firing of three or more atrial foci (Fig. 12–30). The atrial rate exceeds 100 beats/minute and the rhythm usually is irregular. The P waves vary in shape because of the multiple foci. The PR intervals may vary also, depending on the proximity of the focus to the AV node. The QRS complexes are normal unless an impulse is conducted with aberrancy.

Etiology

This rhythm characteristically occurs in patients with severe pulmonary disease. Such patients often exhibit hypoxemia, hypokalemia, alterations in serum pH, or pulmonary hypertension.

Clinical Significance

The patient usually manifests symptoms associated with the underlying disease rather than with the dysrhythmia itself.

Treatment

Treatment is directed toward controlling the underlying pulmonary disease and slowing the ventricular rate if necessary.

Junctional Dysrhythmias

Junctional Premature Beat

Definition

A junctional premature beat (JPB) is defined as an ectopic impulse from a focus in the AV junction, occurring prematurely, before the next sinus impulse (Fig. 12–31). As in all rhythms originating in the AV junction, the QRS

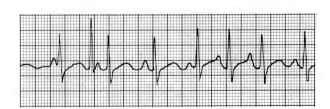

FIGURE 12–30
Multifocal atrial tachycardia. (The atrial rate exceeds 100 beats/minute with three or more different P wave morphologies.)

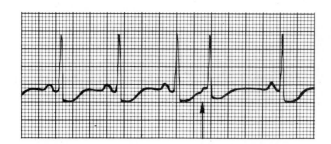

FIGURE 12–31
Junctional premature beat.

will be narrow (<0.12 second), reflecting normal AV conduction. On rare occasions, the QRS may be wide if the impulse is conducted aberrantly. The atria are depolarized in a retrograde fashion at approximately the same time as the ventricles, producing P waves that may occur before, during, or after the QRS complex. These P waves often are inverted in leads II, III, and aVF due to retrograde conduction to the atria.

Etiology

As with PACs, JPBs may occur in normal people or in those with underlying heart disease. Ischemia or infarction may stimulate an ectopic focus in the AV junction, as well as stimulants such as nicotine or caffeine or pharmacologic agents (eg, digitalis).

Clinical Significance

Frequent JPBs may indicate increasing irritability and be a precursor of junctional tachycardia. The patient usually is asymptomatic, although he or she may experience a "skipped beat."

Treatment

No treatment is necessary for JPBs. Increasing irritability may precede junctional tachycardia.

Ventricular Dysrhythmias

Ventricular Premature Beat

Definition

A ventricular premature beat (VPB) is an ectopic beat originating prematurely at the level of the ventricles (Fig. 12–32). This impulse also may be referred to as a PVC (premature ventricular contraction) or a VPC (ventricular premature contraction). Because the beat is ventricular in origin, it will not travel through the normal conduction system. The QRS not only will be premature, but will be

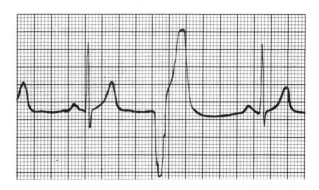

FIGURE 12–32
Ventricular premature contraction.

wide and bizarre with a T wave that is opposite in deflection to the QRS complex. A compensatory pause often follows the premature beat as the heart awaits the next stimulus from the sinus node. The pause is considered fully compensatory if the cycles of the normal and premature beats equal the time of two normal heart cycles.

Ventricular premature beats can be described by both their frequency and pattern. They can be *rare*, *occasional*, or *frequent*, although it is optimal to describe them in number of VPBs/minute. If VPBs occur after each sinus beat, *ventricular bigeminy* is present (Fig. 12–33). *Ventricular trigeminy* is a VPB occurring after two consecutive sinus beats. When VPBs appear in only one form, they are referred to as *uniformed*, versus *multiformed* when there are two or more forms of the QRS complex apparent (Fig. 12–34). Two VPBs in a row is defined as a *couplet* (Fig. 12–35), whereas three in a row is a *triplet*, as well as a short run of ventricular tachycardia.

Etiology

Ventricular premature beats are the most common of all ectopic beats and can occur in any age group, with or without heart disease. They are especially common in a person with myocardial disease (ischemia or infarction) or with myocardial irritability (hypokalemia, increased levels of catecholamines, or mechanical irritation with a wire or catheter).

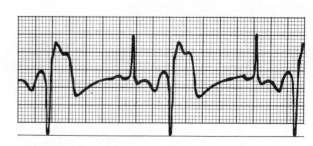

FIGURE 12–33
Ventricular bigeminy. (Every other beat is a VPB.)

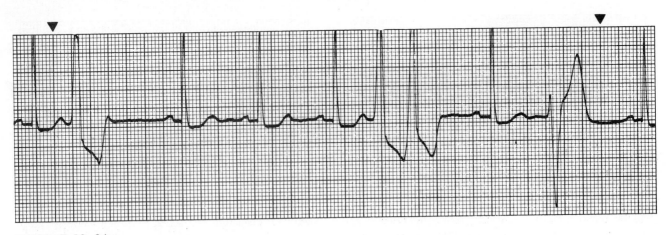

FIGURE 12–34
Multiformed VPBs.

Clinical Significance

The presence of VPBs is a sign of ventricular myocardial irritability and, in some patients, may lead to ventricular tachycardia (VT) or ventricular fibrillation (VF). The nature of the patient's underlying heart disease rather than presence of VPBs as such will determine the prognosis. The presence of numerous and multiformed VPBs in the presence of serious heart disease worsens the prognosis. Ventricular premature beats approaching the apex of the T wave (the R on T phenomenon) do not seem to be any more critical in the development of VT and VF than those that fall away from the T wave in most settings.

Treatment

If infrequent, isolated VPBs require no treatment. Multiple or consecutive VPBs are managed with antiarrhythmic agents. In the emergency setting, lidocaine followed by procainamide are the drugs of choice. Many antiarrhythmic agents are available for chronic therapy (eg, quinidine, procainamide, amiodarone). If the serum potassium is low, potassium replacement may correct the dysrhythmia. If the dysrhythmia is due to digitalis toxicity, withdrawal of the drug may correct it.

Ventricular Tachycardia

Definition

In the previous section, VT was defined as three or more VPBs in a row. It is recognized by wide, bizarre QRS complexes occurring in a fairly regular rhythm at a rate greater than 100 beats/minute (Fig. 12–36). P waves usually are not seen and if seen, are not related to the QRS. VT can present as a short, nonsustained rhythm or be longer and sustained. In the example shown (see Fig 12–36), VT terminates spontaneously, resulting in sinus rhythm.

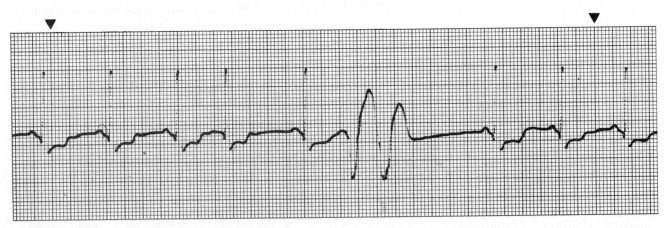

FIGURE 12–35
Couplet (two VPBs in a row).

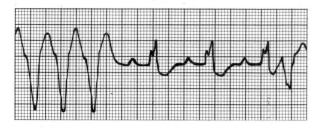

FIGURE 12–36
Ventricular tachycardia. (The first three beats are ventricular tachycardia with the rhythm converting to sinus rhythm with first-degree heart block.)

Etiology

Ventricular tachycardia is rare in adults with normal hearts but is common as a complication of myocardial infarction. Other causes are the same as described for VPBs.

Clinical Significance

Ventricular tachycardia is a precursor of VF; signs and symptoms of hemodynamic compromise (ischemic chest pain, hypotension, pulmonary edema, and unconsciousness) may be seen if the rate is fast and the tachycardia is sustained. Serious dysrhythmia progression depends on the underlying heart disease.

Treatment

If the patient is hemodynamically stable with the dysrhythmia, lidocaine is the treatment of choice. If the patient becomes unstable, synchronized cardioversion (or in emergency situations, unsynchronized cardioversion) is indicated. Long-term treatment for this dysrhythmia may involve the use of an AICD (automatic implantable cardioverter defibrillator).

Torsades de Pointes

Definition

Torsades de pointes ("twisting of the points") is a specific type of ventricular tachycardia (Fig. 12–37). The term refers to the polarity of the QRS complex, which swings from positive to negative and vice versa. The QRS mor-

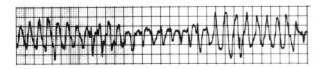

FIGURE 12–37
Torsades de pointes.

phology is characterized by large, bizarre, polymorphous or multiformed QRS complexes of varying amplitude and direction, frequently varying from beat to beat and resembling torsion around an isoelectric line. The rate of the tachycardia is 100 to 180 but can be as fast as 200 to 300 beats/minute. The rhythm is highly unstable; it may terminate in VF or it may revert to sinus rhythm. This form of VT is most likely to develop with severe myocardial disease when the underlying QT interval has been prolonged.

Etiology

Torsades de pointes is favored by conditions that prolong the QT interval. Examples include severe bradycardia, drug therapy, especially with the type IA antiarrhythmic agents (eg, quinidine, procainamide), and electrolyte disturbances, such as hypokalemia and hypomagnesemia. Other factors that can precipitate this dysrhythmia include intrinsic cardiac disease, familial QT prolongation, central nervous system disorders, and hypothermia.

Clinical Significance

Torsades may terminate spontaneously and may repeat itself after several seconds or minutes, or it may transform to VF.

Treatment

Treatment for this dysrhythmia consists of shortening the refractory period (and thus the QT interval) of the underlying rhythm. Both intravenous isoproterenol and overdrive pacing can be used in this setting. In addition, treatment is directed at correcting the underlying problem such as treating the electrolyte deficiency or stopping the offending pharmacologic agent. Emergency cardioversion is indicated if the torsades does not revert spontaneously to sinus rhythm.

Ventricular Fibrillation

Definition

Ventricular fibrillation is defined as rapid, irregular, and ineffectual depolarizations of the ventricle (Fig. 12–38). No distinct complexes are seen. Only irregular oscillations of the baseline are apparent; these may be either coarse or fine in appearance.

Etiology

Ventricular fibrillation may occur in the following circumstances: myocardial ischemia and infarction, catheter manipulation in the ventricles, electrocution, prolonged QT

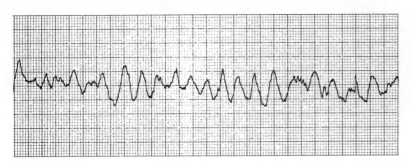

FIGURE 12–38
Ventricular fibrillation.

intervals, or as a terminal rhythm in patients with circulatory failure.

Clinical Significance

As in asystole, loss of consciousness occurs within seconds in the setting of VF. The patient is pulseless and there is no cardiac output. Ventricular fibrillation is the most common cause of sudden cardiac death and is fatal if resuscitation is not instituted immediately.

Treatment

If VF occurs, rapid defibrillation is the management of choice (see the discussion of cardiopulmonary resuscitation in Chapter 13). If the arrest is witnessed, a precordial thump is indicated before the patient is defibrillated. The patient should be supported with cardiopulmonary resuscitation and drugs if there is no response to defibrillation. An AICD may be indicated for long-term management of this problem.

Accelerated Idioventricular Rhythm

Definition

Accelerated idioventricular rhythm is produced by a "speeding up" of ventricular pacemaker cells, which normally have an intrinsic rate of 20 to 40 beats/minute (Fig. 12–39). When the idioventricular rate accelerates above the sinus rate, the ventricular pacemaker becomes the primary pacemaker for the heart. This rhythm is characterized by wide QRS complexes occurring regularly at a

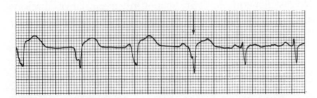

FIGURE 12–39
Accelerated ventricular rhythm. The first three beats are of ventricular origin. The fourth beat (*arrow*) represents a fusion beat. The subsequent two beats are of sinus origin.

rate of 50 to 100 beats/minute. Accelerated idioventricular rhythm may last for a few beats or may be sustained.

Etiology

Typically, this rhythm is seen with acute myocardial infarction, often in the setting of coronary artery reperfusion post-thrombolytic therapy. Less commonly, it may occur as a result of ischemia or digitalis intoxication.

Clinical Significance

The patient usually is not symptomatic with this dysrhythmia. Adequate cardiac output can be maintained and degeneration into a rapid ventricular tachycardia is rare.

Treatment

In most cases, no treatment is necessary.

Atrioventricular Blocks

Atrioventricular block results from a disturbance in some portion of the AV conduction system. The sinus-initiated beat is delayed or completely blocked from activating the ventricles. The block may occur at the level of the AV node, bundle of His, or the bundle branches because the AV conduction system contains all of these structures. In first- and second-degree AV block, the block is incomplete—that is, some or all of the impulses eventually are conducted to the ventricles. In third-degree or complete heart block, none of the sinus initiated impulses are conducted.

First-Degree AV Block

Definition

In first-degree block, AV conduction is prolonged but all impulses eventually are conducted to the ventricles (Fig. 12–40). P waves are present and precede each QRS in a 1:1 relationship. The PR interval is constant but exceeds the upper limit of 0.20 second in duration.

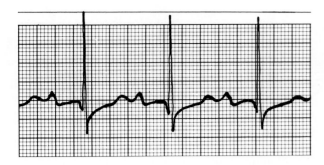

FIGURE 12–40
First-degree AV block (PR interval = 0.36 second.)

Etiology

This type of block occurs in all ages and in both normal and diseased hearts. PR prolongation may be caused by drugs, such as digitalis, β-blockers, or calcium channel blockers, as well as coronary artery disease, a variety of infectious diseases, and congenital lesions.

Clinical Significance

First-degree block is of no hemodynamic consequence to the patient but should be seen as an indicator of a potential AV conduction system disturbance. It may progress to second- or third-degree AV block.

Treatment

No treatment is indicated for first-degree heart block. The PR interval should be monitored closely, watching for further block. The possibility of drug effect also should be evaluated.

Second-Degree AV Block— Mobitz I (Wenckebach)

Definition

In this type of second-degree block, AV conduction is delayed progressively with each sinus impulse until eventually the impulse is completely blocked from reaching the ventricles. The cycle then repeats itself (Fig. 12–41).

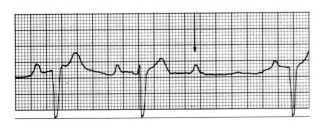

FIGURE 12–41
Second-degree block—Mobitz I (Wenckebach). The arrow indicates the nonconducted P wave in this sequence.

On the ECG tracing, P waves are present and related to the QRS in a cyclic pattern. The PR interval progressively lengthens with each beat until a QRS complex is not conducted. The QRS complex has the same configuration as the underlying rhythm. The interval between successive QRS complexes shortens until a dropped beat occurs.

Etiology

A Wenckebach or Mobitz type I block usually is associated with block above the bundle of His. Therefore, any drug or disease process that affects the AV node, such as digitalis or an inferior wall myocardial infarction, may produce this type of second-degree block.

Clinical Significance

The patient rarely is symptomatic with this type of second-degree AV block because the ventricular rate usually is adequate. It often is temporary in nature and if it progresses to third-degree block, a junctional pacemaker at a rate of 40 to 60 beats/minute usually will take over to pace the ventricles (Table 12–6). Of the two types of second-degree block, Mobitz I is the more common.

Treatment

No treatment is required for this rhythm except to discontinue a drug if it is the offending agent. The patient should be monitored for further progression of block.

Second-Degree AV Block—Mobitz II

Definition

Mobitz type II block is described as an intermittent block in the AV conduction without prior prolongation of the PR interval. It is characterized by a fixed PR interval when AV conduction is present and a nonconducted P wave when the block occurs (Fig. 12–42). This block in conduction can occur occasionally or be repetitive with a 2:1, 3:1, or even 4:1 conduction pattern. Because there is no disturbance in the sinus node, the PP interval will be regular. Often there is accompanying bundle branch block (BBB), so the QRS will be wide.

Etiology

Presence of a Mobitz II pattern implies block below the bundle of His. It is seen in the setting of an anterior wall myocardial infarction and various diseases of the conducting tissue.

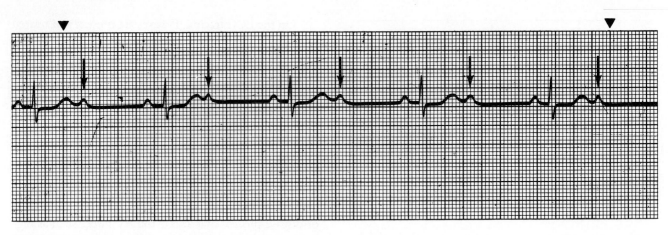

FIGURE 12–42
Second-degree block—Mobitz II. Arrows denote blocked P wave (2:1 block).

Clinical Significance

Mobitz II block is potentially more dangerous than Mobitz I (see Table 12–6). It often is permanent in nature, and it may deteriorate rapidly to third-degree heart block with a slow ventricular response of 20 to 40 beats/minute.

Treatment

Constant monitoring and observation for progression to third-degree heart block is required. Medications, such as atropine or isoproterenol, or cardiac pacing may be required if the patient becomes symptomatic or if this block occurs in the setting of an acute anterior wall myocardial infarction.

Third-Degree (Complete) AV Block

Definition

In third-degree or complete heart block, the sinus node continues to fire normally, but none of the impulses reaches the ventricles (Fig. 12–43). The ventricles are stimulated from escape pacemaker cells either in the junction (at a rate of 40–60 beats/minute) or in the ventricles (at a rate of 20–40 beats/minute), depending on the level of the AV block.

On the ECG tracing, P waves and QRS complexes are both present but there is no relationship between the two. The PP and RR intervals will each be regular but the PR interval will be variable. If a junctional pacemaker paces

TABLE 12–6
Comparison of Second-Degree Atrioventricular (AV) Block

Mobitz I (Wenckebach)	Mobitz II
AV lesion is above bundle of His	Lesion is below bundle of His, in bundle branch system
Associated with inferior MI, digitalis toxicity, chronic lesion of conduction system	Associated with anterior MI, chronic lesion of conduction system
Described as ischemic, reversible, and transient in nature	Described as necrotic in nature
Dropped QRS complex preceded by progressive prolongation of the PR interval	Dropped QRS complex preceded by a fixed PR interval
Regular PP intervals	Regular PP intervals
QRS usually narrow	QRS usually wide
Usually responds well to pharmacologic intervention	Usually not responsive to pharmacologic intervention
May require temporary pacing in symptomatic patients	Often requires cardiac pacing

MI, myocardial infarction.
Adapted from Vinsant MO, Spence MI: Commonsense Approach to Coronary Care, 4th ed, p 310. St. Louis, CV Mosby, 1985.

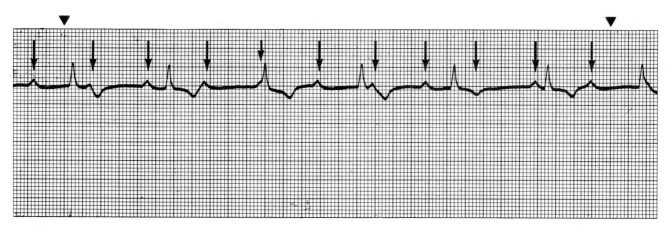

FIGURE 12–43
Third-degree block (complete AV block). Arrows denote P waves. Note the lack of relationship between the atria (P wave) and ventricles (QRS).

the ventricles, the QRS will be narrow. An idioventricular pacemaker will produce a wide QRS complex.

Etiology

The causes of complete heart block are the same as for lesser degrees of AV block.

Clinical Significance

Complete heart block is poorly tolerated if the escape rhythm is ventricular in origin, usually slow and unreliable. The patient may remain asymptomatic if the escape rhythm supports a normal cardiac output.

Treatment

Therapy includes administration of atropine or isoproterenol, but temporary or permanent pacing often is required.

Bundle Branch Block

Definition

A BBB develops when there is either a functional or pathologic block in one of the major branches of the intraventricular conduction system. As conduction through one bundle is blocked, the impulse travels along the unaffected bundle and activates one ventricle normally. The impulse is delayed in reaching the other ventricle, because it travels outside of the normal conducting fibers. The right and left ventricles are thus depolarized sequentially instead of in the normal simultaneous pattern. The abnormal activation produces a wide QRS complex (Fig. 12–44).

Right bundle branch block (RBBB) and *left bundle branch*

block (LBBB) are diagnosed on the 12-lead ECG but also can be identified on the bedside monitor using a V_1 or MCL_1 tracing (see section on Electrocardiographic Monitoring for description of lead). To identify the presence of a BBB, the QRS duration must be prolonged to 0.12 second or greater. A RBBB will have an rSR[1] configuration in V_1, whereas a LBBB will reflect a deep, broad qS or rS complex (Table 12–7). T wave changes are secondary

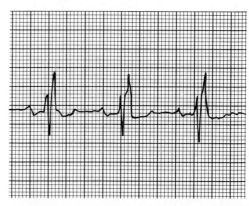

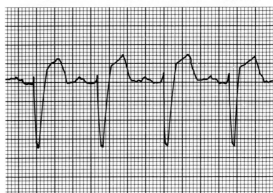

FIGURE 12–44
Right bundle branch block (*top*) and left bundle branch block (*bottom*) in an MCL_1 tracing.

TABLE 12–7
Identification of Bundle Branch Block on MCL₁ Tracing

RBBB
1. QRS ≥ 0.12 sec
2. rSR^1 configuration in V₁

LBBB
1. QRS ≥ 0.12 sec
2. Large negative qS or rS configuration in V₁

to abnormalities in ventricular depolarization and they occur opposite in direction of the QRS complex. The reader is referred to an ECG text for additional criteria for interpretation on the 12-lead ECG.

Etiology

The most common causes of BBB are myocardial infarction, hypertension, and cardiomyopathy. Right bundle branch block is seen more commonly and also may be found in normal people with no clinical evidence of heart disease and with congenital lesions involving the septum. Left bundle branch block is less common and usually associated with some type of underlying heart disease.

Clinical Significance

Bundle branch block signifies underlying disease of the intraventricular conduction system. The patient should be monitored for involvement of the other bundles or fascicles or for progression to complete heart block. Progression of block may be very slow or rapid, depending on the clinical setting.

Treatment

The underlying heart disease determines treatment and prognosis.

Nursing Care Plan

Potential for or actual decrease in cardiac output is a nursing diagnosis that may be ascribed to patients exhibiting serious dysrhythmias. If a dysrhythmia occurs, the nurse should assess the patient for any hemodynamic change and possible cause of the rhythm disturbance, notify the physician, and treat the dysrhythmia as directed. Assessment of the response to treatment must be documented by physical assessment and rhythm strip analysis. The expected outcome would be the elimination or control of the dysrhythmia without hemodynamic compromise to the patient (see Nursing Care Plan 12–1).

Effects of Serum Electrolyte Abnormalities on the Electrocardiogram

Behavioral Objectives

Description

Potassium

Hyperkalemia

Hypokalemia

Calcium

Hypercalcemia

Hypocalcemia

Summary

BEHAVIORAL OBJECTIVES

Based on the content of this section, the reader should be able to:

1. Identify common causes of potassium and calcium imbalances in critically ill patients.
2. Describe the ECG changes associated with serum potassium and calcium abnormalities.

Description

The maintenance of adequate fluid and electrolyte balance assumes high priority in the care of patients in any medical, surgical, or coronary intensive care unit. Patients being treated for renal or cardiovascular diseases are especially vulnerable to electrolyte imbalances. The cure may well be worse than the disease if electrolyte abnormalities go un-

NURSING CARE PLAN 12–1:
The Patient with Dysrhythmia

NURSING DIAGNOSIS	OUTCOME CRITERIA/ PATIENT GOALS	NURSING INTERVENTIONS
Decreased cardiac output: related to electrical instability affecting rate, rhythm, or conduction that affects tissue perfusion	• Cardiac rhythm with adequate systemic perfusion will be maintained	1. Conduct continuous cardiac monitoring in lead II, MCL_1, or optimal lead for waveform analysis. (See Lead Selection in Chapter 12, section on Electrocardiographic Monitoring).
		2. Evaluate and document frequency, morphology, and complexity of dysrhythmia. Obtain 12-lead ECG if unable to evaluate rhythm strip.
		3. Determine effect of dysrhythmia on patient status: assess hemodynamic status (BP), neuro status, skin, renal function, and for evidence of cardiac ischemia.
		4. O_2 2–4 liters per nasal cannula.
		5. Assess patient for presence of predisposing factors: a. Electrolyte imbalance b. Hypoxemia c. Pain d. Fever e. Hypovolemia f. Anxiety g. Drug toxicity h. Increased vagal tone i. Decreased cardiac output/congestive heart failure
		6. Administer antiarrhythmic medication, cardioversion, or life support measures, as ordered.
		7. Document response of dysrhythmia to newly instituted or altered therapy.

detected or ignored because they frequently are caused by the treatment rather than by the disease itself.

Dialysis can very quickly cause major shifts in electrolytes. Certainly, the often insidious drop of serum potassium levels in the digitalized cardiac patient who received diuretics is well known. Diuretics also are used frequently as part of the medical regimen for the control of hypertension. Any addition, deletion, or change in diuretic therapy warrants close following of serum electrolytes.

A history of any of the aforementioned problems should alert the nurse to check the patient's serum electrolytes on an ongoing basis.

Potassium and calcium are probably the two most important electrolytes involved in the proper function of the heart. Because of their effects on the electrical impulse in the heart, excess or insufficiency of either electrolyte frequently causes changes in the ECG. The nurse who is aware of and is able to recognize these changes may well

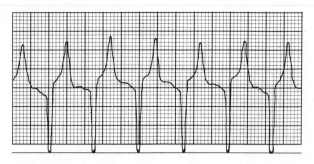

FIGURE 12–45
Hyperkalemia and the presence of peaked T waves.

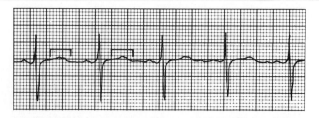

FIGURE 12–47
Fusion of T and U waves (hypokalemia).

suspect electrolyte abnormalities before laboratory findings or clinical symptoms appear and hazardous dysrhythmias occur.

Potassium

Potassium is the primary intracellular cation found in the body. Inside the cardiac cell, potassium is important for repolarization and for maintaining a stable, polarized state.

Hyperkalemia

The earliest sign of hyperkalemia on the ECG is a change in the T wave. It usually is described as tall, narrow, and "peaked" or "tenting" in appearance (Fig. 12–45). As the serum potassium level rises, the P wave amplitude decreases and the PR interval prolongs. Atrial asystole occurs, along with a widening of the QRS. At high, near-lethal potassium levels, the widened QRS merges with the T wave and starts resembling a sine wave. Various dysrhythmias can occur during this time, with progression to VF and asystole. Clinically, the described changes in T waves begin to appear at serum levels of 6 to 7 mEq/liter; QRS widening is seen at serum levels of at 8 to 9 mEq/liter. Vigorous treatment must be instituted to reverse the condition at this point because sudden death may occur at any time after these levels are reached.

The ECG changes in hyperkalemia also may be associated with other conditions. Tall, peaked T waves may be a normal finding or may occur in the early stages of myocar-

dial infarction. QRS widening may be seen with quinidine and procainamide toxicity.

Hypokalemia

Hypokalemia is associated with the appearance of U waves. Although the presence of U waves can be normal for many people, they also may be an early sign of hypokalemia (Fig. 12–46). Usually easily recognized (best seen in lead V_3), the U wave may encroach on the preceding T wave and go unnoticed (Fig. 12–47). The T wave may look notched or prolonged when it is hiding the U wave, giving the appearance of a prolonged QT interval. With increased potassium depletion, the U wave may become more prominent as the T wave becomes less so. The T wave becomes flattened and may even invert. The ST segment tends to become depressed, somewhat resembling the effects of digitalis on the ECG. Only at very low serum levels is there reasonable correlation between ECG changes and serum potassium concentrations.

Changes seen in hypokalemia are observed with other conditions also. The U wave may be accentuated in association with digitalis, quinidine, left ventricular hypertrophy, and bradycardia.

Untreated hypokalemia enhances instability in the myocardial cell. Ventricular premature beats are the most common manifestation of this imbalance, but supraventricular dysrhythmias, conduction problems, and eventually VT and VF can be seen. Hypokalemia also increases the sensitivity of the heart to digitalis and its accompanying dysrhythmias, even at normal serum levels of the drug.

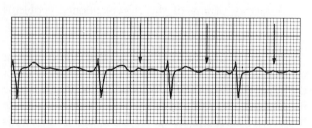

FIGURE 12–46
Presence of U waves (hypokalemia).

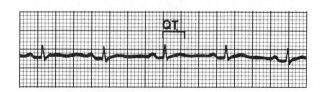

FIGURE 12–48
Shortened QT interval (hypercalcemia). The normal QT interval for the above heart rate of 88 beats/minute is 0.28 second to 0.36 second. This patient's serum calcium level is 12.1 mg/dl, and the QT interval measures 0.24 second.

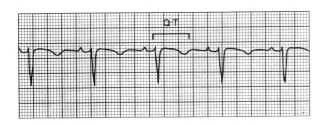

FIGURE 12–49
Prolonged QT interval (hypocalcemia). For this heart rate of 70 beats/minute, the QT interval should be between 0.31 and 0.38 seconds. This patient's QT interval measures 0.50 seconds because his serum calcium level is 5.4 mg/dl. (Normal serum calcium is 8.5–10.5 mg/dl.)

The severity of the dysrhythmias associated with hypokalemia requires early recognition of this problem.

Calcium

Like potassium, calcium is important in normal cardiac function. It is essential for the initiation and propagation of electrical impulses and for myocardial contractility. Abnormal calcium levels are not commonly seen unless they are associated with an underlying disease, and therefore they are not as common as serum potassium abnormalities.

Hypercalcemia

The major ECG finding associated with this disorder is shortening of the QT interval (Fig. 12–48). Because the QRS and T waves usually are unaffected by changes in serum calcium levels, the shortened QT is a result of shortening of the ST segment. QT shortening also is seen in patients taking digitalis. In addition, the ST segment occasionally becomes depressed and T wave inversion may be seen.

Hypocalcemia

On the ECG, low serum calcium levels prolong the QT interval due to a lengthening of the ST segment (Fig. 12–49). The T wave itself does not prolong but may be inverted in some cases. The prolongation of the QT interval in hypocalcemia should not be mistaken for a prolonged QTU interval seen in hypokalemia. Hypocalcemia may be associated with decreased potassium in the patient with chronic renal failure.

In addition to hypocalcemia, QT prolongation may be seen with cerebral vascular disease and after a cardiac arrest. Several antiarrhythmic agents produce prolonged QT intervals and always should be considered when evaluating the ECG for hypocalcemic changes.

Summary

Just as the patient who sustains myocardial infarction may not have chest pain, the patient who has electrolyte abnormalities may not exhibit any of the ECG changes described (Table 12–8). Conversely, a patient with normal serum electrolytes may show some of these ECG changes for other reasons. None of the ECG manifestations described here even approaches being diagnostic. They are valuable primarily in arousing suspicion of electrolyte abnormalities. It is appropriate for the nurse, especially one who cares for the critically ill, to be alert to ECG changes and to interpret observations in the context of known data on the patient.

TABLE 12–8
Electrocardiogram (ECG) Changes Associated with Electrolyte Imbalances

Electrolyte Imbalance	Major ECG Changes	Associated Dysrhythmias
Hyperkalemia	Tall, narrow, peaked T waves; flat, wide P waves; widening QRS	Sinus bradycardia; sinoatrial block; junctional rhythm; idioventricular rhythm; ventricular tachycardia; ventricular fibrillation
Hypokalemia	Prominent U waves; ST segment depression; T wave inversion	Ventricular premature beats; supraventricular tachycardia; ventricular tachycardia; ventricular fibrillation
Hypercalcemia	Shortened QT interval	Rare
Hypocalcemia	Lengthened QT interval; T wave lowering and inversion	Rare

Hemodynamic Monitoring

BEHAVIORAL OBJECTIVES

Based on the content in this section, the reader should be able to:

1. Describe the characteristics of a normal systemic arterial, right atrial, right ventricular, pulmonary artery, and pulmonary capillary wedge waveform.
2. Discuss the basic components necessary to monitor pressure invasively.
3. State nursing interventions that ensure accuracy of pressure readings.
4. Discuss the major complications that can occur with an indwelling arterial line and pulmonary artery catheter.
5. Identify nursing interventions to be taken to prevent the above complications.
6. List possible catheter or machine problems that can occur when monitoring pulmonary artery pressures.
7. Describe nursing interventions for troubleshooting equipment problems.
8. Describe the thermodilution method of measuring cardiac output.

Description

Advances made in medical technology during recent years are most evident in the equipment used to measure hemodynamic parameters. Hemodynamic monitoring of the critically ill patient no longer is an exception but is now the standard of care. The critical care nurse must understand: (1) physiology; (2) basic components necessary to measure pressures; (3) management of the patient; (4) potential complications; and (5) how to troubleshoot problems. All of this knowledge must be integrated and used at the bedside, considering the total patient picture: "Don't just look at the numbers, look at the patient." Clinical assessment of the patient's physiological and psychological status and needs remains imperative. Prioritize those needs but never forget that a person is attached to the other end of all that equipment.

Arterial Pressure Monitoring

Critically ill patients whose hemodynamic status is unstable or who require frequent blood pressure determinations to titrate vasoactive medications may benefit from an indwelling arterial catheter. In low-flow states, the pressure obtained from an indwelling arterial catheter is more accurate than that obtained by indirect auscultation. The availability of continuous pressure measurements saves valuable time for the critical care nurse and provides essential assessment data. In addition, an intra-arterial catheter provides access for frequent sampling of arterial blood gases. Providing a patient with indwelling arterial access reduces the discomfort and risks associated with frequent arterial punctures.

Equipment

Basic Components

The basic equipment necessary to measure pressure directly consists of a transducer, an amplifier, and some means of recording or displaying the information collected (Fig. 12–50).

A transducer is a device that converts one form of energy into another. Transducers can sense changes in flow, temperature, concentration, pressure, light intensity, and other physiological variables. The most commonly used transducer is an external, disposable, strain gauge and pressure transducer. When pressure is applied to the diaphragm of this type of transducer, the sensitive wires attached to the inferior surface of the diaphragm are compressed, increasing the amount of electrical flow to the amplifier–monitor. The amplifier–monitoring system then converts the small electrical signal generated by the transducer to a readable level. Many types of amplifier–monitoring systems are in use, but all have the same basic functions. They contain an on-off switch, a digital readout and oscilloscope to display the pressures, indicators to display systolic, diastolic, or mean pressure values, an audible alarm system with adjustable high and low limits, waveform size or gain control, and zeroing and calibration controls.

Plumbing System

Transmission of pressure from the patient to the transducer occurs through a fluid-filled system. The flush solution or fluid is heparinized saline. The saline solution is placed in a pressure bag, which is pumped up to 300 mm Hg and clamped to maintain that pressure. This is done to prevent backflow of blood through the vascular catheter and to assure a continuous fluid flow of 3 to 5 ml/hour through a continuous-flush device located within the plumbing system. The continuous-flush device maintains patency of the indwelling catheter, preventing clot formation at the catheter tip, and allows for the system to be

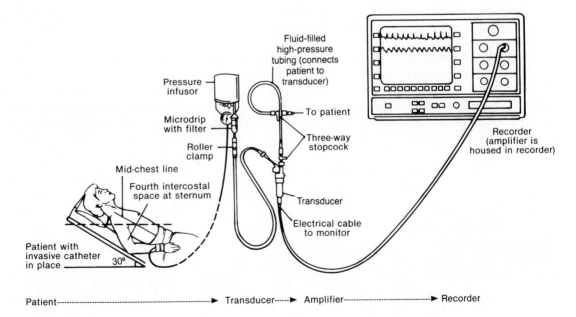

Pressure infusor
Microdrip with filter
Roller clamp
Mid-chest line
Fourth intercostal space at sternum
Patient with invasive catheter in place — 30°
Fluid-filled high-pressure tubing (connects patient to transducer)
To patient
Three-way stopcock
Transducer
Electrical cable to monitor
Recorder (amplifier is housed in recorder)

Patient------------------------------------► Transducer------► Amplifier------------------------------► Recorder

FIGURE 12–50
The indwelling arterial catheter is attached by specialized pressure tubing to a transducer. The transducer is connected to an amplifier/monitor that visually displays a waveform and systolic, diastolic, and mean pressure values. The plumbing system comprises a flush solution under pressure, a continuous flush device, and a series of stopcocks. The stopcocks closest to the insertion site are used to draw blood samples from the artery; the stopcocks located near the transducer are used for zeroing.

flushed manually if necessary. Air bubbles or blood within the plumbing system will distort pressure readings and must be detected and eliminated continually.

The flush solution bag is attached to the indwelling catheter and transducer by a series of tubings and stopcocks. Stiff, noncompliant pressure tubing connects the indwelling catheter to the transducer. The use of soft, distensible tubing may distort and reduce the amplitude of the pressure waveforms. The length of the pressurized tubing should be kept to a minimum to ensure accuracy of readings. Stopcocks are placed in the plumbing system to allow blood samples to be obtained and to permit "zeroing" of the transducer.

The exact location of the transducer, continuous-flush device, stopcocks, and pressurized tubing within the plumbing system will vary. Most institutions use preassembled monitoring kits to avoid gathering and assembling multiple individual pieces.

Procedure

Zeroing and Calibrating the System

Before the system is calibrated and set at zero, all air bubbles must be eliminated. This is done by manually flushing fluid through the plumbing system or transducer. The transducer then must be placed at a preestablished or zero reference point. Because pressure is being measured through a fluid-filled column, any difference between the level of the catheter tip and the transducer will alter the pressure readings obtained. A transducer placed above the level of the catheter tip will produce erroneously low readings, and, conversely, a transducer below the catheter tip will yield falsely elevated readings. The catheter tip is considered to be at the right atrial level. This corresponds to a point 10 cm from the patient's dorsal spine or at the level of the fourth intercostal space in the midaxillary line (see Fig. 12–50). This point also is known as the phlebostatic reference point and the zero reference point. Once the zero reference point has been established, the patient's chest should be marked to ensure consistent transducer placement when subsequent pressure readings are obtained.

"Zeroing" the system negates any effect of atmospheric pressure on the pressure readings obtained, thus ensuring that the measurements reflect only the pressure values in the vessel or heart chamber being monitored. To "zero" the system, adjust the stopcock nearest the transducer *off* to the patient; the transducer then will be open to air. The digital and oscilloscope monitor displays both should be adjusted to read zero.

The transducer and monitoring system then should be calibrated. This procedure ensures that the system accurately reflects the pressure exerted on the transducer. Open the transducer to air, then press the "CAL" button on the monitor system. The digital display and oscilloscope then should be adjusted to the appropriate value (ie, 200 mm Hg). Zeroing and calibrating should be done at least once every 8 hours.

After these two procedures are completed, the stopcock should be adjusted so that the transducer is *open* to the patient and closed to air. Continuous pressure monitoring can then begin.

Arterial Line Insertion

The most common sites for arterial catheter insertions are the radial, brachial, femoral, or dorsalis pedis arteries. Alternate and less frequent sites include the axillary and temporal arteries and the umbilical artery in neonates. Artery selection should be made after several factors are considered. The size of the artery in relation to the size of the catheter should be considered. The artery should be large enough to accommodate the catheter without occluding or significantly impeding flow. The site chosen should be easily accessible and free from contamination by

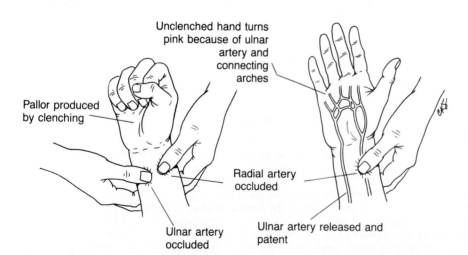

Unclenched hand turns pink because of ulnar artery and connecting arches

Pallor produced by clenching

Radial artery occluded

Ulnar artery occluded

Ulnar artery released and patent

FIGURE 12–51
The modified Allen's test. The patient's hand is clenched into a tight fist, and the nurse compresses the ulnar and radial arteries. The patient then unclenches and clenches the fist until the hand is blanched. The nurse releases the pressure on the ulnar artery and watches for return of color to the hand.

body secretions. Accessibility of the artery is especially important if the patient is on anticoagulants. Finally, the limb distal to the insertion site should have adequate collateral flow in the event that the cannulated artery becomes occluded.

The radial artery is the most frequent site for an arterial catheter. It not only meets the above criteria but it also is superficially located and therefore easy to palpate. Cannulation of this artery also generally poses the least limitation on the patient's mobility.

Before a catheter is inserted into the radial artery, the presence of adequate collateral circulation to the hand by the ulnar artery must be assessed. This is done by performing Allen's test (Fig. 12–51). Both the ulnar and radial arteries are occluded. The patient should then clench and unclench the fist until the hand is blanched. Release pressure on the ulnar artery *only* and observe for color return to the hand. If color returns within 5 to 7 seconds, the ulnar circulation is adequate. If it takes 7 to 15 seconds for color to return, ulnar filling is impaired. Ulnar circulation is considered inadequate if the hand remains blanched for longer than 15 seconds, in which case the radial artery should not be cannulated.

Regardless of the site chosen for arterial catheter placement, the insertion should be performed under sterile technique. The connecting tubing should be assembled and flushed and the transducer zeroed and calibrated before the catheter is inserted. Once the catheter is in place, it should be secured, the site dressed according to the policy of the institution, and the extremity immobilized.

Interpretation of Results

Arterial Pressure Waveform

The normal arterial waveform should have a rapid upstroke, a clear dicrotic notch, and a definite end-diastole (Fig. 12–52). The initial sharp upstroke of the waveform represents the rapid ejection of blood from the ventricle into the aorta. Note that the QRS complex precedes the rapid rise in arterial pressure. Ventricular depolarization causes ventricular contraction and the sharp rise in pressure. This increase in pressure is caused by and therefore follows the QRS complex. The dicrotic notch, closure of the aortic valve, occurs at the end of ventricular repolarization, indicated by the T wave on the ECG (see Fig. 12–52A).

The value measured at the peak of the waveform is the systolic pressure. A normal systolic pressure is 90 to 140 mm Hg. As the pressure in the ventricle falls below the pressure in the aorta, the aortic valve closes. The sudden closure of the aortic valve produces a characteristic dicrotic notch in the descending portion of the waveform. The dicrotic notch then indicates the end of ventricular systole or the beginning of diastole. As blood continues to flow to the periphery, the pressure in the arterial system continues

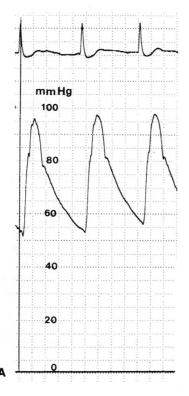

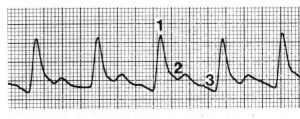

FIGURE 12–52

(**A**) Comparison of arterial waveform with ECG. Note that the rapid rise in arterial pressure follows the QRS complex. The dicrotic notch occurs at the end of the T wave. (**B**) A normal arterial waveform has three components: 1) systolic peak, 2) dicrotic notch, and 3) end-diastole. Normal systolic pressure is 90 to 140 mm Hg, diastolic pressure 60 to 90 mm Hg, MAP 70 to 105 mm Hg.

to fall. The lowest point of the waveform is the diastolic pressure, normally between 60 and 90 mm Hg.

Mean arterial pressure (MAP) and perfusion of vital body organs are directly related. The following equation can be used to calculate MAP:

$$MAP = \frac{systolic + (diastolic \times 2)}{3}$$

Normal MAP is 70 to 105 mm Hg.

The configuration of the arterial waveform and the actual systolic and diastolic pressures may vary depending on the catheter insertion site. The more peripheral the artery used, the steeper the ascending limb of the waveform and the less defined is the dicrotic notch. The systolic pressure is higher and the diastolic pressure lower; however, MAP is unchanged.

Management

The nursing management of the patient with an indwelling arterial catheter should ensure that the readings obtained are accurate and should center around prevention or early detection of complications (Table 12–9).

Before pressure readings are obtained from an arterial line, the nurse should make certain that the transducer is placed at the zero reference point. The quality of the waveform also should be evaluated before readings are taken. The tracing should be clear, with the components of the pressure waveform easily identifiable. Any damping should be corrected. The system should be zeroed and calibrated at least every 8 hours and whenever readings significantly change. The pressure values obtained from an indwelling arterial line should be compared to auscultated cuff pressure at least every 8 hours and whenever the accuracy of the arterial line pressures is questioned. These two methods of measuring arterial pressure will not produce the same values. A disparity of 5 to 20 mm Hg is normal between invasively monitored pressure and auscultated pressure, with values obtained by an indwelling catheter usually *higher* than cuff pressures.

Complications

The major complications associated with indwelling arterial lines are infection, accidental blood loss, and compromised flow to the extremity.

Infection

Proper attention to insertion technique and proper care of the insertion site and plumbing system will reduce the risk of infection. The insertion site should be assessed fre-

quently for signs of infection. Sterile dressing changes, tubing changes, and flush solution changes should be done according to institutional policy. The integrity of the system never should be broken. Blood or air in the system should be removed by aspirating through the stopcocks. The stopcocks should be flushed or cleaned of any blood residue each time a blood sample is withdrawn from the line. Sterile caps may be used to cover the stopcock ports between use.

Accidental Blood Loss

Accidental blood loss from an indwelling arterial line is preventable if basic nursing actions are followed. All connections within the plumbing system should be Luer-Lok and fastened securely together. The extremity in which the line is placed should be immobilized and completely visible at all times. If some type of restraint must be used, never place the restraint over the insertion site. Easy access to the insertion site and connections is imperative. The monitoring system should have an alarm with high and low pressure limits that can be set individually for each patient. The alarms should be inactivated only when someone is working directly with the line (ie, obtaining blood samples or zeroing–calibrating). Assuring that the alarm system remains activated and the limits are appropriately set for the patient's pressure will alert the nurse if damping or disconnection occurs so that immediate action can be taken.

Impaired Circulation to Extremity

Circulation to the extremity in which the arterial line is placed must be monitored continually. Color, sensation, and movement of the extremity should be assessed initially after insertion of the arterial catheter and at least every 8 hours for as long as the catheter is in place. Any indication of impaired circulation should be reported immediately to the physician and may be an indication for catheter removal.

Pulmonary Artery Pressure Monitoring

The pulmonary artery, flow-directed, balloon-tipped catheter (Swan–Ganz) has made possible the safe, easy assessment of left ventricular function. Cardiac output, right atrial (RA), right ventricular (RV), and pulmonary artery (PA) pressures, and pulmonary capillary wedge pressure (PCWP) all are measured using this catheter. In addition to assessing left ventricular function, the pressures obtained using this catheter allow the clinician to determine the therapy needed and to evaluate the effectiveness of the therapy chosen.

TABLE 12–9
Troubleshooting Arterial Pressure Monitoring

Problem	Cause	Prevention	Treatment
Damped pressure tracing	Catheter tip against vessel wall	Usually cannot be avoided	Pull catheter hub back
			Rotate or reposition extremity while observing pressure waveform
	Partial occlusion of catheter tip by clot	Use continuous flush device	Aspirate clot with syringe and manually flush system with heparinized flush solution
		Maintain heparinized saline flush solution under pressure (>300 mm Hg)	
	Clotting in stopcock or transducer	Thoroughly flush catheter after blood withdrawal	Flush stopcock and transducer; if no improvement, change stopcock and transducer
		Use continuous flush device	
Abnormally high or low readings	Change in transducer level	Maintain transducer at mid-chest level for serial pressure measurements	Recheck patient and transducer positions
Damped pressure without improvement after flushing	Air bubbles in transducer or connecting tubing	Carefully flush transducer and tubing when setting up system and attaching to catheter	Check system; flush manually; flush air bubbles out of transducer
	Nonpressure tubing used		
		Use stiff, short pressure tubing	Shorten tubing or replace softer tubing with stiff pressure tubing
No pressure available	Transducer not open to catheter	Follow routine, systematic steps for setting up system and turning stopcocks	Check system—stopcocks, monitor/amplifier setup
	Monitor/amplifier off		
	Incorrect scale selection on monitor	Select scale appropriate to expected range of pressure to be measured	Select appropriate scale

From Daily EK, Schroeder JS: Techniques in Bedside Hemodynamic Monitoring, 4th ed. St. Louis, CV Mosby, 1989.

Equipment

The basic equipment necessary to monitor pulmonary artery pressures is the same used in monitoring a systemic artery pressure. This was discussed earlier in this chapter; refer to that section for a review.

Plumbing System

Likewise, the supplies and set-up for monitoring pulmonary artery pressures are similar to those used for peripheral artery pressure monitoring, also discussed earlier in this chapter.

There are several types of flow-directed, balloon-tipped catheters with different options that warrant discussion. In addition, the use of a fiberoptic pulmonary artery catheter will be discussed to highlight the significance of monitoring mixed venous oxygen saturation.

Swan–Ganz Catheter

The exact type of catheter used is determined by the parameters to be monitored and additional requirements governed by the patient's condition. The 7.5-French (Fr; indicates catheter size) thermodilution catheter is the type most commonly used (Fig. 12–53). This catheter has a proximal port, distal port, balloon inflation valve, and thermistor connector. The proximal or RA port can be used for the infusion of fluids or medications. The outflow tract of this port is located in the RA, so, if connected to a transducer, RA pressure can be measured. The RA port also is used as the injectate infusion port for measuring cardiac outputs. The distal or PA port always is attached to a transducer and a continuous flush system. This allows the PA waveform to be displayed continuously and PA pressures measured. The balloon inflation valve allows the balloon at the catheter tip to be inflated with air and pulmonary artery wedge pressure (PAWP) to be mea-

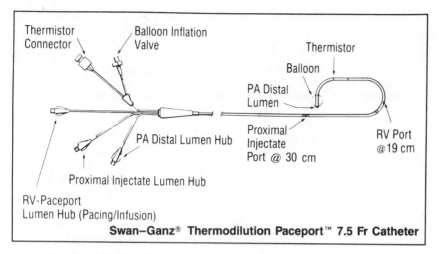

Swan–Ganz® Thermodilution Paceport™ 7.5 Fr Catheter

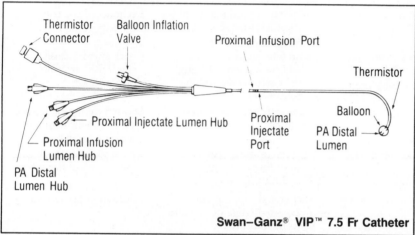

Swan–Ganz® VIP™ 7.5 Fr Catheter

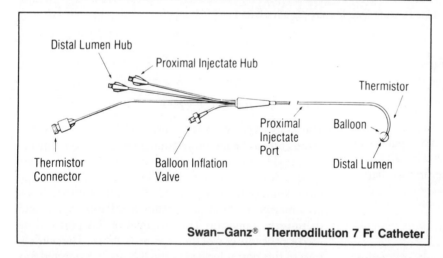

Swan–Ganz® Thermodilution 7 Fr Catheter

FIGURE 12–53
Types of commonly used 7.5-Fr and 7-Fr Swan–Ganz catheters. (Copyright © 1988 by Baxter Healthcare Corp.)

sured. The balloon capacity of a 7-Fr and 7.5-Fr catheter is 1.5 cc, and it never should be inflated with more than this amount of air. The thermistor connector can be connected to a computer, which permits cardiac outputs to be measured directly.

The VIP catheter (Baxter Healthcare Corp., Deerfield, IL) has an additional proximal lumen that serves as another infusion port; the Paceport catheter (Baxter Healthcare Corp.) has an RV lumen through which a pacing probe may be inserted if temporary ventricular pacing is required.

Procedure

Catheter Insertion

Before the catheter is inserted, all necessary equipment should be assembled. The exact set-up and the equipment used will vary depending on the institution. The flush system should be connected to the transducer, which is then placed at the zero reference point, zeroed, and calibrated. Each port of the Swan–Ganz catheter is flushed with sterile saline, and the balloon is inflated with air to check for leaks before the catheter is inserted. The PA port is then connected to the prepared transducer with high-pressure tubing and threaded into the venous access.

The Swan–Ganz catheter is inserted into the venous circulation either through a direct cutdown on a vein or percutaneously through an introducer placed in the vessel of choice. The common insertion sites are the internal or external jugular veins, subclavian or femoral veins, or a vein in the antecubital fossa. An antecubital vein is used only when a direct cutdown is being done. Once the introducer is in place, the PA catheter is inserted by a physician using sterile technique.

Nursing responsibilities during the insertion procedure include recording the pressures in each chamber of the heart as the catheter is passed through and monitoring for ventricular dysrhythmias as the catheter passes through the RV. Ventricular dysrhythmias are a common complication during Swan–Ganz insertion. It therefore is advisable to have a lidocaine bolus and defibrillator available.

The pressure waveform displayed on the monitor indicates the placement of the catheter tip. Final catheter placement always is verified with a chest radiograph.

Interpretation of Results

Waveforms

Right Atrial Pressure

The RA waveform has three positive waves: a, c, and v (Fig. 12–54) The a wave represents RA systole. The v wave represents RA diastole. After RA systole, the tricuspid valve closes. The RA is filling with blood, and the RV is beginning to contract. At this point, the pressure within the RA briefly increases because the force of RV contraction causes the tricuspid valve to balloon into the RA, producing the c wave. Thus, the c wave is caused by the closed tricuspid valve's pushing into the RA during RA diastole. Sometimes, the c wave is superimposed on the a wave and is not distinguishable, or it appears as a notch in the a wave.

In an effort to identify accurately the waves in each of the waveforms, it is helpful to compare the waveform to the ECG. The electrical energy of the heart, illustrated by the ECG, causes and therefore precedes the mechanical events that are illustrated by the waves in each waveform.

On the ECG, the P wave represents electrical discharge of the SA node. After electrical activation, the atria respond by contracting. In comparing the electrical and mechanical events, one can see that the P wave precedes the a wave on the pressure tracing. The QRS complex illustrates ventricular depolarization and serves as the energy source for ventricular contraction. Simultaneous with ventricular contraction, the RA is relaxing and filling with blood. On the hemodynamic tracing, the QRS complex precedes the v wave, indicating atrial relaxation. The v wave often extends beyond the T wave, which illustrates ventricular repolarization on the ECG. If the c wave is visible, it occurs between the a and v waves.

When compared to the ECG, the c wave occurs immediately after the QRS complex. Early in ventricular systole, the pressure within the ventricle pushes the closed tricuspid value toward the RA, causing a slight increase in pressure, as demonstrated by the positive deflection of the c wave (see Fig. 12-54A).

The RA pressure tracing has three negative waves or descents: x, x[1], and y. The descents are of less significance

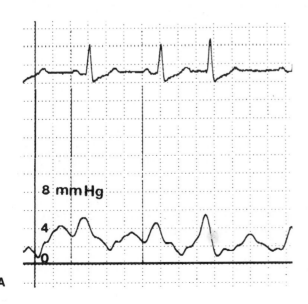

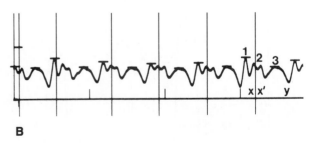

A

B

FIGURE 12–54
(**A**) Comparison of right atrial waveform with ECG. Note that the positive deflection, *a* wave, follows the P wave, the *c* wave is visible and the tall narrower *v* wave follows the T wave. (**B**) Right atrial pressure waveform: 1) *a* wave, 2) *c* wave, 3) *v* wave.

and will be mentioned briefly here. The x descent follows the *a* wave and represents right atrial relaxation. The x^1 descent follows the c wave and represents AV movement during ventricular contraction. The y descent follows the v wave and represents passive RA emptying immediately after opening of the tricuspid valve just before RA systole.

The RA is a low-pressure chamber; the significant RA pressure is the mean. Normal RA pressure is 6 to 2–6 mm Hg.

Right Ventricular Pressure

The RV waveform has an initial rapid rise in pressure that represents isovolumetric contraction (Fig. 12–55) That is, the tricuspid and pulmonary valves are closed, and the volume of blood within the RV remains constant while the pressure increases. When RV pressure exceeds PA pressure, the pulmonary valve opens. Blood is then ejected from the RV into the PA. Right ventricular systolic pressure is represented by the peak of the waveform. The pulmonary valve closes, and the RV pressure rapidly decreases. The tricuspid valve opens, and the RV passively fills with blood from the RA. The lowest point on the waveform represents RV end-diastole.

In comparing the right ventricular waveform with the ECG, notice that after the P wave there is a slight increase in RV filling pressure. This occurs immediately before the steep rise in pressure on the waveform. The increase in RV diastolic pressure represents initial passive filling of the RV and then the impact of atrial contraction, which occurs late in ventricular diastole. On the ECG, the QRS complex precedes the rapid and sharp rise in RV pressure. This steep increase in RV pressure corresponds with ventricular contraction (see Figure 12–55A).

Significant RV pressures are systolic and end-diastolic. Right ventricular systolic pressure is 15 to 30 mm Hg, and RV end-diastolic pressure is less than 6 mm Hg.

Pulmonary Artery Pressure

The rapid rise in the PA waveform represents RV ejection. The dicrotic notch in the downward slope corresponds with pulmonary valve closure. Note that the PA waveform always has a positive pressure; at no time does the pressure wave fall to zero or reach baseline.

After the QRS complex, the PA pressure tracing shows a rapid rise in pressure. This occurs because after the ventricle is electrically activated, the ventricle responds to this stimulation by contraction. When the pressure in the ventricle exceeds the pressure in the PA, the pulmonic valve opens, blood is ejected into the PA, and there is a rapid rise in PA pressure. Maximum PA pressure is reached during ventricular repolarization, the T wave on the ECG. Closure of the pulmonic valve, dicrotic notch, corresponds with the end of ventricular repolarization (Fig. 12–56).

Normal PA pressures are systolic 15 to 30 mm Hg, diastolic 8 to 15 mm Hg, and mean 10 to 22 mm Hg.

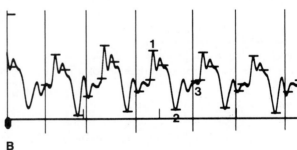

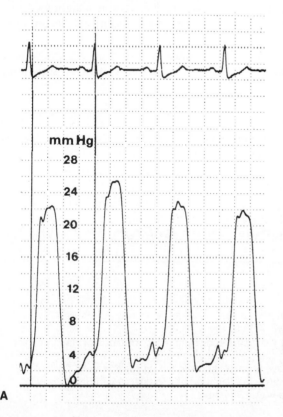

FIGURE 12–55
(**A**) Comparison of right ventricular waveform with ECG. Note that the rapid rise in ventricular pressure follows the QRS complex and the increase in RV diastolic pressure occurs after the P wave. Artifact in tracing is due to catheter movement. (**B**) Right ventricular tracing: 1) systolic pressure, 2) early diastolic dip, 3) end-diastolic pressure.

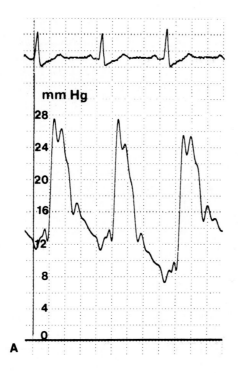

A

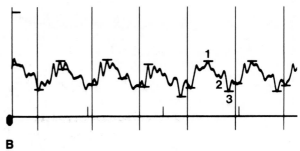

Pulmonary Artery Pressure

B

FIGURE 12–56

(**A**) Comparison of pulmonary artery waveform with ECG. Note the delay in PA rise in pressure after the QRS complex; pressure in the RV must exceed pressure in the PA for the valve to open and ejection to occur. (**B**) Pulmonary artery pressure waveform: 1) systolic pressure, 2) dicrotic notch, 3) diastolic pressure.

Pulmonary Capillary Wedge Pressure

When the tip of the Swan–Ganz catheter is properly positioned in the PA, a PCWP can be obtained by inflating the balloon at the catheter tip. This allows the tip to float into a smaller branch of the PA, occluding forward flow. A change in the waveform from a PA tracing to a PCWP tracing indicates when the catheter is wedged (Fig. 12–57). The PCWP tracing has an a wave, c wave, and a v wave. The a wave reflects left atrial (LA) contraction, the c wave isovolumetric ventricular contraction, and the v wave LA filling.

When comparing the ECG to the PCWP, the P wave will precede the a wave. The P wave is the electrical energy that produces atrial contraction and is reflected as the a wave in the PCWP tracing. In theory, atrial relaxation, the v wave, occurs simultaneously with ventricular contraction, which follows the QRS complex on the ECG. Because of delay in PCWP transmission, both the a and v waves follow the QRS complex (see Figure 12–57A).

When the balloon is inflated and the catheter occludes a branch of the PA, an unrestricted vascular channel extends from the PA through the pulmonary vascular bed, the pulmonary vein, the LA, the open mitral valve, and into the left ventricle (LV) (Fig. 12–58). Thus, the pressure in the PA branch distal to the occluding balloon is essentially the same as the pressure in the pulmonary vein, the LA, and the LV during diastole. The PCWP is thus a reflection of the pressure in the open channel between the balloon tip and the LV at end-diastole. This pressure is an important indication of how well the LV is functioning. Normal PCWP is 6 to 12 mm Hg. This pressure is nearly the same as the PA diastolic pressure in most cases.

Mixed Venous Oxygen Saturation

Mixed venous oxygen saturation ($S\bar{v}O_2$) reflects the balance between oxygen supply and demand needs. Normal oxygen delivery (DO_2) at rest is 1,000 cc/minute, and tissue oxygen consumption (VO_2) is 250 cc/minute. Arterial oxygen saturation is normally 98% to 99%, whereas venous oxygen saturation is about 75%, with a range of 60% to 80%. Under normal conditions, 25% of the oxygen delivered is extracted. With an increased demand for oxygen, the healthy heart can respond by increasing cardiac output to increase oxygen delivery. Venous oxygen saturation is maintained at 75%, and the supply–demand ratio is kept in balance.

$S\bar{v}O_2$ can be measured at the bedside by using a pulmonary artery catheter with fiberoptics that emit light that is reflected by the red blood cells according to the oxygen saturation of the hemoglobin. A decrease in cardiac output, hemoglobin, or oxygen saturation of arterial blood from any cause can result in reduced oxygen delivery and an imbalance between oxygen supply and demand. For example, in the failing heart the cardiac muscle cannot respond to the increased demand for more oxygen by increasing cardiac output. The tissues respond by extracting more oxygen which decreases venous oxygen saturation.

$S\bar{v}O_2$ values are used by the nurse to determine appropriateness and timing of patient care. When $S\bar{v}O_2$ is low (50% or lower), the nurse may choose to modify the plan of care so that additional oxygen will not be demanded when it is not available. Individualized care can be planned and determined by using $S\bar{v}O_2$ values so that oxygen supply and demand are in balance.

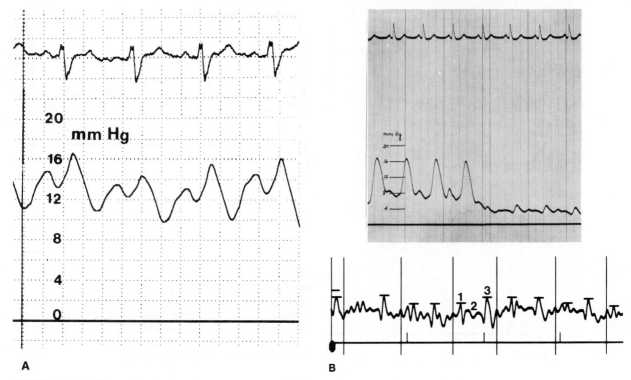

A

B

FIGURE 12–57

(**A**) Comparison of pulmonary capillary wedge tracing with the ECG. The first complete wave after the P wave is the *a* wave, the narrower, taller wave on this tracing. The *v* wave follows the T wave and is shorter and broader. (**B**) Pulmonary artery pressure tracing and pulmonary capillary wedge tracing obtained on balloon inflation (*top*). Pulmonary capillary wedge pressure tracing: 1) *a* wave, 2) *c* wave, 3) *v* wave (*bottom*).

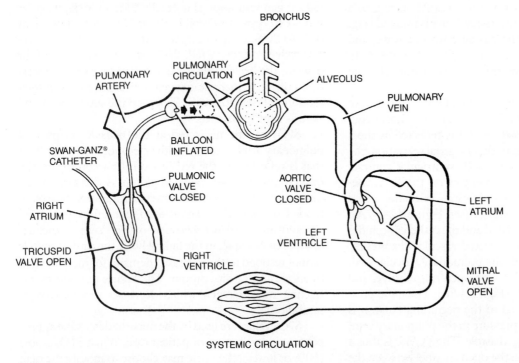

FIGURE 12–58

When the balloon is inflated and the catheter is in the wedge position, there is an unrestricted vascular channel between the tip of the catheter and the left ventricle in diastole. PCWP thus reflects left ventricular end-diastolic pressure, an important indicator of left ventricular function. (Courtesy of Hewlett–Packard.)

Management

Nursing care of the patient undergoing PA pressure monitoring is complex. The critical care nurse must be able to interpret the data obtained as well as be alert to potential complications.

The interventions outlined in the section on arterial pressure monitoring to ensure accurate readings and to prevent infection also apply to the patient with a Swan–Ganz catheter. Troubleshooting of the monitoring system as outlined in Table 12–9 also is applicable to PA pressure monitoring.

The position of the tip of the PA catheter may change after the catheter has been inserted and secured into place. The catheter may migrate forward into a branch of the PA or it may flip back through the pulmonary valve into the RV. Forward migration will be indicated by the pressure of a PCWP tracing without the balloon being inflated (spontaneous wedging). Persistent wedging of the catheter occludes forward flow through a branch of the PA and may cause pulmonary infarction. The PA pressure tracing should be displayed at all times so that spontaneous wedging may be corrected immediately. If the catheter does become spontaneously wedged, make certain the balloon is fully deflated. After doing so, the physician must be notified and the catheter pulled back until a PA tracing once again is present.

The presence of an RV tracing on the monitor indicates that the catheter tip has flipped back into the RV (Fig. 12–59). The change in the waveform also may be accompanied by ventricular ectopy (ventricular premature contractions) due to catheter irritation of the ventricular wall. Inflation of the balloon may protect the ventricle from irritation and decrease the ventricular premature contractions until the catheter tip can either be advanced into the PA or pulled back into the RA.

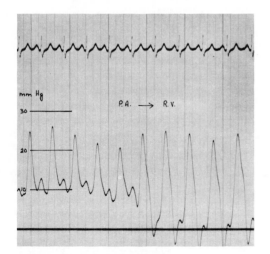

FIGURE 12–59
The appearance of a right ventricular pressure tracing on the monitor indicates that the catheter tip has flipped through the pulmonary valve into the right ventricle.

Proper technique always must be followed when the balloon is inflated to obtain a PCWP. Overinflation may cause PA rupture, prolonged inflation may cause pulmonary infarction, and injection of air into a ruptured balloon may cause air embolization. As mentioned, the balloon capacity of a 7-Fr and 7.5-Fr Swan–Ganz catheter is 1.5 cc. Never insert more air than maximum balloon capacity. Overinflation of the balloon will predispose it to rupture and may cause increased pressure on the walls of the PA, which may damage or rupture the vessel. Inflation of the balloon should be done slowly, while the pressure tracing on the monitor is observed. When the pressure tracing changes from a PA waveform to a PCWP waveform, no more air should be inserted. The amount of air required to obtain a PCWP tracing should then be documented.

When the balloon is being inflated, a slight resistance should be felt. If no resistance is felt and a PCWP tracing cannot be obtained after the maximal volume of air is inserted, balloon rupture should be suspected; in this case, attach a syringe to the balloon valve and withdraw the plunger. The ability to aspirate fluid or blood back into the syringe or the loss of negative pressure will confirm that the balloon is no longer intact. No further air should be injected. Attach a dead-ender cap to the balloon port and apply a piece of tape labeled "balloon rupture" to the inflation port to alert other personnel.

Prolonged inflation of the balloon when obtaining PCWP readings also may cause pulmonary infarction or ischemic injury. The balloon should be inflated for no longer than 30 seconds at a time. Once a PCWP reading is obtained, remove the syringe from the balloon inflation port, allowing the air to escape. Do not manually aspirate the air; this may damage the integrity of the balloon, predisposing it to rupture. After wedging the catheter, always observe the monitor for the return of a clear, undampened PA tracing.

The clinical information obtained from invasive pressure monitoring is truly beneficial in the care of critically ill patients. The role of the critical care nurse in the prevention and early detection of complications is pivotal.

Nursing management of these patients does not end with hemodynamic monitoring. It also must address the psychological needs of patients and their families suddenly placed in a life-threatening situation.

Central Venous Pressure Monitoring

Description

Central venous pressure (CVP) refers to the pressure of blood in the RA or vena cava. It provides information about three parameters—blood volume, the effectiveness of the heart as a pump, and vascular tone. Central venous pressure is to be differentiated from a peripheral venous pressure, which may reflect only a local pressure. Although isolated CVP recordings generally have been replaced by more sophisticated hemodynamic monitoring techniques, an understanding of the physiological principles of CVP is valuable in the critical care setting.

Procedure

For CVP recordings, a long intravenous catheter is inserted into an arm vein, leg vein, or the subclavian vein and threaded into position in the vena cava close to the right atrium. Occasionally, the catheter may advance into the right atrium, which is indicated by rhythmic fluctuations in the pressure manometer corresponding to the patient's heartbeat. In this situation, the catheter may simply be withdrawn to the point at which the pulsations cease.

Figure 12–60 illustrates a typical set-up for measuring the CVP. A manometer with a three-way stopcock is introduced between the fluid source and the patient's intravenous catheter. In this way, three separate systems can be created by manipulating the stopcock.

System 1 connects the fluid source with the patient and can be used for routine administration of intravenous fluids or as an avenue to keep the system patent.

System 2 runs from the fluid source to the CVP manometer and is opened to raise the fluid column in the manometer before venous pressure is measured.

System 3 connects the patient's intravenous catheter

with the manometer, and it is this pathway that must be open to record the CVP. Pressure in the vena cava displaces or equilibrates with the pressure exerted by the column of fluid in the manometer. The point at which the fluid level settles is recorded as the CVP.

To obtain an accurate measurement, make sure that the patient is flat, with the zero point of the manometer at the level of the fourth intercostal space (Fig. 12–61). This level corresponds to the midaxillary line of the patient and can be determined by measuring approximately 5 cm below the sternum. This point is referred to as the phlebostatic axis. Consistency is important, and all readings should be taken with the patient in the same position and the zero point calculated in the same manner. If deviations from the routine procedure must be made, as when the patient cannot tolerate being flat and the reading must be taken with the patient in a semi-Fowler's position, it is valuable to note this on the patient's chart or care plan to provide for consistency in future readings.

A patent system is assured when the fluid column falls freely and slight fluctuation of the fluid column is apparent. This fluctuation follows the patient's respiratory pattern and will fall on inspiration and rise on expiration due to changes in interpulmonary pressure. If the patient is being ventilated on a respirator, a falsely high reading will result. The nurse should check with institutional standards of practice to determine whether or not to take the CVP reading with the patient on or off the ventilator. If it is deemed appropriate to take readings with the patient on the ventilator, significant trends in the CVP still can be determined if consistency in taking the readings is followed.

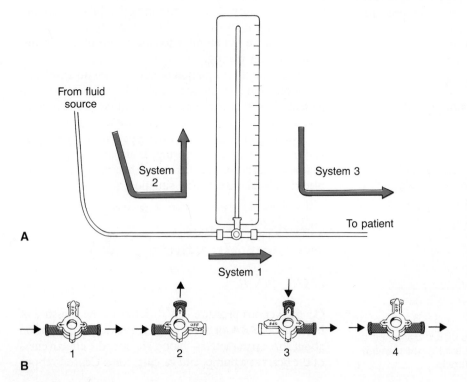

FIGURE 12–60
(**A**) Central venous pressure set-up. System 1 allows for fluid administration. System 2 fills the manometer with fluid. System 3 allows the flow of fluid from the manometer to the patient and determines the CVP reading. (**B**) Steps in measuring central venous pressure. 1, Stopcock turned so that IV fluid flows to patient. 2, Stopcock in position to fill manometer with fluid. 3, Stopcock turned so that it is open from manometer to patient, to obtain reading. 4, Stopcock returned to first position so that IV fluid flows to patient.

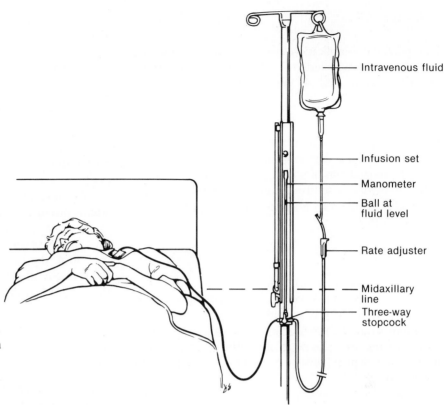

Intravenous fluid

Infusion set

Manometer

Ball at fluid level

Rate adjuster

Midaxillary line

Three-way stopcock

FIGURE 12–61
A typical CVP set-up has a hard plastic manometer that is placed midline on an intravenous infusion set. When read from the midaxillary line with the patient supine, a CVP reading can be obtained.

Interpretation of Results

Central venous pressure is measured in centimeters of water or millimeters of mercury. Considerable variation exists in the range of normal values cited. Normal pressure in the RA is less than 8 cm H_2O, and pressure in the vena cava is approximately 5 to 8 cm H_2O. A CVP reading or an RA pressure reading also can be measured by a pressure transducer. The normal CVP range in this case is 4 to 6 mm Hg mm Hg.

It is the *trend* of the readings that is most significant, regardless of the baseline value. The upward or downward trend of the CVP, combined with clinical assessment of the patient, will determine appropriate interventions.

For example, a patient's CVP may rise gradually from 6 cm H_2O to 8 cm H_2O and then to 10 cm H_2O. This change along with other parameters assessed by the nurse may indicate ensuing complications. For example, auscultation of breath sounds may reveal basilar crackles; an S_3 may be audible; or the pulse and respiratory rate may be increasing insidiously. In this context, the trend of a gradual rise in CVP is more significant than the actual isolated value.

When interpreting CVP data in conjunction with other clinical observations, the nurse has a better understanding of the patient's physiology and will recognize the outcome at which nursing interventions must be aimed. In the example cited in the previous paragraph, the nurse should be aware that too much fluid administration would further compromise the patient's circulatory status, and should act accordingly to reduce this risk.

Sometimes, rate of fluid administration is titrated according to the patient's CVP and urinary output. As long as the urinary output remains adequate and the CVP does not change significantly, this is an indication that the heart can accommodate the amount of fluid being administered. If the CVP begins to rise and the urine output drops, indicating a decreased cardiac output, circulatory overload must be suspected and either ruled out or validated in view of other clinical symptomatology.

The patient who is started on a vasopressor agent will show a rise in CVP due to the vasoconstriction produced. In this situation, the blood volume is unchanged, but the vascular bed has become smaller. Again, this change must be interpreted in conjunction with other assessments that the nurse makes about the patient. Alone, a CVP value can be meaningless, but used with other clinical data, it is a valuable aid in managing and predicting the patient's clinical course.

Some situations commonly produce an elevated CVP. These include CHF, when the heart can no longer effectively handle the venous return, cardiac tamponade, a vasoconstrictive state, or states of increased blood volume such as overtransfusion or overhydration.

A low CVP usually accompanies a hypovolemic state due to blood or fluid loss or drug-induced vasodilation. Increasing the rate of fluid administration or replacing blood loss is indicated in this situation.

Complications

Four potential complications may arise in a patient with a central line. They include (1) infection, (2) thrombosis, (3) air embolism, and (4) line displacement.

Infection

Infection can occur within the catheter or around the insertion site and is diagnosed and verified by blood cultures. Signs and symptoms of infection will appear as with any pyrogenic source. Frequent catheter and tubing changes, as outlined by hospital policy, are primary preventive measures.

Thrombosis

Thromboses can vary in size from a thin fibrin sheath over the catheter tip to a full-sized thrombus. The minor thrombosis can be flushed away without sequela, whereas a thrombus would be nonflushable. The patient may have edema of the arm closest to the catheter site, varying degrees of neck pain (which may radiate), and jugular vein distension.

A full-sized thrombus is classified as an emergency because it may impair circulation to a limb. A properly trained nurse may attempt to aspirate this clot, but only if hospital policy permits. The nurse, at the very least, is responsible for reporting the findings to a physician.

Air Embolism

Air embolism occurs as a result of air entering the system and traveling to the right ventricle via the vena cava. Decreased cardiac output may be the first indicator of this problem.

It is estimated that at least 10 to 20 cc of air must enter the system before the patient becomes symptomatic. Signs of such an emergency may include confusion, light-headedness, anxiety, and unresponsiveness. The physiological event is the creation of foam within the ventricle with each heart contraction, causing a sudden decrease in cardiac output.

If this problem is suspected, the nurse must turn the patient on the left side in the Trendelenburg position. This will cause the air to rise to the wall of the right ventricle and improve blood flow. Oxygen should be started on the patient unless contraindicated.

Line Displacement

Many hospitals have policies that require Luer-Lok connections on all central line tubings. The use of such a connection has proven to be an inexpensive way to prevent a potentially fatal complication. There is no substitute, however, for close observation by skilled and educated nursing staff.

Direct Cardiac Output Measurement

Description

Cardiac output refers to the amount of blood that is pumped out of the heart, and is expressed in liters/minute. It is a function of stroke volume and heart rate. Flow is determined by the ratio of pressure to resistance; thus, cardiac output is determined by the ratio of MAP to total peripheral resistance.

Any condition that causes uncompensated changes in arterial pressure or peripheral resistance will cause a change in cardiac output. Because many disease states, as well as their modes of therapy, affect arterial pressure, peripheral resistance, and cardiac output, it often is important that the critically ill patient's cardiac output be measured so that optimal medical and nursing care can be provided.

Procedure

Methods

The *Fick method* of measuring cardiac output involves determination of the difference in oxygen concentration of mixed venous blood and arterial blood and measurement of oxygen consumption in the lungs. The cardiac output is then calculated from a formula. In the *indicator dilution method*, dye is injected into a large vein or into the right side of the heart, a time-concentration curve from peripheral artery sampling is obtained, and cardiac output is calculated. Neither of these methods is feasible in the clinical setting.

With the advent of the four-lumen Swan–Ganz thermodilution catheter and cardiac output computers, it is now a relatively simple procedure for the critical care nurse to measure cardiac output at the patient's bedside. The *thermodilution method* is similar to the indicator dilution method. When thermodilution is used, the indicator is a solution, either cold or at room temperature, injected into the RA. The sampling device is a thermistor near the end of the catheter in the PA (Fig. 12–62). The thermistor continuously measures the temperature of the blood flowing past it. The catheter is connected to a cardiac output computer that determines the cardiac output from the time–temperature curve resulting from the rate of change in temperature of the blood that flows past the thermistor. Because of the number of variables inherent in the procedure, computation of the average of several consecutive cardiac output determinations will ensure greater accuracy.

The Swan–Ganz thermodilution catheter should be checked for proper functioning before beginning the procedure (Fig. 12–63). If the proximal lumen of the catheter is not fully patent, the cardiac output measurement will be inaccurate. The proximal lumen should be flushed before

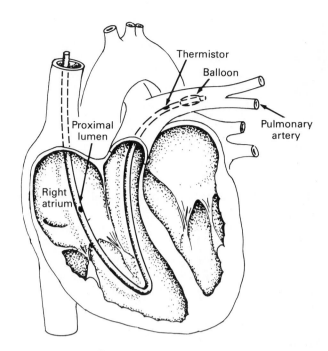

FIGURE 12–62
Swan–Ganz thermodilution catheter in place.

the solution is injected. If the proximal lumen is being used for the administration of intravenous medications, slow flushing before injection also will preclude the administration of a bolus of the infusing medication.

The thermistry circuit in the catheter and the cardiac output computer should be checked for proper functioning before each set of cardiac outputs is determined. This requires connection of the catheter thermistry circuit to the computer cable. Care must be taken to avoid damaging or breaking the relatively fragile connector mechanism. Follow the directions in the cardiac output computer operator's manual for checking the catheter and computer. This also should be done any time a cardiac output determination does not correlate with the patient's clinical condition.

The computation constant should be checked and set on the cardiac output computer to reflect the volume and temperature of the injectate being used. This number also takes into account catheter size and the rise in temperature of the injectate as it is being injected through the catheter. A table of computation constants can be found in the cardiac output computer operator's manual.

Injectate

The injectate solution used for the procedure usually is sterile 5% dextrose in water, although sterile normal saline may be used. Either 5 or 10 ml may be used, although 10 ml allows for more accuracy in the cardiac output determination.

Either glass or plastic Luer-Lok syringes may be used; "control" syringes, which have two finger rings attached to the barrel and a thumb ring at the end of the plunger, facilitate the speed of injection and also allow the nurse to hold the syringe without handling the barrel (Fig. 12–64). It is a common and acceptable practice to measure cardiac output with a room temperature injectate solution of D_5W. Studies have shown little difference in terms of accuracy when comparing room-temperature and iced injectate.

When room-temperature injectate is used, a simple set-up can be attached to a second three-way stopcock attached to the proximal lumen. The principle is the same as with iced injectate except that it remains a closed system (Fig. 12–65).

Iced injectate may be preferred in conditions known to elevate cardiac output, such as sepsis. The injectate should be at 0°C to 4°C to obtain the greatest accuracy. The injectate can be cooled by a variety of methods. Electric coolers manufactured for this purpose are available. An ice bath also may be used, and alcohol may be added to the ice bath for faster cooling. (Care should be taken when using an electric cooling plate or when adding alcohol to the ice bath that the solution in the syringes does not freeze.) Refrigeration of the injectate solution also will allow for faster cooling.

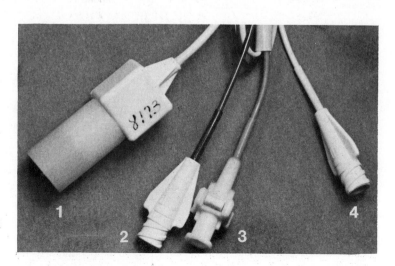

FIGURE 12–63
Entry sites for the four lumens of the Swan–Ganz thermodilution catheter. 1, Thermistor. 2, Proximal (right atrium). 3, Balloon inflation. 4, Distal (pulmonary artery).

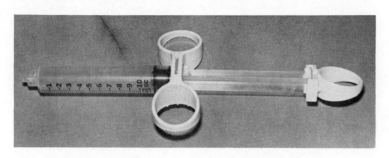

FIGURE 12–64
"Control" syringe.

Each syringe should be filled with sterile injectate, and the sterile cap should be replaced over the tip of the syringe. The syringes can be placed in a container that is then immersed in the ice bath or placed directly into the cooler.

An extra syringe must be filled with the same amount of injectate, the sterile cap replaced, and the plunger removed from the barrel. This syringe is placed in the container with the other syringes, and the injectate temperature probe is placed into the solution in this syringe. The probe is connected to the computer, which measures the temperature of the injectate. All the syringes, including the one containing the temperature probe, should be filled from the same container of solution so that the initial temperature of the injectate in each will be the same. Because the temperature of the solution actually being injected is not measured, the solution in which the temperature *is* being measured should simulate the injectate as closely as possible. The assumption

is that the temperature of the solution in all the syringes is the same.

After the cardiac output determinations have been made, it is helpful to fill a new set of syringes to cool in preparation for the next set of determinations. One should be sure to replace the temperature probe syringe along with the injectate syringes because they all must have the same initial temperature.

Injection

When the injectate solution has cooled to 0°C to 4°C, as indicated by the cardiac output computer, injection can be accomplished with greatest accuracy. Although automatic injectors are available, accurate measurements can be obtained with manual injection.

Significant warming of the injectate can result from

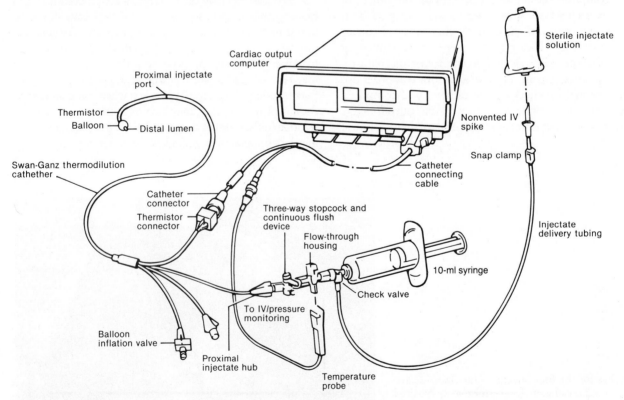

FIGURE 12–65
Sample of a closed injectate delivery system for room-temperature injectate.

holding the syringe in the hand. The syringe should be handled using the finger and thumb rings, avoiding contact of the hands with the syringe barrel. Whether iced or room-temperature injectate is used, it must be made certain that the syringe has been filled to the *exact* volume indicated by the computation constant used, usually 10 ml. Use of inaccurately measured injectate volume will result in inaccurate cardiac output measurements. The cardiac output computer manufacturer's directions should be followed when operating the computer.

The injectate syringe is attached to the proximal lumen of the Swan–Ganz catheter. A three-way stopcock between the proximal lumen and intravenous tubing allows maintenance of a closed system and facilitates rapid attachment of the syringe (Fig. 12–66). Inject the solution into the proximal line at the time the computer indicates readiness. Injection should be accomplished during the end-expiratory phase of the respiratory cycle to minimize the effects of blood temperature variations from respirations. Injection time for 10 ml of solution should be 4 seconds or less. The elapsed time from removal of syringe from the cooling mechanism until injection should be as short as possible so that environmental warming of the injectate is avoided.

The cardiac rhythm should be observed immediately after injection because the sudden bolus of cold solution into the RA may precipitate atrial or ventricular dysrhythmias. The PA pressure waveform also should be observed after injection for migration of the catheter into the wedge position or retrograde into the right ventricle.

Measurements may be repeated when the computer signifies readiness. The catheter thermistry circuit is disconnected from the computer cable after the entire procedure is completed. The protective cap is replaced over the end of the thermistry circuit "tail" of the Swan–Ganz catheter.

Some cardiac output computers are equipped with strip chart recorders, so that the thermodilution curve can be observed and recorded. The curve should have a smooth upstroke, peak, and smooth downstroke. If the curve is distorted because of poor injection technique or improper catheter positioning, that cardiac output measurement should be rejected (Fig. 12–67).

Serial Readings

The average of several cardiac outputs is more accurate than one isolated determination because of the number of possible variables in the patient and procedure performance. Three consecutive determinations should be obtained, if possible. If one measurement is unduly high or low relative to the others in the series, it should be discarded as inaccurate. To ensure optimal accuracy, the measurements should be obtained within 0.5 liter/minute of each other. The remaining determinations are then averaged for the measurement to be recorded in the patient's chart. The cardiac index is calculated as described earlier, and also recorded in the chart.

Interpretation of Results

Normal Cardiac Output and Cardiac Index

Normal cardiac output at rest is considered to be 4 to 8 liters/minute. The determinants of cardiac output are afterload, preload, contractility, and heart rate. Refer to Chapter 11 for a detailed discussion of the first three determinants identified. Actual cardiac output is related to body size. The cardiac index is a more realistic guide for evaluating the cardiac output of any one person. The cardiac index is obtained by dividing cardiac output by the body surface area. Body surface area can be determined with the Dubois body surface chart (Fig. 12–68). A straight line drawn between the patient's height in the left-hand column will cross the number in the middle column that represents body surface area in square meters. Normal cardiac index is 2.5 to 4 liters/minute/m^2.

The cardiac output and index always should be evaluated in conjunction with other assessed parameters and the clinical status of the patient. For example, one would expect the patient in cardiogenic shock to have a low cardiac output and cardiac index and a high PCWP and PA diastolic pressure. With improvement in the patient's clinical status, the cardiac output and index should rise, and the PCWP and PA

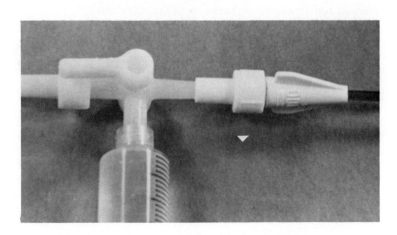

FIGURE 12–66
Attachment of injectate syringe to three-way stopcock between proximal lumen of Swan–Ganz thermodilution catheter on right and intravenous tubing on left. Handle on stopcock points to "off."

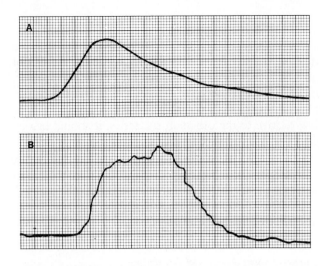

FIGURE 12–67
Examples of accurate and distorted thermodilution curves as produced on strip chart recorder. (**A**) Smooth recording is accurate. (**B**) Irregular recording is distorted, probably from an irregular or uneven emptying of the injectate syringe.

diastolic pressure should decrease. If one of the preceding measurements does not reflect the trend of the others and the patient's clinical status, the nurse should suspect an error in technique or equipment malfunction and begin troubleshooting or repeating measurements. One of the reasons for determining multiple hemodynamic measurements is to use each determination to verify the others.

The gamut of measured hemodynamic parameters can be used to calculate other parameters that cannot be measured directly. Calculators that can be programmed to calculate such information as stroke volume, right and left ventricular stroke work, and systemic and pulmonary vascular resistance from measured parameters are available. Systemic vascular resistance can be hand-calculated as follows:

$$\frac{(\text{mean arterial pressure} - \text{RA pressure}) \times 80}{\text{cardiac output}}$$

In the clinical setting, the nurse determines systemic vascular resistance, which measures afterload of the LV, and pulmonary vascular resistance, which measures afterload of the RV. By assessing these values, the nurse knows the effectiveness of the therapy being instituted.

The patient who has a low MAP, high cardiac index, and low systemic vascular resistance (as seen in septic shock) may be treated best with additional circulatory volume and vasoconstrictor therapy. The patient who has cardiogenic shock may demonstrate a low MAP, low cardiac index, and high systemic vascular resistance because of maximal vasoconstriction. and may be treated best with vasodilator therapy and inotropic agents.

In the patient with acute myocardial infarction, cardiac outputs can be decreased, and PCWP increased. These

pressure changes indicate damage to the LV and poor LV emptying. By relating these two measurements, one may be able to modify therapy to obtain a PCWP that will result in optimal cardiac output and arterial pressure for that patient.

It is obvious that these hemodynamic parameters can be very useful in assessing the efficacy of vasodilators, vasoconstrictors, additional volume, diuretics, and inotropic agents.

Low Cardiac Output

Many disease states may decrease the pumping effectiveness of the LV, resulting in a decrease in the pressure generated within the ventricle. This in turn will cause the cardiac output to fall. Myocardial infarction is the most common cause of compromised pumping ability of the LV. Other causes include valvular heart disease, CHF, myocarditis, cardiac tamponade, and some congenital anomalies. In monitoring therapy in patients who are critically ill because of these disease states, cardiac output determinations, in conjunction with various intracardiac and pulmonary pressure measurements, can be very helpful.

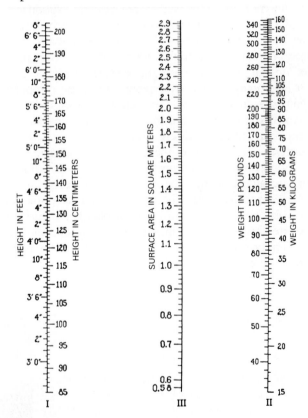

FIGURE 12–68
Dubois body surface chart (as prepared by Boothby and Sandiford of the Mayo Clinic). To find body surface of a patient, locate the height in inches (or centimeters) on scale I and the weight in pounds (or kilograms) on scale II and place a straightedge (ruler) between these two points, which will intersect scale III at the patient's surface area.

Venous return to the right side of the heart is a major factor in determining cardiac output. The heart can pump out only the volume presented to it. If inadequate blood volume is present, the cardiac output must, of necessity, fall. In the critical care unit, low cardiac output due to decreased venous return commonly is caused by severe hemorrhage and dehydration.

It must be remembered that any patient who receives mechanical ventilation with positive-pressure breathing may have a decreased cardiac output because of increased intrathoracic pressure and decreased venous return. In the patient with acute respiratory distress syndrome who is being treated with positive end-expiratory pressure (PEEP), cardiac output monitoring may help determine the level of PEEP that will produce the optimum PO_2 with minimal decrease in cardiac output.

High Cardiac Output

Normally, the cardiac output increases with exercise as a result of increased oxygen consumption at the cellular level. The trained athlete may raise his or her cardiac output to several times normal during strenuous exercise. Stimulation of the sympathetic nervous system also will increase cardiac output by increasing heart rate and the contractile force of the LV.

In the critical care unit, septic shock is one of the causes of abnormally high cardiac output. This occurs because of massive vasodilation, probably from the toxic substances produced by sepsis, thus decreasing peripheral resistance. The cardiac output in septic shock may increase to three or four times normal.

The thiamine deficiency associated with beriberi also may cause vasodilation and high cardiac output.

Because of their effects on peripheral resistance, many of the potent antihypertensive drugs used in the critical care unit should be titrated by monitoring the pressures obtained from a Swan–Ganz catheter and cardiac output determinations.

A high rate of metabolism, as found in thyrotoxicosis, fever, and certain tumors, also may cause an increase in cardiac output because of increased oxygen consumption.

Management

Nursing Considerations

It is important for the critical care nurse to eliminate as many potential sources of error as possible to obtain an accurate cardiac output. The procedure should be done at a time when the patient is in a quiet, steady state. Agitation increases the cardiac output, and the measurement will not be meaningful relative to the resting output or those obtained during various degrees of agitation. It is thought by some that respiratory variations may cause changes in the temperature of the blood in the pulmonary circulation

and thus render the cardiac output measurement something less than accurate. This possible source of error may be avoided if the determination is done when the patient is breathing quietly.

Each cardiac output measurement should be obtained with the patient in the same position, either supine or semierect. Although accurate measurements can be obtained in either position, the actual cardiac output may change significantly with change in position, usually decreasing when the patient is semierect.

Electrical Safety

An electrically safe environment must be maintained at all times for the critical care patient. This is especially important when cardiac output determinations are being made by the Swan–Ganz catheter, which traverses the heart.

The following guidelines should be used to maintain electrical safety for the patient with a Swan–Ganz thermo-dilution catheter:

- The patient should be in a nonelectric bed. If an electric bed must be used, it should be unplugged from the wall outlet or properly grounded.
- Bed linens should be changed immediately when wet.
- The amount of electrical equipment in the immediate environment should be minimal and properly grounded.
- The cardiac output computer cable should be inspected for continuity before use.
- The protective cap should be in place over the thermistry tail on the catheter when not in use.
- The catheter should not be connected to the computer cable during insertion procedure.
- The computer should be on battery power, not AC power, when connected to the catheter.
- The electrical cooler should be disconnected from the wall outlet or the temperature probe removed from the cooler while the catheter is connected to the computer cable.
- Personnel handling the catheter should not be in simultaneous contact with any other electrical equipment.
- The computer and the cable should be kept dry and clean.
- The computer should not be operated in the presence of explosive anesthetic agents.

Summary

It is important that the critical care nurse be adept at setting up, maintaining, and troubleshooting all types of hemodynamic and cardiac monitoring equipment in the critical care unit. Measurements of the various parameters must be made with accuracy and evaluated in conjunction with one another and with the patient's clinical status. Appropriate use of these determinations will aid in medical diagnosis, choice of therapy, monitoring of therapy, and anticipation of prognosis. The ultimate goal in the use of these hemodynamic parameters is the reduction of morbidity and mortality in critically ill patients.

REFERENCES

Cardiac Enzyme Studies

1. Puelo PR, Guadagno PA, et al: Early diagnosis of acute myocardial infarction based on assay for subforms of creatine kinase-MB. Circulation 82:759–764, 1990
2. Lee TH, Goldman L: Serum enzyme assays in the diagnosis of acute myocardial infarction: Recommendations based on a quantitative analysis. Ann Intern Med 105:221–233, 1986

Cardiovascular Diagnostic Procedures

3. Schactman M, Greene JS: Signal-averaged electrocardiography: A new technique for determining which patients may be at risk for sudden cardiac death. Focus on Critical Care 18(3):202–210, 1991
4. Burek KA, Kirscht J, Topol E: Exercise capacity in patients 3 days after acute, uncomplicated myocardial infarction. Heart Lung 18:575–580, 1989
5. Dilsizian V, Rocco T, et al: Enhanced detection of ischemic but viable myocardium by the reinjection of thallium after stress-redistribution imaging. N Engl J Med 323:141–146, 1990

BIBLIOGRAPHY

Auscultation of the Heart

Bates B: A Guide to Physical Examination and History Taking. Philadelphia, JB Lippincott, 1991
Henning RJ, Grenik A: Critical Care Cardiology. New York, Churchill-Livingston, 1991
Seidel HM, Ball JW, et al: Mosby's Guide to Physical Examination. St. Louis: Mosby-Year Book, 1991

Cardiac Enzyme Studies

Apple FS: Creatine kinase-MB. Laboratory Medicine 23(5):298–302, 1992
Goe MR: Laboratory tests using blood and urine. In Underhill SL, Woods SL, et al (eds): Cardiac Nursing, 2nd ed, pp 280–288. Philadelphia, JB Lippincott, 1989
Pasternak RC, Braunwald E, Sobel BE: Acute myocardial infarction. In Braunwald E (ed): Heart Disease: A Textbook of Cardiovascular Medicine, 4th ed, pp 1218–1220. Philadelphia, WB Saunders, 1992
Wu AHB: Creatine kinase MM and MB isoforms. Laboratory Medicine 23(5):303–305, 1992

Cardiovascular Diagnostic Procedures

Apple S, Thurkauf GE: Preparing for and understanding transesophageal echocardiography. Critical Care Nurse 12(6):29–34, 1992
Chaitman B: Exercise stress testing. In Braunwald E (ed): Heart Disease: A Textbook of Cardiovascular Medicine, 4th ed, pp 161–179. Philadelphia, WB Saunders, 1992
Chen JTT: Radiographic diagnosis of heart failure. Heart Disease and Stroke 1:58–63, 1992
Chyun D, Ford CF, Yursha-Johnston M: Silent myocardial ischemia. Focus on Critical Care 18(4):295–306, 1991
Cimini DM: Indium-111 antimyosin antibody imaging: A promising new technique in the diagnosis of MI. Critical Care Nurse 12(6):44–51, 1992
Feigenbaum H: Echocardiography. In Braunwald E (ed): Heart Disease: A Textbook of Cardiovascular Medicine, 4th ed, pp 64–115. Philadelphia, WB Saunders, 1992
Hendel RC, Leppo JA: Myocardial perfusion imaging with technetium-99m sestamibi and teboroxime. Journal of American College of Cardiology 6:53–74, 1990
Kinney MR, Packa DR, et al: Comprehensive Cardiac Care, 7th ed. St. Louis, CV Mosby, 1991
McNulty SA: Pharmacological interventional testing for myocardial perfusion: A new application for adenosine. Cardiovascular Nursing 28(4):24–28, 1992
Popp RL: Echocardiography (first of two parts). N Engl J Med 323:101–109, 1990
Popp RL: Echocardiography (second of two parts). N Engl J Med 323:165–172, 1990
Task Force Committee of the European Society of Cardiology, the American Heart Association, and the American College of Cardiology: Standards for analysis of ventricular late potentials using high-resolution or signal-averaged electrocardiography. Circulation 83:1481–1488, 1991
Underhill SL, Woods SL, et al: Cardiac Nursing, 2nd ed. Philadelphia, JB Lippincott, 1989
Zaret BL, Wackers FJTh: Established and developing nuclear cardiology techniques, Part 1. Modern Concepts of Cardiovascular Disease 60(7):37–42, 1991
Zaret BL, Wackers FJTh: Established and developing nuclear cardiology techniques, Part 2. Modern Concepts of Cardiovascular Disease 60(8):43–47, 1991

Electrocardiographic Monitoring

Conover MB: Understanding Electrocardiography, 6th ed. St. Louis, CV Mosby, 1992
Frye SJ, Lounsbury P: Cardiac Rhythm Disorders: An Introduction Using the Nursing Process. Baltimore, Williams & Wilkins, 1988
Kinney MR, et al: Comprehensive Cardiac Care, 7th ed. St. Louis, CV Mosby, 1991
Vinsant MO, Spence MI: Commonsense Approach to Coronary Care, 5th ed. St. Louis, CV Mosby, 1988

Dysrhythmias and Conduction Disturbances

Braunwald E (ed): Heart Disease, 4th ed. Philadelphia, WB Saunders, 1992
Chou T: Electrocardiography in Clinical Practice, 3rd ed. Philadelphia, WB Saunders, 1991

Conover MD: Understanding Electrocardiography, 6th ed. St. Louis, CV Mosby, 1992

Frye SJ, Lounsbury P: Cardiac Rhythm Disorders. Baltimore, Williams & Wilkins, 1988

Goldschlager N, Goldman MJ: Principles of Clinical Electrocardiography, 13th ed. Norwalk, CT, Appleton & Lange, 1989

Kinney MR, et al: Comprehensive Cardiac Care, 7th ed. St. Louis, CV Mosby, 1991

Marriott HJL: Practical Electrocardiography, 8th ed. Baltimore, Williams & Wilkins, 1988

Underhill SL, et al: Cardiac Nursing, 2nd ed. Philadelphia, JB Lippincott, 1989

Vinsant MO, Spence MI: Commonsense Approach to Coronary Care, 5th ed. St. Louis, CV Mosby, 1988

Effects of Serum Electrolyte Abnormalities on the Electrocardiogram

Braunwald E (ed): Heart Disease, 4th ed. Philadelphia, WB Saunders, 1992

Conover MB: Understanding Electrocardiography, 6th ed. St. Louis, CV Mosby, 1992

DeAngelis R, Lessig ML: Hyperkalemia. Critical Care Nurse 12(3):55–59, 1992

DeAngelis R, Lessig ML: Hypokalemia. Critical Care Nurse 11(7):71–75, 1991

Hurst JW (ed): The Heart, Arteries, and Veins, 7th ed. New York, McGraw-Hill, 1990

Kinney MR, et al: Comprehensive Cardiac Care, 7th ed. St. Louis, CV Mosby, 1991

Hemodynamic Monitoring

Bumann R, Speltz M: Decreased cardiac output: A nursing diagnosis. Dimensions of Critical Care Nursing 8:6–15, 1989

Clark AP, Winslow EH, et al: Effects of endotracheal suctioning on mixed venous oxygen saturation and heart rate in critically ill adults. Heart Lung 19:552–557, 1990

Cline JK, Gurka AM: Effect of backrest position on pulmonary artery pressure and cardiac output measurements in critically ill patients. Focus on Critical Care 10:383–389, 1991

Daily EK, Schroeder JJ: Techniques in Bedside Hemodynamic Monitoring. St. Louis, CV Mosby, 1989

Dolter KJ: Increasing reliability and validity of pulmonary artery measurements. Dimensions of Critical Care Nursing 8:183–191, 1989

Gawlinski A, Henneman EA: Evaluation of oxygen delivery and oxygen utilization with mixed venous oxygen saturation monitoring: A case study approach. Heart Lung 19:566–570, 1990

Guyton AC: Textbook of Medical Physiology. Philadelphia, WB Sanders, 1991

Henning RJ, Grenik A: Critical Care Cardiology. New York, Churchill-Livingston, 1991

Mark JB: Central venous pressure monitoring: Clinical insights beyond the numbers. Journal of Cardiothoracic and Vascular Anesthesia 4:163–173, 1991

Master S: Complication of pulmonary artery catheters. Critical Care Nurse 9(9):82–90, 1990

Pinsky MR: The meaning of cardiac output. Intensive Care Med 16:415–417, 1990

Proctor M: Continuous monitoring of mixed venous saturation ($S\bar{v}O_2$): An adjunct to nursing assessment? Intensive and Critical Care Nursing 8:66–70, 1992

Tyler DO, Winslow EH, et al: Effects of a 1-minute back rub on mixed venous oxygen saturation and heart rate in critically ill patients. Heart Lung 19:562–565, 1990

White KM, Winslow EH, et al: The physiologic basis for continuous mixed venous oxygen saturation monitoring. Heart Lung 19(Suppl):548–551, 1990

Winslow EH, Clark AP, et al: Effects of a lateral turn on mixed venous oxygen saturation and heart rate in critically ill adults. Heart Lung 19:557–561, 1990

Woo MA, Hamilton M, et al: Comparison of thermodilution and transthoracic electrical bioimpedance cardiac output. Heart Lung 20:357–362, 1991

STUDY QUESTIONS

Auscultation of the Heart

1. The following is true about a good-quality stethoscope

   a. short tubing
   b. a head with both a bell and a diaphragm
   c. two separate tubes from the head leading to each ear piece
   d. all of the above

2. S_1 and S_2 are important to recognize because they are timed with

   a. the beginning of systole and diastole, respectively
   b. the closure of the mitral and tricuspid valves and closure of the aortic and pulmonic valves
   c. contraction of the ventricles followed by relaxation and filling of the ventricles
   d. all of the above

3. Which of the following is an important sign of congestive heart failure in the adult?

   a. systolic ejection murmur
   b. holosystolic murmur
   c. S_3
   d. S_4

Cardiac Enzyme Studies

1. Which of the following organs contains the greatest percentage of creatine kinase-MB?

   a. skeletal muscle
   b. cerebral cortex
   c. heart
   d. liver

2. Within 12 hours after acute myocardial infarction, which of the following cardiac enzymes is most likely to be abnormal?

   a. creatine kinase (CK)
   b. serum glutamic-oxaloacetic transaminase (SGOT)
   c. lactic dehydrogenase (LDH)
   d. creatine kinase-BB (CK-BB)

Cardiovascular Diagnostic Procedures

1. All of the following diagnostic tests are used in the assessment of patients for coronary artery disease *except*

   a. thallium exercise perfusion study
   b. coronary angiography
   c. signal-averaged ECG
   d. exercise ECG

2. Holter monitoring, signal-averaged ECG, and electrophysiology studies are diagnostic tests that are most likely to be used in which of the following cardiac conditions?

   a. myocardial infarction
   b. ventricular tachycardia
   c. congestive heart failure
   d. myocardial ischemia

3. "Hot spot" radionuclide imaging studies are so named because

   a. the radiotracer passes through a septal defect
   b. the radiotracer uptake is concentrated in an area of normal myocardium
   c. the radiotracer uptake is concentrated in an area of myocardial ischemia
   d. the radiotracer uptake is concentrated in an area of myocardial necrosis

Electrocardiographic Monitoring

1. In an MCL_1 monitoring system, which of the following statements are true?

   1. negative electrode is below the left clavicle
   2. negative electrode is below the right clavicle
   3. positive electrode is the midaxillary line, 5th ICS
   4. positive electrode is the right sternal border, 4th ICS

      a. 1 and 3
      b. 1 and 4
      c. 2 and 3
      d. 2 and 4

2. Lead II should be used for bedside cardiac monitoring in which of the following situations?

   a. to correct respiratory artifact from a patient in acute respiratory distress
   b. to differentiate right from left bundle branch block
   c. to obtain tall upright P waves
   d. to differentiate ventricular ectopy from aberrancy

3. Which of the following statements is/are true about cardiac monitoring?

   a. before an ECG electrode is applied to the skin, it is necessary to remove excess skin oil to obtain an optimal tracing
   b. to avoid disturbing the patient, the monitor alarm should be turned off when excessive artifact is present
   c. an acute myocardial infarction can be diagnosed accurately on the cardiac monitor
   d. all of the above

Dysrhythmias and Conduction Disturbances

1. Which of the following electrical events occur during the PR interval?

   1. atrial depolarization
   2. AV node conduction
   3. bundle of His transmission
   4. ventricular depolarization

      a. 1
      b. 1 and 2
      c. 1, 2, and 3
      d. all of the above

2. All of the following are ECG characteristics of a premature atrial contraction (PAC) except

   a. the P wave looks different from the sinus P wave
   b. the P wave is premature
   c. it produces an irregular rhythm
   d. the QRS usually is wide and bizarre

3. You are caring for a patient who experiences a run of ventricular tachycardia (VT). All of the following statements are true about this dysrhythmia except

   a. immediate treatment with electrical cardioversion always is indicated
   b. the patient may maintain consciousness during the episode of VT
   c. VT is defined as three or more ventricular premature beats (VPBs) in a row
   d. VT can deteriorate into ventricular fibrillation if not treated promptly

4. Which of the following statements characterize Wenckebach or a Mobitz type I second-degree AV block?

   1. it often has a wide QRS
   2. it is characterized by a fixed PR interval when the sinus impulses are conducted
   3. it is characterized by a gradual prolongation of the PR interval
   4. indicates pathology above the bundle of His

      a. 1 and 2
      b. 3 and 4
      c. 1 and 3
      d. 2 and 4

Effects of Serum Electrolyte Abnormalities on the Electrocardiogram

1. Which of the following electrolyte abnormalities increases the sensitivity of the heart to digitalis and its accompanying dysrhythmias?

   a. hyperkalemia
   b. hypercalcemia
   c. hypokalemia
   d. hypocalcemia

2. Hypercalcemia produces which type of change on the ECG?

   a. prolonged QT interval
   b. shortened QT interval
   c. prominent U waves
   d. tall, peaked T waves

Hemodynamic Monitoring

1. An elevated a wave may be associated with which of the following?

   a. mitral regurgitation
   b. atrial contraction against a closed valve
   c. bulging of the tricuspid valve into the right atrial
   d. dehydration

2. The pulmonary capillary wedge pressure values indicate the

   a. function of the left ventricle
   b. type of therapy needed
   c. effectiveness of the therapy
   d. all of the above

3. Normal pulmonary capillary pressure is

   a. >12 mm Hg
   b. <12 mm Hg
   c. 18–22 mm Hg
   d. >6 mm Hg

4. Which of the following will result in a low central venous pressure?

   a. hypervolemia
   b. biventricular failure
   c. hypovolemia
   d. left ventricular failure

5. Which of the following will result in an increased venous return to the right side of the heart?

   a. fever
   b. septic shock
   c. thyrotoxicosis
   d. all of the above

6. Which of the following is the basis for the thermodilution method in determining cardiac output?

   a. dye concentration
   b. blood temperature change
   c. venous oxygen saturation
   d. pulmonary oxygen consumption

Cardiac Pacing

(continued)

CHAPTER 13

*Management
Modalities:
Cardiovascular
System*

Hudak: Critical Care Nursing:
A Holistic Approach, 6th ed. © 1994
J. B. Lippincott Company.

Procedure

Methods of Pacing
    External Transcutaneous Pacing
    Transthoracic Pacing
    Epicardial Pacing
    Endocardial Transvenous Pacing

Management

Safety Issues With a Pacemaker

Patient Teaching Regarding a Pacemaker

Complications of Pacing

    Failure to Discharge
    Failure to Capture
    Failure to Sense Spontaneous Beats
    Ventricular Irritability
    Perforation of Ventricular Wall or Septum
    Tamponade
    Retrograde Migration of Right Ventricular Catheter
    Abdominal Twitching or Hiccoughs
    Infection and Phlebitis
    Permanent Generator Migration
    Malfunction Due to Defibrillation

Nursing Care Plan: The Patient with a Cardiac Pacemaker

BEHAVIORAL OBJECTIVES

Based on the content in this section, the reader should be able to:

1. Describe the functions of each of the three pacemaker components: pulse generator, lead wire, electrode.
2. Define fixed-rate pacing, demand pacing, synchronous pacing, and rate-modulated pacing.
3. Define AAI, VVI, DVI, DDD, and DDDR pacing.
4. List the indications for pacemaker therapy.
5. Discuss the potential complications of pacemaker therapy and possible treatments.
6. Describe the nursing care of a patient with both a temporary and permanent pacemaker.

Description

Electrical stimulation of the heart was tried experimentally as early as 1819. In 1930, Hyman noted that he could inject the right atrium with a diversity of substances and restore a heartbeat. He devised an "ingenious apparatus" that he labeled an *artificial pacemaker*, which delivered a rhythmical charge to the heart. In 1952, Zoll demonstrated that patients with Stokes–Adams syndrome could be sustained by the administration of current directly to the chest wall. In 1957, Lillehei affixed electrodes directly to the ventricles during open heart surgery.

From 1958 to 1961, implantable pacemakers became accepted treatment for complete heart block. In the 1970s and 1980s, atrioventricular (AV) synchrony and "physiological" pacing became available. Currently, technologic advances have resulted in smaller pacemakers with longer battery life and numerous programmable options. The goal of individualized, physiological pacing is achievable, but will require additional skill and sophistication on the part of health professionals.

Physiological Principles

Pacemaker Components

Every pacemaker, whether implanted permanently or temporarily, has three basic components: the pulse generator, the electrode(s), and the lead wire or catheter.

The Pulse Generator

This contains the power source (lithium battery) and electronic circuitry. Most pulse generators have circuits for pacemaker discharge, timing of functions, sensing of intrinsic heart activity, memory, programmability, telemetry, and interrogation. In an attempt to meet more adequately the physiological needs of the patient, many pulse generators include sensors to detect motion that would cause an increase in heart rate during exercise.

Other sensing parameters such as venous oxygen saturation, pH, temperature, right ventricular stroke volume, minute ventilation, respiratory rate, tidal volume, and QT interval are all being evaluated to determine their ability to detect a patient's metabolic need.[1]

Electrodes

All electrical circuits must have a negative electrode (cathode) and a positive electrode (anode) to complete the circuit. In a bipolar catheter, the negative pacing electrode is at the tip and the positive sensing electrode is approximately 1 cm proximal to the tip (Fig. 13–1), whereas a unipolar catheter contains only a negative pacing electrode at its tip and uses a positive electrode outside of the catheter. In permanent pacing, the generator case is the positive electrode. Clinical research in the area of electrode design is focused on achieving reliable pacing over time while conserving battery life in the permanent pacemaker. Electrodes with steroid-eluding tips and carbon-covered titanium both have demonstrated low chronic pacing thresholds. There still is much to be learned to understand fully what components affect pacing thressholds.

Lead Wire or Catheter

This component provides the communication network between the pulse generator and the heart muscle. The

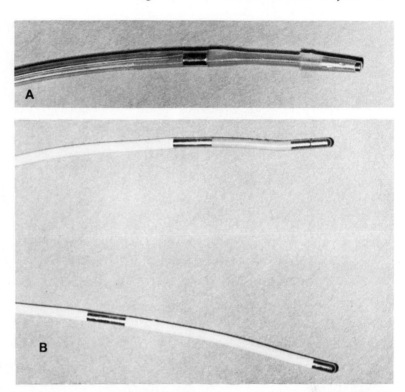

FIGURE 13–1
(**A**) Permanent bipolar pacing catheter. (**B**) Temporary bipolar pacing catheters.

lead is affixed to the myocardium with a lead fixation device. These devices include screws, barbed tips, tines, or coils (Fig. 13–2). Electrical cardiac activity travels to the sensing electrode and, when required, the pulse generator emits an electrical stimulus to the heart muscle through the lead. The catheter must provide adequate electrical conduction, sufficient insulation, and the endurance to withstand pulsatile turbulence. In addition, there is a demand to decrease the lumen size of the catheter. The catheter can either be unipolar or bipolar, containing one or two electrodes. (Table 13–1 compares the differences between the unipolar and bipolar catheters.)

Temporary Versus Permanent Pacing

Temporary Pacing

Temporary pulse generators are used for short-term pacing performed in critical care areas or during a procedure. They are capable of pacing one or both chambers (Fig. 13–3). The temporary transvenous lead system is usually a bipolar catheter. If a bipolar catheter is used, the negative (distal) electrode is attached to the negative generator terminal and the positive proximal electrode is attached to the positive generator terminal. Occasionally, improper sensing can be corrected by reversing the attachment of the catheter tips to the generator terminals (reversed polarity). When reversing the polarity of a bipolar catheter does not correct faulty sensing, conversion to a unipolar system may solve the problem. This is accomplished by disconnecting the bipolar positive electrode from the generator and replacing it with the wire from a monitoring electrode on the anterior chest, arm, or leg (Fig. 13–4). When the chest electrode is used as part of the pacing system, it should be labeled as such so that it will not be confused with other chest electrodes that are being used for monitoring cardiac rhythm.

Permanent Pacing

Most permanent pulse generators are inserted into subcutaneous tissue below the left clavicle. The catheter is placed via a central vein, and the pacing electrodes are connected subcutaneously to the implanted generator.

Permanent pacemaker catheters may be either unipolar or bipolar. Great strides have been made in prolonging electrode and catheter life so that multiple pulse generator replacements can be done while using the same lead system. The permanent steroid-eluding electrodes and abrasive electrodes are achieving stable chronic pacing thresholds. Most permanent pulse generators are powered by lithium batteries that have a life expectancy of 7 to 12 years. Although the generators are much smaller than those used a few years ago, researchers are continuing their efforts to increase the effective life span and decrease the size of permanent generators (Fig. 13–5).

Pacing and Sensing Thresholds

The pacing electrodes should be positioned so that the generator can be set at a relatively small amount of electrical energy and low degree of sensitivity and still allow successful pacing.

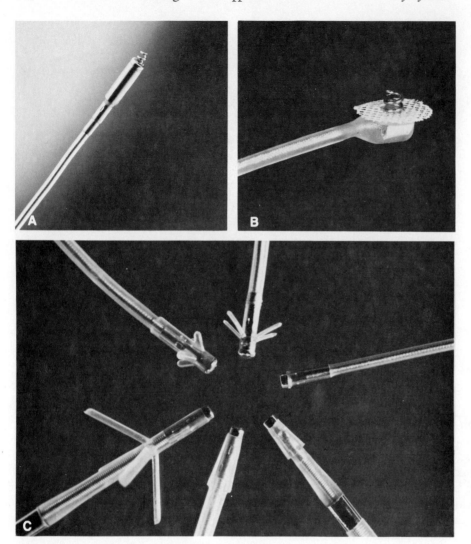

FIGURE 13–2
Lead wires with screws, barbs, or tines ensure fixation to the myocardium.

TABLE 13–1
Advantages and Disadvantages of Bipolar and Unipolar Lead Systems

	Unipolar	Bipolar
Distance between electrical poles	30–50 cm	1–3 cm
Sensitivity	More sensitive to intracardiac electrical activity (may sense depolarization from a different chamber)	Less sensitive to intracardiac/extracardiac electrical activity (less likely to oversense)
	More sensitive to extracardiac electrical activity (may sense myopotentials)	
Muscle twitching	May occur due to electric signals picked up near the pulse generator	Rare occurrence because both electrodes are intracardiac
Pacemaker artifact	Large; may distort QRS complex	Small; less distortion of QRS complex
Insertion	Easier to place	More difficult to place
Uses	Bipolar systems can be converted to unipolar if needed	Temporary/permanent systems
		Must be used in conjunction with the internal cardioverter–defibrillator

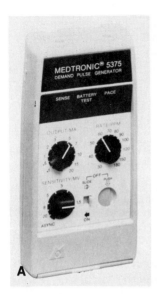 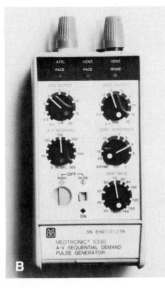

FIGURE 13-3
(**A**) Single-chamber and (**B**) dual-chamber pulse generators.

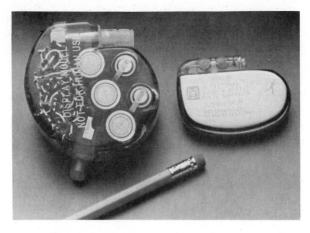

FIGURE 13-5
Permanent pulse generators, old and new. Note the decrease in size and weight that has been achieved over the years. The smaller unit is an example of an activity-responsive pulse generator and is four times smaller than the larger 1968 unit.

The lowest level of electrical energy that is required to initiate consistent capture at the pacing electrode site is called the *pacing threshold*. This threshold level is determined by establishing successful pacing at higher energy and then gradually decreasing the energy output of the generator until capture ceases. The threshold is expressed as milliamperes at this level. The generator output is then set at several milliamperes above the threshold to allow for the usual increase in threshold level that occurs over a period of time after pacing has been initiated.

Many factors affect the pacing threshold. The pacing threshold usually is increased during hours of sleep, possibly due to lowered catecholamine levels. Other factors that may increase pacing thresholds include hypoxia, hyperkalemia, β-blocking drugs, and type I antiarrhythmic drugs. In contrast, thresholds may be decreased with increased catecholamines, digoxin toxicity, and corticosteroids.

Sensing threshold also is determined for permanent pacemakers. The amplitude of the intrinsic depolarization wave at the site of the sensing electrode is measured. The sensitivity setting should allow for adequate sensing without oversensing artifact.

Overdrive and Underdrive Pacing

Occasionally, pacing is used to interrupt tachyarrhythmias that are unresponsive to other forms of therapy. These dysrhythmias may be of either ventricular or supraventricular origin. A temporary transvenous pacemaker catheter electrode is placed in the chamber of dysrhythmia origin. Because most supraventricular tachycardias are of the re-entry type, a pacemaker stimulus is initiated at such time as to enter the reentry circuit, thus interrupting completion of the circuit and terminating the dysrhythmia.

The same principle can be applied to reentrant ventricular tachycardias. One may accomplish overdrive pacing by increasing the pacing rate until pacemaker capture occurs during the nonrefractory period between sponta-

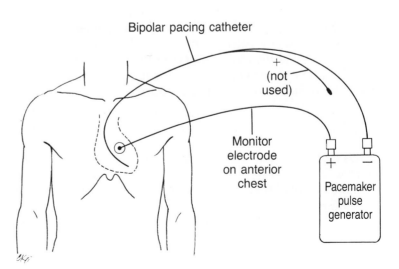

FIGURE 13-4
Conversion of bipolar pacing system to unipolar. The monitoring electrode on anterior chest is used as positive pole in pacemaker system.

neous beats. Once the ectopic focus has been suppressed, the pacing rate usually can be decreased gradually, and the pacing stimulus will continue to maintain control of the ventricles.[2]

When overdrive pacing fails to terminate the ventricular dysrhythmia, underdrive pacing may be attempted. The pacing rate is set at less than the ectopic discharge rate in an attempt to accomplish ventricular capture by the pacing stimulus.

Equipment Features

Modes of Pacing

Four modes of pacing generally are recognized, and some pacemakers can operate in more than one mode in response to changing patient requirements such as age, activity level, and type of heart disease.[3] Leads can be placed in the atria, ventricles, or both.

Asynchronous

This pacing mode stimulates the heart at a preset interval and does not respond to intrinsic heart activity. It was the first mode of pacing developed but is virtually obsolete today due to the development of pacemakers that do respond to the patient's heart activity.

It is important to understand this concept, however, because permanent pacemakers may be switched over to this mode temporarily (by the use of a specialized magnet) to determine if the pacemaker is properly capturing (causing depolarization).

Demand

This pacemaker mode initiates an impulse only when a preset PR, RR interval has elapsed without any spontaneous electrical activation of the ventricle. This escape interval is determined by the rate at which the pacemaker is set; that is, if the ventricular rate is set at 60 beats/minute, the pacemaker will discharge only when the patient's ventricular heart rate drops below 60 beats/minute (Fig. 13–6). Thus, the pacemaker is inhibited by intrinsic heart activity, and there is no danger of the pacemaker firing at a time that could initiate a dangerous cardiac dysrhythmia such as ventricular tachycardia.

Synchronous

In this type of demand pacing mode, one chamber of the heart is triggered to fire or is inhibited by the other chamber's activity.[4] For example, a sensing lead is placed in the atria and a pacing lead in the ventricles. When the patient's sinoatrial (SA) node fires, resulting in atrial depolarization, this is sensed and results in a pacemaker discharge to the ventricles.

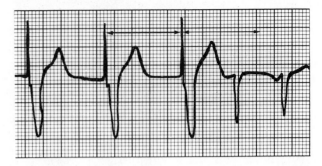

FIGURE 13–6
Demand pacing. Pacemaker is inhibited by each spontaneous beat that appears at a shorter interval than that indicated on the pacemaker rate settings.

Because atrial contraction contributes 15% to 20% to ventricular stroke volume, without this "atrial kick," hypotension or congestive heart failure will develop in patients who have low cardiac reserve. When a ventricular pacemaker is used, either AV dissociation or retrograde atrial conduction can result (Fig. 13–7). In either case, the atria and ventricles do not contract in proper sequence, and atrial kick is lost. With the use of synchronous modes, this atrial contribution to cardiac output can be maintained and various problems avoided (Fig. 13–8).

Rate-Modulated

The rate-modulated sensing mode may be used in conjunction with those modes discussed above. Rate modulation refers to an increase or decrease in heart rate in response to the "sensor." The sensor variable is independent of the intrinsic or paced electrical activity of the heart. Instead, it is tracking a variable that has been associated with the metabolic increases and decreases of the body during exercise (eg, vibration, venous oxygen saturation, stroke volume, and several others). The sensor-driven heart rate variation is designed to meet adequately the physical demands of exercise when patients are pacemaker dependent.[5]

Pacemaker Functional Capabilities Based on the ICHD Code

For many years, pacemaker usage had been limited to fixed-rate (asynchronous) and demand pacing of the ventricles. The successful use of AV sequential pacemakers and increased pacemaker programmability have greatly broadened the functional capabilities of pacemakers currently in use. The Inter-Society Commission for Heart Disease Resources (ICHD) developed a code for differentiation of the various functional capabilities of pacemakers. The letter ICHD code includes the paced chamber(s), the sensing chamber(s), the mode of response to sensed electrical impulses (inhibited or triggered), programmable functions, and special tachycardia functions.

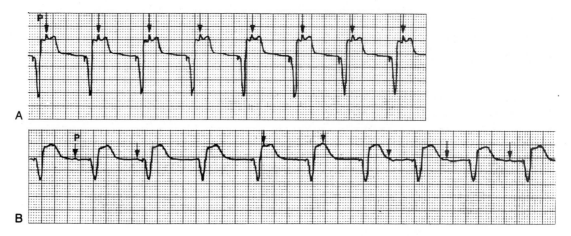

FIGURE 13–7
(**A**) Pacing with retrograde conduction. Each pacemaker stimulus is conducted retrograde through the atria as well as antegrade through the ventricles. Retrograde atrial conduction produces a P wave after each paced QRS. (**B**) Pacing with AV dissociation. P waves are dissociated from paced QRSs, indicating that pacemaker stimulus is not conducted retrograde to atria.

Commonly Used Pacemaker Modes

Although the VVI (ventricular demand) pacemaker is the mode most commonly used in temporary pacing, other modes will be encountered by the critical care nurse owing to advances in dual-chambered temporary pacing and the multiprogrammability in permanent pacemakers.

Most of the permanently implanted pacemakers can be externally programmed by using a special programmer. Changes can be made in rate, energy output, sensitivity, mode, refractory period (period after the QRS during which the pacemaker cannot discharge an impulse), and hysteresis. For troubleshooting purposes, it is essential that the critical care nurse understand the pacing mode, so that the paced rhythm can be interpreted correctly and misdiagnosis can be avoided.

Single-Chamber Modes
VVI. This is the ventricular demand, ventricular sensed and inhibited mode. This mode really is the standard against which all others are compared. The pacemaker senses electrical activity in the ventricle and an RR interval is programmed. If no electrical depolarization is sensed, the pacemaker will fire. But, if ventricular depolarization occurs, the pacemaker will be inhibited. It is used in relatively inactive patients for whom the hemodynamic benefits of atrial activity are absent or unnecessary. It also is the most commonly used mode for temporary cardiac pacing.

AOO or VOO. This is the atrial or ventricular fixed-rate pacemaker mode used when evaluating pacemaker function. Regardless of intrinsic electrical stimulus, the pacemaker will pace.

AAI. This is similar to the VVI mode except that the electrodes are placed in the atrium. Thus, this system paces the atrium when the patient's atria do not depolarize on their own. It is used in patients with atrial bradycardia and intact AV conduction systems.

Dual-Chamber Modes
DVI. This is the AV sequential demand pacemaker mode that paces both the atria and ventricles in sequence. The atria are not sensed, but the ventricles are sensed. Pacing occurs only when the ventricular rate slows (atrial activity is ignored; Figs. 13–9 and 13–10). Thus, the benefit of the paced *atrial* activity is lost if the patient's inherent *ventricular* rate is fast enough. It was used in patients with slow sinus rates, but the addition of rate modulation has made DVIR or DDIR more appropriate pacing modes for these patients.[6]

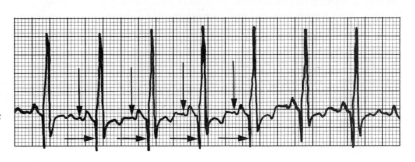

FIGURE 13–8
AV sequential pacemaker stimulating both the atria and the ventricles. Vertical arrows indicate atrial pacing spikes; horizontal arrows indicate ventricular pacing spikes.

ICHD Code for Differentiation of Pacemaker Functional Capabilities

Paced Chamber	Sensing Chamber	Response to Sensing	Programmable Function	Special Antitachycardia Functions
V = Ventricle	V = Ventricle	I = Inhibited	P = Program (rate and/or output)	P = Standard pacer technology
A = Atrium	A = Atrium	T = Triggered	M = Multiprogrammable	S = Shock
D = Dual chambers	D = Dual	D = Dual	C = Communicating	D = Paces and shocks
0 = None	0 = None	0 = None	R = Rate modulation	
			0 = None	

VDD. In this atrial synchronous mode, the pacemaker stimulates the ventricles in response to intrinsic atrial activity. It is inhibited by ventricular depolarization, and pacing does not occur in the atria regardless of atrial or ventricular activity. It is most appropriate for patients with good or normal sinus node function and AV block, who would benefit from heart rates that change with changes in metabolic demands.

DDD. This is the extremely flexible, fully automatic pacemaker mode that can switch to DVI, AAI, or VDD modes as needed. Both atria and ventricles can be paced and sensed. It is indicated in patients having a combination of rhythm disturbances that would benefit from AV synchrony.

DDDR. This mode allows both atrium and ventricles to be sensed and paced; however, rather than simply relying on atrial depolarization or atrial pacing for heart rate control, the pacemaker will be sensitive to the sensor, which may increase the heart rate to meet the patient's metabolic needs. The complexity of the pacemaker intervals in this mode requires advanced training to troubleshoot pacemaker function.

The Internal Cardioverter–Defibrillator

In the 1980s, a device for the treatment of episodes of sudden death syndrome and resistant ventricular dysrhythmias became available.[7] The internal cardioverter–defibrillator (ICD) is capable of interrupting episodes of ventricular tachycardia or fibrillation by delivering an internal shock. Although the pulse generator is several times larger and heavier than a typical dual-chamber pulse generator, the ICD functions in a fashion similar to that of other permanent pacemakers. The sensing leads connect the pulse generator to the heart and continuously sense

heart rate. When ventricular tachycardia or fibrillation is sensed, the ICD discharges 0.05 to 34 joules of electricity, depending on the programmed energy level. It repeats this up to four times if the dysrhythmia persists.

Similar to the initial pacemakers, the defibrillation patches and sensing electrodes are applied to the epicardium and require a sternotomy or thoracotomy. The new-generation ICDs that are under clinical investigation include a transvenous lead system that would abolish the need for a thoracotomy and offer additional programmability.[8] The programmable options include VVI pacing for bradycardia, antitachycardia pacing, and variable energies for cardioversion and defibrillation. Internal cardioverter–defibrillators are undergoing many of the same advances that were seen in permanent pacemakers—for example, multiprogrammability, smaller pulse generators, and transvenous lead systems. Additional knowledge and expertise will be required by health professionals caring for patients with ICDs because of the sophistication available in programming therapy.

Indications for Pacing

Cardiac pacing is indicated for conditions that result in failure of the heart to initiate or conduct an intrinsic electrical impulse at a rate normally adequate to maintain body perfusion. It may be used prophylactically when certain dysrhythmias or conduction defects warn of such failure. It also may be used to interrupt tachyarrhythmias that are unresponsive to other forms of therapy. The critical care nurse should anticipate dysrhythmias that may require pacing in patients with atherosclerotic heart disease, an acute myocardial infarction, or digitalis toxicity.

There are limited resources available for the use of technology in health care delivery. To assist medical professionals in determining the clinical criteria for implanta-

FIGURE 13–9
AV sequential (DVI) pacemaker. Because pacemaker does not sense spontaneous atrial activity, sinus P waves may be found that are unrelated to pacemaker activity. Lack of paced P waves in complexes 2 and 5 results from atrial pacemaker discharge during atrial refractory period following sinus P waves.

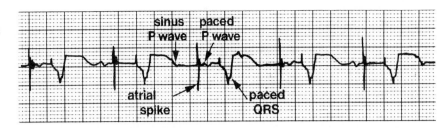

tion, a Joint Committee of the American College of Cardiology and the American Heart Association was formed to establish uniform criteria for pacemaker implantation. The revised 1991 Committee recommendations include guidelines for specific conduction disturbances associated with "symptomatic bradycardia."[9] Symptomatic bradycardia refers to the clinical manifestations of transient dizziness, lightheadedness, near syncope, frank syncope, and generalized symptoms such as exercise intolerance or congestive heart failure. The committee has divided its recommendations into class I (condition under which a pacemaker implantation is necessary), class II (condition under which pacemaker implantation may be necessary, but there is some divergence of opinion), and class III (condition under which pacemaker implantation is not necessary). The following sections include only the class I recommendations for pacemaker implantation.

Bradyarrhythmias

The dysrhythmias that may preclude adequate cardiac output include *symptomatic* sinus bradycardia, sinus arrest, sick sinus syndrome, and symptomatic second- and third-degree heart blocks. One must evaluate the effect on the patient and the underlying cause of each of these rhythms when considering artificial pacing as a mode of therapy or when considering the need for permanent pacing. Pacing has been used successfully to prevent symptoms of severe bradycardia due to hypersensitive carotid body.

Heart Block

There is no evidence to suggest that pacemakers are indicated in first-degree heart block. Patients who have symptomatic bradycardia with second-degree heart block, how-

ever, should receive pacemakers. Complete heart block always requires a pacemaker, unless there is a ventricular rate greater than 40 beats/minute and the patient is asymptomatic. Pacemaker implantation in patients with AV block associated with a myocardial infarction is not as clearly defined because it is dependent on the extent of the myocardial injury. Therefore, postinfarction patients with persistent second-degree AV block, complete heart block, or AV block associated with bundle branch block (BBB) should receive pacemakers. Bifascicular block (right BBB and hemiblock of left BBB) with intermittent, symptomatic complete heart block or with asymptomatic, intermittent second-degree heart block (type II) also should have a pacemaker implanted.

Persistent Tachycardias

Supraventricular and ventricular tachycardias sometimes are suppressed successfully by pacing faster than the intrinsic tachycardia (overdrive pacing). This method often is used temporarily during an electrophysiology study and now is available in the new generation of ICDs.

Procedure

Methods of Pacing

Various methods of pacing have been used over the years, including external pacing, transthoracic pacing, epicardial pacing, and endocardial or transvenous pacing.

External Transcutaneous Pacing

This method involves pacing directly on the chest wall through large gelled electrode patches placed anteriorly

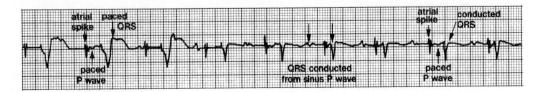

FIGURE 13–10
AV sequential (DVI) pacemaker with QRSs resulting from ventricular pacing, from conduction of sinus impulse, and from conduction of paced P waves.

and posteriorly. The electrodes are connected to an external transcutaneous pacemaker (Fig. 13–11).[10] When first developed, transcutaneous pacing required higher amounts of electricity for pacing, resulting in pain, burns, and skeletal muscle twitching. Because of these problems, the method was abandoned. New technology, however, has permitted the use of lower amounts of electricity, nearly eliminating many of these earlier problems. This technique is becoming more widely used in emergency situations while the patient awaits the insertion of a temporary transvenous pacemaker or as prophylaxis against warning dysrhythmias.

Transthoracic Pacing

This method involves introduction of a pacing lead into the heart through a needle in the anterior wall. Because of its limited success rate and its potential for complications, this method is used as a last resort in emergency situations. Transthoracic pacing is not suitable for long-term pacing or as prophylaxis against warning dysrhythmias.

Epicardial Pacing

This method can be accomplished by thoracotomy or through a subxyphoid incision with the placement of pacing electrodes directly on the surface of the heart. It often is used as a temporary adjunct during and after open heart surgery. The pacing wires are sutured to the epicardial surface of the heart, brought outside through the chest incision, and either connected to a temporary pacemaker generator or capped and then connected if the need

arises. The wires may be removed without reopening the incision, even after scar tissue has formed over the tips.

Permanently implanted epicardial leads rarely are used due to the extensive surgical procedure required, unless a thoracotomy is warranted for concomitant surgery. Many physicians prefer to use the "screw-in" type electrodes, the tips of which can be rotated into the epicardium (Fig. 13–12). The main advantage of permanent epicardial leads is the stability of the electrodes, resulting in a low incidence of displacement.

Endocardial Transvenous Pacing

This method, which involves a transvenous pacing catheter, is the most common type of pacing. It can be used for either temporary or permanent pacing. For temporary pacing, the catheter is introduced into a superficial vein, using local anesthesia. The brachial, femoral, internal jugular, or subclavian veins may be used. The subclavian and internal jugular sites afford catheter stability and allow for patient mobility; however, pneumothorax may occur as a complication of catheter insertion. The femoral vein affords easy access, but use of this site markedly reduces patient mobility.

The pacing catheter is threaded through the vein, the vena cava, the right atrium, and into the right ventricle. It is placed in contact with the endocardial surface of the right ventricle (Fig. 13–13). The insertion procedure may be done with or without fluoroscopy. When fluoroscopy is not available, the electrocardiogram (ECG) complex may be used as an alternative guide for catheter position-

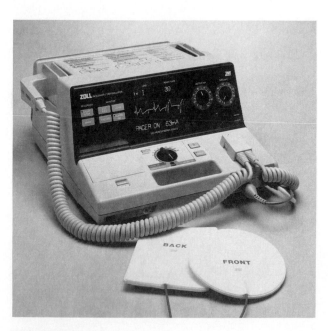

FIGURE 13–11
Commercially available transcutaneous cardiac pacing generator and surface patch electrodes.

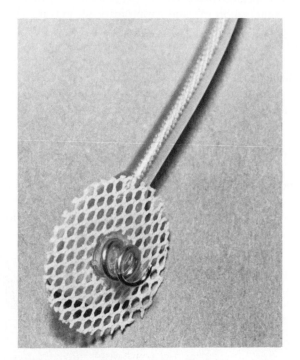

FIGURE 13–12
Screw-in type electrode for permanent epicardial pacing.

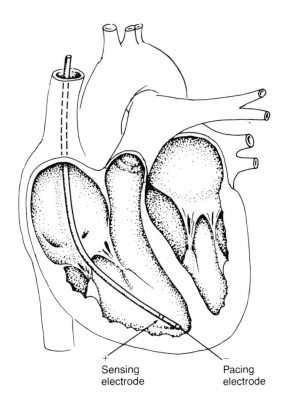

FIGURE 13–13
Transvenous bipolar pacing catheter in place.

ing. The limb leads of a 12-lead ECG are applied to the appropriate limbs and the V lead is connected to the proximal end of the pacing (negative) electrode with an alligator clamp (Fig. 13–14). The distal catheter electrode becomes an "exploring" ECG electrode, and catheter position can be determined by analysis of ECG complex changes as the catheter is advanced. The ECG will reveal large P waves when the electrode touches the atrium. As the catheter tip is advanced into the right ventricle, the QRS complexes become large and the P waves diminish.

The experienced clinician often can accomplish "blind" insertion, using only the standard ECG monitor to indicate successful pacing. Many physicians prefer to use the balloon-tipped, flow-directed pacing catheter to facilitate insertion. The balloon is inflated with air in the vena cava and carries the catheter in the direction of blood flow through the right atrium, the tricuspid valve, and into the right ventricle. The balloon is then deflated and lodged against the right ventricular wall. Also, temporary pacing may be done in conjunction with specific pulmonary artery catheters. The pacing leads are attached to the pulmonary artery catheter or a lumen is provided for the introduction of a pacing wire into the right ventricle.

The transvenous approach is the most widely used for permanent pacemaker implantation. This procedure may be performed under general anesthesia by a surgeon, or

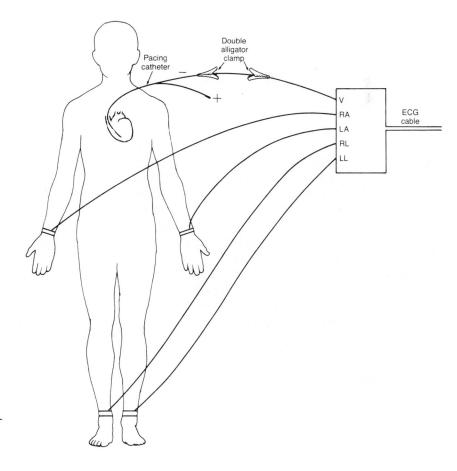

FIGURE 13–14
Set-up for using the distal (negative) pacing electrode as an "exploring" electrode during transvenous pacemaker catheter placement.

implantation can be done under local anesthesia by the cardiologist in the catheterization laboratory. In either case, fluoroscopy would be used for lead positioning. The lead is introduced into the subclavian, cephalic, or internal or external jugular vein. This allows access to the right side of the heart for atrial or ventricular lead placement. The leads are connected to the pulse generator and tucked into the generator pocket, commonly in the left infraclavicular region.

Management

Safety Issues With a Pacemaker

Electrical safety precautions must be observed when the patient has a temporary pacemaker. Electrical equipment in the room should be kept at a minimum and must be properly grounded. Use of a nonelectric bed is preferable. If an electric bed is used, it should remain disconnected from AC current. A tap bell should be provided for the patient, and the electric call light should be disconnected. Only battery-operated electric shavers, toothbrushes, or radios may be used. An AC-powered television may be used if it is operated by someone who is not in contact with the patient. The nurse should avoid simultaneous contact with the patient and any electrical equipment. The patient's bed must be kept dry at all times. Diathermy and electrocautery equipment should not be used because their waves may be sensed by and inhibit the demand pacemaker. See Nursing Care Plan 13–1 for a thorough discussion of nursing care.

If an older-model temporary pacemaker generator with exposed metal catheter tips or terminals is in use, these metal parts must be insulated. A rubber glove can be cut and taped over the exposed metal to provide insulation from external current sources.

The plastic cover supplied with the temporary generator must be kept in place over the dials to prevent inadvertent change in settings. The generator should be attached securely to the patient's arm or abdomen. The catheter should be taped securely to the patient's skin without direct tension on the catheter. Motion of the extremity nearest the catheter entry site should be minimized, especially if the femoral site has been used.

According to manufacturers of permanent pacemaker generators, there are very few electrical hazards associated with the permanent generators currently in use. These generators are shielded from external electrical sources and are not affected by microwave ovens or small appliances. There have been rare reports of unipolar pacemakers being affected by large electromagnetic fields, such as radio transmitters. Defibrillator paddles should not be placed directly over or adjacent to the implanted generator. Internal cardioverter–defibrillator patients must avoid large electromagnetic fields because they can disable the detection capability of the device.

Patient Teaching Regarding Pacemakers

A planned and systematic approach to teaching the patient to live with a pacemaker is a vital part of nursing care. A helpful tool in patient teaching is a progress report accessible to the physician and other members of the team, along with written guidelines for the nurse who is instructing the patient.[11] The patient's family also should be involved in the learning process.

Patient teaching relative to pacemakers begins at the time the decision for pacemaker insertion is made. The patient and family should be told why the pacemaker is necessary. The insertion procedure should be explained, as well as the immediate postinsertion care that can be expected.

Many booklets and media presentations are available to aid the nurse in teaching the pacemaker patient. It is helpful to have written guidelines for the patient to review after discharge from the hospital.[12]

The depth of teaching that is appropriate and the teaching tools used depend on such variables as the patient's age, intellect, attention span, vision, and interest in learning. An occasional patient will demonstrate difficulty in accepting the prospect of living with a pacemaker. Initial teaching should be confined to the positive aspects of life with a pacemaker. Knowledge of the function and care of the pacemaker are of no interest until this patient is able to accept it as part of life. Many misconceptions can be negated by asking the patient what is already known about pacemakers or ICDs, and if there are any preconceived expectations relative to them.

The teaching areas listed in Table 13–2 should be covered with the patient during hospitalization.

Complications of Pacing

Failure of proper function in the demand pacemaker can be determined on the cardiac monitor ECG. The pacemaker may malfunction because of failure to discharge a stimulus, failure to capture the chamber(s) involved, or failure to sense intrinsic depolarizations.

Failure to Discharge

Because stimulus discharge from the pacemaker causes an artifact, or "spike," to appear on the ECG, failure to discharge results in absence of the artifact (Fig. 13–15). This failure may be within the generator itself (either mechanism or battery failure), at the site of lead attachment to the generator, or within the lead due to wire fracture. When failure occurs in the temporary pacemaker, check the connections at the generator terminals, replace the batteries in the generator, or replace the generator. If

(*Text continues on page 228*)

NURSING CARE PLAN 13–1:
The Patient With a Cardiac Pacemaker

NURSING DIAGNOSIS	OUTCOME CRITERIA/ PATIENT GOALS	NURSING INTERVENTIONS
Preoperative *Decreased cardiac output: related to abnormal cardiac rate, rhythm, or conduction.*	• Maintenance of a cardiac rhythm with adequate systemic perfusion.	1. Monitor cardiac rhythm continuously in MCL or "lead II." 2. Document and report changes in cardiac rhythm. 3. Obtain 12-lead ECG, as ordered. 4. Assess for and report signs of reduced cardiac output such as low BP, reduced level of consciousness, absent peripheral pulses, reduced urine output, cyanosis, dyspnea. 5. Facilitate measures to decrease myocardial O_2 demand such as bed rest, elevate the head of bed, restrict activities. 6. Facilitate measures to avoid the Valsalva response such as avoidance of straining, breath holding. 7. Maintain IV line, as ordered. 8. Administer atropine or isoproterenol, as ordered. 9. Assist with the insertion of external cardiac pacemaker or temporary transvenous cardiac pacemaker, as ordered.
Anxiety: related to life-threatening cardiac disease requiring pacemaker and its future implications.	• Patient will use effective coping mechanisms.	1. Initiate nurse–patient relationship. 2. Explain critical care environment, procedures, etc. 3. Use communication techniques that foster verbalizations, such as silence, open-minded statements, etc. 4. Encourage decision-making regarding care. 5. Sedate as needed and if ordered. 6. Encourage family support. 7. Document the patient's response to illness. 8. Refer to teaching plan for more details.

(continued)

NURSING CARE PLAN 13–1: (Continued)
The Patient With a Cardiac Pacemaker

NURSING DIAGNOSIS	OUTCOME CRITERIA/ PATIENT GOALS	NURSING INTERVENTIONS
Knowledge deficit: related to impending pacemaker insertion.	• Patient will describe why a pacemaker must be inserted and how it works. • Patient will describe a normal postoperative course.	1. Include family in the teaching process about permanent pacemakers. 2. Describe all therapies such as IV medications and temporary pacemaker insertion. 3. Describe, in brief terms, the operative process and procedure. 4. Use general preoperative teaching techniques. 5. Aim all teaching at the appropriate level for the individual patient. 6. Evaluate the patient's understanding. 7. Document the patient's response. 8. Refer to teaching plan.
Postoperative *Alteration in comfort: incisional pain related to surgical procedure.*	• Patient will be comfortable.	1. Assess degree of pain on a scale of 1–10. 2. Administer pain medications when needed, as ordered. 3. Assess and document pain relief. 4. Assist with ADLs. 5. Promote periods of uninterrupted rest.
Knowledge deficit: related to daily living with a permanent pacemaker.	• Patient will articulate information taught, in own words.	1. Initiate nurse–patient relationship. 2. Include family in the teaching process. 3. Describe at the appropriate level the following topics (see teaching plan for more details); condition, activity, signs of malfunction, infection, pulse generator replacement, medications, safety, follow-up care. 4. Evaluate the patient's understanding. 5. Document the patient's response.
Decreased cardiac output: related to pacemaker system failure.	• Mechanical aspects of pacemaker systems will be stable.	1. Monitor cardiac rhythm in lead that best displays pacemaker artifact.

(continued)

NURSING CARE PLAN 13–1: (Continued)
The Patient With a Cardiac Pacemaker

NURSING DIAGNOSIS	OUTCOME CRITERIA/ PATIENT GOALS	NURSING INTERVENTIONS
		2. Monitor vital signs every 4 hr for 24 hr.
		3. Assess for and report signs of failure to pace, capture and sense (see text and examples).
		4. Assess for and report signs of congestive heart failure.
		5. Assess for and report signs of increasing ectopy, perforation, tamponade, migration of catheter, muscle twitching, migration of pulse generator, or lead dislodgement.
		6. Maintain activity restrictions as ordered.
		7. Provide for gradual increase in activity once it has been determined that pacemaker system is stable.
		8. Monitor rhythm strip with changes in activity.
		9. Document type of insertion approach, unipolar or bipolar, mode, pacing rate, intrinsic rhythm and paced rhythm.
High risk for infection: related to surgical procedure and presence of foreign body.	• Signs and symptoms of infection will be absent.	1. Patient and nurse will wash hands frequently.
		2. Keep occlusive dressing intact for at least 24 hr after surgery.
		3. Use sterile technique with dressing changes every 24 hr thereafter.
		4. Monitor for signs of infection such as fever, redness, and swelling and unusual pain or tenderness at incision site.
High risk for impaired physical mobility: related to pain and effects of bed rest.	• Patient will steadily increase activity.	1. Initiate passive ROM every 2 hr for unaffected arm while patient is still on bedrest.
		2. Initiate passive ROM every 2 hr for affected arm 24 hr after insertion.
		3. Encourage active leg exercises while patient is on bed rest.
		4. Be present when patient initially gets out of bed and monitor rhythm strip for changes.

(continued)

NURSING CARE PLAN 13–1: *(Continued)*
The Patient With a Cardiac Pacemaker

NURSING DIAGNOSIS	OUTCOME CRITERIA/ PATIENT GOALS	NURSING INTERVENTIONS
High risk for ineffective individual coping: related to change in body image and dependence on pacemaker.	• Patient will demonstrate effective coping mechanisms.	1. Assess for and report fear, depression, and reduced mobility. 2. Portray a positive and healthy image. 3. Use appropriate communication techniques. 4. Mobilize hospital and community resources, as needed.

these efforts do not solve the problem, it must be assumed that wire fracture is the culprit. If only one wire is fractured, conversion to a unipolar system, with a chest electrode to replace the fractured wire, may provide successful pacing. When the permanent pacemaker fails to discharge a stimulus, the problem must be solved operatively. If the situation is emergent, the physician may insert a temporary transvenous pacemaker to support the patient hemodynamically until the permanent pacemaker problem can be corrected.

Failure to Capture

Failure of the pacing stimulus to capture the ventricles or atria will be noted by the absence of the QRS or P wave immediately after the pacemaker artifact on the ECG (Fig. 13–16). If the pacing threshold has increased, the milliamperage may need to be increased until ventricular capture occurs. Displacement of the pacing electrode also may cause failure to capture. It sometimes is possible to regain capture by repositioning the patient, often in the left lateral decubitus position, until the electrode can be repositioned.

Battery failure also can cause failure to capture. If the patient is pacemaker dependent and becomes symptomatic, drug therapy (atropine, isoproterenol), external

pacing, or cardiopulmonary resuscitation may be required until the cause of the problem is found and corrected.

Failure to Sense Spontaneous Beats

Failure of the pacemaker to sense spontaneous beats results in inappropriately placed pacemaker artifacts on the ECG (Fig. 13–17). This may be caused by improper electrode placement, battery or component failure, or lead wire fracture. Ventricular dysrhythmias caused by occurrence of the pacemaker stimulus during the vulnerable phase of the T wave are most likely to occur in the patient who has an acute cardiac disease process, electrolyte imbalance, or drug toxicity, but seldom are seen in the patient who is hospitalized for battery replacement rather than acute illness. The most likely cause for sensing failure in the temporary pacemaker is electrode displacement. If nonsensing renders the pacemaker totally ineffective, it may be advantageous to turn the pacemaker off until the electrode can be repositioned. Again, it may be necessary to institute emergency measures in the interim.

Failure of proper function in pacemakers with dual leads is not detected as easily on the ECG as in the single-lead pacemakers. The nurse must know the functional capabilities and the parameters that have been programmed into the particular pacemaker in use. The ECG strip can

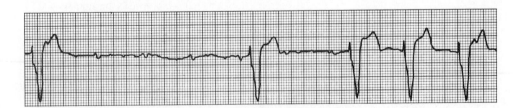

FIGURE 13–15
VVI pacemaker. Failure to discharge is indicated by lack of pacemaker spikes at appropriate intervals.

TABLE 13–2
Teaching the Patient With a Pacemaker

1. Knowledge of Condition

- Elicit the patient's previous knowledge of pacemakers and clarify any misconceptions.
- If appropriate, clarify the difference between heart block and heart attack. (A patient may confuse cardiac monitoring with pacing and become very anxious when the monitoring electrodes are removed.)
- Don't assume *anything* about the patient's understanding.
- The anatomy of the heart should be discussed in general terms when explaining the need for pacing and how the pacemaker takes the place of or complements spontaneous rhythm.
- The difference between temporary and permanent pacing also should be discussed.

2. Patient Activity

- Passive and active range-of-motion exercises should be started on the affected arm 48 hr after pacemaker implantation in the pectoralis major muscle to avoid "frozen shoulder."
- The patient should be instructed to repeat these exercises several times daily until the implantation site is completely free of discomfort through all ranges of arm motion.
- Explain that the pacemaker is relatively sturdy and that touching or bathing the implantation site will not damage it.
- The patient's activities of daily living and recreational activities should be discussed *before* permanent pacing to ascertain an appropriate site for implantation; for example, the right pectoralis muscle should not be used in the right-handed rifle hunter.
- Abdominal implantation may be preferable for the avid swimmer because of the strenuous arm activity.
- Activities that may result in high impact or stress at the implantation site should be avoided. This includes all contact sports.
- Instruct the patient to report any activity that may have damaged his pacemaker.
- The patient can return to work at the discretion of his physician.
- Discuss the type of work he will do and what his job entails. He may return to whatever degree of sexual activity he prefers.
- The patient should be aware that his pacemaker may set off the alarm on metal-detector devices in airports.

3. Signs of Pacemaker Malfunction

- The symptoms of pacemaker malfunction are those associated with decreased perfusion of the brain, heart, or skeletal muscles.
- The patient should be instructed to report any dizziness, fainting, chest pain, shortness of breath, undue fatigue, or fluid retention.

- Fluid retention should be described in terms of sudden weight gain, "puffy ankles," "tightness of rings," and so forth.
- Patient should be instructed to take pulse once daily upon awakening. Patient should report a pulse rate that is more than 5 beats/min slower than that at which pacemaker is set.
- Patient should be aware that pulse may be somewhat irregular if it is a demand pacemaker and has some spontaneous beats as well as paced beats. It must be stressed that this does not signify pacemaker malfunction.

4. Signs of Infection

- The patient should report any redness, swelling, drainage, or increase in soreness at the implantation site.

5. Pulse Generator Replacement

- Instruct the patient regarding the expected life of pacemaker battery.
- Patient should know that generator replacement requires hospitalization for about 1 day and that usually only the generator will need to be replaced.

6. Medications

- The patient should be instructed regarding any medication needed.
- Patient should know the name of the medication, as well as the dose, frequency of administration, side effects, and use of each medication.

7. Safety Measures

- The patient should inform any physician or dentist of the pacemaker and of the medications being taken.
- Patient should carry a pacemaker identification card at all times. This card shows the brand and model of pacemaker, the date of insertion, and the programmed settings.
- It also is advisable to wear a medical alert bracelet or necklace stating that patient has a pacemaker.

8. Follow-up Care

- The importance of physician or clinic follow-up visits should be stressed.
- The follow-up visit will include an interval history and physical examination and a 12-lead ECG.
- Many pacemaker clinics have specialized equipment available to measure the rate, amplitude, duration, and contours of the pacemaker artifact. This information is very helpful in predicting battery depletion. Some clinics have the capability for obtaining this information by telephone, reducing the necessity for travel to the clinic.

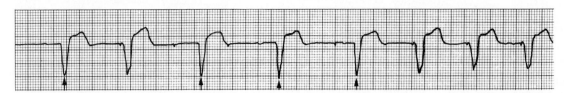

FIGURE 13-16
Ventricular demand pacemaker. Lack of QRS after each pacemaker spike indicates failure to capture. Complexes 1, 3, 4, and 5 result from a spontaneous ventricular escape focus.

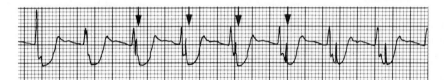

FIGURE 13-17
Ventricular demand pacemaker. Failure to sense is indicated by pacemaker spikes at inappropriate intervals after spontaneous QRSs.

then be examined with consideration of programmed parameters for each pacemaker function. Each electrical event, both paced and intrinsic, must be examined in relation to the preceding electrical event to determine whether pacing, sensing and inhibition, or triggering are occurring, and whether they are occurring at the appropriate programmed intervals. Those pacemakers with sensor-driven rates will complicate the rate limit settings even further. Thus, it is essential to understand the basics of rhythm strip analysis before undertaking the complicated task of evaluating dual-chamber pacemaker strips, especially those with rate modulation.

Ventricular Irritability

Ventricular irritability at the site of the endocardial catheter tip is a frequent occurrence after initial catheter insertion. The premature ventricular complexes usually appear similar in configuration to the pacemaker complexes (Figs. 13–18 and 13–19). Irritability from the catheter as a foreign body usually disappears after 2 or 3 days.

Perforation of Ventricular Wall or Septum

Perforation of the ventricular wall or septum by the transvenous catheter occurs in a small number of patients. This may or may not result in noncapture. It can be suspected on cardiac monitoring if the patient is monitored in a modified V1 lead. Right ventricular pacing should provide a negative QRS in this lead. Often, ventricular per-

foration results in pacing from the left ventricle, and the QRS becomes positive in polarity. Pericardial tamponade, causing a decrease in blood pressure and increase in sinus node discharge rate, must be watched for after ventricular wall perforation.

Tamponade

Tamponade occurs infrequently because of the ability of myocardial fibers to regain their integrity after the catheter has been pulled back into the ventricle; however, anticoagulation therapy should be discontinued after perforation.

Retrograde Migration of Right Ventricular Catheter

Retrograde migration of the right ventricular pacing catheter into the right atrium may result in atrial pacing (pacing artifact followed by P wave) or inhibition of the pacemaker by atrial depolarizations. The effects on the patient depend on the ability of the AV node to conduct atrial impulses and on the ability of a lower escape focus to emerge at an adequate rate.

Abdominal Twitching or Hiccoughs

Abdominal twitching or hiccoughs occur occasionally as a result of electrode placement against a thin right ventricular wall and resultant electrical stimulation of the abdominal

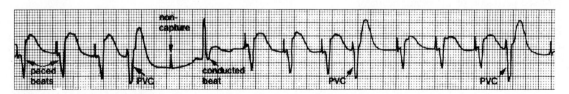

FIGURE 13-18
Ventricular demand pacemaker with PVCs. This strip also shows one noncaptured pacemaker spike followed by a spontaneous conducted beat.

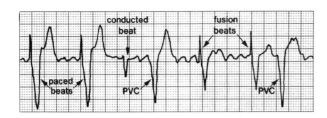

FIGURE 13–19
Ventricular demand pacemaker with PVCs and with fusion beats that result from ventricular depolarization by both the pacemaker and a spontaneous beat.

muscles or diaphragm. This usually is very uncomfortable for the patient, and the electrode should be repositioned as soon as possible.

Infection and Phlebitis

Infection and phlebitis can occur at the temporary pacemaker insertion site, and infection or *hematoma* may occur at the site of permanent generator implantation. These sites must be inspected for swelling and inflammation, and kept dry. Sterile technique must be used when dressings are being changed.

Permanent Generator Migration

Migration of the permanent generator from its initial site of implantation may occur in patients who have very loose connective tissue. This may or may not require reimplantation. *Erosion* at the implantation site occurs rarely.

Malfunction Due to Defibrillation

Defibrillation of the patient while the temporary pacemaker system is intact may affect various components of the generator and cause it to malfunction. The temporary generator should be turned off *and* the catheter wires disconnected from the generator, if at all possible, before defibrillating.

Nursing Care Plan

The nurse who cares for the patient with a pacemaker or ICD must have thorough knowledge of the heart, the pacemaker, and the patient as a person. This knowledge must be applied continuously from the time the decision for device insertion is made until the patient is discharged from the hospital, and sometimes beyond, to follow-up care. The nurse plays a vital role in ensuring success after implantation and in reassuring the patient, whose well-being depends on the device. Caring for the pacemaker/ICD patient is a challenging but most rewarding experience when the nurse is secure in his or her knowledge of the subject.

See Nursing Care Plan 13–1 for a thorough discussion of nursing care for the patient with a cardiac pacemaker.

Commonly Used Antiarrhythmic Agents and Cardioversion

Behavioral Objectives

Pharmacologic Agents

Description

Digitalis Preparations
  Digoxin
  Ouabain
  Digitoxin

Digitalis Toxicity

Class IA Antiarrhythmic Agents
  Quinidine
  Quinidine Toxicity
  Procainamide

Procainamide Toxicity
Disopyramide
Disopyramide Toxicity

Class IB Antiarrhythmic Agents
  Lidocaine
  Phenytoin
  Tocainide
  Mexiletene

Class IC Antiarrhythmic Agents
  Encainide and Flecainide
  Propafenone
  Moricizine

(*continued*)

BEHAVIORAL OBJECTIVES

Based on the content in this section, the reader should be able to:

1. Name the most commonly used agents in the treatment of dysrhythmias.
2. State the normal dose and side effects of these common antiarrhythmic agents.
3. Describe the indications and procedure for cardioversion.

Pharmacologic Agents

Description

In 1969, Vaughan Williams proposed a way of classifying antiarrhythmic agents based on their effect on action potential and conduction. Table 13–3 lists the agents commonly used. The reader might find it helpful to review the section on action potential (Chapter 11). Features of those agents most commonly used for management of dysrhythmias are listed in Tables 13–4 and 13–5.

Digitalis Preparations

Digoxin

This agent often is the first selected for patients with supraventricular dysrhythmias, such as paroxysmal atrial tachycardia, atrial fibrillation, and atrial flutter. Digoxin

TABLE 13–3
Commonly Used Antiarrhythmic Agents

Class	Action	Drug
I	All class I antiarrhythmic agents block sodium movement into the tissue, resulting in a reduced maximal velocity of phase 0 depolarization	
IA	Slows depolarization at all heart rates and increases the duration of action potential	Quinidine Procainamide Disopyramide
IB	Slows phase 0 depolarization at fast heart rates	Lidocaine Tocainamide Phenytoin Mexilitene
IC	Slows phase 0 depolarization at normal rates, does not affect the action potential duration	Encainide Flecainide Propafenone Moricizine
II	Blocks sympathetic stimulation of the conduction system	β-Blockers (propranolol) Acebutolol Esmolol
III	Prolongs the action potential duration	Amiodarone Bretylium Sotalol
IV	Blocks influx of calcium into the cell and decreases conduction velocity	Calcium channel blockers (verapamil, diltiazem)

has little effect on multifocal atrial tachycardia. Digitalization often produces reversion to a normal sinus rhythm or, in the case of atrial fibrillation or flutter, slowing of the ventricular rate to a more satisfactory level. Digoxin should not be used to treat sinus tachycardia except when the tachycardia is secondary to congestive heart failure. The reduction in heart rate in such instances results from improved cardiac output.

Table 13–6 lists the chief characteristics of three digitalis preparations. Because digoxin receives the widest use, it merits further discussion.

Seventy percent to 80% of an oral dose of digoxin is absorbed. Digoxin also is absorbed when given intramuscularly, but this route is painful and has few advantages. When given intravenously (IV; preferable for many seriously ill patients), the usual starting dose is 0.5 mg, followed by 0.25 mg every 2 to 4 hours. Total dosage requirements vary widely, although most patients will respond to a total dose of 1.0 to 1.5 mg IV. Some patients will not respond to customary doses of digoxin.

In order to minimize the risks of *digitalis toxicity*, a serious and sometimes lethal complication, the following

TABLE 13–4
Pharmacokinetics of Most Commonly Used Antiarrhythmic Drugs

Drug	Effect on ECG	Dose and Interval	Route	Adverse Effects	Therapeutic Plasma Level
Digoxin	Prolongs PR ($\pm$) ST depression	0.5 mg initially; 0.25 mg q2–4h total 1.0–1.5 mg first 24 hr	IV or PO	Nausea, vomiting, abdominal pain, blurred or colored vision, weakness, psychosis, VPCs, heart block	0.8–1.8 ng/ml
Quinidine	Prolongs QRS, QT, and PR ($\pm$)	100–600 mg q4–6h	PO	GI symptoms, cinchonism, thrombocytopenia, hypotension, heart block, ventricular tachycardia	2.3–5.0 μg/ml
Procainamide (Pronestyl)	Prolongs QRS, QT, and PR ($\pm$)	500 mg–1 g; then 2–5 g/day 250–500 mg q3–6 h 100 mg q5 m to 1 g total Maintenance: 2–4 mg/min	PO IM IV	GI symptoms, psychosis, hypotension, rash, lupus-like syndrome	4–10 μg/ml
Disopyramide (Norpace)	Prolongs QRS, QT, and PR	Loading: 200–300 mg Maintenance: 100–200 mg q6h	PO	Anticholinergic effects, hypotension, heart failure, heart block, tachyarrhythmias	2–8 μg/ml
Lidocaine	None	1 mg/kg; may repeat at 0.5 mg/kg	IV	Drowsiness, seizures	1.5–6 μg/ml
Propranolol (Inderal)	Prolongs PR, no change QRS, shortens QT	10–80 mg q6h 0.3–5 mg total (not >1 mg/min)	PO IV	Hypotension, heart failure, heart block, asthma	Not established; 50–100 ng/ml needed for β-blockade
Verapamil	Prolongs PR	5–10 mg 80–120 mg tid–qid	IV PO	Hypotension, bradycardia, dizziness, GI disturbance	Not established

ECG, electrocardiogram; VPC, ventricular premature contraction; GI, gastrointestinal.

options should be considered for the patient with a supraventricular tachycardia:

- Stop treatment if the heart rate has reached a satisfactory, although not ideal, level and further doses of digoxin produce no further slowing (an example is atrial fibrillation with a ventricular rate of 100–120 beats/minute)
- Choose a second drug for control of heart rate, such as propranolol or verapamil
- Attempt electrical cardioversion
- Use an agent such as quinidine, procainamide, or disopyramide, which may reestablish normal sinus rhythm

Alternate forms of digitalis are useful in specific circumstances.

Ouabain

Given only IV, ouabain exerts an effect on atrial dysrhythmias within minutes. Its chief benefits are for the two following types of patients: those in whom speed of rhythm control is important and those in whom the status of digitalization is uncertain. In each group, small increments of ouabain (0.1 mg IV, every 30 minutes) may produce either a favorable response or evidence of toxicity, such as the development of ventricular premature beats. The latter indicates that safe levels of digitalization have been exceeded. The small, stepwise doses and the shorter half-life make this approach somewhat safer than the use of digoxin for this purpose.

Digitoxin

By virtue of its relatively slow excretion, digitoxin is especially useful in some patients with chronic atrial fibrillation or atrial flutter who continue to exhibit rapid ventricular rates. The vagotonic action of digitoxin on the AV node is more consistent than that of digoxin, leading to more dependable rate control.

Digitalis Toxicity

All digitalis glycosides should be used with great caution in patients with Wolff–Parkinson–White (WPW) syndrome in whom atrial fibrillation or flutter develops. Digitalis reduces the refractory period of the accessory path-

TABLE 13–5
Pharmacokinetics of Newer Antiarrhythmic Drugs

Drug	Effect on ECG	Dose and Interval	Route	Adverse Effects
Tocainide	No effect on PR, QRS, QT	400–600 mg q8h	Oral	Nausea, vomiting, abdominal pain, dizziness, tremor
Mexilitene	No effect on PR, QRS, QT	150–400 mg 3–4 times/day	Oral	Nausea, vomiting, dizziness, tremor
Encainide	Prolongs PR, QRS, may slightly prolong QT	25–50 mg q8h	Oral	Exacerbation of ventricular ectopy, visual disturbances, tremors, nausea
Flecainide	Prolongs PR, QRS, may slightly prolong QT	100–200 mg twice daily	Oral	Dizziness, blurred vision
Amiodarone	Prolongs QRS, QT; may slightly prolong PR	Loading dose— 800–1200 mg/day for 10–14 days; then 200–400 mg/day	Oral	Corneal microdeposits, hyper/hypothyroidism, pulmonary fibrosis, skin sensitivity (blue skin), nausea, tremor, headache, ataxia
Bretylium	None	5–10 mg/kg	IV	Hypotension, nausea, vomiting
Propafenone	Prolongs PR and QRS	150–300 mg every 8 hr	Oral	Nausea, bitter taste, hypotension, exacerbation of ventricular ectopy
Moricizine	Prolongs PR and QRS	200–300 mg every 8 hr	Oral	Dizziness, headache, nausea, exacerbation of ventricular ectopy
Adenosine	Prolongs PR	6–12 mg	IV	Hypotension, facial flushing, dyspnea

ECG, electrocardiogram.

way. This action leads to transmission of potentially very rapid atrial rates to the ventricle; ventricular fibrillation may result.

Excessive doses of digitalis can be avoided if consideration is given to some principles of its metabolism. When renal function is normal, one-third of the digoxin stored in the body is excreted daily. The renal clearance of digoxin directly relates to the creatinine clearance. When serum creatinine is elevated to 2 to 5 mg/dl, the mainte-

nance dose of digoxin should be reduced by at least one-half. More severe levels of renal failure require an even further reduction of dosage. Because creatinine levels rise only after considerable loss of renal function, a normal serum creatinine does not ensure a normal clearance of digoxin.

It is prudent to reduce the maintenance dose of digoxin in the elderly patient. Creatinine clearance declines with age. A second factor that favors accumulation of

TABLE 13–6
Digitalis Preparations

Agent	Onset of Action (min)	Peak Effect (hr)	Average Half-life	Principal Excretory Path	Average Digitalizing Dose		Usual Daily Oral Maintenance Dose
					Oral	*IV*	
Ouabain	5–10	$1/2$–2	21 hr	Renal; some GI	—	0.3–0.5 mg	—
Digoxin	15–30	1–2	33 hr	Renal	1.25–1.5	0.75–1.0 mg	0.25–0.5 mg
Digitoxin	25–120	4–12	4–6 days	Hepatic	0.7–1.2 mg	1.0 mg	0.1 mg

GI, gastrointestinal.

digoxin in this age group is the age-related decrease in muscle mass. Skeletal muscle is the major body depository for digoxin; a decrease in muscle mass is reflected in increased glycoside concentration in the serum and in the heart. Features of digitalis toxicity are listed in the accompanying chart.

Other conditions that may lead to digitalis toxicity include hypokalemia, hypomagnesemia, hypothyroidism, pulmonary hypertension, and severe heart disease of any etiology. Concomitant therapy with quinidine or verapamil also is known to increase the serum digoxin level. Certain of these states, such as severe heart failure, are themselves associated with atrial dysrhythmias. The utmost care is required in choosing the dose of digitalis for these patients.

Cases of life-threatening digoxin or digitoxin intoxication or overdose may be treated with Digibind Digoxin Immune Fab (Burroughs Wellcome, Research Triangle Park, NC), an antibody that binds with digoxin, rendering it unable to react at receptor sites on the myocardium and allowing for its elimination through the kidneys.[13] It has been demonstrated to be effective in reversing the cardiac effects of toxicity. Dosing is based on how much drug was ingested, serum levels, and body weight. Digibind should be administered over 30 minutes through a 0.22-μm filter; however, in the case of cardiac arrest, it may be administered as an IV bolus. Average dosing during clinical trials was 6 to 10 vials (40 mg/vial).[14] An initial response to treatment can be expected to occur within 1 hour. Serum potassium levels should be monitored because as the digoxin level is lowered hypokalemia may result.

Manifestations of Digitalis Toxicity

Gastrointestinal

Anorexia
Vomiting
Abdominal pain
Diarrhea
Unexplained weight loss

Neurologic

Weakness
Blurred or colored vision
Psychosis

Cardiac (entirely manifest as dysrhythmias)

Atrial tachycardia, commonly with AV block
Junctional tachycardia
Ventricular ectopic rhythm
SA node depression
AV block
Bidirectional tachycardia

Measurements of serum digoxin levels have assisted in many cases in dysrhythmia management. The normal range is 0.8 to 1.8 ng/ml. It cannot be stressed too strongly that the serum level is only a guide and not an absolute indicator of the adequacy of digitalization. The clinical status of the patient, in particular the adequacy of rate control, often provides more useful information about the status of digitalization than absolute serum levels. As a common clinical example, a patient with chronic atrial fibrillation may require larger than customary doses of digoxin for maintenance of a satisfactory ventricular rate. A serum level above the "therapeutic range" in this instance may be misleading as an indicator of toxicity.

Class IA Antiarrhythmic Agents

Quinidine

Quinidine is highly effective in the management of atrial and ventricular ectopic rhythms. These include supraventricular tachycardia, atrial fibrillation, atrial flutter, multifocal atrial tachycardia, ventricular premature contractions, and ventricular tachycardia. Quinidine has been found superior to placebo treatment in maintaining sinus rhythm after cardioversion from atrial fibrillation or flutter.

Quinidine has two modes of action. First, it is vagolytic, and thus enhances conduction through the AV node. This action tends to speed the ventricular rate in atrial fibrillation or flutter; prior digitalization prevents this undesirable effect. Second, quinidine exerts a direct myocardial effect that prolongs AV conduction, His–Purkinje conduction times, and the duration of repolarization (the QT interval on the ECG).

Quinidine sulfate is well absorbed orally and reaches a peak serum level at about 1.5 hours. In contrast, quinidine gluconate is absorbed more slowly, with a peak level occurring at about 4 hours. It would be expected that quinidine gluconate could be given less frequently (every 8–12 hours) than the sulfate compound (every 6–8 hours) because of the more prolonged absorption of the gluconate salt, which also results in lower peak levels. The effective dose in any given patient will vary quite widely as a result of patient variation, the disease state, the presence of other drugs, and differences in composition of other products. An initial total dose of 600 to 900 mg daily usually is given. The dose should be increased gradually as needed with attention directed to ECG signs of toxicity (prolonged QRS and QT intervals).

Blood levels offer a guideline for management and should be obtained after the first six to eight doses. With current techniques, the therapeutic levels range from 2.3 to 5.0 μg/ml. An occasional patient may show signs of toxicity with "therapeutic" serum levels. In some of these patients, the QT interval may show considerable prolongation over the pretreatment ECG and warn of impending toxicity. Excessive serum levels are associated with a high frequency of toxicity. Conversely, some patients may be controlled at "subtherapeutic" blood levels. The dosage of the drug should not be raised further in this situation. Concomitant administration of quinidine with digoxin can raise digoxin levels.

Quinidine should not be given intramuscularly because of erratic absorption and the tendency to produce pain at the injection site. The IV route is hazardous because quinidine produces vasodilation and sometimes circulatory collapse. Intravenous quinidine, given by slow drip, should be reserved for patients with serious rhythm disorders that have not responded to other modes of therapy.

Quinidine Toxicity

About 30% of the patients on quinidine cannot tolerate the drug because of troublesome side effects. Diarrhea is the most common, is unrelated to plasma concentrations, and often is associated with nausea and vomiting. Cinchonism (headache and visual, auditory, and vestibular symptoms) occurs with increased plasma concentrations. Dysrhythmias, especially ventricular ectopic rhythms, occur more frequently in patients with advanced cardiac failure. A very slow ventricular rate in patients with atrial fibrillation or flutter also predisposes to ventricular dysrhythmias. Transient ventricular flutter or fibrillation may produce the entity known as "quinidine syncope." This proarrhythmic effect—a worsening of ventricular arrhythmias—has been seen in the class IA and IC agents.

Sudden death occurs in a small percentage of patients on maintenance quinidine. A retrospective look at patients with quinidine syncope reveals a prolonged QT interval in many cases. Other patients may show AV block. Finally, idiosyncratic reactions occur in some patients; these include fever, rash, thrombocytopenia, hemolytic anemia, and hepatic dysfunction.

As a rule, the maintenance dose of quinidine should be reduced to 70% in the presence of congestive failure and to 50% with renal failure. The blood level should be checked at the peak serum concentration (1.5 hours after oral use) and at the trough (1 hour before the next dose).

Procainamide

Procainamide (Pronestyl, E. R. Squibb and Sons, Princeton, NJ) is highly effective for atrial and ventricular ectopic rhythms, whether given orally, intramuscularly, or IV. Like quinidine, procainamide has a mild vagolytic effect on the AV node, which in some patients will prove deleterious by increasing the ventricular rate. Procainamide has the potential for myocardial depression. It decreases conduction throughout the heart and can prolong the QRS and QT intervals. A reduced cardiac output and hypotension may occur after rapid IV use or when the oral dose accumulates as a result of renal failure.

A metabolite of procainamide, N-acetylprocainamide

(NAPA), also has antiarrhythmic activity. N-Acetylprocainamide has a longer serum half-life than procainamide. Renal failure produces a toxic level of NAPA that is not detected by the usual serum measurements. Patients with renal failure therefore should be treated with lower doses of procainamide and followed closely to detect QRS prolongation.

Procainamide is well absorbed orally, reaching a peak level at 1 hour. The usual dose ranges from 250 to 500 mg every 3 to 6 hours. Therapeutic plasma levels range between 4 to 10 μg/ml. Earlier investigations indicated that the serum level fell to subtherapeutic levels after 3 to 4 hours. Many patients, however, exhibit a continued response for longer periods. This effect probably results from the more prolonged antiarrhythmic action of NAPA.

Procainamide is given IV in initial doses of 100 mg by slow infusion and repeated every 5 minutes until either a therapeutic effect is obtained or toxicity (hypotension or widening of the QRS complex) is noted. The total IV dose should not exceed 1 g. The loading dose is followed by a maintenance infusion of 2 to 3 mg/minute. The dose should be reduced in patients with heart failure or hepatic or renal insufficiency.

Procainamide Toxicity

Commonly encountered side effects of procainamide include nausea, vomiting, and diarrhea with the oral route. Rash, fever, agranulocytosis, and frank psychosis are seen occasionally. Long-term use leads to a very high incidence (80%) of antinuclear antibodies. Thirty percent of patients manifest a lupus-like syndrome characterized by high antinuclear antibody titer, fever, pleuropericarditis, and arthritis. Cessation of the drug usually reverses these findings.

Disopyramide

Disopyramide (Norpace, Searle Laboratories, Chicago, IL) is effective for both atrial and ventricular dysrhythmias. By prolonging the refractory period of the accessory pathway, disopyramide may be especially effective in patients with WPW syndrome in whom supraventricular tachyarrhythmias develop. Although disopyramide is used less than quinidine and procainamide, it has been useful in treating the arrhythmias associated with hypertropic cardiomyopathy and neurally mediated syncope.[15]

Disopyramide is well absorbed by the oral route. Peak plasma levels occur in 2 hours; plasma half-life approximates 6 hours. Excretion occurs mainly by the renal route. Oral doses range from 100 to 300 mg every 6 hours. Effective plasma levels occur at about 2 to 8 μg/ml. The IV route has not been approved for general use.

Disopyramide Toxicity

Disopyramide causes a slight to moderate decrease in cardiac output. It may precipitate overt cardiac failure in patients with limited myocardial reserve. The drug should be avoided in patients with advanced heart block. The most frequent side effects of this drug are anticholinergic, namely, dry mouth, blurred vision, and, especially in men with prostatic enlargement, urinary retention.

Disopyramide, like quinidine and procainamide, can prolong the QT interval. Patients with marked prolongation of this interval appear especially susceptible to malignant ventricular rhythms and sudden death.

Class IB Antiarrhythmic Agents

Lidocaine

Lidocaine (Xylocaine, Astra Pharmaceutical Products, Inc., Westboro, MA) is of great value in the management of ventricular ectopic rhythms in the critically ill. It has the advantages of rapid effectiveness and minimal effect on cardiac contractility.

An initial intravenous bolus of 50 to 100 mg or 1 mg/kg usually will suppress ectopic activity for approximately 20 minutes. Recurrence of ventricular premature contractions calls for a repeat IV bolus followed by a sustained IV infusion of 1 to 4 mg/minute. The dosage is adjusted to control ventricular ectopic beats. Care is taken to avoid excessive doses, which produce agitation or seizures. As a rule, lidocaine is not helpful in the management of supraventricular dysrhythmias.

Evidence indicates that the usual protocol of lidocaine use may not provide adequate plasma levels during the early hours of therapy. Some authorities have recommended giving multiple doses of lidocaine to a total of 225 mg over 16 minutes followed by a constant infusion of 2 to 4 mg/minute.

Because lidocaine is metabolized by the liver, the dose should be reduced when hepatic blood flow is decreased, as in congestive heart failure. Atrioventricular block with a slow junctional or ventricular focus also is a contraindication to the use of lidocaine. Therapeutic levels range from 1.5 to 6 μg/ml.

Phenytoin (Dilantin)

Phenytoin (Dilantin, Parke-Davis, Morris Plains, NJ) usually is ineffective for atrial dysrhythmias. It is reserved largely for digitalis toxicity rhythms, in which it has moderate success. Such rhythms include atrial tachycardia, with or without block, and atrial fibrillation or flutter with a very slow ventricular rate and multiple ventricular premature contractions. In this setting, phenytoin may increase the ventricular rate to a more normal range and abolish the ventricular ectopic activity.

Phenytoin should be given IV, slowly and undiluted from the vial because it can cause severe bradycardia or asystole. The rate of administration should not exceed 50 to 100 mg every 5 minutes. The drug should be given until the dysrhythmia is controlled or a maximal dose of 1 g is given. Phenytoin seldom is used in maintenance by the oral route.

Tocainide

This drug is an analogue of lidocaine, but unlike lidocaine, it is effective orally. Tocainide is useful primarily in the therapy of ventricular dysrhythmias. The dose ranges from 400 to 600 mg every 8 hours. Adverse effects involve the gastrointestinal tract (nausea, vomiting, abdominal pain, or constipation) and the central nervous system (dizziness, tremor, or paresthesias). Half-life of this drug is 9 to 20 hours. Because tocainide is excreted through the kidneys, the dose should be reduced in patients with renal impairment.

Mexiletene

Mexiletene also is structurally similar to lidocaine. It may be given IV or orally. The oral dose is 150 to 400 mg given three to four times daily. Half-life of mexiletine is 12 to 13 hours. Effectiveness has been established for ventricular dysrhythmias, whether given IV in the setting of acute myocardial infarction or administered orally for chronic symptomatic ventricular dysrhythmias. Dose-related neurologic and gastrointestinal adverse effects are common, but hemodynamic reactions are minor. Periodic blood counts should be obtained because mexiletene has been shown to cause agranulocytosis. This side effect decreases its use in the treatment of arrhythmias.

Class IC Antiarrhythmic Agents

Encainide and Flecainide

Encainide and flecainide both have been shown to be effective in the treatment of ventricular arrhythmias, but currently are used only in the treatment of life-threatening arrhythmias. During the Cardiac Arrhythmia Suppression Trial (CAST), both were removed due to an increase in mortality in the patients treated with these agents. Both were shown to exhibit a proarrhythmic effect, a worsening of ventricular arrhythmias.[16] Encainide is available on a limited basis. Flecainide has proven to be effective in the treatment of supraventricular arrhythmias but still is under investigation.

Encainide is administered in doses of 75 to 300 mg/day given in divided doses every 4 to 6 hours. Its half-life is about 12 hours. In addition to its proarrhythmic effects, both neurologic and gastrointestinal side effects have been reported.

Flecainide has a long half-life of 12 to 27 hours. Doses of 100 to 200 mg/day can be given with slow increases every 4 to 7 days up to 400 mg/day. The drug exerts a negative effect on cardiac performance, probably of importance only in patients with markedly compromised ventricular function. Other major side effects include dizziness and blurred vision.

Propafenone

This drug is approved for the treatment of life-threatening ventricular arrhythmias. In addition to its class IC properties, it also exhibits a β-blocking effect and calcium channel-blocking effect.[17] Dosing ranges from 150 to 300 mg every 8 hours. Its half-life is from 2 to 10 hours. The chief adverse effects include nausea, bitter taste, hypotension, and, in susceptible patients with AV nodal disease, heart block. Due to its β-blocking and calcium channel-blocking effects, it can lower heart rate and depress cardiac function. There is a risk of proarrhythmic activity, as with the other class IC agents.

Moricizine

Moricizine (Ethmozine) is classified mainly as a IC agent because it slows atrial, AV nodal, and intraventricular conduction.[18] It is used in the treatment of severe, life-threatening ventricular arrhythmias. Moricizine is metabolized in the liver and excreted in the feces and kidney. Dosing ranges from 200 to 300 mg every 8 hours, but should be decreased in the presence of hepatic and kidney dysfunction. Its half-life is 10 hours. The most common side effects are central nervous system (dizziness and headache) and gastrointestinal (nausea). Moricizine also has been shown to be proarrhythmic, thus causing new, or worsening existing ventricular arrhythmias.

Class II β-Blocking Agents

β-Blocking adrenergic agents interfere with stimulation of the sympathetic nervous system, thus slowing heart rate and conduction through the AV node, and decreasing automaticity. β-Blockers have been effective in the treatment of both ventricular and supraventricular dysrhythmias. They are categorized as cardioselective (inhibition of β_1 receptors) or nonselective (inhibition of β_1 and β_2 receptors).[19] Inhibition of β_1 receptors causes a slowing of heart rate, decreases conduction through the AV node, and depresses cardiac function. Inhibition of β_2 receptors causes bronchoconstriction, vasoconstriction, and a decrease in glycogenolysis. Table 13–7 indicates the β activity of the various β-blocking agents. Although these agents can be used in the treatment of angina and hypertension, only three of them are used in the treatment of arrhythmias: propranolol, acebutolol, and esmolol.

Propranolol (Inderal)

Propranolol (Inderal, Ayerst Laboratories, New York, NY) is the most commonly used β-blocker for treatment of dys-

TABLE 13–7
β-Blocking Agents

Drug	Cardioselective	Nonselective
Propranolol		X
Acebutolol	X	
Esmolol	X	
Atenolol	X	
Labetalol		X
Metoprolol	X	
Nadolol		X
Timolol		X

rhythmias in the United States. It is useful for a variety of atrial and ventricular tachyarrhythmias. Propranolol increases the degree of block at the AV node and reduces the heart rate in patients with atrial fibrillation or flutter. In some, these rhythms may revert to a sinus rhythm. Propranolol may be useful alone or as an adjunct to digitalis or quinidine. β-Blockade is especially helpful in some patients with chronic atrial fibrillation or flutter in whom digitalization is insufficient to control the ventricular rate. Propranolol is the agent of choice for rapid atrial dysrhythmias due to hyperthyroidism.

The oral dose of propranolol varies over a wide range owing to differences in the rate of removal by the liver. The usual dose is between 80 and 320 mg/day given in three or four divided doses. On occasion, however, even low doses of propranolol (10–20 mg/day) increase the degree of block at the AV node and provide satisfactory control of the heart rate. The dose in each situation must be "titrated," beginning with small amounts of the drug and adjusting further doses according to the degree of response. Therapeutic serum level measurements have not been established. β-Blockade usually is present at 50 to 100 ng/ml.

The IV use of propranolol requires great caution. Hypotension, acute pulmonary edema, and cardiovascular collapse may occur with IV doses as low as 1 mg. Doses of 0.3 to 0.5 mg IV should be used initially with close ECG and blood pressure monitoring. The dose should be repeated every 1 to 2 minutes and increased slowly as needed. The total IV dose should not exceed 7 to 10 mg in the first 2 to 3 hours.

Propranolol Toxicity

Side effects are common. Sinus bradycardia, usually well tolerated, need *not* be regarded as a complication. Fatigue, depression, nausea, diarrhea, alopecia, impotence, increased peripheral vascular insufficiency, and hypoglycemia have been noted.

Propranolol depresses cardiac output in patients with preexisting congestive heart failure and therefore is contraindicated in such patients. An exception to this statement is the patient with heart failure due to atrial fibrillation or flutter with a very rapid ventricular response. Reduction of the ventricular rate in this instance may improve cardiac output and offset the depressant action of propranolol on the heart.

The drug should be used with great caution in patients with asthma, in whom it may induce irreversible and fatal bronchospasm. Finally, in the insulin-dependent diabetic patient, propranolol may mask the symptoms of hypoglycemia and therefore should be given with great care.

Acebutolol

Acebutolol (Sectral, Wyeth Laboratories, Philadelphia, PA) is a cardioselective β-blocker used in the treatment of ventricular dysrhythmias.[20] Its effectiveness in the treatment of supraventricular dysrhythmias still is under investigation. Acebutolol exhibits intrinsic sympathomimetic activity properties, which allow it to have a lesser effect on slowing of heart rate and depression of cardiac function than propranolol. Dosing ranges from 600 to 1,200 mg orally per day. Its half-life ranges from 9 to 20 hours. Major adverse effects include bradycardia, hypotension, heart failure, anxiety, dizziness, nausea, and abdominal pain.

Esmolol (Brevibloc)

Esmolol (Brevibloc, DuPont, Wilmington, DE) is an ultra-short—acting, cardioselective β-blocker effective in slowing the ventricular rate in supraventricular dysrhythmias, and to a lesser extent conversion to sinus rhythm. Due to its short half-life of 9 minutes, adverse effects resolve quickly. Adverse effects include hypotension, bradycardia, and pulmonary edema. Esmolol is administered by the IV route and titrated to the desired effect. A loading dose of 500 μg/kg/minute is administered over 1 minute, followed by 50 μg/kg/minute over 4 minutes. After 30 minutes, if the desired effect is not achieved, the dose may be doubled. An infusion of 25 to 50 μg/kg/minute may be used to maintain the desired effect for 24 to 48 hours. Esmolol has proven to be effective in treating the cardiovascular hyperactivity exhibited during surgery and anesthesia.[17]

Class III Antiarrhythmic Agents

Amiodarone

Initially introduced in the 1960s as an antianginal agent, amiodarone has shown great promise as an antiarrhythmic drug. A unique feature of amiodarone is that it has an extraordinarily long duration of action, with a half-life of 14 to 52 days. This characteristic makes less frequent

dosing possible but increases the duration of toxic effects when they occur.

Amiodarone is useful for recurrent supraventricular and ventricular tachyarrhythmias not responsive to conventional agents. The oral dose ranges from 200 mg 5 days a week to 600 mg once a day. Adverse effects are seen commonly and sometimes are life-threatening. When looked for, corneal microdeposits are found in nearly all cases; impaired vision occasionally is present. Hyperthyroidism and hypothyroidism both have been reported. Cutaneous problems include photosensitivity and skin pigmentation. Other problems include neurologic toxicity and an increase in hepatic enzyme levels. The most dreaded complication is pulmonary fibrosis, which may reverse when the drug is discontinued but progresses in some instances to respiratory impairment and death.

Bretylium

Intravenous bretylium tosylate has been approved for those life-threatening ventricular dysrhythmias (recurrent ventricular tachycardia or fibrillation) occurring during myocardial infarction that fail to respond to lidocaine or procainamide. The recommended dose, 5 to 10 mg/kg, is delivered IV over 10 to 12 minutes and is followed by an IV infusion of 1 to 2 mg/minute. Hypotension, which may occur even when the patient is supine, and nausea and vomiting are the most common adverse effects.

Sotalol

Sotalol is an investigational agent that exhibits properties of class III agents (prolonged repolarization) and β-blockade (noncardioselective).[21] Studies have reported its effectiveness in the treatment of both supraventricular and ventricular dysrhythmias; however, further studies are warranted.

Class IV Calcium Channel Blockers

Verapamil

Given IV, verapamil has become the drug of choice in the treatment of paroxysmal supraventricular tachycardia (PSVT). The drug also has antianginal and antihypertensive properties. Verapamil has a potent depressant action on the AV node, thereby slowing conduction and prolonging the effective refractory period in the AV node. Verapamil interrupts the pathways used by reentrant atrial rhythms such as PSVT, and, when given IV, causes reversion to normal sinus rhythm in most cases. The agent also is useful in retarding the ventricular response in patients with atrial fibrillation or atrial flutter and often is used alone or in conjunction with digoxin for this purpose. Verapamil is less successful in restoring sinus rhythm in patients with atrial fibrillation or flutter.

The usual dose of verapamil is 5 to 10 mg IV given over 1 to 3 minutes. The dose may be repeated in 20 minutes if necessary. When administered orally, the dose ranges from 80 to 120 mg given three to four times daily.

Verapamil Toxicity

Adverse effects include hypotension (especially with IV use), bradycardia, gastrointestinal intolerance, headache, anxiety, and edema. In susceptible patients with SA or AV nodal disease, verapamil should be avoided. It also should not be given to patients on β-blocking agents if such patients exhibit left ventricular dysfunction or significant bradyarrhythmias. Verapamil may be used safely in combination with digoxin, but because verapamil increases the serum level of digoxin by 50% to 70%, the maintenance dose of digoxin should be adjusted downward.

Diltiazem

Diltiazem is a calcium channel blocker that has actions similar to those of verapamil. It recently has been approved for treatment of supraventricular dysrhythmias. It has been shown to decrease the ventricular rate in atrial flutter and atrial fibrillation, and in some cases convert PSVT to sinus rhythm by slowing conduction through the AV node. Plasma half-life ranges from 3.5 to 6 hours. Adverse effects include hypotension, flushing, and junctional dysrhythmias. It is metabolized by the liver and excreted through the kidneys. The initial dose is 0.25 mg/kg administered over 2 minutes. If the response is not sufficient, then it may be repeated at 0.35 mg/kg. An infusion of 5 to 15 mg/hour may be infused for a period of 24 hours to maintain the desired effect. Further studies are needed to show effectiveness beyond this time frame.[22]

Other Antiarrhythmic Agents

Adenosine

Adenosine (Adenocard) is a new antiarrhythmic agent that is effective in converting PSVT to normal sinus rhythm by slowing conduction through the AV node. It has not shown to be effective in converting atrial flutter or fibrillation to sinus rhythm, but may slow the ventricular rate.[23] Adenosine has a half-life of 10 seconds; thus, side effects are short-lived. A dose of 6 mg is administered rapidly IV, followed by a saline flush. The dose can be repeated at 12 mg in a few minutes if the desired effect is not obtained. Adverse effects include a brief period of hypotension, facial flushing, and dyspnea. As the rhythm is converted, various degrees of AV block, sinus bradycardia, or ectopic beats may be seen before sinus rhythm is established.

Atropine

Atropine is a parasympatholytic agent used for treatment of symptomatic bradycardias and slowed conduction at the AV node. It reduces the effects of vagal stimulation, thus increasing the heart rate and improving cardiac function. Doses of 0.5 to 1 mg given IV are recommended. The dose can be repeated in a few minutes, but not to more than a total of 2 mg. It is important not to increase the heart rate to an excessive degree in patients with ischemic heart disease because myocardial oxygen consumption can be increased and the ischemia worsened.

Assessment and Management

As can be seen, there are a number of antiarrhythmic agents used for the the treatment of supraventricular and ventricular dysrhythmias. Each has its own mode of action as well as potential side effects. Nurses need to be knowledgeable about these agents, including the goal of treatment, recommended dose, effects on the body systems, and potential side effects.

Knowledge deficit is a nursing diagnosis that may be ascribed to patients taking these agents. Therefore, education is important to help ensure proper administration, as well as knowledge of when to report side effects, when the patient is discharged.

Cardioversion

Description

Electric countershock therapy is useful in converting supraventricular and ventricular dysrhythmias to sinus rhythm. As opposed to defibrillation, which delivers an unsynchronized current to the heart through the chest wall in an attempt to convert pulseless ventricular tachycardia/fibrillation to sinus rhythm (see section on Cardiopulmonary Resuscitation), cardioversion delivers a shock that is synchronized with the heart's activity, that is, it is delivered on the R wave. Indications for cardioversion and recommendations for initial joules (J) used are listed in Table 13–8.[24]

The energy needed to convert unstable ventricular tachycardia with a pulse may be as low as 10 J, but often the use of 50 J initially, followed by 100, 200, 300, or 360 J is necessary for conversion. The energy required for

TABLE 13–8
Energy Requirements for Cardioversion

Indications	Energy in Joules (J)
Unstable VT with a pulse	50–360
Supraventricular tachycardia	75–100
Atrial flutter	25 initially
Atrial fibrillation	100 initially

VT, ventricular tachycardia.

conversion of PSVT and atrial flutter ranges from 25 to 75 joules initially. Further increases in energy may be needed for conversion. The energy required to convert atrial fibrillation is greater, starting at 100 J with increases to 360 J if necessary. After conversion to sinus rhythm, further antiarrhythmic therapy should be initiated.

Procedure

The technique for cardioversion is as follows:

1. Before conversion of supraventricular tachycardia, it is helpful to begin the patient on quinidine 0.2 g every 6 to 8 hours for 24 hours before conversion. This will produce reversion to sinus rhythm in up to 15% of such patients.
2. The patient is maintained in a fasting state for 6 to 8 hours before cardioversion, unless emergency cardioversion is required. The procedure should be explained to the patient.
3. An IV line is inserted, the patient is placed on the monitor, and all necessary resuscitation apparatus is readily available.
4. Ideally, digitalis should be withheld for 24 hours before cardioversion, although cardioversion may be attempted in an emergency situation without this precaution.
5. Sedation is accomplished with the use of intravenous diazepam or midazolam (Versed, Roche Laboratories, Nutley, NJ).
6. Turn on the defibrillator/monitor.
7. Obtain a good ECG pattern with a tall R wave.
8. Turn on the synchronizer button.
9. Remove paddles and apply a generous amount of electrode jelly to them or apply gel pads to the chest wall. This is done to prevent skin burns and to decrease electric resistance.

10. Apply paddles, one just below the right clavicle and the other over the apex of the heart. If anterior–posterior paddles are used, place the anterior paddle over the precordium and the posterior one on the back opposite the anterior one. Make sure the paddles are away from electrode wires and any pacemaker battery.
11. Set desired energy level.
12. Press charge button. A light will flash until paddles are fully charged.
13. Call out "clear" to make sure no one is touching the patient or the bed.
14. Discharge the paddles while applying 25 to 30 pounds of pressure. Maintain contact on the chest wall until the machine has delivered the shock. There will be a momentary delay from the pressing of the discharge button to delivery of the shock because of the synchronization with the R wave. Failure to keep the paddles on the chest can result in failure to cardiovert and burns to the chest.
15. Remove paddles and check status of the patient.
16. Subsequent shocks may need to be delivered.
17. After cardioversion, the patient should be observed for changes in rhythm, blood pressure, and respirations. Further antiarrhythmic agents may need to be administered to maintain sinus rhythm. The patient's respiratory status and level of consciousness should be monitored because sedation was delivered before the procedure. The chest wall should be inspected for any signs of burns and treated appropriately.
18. If the patient's rhythm deteriorates to ventricular fibrillation, the synchronizer should be turned off and the patient immediately defibrillated, starting with 200 J and increasing to 360 J as needed.

Percutaneous Transluminal Coronary Angioplasty and Percutaneous Balloon Valvuloplasty

BEHAVIORAL OBJECTIVES

Based on the content in this section, the reader should be able to:

1. Describe indications and contraindications for percutaneous transluminal coronary angioplasty (PTCA) and percutaneous balloon valvuloplasty (PBV).
2. Discuss interventions for complications associated with PTCA and PBV.
3. List five potential nursing diagnoses and the interventions for each diagnosis in the patient undergoing PTCA.

Percutaneous Transluminal Coronary Angioplasty

Description

In PTCA, a coaxial catheter system is introduced into the coronary arterial tree and advanced into an area of coronary artery stenosis. A balloon attached to the catheter is then inflated, increasing the luminal diameter and improving blood flow through the dilated segment. Percutaneous transluminal coronary angioplasty is a nonsurgical technique applied as an alternative to coronary artery bypass surgery in the treatment of obstructive coronary artery disease (CAD). When indicated and if successful, PTCA can alleviate myocardial ischemia and relieve angina pectoris.

History

Cardiovascular disease is the number one cause of death in the United States. In 1992, the American Heart Association estimated 1,500,000 Americans would have a heart attack and about 500,000 of them would die.

The first major advance in the palliative treatment of CAD was the implantation of an aortocoronary saphenous vein bypass graft in 1967. Since that time, coronary artery bypass graft surgery (CABG) has been refined continually and has been the treatment of choice for many patients with CAD. The first PTCA, however, performed by Gruentzig in 1977, marked another major innovation in the treatment of coronary artery disease.

The path to PTCA began in 1964, when Dotter and Judkins introduced the concept of mechanically dilating a stenosis in a blood vessel with a technique of inserting a series of progressively larger catheters to treat peripheral vascular disease. After experimenting with this technique, Gruentzig modified the procedure by placing on the tip of a catheter a polyvinyl balloon, which was passed into a narrowed vessel and then inflated. Because it produced a smoother luminal surface with less trauma than the Dotter–Judkins approach, this new method reduced the risk of complications such as vessel rupture, subintimal tearing, and embolism. At first, Gruentzig continued to apply his technique only to peripheral vascular lesions. Then, after successful dilation of more than 500 peripheral lesions, he designed a smaller version of the dilation catheter for use within the coronary arterial tree. This new design was tested initially on dogs with experimentally induced coronary artery stenoses. After extensive canine experimentation, Gruentzig performed the first human PTCA in 1977. Since then, considerable improvements in technique and equipment have made PTCA the treatment of choice for appropriate cases of CAD.

Physiological Principles

Mechanisms of Action

The process that leads to successful dilation is complex and is not clearly defined. Angiographic evaluation as well as animal and human histologic studies indicate that PTCA stretches the vessel wall, often leading to fracture of the inelastic atheromatous plaque and to tearing or cracking within the intima and media. This cracking or slight dissection of the inner lumen of the vessel may be necessary for successful dilation.[25]

Comparisons Between PTCA and CABG

As an alternative treatment in appropriate cases of CAD, angioplasty compares favorably to bypass surgery in terms of risk, success rate, the patient's physical capacity after the procedure, and cost.

Mortality rates associated with first-time angioplasty and CABG are quite similar. The in-hospital death rate for patients undergoing angioplasty ranges from 0% to 2%; the CABG mortality rate ranges from 1.5% to 4%. If a second surgical operation becomes necessary to alleviate the symptoms of progressive disease, the mortality and complication rates for the bypass procedure are significantly greater than for second angioplasty.

Successful PTCA, which often is defined as a significant reduction of the luminal diameter stenosis without in-hospital death, myocardial infarction, or CABG surgery, ranges from 80% to 95%, depending on the severity of the patient's angiographic and clinical presentation. Long-term survival also is excellent. In a study by Bentivoglio et al, cumulative 2-year survival was 96% and 95% among patients with stable and unstable angina, respectively, with event-free survival (ie, no death, myocardial infarction, or CABG) in 79% and 76%, respectively.[26] Among patients with multivessel PTCA, actuarial survival was 97% at 1 year and 88% at 5 years in a study by O'Keefe et al.[27] At 7 years after PTCA, Dorros et al reported a survival rate of 90% in patients with simple single-vessel angioplasty and 95% in patients with simple multivessel angioplasty.[28]

In the Coronary Artery Surgery Study, graft patency after CABG was 90% at 2 months, 82% at 18 months, and 82% at 5 years.[29] Ten-year survival was 82%.

Restenosis or patency data differ greatly between CABG and PTCA. Within 6 months after angioplasty, 20% to 30% of lesions recur or restenose. The mean occlusion rate for bypass grafts is approximately 18% during the first 5 years and 4% to 5% between 5 and 10 years.[29]

Psychological advantages of PTCA over surgery may argue favorably for the procedure. The emotional stress of awaiting dilation is less than that of awaiting surgery. This reduction in anxiety, however, is partly offset by the risk of psychological crisis if the angioplasty fails and surgery—especially immediate surgery—is needed. The psychological impact of this discouraging situation is significant, but it occurs in a relatively low percentage of cases (1%–5%).

If there are no complications with either procedure, PTCA requires a hospital stay of 2 to 3 days, whereas CABG requires a stay of 7 to 10 days. Because the average hospital stay is shorter with PTCA and because PTCA is performed in the cardiac catheterization laboratory under local anesthesia, the average cost of PTCA is substantially lower than that of CABG. The following factors, however, can increase the cost of PTCA: (1) complications occurring during the procedure requiring emergency surgery; (2) lesions that recur requiring repeat dilation or bypass surgery; and (3) surgical standby, which is provided in different levels to correspond to the risk associated with each PTCA.

A factor in favor of PTCA is the lower morbidity after the procedure compared to CABG. Percutaneous transluminal coronary angioplasty patients often return to work within 7 to 10 days after angioplasty, whereas bypass patients return to work within 8 weeks.

In short, the major advantages of angioplasty over bypass surgery include reduced mortality and morbidity, shorter convalescence, and lower cost to the patient.

Diagnostic Tests for PTCA and CABG Patient Selection

Before deciding between PTCA and bypass surgery, all objective evidence of coronary insufficiency must be documented. Noninvasive methods of evaluation that may be used before and after PTCA include standard *treadmill stress testing* and *thallium stress and redistribution myocardial imaging*. These tests allow the physician to discover the areas of ischemia in the myocardium when the patient is subjected to stress (ie, exercise; see Chapter 12 for a discussion of these tests). The nurse should be familiar with the results of the thallium stress test indicated on the examination report because an understanding of the patient's diagnosis and related symptoms, and thus of the reasons for interventional angioplastic therapy, promotes more informed patient care.

Coronary arteriography with cardiac catheterization, another method of documenting coronary insufficiency, is done if the previous tests indicate coronary disease. Although this procedure is more invasive than treadmill testing and thallium imaging, it is required to pinpoint the location of any stenoses and the degree of involvement of the artery or arteries (see Chapter 12 for a discussion of this test). This procedure yields a 35-mm cineangiogram of the coronary artery anatomy. The physician can then analyze closely areas of narrowing, gaining precise information with which to decide the mode of treatment (Figs. 13–20 and 13–21).

Equipment Features

Since the introduction of PTCA, there has been continual refinement of the equipment, resulting in fewer contraindications, and lower rates of mortality and emergency bypass surgery.

The guiding catheters used to direct and support the advancement of the dilation catheter into the appropriate coronary artery ostium have an outer diameter of 6 to 9 Fr. Like the Judkins and Amplatz coronary angiography catheters, the tips of the guiding catheters have curves that are preshaped for selective access to either the right or the left coronary artery (Fig. 13–22).

Balloon dilation systems have evolved since Gruentzig's original design, in which the guidewire tip and catheter shaft were integral. In the early days of angioplasty, physicians were limited by catheter performance and could address lesions only in the proximal anatomy. In 1982, Simpson introduced a coaxial "over-the-wire" system, an improvement that has become predominant in current catheter designs. The main innovation is an independently movable guidewire within the balloon dilation catheter. This guidewire can be manipulated to select the correct vessel despite side branches and permits safe advancement of the dilation catheter across the lesion. Currently, the

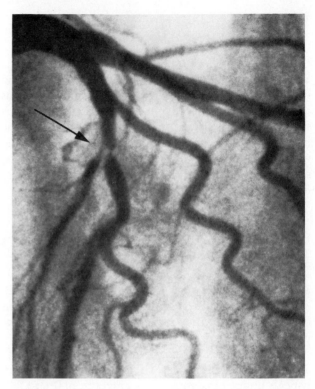

FIGURE 13–21
A coronary arteriogram of the circumflex artery (CX) illustrating a concentric stenosis. The term "concentric" defines a plaque involving the intraluminal wall circumferentially, giving a dumbbell appearance. (Courtesy of John B Simpson, MD, Palo Alto, CA.)

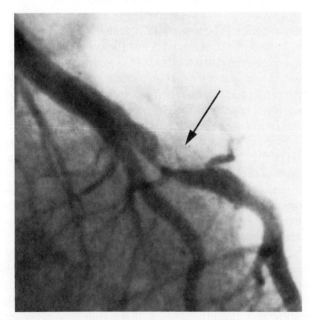

FIGURE 13–20
An eccentric stenosis in the left anterior descending (LAD) artery. The term "eccentric" defines a plaque involving only one side of the intraluminal wall. (Courtesy of John B Simpson, MD, Palo Alto, CA.)

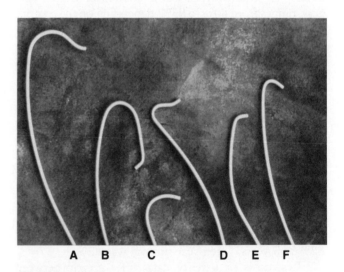

FIGURE 13–22
A variety of guiding catheters with preshaped tips suitable for selectively engaging the appropriate coronary ostia, from left to right: (**A**) Left Amplatz guiding catheter; (**B**) Left Judkins guiding catheter; (**C**) Hockey Stick guiding catheter; (**D**) Right Amplatz guiding catheter; (**E**) Right Judkins guiding catheter; (**F**) Left internal mammary guiding catheter. (Reprinted with permission of Advanced Cardiovascular Systems [ACS] Inc., Santa Clara, CA.)

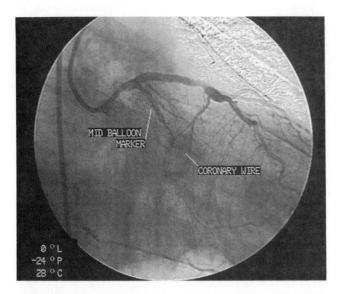

FIGURE 13–23
Contrast injection through the guiding catheter to verify position. The coronary guidewire tip is located at the occlusion of the circumflex artery, and the coronary balloon is positioned in the proximal vessel. (Reprinted with permission of Advanced Cardiovascular Systems [ACS] Inc., Santa Clara, CA.)

available guidewires measure between 0.010 and 0.018 inches in diameter, and thus usually pose little threat of interference with the blood flow through a stenosis.

Coronary dilation catheter shafts range in size from 1.9 to 4.2 Fr, small enough for easy passage through the guiding catheter and for visualization around the catheter during contrast injection (Fig. 13–23). The dilation catheter has a radiopaque gold marker that can be imaged by fluoroscopy (Fig. 13–24). Thus, the physician can position the balloon accurately across the lesion. The inflated balloon size ranges from 1.5 to 4.0 mm in diameter and from 10 to 40 mm in length. The size (inflated diameter) of the balloon to be used for a particular PTCA is usually the same as the smallest-diameter segment of the coronary artery proximal or distal to the stenosis (eg, 3-mm vessel, 3-mm balloon). Lesion and balloon length also are approximated.

The physician manually inflates the balloon with a contrast-filled, disposable inflation–deflation device that connects to the side arm or balloon lumen of the coronary dilation catheter (see Figure 13–24). The device incorporates a pressure gauge that indicates the amount of pressure exerted against the balloon wall during balloon infla-

tion. Balloon pressure is measured in pounds per square inch (psi) or atmospheres (atm). The average initial inflation is between 60 and 80 psi or 4 to 6 atm, and lasts from 1 to 3 minutes. Inflations up to 30 minutes or longer have shown promising results. Longer inflations seem to promote a smoother, more regular vessel wall as assessed by angiography, and are used primarily for the treatment of major dissections and abrupt closure. Extended inflations are performed safely with perfusion catheters that simultaneously dilate and perfuse.

Many factors must be considered in selecting the most appropriate equipment for performing PTCA. Technologic advances in angioplasty equipment have made available several dilation catheter systems that have been developed to improve the success and safety associated with any PTCA.

The coaxial "over-the-wire" system is considered a workhorse catheter by many physicians because it can approach any anatomy well. A physician also might select a "rapid-exchange" system to accomplish more easily the dilation of a bifurcation lesion. This type of device incorporates a "rail" system that facilitates the exchange process. A "fixed-wire" catheter is used to reach and dilate lesions in distal, tortuous anatomy, and its small shaft also makes it an option for the use of two coronary dilation catheters in one guiding catheter when the strategy calls for side-by-side balloons.

Each strategy also encompasses an inflation strategy. The main elements of an inflation strategy are the duration and pressure of balloon inflation required to open a lesion. Today, balloons are available that can withstand greater pressure for the treatment of calcific lesions.

The outcome of any PTCA is greatly affected by: (1) the selection of a guiding catheter that provides a platform for the advancement of the dilation system while preserving flow to the coronary artery; and (2) the selection of a dilation system that best addresses the vessel's anatomy and the lesion's location. In making appropriate choices of equipment, there is no substitute for a physician's expertise.

Indications and Contraindications for PTCA

Indications

In choosing to treat with PTCA (as with CABG), the physician's purpose is to alleviate angina pectoris unrelieved by maximal medical treatment and to reduce the risk

FIGURE 13–24
PTCA balloon dilation catheter illustrating the key components of the system. (Reprinted with permission of Advanced Cardiovascular Systems [ACS] Inc., Santa Clara, CA.)

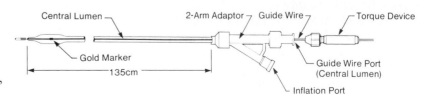

of myocardial infarction in symptomatic patients and asymptomatic patients with severe stenosis. The indications for PTCA have expanded as equipment, technique, and operator experience have improved. In fact, there are at present no absolute contraindications in selection of patients for PTCA, and each case should be evaluated on the basis of the indications presented by the current condition, the physician's experience, and the sophistication of the catheterization laboratory.

Percutaneous transluminal coronary angioplasty is indicated for patients with coronary arteries that have at least a 50% narrowing. Lesions with less narrowing are not considered appropriate for PTCA because they are equally at risk for abrupt closure, which can have serious consequences. Patients with severe surgical risk factors, such as severe underlying noncardiac diseases, advanced age, and poor left ventricular function, are particularly suited for PTCA because successful dilation obviates the need for an operation that would be poorly tolerated.

An example of the wide spectrum of candidacy for PTCA is the accepted practice of treating patients with multivessel disease. The common technique for dilating multiple lesions is to dilate the most critical stenosis first. With successful dilation of this "culprit" lesion, remaining lesions are dilated in stages (ie, at different intervals during the procedure or over several days). Dilation of multiple vessels, however, is technically more demanding and carries a higher risk of complications.

Another expanded indication is the approach to treating the patient with a totally occluded vessel. Early in PTCA practice, total occlusion disqualified a patient for the procedure because the stenosis could not be crossed with the guidewire and dilation catheter without causing severe trauma to the artery. Currently, due to refinement of equipment, technical advances, and greater physician experience, dilation of total occlusions may be attempted in appropriate candidates. Total occlusions of a short duration (eg, 3 months or less) are easier to cross and dilate successfully than total occlusions of a longer duration. Therefore, dilation of chronic total occlusions should be attempted only in selected patients.

Other candidates for PTCA are those who have undergone CABG in whom symptoms have recurred due to stenosis and graft closure or progression of coronary disease in the native vessels. For these candidates, successful angioplasty makes second surgery, with its increased potential for complications, unnecessary. It is thought that the proliferative disease in the graft wall generates fibrous stenosis that is much less dense than most fibrotic tissue in the native vessels, and so certain vein graft stenoses respond favorably to dilation.

In the past, if a patient had an acute myocardial infarction documented by significant ST segment elevation, increased cardiac enzyme levels, and pain unrelieved by medication, surgery or pharmacologic treatment with complete bed rest in a coronary care unit were the only

treatment alternatives. Now, if thrombosis and underlying stenosis are causing the infarction, thrombolytic therapy, PTCA, or both offer other alternatives. When a blood clot has impeded flow to the distal myocardium and thus caused an ischemic episode, a thrombolytic agent (eg, streptokinase, urokinase, tissue-type plasminogen activator) can be administered IV. On successful lysis of the thrombus, delayed dilation of the underlying stenosis often further enhances blood flow to the reperfused myocardium, reducing the risk of rethrombosis or critical narrowing caused by normal or spastic vasomotion superimposed on an organic stenosis.

Rescue PTCA after thrombolytic therapy is appropriate in patients with a persistently occluded infarct-related artery. Primary PTCA (ie, PTCA without prior thrombolytic therapy) also has been shown to be an effective intervention in patients with acute myocardial infarction, either as an alternative to thrombolytic therapy or in patients contraindicated for thrombolytic therapy (the latter account for 67% of infarct patients, according to Muller and Topol[30]). Among patients with acute myocardial infarction complicated by cardiogenic shock, direct PTCA has resulted in a significant increase in survival compared to conventional medical therapy or thrombolytic therapy.

TABLE 13–9
Indications and Contraindications for PTCA

Indications	Contraindications
Clinical	
Symptomatic (angina unrelieved by medical therapy)	Presence of coronary artery spasm
Asymptomatic but with severe underlying stenosis	
Stable/unstable angina	
Acute myocardial infarction	
High-risk surgical candidates	
Anatomic	
Severe stenosis (≥50%)	Mild stenosis (<50%)
Proximal and distal lesions	Diffuse "cheesy" atheroma in grafts
Single and multivessel disease	Evidence of preexisting dissection or thrombosis
Bifurcation lesions	"Unprotected" left main coronary artery
Ostial lesions	
Totally occluded vessels	
Bypass graft lesions	
"Protected" left main coronary artery (previous LAD or CIRC CABG)	

LAD, left anterior descending artery; CIRC, circumflex artery; CABG, coronary artery bypass graft.

Contraindications

There are very few contraindications for PTCA. Patients with left main CAD generally are not considered candidates for angioplasty. The obvious drawback of PTCA in left main artery disease is the possibility of acute occlusion or spasm of the left main artery during the procedure, which would result in severe left ventricular dysfunction. The only exception to this rule is the patient who has a "protected" left main (ie, has had previous bypass surgery to the left anterior descending or circumflex arteries with patent grafts present). Only then might a physician consider dilating a left main artery stenosis. At present, however, most of these patients still are considered surgical candidates.

For high-risk patients (eg, patients with left main vessel disease, or severe left ventricular dysfunction, or dilation of the last remaining patent artery), percutaneous support devices may improve the safety of PTCA. Among the devices and techniques being investigated are perfusion balloons, intra-aortic balloon counterpulsation, coronary sinus retroperfusion, cardiopulmonary support, and partial left heart bypass.[31]

Table 13–9 summarizes the indications for PTCA and lists those factors that usually would contraindicate the procedure.

Procedure

The PTCA procedure is carried out in a sterile fashion, with the use of local anesthesia and either the Judkins (percutaneous femoral) approach or, less often, the Sones (brachial cutdown) approach (Fig. 13–25).

With the Judkins approach, the physician cannulates the femoral vein and artery percutaneously by inserting a needle (usually 18-gauge) containing a removable obturator. The obturator then can be removed to confirm by the presence of blood flow that the outer needle is within the lumen of the vessel. Once proper placement is established, a guidewire is introduced through the needle into the artery to the level of the diaphragm. The needle then is removed, and replaced by a valved introducer sheath. The sheath provides support at the puncture site in the groin as well as hemostasis, and reduces potential arterial trauma if multiple catheter exchanges are necessary. The guiding catheter is preloaded with a 0.038-inch J wire and introduced into the sheath. The 0.038-inch J wire is advanced over the arch and the guiding catheter is advanced over the wire. The 0.038-inch J wire is removed and the guiding catheter is rotated precisely to the appropriate coronary ostium. The procedure also may be accomplished by the Sones approach, in which a brachial cutdown is used to isolate the brachial vein and artery. A small arteriotomy is made, and the catheter is passed to the level of the aortic arch.

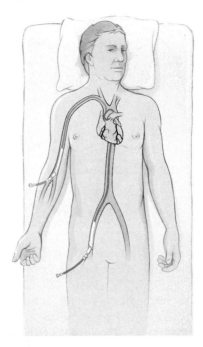

FIGURE 13–25
Two approaches to left heart catheterization. The Sones technique uses the brachial artery, and the Judkins technique uses the femoral artery. With either method, the catheter is passed retrograde through the ascending aorta to the left ventricle. (Reprinted with permission of Advanced Cardiovascular Systems [ACS] Inc., Santa Clara, CA.)

Regardless of the mode of access, repeat coronary arteriography is then carried out in both the left anterior oblique (LAO) and right anterior oblique (RAO) views. These views (LAO 30° and RAO 60°) allow for visualization of the heart along its transverse and longitudinal planes. Opposing views provide a thorough assessment of both the lesion and the anatomic approach. A "freeze frame" of each view is obtained as a "road map" or guide throughout the procedure. A final lesion assessment is made, confirming lesion severity and vessel diameter for appropriate balloon sizing.

If PTCA is indicated, surgical standby is confirmed, and the patient is anticoagulated with 10,000 U heparin to prevent clots from forming on or in the catheter system during the procedure. A continuous IV nitroglycerin drip is started just before the procedure, and titrated to maintain blood pressure for adequate perfusion. Intracoronary nitroglycerin is kept on the sterile field throughout the procedure and given intermittently as needed for vasospasm. A temporary pacing electrode may be positioned in the apex of the right ventricle and placed on standby in case emergency pacing is required.

The dilation catheter is introduced into the guiding catheter through a bifurcated adapter that provides access, as well as a port for contrast injections and aortic pressure measurement. The dilation catheter and guidewire are advanced to the tip of the guiding catheter while their

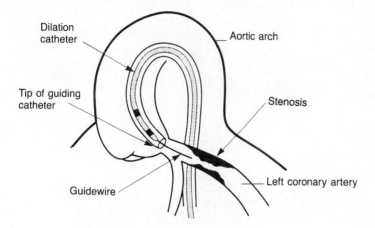

FIGURE 13–26
The advancement of the coronary dilation catheter to the tip of the guiding catheter, which is positioned in the left coronary artery, is facilitated by fluoroscopy. (Reprinted with permission of Advanced Cardiovascular Systems [ACS] Inc., Santa Clara, CA.)

position is checked by fluoroscopy (Fig. 13–26). The guidewire then is advanced and manipulated to negotiate branch vessels. Proper advancement can be confirmed by injecting contrast through the guiding catheter and fluoroscopically visualizing the coronary tree.

Once the guidewire is positioned safely beyond the stenosis, the dilation catheter can be advanced slowly over the guidewire into the narrowing without risk of injury to the intima (Fig. 13–27).

Exact placement of the dilation balloon within the stenosis is facilitated under fluoroscopy by the radiopaque marker on the balloon as well as by contrast injections for visualization. Initially, the balloon is inflated at 1 to 2 atm to confirm its position. At first, it expands at both ends and not in the center, where it is pinched in by the stenosis (Figs. 13–28 and 13–29). The central indentation usually disappears as the stenosis is dilated. After each inflation, the physician injects a small bolus of contrast medium to assess any changes in coronary blood flow through the stenosis and to assess any increase in luminal diameter. At this time, the need for additional inflations is determined and a waiting period of 10 to 15 minutes is observed. Complications such as vessel recoil and abrupt closure occur most often during this early phase; however, their incidence is low, and redilation can be done readily at this time. After dilation is complete, the guiding catheter and the dilation catheter are removed. Postdilation arteriography is performed to define more clearly the results of the PTCA.

According to Kahn and Hartzler,[32] the reasons for failure to complete a PTCA procedure include (1) inability to cross the target lesion with a guidewire or dilation catheter, due primarily to chronic total occlusions; (2) inability to dilate the lesion due to rigid lesions or severe dissection; and (3) embolization of friable vein graft material or embolization of thrombus.

Successful dilation of a lesion commonly is defined as a reduction of the luminal diameter stenosis by about 40% or 50%. Clinical success commonly is defined as angiographic success with clinical improvement and without significant in-hospital complications, such as death, myocardial infarction, or CABG.

Angiography after successful angioplasty demonstrates an immediate increase in the intraluminal diameter of the involved vessel (Fig. 13–30). Clinical improvement of the patient is demonstrated by improved or normalized myocardial perfusion deficits, as shown by comparison of a post-PTCA thallium stress image to the pre-PTCA stress image. Postangioplasty treadmill test results compared to the preprocedure test results reveal increased exercise endurance and a decrease in exercise-induced chest pain.

Results

Excellent short- and long-term results have been achieved in patients undergoing coronary angioplasty. The results vary depending on the patient's clinical presentation (eg,

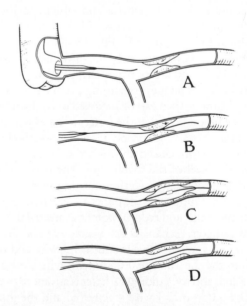

FIGURE 13–27
(**A**) PTCA dilation catheter and guidewire exiting the guiding catheter. (**B**) Guidewire advanced across the stenosis. (**C**) Dilation catheter advanced across the stenosis and inflated. (**D**) Dilation catheter pulled back to assess luminal diameter. (Reprinted with permission of Advanced Cardiovascular Systems [ACS], Inc., Santa Clara, CA.)

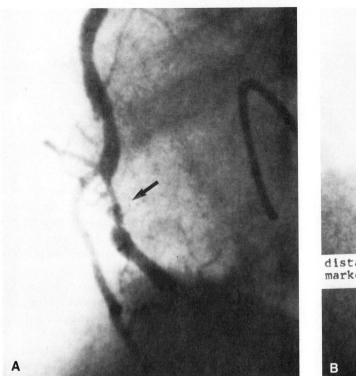
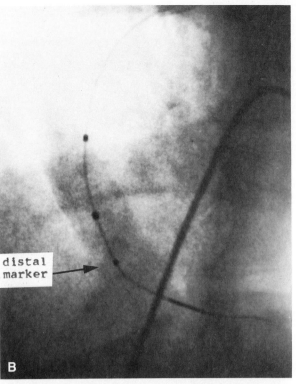

FIGURE 13–28
Thirty-five–spot frames showing (**A**) stenosis involving the midright coronary artery (RCA), and (**B**) the first and second radiopaque markers revealing the position of the dilation balloon across the stenosis, with the distal marker referring to the tip of the catheter beyond the narrowing. (Courtesy of John B Simpson, MD, Palo Alto, CA.)

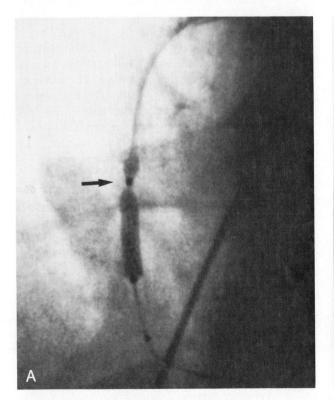
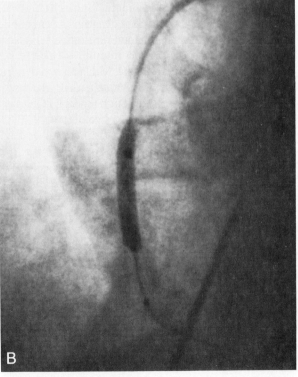

FIGURE 13–29
Thirty-five–spot frames showing (**A**) inflation of the balloon, revealing the position of the stenosis by the "dumbbell" effect, and (**B**) absence of stenosis after dilation. (Courtesy of John B Simpson, MD, Palo Alto, CA.)

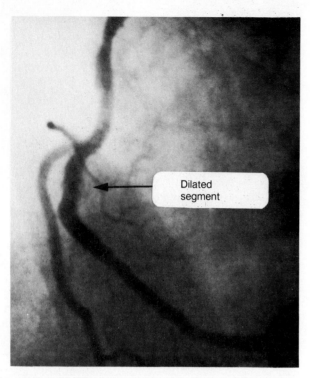

FIGURE 13–30
Repeat angiography after PTCA of a right coronary artery stenosis showing increased flow and increased diameter of the dilated segment. (Courtesy of John B Simpson, MD, Palo Alto, CA.)

stable or unstable angina) and angiographic characteristics (eg, subtotal or total occlusion). Among patients undergoing either single-vessel dilation or multivessel dilation, in-hospital clinical success ranges from 85% to 95%.[27,28,33] In-hospital complications are low, with a reported mortality rate of 1% to 2% in both these patient groups.[27,33] Long-term survival is high, although repeat PTCA may be necessary for recurrent or progressive disease.

Among patients with higher-risk clinical or angiographic presentations, success rates may be lower; however, PTCA often is preferable to surgical revascularization owing to the latter's increased risk in such patients as the elderly or patients with depressed left ventricular function.

Assessment and Management

Patient Preparation

Evaluate Laboratory Tests

Once the decision has been made to proceed with coronary angioplasty, the patient usually is admitted to the hospital the day before the procedure. The nurse should monitor all preliminary laboratory tests, such as evaluations of cardiac enzymes, serum electrolytes, and prothrombin time (assessing coagulability), and should notify the physician of any abnormalities. The serum levels of potassium, creatinine, and blood urea nitrogen (BUN) are particularly important.

It is essential that potassium levels be within normal limits because low levels result in increased sensitivity and excitability of the myocardium. The cardiac muscle also is sensitive and becomes irritable when the flow of oxygen-rich blood decreases, as happens for a controlled period of time during placement and inflation of the dilation balloon across the lesion. The irritability arising from hypokalemia or ischemia or both can give rise to ventricular dysrhythmias that pose a threat to the patient.

Elevation in the levels of serum creatinine, BUN, or both may indicate problems in kidney function. Good kidney function is important because during angioplasty, radiopaque contrast material (which allows fluoroscopic visualization of the coronary anatomy and of catheter placement) is introduced into the bloodstream. This contrast material is a hyperosmotic solution that the kidneys must filter from the blood and excrete. High levels of creatinine and BUN may reflect decreased renal filtration capability and vulnerability of the kidney in processing the extra load of radiopaque solution. Instances of acute renal failure have resulted from high doses of radiopaque contrast. Because false high serum levels may result from hypovolemia, however, the nurse should take care to keep the patient adequately hydrated, either by mouth with clear liquids or by means of IV solutions. If the efficacy of kidney function is in question, it can be monitored best by trends in creatinine and BUN levels, in conjunction with measurement and documentation of urine output.

Obtain Informed Consent

Once it is determined that the physical condition permits angioplasty, the physician must obtain from the patient an informed consent to the procedure. The physician will explain how the angioplasty is done, the reasons for the treatment, and the risks and potential benefits of PTCA and of the available alternative, surgery. The nurse should answer any questions that the patient may have and should explain the course of post-PTCA care.

Preoperative Medications

Twenty-four hours before the procedure, the patient's medications may include aspirin, 325 mg three times a day; dipyridamole (Persantine, Boehringer Ingelheim, Ridgefield, CT), 75 mg three times a day; or sulfinpyrazone (Anturane, Ciba Pharmaceutical Co., Summit, NJ), 200 mg three times a day for their antiplatelet effect. Also prescribed to reduce vasospastic events are nitroglycerin and calcium-blocking agents, such as nifedipine (Procardia, Pfizer Laboratories, New York, NY), 10 mg three times a day, and diltiazem (Cardizem, Marion Laboratories, Inc., Kansas City, MO), 30 mg three times a day.

Arrange Surgical Standby

Surgical standby for PTCA is arranged before the procedure. Surgical availability is required, but the degree to which the operating room is held for availability varies according to patient's risk factors, hospital policies, or both.

Nursing Management During PTCA

During the preparation for angioplasty and throughout the procedure, the nurses in the cardiac catheterization laboratory are responsible for understanding all aspects of equipment use and patient care. They should be experienced in advanced life support and knowledgeable about the proper administration of emergency medications and the correct application of emergency equipment, including the defibrillator, the ventilator, and the pacemaker. They should observe and communicate with the patient intermittently and report any changes in patient status to the physician. The nurse monitors the ECG and arterial pressure scopes constantly and is aware of changes in tracing that may accompany the administration of drugs, symptoms of ischemia, or chest pain. The nurse must recognize signs and symptoms of contrast sensitivity, such as urticaria, blushing, anxiety, nausea, and laryngospasm. The nurse should understand the proper assembly and use of all angioplasty equipment and should be able to "troubleshoot" any malfunction that might arise.

After the PTCA is complete, the nurse instructs the patient in the precautions necessary *to prevent bleeding from the puncture site*. These include the following:

- Six to eight hours of bed rest
- Maintenance of the involved leg in a straight position (for Judkins technique)
- Avoidance of the upright position
- Avoidance of vigorous use of the abdominal muscles, as in coughing, sneezing, or moving the bowels

The patient then is transferred to a telemetry unit for observation.

Nursing Assessment and Management Post-PTCA

Once the patient has returned to the coronary care or telemetry unit, the nurse plays an important role in observing and assessing his or her recovery. Postangioplasty care is designed to monitor the patient closely for signs and symptoms of myocardial ischemia. The most overt symptom of a possible complication—early recurrence of angina pectoris after PTCA—requires swift nursing action.

As soon as possible on receiving the patient from the cardiac catheterization laboratory, the nurse should attach the ECG monitor, which allows a quick initial cardiac assessment and establishes a baseline to refer to if the patient's condition should change suddenly. While the patient is transferred from the gurney to the bed, the nurse should assess the patient's status from head to toe, noting the overall skin color and temperature and carefully observing the level of consciousness. After the patient is transferred to the bed and attached to the monitor, the nurse should listen closely to the heart and breath sounds. The nurse should evaluate the peripheral circulation by noting peripheral skin color and temperature and the presence and quality of dorsalis pedis and posterior tibialis pulses in the limbs.

Because the Judkins technique is used most often in PTCA to access the vasculature, most patients will have an entry port in either the right or the left groin through which sheaths will have been placed percutaneously in a vein and artery to allow catheterization. (If the Sones technique was used, there will be an arterial catheter in the brachial area—see Figure 13–25.) The sheaths are not removed immediately after PTCA because the patient was anticoagulated at the start of the procedure to avoid complications of clot formation; consequently, the effects of the warfarin or heparin are not reversed but allowed to dissipate naturally, over 3 to 4 hours. The nurse should pay careful attention to the area distal to the puncture site, checking pulses frequently and reporting immediately to the physician any changes that may indicate clotting. Bleeding at the sheath site may result in a major hematoma that can require surgical evacuation or compromise distal blood flow to the lower extremity. To prevent excessive bleeding and to aid hemostasis, the physician may order a 5-lb sandbag placed over the puncture site.

The nurse should impress on the patient the importance of keeping the involved leg straight and the head of the bed angled up no more than 45°. To prevent clotting within the lumens of the introducing sheaths, an IV infusion is attached to the venous sheath, and a pressurized arterial flush is attached to the arterial line. This arrangement also ensures patency should an immediate return to the cardiac catheterization laboratory be necessary because of a complication. The physician chooses both the type of solution infused (via the venous sheath) and the rate of infusion, which depends on the patient's fluid volume state.

Initial post-PTCA laboratory blood tests should include (1) prothrombin time, to assess the patient's coagulability; (2) cardiac enzymes, with particular attention to creatine kinase (CK) and CK isoenzymes; and (3) serum electrolytes. Elevation of the cardiac enzymes can indicate that a silent myocardial infarction has occurred (ie, infarction unannounced by prolonged chest pain). If an abnormal cardiac enzyme laboratory value appears, the nurse should notify the physician immediately because the patient's postoperative care might need to be modified to prevent further injury.

The nurse plays a significant role in observing and assessing angina that recurs soon after PTCA. Any chest pain demands immediate and careful attention because it may indicate either the start of vasospasm or impending occlusion. The patient may describe angina as a burning, squeezing heaviness or as sharp midsternal pain. Other signs and symptoms of myocardial ischemia include (1) ischemic ECG changes (elevation of the ST segments or T wave inversion); (2) dysrhythmias; (3) hypotension; and (4) nausea. The nurse should notify the physician immediately of any such change in the patient's condition because it is impossible to tell merely by observation whether the change indicates a transient vasospastic episode, which can be resolved with vasodilation therapy, or an acute occlusion requiring emergency surgery.

If vasodilation therapy is indicated, it may be administered as described subsequently unless the patient is severely hypotensive; in that case, vasodilation is contraindicated. At the first sign of vasospasm, first give oxygen by mask or nasal cannula. For fast, temporary (and possibly permanent) relief, 0.4 mg of nitroglycerin, 5 mg of isosorbide, or 10 mg of nifedipine should be administered sublingually. In addition, the IV drip of nitroglycerin should be titrated to maintain a blood pressure adequate to ensure coronary artery perfusion and to alleviate chest pain.

In conjunction with the onset of the chest pain, a 12-lead ECG reading should be taken to record any acute changes. If the angina resolves and any acute ECG changes caused by medical therapy disappear, it is safe to assume that a transient vasospastic episode occurred; however, if the angina continues and the ECG changes persist, redilation or emergency bypass surgery should be considered.

If the postangioplasty course is uncomplicated, the sheaths are removed after 3 to 4 hours and a mild pressure dressing is applied to the site. The patient must continue complete bed rest for 6 to 8 hours after the sheaths are removed. A normal, low-sodium or low-cholesterol diet may be resumed, depending on the preference of the physician and the needs of the patient.

During the recovery period, the nurse can introduce the patient to the rehabilitation process, emphasizing ways to combat the advance of CAD. Efforts should be made during this instruction to reinforce the importance of aerobic conditioning with regular, moderate exercise with reasonably paced increases. Also, the nurse should explain that such abuses as frequent stress, excessive weight, and smoking promote CAD and that the patient has the power and responsibility to avoid these abuses by behavior modification.

As preventive therapy, the patient will, for 6 months after angioplasty, take medications that help prevent thrombus formation and maintain maximal dilation at the angioplasty site. The patient routinely is sent home on aspirin; dipyridamole, 75 mg given orally three times a day; or sulfinpyrazone, 200 mg given orally four times a day, for the antiplatelet effect, and a calcium channel blocker. Occasionally, long-acting nitrates are added to the medical regimen. The nurse ultimately is responsible for explaining to the patient the indications for the specific medications ordered by the physician, including side effects and signs of overdose, and should answer any questions the patient may have on the follow-up care, making sure that all aspects are clearly understood. Table 13–10 lists medications currently associated with PTCA and PBV.

Before the patient's discharge, an exercise treadmill stress test and a thallium rest–stress imaging study are done to test the efficacy of the PTCA. In comparison to the pre-PTCA tests, an increase in exercise capacity and a decrease in or disappearance of exercise-induced chest pain (without ST segment changes) suggest improved blood flow and normalization of cardiac function in the previously hypoperfused muscle. Treadmill stress testing should be repeated at 1 month, 3 months, 6 months, and 1 year after angioplasty.

Complications

Although indications for PTCA have expanded to include patients with more severe CAD (eg, total occlusions, multivessel disease, recent or ongoing myocardial infarction, poor left ventricular function), the rate of complications associated with dilation has not increased. Complications from angioplasty can occur during the procedure or after it is completed. Thus, close observation and monitoring of the patient are imperative after successful PTCA. Major complications that can result in ischemia and possible severe left ventricular dysfunction necessitating emergency surgery include (1) angina unrelieved by maximal administration of nitrates and calcium channel blockers (see Table 13–10); (2) myocardial infarction; (3) coronary artery spasm; (4) abrupt reclosure of a dilated segment; (5) coronary artery dissection leading to occlusion; and (6) restenosis.

Angina, Infarction, and Vasospasm

Normally, angina is an anticipated complication during coronary angioplasty due to the temporary occlusion of the involved vessel during dilation. Such incidence of angina is handled with intracoronary nitroglycerin or removal of the dilation catheter while the guidewire is left across the lesion. Evidence of persistent chest pain after PTCA, reflected in changes in heart rate and blood pressure and elevated ST segments, indicates ischemia predisposing to an insult to the myocardium and requiring immediate intervention.

Coronary artery spasm sometimes requires surgical intervention when the vasoconstriction, occlusion, and ischemia cannot be reversed through the administration of nitrates.

Abrupt Reclosure of Dilated Segment

Abrupt reclosure is a serious complication of coronary artery dilation that occurs in approximately 7% of those undergoing angioplasty.[34, 35] An estimated 70% to 80% of

TABLE 13–10
Summary of Medications Most Often Associated with PTCA and PBV

Anticoagulants/Antiplatelets

Aspirin

Indications: Prophylaxis of coronary and cerebral arterial thrombus formation
Actions: Blocks platelet aggregation
Dosage: 80–325 mg qid
Adverse effects: Well tolerated. Nausea, vomiting, diarrhea, headache, and vertigo occasionally

Dipyridamole (Persantine)

Indications:
1. Unstable angina pectoris
2. Prophylaxis in thromboembolic disease by decreasing platelet aggregation
Actions: Antiplatelet effect, mild vasodilatation
Dosage: 25–75 mg tid
Adverse effects: Well tolerated. Nausea, vomiting, diarrhea, headache, and vertigo occasionally

Heparin

Indications: Prophylaxis of impending coronary occlusion and prophylaxis of peripheral arterial embolism
Actions: Inhibits clotting of blood and formation of fibrin clots. Inactivates thrombin, preventing conversion of fibrinogen to fibrin. Also prevents formation of a stable fibrin clot by inhibiting the activation of fibrin stabilizing factor. Inhibits reactions that lead to clotting but does not alter normal components of blood. Prolongs clotting time but does not affect bleeding time. Does not lyse clots.
Dosage: Varies with indications. IV or IA: 10,000 U at start of PTCA
Adverse effects: Uncontrollable bleeding, hypersensitivity

Sulfinpyrazone (Anturane)

Indications: Prophylaxis in thromboembolic disease
Actions: Blocks platelet aggregation
Dosage: 100–200 mg qid
Adverse effects: GI irritation (lessened if taken in divided doses with meals), hypersensitivity (rash and fever), blood dyscrasias

Coronary Vasodilators

Isosorbide dinitrate (Isordil, Sorbitrate)

Indications: Prophylaxis of angina
Actions: A nitrate that acts as a smooth muscle relaxant. Causes coronary vasodilation without increasing myocardial oxygen consumption. Secondary to general vasodilation, blood pressure decreases.
Dosage:
1. Sublingual: 2.5–10 mg q2–3 h prn angina
2. Oral: 5–40 mg qid
3. Sustained action oral: 40 mg q6–12 h
Adverse effects:
1. Cutaneous vasodilation that can cause flushing
2. Headache, transient dizziness, and weakness
3. Excessive hypotension

Nitroglycerin

Indications: Control of blood pressure and angina pectoris
Actions: Potent vasodilator that affects primarily the venous system. Selectively dilates large coronary arteries increasing blood flow to ischemic subendocardium.
Dosage:
1. Sublingual: 0.3–0.4 mg prn chest pain
2. Topical (patch): 2.5–10 mg/day. Indicated for primary, secondary, or nocturnal angina due to more sustained effect.
3. IV: 5 μg/min to start—titrate to patient response. (No fixed dose due to variable response in different patients.)
Adverse effects:
1. Excessive and prolonged hypotension
2. Headache
3. Tachycardia, palpitations
4. Nausea, vomiting, apprehension
5. Retrosternal discomfort

(continued)

TABLE 13-10
Summary of Medications Most Often Associated with PTCA and PBV (Continued)

Calcium Channel Blockers

Nifedipine, Diltiazem

Indications:
1. Angina pectoris due to coronary artery spasm and fixed vessel disease
2. Hypertension
3. Dysrhythmias
Actions: Inhibits calcium ion flux across the cell membrane of the cardiac muscle and vascular smooth muscle without changing serum calcium concentration. Decreases afterload through peripheral arterial dilation and
1. Reduces systemic and pulmonary vascular resistance
2. Vasodilates coronary circulation
3. Decreases myocardial oxygen demands and increases myocardial oxygen supply
Dosage:
1. Nefidipine (Procardia): 10–30 mg tid-qid
2. Diltiazem (Cardizem): 30–90 mg tid-qid
Adverse effects:
1. Contraindicated in patients with sick sinus syndrome
2. Hypertension after IV use
3. GI distress
4. Headache, vertigo, flushing
5. Peripheral edema, occasional increase in angina, tachycardia

---

Vasopressors

Levophed (norepinephrine)

Indications: Restoration of a normal systemic blood pressure in acute hypotensive states
Actions: α-Adrenergic action causes an increase in systolic and diastolic pressures. Peripheral vascular resistance also increases in most vascular beds and blood flow is reduced through the liver, kidney, and usually skeletal muscle.
Dosage: IV concentration: 2 mg Levophed/250 ml solution. Initial IV infusion of 2–3 ml (8–12 μg/min), adjust rate of infusion to reestablish and maintain a normal blood pressure (80–100 mm Hg) sufficient to maintain blood flow to vital organs.
Note: Before administering, hypovolemia should be corrected.
Adverse effects:
1. Anxiety, bradycardia, severe hypertension, marked increase in peripheral vascular resistance, headache, decreased cardiac input
2. Necrosis and sloughing can occur with extravasation at infusion site.
3. Reduced blood flow to vital organs (kidney, liver)

See text for full discussion of antiarrhythmics.
PTCA, percutaneous transluminal coronary angioplasty; PBV, percutaneous balloon valvuloplasty; GI, gastrointestinal.

abrupt reclosures occur while the patient still is in the cardiac catheterization laboratory. Approximately one-third to one-half of those patients whose vessel recloses undergo a successful repeat dilation. Abrupt reclosure can be caused by coronary artery dissection, coronary artery spasm, and thrombus formation. Treatment options include immediate repeat dilation, emergency surgery, or pharmacologic therapy. To maintain blood flow through the occlusion while the patient is being prepared for emergency surgery, the physician can use a perfusion balloon catheter, which has side holes along its shaft to allow blood to flow through the catheter at the site of occlusion and perfuse the distal myocardium.

Coronary Artery Dissection

Coronary artery dissection or an intimal tear in the inner lining of the artery can be visualized in the form of intra-

luminal filling defects or extraluminal extravasation of contrast material. Mild interruptions in the intraluminal wall are an expected result of the splitting and stretching of the intima on inflation of the dilation balloon at the lesion site. Therefore, in the absence of adverse effects early after PTCA, angiographically apparent dissection usually does not represent a major complication. A dissection sometimes may cause a major luminal obstruction associated with coronary artery occlusion, however, leading to a deterioration in blood flow with resultant severe ischemia or myocardial infarction that requires emergency bypass surgery.

Restenosis

Restenosis of a dilated lesion occurs in about 20% to 30% of PTCA cases within the first 6 months after angioplasty.

Various pharmacologic agents that reduce restenosis

Table 13–11 is a summary of complications that may result from PTCA, including general signs of the complications and possible interventional actions.

Table 13–11 is a summary of complications that may result from PTCA, including general signs of the complications and possible interventional actions.

Nursing Care Plan

See Nursing Care Plan 13–2 for a complete outline of nursing care for the patient undergoing PTCA or PBV.

The Future of Interventional Cardiology

The immediate and long-term efficacy of coronary angioplasty in treating symptomatic patients with single-vessel disease has been well established. In many centers, PTCA also is routinely and successfully applied to patients with multivessel disease. The safety and efficacy with which angioplasty has been applied has fostered research into treating patients with unstable angina, acute myocardial infarction, and cardiogenic shock.

New technologies are being developed to address the challenges associated with complex angioplasty and to expand physicians' options and patient selection for PTCA. Percutaneous removal of plaque using directional or rotational atherectomy catheters has been used in coronary arteries with good results. Laser technology has progressed and is being used to ablate plaque or as an adjunct to PTCA to make a pathway in total occlusions. Implantations of intravascular stents to reinforce arterial walls has been successful and is well suited for repairing acute occlusive dissection. In a study by Leon et al, 1,256 lesions were treated with various investigational interventional devices using a lesion-specific approach.[36] They reported an overall success in unfavorable coronary anatomy of 94%.

Also under development are devices for viewing the vasculature directly, such as angioscopy and intravascular ultrasound, to assess lesion severity and type before inflation and to determine change in lesion diameter and arterial structure after deflation. Angioscopy and ultrasound also may provide information to help determine which interventional technology (eg, PTCA, atherectomy, stent implantation) is best suited to the lesion.

A major factor limiting the expansion and long-term efficacy of PTCA is the problem of restenosis. Unfortunately, none of these newer technologies has resulted in a restenosis rate lower than that in PTCA alone. Pharmacologic treatment before and after dilation, procedure techniques, and patient identification continue to be investigated as ways to reduce the recurrence rate.

With the various tools and technologies available to the interventional cardiologist, as well as improved pharmacologic adjunctive therapy, the future should bring further improvement in the efficacy and predictability of

(*Text continues on page 263*)

Factors Associated With Increased Incidence of Restenosis

Clinical Factors

Severe angina
Absence of prior myocardial infarction
Diabetes
Smoking cigarettes

Angiographic Factors

Lesion location
Lesion length
Lesion severity before and after PTCA
Adjacent arterial diameter

---

are being investigated. These include fish oil, prostacyclins, anticoagulants, platelet antibodies, and corticosteroids.

The development of new devices to remove atherosclerotic plaque (atherectomy catheters) and implantable devices to maintain the opening mechanically (stents) may provide effective adjuncts or alternatives to angioplasty for the problem of recurring lesions. Restenosis of previously nondilated stenoses after both atherectomy and intracoronary stent implantation is similar in character and prevalence to that in PTCA, however.

The cause of restenosis still is unclear, although many studies have been and are being conducted. It appears to be the result of an excessive healing response to balloon dilation that exposes the subintimal structures of the vessel to circulating blood. These exposed areas are then potential sites for platelet adhesion and aggregation, and for thrombus formation. The degree of this "healing" response varies from lesion to lesion and may be influenced by the clinical and angiographic factors associated with restenosis that were discussed earlier. The restenosis rate remains at a discouraging 20% to 30% despite a clearer understanding of its mechanism.

Other Complications

Other major complications of PTCA requiring medical intervention are (1) bradycardia, which requires temporary pacing; (2) ventricular tachycardia or ventricular fibrillation, which requires immediate defibrillation; and (3) a central nervous system event causing transient or persistent neurologic deficit.

Peripheral vascular complications occurring primarily at the catheter site include (1) arterial thrombosis, (2) excessive bleeding that causes a significant hematoma, (3) pseudoaneurysm, (4) femoral arteriovenous fistula, and (5) arterial laceration. If any of these complications persists or compromises distal blood flow to the involved extremity, surgical intervention may be required.

TABLE 13–11
Complications of PTCA

Complications	General Signs/Symptoms	Possible Interventions
Prolonged angina Myocardial infarction	Angina pectoris Dysrhythmias: tachycardia, bradycardia, ventricular tachycardia/fibrillation	CABG Redo PTCA Oxygen Medications: vasodilators (nitrates), calcium channel blockers, analgesics, anticoagulants, vasopressors
Abrupt reclosure Dissection/intimal tear	Marked hypotension Acute ECG changes (ST segment change)	
Hypotension Coronary branch occlusion Coronary thrombosis	Nausea/vomiting Pallor Restlessness Cardiac/respiratory arrest	Complete bed rest Increase IV fluid volume within patient tolerance
Restenosis	Angina pectoris	Redo PTCA
Marked change in heart rate: bradycardia, ventricular tachycardia, ventricular fibrillation	Positive exercise test Rate below 60/min Rate above 250/min No discernible cardiac rhythm Pallor Loss of consciousness Hypotension	CABG Temporary pacemaker Defibrillation Medications: antiarrhythmics, vasopressors
Vascular: excessive blood loss	Hypotension Decreased urine output (from hypovolemia) Decreased hemoglobin/hematocrit Pallor Hematoma at puncture site	Possible surgical repair Fluids Transfusion Oxygen Flat in bed or in Trendelenburg position
Allergic	Hypotension, urticaria, nausea/vomiting, hives, laryngospasm, erythema, shortness of breath	Medications: antihistamines, steroids, antiemetics Clear liquids/NPO Oxygen With anaphylaxis: fluids for volume expansion, epinephrine, vasopressors for hypotension
Central nervous system events	Changes in level of consciousness Hemiparesis Hypoventilation/respiratory depression	Oxygen Discontinue/hold sedatives Medication: narcotic antagonist as a respiratory stimulant

Miscellaneous complications: conduction defects, pulmonary embolism, pulmonary edema, coronary air embolism, respiratory arrest, febrile episode, nausea, minor bleeding.
PTCA, percutaneous transluminal coronary angioplasty; CABG, coronary artery bypass graft; ECG, electrocardiogram.

NURSING CARE PLAN 13–2:
The Patient With PTCA/PBV

NURSING DIAGNOSIS	OUTCOME CRITERIA/ PATIENT GOALS	NURSING INTERVENTIONS
High risk for decreased cardiac output: related to mechanical factors that affect preload, afterload, and left ventricular failure.	• Reduce cardiac workload and maintain hemodynamic stability.	1. Assess and record vital signs: • BP (note narrowing of arterial pulse pressure). After procedure: q15m × 4, q30m × 4, q1h × 4, then q4h × 24 hr • HR (note more frequent increase during activity) • RR (note tachypnea or orthopnea) • Procedure site and distal pulses, distal CMS 2. Monitor cardiac rhythm. 3. Obtain baseline laboratory tests (serum electrolytes, BUN, enzymes, creatinine). Type and crossmatch for potential blood replacement. 4. Notify physician of results not within normal limits. 5. Assess blood gases, note hypoxemia, administer supplemental oxygen as needed. 6. Auscultate lung fields for presence of crackles, and heart sounds for S₃ gallop. 7. Record presence of cough or complaints of dyspnea. 8. Observe for peripheral edema, jugular vein distention. 9. Obtain baseline neurologic status. 10. In the presence of chronic atrial fibrillation, if anticoagulant therapy is discontinued, observe for signs and symptoms of embolism (stroke). 11. Note skin color and temperature. 12. Obtain baseline body weight. 13. Maintain bed rest with assistance in ADL. 14. Measure baseline urine specific gravity.

(continued)

NURSING CARE PLAN 13–2: (Continued)
The Patient With PTCA/PBV

NURSING DIAGNOSIS	OUTCOME CRITERIA/ PATIENT GOALS	NURSING INTERVENTIONS
		15. Monitor fluid intake and output.
		16. Maintain parenteral fluids.
		17. Administer prescribed cardiotonics (digoxin), diuretics, nitrates, or vasopressors, as ordered.
		18. Be prepared for repeat PTCA or cardiac surgery.
High risk for decreased cardiac output: related to electrical factors affecting rate, rhythm, or conduction.	• Maintenance of cardiac rate and rhythm for optimal coronary artery perfusion and cardiac output as demonstrated by optimal systemic perfusion.	1. Record baseline ECG rhythm.
		2. During and after procedure continuously assess and record:
		• BP, HR, RR
		• ECG rhythm
		3. Note presence and frequency of dysrhythmias.
		4. Administer antiarrhythmic medications, as ordered.
		5. Be prepared to alert OR if surgery is indicated.
		6. Administer oxygen, as ordered.
		7. Maintain patient IV.
		8. Have temporary pacemaker or external pacemaker available.
High risk for decreased cardiac output: related to acute structural changes (dissection, thrombus, or arterial spasm at PTCA site), resulting in myocardial ischemia and/or infarction.	• Maintenance of hemodynamic stability.	1. Continuously assess and record:
		• BP, HR, RR (CVP, PAP, PCWP, as available)
		• ECG rhythm (monitor in leads most reflective of myocardial ischemia associated with PTCA site)
		2. Maintain patent IV and oxygen setup.
		3. Administer medications to treat coronary artery spasm, angina, and clotting (eg, nifedipine and heparin) as required.
		4. Evaluate severity and location of angina by talking with patient and observing ECG.
		5. Instruct patient to verbalize recurrence of angina.
		6. Observe for hypotension and pulmonary edema.

(continued)

NURSING CARE PLAN 13–2: (*Continued*)
The Patient With PTCA/PBV

NURSING DIAGNOSIS	OUTCOME CRITERIA/ PATIENT GOALS	NURSING INTERVENTIONS
		7. Administer vasopressors (dopamine), as ordered.
		8. Assess level of consciousness.
		9. Have access to arrest cart with emergency medications, defibrillator, temporary pacemaker, and intra-aortic balloon pump.
		10. Be prepared for emergency CABG surgery.
		11. After procedure: VS q15m × 4, q30m until stable, q4h × 24 hr.
		12. Auscultate heart sounds and breath sounds every 4 hr.
		13. Record I & O.
		14. Administer analgesics, as ordered.
		15. Administer oxygen, as ordered.
High risk for decreased cardiac output: related to increased preload and pulmonary congestion related to temporary mechanical factors (eg, balloon inflation during PBV).	• Return to hemodynamic stability after balloon deflation.	1. Continuously assess and record during and after balloon inflation: • BP (observe for continued hypotension) • HR • ECG rhythm • PAP, PCWP
		2. Observe for progressive signs and symptoms of pulmonary edema.
		3. Maintain patent IV.
		4. In the case of severe hypotension, administer vasopressors, as ordered (eg, dopamine, Levophed).
		5. Administer antiarrhythmics as required (eg, lidocaine).
		6. In the case of severe bradycardia, administer an anticholinergic (eg, atropine).
		7. Have temporary pacemaker or external pacemaker on standby.

(*continued*)

NURSING CARE PLAN 13–2: (Continued)
The Patient With PTCA/PBV

NURSING DIAGNOSIS	OUTCOME CRITERIA/ PATIENT GOALS	NURSING INTERVENTIONS
		8. Have access to cardiac arrest cart with emergency medications, endotracheal intubation tray, and defibrillator.
		9. Be prepared to alert OR if surgery is indicated.
High risk for decreased cardiac output: related to left-to-right shunt with mitral PBV and/or late cardiac tamponade.	• Maintenance of hemodynamic stability, as evidenced by normal BP, CVP, PA, and PCWP.	1. Monitor and record BP, CVP, PAP, and PCWP qh.
		2. Notify physician of continued elevation in pressures.
	• Absence of pulmonary congestion.	3. Record fluid intake and measure urine output (if Foley catheter in place) qh. Urine output of less than 30 ml/hr should be reported to physician.
		4. Maintain patent IV.
High risk for altered peripheral perfusion: related to hematoma, thrombus formation, or infection associated with cannulation site.	• Pulses distal to arterial puncture site will be palpable and strong.	1. Palpate pulses distal to arterial puncture site for presence and strength q15m × 4, q30m × 4, then q4h × 24 hr.
		2. Assess extremity distal to arterial puncture site for coolness, pallor, mottling, cyanosis, tingling, numbness, pain, and report changes to physician.
	• Arterial puncture site will not be erythemic or tender to touch.	3. Elevate and note arterial puncture site and dressings for presence of hematoma, tenderness, ecchymosis, warmth, and drainage.
		4. Maintain a pressure dressing to arterial puncture site.
		5. Instruct patient of need for complete bed rest.
		6. Apply 5-lb sandbag over arterial puncture site, if required.
		7. Keep involved extremity straight.
		8. Keep head of bed at a level no greater than 45° for first 8 hr post-PTCA.
		9. Obtain coagulation tests and report any abnormal results to physician.

(continued)

NURSING CARE PLAN 13–2: (Continued)
The Patient With PTCA/PBV

NURSING DIAGNOSIS	OUTCOME CRITERIA/ PATIENT GOALS	NURSING INTERVENTIONS
	• Patient will remain afebrile.	10. Obtain oral or rectal temperature, q4h. Notify physician, if febrile. Physician may request blood cultures.
		11. Assess and report to physician diaphoresis and/or chilling.
		12. Dispense antibiotic and antipyretic medications as ordered.
High risk for altered cerebral perfusion: related to embolism from procedure site, left ventricle, or left atrium.	• Patient will demonstrate usual level of consciousness with intact motor and sensory function.	1. Assess if patient is awake, alert, and oriented to time, place, and person.
		2. Assess motor function: able to move all extremities with equal strength.
		3. Assess if PERRL.
High risk for potential for alteration in comfort: related to angina, or stretching of the valve during dilation.	• Chest pain will be relieved.	1. Continuously assess and record: • BP, HR, RR, PA, PCWP • ECG rhythm (if occlusive disease present, monitor leads most reflective of coronary artery[s] having disease)
		2. Evaluate severity and location of angina by talking with patient and observing ECG.
		3. Assess skin color and temperature.
		4. Maintain patent IV and oxygen setup (2–4 L/min.)
		5. Administer pain medications to treat angina (eg, nitrates or narcotics) as required.
		6. Assess relief of pain.
		7. Instruct patient to verbalize recurrence of angina.
High risk for altered fluid volume: related to renal sensitivity to contrast material, or diuretic therapy.	• Maintenance of normal serum creatinine, BUN, electrolyte levels, and body weight.	1. Obtain serum creatinine, BUN, and electrolyte levels. Report changes from baseline to physician.
		2. Monitor and record 24-hr intake and output. Record urine output qh if catheterized; report if less than 30 ml/hr.
		3. Assess and report signs and symptoms of hypovolemia such as decreased BP and urine output, tachycardia, complaints of thirst.

(continued)

NURSING CARE PLAN 13–2: (Continued)
The Patient With PTCA/PBV

NURSING DIAGNOSIS	OUTCOME CRITERIA/ PATIENT GOALS	NURSING INTERVENTIONS
		4. Encourage oral fluids and administer IV fluids, as ordered.
		5. Assess and report signs and symptoms of hypervolemia such as dyspnea, crackles, development of peripheral edema, and jugular vein distention.
		6. Deliver osmotic diuretics, as ordered.
		7. Administer maintenance diuretics, as ordered.
Knowledge deficit: related to illness and impact on patient's future.	• Patient will verbalize understanding of coronary artery disease process and begin to identify possible changes in lifestyle.	1. Begin cardiac rehabilitation education: risk factors, pathophysiology, when to seek medical consultation, proper administration of medications, progressive ADL, diet, stress reduction. May include family in cardiac rehabilitation.
		2. Evaluate patient's understanding. Document teaching and response.
Anxiety/fear: related to lack of knowledge of PTCA/PBV, acute care environment, and potential for surgery.	• Patient will verbalize an understanding of procedure and treatment.	1. Provide the patient with an explanation of the procedure.
		2. Orient patient to catheterization lab, ICU, or post-PBV room.
		3. Explain rationale behind preliminary tests which will include: blood tests, chest radiograph, and temporary change in medications.
		4. Explain sensations so the patient can become familiar with expectations during the procedure.
		5. Explain activities to be expected of physician and nurse during the procedure.
		6. Administer prescribed sedatives, as ordered.
		7. Include family or significant other in teaching and explanations of procedures.

PTCA and in the long-term patency of involved atherosclerotic vessels.

Percutaneous Balloon Valvuloplasty

Description

Percutaneous balloon valvuloplasty is a nonsurgical technique for increasing blood flow through stenotic cardiac valves using dilation catheters. This relatively new procedure is similar to PTCA in that a catheter system is inserted percutaneously and advanced to the region of narrowing using fluoroscopic guidance. A dilation catheter then is inflated to increase the valvular opening and improve blood flow.

History

The first cases of balloon dilation of stenotic cardiac valves were reported in 1979 and 1982, when physicians successfully dilated pulmonary valve stenoses. This technique was considered an effective alternative to open heart surgery, although long-term results could not yet be evaluated. Because surgical commissurotomy was successful in treating mitral valve stenoses and because of the initial success with pulmonary valve dilation, physicians began percutaneous dilation of mitral valves in 1984, to avoid the need for thoracotomy. In 1984 and 1985, physicians successfully dilated congenital aortic valve stenoses (AVS). A calcific AVS was first dilated in 1985. These procedures improved cardiac function with no serious procedural complications.

The number of cases performed in 1992 does not approach the volume of coronary angioplasty. This is due partly to the lesser incidence of valve disease compared to CAD and partly to the limitations of this new procedure, which is indicated primarily for inoperable candidates. Percutaneous balloon valvuloplasty is considered the treatment of choice for children with pulmonary valve stenosis, however.

Assuming patients have long-term clinical improvement associated with PBV, the advantages compared to surgery are similar to PTCA versus CABG surgery. Percutaneous balloon valvuloplasty (1) is less traumatic, (2) requires no anesthesia, (3) is associated with lower morbidity and shorter hospital stay, (4) causes no scarring, and (5) is less expensive.

Pathophysiology of Stenotic Valves

Stenotic valves are caused by (1) calcific degeneration, (2) congenital abnormalities, or (3) rheumatic heart disease. Calcific aortic valve degeneration now appears to be the most frequent cause of AVS requiring surgical treatment. Refer to Chapter 16 for a discussion of the pathophysiology and clinical manifestations of specific stenotic values.

Diagnostic Tests for PBV and Valve Replacement

Before deciding the appropriate intervention, the physician evaluates the patient for evidence and severity of valvular stenosis. A variety of noninvasive tests allow the physician to determine the degree of left atrial or left ventricular hypertrophy, pulmonary venous congestion or hypertension, valvular rigidity, and transvalvular gradient. In a 12-lead ECG, the magnitude of the R wave in the precordial leads reflects the presence of left ventricular hypertrophy associated with AVS. The presence of peaked P waves reflects left atrial hypertrophy associated with mitral valve stenosis. A chest radiograph illustrates the presence of calcium within or around the valve, left ventricular or atrial hypertrophy, and pulmonary venous congestion or congestive heart failure. A two-dimensional echocardiogram is used to scan the cardiac valves and chambers. A Doppler ultrasound study allows measurement of the transvalvular gradient, indirect calculation of valve area, and assessment of valvular regurgitation. With this information, the physician is able to (1) estimate the size of the valve orifice, (2) visualize the degree of valve leaflet movement, and (3) determine the extent of left ventricular or atrial hypertrophy.

Right and left heart catheterization is done if the previous tests indicate valvular disease. Although this procedure is invasive, it is required to determine the pressures within each of the cardiac chambers and to confirm transvalvular gradients. Once the pressures and gradients are obtained, a series of radiographs may be taken by injecting radiopaque contrast medium, either in the aorta to visualize aortic regurgitation, or in the left ventricle to visualize mitral regurgitation. This procedure yields a cineangiogram illustrating the function of the cardiac valves and chamber sizes.

After this series of tests, the physician can analyze the valves closely, gaining precise information with which to decide the mode of treatment. The nurse should be familiar with the results of these tests because a better understanding of the patient's diagnosis and related symptoms, and thus of the reasons for intervention, promotes better care.

Equipment Features

Although PBV and PTCA catheters are based on similar designs, there are important differences, primarily because of the larger diameters of heart valves compared to coronary arteries. One major difference is the outer diameter of the catheters. Percutaneous balloon valvuloplasty catheter shafts range from 7 to 9 Fr (versus 2–4 Fr for PTCA catheters); PBV balloons range from 15 to 25 mm in diameter when inflated (versus 1.5–4.0 mm for PTCA balloons). Guiding catheters, which are necessary during PTCA, cannot be used for PBV because of the large diameter of PBV dilation catheters. A 10- to 14-Fr introducing sheath may be used at the arterial or venous puncture site to allow for introduction of the valve dilation catheter. A larger guide wire, 0.035 to 0.038 inches, also is used to provide the added stiffness and support required to introduce the dilatation catheter. Percutaneous balloon valvuloplasty dilation catheters have radiopaque markers similar to PTCA dilation catheters for fluoroscopic imaging.

A major complication associated with PBV is excessive bleeding at the puncture site due to the large catheters required to perform dilation. The development of smaller catheters may reduce this bleeding. As with PTCA, PBV catheters are being refined continually to increase procedural safety, time, and efficacy.

Indications and Contraindications for PBV

The use of PBV initially was limited by the fear of embolization of calcific debris, disruption of the valve ring, acute valvular regurgitation, and valvular restenosis. The incidence of these complications continues to be a concern. Both major and minor complications have been reported in numerous early studies; however, it is important to assess these complications in terms of the patient population in which the procedure is performed. Restenosis remains a limitation of both PBV and PTCA.

Although surgical valve replacement is an effective treatment for those with AVS, and operative mortality is low, operative mortality significantly increases in patients with multisystem disease (who often are elderly). Percutaneous balloon valvuloplasty initially has proven to be a safe and efficacious alternative for these patients. It also is an effective therapy for children who are high surgical risks, because it delays the need for surgery until the child is older and better can tolerate an operation. In addition, the longevity of both mechanical and bioprosthetic valves is approximately 10 years, so PBV delays or prevents the need for a second operation. Also, the long-term anticoagulation therapy required with mechanical valve prostheses is undesirable in younger patients and pregnant women. Percutaneous balloon valvuloplasty also is effective for stabilizing those with poor left ventricular function before surgery; it is contraindicated in patients with moderate to severe valvular regurgitation due to a small but significant risk of increasing valvular insufficiency with the procedure (see Display Box 13–1).

Procedure

Percutaneous balloon valvuloplasty is performed in the cardiac catheterization laboratory and involves many of the same steps as PTCA (see earlier section on PTCA Procedure). Right and left heart catheterization is repeated to evaluate hemodynamic status and to obtain baseline transvalvular gradients. Coronary angiography, when indicated, is repeated to determine whether the patient still meets the criteria for valvuloplasty. Thorough repeat evaluation is necessary because a patient's status can change, precluding treatment with this intervention. Factors that might be grounds for canceling PBV are (1) progression of mild valvular regurgitation, (2) previously unapparent stenotic coronary artery lesions, or (3) progression of coronary artery lesions.

If PBV still is indicated, the angiographic catheter is replaced either by an introducing sheath or a dilatation catheter. In mitral PBV, a venous puncture is made in the right femoral vein. During both aortic and mitral PBV, maintaining patent intravenous and radial or femoral arterial lines is important to administer medications and to draw blood samples.

In aortic PBV, once the sheaths are in place, the patient is anticoagulated with 5,000 to 10,000 U heparin to prevent clot formation within the catheter system. The dilation catheter and guidewire then are advanced to the root of the ascending aorta. The guidewire is advanced across the stenotic aortic valve and the dilation catheter is advanced over the guidewire (Fig. 13–31). Exact placement of the dilation catheter is facilitated by fluoroscopy and radiopaque markers on the balloon.

DISPLAY BOX 13–1
Indications and Contraindications for PBV

Clinical Indications

High-risk surgical patients (advanced age, severe pulmonary hypertension, renal failure, pulmonary dysfunction, left ventricular dysfunction)
Unstable presurgical patients
Patients not candidates for chronic anticoagulation

Anatomic Indications

Moderate to severe valvular narrowing
Moderate to severe valvular calcification
Mild valvular regurgitation

Anatomic Contraindications

Inability to access vasculature
Thrombus
Severe valvular regurgitation
History of embolic events

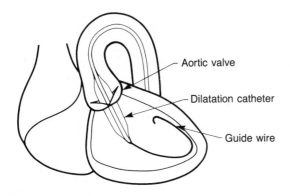

FIGURE 13–31
Cross-sectional view of heart illustrating guidewire and dilation catheter positions across the aortic valve. The guidewire is curved to prevent ventricular dysrhythmias or puncture.

In mitral PBV, a pacing catheter may be positioned through a separate venous sheath at the level of the inferior vena cava or right atrium and placed on standby. The mitral valve then is approached either by way of the femoral artery and aortic valve, or in most cases through the right heart by perforating the atrial septum to enter the left atrium. Once the mitral valve has been accessed, the patient is anticoagulated with 5,000 to 10,000 U heparin. The dilation catheter is then advanced over the guidewire through the atrial septal puncture and across the mitral valve (Fig. 13–32). Again, exact placement of the dilation catheter within the valve is facilitated by fluoroscopy and radiopaque markers on the balloon. In both aortic and mitral PBV, dual balloons sometimes are used to increase the potential capacity for dilation.

Average inflation time of the dilation catheter is 15 to 60 seconds in aortic valvuloplasty and 10 to 30 seconds in mitral valvuloplasty. During dilation of either valve, the nurse should monitor blood pressure closely because of the imposed decrease in cardiac output. Once the dilation

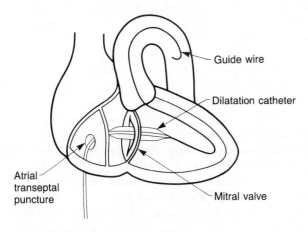

FIGURE 13–32
Cross-sectional view of heart illustrating guidewire and dilation catheter placed through an atrial transseptal puncture and across the mitral valve. The guidewire is extended out the aortic valve into the aorta for catheter support.

catheter has been deflated, blood pressure should return to normal. During dilation of the mitral valve, there is a temporary increase in the pulmonary capillary wedge pressure (PCWP), which the nurse should monitor. Once the dilation catheter has been deflated, the PCWP should return to baseline. Sinus bradycardia also may occur, especially during mitral dilation.

Once maximum dilation has been obtained, the catheter is removed. Hemodynamic measurements, including transvalvular gradients, are repeated to determine efficacy of the procedure. Repeat angiography is done to assess for valvular regurgitation. When the procedure is complete, to prevent bleeding complications associated with the large puncture site, the anticoagulant effects of heparin are reversed.

Results

Aortic PBV is associated with a decrease in pressure gradient and end-systolic volume and an increase in aortic valve area, ejection fraction, and cardiac output. In-hospital mortality ranges between 2% and 5%. Although there is an increase in the aortic valve area, it is not as great as with surgical valve replacement. Additionally, the restenosis rate associated with PBV is high. Therefore, aortic valvuloplasty is indicated primarily for elderly and high-risk surgical patients, and generally is considered a palliative, not a curative procedure.

Results of mitral valvuloplasty are more dramatic. There is a more significant increase in valve area and cardiac output, and a decrease in valve gradient, PCWP, and mean pulmonary arterial pressure. Operative mortality has been reported as 1.5% and sustained clinical improvement has been reported in 63% to 90% of cases. Late deaths occur in approximately 5% to 10%.

Three mechanisms have been postulated for the improvement of valvular function due to PBV: (1) fracture of calcific nodules adherent to leaflets (most frequent); (2) separation of fused commissures; and (3) stretching of the anulus and leaflet structure.

Assessment and Management

Patient Preparation

Once the decision has been made to proceed with PBV, the patient is admitted to the hospital 1 to 2 days before the procedure. The goal of nursing care is to (1) reduce the cardiac workload, (2) monitor fluid and electrolyte balance, and (3) reduce psychological stress so the patient remains hemodynamically stable.

In most cases, the patient will not have invasive pressure monitoring lines in place before the procedure. The nurse, therefore, carefully should monitor signs and symptoms of congestive heart failure: narrowing in the arterial pulse pressure, more frequent increases in heart rate during activity, peripheral edema, presence of a cough, complaints of dyspnea, or rales in lung fields. The nurse also must note any changes in sensorium, color, skin temperature, pulse volume, and any decrease in urinary output.

To monitor fluid and electrolyte balance, the nurse should obtain a baseline serum electrolyte level and baseline body weight. In addition, daily fluid intake and output should be recorded.

The patient's medications before admission may have included diuretics, digoxin, and anticoagulants. Before the procedure, any anticoagulant medication will be discontinued owing to the possibility of emergency surgery. Therefore, patients with chronic atrial fibrillation who have the potential for systemic embolization due to thrombus should be monitored closely. The nurse also should monitor preliminary laboratory tests and notify the physician of any abnormalities. (See the section on PTCA Patient Preparation for further information on these tests.)

The physician will explain to the patient how the valvuloplasty is performed and the potential risks and benefits. To decrease stress and anxiety, the nurse may need to reinforce the physician's explanation and answer any further questions.

After the patient fully understands the procedure, the physician must obtain an informed consent for PBV, anesthesia, and surgery. Surgical standby usually is provided during PBV due to possible complications requiring emergency valve replacement. Because all patients are not surgical candidates, surgical standby is not provided for everyone; however, those who are surgical candidates must be surgically prepared as if for elective valve replacement.

Nursing Assessment and Management

During PBV

Patient care during PBV is similar to care during PTCA (see section on Nursing Management During PTCA). In addition, the nurse continuously monitors pulmonary artery pressure and PCWP, and is aware of changes in tracings that may suggest symptoms of congestive heart failure or pulmonary edema.

In the presence of severe hypotension, the nurse should be prepared to start an IV infusion of dopamine or Levophed. In the case of ventricular dysrhythmias, a lidocaine drip should be available for infusion. A summary of medications most often associated with PTCA and PBV is given in Table 13–10.

Post-PBV

Once the patient has returned to the coronary care or telemetry unit, the nurse plays an important role in recovery. The goal of postvalvuloplasty nursing care is to maintain adequate cardiac output, maintain fluid and electrolyte balance, and verify hemostasis at the puncture site.

Alterations in cardiac output can be caused by (1) dysrhythmias secondary to valve manipulation, resulting in edema near the bundle of His, (2) left-to-right atrial shunt through the transseptal puncture created during mitral valvuloplasty, (3) cardiac tamponade, (4) alteration in circulating fluid volume, or (5) blood loss. Alteration in fluid and electrolyte balance results from diuretic therapy and contrast medium used during catheterization. Bleeding at the puncture site is secondary to the combined effect of systemic anticoagulation and the large diameter of catheters used.

To begin, the nurse should attach the ECG monitor, which allows a quick initial cardiac assessment and establishes a baseline rhythm for reference if the condition changes. The presence of either atrial or ventricular dysrhythmias can affect optimal cardiac output and may necessitate either parenteral administration of antiarrhythmia medications such as lidocaine or the insertion of a temporary transvenous pacemaker. If the patient has a pulmonary artery or central venous pressure monitoring line in place, these also should be checked after initial baseline recordings are obtained. One indicator that the atrial septal puncture site has failed to close after PBV is a left-to-right shunt, as documented by an elevated central venous pressure.

Because fluids are important in the hemodynamic balance of the patient with valvular disease, the volume of IV fluids should be recorded to establish an accurate intake and output. The decreased circulating volume from diuretic medications given before PBV combined with improved stroke volume after successful PBV can be reflected as a decrease in cardiac output. Therefore, careful monitoring of central venous pressure, pulmonary artery pressure, PCWP, and blood pressure, in addition to heart rate, urinary output, and electrolyte balance, are essential in the evaluation and assessment of circulating fluid volume and cardiac pumping status.

Additionally, the nurse should assess the patient's status from head to toe, noting overall skin color and temperature and carefully observing the level of consciousness and neurologic signs. The nurse also should listen closely to heart and breath sounds. Circulation distal to the puncture site should be evaluated by noting peripheral skin color and temperature in addition to the presence and quality of the dorsalis pedis and posterior tibial pulses.

Finally, the presence of any drainage on the puncture site dressing or tenderness during palpation should be noted to establish a baseline for the possibility of increased pericatheter bleeding. The nurse should report immediately any changes that may indicate excessive bleeding. Bleeding at the sheath site may result in a hematoma requiring surgical evacuation. To prevent excessive bleeding and to aid hemostasis, the physician may order a sandbag or clamp placed over the puncture site.

If the patient has documented CAD, the physician also may request a serum cardiac enzyme panel. Particular attention should be paid to CK and CK isoenzymes (see section on Nursing Assessment and Management Post-PTCA). The nurse should be aware of the signs and symptoms of myocardial ischemia in addition to the appropriate interventions.

The nurse should impress on the patient the importance of keeping the involved leg straight and the head of the bed flat for the first 6 hours after valvuloplasty.

Post-PBV evaluation may include prothrombin time, hemoglobin and hematocrit, coagulation studies, serum electrolytes, CK, ECG, and chest radiograph.

Complications

A common in-hospital complication associated with PBV is bleeding at the arterial puncture site due to the large diameter of the catheters needed to dilate the valve anulus. Additionally, in mitral PBV, a common complication is left-to-right shunting secondary to septal dilation, again due to the large diameter of the dilation catheters. Systemic embolization in both mitral and aortic PBV is a potential and significant complication, although its incidence is low. There have been few reports of significant increase in valvular regurgitation. A long-term complication related to the procedure is restenosis. Other complications associated with PBV are listed in Display Box 13–2.

Nursing Care Plan

Nursing Care Plan 13–2 discusses the nursing diagnoses, patient goals, and nursing interventions for the patient undergoing PBV.

DISPLAY BOX 13–2
Complications Associated With PBV

- Embolization of calcific debris
- Valve ring disruption
- Valvular regurgitation
- Valvular restenosis
- Bleeding at arterial puncture site
- Left ventricular perforation
- Severe hypotension
- Transient ischemia
- Vascular trauma
- Atrial septal defect (with mitral PBV)
- Aortic dissection
- Aortic rupture
- Cardiac tamponade
- Chordae tendineae rupture

Summary

Percutaneous balloon valvuloplasty is a relatively new procedure that can be performed successfully in both children and adults. Long-term clinical outcome and restenosis rates continue to be assessed to determine the efficacy of this treatment as compared to surgery. Percutaneous balloon valvuloplasty appears to be an alternative for inoperable patients, and with more advanced catheter technology, may be performed in the future more easily and with less complications. More research is indicated to define which surgical candidates should be considered for PBV.

Intra-Aortic Balloon Pump Counterpulsation and Other Ventricular Assist Devices

Behavioral Objectives

Intra-Aortic Balloon Pump Counterpulsation

Description

Physiological Principles
   Afterload
   Preload
   Contractility
   Heart Rate

Equipment Features

Indications
   Cardiogenic Shock
   Response Patterns
   Postoperative Left Ventricular Failure
   High-Risk Cardiac Surgery
   Septic Shock
   General Surgery for High-Risk Patient

(continued)

BEHAVIORAL OBJECTIVES

Based on the content in this section, the reader should be able to:

1. Describe the physiological effect of intra-aortic balloon pump (IABP) counterpulsation therapy.
2. List indications and contraindications for IABP therapy.
3. Draw and describe the components of an IABP augmented arterial waveform.
4. List five vital assessments the nurse must make during care of the patient receiving IABP therapy.
5. List and describe five potential nursing diagnoses and interventions for each diagnosis.
6. Describe a ventricular assist device that totally supports left ventricular function.

Intra-Aortic Balloon Pump Counterpulsation

Description

Intra-aortic balloon pump counterpulsation was first introduced clinically by Kantrowitz and associates in 1967. This therapeutic approach was instituted for treatment of two patients with left ventricular failure following acute myocardial infarction. Since that time, IABP has become a standard treatment for medical and surgical patients with acute left ventricular failure that is unresponsive to pharmacologic and volume therapy.

Therapeutic goals are directed toward (1) increasing oxygen supply to the myocardium, (2) decreasing left ventricular work, and (3) improving cardiac output. Before IABP, no single therapeutic agent was capable of meeting these three goals.

Intra-aortic balloon pump counterpulsation is designed to increase coronary artery perfusion pressure and blood flow during the diastolic phase of the cardiac cycle by inflation of a balloon in the thoracic aorta. Deflation of the balloon, just before systolic ejection, decreases the impedance to ejection and thus left ventricular work. Inflation and deflation counterpulse each heart beat. With improved blood flow and effective reduction in left ventricular work, the hoped-for results are improved myocardial pump function and increased cardiac output.

Physiological Principles

In the failing heart, greater work is required to maintain cardiac output. With this added work requirement, oxygen demand increases. This may occur at a time when the myocardium already is ischemic and coronary artery perfusion is unable to meet the oxygen demands. As a result, left ventricular performance diminishes even further, resulting in decreased cardiac output. A vicious cycle ensues that is difficult to interrupt (Fig. 13–33). Without interruption of the cycle, cardiogenic shock may be imminent. This cycle can be broken with IABP by increasing aortic root pressure during diastole through inflation of the balloon. With increased aortic root pressure, the perfusion pressure of the coronary arteries will be increased.

Effective therapy for the patient in left ventricular failure also involves decreasing myocardial oxygen demand. Four major determinants of myocardial oxygen demand are (1) afterload, (2) preload, (3) contractility, and (4) heart rate. Intra-aortic balloon pump counterpulsation therapy can have an effect on all these factors. It will

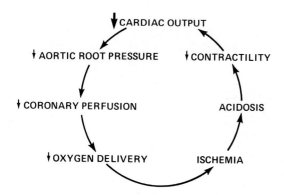

FIGURE 13–33
Cycle leading to cardiogenic shock.

decrease afterload directly and will affect the other three determinants indirectly as cardiac function improves.

Afterload

This is the amount of muscle tension that must be generated by the ventricle to raise intraventricular pressure, allowing the ventricle to overcome impedance to ejection. When adequate intraventricular pressure is reached, the semilunar valve is forced open and ejection occurs. This occurs in either ventricle. Because IABP assists the left heart, only the left ventricle will be discussed. Impedance to ejection is caused by the aortic valve, aortic end-diastolic pressure, and vascular resistance. With greater impedance, afterload increases, and thus more oxygen is demanded by the ventricle. The aortic valve is a factor that does not change beat-to-beat, so its contribution to the level of afterload is fixed. Greater aortic end-diastolic pressures require higher afterload to overcome impedance to ejection. Vascular resistance will increase impedance when vessels become vasoconstricted. Vasodilation or lower vascular resistance will decrease impedance to ejection, and thus afterload decreases.

Deflation of the balloon in the aorta, just before ventricular systole, lowers aortic end-diastolic pressure, which decreases impedance. The greatest amount of oxygen required during the cardiac cycle is for the development of afterload. With decreased impedance, the workload of the ventricle also decreases. In this way, IABP can decrease effectively the oxygen demand of the heart.

Preload

Preload is the volume or pressure in the ventricle at end-diastole. Volume in a chamber creates pressure. A person in acute left ventricular failure has increased volume in the ventricle at end-diastole due to the heart's inability to pump effectively. This excessive increase in preload also increases the workload of the heart. Clinically, preload of the right heart is measured by central venous pressure or

right atrial pressure, and preload of the left heart is measured with the PCWP or left atrial pressure. These pressures increase when the ventricles are in failure.

IABP therapy helps decrease excessive preload in the left ventricle by decreasing impedance to ejection. With decreased impedance, there is a more effective forward flow of blood. Preload is decreased, with more efficient emptying of the left ventricle during systole.

Contractility

Contractility refers to the velocity and vigor of contraction during systole. Although vigorous contractility requires more oxygen, it is a benefit to cardiac function because it ensures good, efficient pumping, which serves to increase cardiac output. In failure, contractility is depressed. The biochemical status of the myocardium directly affects contractility. Contractility is depressed when calcium levels are low, when catecholamine levels are low, and when ischemia is present with resultant acidosis.

Intra-aortic balloon pump counterpulsation can increase oxygen supply, thereby decreasing ischemia and acidosis. In this way, IABP contributes to improved contractility and better cardiac function (see Figure 13–33).

Heart Rate

Heart rate is a major determinant of oxygen demand because the rate determines the number of times per minute the high pressures must be generated during systole. Normally, myocardial perfusion takes place during diastole. Coronary artery perfusion pressure is determined by the gradient between aortic diastolic pressure and myocardial wall tension. It can be expressed by the following equation:

$$\text{Coronary perfusion pressure} = \text{Aortic diastolic pressure} - \text{Myocardial wall tension}$$

Tension in the muscle retards blood flow, which is why approximately 80% of coronary artery perfusion occurs during diastole. With faster heart rates, diastolic time becomes shortened, with very little change occurring in systolic time. A rapid heart rate not only increases oxygen demand but also decreases the time available for delivery of oxygen. In acute ventricular failure, a person may not be able to maintain cardiac output by increasing the volume of blood pumped with each beat (stroke volume) because contractility is likely to be depressed. Cardiac output is a function of both stroke volume and heart rate.

$$\text{Cardiac output} = \text{Stroke volume} \times \text{Heart rate}$$

If stroke volume cannot be increased, heart rate must increase to maintain cardiac output. This is very costly in terms of oxygen demand.

By improving contractility, IABP helps improve myocardial pumping and the ability to increase stroke volume. Decreasing afterload also increases pumping efficiency. With improved myocardial function and cardiac output, the need for compensatory tachycardia diminishes. Intra-aortic balloon pump counterpulsation also will increase coronary artery perfusion pressure by increasing aortic diastolic pressure during inflation of the balloon, resulting in improved blood flow and oxygen delivery to the myocardium.

Physiological effects of IABP are summarized in Display Box 13–3. Proper inflation of the balloon will increase oxygen supply, and proper deflation of the balloon will decrease oxygen demand. Timing of inflation and deflation is crucial and must coincide with the cardiac cycle.

Equipment Features

The intra-aortic balloon catheter is constructed of a biocompatible polyurethane material. Polyurethane also is used to make the balloon that is mounted on the end of the catheter. Filling of the balloon is achieved with pressurized gas that enters through the catheter. A standard adult-size balloon holds 40 cc of gas. With inflation, the addition of 40 cc of volume into the aorta acutely increases aortic pressure and retrograde blood flow back toward the aortic valve. With deflation, the sudden evacuation of 40 cc of volume out of the balloon acutely decreases aortic pressure. Because of its low molecular weight, helium is the pressurized gas of choice. Catheters may have a central lumen with which aortic pressure can be measured from the tip of the balloon, or they may come with a guidewire centered in the the balloon and no central lumen.

Indications

Two major applications of IABP therapy are for treatment of cardiogenic shock after myocardial infarction and for acute left ventricular failure after cardiac surgery. In addition, other applications have been made for other types of patients with cardiac pathophysiological conditions (see Display Box 13–4). Successful support of the septic shock patient and the cardiovascular patient undergoing general surgery also has been reported.

Cardiogenic Shock

Treatment of cardiogenic shock is complicated, and the mortality remains high. Cardiogenic shock will develop in approximately 15% of patients with myocardial infarction. The presence of cardiogenic shock is confirmed by the following accepted criteria:

- Low cardiac output syndrome
- Cardiac index of 2.0 L/minute/m² or less

DISPLAY BOX 13–3
Direct Physiological Effects of IABP

Inflation
↑ aortic diastolic pressure
↑ aortic root pressure
↑ coronary perfusion pressure
↑ oxygen supply

Deflation
↓ aortic end-diastolic pressure
↓ impedance to ejection
↓ afterload
↓ oxygen demand

- Systolic blood pressure less than 80 mm Hg or less than 100 mm Hg in a formerly hypertensive patient
- Urine output less than 20 ml/hour

Patients first will be given a short period of treatment with various inotropic drugs, vasopressors, and volume. A lack of or minimal response in cardiac output, arterial pressure, urine output, and mental status after this therapy will indicate a need for assisted circulation with IABP. Once hypotension is present, the self-perpetuating process of injury will be in effect. Control of further injury and improvement in survival require early reversal of the shock state.

Most research centers agree that patients who hemodynamically exhibit left ventricular end-diastolic pressures or PCWPs greater than 18 mm Hg with cardiac indexes less than 2.0 to 2.2 L/minute/m² are prone to high mortality and should be considered for IABP if they are unresponsive to a short period of pharmacologic and volume therapy.

DISPLAY BOX 13–4
Indications for IABP

- Cardiogenic shock after acute infarction
- Left ventricular failure in the postoperative cardiac surgery patient
- Severe unstable angina
- Postinfarction ventricular septal defect or mitral regurgitation
- Septic shock
- General surgery for the patient with cardiovascular disease
- Bridge to cardiac transplantation

Response Patterns

Once IABP therapy is instituted, improvement should be seen in 1 to 2 hours. At this time, steady improvement should be seen in cardiac output, peripheral perfusion, urine output, mental status, and pulmonary congestion. With improved cardiac function, a decrease in central venous pressure and PCWP also should be seen. Average peak effect should be achieved within 24 to 48 hours.

There are three general responses to IABP therapy. One group of patients will achieve hemodynamic stabilization and survive with the support of medical therapy and IABP. The second group of patients will continue to deteriorate with the support of IABP and will die from irreversible cardiogenic shock. The third group of patients will become dependent on IABP for circulatory support. Attempted withdrawal of IABP in this group results in hemodynamic deterioration. Patients who are awaiting heart transplantation will fall into this category. The condition will be relieved only by replacement of the failing heart or more aggressive forms of circulatory support. Some of the patients in this group may achieve some benefit from cardiac surgical intervention. There are centers that advocate early CABG for this group of patients. Surgery on patients in cardiogenic shock carries extremely high risk; however, many of the nonoperated patients will die from complications of their illness.

Postoperative Left Ventricular Failure

Successful reduction in mortality has been achieved by using IABP for patients with acute left ventricular failure or cardiogenic shock after cardiac surgery. There are two major conditions that might lead to postoperative pump failure: (1) severe preoperative left ventricular dysfunction, and (2) intraoperative myocardial injury.

Intra-aortic balloon pump counterpulsation therapy can be used to wean patients from cardiopulmonary bypass and to provide postoperative circulatory assistance until left ventricular recovery occurs. In these situations, early recognition of failure is evidenced by the heart's inability to support circulation after cardiopulmonary bypass.

Early recognition and treatment is crucial if left ventricular failure is to be reversed. Later development and recognition of failure after cardiac surgery results in much higher mortality, even with the assistance of IABP support.

High-Risk Cardiac Surgery

Intra-aortic balloon pump counterpulsation therapy has been used in the high-risk cardiac surgery patient for safer induction of anesthesia. Patients who develop signs of acute cardiac ischemia unresponsive to pharmacologic therapy may benefit from IABP support during anesthesia induction and for support before cardiopulmonary bypass.

Intra-aortic balloon pump counterpulsation therapy also may be used during cardiac catheterization for this same group of high-risk patients. In this situation, cardiac catheterization studies generally are followed by emergency cardiac surgery. Patients in this category include those with unstable angina, postinfarction angina and postinfarction ventricular septal defects, or mitral regurgitation from papillary muscle injury with resultant cardiac failure. Intra-aortic balloon pump counterpulsation therapy has been used successfully to control the severity of angina in patients in whom previous medical therapy has failed. The use of IABP therapy for patients with cardiac failure after ventricular septal rupture or mitral valve incompetence will aid in the promotion of forward blood flow, which will decrease shunting through the septal defect and decrease the amount of mitral regurgitation.

Septic Shock

Another application of IABP is for the support of patients in septic shock. These patients have very low systemic vascular resistance due to vasodilation caused by the endotoxin. To review, mean arterial blood pressure is a function of cardiac output and systemic vascular resistance. To maintain adequate perfusion pressure to vital organs, the patient in septic shock must maintain a very high cardiac output. Intra-aortic balloon pump counterpulsation therapy has been used when traditional vasopressor support fails to maintain adequate mean arterial pressure. Prolonged, inadequate perfusion pressure will result in possible renal failure or myocardial infarction. Intra-aortic balloon pump counterpulsation support is advocated by some clinicians to assist blood pressure maintenance and increase coronary perfusion when traditional support fails. The need for extra support may be very important in patients with preexisting cardiac disease.

General Surgery for High-Risk Patient

Another application of IABP is for the high-risk cardiovascular patient undergoing a general surgical operation. Any patient with ischemic heart disease will be at higher risk during general anesthesia and the surgical procedure. Intra-aortic balloon pump counterpulsation is used to ensure adequate coronary artery perfusion pressure during the procedure.

Contraindications

Few contraindications are associated with the use of IABP therapy.

A competent aortic valve is necessary if the patient is to benefit from IABP. With *aortic insufficiency*, balloon inflation would only increase aortic regurgitation and offer little, if any, augmentation of coronary artery perfusion pressure. In fact, the patient's heart failure could be expected to become worse.

Severe peripheral vascular occlusive disease also is a contraindication to use of IABP. Occlusive disease would make insertion of the catheter difficult and possibly interrupt blood flow to the distal extremity or cause dislodgement of plaque formation along the vessel wall, resulting in potential emboli. In patients who absolutely require IABP therapy, insertion can be achieved through the thoracic aorta, thus bypassing diseased peripheral vessels.

Any previous aortofemoral or aortoiliac *bypass graft* would contraindicate femoral artery insertion.

The presence of an *aortic aneurysm* also is a contraindication to the use of IABP therapy. A pulsating balloon against an aneurysm may predispose the patient to dislodgement of aneurysmal debris with resultant emboli. A more serious complication would be rupture of the aneurysm. It also is possible that the catheter could perforate the wall of the aneurysm during insertion. Display Box 13–5 lists the contraindications to IABP.

Procedure

Insertion

Proper position of the balloon is in the thoracic aorta just distal to the left subclavian artery and proximal to the renal arteries (Fig. 13–34). Insertion of the catheter may be achieved through a Dacron graft that has been anastomosed to either a femoral or iliac artery. The catheter is advanced until proper position is achieved. End-to-side anastomosis of the graft to the artery allows for proper securing of the catheter without obliteration of blood flow to the extremity. Suture is used around the graft to secure the catheter so that it will not slip out of proper position. This method is used most often in small children who require IABP therapy. The most commonly used method of catheter placement is percutaneous insertion using a Seldinger technique, although other approaches have been described. The most common alternative is direct insertion into the thoracic aorta. Because this requires a median sternotomy incision, it is restricted essentially to cardiac surgery patients whose chests have been opened for the surgery.

Once in place, the catheter is attached to a machine console that has three basic components: (1) a monitoring

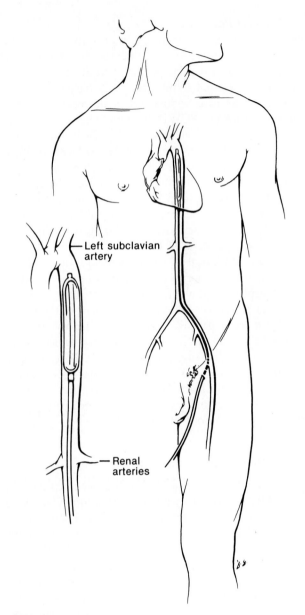

FIGURE 13–34
Proper position of the balloon catheter, illustrating percutaneous insertion.

system, (2) an electronic trigger mechanism, and (3) a drive system that moves gas in and out of the balloon. Monitoring systems have the capability of displaying the patient's ECG and an arterial waveform showing the effect of balloon inflation–deflation. Some consoles also are capable of displaying a balloon waveform that illustrates the inflation and deflation of the balloon itself. The standard trigger mechanism for the balloon pump is the R wave that is sensed from the patient's ECG. This trigger will signal the beginning of each cardiac cycle for the drive system. Other possible triggers include systolic arterial pressure or pacemaker spikes on the ECG. Adjustment of exact timing is controlled on the machine console. Inflation of the balloon will have to be delayed until the end of

---

DISPLAY BOX 13–5
Contraindications to IABP

- Aortic valve incompetence
- Severe peripheral vascular occlusive disease
- Previous aortofemoral or aortoiliac bypass grafts
- Aortic aneurysm

systole. The drive system is the actual mechanism that drives gas into and out of the balloon by alternating pressure and vacuum.

Timing

The first step to proper timing of the balloon pump is the identification of the beginning of systole and diastole on the arterial waveform. Every patient must have an arterial catheter in place to monitor timing. Central aortic pressure waveforms may be used if a balloon catheter with a central lumen is in place. The cycle of the left heart will be used to describe the events of the cardiac cycle. Systole begins when left ventricular pressure exceeds left atrial pressure, forcing the mitral valve closed.

There are two phases to systole: (1) isovolumic contraction, and (2) ejection. Once the mitral valve is closed, isovolumic contraction begins and continues until enough pressure is generated to overcome impedance to ejection. When ventricular pressure exceeds aortic pressure, the aortic valve is forced open, initiating ejection, or phase two. Ejection continues until pressure in the left ventricle falls below pressure in the aorta. At this point, the aortic valve closes and diastole begins.

Closing of the aortic valve creates an artifact on the arterial waveform that is called the dicrotic notch. The dicrotic notch is used as a timing reference to determine when balloon inflation should occur. Inflation should not occur before the notch because systole has not been completed.

After aortic valve closure, two phases of diastole begin: (1) isovolumic relaxation, and (2) ventricular filling. After aortic valve closure, there is a period of time in which neither the aortic nor mitral valve is open. The mitral valve remains closed because left ventricular pressure still is higher than left atrial pressure. This phase is isovolumic relaxation. When left ventricular pressure falls below left atrial pressure, the mitral valve is forced open by the higher pressure in the left atrium. This begins the filling phase of diastole. Balloon inflation should continue throughout diastole. Deflation should be timed to occur at end-diastole, just before the next sharp systolic upstroke on the arterial waveform.

Figure 13–35 illustrates the cardiac cycle with left atrial, left ventricular, and aortic pressure superimposed on one another. Note the systolic upstroke seen on the aortic tracing and the appearance of the dicrotic notch.

Figure 13–36 illustrates a radial artery waveform with the beginning of systole and diastole marked. The amount of time balloon inflation should last can be estimated by knowing the patient's heart rate. Systole is roughly one-third of the cardiac cycle, and diastole is approximately two-thirds. Each RR interval on the ECG represents one cardiac cycle. Heart rate per minute is actually the number of cardiac cycles per minute. With each minute equaling 60,000 milliseconds, 60,000 milliseconds divided by heart

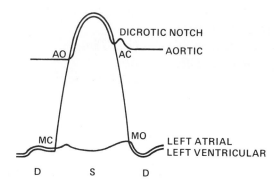

FIGURE 13–35
Cardiac cycle of the left heart with aortic, left ventricular, and left atrial pressure waveforms. AO, aortic valve opening; AC, aortic valve closure; D, diastole; MO, mitral valve opening; MC, mitral valve closure; S, systole.

rate equals the total milliseconds in each cardiac cycle, or RR interval. Approximately one-third of the RR interval will be systole, or the number of milliseconds the balloon is deflated, and two-thirds will be diastole, or the balloon inflation interval. It is wise to add extra time to the deflation period until fine adjustment of the waveform can be made.

Display Box 13–6 outlines the mathematic calculation that determines inflation and deflation time for a patient with a heart rate of 60 beats/minute. This calculation illustrates approximate times in which the balloon will be inflated and deflated in one cardiac cycle.

Interpretation of Results

Waveform Assessment

An important nursing function is the analysis of the arterial pressure waveform and the effectiveness of IABP therapy. Nurses must be able to recognize and correct problems in balloon pump timing.

Step 1. The first step in timing assessment is the ability to recognize the beginnings of systole and diastole on the

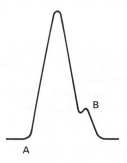

FIGURE 13–36
Arterial waveform, with A representing the point of balloon deflation before the systolic upstroke, and B representing balloon inflation at the dicrotic notch, at diastole.

DISPLAY BOX 13–6
*Calculation of Inflation Time
for a Heart Rate of 60*

---

msec in RR interval

$$+ \ \frac{60,000 \text{ msec/min}}{\text{patient's heart rate (60 beats/min)}}$$

one RR interval = 1,000 msec
systole ($^1\!/_3$) ~ 400 msec
diastole ($^2\!/_3$) ~ 600 msec

---

arterial waveform, as shown in Figure 13–36. Systole begins at point A, where the sharp upstroke begins. Point B marks the dicrotic notch, which represents aortic valve closure. It is at this point that diastole begins and the balloon should be inflated. Balloon deflation occurs just before point A, at end-diastole.

Display Box 13–7 lists five criteria that can be used to measure the effectiveness of IABP on the arterial pressure waveform. To evaluate the waveform effectively, the patient's unassisted pressure tracing must be viewed alongside the assisted pressure tracing. This can be accomplished through adjustment of the console so that the balloon inflates and deflates on every other beat (ie, a 1:2 assist ratio). Most patients will tolerate this well for a brief period of time. Many machine consoles are capable of freezing the waveform on the console monitor so that it would be necessary to assist 1:2 only for one screen. The machine can then return to 1:1 assistance while the nurse assesses the tracing. Another alternative would be to obtain a strip recording of the 1:2 assistance for analysis. These two approaches might be necessary if the mean

---

DISPLAY BOX 13–7
*Criteria for Assessment of Effective IABP
on the Arterial Pressure Waveform*

- Inflation occurs at the dicrotic notch.
- Inflation slope is parallel to the systolic upstroke and is a straight line.
- Diastolic augmentation peak is greater than or equal to the preceding systolic peak.
- An end-diastolic dip in pressure is created with balloon deflation.
- The following systolic peak (assisted systole) is lower than the preceding systole (unassisted systole).

---

arterial blood pressure (MAP) drops significantly on 1:2 assistance.

Step 2. Using the first criterion, the patient's dicrotic notch should be identified. Comparison is then made with the assisted tracing to see that inflation occurs at the point of the dicrotic notch. Inflation before the dicrotic notch will shorten systole abruptly and increase ventricular volume as ejection is interrupted. Late inflation, past the dicrotic notch, will not raise coronary artery perfusion pressure as effectively. The peak-diastolic pressure may not be as high as it would be with proper timing. Also, the duration of assistance during diastole will be unnecessarily shortened.

Step 3. Next, the slopes of systolic upstroke and diastolic augmentation should be compared. The diastolic slope should be sharp and parallel the systolic upstroke. The slope always should be a straight line. A diastolic slope that reaches its peak slowly indicates that the increase in aortic root pressure rises slowly and is not as effective in immediately increasing coronary perfusion pressure. The greater the peak in diastolic pressure, the greater the increase in aortic root pressure. For this reason, balloon assistance is adjusted until the highest peak possible is achieved. The method of doing this will vary with different brands of consoles. The nurse should be familiar with the particular console used by the institution.

Step 4. Deflation should occur just before systole, causing an acute drop in aortic end-diastolic pressure. This quick deflation displaces approximately 40 cc of volume, depending on the size of the balloon. This displacement of volume causes a drop in pressure because the volume was contributing to pressure. The result is an end-diastolic dip in pressure that reduces the impedance to the next systolic ejection. The end-diastolic pressure without the balloon assistance should be compared to the end-diastolic pressure with the dip created by balloon deflation. Optimally, a pressure difference of at least 10 mm Hg should be obtained. Better afterload reduction is achieved with the lowest possible end-diastolic dip.

The point of deflation also is crucial. Deflation that is too early will allow pressure to rise to normal end-diastolic levels preceding systole. In this situation, there will be no decrease in afterload. Very early deflation actually may have a "sink-like" effect on the aortic root, impairing coronary perfusion because blood is distracted to the area of the pressure drop. Late deflation will encroach on the next systole and actually increase afterload owing to greater impedance to ejection from the presence of the still inflated balloon during systolic ejection.

Step 5. Finally, if afterload has been reduced, the next systolic pressure peak will be lower than the unassisted systolic pressure peak. This implies that the ventricle did not have to generate as great a pressure to overcome impedance to ejection. This may not be seen always because the systolic pressure peak also represents the compliance of the vasculature. If the vasculature is noncompliant due to atherosclerotic disease, the systolic peak may not change very much. Figure 13–37 illustrates the five points that are assessed on the waveform; Figure 13–38 demonstrates possible errors in timing.

Balloon fit. The fit of the balloon to any particular patient's aorta will determine how well these criteria are met. Ideally, approximately 80% of the aorta is occluded with balloon inflation. Any occlusion greater than this may damage aortic tissue. Occasionally, the larger balloon cannot be threaded through the femoral or iliac arteries, so a smaller balloon must be used. In this situation, the effect of inflation and deflation will not be as dramatic on the waveform. When a patient is hypotensive or hypovolemic, the balloon will not have as pronounced an effect on the waveform because there is less volume displacement as the balloon inflates or deflates.

Assessment and Management

Patients requiring IABP are managed much like any other critically ill patient in cardiogenic shock or acute left ventricular failure. Nursing assessment and management of these conditions are discussed in Chapters 14 and 15. There are additional nursing skills and assessment considerations specific to IABP therapy that must be included in the care of these patients. Nursing Care Plan 13–3 outlines interventions unique to patients receiving IAPB therapy. Other diagnoses common to patients in heart failure or cardiogenic shock also may be appropriate.

Cardiovascular System

Monitoring the cardiovascular system is extremely important in determining the effectiveness of balloon pump therapy. The basis for this assessment includes vital signs,

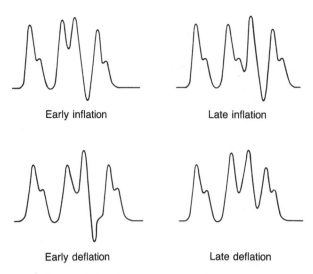

FIGURE 13–38
Illustration of possible errors occurring with timing.

cardiac output, heart rhythm and regularity, urine output, color, perfusion, and mentation.

Vital Signs

Three important vital signs with respect to IABP are heart rate, MAP, and PCWP.

Because timing of the balloon pump is based on *heart rate*, any variation of heart rate may affect the performance of the balloon pump significantly. Any variation in heart rate of 10 or more beats necessitates an evaluation and possible readjustment of inflation and deflation timing. Large variations in heart rate also may indicate a change in the overall clinical status. Newer balloon pump consoles have the capability to self-adjust for changes in heart rate, but the nurse needs to be aware that changes are occurring as fine adjustments may be required.

Mean arterial blood pressure should improve with effective IABP support. An acute change in MAP may require a quick evaluation of timing and then a further assessment of other vital signs. In such cases, patients tolerate very little change in volume status, and an acute drop in MAP also may indicate volume depletion.

The *PCWP* is an important parameter for monitoring volume status. It will provide an early indication of volume depletion or volume overload.

Blood pressure readings require special consideration. Because the balloon inflates during diastole, peak-diastolic pressure may be higher than peak-systolic pressure. It is important to remember that some monitoring equipment cannot distinguish systole from diastole, but only peak pressures from low-point pressures. For this reason, a monitor digital display of systolic pressure actually may represent peak-diastolic pressure. It is advisable to record blood pressure as systolic, peak-diastolic, and end-diastolic—that is, 100/110/60. These pressures can be read from a strip recording of the arterial waveform. Most

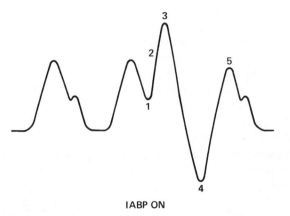

FIGURE 13–37
Inspection of the arterial waveform with intra-aortic balloon assistance should include observation of 1) inflation point; 2) inflation slope; 3) diastolic peak pressure; 4) end-diastolic dip; 5) next systolic peak.

recent-model IABP consoles have monitoring systems capable of distinguishing systole from peak diastole.

Heart Rhythm and Regularity

Heart rhythm and regularity also are important considerations. Early recognition and treatment of *dysrhythmias* are crucial not only for safety but also for effective IABP support. Irregular dysrhythmias may inhibit efficient IABP therapy because timing is set by the regular RR interval on the ECG. A safety feature of all balloon pump consoles is automatic deflation of the balloon for premature QRS complexes. Any patient in whom a bigeminal rhythm develops will then lose 50% of the balloon assistance. If the dysrhythmia persists, another alternative might be use of the systolic peak on the arterial waveform as the trigger mechanism for balloon inflation. A key issue to remember with dysrhythmias is that the primary goal is to treat the dysrhythmia. Pacing may be indicated when a heart rhythm is very irregular.

Other Observations

Urine output, *color*, *perfusion*, and *mentation* all are important assessment parameters for determining the adequacy of cardiac output. Any deterioration in these signs also might indicate a fall in cardiac output. If the patient is responding to IABP therapy, these signs also should show improvement. Cardiac output measurement is indicated when deterioration is evident or when a major change in volume or pharmacologic therapy has been instituted. Monitoring the patient's ability to maintain cardiac output also is important during weaning procedures from IABP support.

Special attention should be given to the *left radial pulse*. A decrease, absence, or change in character of the left radial pulse may indicate that the balloon has advanced up the aorta and may be partially obstructing the left subclavian artery, or has advanced into this artery.

The presence of the balloon catheter in the femoral or iliac artery predisposes the patient to impaired circulation of the involved extremity. The extremity cannulated with the catheter will need to be kept relatively immobile. Any flexion of the hip may kink the catheter and impair balloon pumping. Hip flexion also contributes to decreased perfusion to the distal extremity. Extremities should be checked hourly for pulses, color, and sensation. Any deterioration in the affected extremity should be reported to the physician. Severe arterial insufficiency will necessitate the removal of the catheter. Patients should be encouraged to flex their feet frequently every hour to avoid venous stasis. If they are unable to do this, the nurse can do it for them. Another alternative is the use of sequential compression devices.

Some physicians advocate the use of heparin therapy to prevent possible thrombus formation around the catheter and vascular insufficiency. Each physician will determine whether the risks of anticoagulation outweigh the benefits for the specific patient. If anticoagulation is used, it is advisable to perform a guaiac test periodically on nasogastric drainage and stools for the presence of blood. Observation of *urine* for hematuria, *skin* for petechiae, and any *incisions* for oozing of blood also should be part of the assessment. If any of these are noted, the physician should be alerted. Heparin therapy may require adjustment or possible reversal with protamine sulfate. Low-molecular weight dextran is another possible choice of therapy to prevent thrombus formation. This agent impairs platelet function and prevents triggering of the coagulation cascade.

Pulmonary System

Most patients on IABP therapy will require intubation and ventilatory assistance. Many will have some degree of respiratory insufficiency as the result of the fluid overload associated with cardiac failure. Any intubated patient has an increased risk for *respiratory tract infection*. This risk increases greatly in the debilitated patient. Invasive hemodynamic monitoring catheters and the balloon catheter will restrict mobility, requiring modification in turning. This relative immobility may increase the risk of *atelectasis*. Turning is appropriate as long as the extremity with the balloon catheter is kept straight. It may be helpful to use a knee brace on the affected extremity to remind the patient to avoid flexion of the hip. For the same reason, the head of the bed cannot be elevated more than 30°. In addition, elevation may cause the catheter to advance up the aorta.

Some patients might require horizontal lifting for placement of a chest radiography film when portable roentgenograms are taken. Daily chest roentgenograms are needed to follow pulmonary status and to inspect IV catheter placement. The position of the balloon catheter also can be determined in this manner.

Renal System

Patients in cardiogenic shock are at risk for the development of acute renal failure. In the shock state, the kidneys suffer the consequences of a hypoperfused state. Urine output and quality should be monitored closely. Serum levels of blood urea nitrogen and creatine are included in daily laboratory studies to monitor renal function. It is advisable to study creatine clearance in addition to serum creatine. Creatine clearance will indicate renal dysfunction and possible failure much earlier than elevated serum creatine. Serum creatine also does not rise until significant renal function is lost. Any acute, dramatic drop in urine output might be an indication that the catheter has slipped down the aorta and is obstructing the renal arteries. A portable roentgenogram can confirm this suspicion. Predisposition to urinary tract infection is present with indwelling Foley catheters. Good catheter hygiene and maintenance of an acidic urine will help prevent infection.

Psychosocial Problems

Balloon insertion usually is an unplanned, emergent procedure for deteriorating conditions. Abundant monitoring is frightening for both the patient and family. Every effort should be made to explain surroundings and procedures. The goal is to make them feel more secure in their environment and to alleviate anxiety.

Family members need to be prepared for the first visit after balloon insertion. Good preparation helps them deal with the stress of the situation and be more supportive of their loved one. Honest communication with the family is very important. This helps them interpret the situation realistically and view changes in the patient's condition with appropriate significance. Families also will be carrying the responsibility of making decisions about the patient's care. It often is helpful to provide contact with another nonmedical personnel member, such as a social worker or clergyman; these people can provide additional support to the family. Sometimes it is easier to express feelings of hopelessness or fear of the family member's death when dealing with a person who is not directly involved in the care.

Critically ill people often suffer from sleep deprivation and disorientation. Immobility and unfamiliar noises and machinery also increase stress and anxiety. Frequent orientation by staff and family visits can help alleviate some of this stress. Good care planning can help organize procedures such as suctioning, turning, and dressing changes so that patients receive longer periods of uninterrupted rest.

Other Parameters

Nutrition should be an early consideration to promote healing and strength. Hyperalimentation can be instituted to provide nutrients and essential vitamins. Tube feedings also might be considered for those who are able to tolerate them.

Infection is a major problem in the debilitated patient. Thus, it is extremely important to maintain sterile technique, particularly in relation to the dressing over the balloon catheter exit site. In patients with a Dacron graft lying beneath subcutaneous tissue, the risk of wound infection increases. Once bacteria lodge in the graft, infection is relatively impossible to treat. Intravenous antibiotics have little effect because the graft has no blood supply. Once the wound is infected, the graft must be removed for successful treatment. For that reason, dressings should be changed with sterile gloves and, ideally, a sterile mask. Dressings should be kept clean and dry. In some institutions, sterile, occlusive dressings are used for this type of wound care.

Weaning

Indications for Weaning

Weaning patients from balloon assistance generally can begin 24 to 48 hours after insertion. Some patients will require longer periods of support. Weaning can begin when there is evidence of *hemodynamic stability*. A patient should not require excessive vasopressor support to maintain hemodynamic stability. Ideally, vasopressor support is minimal when weaning begins. After the balloon is removed, it is much easier to increase vasopressor support than to reinsert a balloon catheter for hemodynamic support. Each physician will determine his or her own criteria for hemodynamic stability. General guidelines might include a cardiac index greater than 2 L/minute, a PCWP less than 20 mm Hg, and a systolic blood pressure greater than 100 mm Hg.

The patient should exhibit signs of *adequate cardiac function*, demonstrated by good peripheral pulses, adequate urine output, absence of pulmonary edema, and improved mentation. *Good coronary artery perfusion* will be evidenced by an absence of ventricular ectopy and no evidence of ischemia or injury on the ECG.

Complications may require abrupt cessation of IABP. This may or may not result in reinsertion of another balloon catheter. Severe arterial insufficiency evidenced by a loss of pulses in the distal extremity, pain, and pallor is definitely an indication to remove the balloon catheter from that particular insertion site. Any balloon that develops a leak also requires removal, for obvious reasons. The physician may choose to reinsert the balloon catheter in another extremity or to replace the faulty balloon if the patient is hemodynamically unstable. Depending on the philosophy of the institution and physician, a deteriorating, irreversible situation also might be an indication for weaning or discontinuing balloon pump support. Display Box 13–8 lists major indications for weaning from IABP therapy.

Approaches to Weaning

Weaning may be achieved by any combination of the approaches listed in Display Box 13–9. The first likely step would be to decrease the assist ratio from 1:1 to 1:2 and so on, until the minimum assist ratio is achieved on any particular console. A patient might be assisted at the first decrease for up to 4 to 6 hours. The minimum amount of time should be 30 minutes. During this time, the patient must be assessed for any change in hemodynamic status. An increasing heart rate with decreasing

---

DISPLAY BOX 13–8
Indications for Weaning From IABP

- Hemodynamic stability
  Cardiac index >2 L/min
  PCWP <20 mm Hg
  Systolic blood pressure >100 mm Hg
- Minimal requirements for vasopressor support
- Evidence of adequate cardiac function
  Good peripheral pulses
  Adequate urine output
  Absence of pulmonary edema
  Improved mentation
- Evidence of good coronary perfusion
  Absence of ventricular ectopy
  Absence of ischemia on the ECG
- Severe vascular insufficiency
- Balloon leakage
- Deteriorating, irreversible condition

---

blood pressure indicates a deterioration in hemodynamic status. Cardiac output also is assessed at this time. A decrease in cardiac output or any evidence listed previously indicates that the patient is not tolerating the weaning. Weaning should be discontinued temporarily. Therapy may be adjusted before another weaning attempt. If the first decrease in assist ratio is tolerated, the assist ratio is decreased to minimum, with 1 to 4 hours allowed for each new assist ratio. Again, the patient must be assessed continually for any indications of intolerance to the process.

Another approach, which might be used in conjunction with decreasing assist ratio, is decrease of diastolic augmentation. This will result in decreased aortic root pressure, which should be tolerated by the patient who is ready for weaning. At this time, and also during decreasing assist ratio, the ECG is monitored for any ST segment changes. In addition, a return of angina is an indication that this procedure is not being tolerated.

The preceding steps may be all that are required to assess the patient's ability to maintain hemodynamic stability without IABP.

DISPLAY BOX 13–9
Approaches to Weaning From IABP

- Gradually decrease assist ratio
- Decrease diastolic augmentation

Removal of the Balloon Catheter

Before removal, the patient is heparinized if he or she has not been on anticoagulant therapy. After the balloon catheter has been removed, a Fogarty catheter may be passed proximally to the aortic bifurcation and distally to the popliteal artery. The purpose of this procedure is to remove any clot formation that may be present and to prevent thromboembolic complications. If a graft has been used, it is removed, and the arteriotomy is closed with either a Dacron or saphenous vein patch. The patch secures hemostasis and decreases the potential for late femoral artery or iliac artery stenosis. Graft removal will be done in the operating room, whereas removal of a catheter inserted percutaneously can be done at the bedside. If the balloon was inserted percutaneously, direct pressure will be applied for up to 30 minutes, followed by placement of a 5-lb sandbag to the site. The sandbag will be kept in place for at least 1 hour after catheter removal. After removal, the patient will require frequent assessment of perfusion to the distal extremity.

Complications

Compartment Syndrome

Intra-aortic balloon pump counterpulsation patients need to be monitored for development of poor blood flow to the cannulated extremity, which could lead to compartment syndrome. It may occur within the first 24 hours of support or not until several days after catheter insertion. Compartment syndrome is caused by a rise in the tissue pressure in one of the compartments of the affected lower extremity. Bone, muscle, nerve tissue, and blood vessels all are enclosed by a fibrous membrane called the fascia, and this enclosed space is called a compartment. It is nonyielding, so a rise in volume in the compartment will increase the pressure in the compartment. The IABP patient in whom limb ischemia develops from decreased capillary flow can suffer cellular and capillary damage that leads to increased capillary permeability. The resultant transudation of fluid into the closed compartment space increases tissue pressure to a level that can interfere with capillary blood flow. When this degree of tissue pressure is reached, tissue viability may be threatened. Treatment is directed at improving blood flow. Pressure release by fasciotomy may be needed to prevent tissue death.

Blood Count Changes

Decreased circulating platelets in the first 24 hours of IABP and a minimal decrease in red blood cell count have been reported; however, they are not thought to be significant problems. There is a low incidence of balloon leakage and rupture. These complications might result from balloon inflation against a calcific, atherosclerotic plaque in the aorta. This disruption in the balloon surface may be as small as a pinhole or may be a large tear. The associated danger is gas embolism.

Infection

A complication of any catheter insertion is the possibility of infection at the insertion site. This can be a considerable problem in the unstable, critically ill patient because of the necessity of catheter removal. The advantages of IABP, however, clearly outweigh the risks associated with its use for appropriately selected patients.

Other Problems

Insertion of the catheter in the face of severe atherosclerotic vascular disease might result in arterial perforation or occlusion. Iatrogenic dissection of the aorta is rare but has been reported. Arterial insufficiency is the most common complication of IABP. Arterial insufficiency may be permanent, or it may possibly be relieved by aortofemoral or ileofemoral bypass grafting. Neuropathy in the catheterized extremity is another reported complication.

Troubleshooting

Conduction Problems

Some console units require a separate set of ECG leads for input into the trigger mechanism; others can be jacked into the primary bedside monitor, requiring only one set of ECG leads. The nurse should be familiar with the capabilities of the particular console. Maintenance of good conduction through the skin is important.

Any ECG artifact will interfere with the console's ability to recognize the trigger, or R wave, and will result in ineffective assistance. Any interference will cause an automatic deflation of the balloon. If the amplitude of the R wave is too low to trigger effectively, this can be corrected by changing lead placement. Low ECG voltage may necessitate the use of a pacemaker spike as the trigger mechanism. Many newer models of IABP consoles are capable of using ventricular pacemaker spikes even when AV sequential pacing is in use. The console recognizes the ventricular spike by distinguishing between it and the atrial spike. It recognizes that the ventricular spike follows the shortest spike-to-spike interval (atrial spike to ventricular spike versus ventricular spike to atrial spike).

A cardiac arrest due to ventricular fibrillation or asystole will not provide a trigger for IABP. In this situation, the machine can be turned off; however, it should not be left off for more than 5 minutes because this likely will result in platelet aggregation and thrombus formation on the balloon. It is suggested that the arterial systolic peak be used as the trigger. Cardiopulmonary resuscitation will generate a systolic pressure peak that can be used as a trigger. Cardioversion or defibrillation can be performed while the machine remains on. The machines are insulated so that this electric current will not damage the internal mechanisms. Tachycardias also may impair pumping ability. Often, switching the machine to a 1:2 assist will enable it to follow the rapid rate with increased effectiveness. Most newer machines are capable of effectively tracking rates up to 120.

Balloon Problems

A small amount of gas normally will diffuse out of the balloon. This necessitates that the balloon be evacuated and filled periodically. Normally, this is required approximately every 2 hours. Some consoles do this automatically, whereas others require manual refilling by the nurse. Loss of balloon volume will be evident when the diastolic pressure peak and end-diastolic dip begin to decrease. Any increase in frequency required for refilling might suggest a leak in the catheter or balloon. Normal diffusion of gas should be only 1 to 2 cc/hour. Rarely, a balloon may develop a leak. Initially, a loss in balloon effectiveness will be noted; eventually, blood will back up into the catheter. The physician should be notified immediately because the faulty balloon will have to be removed to avoid the possibility of gas embolus. In this situation, it is important to keep the balloon moving slightly. The frequency of inflation should be decreased to the absolute minimum. A major rupture of the balloon, detected by a rush of arterial blood back into the tubing, is an indication to turn the IABP off. Again, it must be remembered that the balloon cannot sit idle because thrombus formation will occur. This situation is an emergency, and immediate balloon removal is indicated.

Vacuum Problems

Each machine will have an alarm system that will alert the nurse to any loss of vacuum. The vacuum is responsible for deflation of the balloon. Any decrease in vacuum will interfere with the balloon's ability to deflate; however, a loss of pressure from the compressor pump will interfere with effective inflation. Any fault in the drive system (the vacuum or compressor) requires that the console be changed. The malfunctioning console then should be inspected by a biomedical engineer or the service representative from the particular manufacturer.

Nursing Care Plan

Nursing Care Plan 13–3 summarizes the important aspects of care for the patient undergoing IABP.

(Text continues on page 283)

NURSING CARE PLAN 13–3:
The Patient Undergoing IABP Therapy

NURSING DIAGNOSIS	OUTCOME CRITERIA/ PATIENT GOALS	NURSING INTERVENTIONS

High risk for decreased cardiac output: related to improper or ineffective IABP timing.	• Maintenance of hemodynamic stability as demonstrated by proper waveforms.	1. Place assist ratio on 1:2 and verify correct IABP timing hourly.
		2. Document IABP settings hourly to illustrate trends and improvement.
		3. Reevaluate timing for any increase or decrease in heart rate greater than 10 beats/min.
		4. Maintain proper balloon volume.
		5. Refill balloon every 2–4 hr as needed. Use automatic filling mode if available.
		6. Maintain good arterial waveform to allow for evaluation of timing. Notify physician if line starts to fail so a new line can be inserted.
		7. Reduce or eliminate situations which will interfere with the IABPs ability to maintain proper assist ratio.
		  • Maintain adequate ECG signal.
		  • Alert physician if irregular heart rhythms or rapid tachycardias occur.
		  • Initiate pacing or antiarrhythmic drug therapy as ordered.
		8. Avoid flexion of hip, which may impair gas movement in and out of IABP catheter.

High risk for altered peripheral perfusion: decreased related to impaired circulation in lower extremity related to presence of catheter, emboli, or thrombosis.	• Patient will have palpable peripheral pulses with skin that is warm, dry, and of normal color.	1. Document quality of peripheral pulses before IABP insertion. 2. Assess peripheral pulses, skin temperature, and color hourly and document. 3. Notify physician of any decrease in pulses. 4. Maintain anticoagulation at prescribed level. 5. Maintain head of bed at a 15° angle or lower to avoid hip flexion, which might obstruct distal flow in the cannulated leg.

(continued)

NURSING CARE PLAN 13–3: (Continued)
The Patient Undergoing IABP Therapy

NURSING DIAGNOSIS	*OUTCOME CRITERIA/ PATIENT GOALS*	*NURSING INTERVENTIONS*
		6. Maintain cannulated leg in a straight position to avoid hip flexion. Restrain or brace as needed.
		7. Maintain balloon motion to prevent thrombus formation on balloon.
		8. Assist patient with ankle flexion and extension hourly to promote venous return and prevent venous stasis and potential deep venous thrombosis.
		9. Immediately evaluate peripheral perfusion with any complaints of leg/foot pain by patient.
High risk for impaired gas exchange: related to immobility, sedation, and secretions.	• Oxygenation will be normal, as evidenced by arterial blood gases.	1. Auscultate breath sounds every 2–4 hr and document.
		2. Assist patient with clearing of secretions by coughing or suctioning as indicated.
		3. If intubated, suction at least every 2 hr.
		4. Turn patient every 2 hr.
		5. Obtain order for pulse oximetry if patient has abnormal blood gases, excessive secretions, or respiratory difficulty.
High risk for sensory–perceptual alterations: sensory overload related to critical care unit environment.	• Patient will maintain orientation to name, time, and date and will be able to communicate appropriately.	1. Maintain alarm volumes and monitor noise to lowest possible levels.
		2. Minimize unnecessary noise in patient's room.
		3. Talk with patient frequently and inform of time and date.
		4. Encourage family visits.
		5. Explain all procedures, noises, and activities so that patient interprets them appropriately.
High risk for impaired skin integrity: related to immobility, debilitated condition, and impaired circulation.	• Maintenance of normal skin integrity.	1. Assess skin integrity every 2–4 hr and document any redness or ulcerations over bony prominences.
		2. Elevate any edematous extremities (only slightly if cannulated extremity is involved).

(continued)

NURSING CARE PLAN 13–3: (Continued)
The Patient Undergoing IABP Therapy

NURSING DIAGNOSIS	OUTCOME CRITERIA/ PATIENT GOALS	NURSING INTERVENTIONS
		3. Place sheepskin or foam pad over mattress. Obtain order for air–fluid bed if needed.
		4. Turn patient every 2 hr.
		5. Massage and lubricate skin exposed to pressure with each repositioning.
		6. Ensure that skin remains clean and dry.
		7. Maintain adequate nutrition by obtaining order for hyperalimentation or nasogastric feedings.
High risk for sleep pattern disturbance: related to critical illness, procedures, and constant monitoring of physiological parameters.	• Patient will have planned blocks of time for undisturbed sleep.	1. Turn down lights in the room during night.
		2. Organize care to allow for progressive increases in uninterrupted time for sleep during night. Amount to be determined by patient condition.
		3. Sedation given patient, as ordered by physician.
High risk for infection: related to a number of indwelling catheters and debilitated condition.	• Patient will remain afebrile, with a normal white blood cell count and negative cultures.	1. Monitor and record temperature every 2 hr.
		2. Observe all insertion sites and incisions daily for signs of infection with dressing changes.
		3. Report any elevation of white blood cell count to physician.
		4. Maintain sterile technique with dressing changes.
		5. Change any dressing that becomes wet or is not intact.
		6. Change all infusion lines, stopcocks, and infusions as per unit protocol.
		7. Culture any site with suspicious drainage, redness, or swelling.
		8. Give antibiotic, as ordered by physician.

Other Ventricular Assist Devices

Description

Since the introduction of IABP therapy, many advances have been made in the development of ventricular assist devices (VADs) that are capable of providing more significant or total support of left ventricular function. Intra-aortic balloon pump counterpulsation therapy is capable of augmenting a patient's cardiac output only by 8% to 12%. In many instances, this level of support will be inadequate and a device capable of temporarily replacing left ventricular function will be needed. Three types of VADs have come into common use in the last decade. These include centrifugal pumps, which are widely used, and pulsatile pumps, which are driven by either a pneumatic or an electrical system. Patients requiring such support include those who have cardiogenic shock after major acute myocardial infarction, cardiac surgery patients who cannot be weaned from cardiopulmonary bypass with the support of IABP therapy alone, and patients with end-stage heart disease who are waiting for donor hearts for transplantation. In the latter group, it is not uncommon for patients to have to wait for periods that exceed 30 days. Since the IABP is designed for short-term support and cannot totally assist the left ventricle, it is not always the best choice for patients in end-stage disease whose condition is deteriorating.

Physiological Principles

Centrifugal Pumps

Centrifugal pumps work by bringing blood from the left atrium through a cannula to a pump located outside the body. The blood in the pump is rotated at high speed by a rotating impeller that is controlled by an opposing rotating magnet. The faster the magnet spins, the more kinetic energy is generated inside the pump, which drives blood forward, back to the patient. Blood returns to the ascending aorta through another, separate cannula. Pumps of this type create linear blood flow with no systole or diastole. They do not generate pulsatile blood flow. A continuous arterial pressure is maintained at an optimal level for organ perfusion. The left ventricle is bypassed totally and is not required to generate its usual high pressures. When the ventricle has been bypassed, it can be given time to recover from injury with minimal work requirements. A commonly used pump in this category is the Biomedicus centrifugal pump (Eden Prairie, MN).

Pulsatile Pumps

Pulsatile pumps can be implanted temporarily in the abdomen or be located outside the body. Pulsatile pumps also are capable of taking over total left ventricular work requirements. Blood is directed to these pumps through cannulas placed in the left atrium or the left ventricular apex. After passing through the pump, blood is returned to the ascending aorta. Pulsatile pumps all will have inflow and outflow valves that keep blood moving in a forward direction. When blood enters the pump, it fills a blood sac inside the rigid housing of the pump. When filled, the blood sac is collapsed by either a pneumatic or electrical mechanism that forces the blood out of the sac and into the return cannula. This action creates a systolic blood pressure. Diastolic pressure is created as blood flows into smaller vessels and the pressure in the aorta falls. Compression and ejection of blood from the blood sac can be timed to synchronize with the patient's cardiac cycle by using the R wave of the ECG or by using the sensing mechanisms in the pump, which are capable of determining when maximal filling of the blood sac has occurred. Most pumps also will have an ability to pump in a fixed-rate mode. The preferred method of pumping is to use the sensing capabilities that detect maximal filling. The ventricle may still contract; however, only minimal pressures from the ventricle are required to fill the pump because the pump offers no resistance to filling when it is empty. During this time of support, the ventricle can rest and potentially recover from its injury. These pumps can operate for several months if necessary and are capable of supporting a patient waiting for transplant for as long as necessary. An example of a pneumatic pulsatile pump that is commonly used is the Pierce-Donachy Thoratec pump (Berkeley, CA). A widely used electrically driven pump capable of being implanted is the Novacor (Novacor Biomedical, Oakland, CA) left ventricular assist system.

Assessment and Management

All patients on VADs have some nursing care issues in common. Because all of these require cardiopulmonary bypass for placement, bleeding is a common problem postinsertion. Patients also must be anticoagulated at some point to prevent thrombus formation in the pump, cannulas, and resting ventricle. Because these patients have extensive invasive monitoring lines and large surgical incisions, and may have their pump located outside the body, they are at extremely high risk for infection. Good aseptic technique for dressing changes and astute observation of wounds and cannula exit sites are important nursing functions for the prevention and early recognition of infection. Patients with more serious left ventricular failure also may have some degree of right ventricular failure. It is important that this is recognized and treated early because the output from the left-sided pump is totally dependent on how well the right ventricle contracts and moves blood forward over to the left side of the heart and to the VAD. Because this patient has undergone a major surgical intervention, pain management will be a major nursing focus during the first several days of assist.

Many other nursing care issues are similar to those encountered with IABP patients. Those issues include potential for thrombus formation, and potential problems related to immobility, sensory alterations, sleep deprivation, and inadequate nutritional intake. The nursing care plan for the IABP patient can be used as a basis for developing a plan of care for the more complicated VAD patient (see Nursing Care Plan 13–3).

Autologous Blood Transfusion

Behavioral Objectives

Description

Physiological Principles

Homologous Blood

Autologous Blood

Equipment Features

Indications and Advantages

Safety

  Elimination of Disease Transmission

  Elimination of Transfusion Reaction

  Absence of Anticoagulants

Availability of Blood

Reduction of Religious Objections

Cost Effectiveness

Contraindications

Procedure

Predeposit Phlebotomy (Autodonation or Predonation)

Intraoperative Autotransfusion

Preoperative Phlebotomy With Hemodilution

Perioperative and Emergency Autotransfusion

  Postoperative Autotransfusion

  Wound Drainage Reinfusion

  Emergency Autotransfusion

Continuous Reinfusion Method

Regional Anticoagulants

Assessment and Management

General Measures

Laboratory Studies

Record Keeping

Anticoagulation

Complications

Coagulopathy

Troubleshooting

Summary

Nursing Care Plan: The Patient Undergoing Autologous Blood Transfusion

BEHAVIORAL OBJECTIVES

Based on the content in this section, the reader should be able to:

1. Define *autologous blood transfusion*.
2. List five indications for autologous blood transfusion.
3. Explain four methods of autotransfusion.
4. Describe the nursing assessments and interventions necessary for the patient undergoing autotransfusion.

Description

Autologous blood transfusion (autotransfusion) is the collection, filtration, and reinfusion of the patient's own (autologous) blood. The purpose of autotransfusion is to avoid or decrease the requirements for bank homologous blood and its potential complications. Autologous blood is the safest type of blood for transfusion when guidelines established by the American Association of Blood Banks are followed. Autotransfusion eliminates risks associated with homologous (bank blood) transfusion, such as the transmission of donor-related diseases, including hepatitis (5%–10% of patients with homologous transfusions), acquired immune deficiency syndrome (AIDS), malaria, syphilis, and immunoviruses (cytomegalovirus and Epstein–Barr viruses).[37–39] Autotransfusion is cost effective and saves bank blood for use when no other alternative is available. Although reported by Blundell in 1818 and performed successfully in 1914, autotransfusion has gained widespread use and acceptance only since technologic advances were made in response to advances in open heart surgery that increased the demand for blood in the 1970s.

Because postoperative bleeding in cardiothoracic surgical patients can be significant, postoperative as well as intraoperative autotransfusion systems were developed. Although associated primarily with perioperative cardiovascular management, autotransfusion is used widely in other areas with requirements for large volumes of blood replacement, such as trauma care. Recent advances include the use of autotransfusion in orthopedic procedures such as hip fractures, spinal fusion, and hip, knee, and shoulder arthroplasty procedures that require an average transfusion volume exceeding 1 unit.

The addition of autologous perioperative plasmapheresis facilitates complete autotransfusion of both washed red blood cells and platelet-rich plasma, significantly reducing the need for supplemental use of homologous components. Both whole blood and component autotransfusion now are well accepted procedures that in many instances are lifesaving.

Physiological Principles

Homologous Blood

Homologous blood transfusion is the transfer or transplantation of living tissue from one person to another. All homologous blood products carry the risk of disease transmission and transfusion reactions. In 1989, the risk of hepatitis transmission was estimated at 1 person in 100, with human immunodeficiency virus transmission ranging between 1 in 40,000 to 1 in one million.[40] Although the development of sensitivity screening of donor blood for the presence of the HTLV-3 antibodies has reduced the incidence of the AIDS virus in bank blood, it has not eliminated transmission of the virus. Patients continue to have a high level of anxiety related to disease transmission by exposure to homologous blood. Reactions to homologous transfusion, which can occur with as little as 10 to 15 ml of incompatible blood, include hemolytic reactions, transfusion-induced graft-versus-host disease, hemoglobinuria, purpura, fever, circulatory overload, thrombophlebitis, urticaria, hyperkalemia, asymptomatic hemoglobinuria, pulmonary edema, and allergic and anaphylactic reactions.[41]

Autologous Blood

Autologous blood is considered the safest type of blood for transfusion in most patients for a variety of reasons, including elimination of disease transmission and elimination of transfusion reaction. In addition, the quality of autologous blood is morphologically, physiologically, and biochemically superior to that of homologous blood.

Because all blood components are damaged to some degree by storage, it is recommended that fresh autologous blood be reinfused within 6 hours of initial collection or discarded.[42]

Platelets in autologous blood remain viable with nearly normal platelet count and function, whereas platelets in stored blood become nonviable within 24 hours.

2,3-Diphosphoglycerate (DPG), which is essential to adequate tissue oxygenation, is within normal levels in fresh autologous blood. Bank blood shows a decreased amount of 2,3-DPG stored in the red blood cells, with blood stored more than 10 days containing no 2,3-DPG. This results in a shift to the left in the oxyhemoglobin dissociation curve that leads to impairment of oxygen transfer at the tissue level.

Fresh autotransfused erythrocytes have a near-normal survival time. Also, levels of clotting factors V (labile factor), VIII (antihemophilic factor), and IX (Christmas factor) remain near normal in autologous blood but not in bank blood. In addition, autologous blood has normal partial thromboplastin time and potassium and ammonia levels, and is near body temperature.

Red blood cells in stored blood lose their wall integrity, causing potassium leakage and an increase in serum potassium.

It has been suggested that patients receiving autologous blood transfusion have a lower incidence of postoperative bacterial infections than those receiving homologous transfusions.[43] This may be attributed to diminished host defenses secondary to immunologic differences between a donor and recipient of homologous transfusion. One study showed a postoperative infection rate of 32% in patients receiving 2 or 3 units of homologous blood, compared to 3% in patients transfused with 2 to 3 units of autologous blood.[43] The use of autologous blood during surgery may provide a means of reducing morbidity due to infection.

Defibrinogenated blood aspirated from the mediastinum, such as during hemothorax drainage or after surgery, is devoid of fibrinogen with prolonged prothrombin (activity 30%–50% of normal) and partial thromboplastin time and increased levels of fibrin split products. Values usually return to normal by the second postoperative day.

Hemolysis, the primary effect of autotransfusion systems on blood, causes a reduction in hematocrit, an increase in serum and urine hemoglobin, and accumulation of erythrocyte debris. Correct collection techniques, filtration, and washing procedures reduce the risk of associated pathophysiology.

Equipment Features

A variety of autologous blood transfusion systems (ATS) are available for whole blood autotransfusion and component (washed or processed) autotransfusion (Figs. 13–39 and 13–40). Whole blood autotransfusion is used most

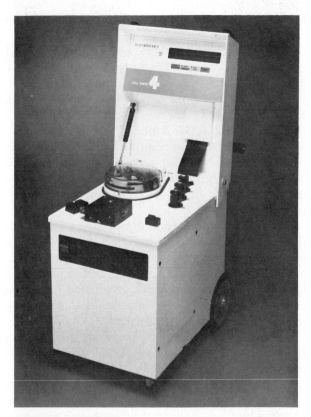

FIGURE 13–39
Cell Saver® 4 system for washed red cell autotransfusion. (Courtesy of Haemonetics® Corporation, Braintree, MA.)

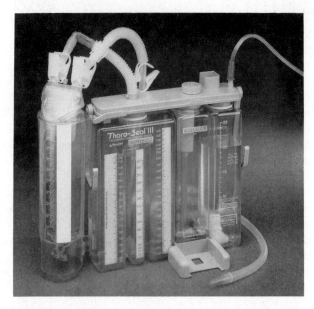

FIGURE 13–40
Blood recovery system for autotransfusion with water-seal chest drainage system for collection and reinfusion of shed mediastinal/pleural cavity blood. (Thora-Seal® III Autotransfusion Chest Drainage System. Courtesy of Sherwood Medical, St. Louis, MO.)

frequently with emergency/trauma patients and during the postoperative management of cardiovascular patients. Whole blood systems are easier to set up and use, provide faster access to blood for reinfusion, and return all blood components.

A sterile autotransfusion chest drainage unit is used to collect whole blood from the mediastinal or pleural cavity after surgery and after emergency hemothorax evacuation. The water seal, usually set to provide a constant negative pressure of 20 cm water to the thoracic cavity, provides a visual confirmation of any air leak. The blood from the chest tubes passes through a gross filter within the chest drainage unit to remove clots and gross debris. Because postoperatively shed mediastinal blood usually is defibrinogenated, regional anticoagulant seldom is added to the collection chamber. Regional anticoagulant is added routinely to mediastinal–pleural blood that is not defibrinogenated, such as with emergency hemothorax or postoperative thoracic hemorrhage, where the blood has not remained in the chest cavity long enough to become defibrinogenated. The blood may be reinfused as whole blood using an intermittent or continuous reinfusion technique, or transferred to a cell washer system for processing before reinfusion.

The cell washer–processor is used most commonly in operating rooms, blood banks, and for postoperative orthopedic drainage. A cell washer–processor is a centrifuge device that separates the plasma from the red blood cells. The red blood cells are washed and resuspended in normal saline by continuous centrifugation. Devices that wash red blood cells remove approximately 90% of the debris, irrigating solutions, activated clotting and complement factors, anticoagulants, free hemoglobin, platelet aggregates, and hemolyzed red cells.[44]

In addition to reducing the risk of microemboli, washed–processed blood provides increased hemoglobin and hematocrit secondary to volume reduction.

Enteric contamination is reduced, but not eliminated, by cell washing. Blood leaving the operating room for processing should be labeled.

Blood parameters that remain relatively unchanged by cell washing include mean corpuscular volume and 2,3-DPG levels. There may be a slight drop in white blood cells.

Disadvantages of washed–processed blood include cost, complexity, and time delay as well as loss of clotting factors, white blood cells, plasma proteins, and platelets. Systems now are available for perioperative recovery of platelet-rich plasma, used in conjunction with washed erythrocytes.

Specially trained operators are required for cell washer–processor autologous blood systems. Smaller portable systems with disposable cassettes that are easier and faster to set up are being used more extensively in PACUs and ICUs (Fig. 13–41).

Although orthopedic surgery often was considered a contraindication for the use of autologous blood transfusion, systems specifically designed for use on orthopedic

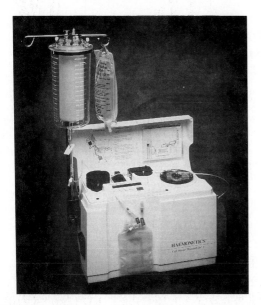

FIGURE 13–41
The availability of compact, portable, easier-to-use, blood-washing equipment has made autotransfusion more accessible in OR, PACU, and ICU areas. This has expanded the use of washed blood in orthopedic and other specialty applications. (HaemoLite® 2. Courtesy of Haemonetics® Corporation, Braintree, MA.)

patients both during surgery and for postoperative wound drainage now are available. It is recommended that blood harvested during orthopedic procedures be washed before reinfusion.[44-46]

Indications and Advantages

Because there are many indications and advantages associated with reinfusing the patient's own blood, candidates for transfusion should be evaluated for autotransfusion. These indications and advantages are discussed subsequently (see Display Box 13–10).

Safety

Elimination of Disease Transmission

The risks of donor-related diseases such as AIDS, hepatitis, malaria, syphilis, cytomegalovirus, and Epstein–Barr virus are avoided.

Elimination of Transfusion Reaction

Autologous blood is type specific and crossmatch compatible. This eliminates the hemolytic, febrile, allergic, or graft-versus-host reactions sometimes associated with homologous (bank) blood. In addition, there is no risk of isoimmunization to erythrocyte, leukocyte, platelet, or protein antigens.

Bank blood is associated with a 5% risk of serious

---

transfusion reaction, including deaths secondary to post-transfusion hepatitis and hemolytic reactions. It is estimated that 5% to 10% of bank blood recipients contract post-transfusion hepatitis, with a significant incidence of cirrhosis.

Absence of Anticoagulants

Whereas all bank blood contains anticoagulants, intraoperative (washed) blood and postoperative shed mediastinal autologous blood contain little or no anticoagulants.

Availability of Blood

Because type-matching and crossmatching are not required on autotransfused blood, the blood often is available immediately for initial stabilization of the patient.

Inexpensive systems are available that are simple and fast to set up, eliminating the need for special operators or technicians.

Reduction of Religious Objections

Religious groups whose beliefs forbid transfusion, such as Jehovah's Witnesses, often permit autotransfusion.

Cost Effectiveness

Autotransfusion eliminates the need for type-matching and crossmatching and reduces or eliminates the need for bank blood in selected patients.

Contraindications

Autotransfusion is contraindicated in patients with malignant neoplasms septicemia, intrathoracic infections or infestations, coagulopathies, and renal failure (see Display

---

DISPLAY BOX 13–11
Contraindications to Autotransfusion

- Malignant neoplasm
- Infections and infestations
- Blood contamination
- Coagulopathies
- Excessive hemolysis
- Renal failure

DISPLAY BOX 13–12
Autologous Transfusion Methods

Predeposit phlebotomy: One or more units are collected before an elective surgical procedure for reinfusion during or after the procedure.

Intraoperative autotransfusion: Pooled blood is aspirated from a body cavity during surgery and reinfused.

Perioperative phlebotomy with hemodilution: Blood is collected before a surgical procedure with concomitant replacement by crystalloid or colloid solutions and reinfused later.

Perioperative and emergency autotransfusion: Shed mediastinal blood is salvaged after open heart surgery and traumatic hemothorax and reinfused usually as whole blood. Wound drainage usually is washed before reinfusion.

Box 13–11). The use of a substance such as an antibiotic not suitable for IV use at the injury site, and excessive hemolysis, such as found in injuries more than 6 hours old, also are contraindications to autotransfusion. Predeposit phlebotomy is not done on patients with an infection or during antibiotic therapy. Sepsis could be induced by bacteria growing in the blood bag before reinfusion.

Contamination of the blood with abdominal contents, such as feces, urine, or bile, is a relative contraindication. If bank blood is available, its use is recommended. Cell washing reduces but does not eliminate enteric contamination. When contamination of the blood is suspected, autologous blood is used only if failure to transfuse would be life-threatening.

Procedure

It is recommended that autologous blood be collected and reinfused within 4 to 6 hours of initiating blood collection. Aseptic technique is used with all autotransfusion procedures. A 20- to 40-μm depth or screen microaggregate filter is used for reinfusion so that microaggregate debris (consisting of degenerating platelets, white cells, red cells, fibrin, and fat particles) can be eliminated. Adult respiratory distress syndrome has been reported less frequently with filtered autotransfusion blood than with bank blood.

Display Box 13–12 outlines the various methods of autologous transfusion.

Predeposit Phlebotomy (Autodonation or Predonation)

One or more units of whole blood, red blood cells, plasma, and/or platelets are collected before an elective surgical procedure for retransfusion into the same person during or after the surgical procedure. Standards for autologous blood donors have been established by the American Association of Blood Banks,[42] and, with the exceptions of the 8-week minimum between phlebotomies and differences in age limits, are similar to those for homologous donation. Some centers for predeposit phlebotomy perform the same tests on autologous blood as on homologous. In this way, unused autologous donations can be transferred to the homologous supply.[47] Autologous donations are made at 4- to 7-day intervals beginning up to 42 days before surgery. The last phlebotomy is performed at least 72 hours before the surgery.

The length of time the blood can be stored unfrozen depends on the type of anticoagulant used. Blood with citrate–phosphate–dextrose–adenine (CPDA-1) can be stored unfrozen for up to 35 days. Blood with ADSOL (Adenine, Dextrose/Sodium Chloride, Mannitol; Baxter Healthcare Corp., Deerfield, IL), Nutricel (Miles Pharmaceutical Division, Berkeley, CA), and CPD (Optisol Solution; Terumo Medical Corp., Somerset, NJ) can be stored unfrozen for up to 42 days. If stored autotransfusion blood is unused by the expiration date, rejuvenation fluids can be added to the blood to restore 2,3-DPG levels, and the blood then can be frozen.[47] Frozen autologous blood may be stored for at least 3 years. Once thawed, frozen autologous blood must be washed and reinfused within 24 hours.

Oral iron supplements usually are begun approximately 1 week before the first donation. Some protocols use daily iron supplements, whereas others have maintained adequate hemoglobin levels of about 11 g/dl with hematocrit greater than 34% with 325 mg of ferrous sulfate, three times a day. Autologous blood donors are encouraged to drink fluids before and after phlebotomy. In some instances, IV fluid, usually 0.9% normal saline, is administered to prevent hypovolemia in elderly, cardiac, or underweight patients.[47] Anemia and hypovolemia are potential adverse reactions. Iron supplements usually are continued after the surgical procedure. Unused blood usually is discarded.

Intraoperative Autotransfusion

Intraoperative autotransfusion usually consists of the collection of anticoagulated blood during surgery, cell processing, and the reinfusion of washed, packed red blood cells in the operating room. In selected patients, whole-blood autotransfusion is used.

Pooled blood is aspirated from a body cavity during surgery and reinfused during or after the procedure. This is used most often during thoracic and cardiovascular surgery. Its use also has been reported with gastric liver resection, orthopedic surgery (hip resection), gynecologic surgery (for ruptured ectopic pregnancy), and neurosurgical (spinal fusion) procedures.

Systemic anticoagulation of the patient is used as medically indicated. Regional anticoagulation of the aspirated blood with citrate–phosphate–dextrose (CPD), acid–citrate–dextrose (ACD), or heparin is performed routinely. To keep the operative field dry, a standard suction wand is used in conjunction with the autotransfusion suction wand. For reduction of hemolysis secondary to air–blood interface, pooled blood is aspirated into the autotransfusion system.

Cell washing removes approximately 90% of the contaminants present in whole blood. The American Association of Blood Banks suggests that the hematocrit in washed blood be in the range of 50% to 60%, with the levels of heparin reduced to 0.1 to 0.2 μg/ml.[42]

The processed blood is reinfused according to the standard protocol for the infusion of packed red blood cells. Depending on the patient's cardiovascular status, a unit of red blood cells may be reinfused through an in-line filter over a period of 1.5 to 4 hours.

Preoperative Phlebotomy With Hemodilution

Used primarily with open heart surgery, 1 or 2 units of blood are withdrawn immediately after induction of anesthesia and before heparinization. The blood is replaced with equivalent amounts of crystalloids or colloids, such as Ringer's lactate, 5% serum albumin, or 5% dextran to produce normovolemic anemia. This decreases the blood viscosity, decreasing the workload on the heart and increasing the microcirculation. All blood removed is reinfused into the patient during surgery, usually after reversal of heparin. Because this blood has not been exposed to air, damaged tissue, or cardiopulmonary bypass equipment, it contains labile plasma coagulation factors, platelets, and fresh red blood cells. The patient may be given a diuretic after surgery to lower plasma volume before reinfusion of the autologous blood.

Perioperative and Emergency Autotransfusion

Postoperative Autotransfusion

Postoperative autotransfusion chest drainage systems are used to collect shed mediastinal blood via chest tubes after cardiac surgery. (see Figure 13–40). Multipurpose systems combine standard water-seal chest drainage with a system for collecting, filtering, and reinfusing autologous blood. The autologous blood may be reinfused as whole blood or washed blood. Before initiation of reinfusion, all air is removed from the blood collection system. Anticoagulation usually is not required because mediastinal blood is defibrinogenated by its contact with serosal surfaces and the beating action of the heart.

Although mediastinal blood usually is defibrinogenated, some clotting may occur. The presence of clots in the gross filter is not a contraindication to reinfusion of the shed mediastinal blood. Reinfusion may be expedited by placement of the blood in a pressure administration cuff inflated to a maximum of 150 mm Hg.

The use of anticoagulants may be indicated in patients with rapid blood loss through chest tubes, as with postoperative hemorrhage or hemothorax. With rapid blood loss, the blood may not be in contact with the serosal surfaces of the lung long enough to defibrinogenate.

Wound Drainage Reinfusion

Orthopedic autotransfusion systems are available for postoperative wound drainage. Various-size wound drains are placed during hip, knee, and spinal surgery. The sanguineous wound drainage usually is washed before reinfusion to prevent platelet or complement activation. Activation of the complement cascade and complement-induced granulocyte aggregation may be a mechanism of noncardiogenic pulmonary edema.

Emergency Autotransfusion

Emergency autotransfusion is categorized as postoperative autotransfusion.

Although most commonly used for hemothorax, emergency autotransfusion also can be used in primary injuries of the lungs, liver, chest wall, heart, pulmonary vessels, spleen, kidneys, inferior vena cava, and iliac, portal, and subclavian veins.

Because the source of bleeding is not always apparent in an emergency situation, a regional anticoagulant, most commonly CPD, is added to the collection device before and during blood collection. Although a 7:1 ratio of blood to CPD usually is used, variations in ratio are reported. If the blood is known to be mediastinal in origin and defibrinogenated, regional anticoagulants such as CPD and ACD sometimes are omitted.

Blood usually is collected through chest tubes into a sterile, disposable liner with a gross particulate filter (170 μm) that has been primed with CPD. A vacuum of 10 to 30 mm Hg is maintained so that hemolysis can be reduced. Should there be a loss of vacuum during blood collection, the chest tube must be clamped immediately. Failure to do so may result in pneumothorax. Before discontinuing autotransfusion vacuum, an underwater seal must be established.

During aspiration of blood, the quantity of added anticoagulant is controlled to provide approximately 100 ml of anticoagulant for every 700 ml of blood. This 1:7 ratio is the same "CPD: blood ratio" used in bank blood.

Reinfusion is initiated when all blood is evacuated from the site, when immediate transfusion is clinically indicated, or when the autotransfusion collection liner is full.

A microaggregate (microemboli) filter and recipient set is attached to the disposable autotransfusion collection container, usually a flexible, sterile liner. All air should be removed from the blood container before initiation of reinfusion so that risk of air emboli is reduced.

Blood pumps or pressure administration cuffs may be used to expedite rapid blood infusion.

Although whole blood is used most commonly in an emergency situation, a cell washer–processor may be used in selected patients to salvage the patient's erythrocytes for reinfusion and discard contaminants and debris in the plasma.

Continuous Reinfusion Method

For continuous autotransfusion, an infusion pump is added to the intraoperative or postoperative system. This provides a continuous reinfusion of blood adjusted to the amount of blood loss and need for volume replacement.[37,48] Continuous autotransfusion systems are used most commonly during short periods of high-volume blood loss. When used with an intraoperative cell-washing system, the blood collected in the reservoir is reinfused continuously through a microaggregate filter located in the collection chamber. A three-way IV system is located between the filter and an infusion pump with a bubble detector. When autologous blood is not available during the reinfusion cycle, saline is given. A typical reinfusion cycle lasts 1 hour.

Defibrinogenated blood may be reinfused directly from the postoperative autotransfusion chest drainage unit chamber being used for collection. An infusion set primed with saline connects the spike port of recollection chamber to a blood-compatible infusion pump. If a regional anticoagulant has been added, it is recommended that the collection unit be separated from the chest drainage unit before reinfusion; this facilitates maintaining the 7:1 ratio between collected blood and anticoagulant. The pump is programmed to reinfuse continuously the amount collected in one collection device, whereas a second device is used to continue collection.

Regional Anticoagulants

Regional anticoagulants such as CPD, CPDA-1, ACD, ADSOL, Nutricel, Optisol, and sometimes heparin are added to the collection system during intraoperative, noncardiovascular postoperative, and emergency autotransfusion systems.[47] Citrate–phosphate–dextrose, the same anticoagulant used in bank (homologous) blood, is the most commonly used regional anticoagulant. The citrate chelates calcium, preventing the blood from coagulating, with the dextrose and phosphate providing metabolic support of the blood. The usual ratio is one part anticoagulant to seven parts blood, the same ratio used in homologous blood.

Cardiovascular patients who are candidates for intraoperative autotransfusion often are systemically anticoagulated during surgery. Heparin prevents clotting by interfering with the formation of thromboplastin and thrombin. When the heparin is reversed during surgery, a regional anticoagulant is added to the autologous blood collection system. Platelet-rich plasma usually is transfused after protamine reversal of the heparin anticoagulation.

Assessment and Management

General Measures

Before using autotransfusion, hospital protocols for infection control, blood anticoagulation, collection, reinfusion, and disposal of blood and ATS devices should be reviewed.

When predeposit or predonation phlebotomy is used, it is important to follow the same procedure used for homologous blood. The clinician should check patient identification and all forms and labels to make certain the patient receives only autologous blood. Mistaken identification has been reported as the primary cause of transfusion reactions.[41]

Laboratory Studies

Laboratory evaluations done before and after autotransfusion include urinalysis, chest radiograph, complete blood count, CO_2 content, and serum levels of NA^+, K^+, Cl^-, Cr, glucose, and BUN. Additional studies on selected patients include calcium levels, blood cultures, arterial blood gases, and IV pyelograms.

Record Keeping

Patient records should include laboratory values such as platelet count and hemoglobin, the amount of whole blood or washed components reinfused, the length of time between initial collection of autologous blood and completion of reinfusion, and disposition of unused blood. Note the type and amount of anticoagulant used in whole blood reinfusion. Record the amount of vacuum used and any complications encountered, such as clots.

Anticoagulation

Regional anticoagulants may be added directly to the ATS collection system for mixture with the harvested blood to prevent or minimize clotting during surgery, after heparin reversal with protamine, and after surgery, during thoracic hemorrhage and evacuation of traumatic hemothorax. The maximum recommended dosage is one part anticoagulant to seven parts blood. Because rapid infusion of anticoagulated blood may cause citrate toxicity and myocardial depression, blood pH and serum calcium levels are analyzed during rapid infusions and the patient monitored for dysrhythmias, stomach cramps, and tingling around the mouth.

Complications

Although autologous blood transfusion has proven to be safe and effective, there are certain risks associated with the procedures. These include hemolysis, air and particulate emboli, coagulation, and thrombocytopenia. Knowledgeable selection of equipment used according to the manufacturer's instructions makes risks negligible.

Coagulopathy

Although the incidence is small, coagulopathy associated with autologous blood collection and reinfusion techniques, multiple transfusions, hypothermia, and shock have been reported.[49] When a preexisting blood dyscrasia or clotting anomaly is present, the risk of hemorrhage and prolonged clotting times is increased by reinfusing autologous blood that lacks the necessary clotting factors.[37] Rapid infusion of anticoagulated blood may cause citrate toxicity and myocardial depression. The acceptable ratio of regional anticoagulants, such as CPD or ACD, to blood is between 1:7 and 1:20.

The incidence of coagulopathy has been reduced by the use of autologous perioperative plasmapheresis. To obtain 600 to 1,000 ml of platelet-rich plasma, approximately 20% of the total blood volume is used. For patients with normal weight, body build, hematocrit, and cardiovascular compliance, this volume usually is well tolerated. Because heparin may activate platelets and cause a hypercoagulable state, ACD is the recommended anticoagulant. The temperature of the platelet-rich plasma should be maintained at 36°C and 37°C before reinfusion.

Troubleshooting

Table 13–12 outlines some guidelines for troubleshooting problems with autotransfusion.

Nursing Care Plan

Nursing Care Plan 13–4 outlines the important aspects of care for the patient undergoing autologous blood transfusion.

Summary

Autotransfusion is a safe, effective method for reducing the risks associated with homologous (bank) blood transfusion in selected patients. It is lifesaving for patients who are bleeding rapidly and for those who have blood types that are unavailable in bank blood. Autologous blood is compatible and often immediately available, and its use allows conservation of bank blood.

One study demonstrated a 48.5% decrease in the use of homologous blood by open heart surgery patients,[39] and another study demonstrated that one-third of the red blood cell requirement for surgical patients was provided by intraoperative autotransfusion.[38]

A comprehensive autotransfusion program uses both perioperative and intraoperative autologous blood transfusion systems to minimize the use of homologous blood. It is important to note that whole-blood autotransfusion is less expensive than most bank blood.

(Text continues on page 295)

TABLE 13–12
Autotransfusion Troubleshooting Guidelines

Complication	Cause	Intervention
Coagulation	Insufficient anticoagulant added	Added regional anticoagulant such as CPD at a ratio of 7:1 blood to CPD
		Shake collection device periodically to mix blood and regional anticoagulant
	Mediastinal blood not defibrinogenated	Check reversal of anticoagulant
		Strip chest tubes PRN
Hemolysis	Blood trauma secondary to turbulence or roller pumps	Avoid skimming operative field during blood harvesting
		Avoid using equipment containing roller pumps
		Maintain vacuum below 30 mm Hg when collecting blood from chest tubes, below 60 mm Hg when aspirating from a surgical site
Coagulopathies	Hypothermia, shock, multiple transfusions	Patients autotransfused with more than 4,000 ml of blood may require transfusion of fresh frozen plasma or platelet concentrate
	Decreased levels of platelets and fibrinogen	
	Platelets trapped in filters	
	Increased levels of fibrin split products	
Particulate and air emboli	Microaggregate debris	Use 20 to 40 μm microaggregate filter during reinfusion
	Air emboli	Use only infusion pumps with a bubble detector system
		Remove air from blood bags prior to reinfusion
	Nonparenteral medication at site	Avoid use of blood containing non-IV medications
		Wash blood as indicated
Sepsis	Breakdown of aseptic technique	Broad-spectrum antibiotics as indicated
		Maintain good aseptic technique
		Reinfuse within 4 to 6 hr of initial collection
	Contaminated blood	Avoid use of blood from infected areas and/or with known contaminants, such as stool and urine
Citrate toxicity (rare and unpredictable)	Chelating effect of citrate in the CPD/ACD on calcium	Monitor for hypotension, dysrhythmias, and myocardial contractility; when more than 2,000 ml of CPD anticoagulated blood is given over a 20-min period, calcium chloride may be given prophylactically
	Hyperkalemia, hypocalcemia, acidosis, hypothermia, myocardial dysfunction, and liver or renal dysfunction are disposing factors	Slow down or stop CPD infusion, correct acidosis
		Monitor toxicity with frequent blood gases and serum calcium levels

CPD, citrate–phosphate–dextrose; ACD, acid–citrate–dextrose.

NURSING CARE PLAN 13–4
The Patient Undergoing Autologous Blood Transfusion

NURSING DIAGNOSIS	OUTCOME CRITERIA/ PATIENT GOALS	NURSING INTERVENTIONS
Fluid volume deficit: related to hemorrhage, anticoagulants, surgical procedure, or complications.	• Vital signs will be maintained within established parameters to maintain systemic perfusion.	1. Monitor and record intake and output. 2. Assess and report signs and symptoms of hypovolemia: decreased BP and urinary output, tachycardia, weak, thready pulse, complaints of thirst, decreased CVP, PCWP. 3. Observe for hemorrhage from chest tubes. 4. Assess and report signs of hypervolemia: tachycardia, dyspnea with moist rales, normal to high BP, excessive, frothy saliva, increased CVP, PCWP. 5. Hb and Hct labs, q4h or as ordered.
High risk for infection: related to vascular access line.	• Prevent nosocomial infections.	1. Use strict sterile technique during collection and reinfusion of autologous blood. 2. Reinfuse autologous blood within 4 to 6 hr of initiating collection of blood. 3. Assess for symptoms of infection: elevated temperature, increased WBC, erythema, drainage at access site. 4. Obtain WBC, blood cultures, as ordered. 5. Administer antibiotics, as ordered.
High risk for poisoning: related to citrate toxicity.	• Toxic responses to anticoagulant will be prevented.	1. Assess patient for increased risk caused by hyperkalemia, hypocalcemia, acidosis, hypothermia, myocardial dysfunction, and liver or renal dysfunction. 2. Monitor for hypotension, dysrhythmias, and myocardial contractility, when more than 2,000 ml of CPD-anticoagulated blood is given over a 20-min period. 3. Calcium chloride may be given prophylactically, as ordered. 4. Slow down or stop CPD infusion, correct acidosis. 5. Monitor toxicity with frequent blood gases and serum calcium levels.

(continued)

NURSING CARE PLAN 13–4 (Continued)
The Patient Undergoing Autologous Blood Transfusion

NURSING DIAGNOSIS	OUTCOME CRITERIA/ PATIENT GOALS	NURSING INTERVENTIONS
High risk for altered body temperature: related to reinfusion of autologous blood or infection.	• Body temperature will stay within normal limits.	1. Maintain aseptic technique within all procedures. 2. Check temperatures before and after reinfusion. 3. Check and record temperature q1h and prn.
High risk for injury: related to reinfusion reaction and particulate or air emboli.	• Transfusion will occur without complications or unusual incidents.	1. Assess patient for preexisting blood dyscrasia or a clotting anomaly. 2. Check patient identification forms and labels before reinfusion. 3. Reinfuse blood within 4 to 6 hr of beginning collection. 4. Filter all blood and wash blood as indicated before reinfusion. 5. Observe for signs of hemolytic reaction: fever, chills; nausea; hypotension; pain at IV access; back pain; dyspnea; flushing; hemoglobinuria; decreased urinary output. 6. Assess ability to maintain patent airway. 7. Assess respirations for rate, depth, regulatory, and chest expansion. 8. Assess ABGs for evidence of adequate gas exchange, prn. 9. Monitor vital signs, hematocrit, prothrombin time, and partial thromboplastin time. 10. Observe for and record signs of coagulopathy: hematuria, increased bleeding from chest tubes, oozing wounds.
Knowledge deficit: related to risks of transfusion.	• Verbalizes knowledge of autologous and homologous transfusion and associated risks.	1. Assess level of knowledge. 2. Provide relevant information on transfusion risks and benefits. 3. Encourage verbalization of concerns regarding risks and procedures. 4. Document patient–family teaching. 5. Assess level of transfusion-related anxiety.

Cardiopulmonary Resuscitation

BEHAVIORAL OBJECTIVES

Based on the content in the section, the reader should be able to:

1. Define the terms *cardiac arrest*, *resuscitation*, *clinical death*, and *biologic death*.
2. List symptoms of a cardiac arrest.
3. Describe the role of each member of the resuscitation team.
4. List, in order, the steps of cardiopulmonary resuscitation (CPR) according to advanced cardiac life support (ACLS) guidelines.
5. Discuss the first line pharmacologic therapy for cardiac arrest, including indications, dose, route, and side effects.

Description

Cardiopulmonary resuscitation has been in use for more than 30 years. Success rates, defined as return of adequate vital signs with long-term survival without disabling complications, remain distressingly low. The procedure is based on external cardiac massage, begun in 1960, and IV drug use, which has been updated continuously over these decades. Many other interventions have been introduced from time to time, but only a few have proven useful.

Out-of-hospital cardiac arrests have gained more attention recently, especially those without acute myocardial infarction. These patients usually are candidates for more intense investigation of their arrhythmia potential and frequently are subjected to electrophysiological studies. Ongoing clinical studies will, it is hoped, clarify the best approach to these patients.

Some of the common terms associated with CPR are defined in the following paragraphs.

Cardiac arrest is the abrupt cessation of effective cardiac pumping activity, resulting in cessation of circulation. There are only two types of cardiac arrest: cardiac standstill (asystole) and ventricular fibrillation (plus other forms of ineffective ventricular contraction, such as ventricular flutter and, rarely, ventricular tachycardia). The condition referred to as "profound cardiovascular collapse" will not be specifically included because its recognition and definition are nebulous and management less specific. One form, referred to as *cardiogenic shock*, is included in Chapters 14 and 15.

Resuscitation, liberally interpreted, is the restoration of vital signs by mechanical, physiological, and pharmacologic means. The application of CPR is made possible by the concept of clinical versus biologic death.

Clinical death is defined as the absence of the vital signs, and *biologic death* refers to irreversible cellular changes. As determined both experimentally and clinically, the interval between clinical and biologic death is approximately 4 minutes.

Indications and Contraindications

It is easier to determine who should *not* be resuscitated than who should be resuscitated. People who should not be resuscitated include those with known terminal illness and those who have been clinically dead for longer than 5 minutes. Both represent situations in which resuscitation likely would prove impossible and survival would be brief and meaningless.

All others should be regarded as candidates for resuscitation. Remember that resuscitation always can be abandoned, but it cannot be instituted after undue delay.

One additional point is that the term *the very elderly* often is used to differentiate likely degrees of vitality and therefore of survival probability. On the surface, this is perhaps reasonable, but age alone should rarely, if ever, determine treatment. Bear in mind that, regardless of chronologic age, a person who is alert and able to carry on any sort of thoughtful conversation is a candidate for resuscitation unless that person has clearly stated otherwise in the presence of witnesses.

Refer to the discussion of Do Not Resuscitate (DNR) in Chapter 8.

Features of the Resuscitation Team

An organized approach to resuscitation is essential. Resuscitation should be approached by a team made up of trained personnel, including nurses, physicians, ECG technicians, respiratory technicians, and people to transport special instruments (eg, defibrillators, pacemakers, and special tray sets).

The team also should include an administrative or secretarial member who can do the legwork, make all necessary phone calls, and perform other miscellaneous duties that are a minor but necessary part of every prolonged resuscitation attempt. A common method of organizing a resuscitation team is to designate specific people who will respond to all cardiac emergencies; this works quite well, but it is not the only method, nor is it always feasible.

The following is an illustration of a successful method of resuscitation geared to an institution with trained resuscitative personnel. The team includes a nurse who serves as the primary member. The first nurse present becomes the initial captain of the team, who also institutes the resuscitation attempt as outlined.

A single call, preferably by the secretary, should immediately summon the entire team and those who will immediately transport the necessary equipment (defibrillator, monitor, and pacemaker instrument) to the site of the emergency.

An important member of the team is the switchboard operator, who must immediately alert the entire team in preference to all other duties. A single digit on the telephone dial should be used to alert the switchboard. The switchboard operator often will know where to find key physician members of the team and can summon them individually.

Hospitals with house officers who carry emergency electronic communication equipment are at an obvious advantage and should have the best resuscitation statistics. Many smaller institutions, however, may be just as successful using only nursing personnel and well trained technicians. Minor variations in approaches may bring the same results.

Two additional factors are crucial to the team's success. The team must have a definite routine that is kept up to date by all members. Furthermore, nursing personnel and other key nonphysician members must be sanctioned to act spontaneously.

Because many episodes of cardiac arrest occur outside a hospital setting, there has been a sharp growth of well trained teams in mobile units who can respond in minutes to emergency calls. The reported success rates vary greatly, with many factors operative, but on the whole they are more effective than many health care personnel predicted. In any case, they have made an impact, and promise to be a more important participant in the future—for example, the potential for more accurate field diagnosis of ischemia and use of thrombolytic agents at an early stage has attracted mounting interest.

Assessment of Cardiac Arrest

The recognition of cardiac arrest depends on the finding of signs of absence of circulation:

- Unconscious state preceded by less profound states of mental obtundation
- Pulselessness
- Dilated pupils
- Minimal or absent respirations

Two things should be noted. First, the pupils require a certain amount of time to dilate, which has been estimated at approximately 45 seconds but may be longer than 1 minute. It therefore occasionally is a valuable sign for pinpointing the time of cardiac arrest. Second, inadequate respiratory excursions may be noted in the early seconds of cardiac arrest, and these should not cause delay in recognition of the other signs.

Pulselessness is best determined by palpation of either the carotid or femoral arteries. Palpation of the carotid almost always is immediately available, whereas palpation of the femoral is not. Brachial or radial pulse palpation is of lesser value. Pulselessness should not be determined by attempting to obtain a blood pressure.

Ideally, coronary care units or well equipped critical care units should include continuous monitoring, electronic warning signals, and the automatic conditioned response of a skilled team, thus obviating the delay of feeling pulses or auscultating over the precordium.

Procedure for CPR

The ACLS guidelines developed by the American Heart Association for adult emergency cardiac care (the Universal Algorithm and the Asystole Treatment Algorithm) are outlined in Table 13–13. Other ACLS guidelines can be found in Appendix III.

There are two hospital settings in which health care personnel may encounter a person in need of CPR: (1) that of a patient whose ECG is being monitored continuously, as in the coronary care unit; and (2) that in an area where the patient is not under continuous monitoring, such as a regular hospital room or unit.

For the continuously monitored patient, the dysrhythmia sets off the alarm, and if it is ventricular fibrillation, the patient is immediately defibrillated (without prior attempts by other means), after which a physician is summoned for evaluation.

In the unmonitored patient, proceed immediately as described in the following.

1. Sharp Blow to the Precordium

A sharp blow to the precordium requires virtually no time and may institute a cardiac rhythm; if so, it may be the only required resuscitation. This is referred to as *thumpversion*

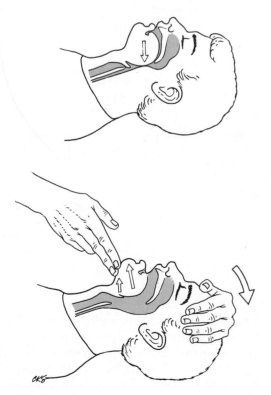

FIGURE 13–42
Opening the airway with back head tilt and chin lift.

and is especially effective in ventricular tachycardia. Some believe that thumpversion may not be appropriate or worthwhile in unwitnessed cardiac arrest. Nonetheless, it is not time-consuming or risky, and others believe it should be applied routinely.

2. Call for Help

To call for help, simply relay the message "code zero" or "red alert," together with the location of the patient to a second individual who then places the emergency call to bring the team together.

3. Achieve Adequate Airway

Artificial ventilation (mouth-to-mouth) is instituted immediately. The head is back-tilted and chin raised to stretch the airway and advance the tongue in preparation for mouth-to-mouth ventilation (Fig. 13–42). Newer techniques advise 1.5-second ventilatory pause and less force and pressure on exhalation so that the esophagus is not opened (which would allow air under pressure into the stomach). Along with this, chest compressions should be done 80 to 100 times/minute.

4. External Cardiac Compression

External cardiac compression is a simple technique performed by standing at either side of the patient, placing the heel of one hand over the lower half of the sternum, and the heel of the other hand over the first. Vigorous compression is applied directly downward, and the sternum is depressed between 1.5 and 2 inches and released abruptly. This rhythm is maintained at the rate of 80 to 100 times/minute. To be effective, this technique must be learned correctly and applied skillfully (Fig. 13–43).

If one person must apply both ventilation and massage, it is best to give two quick inflations mouth-to-mouth or by other readily available means, followed by 15 external cardiac compressions. This routine may be maintained until additional members of the team arrive.

The generally accepted theory underlying CPR maintains that the heart functions as a pump and the valves operate appropriately as one-way passages during external compression. More recent work, involving two-dimensional echocardiography during CPR in animals and humans, indicates that different mechanisms may necessitate some minor alterations in the standard CPR procedure. The new studies emphasize that the heart serves primarily as a conduit, not as a pump, and that the properties of veins as capacitors and arteries as conduits influence cerebral and coronary circulation during CPR. Venous beds may act as reservoirs, whereas some venous circuits func-

TABLE 13–13
ACLS Guidelines: Universal Algorithm and Asystole Treatment Algorithm

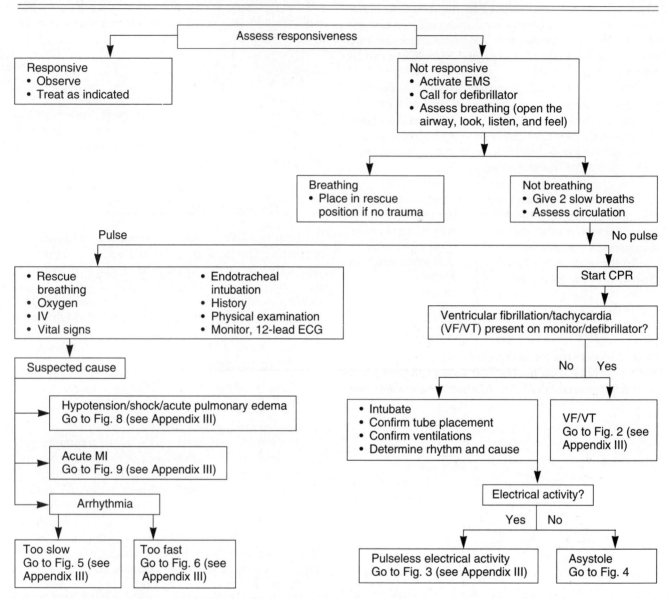

Fig. 1. Universal algorithm for adult emergency cardiac care (ECC). (JAMA 286[16]:2216.)

(continued)

tion as barriers to retrograde flow due to the presence of valves. Arteries show less tendency to collapse and therefore should receive more blood during artificial massage. The splanchnic venous bed, however, may form a large static pool that robs the total circulation during CPR. Some advocate abdominal compression to prevent this. Experiments involving the "thoracic pump model" of CPR have their origin in the known hemodynamic effects of cough, which include augmentation of aortic pressure and flow, carotid flow, and impressive maintenance of consciousness. It involves the basic concept of CPR, which holds that the heart is a passive conduit during chest compression (or cough), with changes in thoracic pressure in a phasic manner responsible for perfusion of portions of the body. At present, cough CPR has limited application (only in the conscious patient, of course); its main value

TABLE 13–13
ACLS Guidelines: Universal Algorithm and Asystole Treatment Algorithm (Continued)

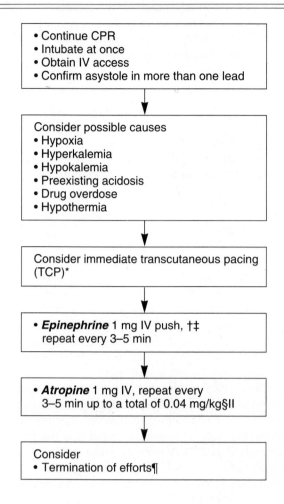

- Continue CPR
- Intubate at once
- Obtain IV access
- Confirm asystole in more than one lead

↓

Consider possible causes
- Hypoxia
- Hyperkalemia
- Hypokalemia
- Preexisting acidosis
- Drug overdose
- Hypothermia

↓

Consider immediate transcutaneous pacing (TCP)*

↓

- *Epinephrine* 1 mg IV push, †‡
  repeat every 3–5 min

↓

- *Atropine* 1 mg IV, repeat every
  3–5 min up to a total of 0.04 mg/kg§‖

↓

Consider
- Termination of efforts¶

Class I: definitely helpful
Class IIa: acceptable, probably helpful
Class IIb: acceptable, possibly helpful
Class III: not indicated, may be harmful
* TCP is a Class IIb intervention. Lack of success may be due to delays in pacing. To be effective TCP must be performed early, simultaneously with drugs. Evidence does not support routine use of TCP for asystole.
†The recommended dose of **epinephrine** is 1 mg IV push every 3–5 min. If this approach fails, several Class IIb dosing regimens can be considered:
- Intermediate: **epinephrine** 2–5 mg IV push, every 3–5 min
- Escalating: **epinephrine** 1 mg–3 mg–5 mg IV push (3 min apart)
- High: **epinephrine** 0.1 mg/kg IV push, every 3–5 min
‡ **Sodium bicarbonate** 1 mEq/kg is Class I if patient has known preexisting hyperkalemia.
§Shorter **atropine** dosing intervals are Class IIb in asystolic arrest.
‖ **Sodium bicarbonate** 1 mEq/kg:
Class IIa
- if known preexisting bicarbonate-responsive acidosis
- if overdose with tricyclic antidepressants
- to alkalinize the urine in drug overdoses
Class IIb
- if intubated and continued long arrest interval
- upon return of spontaneous circulation after long arrest interval
Class III
- hypoxic lactic acidosis
¶If patient remains in asystole or other agonal rhythms after successful intubation and initial medications and no reversible causes are identified, consider termination of resuscitative efforts by a physician. Consider interval since arrest.

Fig. 4. Asystole treatment algorithm. (JAMA 286[16]:2220.)

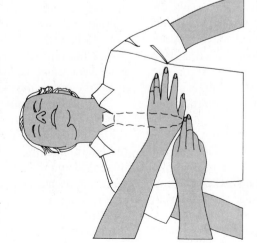

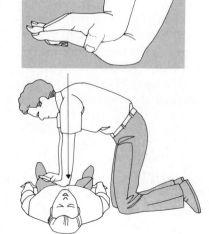

FIGURE 13–43
External chest compression. *Left*, proper hand position over lower portion of sternum; *Right*, correct rescuer position. (From Taylor C, Lillis C, LeMone P: Fundamentals of Nursing: The Art and Science of Nursing Care. Philadelphia, JB Lippincott, 1989)

has been in studies that helped elucidate the mechanism responsible for blood flow in external chest compression. Clinical studies in patients now underway should clarify its role further.

5. External Countershock

External countershock should be applied as soon as the instrument is available. This procedure should be done even if the specific rhythm diagnosis is unknown (eg, if there has been a delay in determining this).

If *cardiac standstill* (asystole) is present, the countershock will take only moments and will do no harm. If *ventricular fibrillation* is present, the earliest possible countershock delivered is the one most likely to be effective and should be done at a time when the rhythm more likely may be maintained.

Any adult is capable of doing this; thus, all personnel involved should be trained in defibrillation techniques and be expected to execute them without need of supervision.

A specific *diagnosis* now is required (the word *recognition* has been used up to now, not diagnosis). As mentioned earlier, this will be either cardiac standstill or ventricular fibrillation (discussed in items 9 and 10 of this section).

6. Intravenous Infusion

Establishing and maintaining IV access is the responsibility of a very important member of the team—the first nurse who is available after two members are applying ventilation and massage. This person will be in charge of the emergency cart and therefore responsible for preparing the drugs and the IV infusion set. The importance of this function cannot be minimized because most drug therapy will require IV access and infusion by the most feasible route.

The simplest method of all is the insertion of a needle, cannula, or scalp needle into an arm vein. If this fails, the femoral vein is readily accessible, or a very large cannula easily can be inserted into the large blood vessel (superior vena cava) by simple puncture. A cutdown on a branch of the basilic system just above the elbow crease on the medial aspect of either arm or on the external jugular vein also may allow insertion of a large cannula into the superior vena cava or right atrium.

Internal jugular or subclavian venupuncture sites are excellent, readily available, and accessible. The internal jugular is used most commonly because it is a simpler approach and recently trained physicians feel more comfortable with it. Both the internal jugular and subclavian sites may be used for rapid infusion, blood withdrawal for laboratory studies, or monitoring of central venous pressure and oxygen saturation. No survival benefit (success rate) has been shown for central lines despite their frequency of use and advantages in other ways.

The *intracardiac route* should be reserved for situations in which urgency takes precedence over availability of the IV route. This should be a rare occurrence.

7. Endotracheal Intubation

Endotracheal intubation is required for the patient in whom spontaneous cardiac rhythm and respiration have not resulted from the measures already outlined.

8. Pharmacologic Therapy

Pharmacologic agents and appropriate preparations to be made ready immediately include the following:

a. *Epinephrine* in a 1:10,000 aqueous solution.

This drug is the most frequently used in cardiac arrest, long thought due to its β-adrenergic effect, but recent evidence suggests that its α-adrenergic effect is the basis for its effectiveness. Thus, pure α drugs are being used more commonly by many (see later).

In this regard, recent experience with high-dose epinephrine has yielded results that support further study. It is now usual, if not routine, to use up to 5 mg IV epinephrine per dose. It should be noted that the 1:1,000 concentration would be more convenient and more rapidly administered.

b. *Lidocaine* should be prepared in an IV solution of varying concentration, but 1 to 4 mg/ml is an adequate solution for continuous infusion. Adequate blood levels are obtained by IV push in 50- to 75-mg bolus increments (or 1 mg/kg, repeated at half the initial dose at 8 minutes, to a total dose of 3 mg/kg) and then a continuous infusion of 2 to 4 mg/minute.

Recent clinical trial results indicate that routine use of lidocaine in acute myocardial infarction is not efficacious and is potentially harmful. Thus, the drug should be used only in the presence of active ventricular ectopy with a bolus followed by infusion of sharply limited duration (4–12 hours). This regimen should provide protection from ventricular tachycardia/ventricular fibrillation and avoid the excess mortality of prolonged infusion.

c. *Bretylium tosylate* (Bretylol, American Critical Care, McGraw Park, IL) is a second-line antiarrhythmic used in ventricular fibrillation when lidocaine has failed to convert the life-threatening dysrhythmia. Bretylium often causes hypotension and has a delayed onset (often 20 minutes), requiring resuscitative efforts to continue until the drug's action is apparent.

Bretylium's actions are complex and include adrenergic influences that give it a modest inotropic effect (unlike other antiarrhythmics). Its major action is a striking anti-fibrillatory effect produced by prolongation of both the action potential duration and the effective refractory period. Occasionally, it causes defibrillation without use of countershock. This sharp rise in threshold for ventricular fibrillation and ventricular tachycardia makes it extremely effective when these rhythm disturbances are recurrent, and it is becoming the drug of choice in this circumstance. It is given by IV bolus, in a usual dose of 5 mg/kg, and it can be repeated one or more times within 1 hour.

d. *Sodium bicarbonate* in a 5% solution may be given in 50-ml prefilled syringes in a dose of 1 mEq/kg and repeated at half the dose every 10 minutes.

It has been argued that giving sodium bicarbonate IV results in a rise in PCO_2 (by the reaction $HCO_3^- + H^+ \rightarrow H_2CO_3 \rightarrow H_2O + CO_2$) and an increase in osmolality. This alkalizing agent has been reexamined recently and is used less frequently today for cardiac arrest. Usually, pH, PO_2, and PCO_2 are followed with arterial blood sampling and often show normal or only moderately abnormal values. Due to the invariably poor perfusion during CPR, venous blood reflects rising PCO_2 from reduced pulmonary perfusion, where CO_2 is normally lost. Thus, adding sodium bicarbonate may worsen this gap, causing deterioration in metabolic status. It is used primarily in patients with hyperkalemia or in those who were in metabolic acidosis at the time of arrest.

Vigorous correction of metabolic acidosis during a cardiac arrest should be attempted by overventilation with a hand-held ventilation bag. This will reduce PCO_2 and hyperinflate the alveoli, while delivering higher levels of PO_2. If sodium bicarbonate is overused, alkalosis may result. Metabolic alkalosis will shift the oxygen dissociation curve and cause less oxygen to be released from hemoglobin at the tissue level (see Chapter 18). The blood levels of PO_2 may remain high, and the tissue level suffers from hypoxemia.

e. *Calcium chloride* is no longer used routinely in CPR. Due to lack of efficacy in clinical studies in cardiac arrest, calcium has fallen into disfavor. It is thought detrimental owing to its raising of plasma levels, and it may even intensify the increased intracellular concentration already present in cardiac arrest victims. Its use is limited largely to instances of hypocalcemia, excessive calcium channel blockage, and hyperkalemia, although it still is used by some in the presence of electromechanical dissociation.

f. *Isoproterenol* is not useful as a routine drug in cardiac arrest and is reserved for "medical pacing" in bradycardia for temporarily maintaining the heart rate.

g. *Magnesium ion* is second only to potassium in intracellular concentration and is vital in energy metabolism (including membrane transport function). Studies have shown its administration to be effective in certain life-threatening dysrhythmias, notably torsades de pointes. Its role in regulating intracellular concentrations of potassium, calcium, and phosphorus suggests its usefulness in cardiac

arrest due to ventricular tachycardia and ventricular fibrillation. Studies using magnesium in cardiac arrest are now underway and should help clarify its role. Also, this cation may be depleted in a manner parallel to potassium depletion, and thus its use may be especially beneficial in patients on diuretics or digitalis or both. In the absence of known hypermagnesemia or renal failure, it is quite safe. It may be given in a 10% solution at a rate of 1 to 2 ml/minute in doses of 3 to 4 mEq and may be repeated, depending on response.

h. *Other IV drugs* such as procainamide (Pronestyl); quinidine; diuretics such as ethacrynic acid (Edecrin, Merck Sharp & Dohme, West Point, PA) and furosemide (Lasix, Hoechst-Roussel Pharmaceuticals, Inc., Somerville, NJ); mannitol; dexamethasone (Decadron, Merck Sharp & Dohme); and β-blockers, such as propranolol and metoprolol, should be available, although they are not prepared routinely for immediate use.

The inotropic and chronotropic agent *glucagon* has gained use in some situations. Its effects are less predictable, and it should not be considered a routine drug. Its inotropic effect is substantial, but less than that of isoproterenol, and it has the advantage of a lesser chronotropic effect and generally induces less hyperexcitability.

The catecholamine *dopamine* has emerged as perhaps the inotropic agent of choice. Its central inotropic effect is comparable to that of isoproterenol, but it has the advantage of augmenting renal blood flow. It largely has replaced isoproterenol and norepinephrine for enhancing perfusion pressure (although isoproterenol still is more effective as a temporary medical "pacemaker").

Other drugs that have become useful in cardiopulmonary emergencies include dobutamine and the class referred to as *calcium antagonists* (eg, verapamil). These drugs have not been fully evaluated but are unlikely to be important except in very special situations (eg, recurrent dysrhythmias associated with variant angina). Animal work suggests that calcium antagonists may prevent microvascular spasm, a potential factor in ischemia and necrosis. Their use in CPR for this purpose is uncertain, although it appears promising, with further work anticipated.

Disopyramide (Norpace) is not yet available for parenteral use and probably will have limited value.

Dobutamine, a derivative of isoproterenol, has the advantage of possessing minimal chronotropic effect. When dopamine produces tachycardia, dobutamine may provide potent inotropy without the harmful effects of excess heart rate.

An additional advantage of dobutamine is its effects in reducing PCWP (preload), which may be important in some patients. Thus, it may be combined with dopamine in certain patients to take advantage of the augmented renal blood flow and reduced PCWP.

Experimental drugs useful in cardiac dysrhythmias are proving effective; it is not anticipated, however, that any currently in trials will be especially useful in CPR.

9. Countering Cardiac Standstill

If cardiac standstill is present, epinephrine (1:10,000) should be given routinely, usually 1 mg IV, and artificial ventilation and circulation should be continued; if unsuccessful, epinephrine should be repeated and an epinephrine drip started.

The available transcutaneous pacemakers have been proven effective. Recent studies describe external pacing as effective and readily available; the patient experiences less pain and skeletal muscle contraction than in the past (external transcutaneous pacing has been available since the late 1950s). This device should be available as part of the routine CPR equipment. Pacing, however, by any method, usually is ineffective and has contributed little to successful resuscitation efforts. The routine use of the newer transcutaneous pacemaker could prove more effective and deserves a concerted trial in CPR, because it obviates the need for insertion of a transvenous or transthoracic pacemaker electrode, thus avoiding delay in applying electrical stimulation to the heart.

10. Ventricular Fibrillation

If ventricular fibrillation is present, epinephrine is given IV. It is important that the continuous artificial ventilation and circulation are maintained and that interruptions not exceed 5 seconds, and external *countershock* is given at the initial setting of 200 J, followed by 200 to 300 J, and 360 J. Immediate resumption of artificial circulation and ventilation should occur after each countershock if no pulse returns.

If ventricular fibrillation persists despite the preceding intervention or if reversion to ventricular fibrillation occurs each time it is applied, IV *antiarrhythmics* should be given without delay. It is here that lidocaine probably is the drug of choice (dosage as given previously), and it should be administered without the delay of first trying other more commonly used agents.

If lidocaine is ineffective, bretylium is given in doses of 5 mg/kg and repeated at 10 mg/kg, to a total of 30 mg/kg. *Procainamide*, if preferred, also may be given by IV push, and either drug may be given by IV drip. β-*Blocking drugs* such as propranolol or metoprolol may be effective here. *Quinidine* is preferred by some, but its tendency to lower peripheral blood pressure and reduce myocardial contractility (resulting in a diminished cardiac output should a rhythm be resumed) constitute important disadvantages.

Regardless of the initial mechanism (whether it be an irritable or a depressive phenomenon), once cardiac arrest has gained a foothold with some duration, it must be assumed that the heart is depressed, making the routine use of depressive drugs unwarranted.

Because uneven tissue perfusion, particularly myocardial perfusion, may be a factor in perpetuating the ventricular fibrillation or standstill, a *vasopressor agent* of the peripheral constrictor type may be of value at this point. Digitalis and potassium chloride rarely are indicated in resuscitative attempts, their use being based on knowledge of special preexisting situations.

As already indicated, depressive cardiac mechanisms often are the cause of repetitive ventricular fibrillation, and, paradoxically, pacing the heart (pharmacologically with isoproterenol or electronically by transvenous pacing catheter) is the treatment of choice in some cases (after resumption of rhythm, of course).

Much has been written about defibrillation with regard to energy level, type of paddles, and so forth. Some believe that instruments should provide greater energy bursts, especially for large patients. Conversely, others have demonstrated that lesser energy (eg, 200 J) is as effective as maximum levels. In my experience, the most important single factor in delivering shocks is the constant and rather heavy-handed pressure applied by the operator at the instant the button is pushed. Remember that all instruments deliver less energy than the setting indicates. Finally, there seems to be no justification for insisting on front-to-back paddles.

11. Pericardial Tap

If the preceding measures fail:

a. Pericardial tap should be performed, preferably by the subxyphoid route, to treat a possible cardiac tamponade. Although an uncommon factor in cardiac arrest, pericardial tap may result in dramatic recovery. Tamponade is hallmarked by electrical–mechanical dissociation, distended jugular veins, absence of central pulses despite adequate CPR, and inadequate physiological responses to all other therapies.

b. Consider further underlying causes subject to treatment, such as pneumothorax (insertion of chest tubes); pulmonary embolism (assisted circulation, surgery, thrombolysis, heparin); ventricular aneurysm or rupture of papillary muscle or interventricular septum (assisted circulation, surgery); subvalvular muscular aortic stenosis with extreme gradients (propranolol, reserpine, etc.).

12. Terminating Resuscitation

If these interventions fail, the decision to terminate resuscitative attempts is imminent, based on central nervous system changes or the assumption of a nonviable myocardium.

At this point, a reminder is in order. Since 1960 (advent of external or closed chest massage), many modifications of the mechanical, pharmacologic, and physiological approach to CPR have been instituted. Only modest, and in many ways disappointing improvement in results has occurred. It would seem that only the availability of on-site defibrillators and widespread training in their use will significantly affect the poor results thus far accomplished. This might be realized through cooperative efforts between health care institutions and industry.

Management

Nursing Care

The nurse plays a vital role in the efforts to resuscitate a patient. As already mentioned, the nurse often is the one who first assesses the patient and initiates CPR and calling of the team. The patient's primary nurse should be present to answer questions about events leading to the arrest. Roles of the nurses who respond to the arrest situation include continued CPR, monitoring heart rhythm and other vital signs, defibrillation, administration of drugs, recording of events, crowd control, and notifying the attending physician as well as family members. Support to the family and friends is very important at this time, and should be given by other nurses and health care professionals until the primary nurse and physician are available to speak to them.

After a successful resuscitation, the nurse along with the physician needs to monitor closely the vital signs and hemodynamics of the patient as well as any signs of complications. Prompt recognition and treatment of abnormalities are important in the care and outcome of the patient.

Postresuscitative Phase

If there is resumption of spontaneous cardiac activity, the situation should be evaluated thoroughly as to the clinical state, underlying causes, and complicating factors to determine proper management. The following routine has been found successful: IV diuretic (eg, furosemide 80–240 mg), a steroid such as dexamethasone for its salutary effect on cerebral edema, and electrical and physiological monitoring in a critical care unit. A portable chest roentgenogram is routine, and arterial blood gases should be obtained as indicated. Continuous oxygen therapy is maintained; an IV infusion is of course essential. Routine measurements other than continuous ECG monitoring include frequent blood pressures (ideally done by intra-arterial cannula), hourly urine volumes, frequent bedside estimates of tissue perfusion, and central venous pressure and O_2 saturation measurements.

If central nervous system damage is evident, additional mannitol or IV urea should be given, and dexamethasone for cerebral edema should be continued. Otherwise, monitoring is continued as already outlined.

If oliguria or anuria is present, massive doses of furosemide should be given immediately. If there is no re-

sponse to these, management like that used in acute renal insufficiency should be instituted (see Chapter 25).

The specific approach in the postresuscitative period will depend not only on the patient's condition at the time but also on the underlying disease process, the previous condition of the patient, and the events in the immediate postresuscitative period. More patients are being studied by catheter techniques acutely to evaluate them for emergency surgical procedures such as saphenous bypass grafts, percutaneous transluminal coronary angioplasty, and thrombolysis. The state of this art is changing rapidly, and it frequently is necessary to transfer the patient to a facility in which these procedures are available.

It has long been known that abnormalities of coagulation may result from, or be aggravated by, cardiac arrest, especially in ischemic heart disease. Antithrombin III activity, fibrinolytic activity, as well as fibrinogen, prothrombin time, and partial thromboplastin time should be evaluated.

Complications of Resuscitation

Resuscitation has come a very long way; it has changed drastically with time and undoubtedly will continue to do so. It has proved its worth beyond doubt. There are complications, of course, including (1) injuries to sternum, costal cartilages, ribs, esophagus, stomach, liver, pleura, and lung, any one of which can be serious; (2) the production, fortunately rare, of permanent central nervous system damage in a live patient, which renders the patient totally dependent; and (3) medicolegal considerations, which originally leaned against the attempt because of the frequency of undignified failures (see Display Box 13–13).

This last, medicolegal considerations, probably should be ignored for the most part, because we are dealing with an earnest and reasonable approach to the treatment of sudden death in reversible situations. Nonetheless, it does emphasize that resuscitation should always be applied by well trained, responsible people. The aim of resuscitation is to reverse the reversible and not to inflict suffering in situations involving the irreversible. The alternative in both, of course, is death. Differentiating between reversible and irreversible requires good judgment, which, as someone has said, "is difficult to learn, impossible to teach."

DISPLAY BOX 13–13
Complications of Resuscitation

- Injuries to: sternum, costal cartilage, ribs, esophagus, stomach, liver, pleura, and lung
- Permanent CNS damage
- Medicolegal problems

REFERENCES

Cardiac Pacing

1. Bellamy CM, Roberts DH, Hughes S, Charles RG: Comparative revaluation of rate modulation in new generation evoked QT and activity sensing pacemakers. Pace 15:993–999, 1992
2. Cavanaugh JA: Overdrive pacing: An approach to terminating ventricular tachycardia. Journal of Cardiovascular Nursing 5(3):58–64, 1991
3. Teplitz L: Cardiac pacing. Journal of Cardiovascular Nursing 5(3):1–8, 1991
4. Kleinschmidt KM, Stafford MJ: Dual-chamber cardiac pacemakers. Journal of Cardiovascular Nursing 5(3):9–20, 1991
5. Fabiszewski R, Volosin KJ: Rate-modulated pacemakers. Journal of Cardiovascular Nursing 5(3):21–31, 1991
6. Oto MA, et al: Improved quality of life in patients with rate responsive pacemakers VVIR vs VVI: Part I. Pace 14:800–806, 1991
7. Horowitz LN: The automatic implantable cardioverter defibrillator: Review of clinical results—1980–1990: Part III. Pace 15:604–609, 1992
8. Block M, et al: Results and realistic expectations with transvenous lead systems: Part III. Pace 15:665–670, 1992
9. Dreifus LS, et al: Guidelines for implantation of cardiac pacemakers and antiarrhythmia devices, Circulation 84:455–467, 1991
10. Pezzella DA: Transcutaneous pacing. Progress in Cardiovascular Nursing 4(1):18–22, 1989
11. Stewart JV, Sheehan AM: Permanent pacemakers: The nurse's role in patient education and follow-up care. Journal of Cardiovascular Nursing 5(3):32–43, 1991
12. Brannon PHB, Johnson R: The internal cardioverter defibrillator: Patient–family teaching. Focus 19(1):41–46, 1992

Commonly Used Anti-Arrhythmic Agents and Cardioversion

13. Marchlinski F, Hook B: Which cardiac disturbance should be treated with digoxin immune fab (Ovine) antibody. Am J Emerg Med 9(2 Suppl 1):24–28, 1991
14. Burroughs Wellcome Co.: Insert: Digoxin Immune Fab Ovine, 1991
15. Clutter C: Neurally mediated syncope. Journal of Cardiovascular Nursing 5(4):65–73, 1991
16. Cardiac Arrhythmia Suppression Trial (CAST): Preliminary report: Effect of encainide and flecainide on mortality in the randomized trial of arrhythmia suppression after myocardial infarction. N Engl J Med 321:406–412, 1989
17. Weiner B: Second generation of antidysrhythmic drugs. Critical Care Nursing Clinics of North America 1(2):417–422, 1989
18. Dunn S: Moricizine hydrochloride: Ethmozine. Critical Care Nurse 12(4):61–63, 1992
19. Sayre M, Nordeman L: Cardiovascular pharmacology. Emergency Medicine 11(2):23–41, 1989
20. McEvoy G, Litvak L: Drug Information, American Hospital Formulary. Bethesda, Maryland, American Hospital Pharmacists, 1992
21. Singh B: Class III activity: The utility of sotalol. Cardiovascular Drugs and Therapy 4:597–602, 1991
22. Marion-Merrill Dow, Inc.: Clinical Monograph: Cardiazem, 1992
23. Grauer K: New developments in cardiopulmonary resuscitation. American Family Physician 43(3):832–844, 1991
24. Albarran-Sotelo R, Atkins J: Textbook of Advanced Cardiac Life Support. Dallas, American Heart Association, 1987

PTCA and PBV

25. Huber MS, Mooney JF, Madison J, Mooney MR: Use of a morphologic classification to predict clinical outcome after dissection from coronary angioplasty. Am J Cardiol 68:467–471, 1991
26. Bentivoglio LG, Holubkov R, Kelsey SF, et al: Short and long term outcome of percutaneous transluminal coronary angioplasty in unstable versus stable angina pectoris: A report of the 1985–1986 NHLBI PTCA registry. Cathet Cardiovasc Diagn 23:227–238, 1991
27. O'Keefe JH Jr, Rutherford BD, McConahay DR, et al: Multivessel coronary angioplasty from 1980 to 1989: Procedural results and long-term outcome. J Am Coll Cardiol 16:1097–1102, 1990
28. Dorros G, Iyer SS, Hall P, Mathiak LM: Percutaneous coronary angioplasty in 1,001 multivessel coronary disease patients: An analysis of different patient subsets. Journal of Interventional Cardiology 4:71–80, 1991
29. Alderman EL, Bourassa MG, Cohen LS, et al, for the CASS Investigators: Ten-year follow-up of survival and myocardial infarction in the randomized coronary artery surgery study. Circulation 82:1629–1646, 1990
30. Muller DWM, Topol EJ: Selection of patients with acute myocardial infarction for thrombolytic therapy. Ann Intern Med 113:949–960, 1990
31. King SB III: Role of new technology in balloon angioplasty. Circulation 84:2574–2579, 1991
32. Kahn JK, Hartzler GO: Frequency and causes of failure with contemporary balloon coronary angioplasty and implications for new technologies. Am J Cardiol 66:858–860, 1990
33. Bell MR, Bailey KR, Reeder GS, Lapeyre AC III, Holmes DR Jr: Percutaneous transluminal angioplasty in patients with multivessel coronary disease: How important is complete revascularization for cardiac event-free survival? J Am Coll Cardiol 16:553–562, 1990
34. DeFeyter PJ, van den Brand M, Jaarman GJ, et al: Acute coronary artery occlusion during and after percutaneous transluminal coronary angioplasty: Frequency, prediction, clinical course, management, and follow-up. Circulation 83:927–936, 1991
35. Detre KM, Holmes DR Jr, Holubkov R, et al: Incidence and consequences of periprocedural occlusion. Circulation 82:739–750, 1990
36. Leon M, Kent K, Lowell SF, et al: A multi-device lesion-specific approach for unfavorable coronary anatomy (abstr). J Am Coll Cardiol 19:93A, 1992

Autologous Blood Transfusion

37. Sympson G: CATR™: A new generation of autologous blood transfusion. Critical Care Nurse 11(4):60–64, 1991
38. Koehler LC, Williamson KR, et al: A comprehensive program to ensure quality in intraoperative blood salvage. Journal of Intravenous Nursing 14:193–197, 1991
39. Tennant DF, Evans MM: Minimizing blood usage after open heart surgery nurses play a key role. Focus On Critical Care AACN 17:308–312, 1990

40. Wood L: Autotransfusion in the postanesthesia care unit. Journal of Post Anesthesia Nursing 6(2):98–101, 1991
41. Gloe D: Common reactions to transfusions. Curriculum in Critical Care 20:506–514, 1991
42. Committee on Standards, American Association of Blood Banks: Standards for Blood Banks and Transfusion, 14th ed. Arlington, VA, American Association of Blood Banks, 1991
43. Murphy P, Heal JM, et al: Infection or suspected infection after hip replacement surgery with autologous or homologous blood transfusions. Transfusion 31:212–217, 1991
44. Clements DH, Sculco TP, et al: Salvage and reinfusion of postoperative sanguineous wound drainage. J Bone Joint Surg [A] 74:646–651, 1992
45. Bovill DF, Norris TR: The efficacy of intraoperative autologous transfusion in major shoulder surgery. Clin Orthop 240:137–140, 1989
46. Woda R, Tetzlaff JE: Upper airway oedema following autologous blood transfusion from a wound drainage system. Can J Anaesth 39:290–292, 1992
47. Drago S: Banking on your own blood. Am J Nurs 92(3):61–64, 1992
48. Martin E, Harris A, et al: Autotransfusion systems (ATS). Critical Care Nurse 9(7):65–73, 1989
49. Tawes RL, Sydorak GR, et al: Avoiding coagulopathy in vascular surgery. Am J Surg 160:212–216, 1990

BIBLIOGRAPHY

Cardiac Pacing

Ellenbogen KA: Cardiac Pacing. Boston, Blackwell Scientific Publications, 1992

Commonly Used Antiarrhythmic Agents and Cardioversion

Antman E, Wender T, et al: Treatment of 150 cases of life threatening digitalis intoxication with digoxin specific fab antibody fragments. Circulation 81:1744–1752, 1990
Belardinelli L, Linden J, Berne R: The cardiac effects of adenosine. Prog Cardiovasc Dis 32:73–79, 1989
Clark R, Shaffhebarger C: Electrical interventions. Topics in Emergency Medicine 11(2):42–51, 1989
Camm AJ (ed): Mexiletine: Pharmacology and therapeutic use. Clin Cardiol 13:349–359, 1990
Horowitz L: Efficacy of moricizine in malignant ventricular arrhythmias. Am J Cardiol 65:41D–46D, 1990
Mahmorian I, Verani M, Pratt C: Hemodynamic effects of intravenous and oral sotalol. Am J Cardiol 65:28A–34A, 1990
Maeden S, Chalay M: Drug corner: Esmolol. Critical Care Nurse 9(10):12–14, 1989
McCollam P, Parker R: Therapy reviews: Evaluation and treatment of ventricular arrhythmias: an update. Clin Pharm 10:195–205, 1991
Nelson G, Driscoll C: Procedures for your practice: Emergency defibrillation and cardioversion. Patient Care 23:193–196, 1989
Roach A: Adenosine–Adenocard: A new intravenous antiarrhythmic agent for supraventricular tachycardia. Critical Care Nurse 11(7):78–79, 1991
Salerno D, Dias V, et al: Efficacy and safety of intravenous diltiazem for treatment of atrial flutter and atrial fibrillation. J Am Coll Cardiol 8(4):891–897, 1991
Weiner B: Hemodynamic effects of antidysrhythmic drugs. Journal of Cardiovascular Nursing 5(4):39–48, 1991
Wolters K, Olin B, Hebel S: Drugs, Facts and Comparisons. Philadelphia, JB Lippincott, 1992

Percutaneous Transluminal Coronary Angioplasty and Percutaneous Balloon Valvuloplasty

PTCA

American Heart Association: 1992 Heart and Stroke Facts. Dallas, American Heart Association, 1992
Brodie BR, Weintraub RA, Stuckey TD, LeBauer EJ, Katz JD, Kelly TA, Hansen CJ: Outcomes of direct coronary angioplasty for acute myocardial infarction in candidates and non-candidates for thrombolytic therapy. Am J Cardiol 67:7–12, 1991
Califf RM, Fortin DF, Frid DJ, et al: Restenosis after coronary angioplasty: An overview. J Am Coll Cardiol 17:2B–13B, 1991
Hibbard MD, Holmes DR Jr, Gersh BJ: Coronary angioplasty in cardiogenic shock. Journal of American College of Cardiology 17:52–64, 1991
Hirshfeld JW Jr, Schwartz JS, Jugo R, et al: Restenosis after coronary angioplasty: A multivariate statistical model to relate lesion and procedure variables to restenosis. J Am Coll Cardiol 18:647–656, 1991
Hlatky MA, Lipscomb J, Nelson C, et al: Resource use and cost of initial coronary revascularization: Coronary angioplasty versus coronary bypass surgery. Circulation 82:208–212, 1990
Lincoff AM, Popma JJ, Ellis SG, Vogel RA, Topol EJ: Percutaneous support devices for high risk or complicated coronary angioplasty. J Am Coll Cardiol 17:770–780, 1991
Meester BJ, Samson M, Suryapranata H, et al: Long-term follow-up after attempted angioplasty of saphenous vein grafts: The Thoraxcenter experience 1981–1988. Eur Heart J 12:648–653, 1991
Muller DWM, Topol EJ: Thrombolytic therapy: Adjuvant mechanical intervention for acute myocardial infarction. Am J Cardiol 69:60A–70A, 1992
Myler RK, Stertzer SH, Shaw RE: Coronary angioplasty and coronary bypass surgery. Journal of Invasive Cardiology 3:180–190, 1991
O'Connor GT, Plume SK, Olmstead EM, et al: A regional prospective study of in-hospital mortality associated with coronary artery bypass grafting. JAMA 266:803–809, 1991
Parisi AF, Folland ED, Hartigan P: A comparison of angioplasty with medical therapy in the treatment of single-vessel coronary artery disease. N Engl J Med 326:10–16, 1992
Waller BF, Pinkerton CA, Orr CM, Slack JD, Van Tassel JW, Peters T: Morphological observations late (> 30 days) after clinically successful coronary balloon angioplasty. Circulation 83: I28–I41, 1991
Weintraub WS, Craver JM, Cohen CL, Jones EL, Guyton RA: Influence of age on results of coronary artery surgery. Circulation 84:III226–III235, 1991

PBV

Barden C, Austin JH, Burgman V, Wood MK: Balloon aortic valvuloplasty: Nursing care implications. Critical Care Nurse 10(6):22–30, 1990

McKay CR: Should patients with mitral stenosis who are acceptable surgical commissurotomy candidates now have balloon valvuloplasty treatment? Cardiovasc Clin 21:175–195, discussion 196–197, 1990

The National Heart, Lung, and Blood Institute Balloon Valvuloplasty Registry Participants: Multicenter experience with balloon mitral commissurotomy: NHLBI Balloon Valvuloplasty Registry Report on immediate and 30-day follow-up results. Circulation 85:448–461, 1992

Safian RD, Kuntz RE, Berman AD: Aortic valvuloplasty. Clin Cardiol 9:289–299, 1991

Shaw TR, Elder AT, Flapan AD, Essop AR: Mitral balloon valvuloplasty for patients aged over 70 years: An alternative to surgical treatment. Age Ageing 20:299–303, 1991

Strauss B, Marquis JF: Percutaneous valvuloplasty as a treatment for aortic and mitral valve disease. Am Heart J 119:1184–1192, 1990

Waller BF, Dorros G, Lewin RF, King JF, McKay C, VanTassel JW: Catheter balloon valvuloplasty of stenotic aortic valves: Part II. Balloon valvuloplasty during life subsequent tissue examination. Clin Cardiol 14:924–930, 1991

Waller BF, McKay C, VanTassel JW, Talierco C, Howard J, Green F: Catheter balloon valvuloplasty of stenotic aortic valves: Part 1. Anatomic basis and mechanisms of balloon dilatation. Clin Cardiol 14:836–846, 1991

Intra-Aortic Balloon Pump Counterpulsation and Other Ventricular Assist Devices

Curtiss J, Boland M, Bliss D, et al: Intra-aortic balloon cardiac assist: Complication rates for the surgical and percutaneous insertion technique. Am Surg 54:142–147, 1988

Freed PS, Wasfie T, Zado B, et al: Intra-aortic balloon pumping for prolonged circulatory support. Am J Cardiol 61:554—559, 1988

Goran SF: Vascular complications of the patient undergoing intra-aortic balloon pumping. Critical Care Nursing Clinics of North America 1:459–467, 1988

Gould KA: Perspectives on intra-aortic balloon pump timing. Critical Care Nursing Clinics of North America 1:469–473, 1988

Quaal S: Mechanical treatment of the failing heart. In Kern L (ed): Cardiac Critical Care Nursing, pp 397–452. Rockville, MD, Aspen Publishers, 1988

Shinn JA: Novacor left ventricular assist system. AACN Clinical Issues 2:575–586, 1991

Reedy JE, Ruzevich SA, Swartz MT, et al: Nursing care of a patient requiring prolonged mechanical circulatory support. Progress in Cardiovascular Nursing 4:1–9, 1989

Shoulders-Odom B: Managing the challenge of IABP Therapy. Critical Care Nurse 11(2):60–76, 1991

Teplitz L: Patients with ventricular assist devices: Nursing diagnoses. Dimensions in Critical Care Nursing 9(2):82–87, 1990

Cardiopulmonary Resuscitation

Anderson M, Atkins JM, et al: Textbook of Advanced Cardiac Life Support. Dallas, TX, American Heart Association, 1990

Grauer K, Cavallaro D, Gums J: New developments in cardiopulmonary resuscitation. American Family Physician 43(3):832–844, 1991

Wesley R, Rash W, Zimmerman D: Reconsideration of the routine and preferential use of lidocaine in the emergent treatment of ventricular arrhythmias. Crit Care Med 19:1439–1443, 1991

STUDY QUESTIONS

Cardiac Pacing

1. The VVI pacemaker is

   a. atrial demand
   b. AV sequential
   c. ventricular demand
   d. ventricular fixed rate

2. All of the following electrical safety precautions should be adhered to except

   a. use of a nonelectric bed
   b. use of a tap bell rather than electric call light
   c. use of a plug in electric shaver
   d. use of a battery-operated radio

3. All of the following statements about bipolar lead systems are true except

   a. they are less likely to oversense than unipolar systems
   b. muscle twitching is a rare occurrence
   c. they are easier to place
   d. there is less distortion of the QRS

Commonly Used Antiarrhythmic Agents and Cardioversion

1. Which of the following drugs decreases the contractility of the heart muscle?

   a. digitalis
   b. glucagon
   c. propranolol
   d. calcium

2. Which of the following antiarrhythmic drugs has a half-life of 14 to 52 days, making less frequent dosing a possibility?

   a. amiodarone
   b. encainide
   c. propafenone
   d. digoxin

3. Which of the following can be used in the treatment of severe digoxin toxicity?

   a. calcium
   b. Digibind
   c. verapamil
   d. epinephrine

4. Which antiarrhythmic agent has a short half-life of 10 seconds and can be used to treat supraventricular arrhythmias?

   a. procainamide
   b. encainide
   c. verapamil
   d. adenosine

Percutaneous Transluminal Coronary Angioplasty and Percutaneous Balloon Valvuloplasty

1. All of the following comparisons between PTCA and CABG are true except

   a. restenosis occurs in 20% to 30% of lesions within 6 months after PTCA and 18% of bypass grafts occlude within 18 months of CABG
   b. PTCA is less psychologically stressful than CABG
   c. mortality rates for first-time CABG patients are higher than for first-time PTCA patients
   d. morbidity rates are lower after PTCA than CABG

2. PTCA is indicated for individuals with the following degree of vessel narrowing

   a. 50%
   b. 60%
   c. 70%
   d. 40%

3. After PTCA, the most obvious symptom of a complication is

   a. elevated temperature
   b. recurrence of angina
   c. cool, moist skin
   d. nausea

4. Complications resulting from PBV include all of the following except

    a. bleeding at the arterial puncture site
    b. systemic embolization
    c. restenosis
    d. right ventricular perforation

Intra-Aortic Balloon Pump Counterpulsation and Other Ventricular Assist Devices

1. The following arterial waveform illustrates an IABP that is

    a. inflating too early
    b. deflating too early
    c. deflating too late
    d. is timed correctly

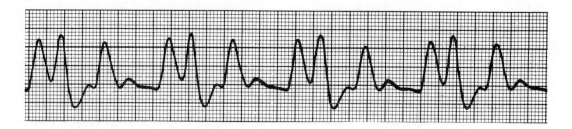

2. Which of the following are important nursing functions when caring for an IABP patient?

    1. evaluation of pedal pulses
    2. decompression of the stomach
    3. keeping the patient flat in bed
    4. monitoring the effect of IABP therapy on the patient's need for inotropic support

        a. 1, 3, and 4
        b. 1, 2, and 4
        c. 1 and 4
        d. 1, 2, 3, and 4

3. All of the following are contraindications to IABP therapy except

    a. aortic aneurysm
    b. previous aortofemoral bypass graft
    c. terminal cancer
    d. aortic valve incompetence

Autologous Blood Transfusion

1. Indications for autotransfusion include

    a. hypovolemia
    b. coagulopathy
    c. prevention of donor-related disease transmission
    d. prevention of allergic and anaphylactic reactions to transfusion

2. Autologous blood may be

    a. collected in the OR, ER, PACU, and ICU
    b. administered within 6 hours of collection
    c. contraindicated in some patients
    d. reinfused as whole and/or washed–processed blood

3. Major hematologic differences between homologous and autologous blood include the following

   a. autologous blood has normal levels of 2,3-DPG, a higher platelet count, and a higher hematocrit than homologous blood
   b. homologous blood has normal levels of 2,3-DPG, a higher platelet count, and a higher hematocrit than autologous blood
   c. autologous blood has normal levels of 2,3-DPG, a lower platelet count, and a higher hematocrit than homologous blood
   d. bank blood has normal levels of 2,3-DPG, a higher platelet count, and a lower hematocrit

4. The most frequent complication associated with autotransfusion is

   a. citrate toxicity
   b. hemolysis
   c. microaggregate emboli
   d. hepatitis

Cardiopulmonary Resuscitation

1. All of the following *except* which one are major drugs used to treat ventricular fibrillation?

   a. epinephrine
   b. atropine
   c. lidocaine
   d. bretylium

2. All of the following except *which* are true of bretylium?

   a. can cause hypotension
   b. a major action is an antifibrillatory effect
   c. is administered by IV bolus
   d. has an immediate effect on administration

3. All of the following *except* which one are signs of absence of circulation?

   a. unconscious state
   b. pulselessness
   c. reactive pupils
   d. absent respirations

CHAPTER 14

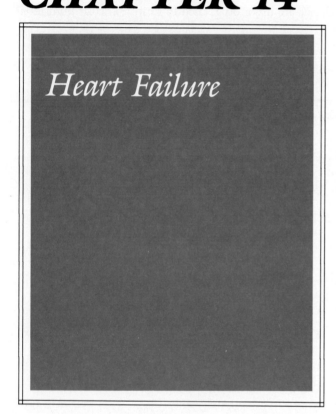

Heart Failure

BEHAVIORAL OBJECTIVES

Based on the content in this chapter, the reader should be able to:

1. Describe each of the four reserve mechanisms of the heart.
2. Compare and contrast the etiologies and clinical symptoms of left ventricular failure and right ventricular failure.
3. List the four Killip classifications of heart failure.
4. Explain the vicious cycle of heart failure.
5. Outline the treatment plan for heart failure, including three anticipated pharmacologic interventions and three nursing diagnoses.

Hudak: Critical Care Nursing:
A Holistic Approach, 6th ed. © 1994
J. B. Lippincott Company.

Description

The heart, a complex structure composed of fibrous tissue, cardiac muscle, and electrical conducting tissue, has a single function: to pump blood. To do its job well, a good heart pump requires good functioning muscle, a good valve system, and an efficient pumping rhythm. An abnormality of sufficient severity of any component of the pump can affect its pumping efficiency and may cause the pump to fail.

Physiological Principles

Reserve Mechanisms of the Heart in Response to Stress

When the heart is stressed, several reserve mechanisms can be called on to maintain good pumping function—that is, to provide a cardiac output sufficient to meet the demands of the body. These mechanisms are increased heart rate, dilation, hypertrophy, and increased stroke volume.

Increased Heart Rate

The first response is an increase in *heart rate*. This adjustment is rapid and has been experienced by everyone during periods of exercise or anxiety. Increasing the heart rate is an excellent way of quickly increasing the cardiac output and meeting the demands of the body for blood. Its utility and effectiveness, however, are functions of age, the functional state of the myocardium, and the amount of obstructive coronary artery disease (CAD).

The maximum heart rate that can be achieved is related to age (Table 14–1). For example, heart rate in a 20-year-old person will plateau at approximately 200 beats/minute at maximum effort, whereas at 65 years of age, maximum heart rate is about 150 beats/minute. After 25 years of age, maximum heart rate capability drops approximately six beats for each 5 years. There is, of course, considerable spread around these mean maximum heart rates for each age—some people will exceed the average value, whereas others will fail to achieve it. As heart rate increases, the time for diastolic ventricular filling decreases, and at high heart rates the time available for ventricular filling may be so small that filling is inadequate and cardiac output starts to fall.

In addition to advancing age, the functional state of the heart muscle (how capable it is of maintaining repeated rapid contractions) and the state of the coronary circulation are important determinants of the effectiveness of heart rate as a response to stress. In people with coronary artery disease and significant obstruction to one or more coronary arteries, a substantial increase in heart rate can be a potentially dangerous event. Coronary artery blood flow to the left ventricle takes place primarily in

TABLE 14–1
Maximum Heart Rate According to Age

Age (yr)	Maximum Heart Rate (beats/min)
20	200
22	198
24	196
26	194
28	192
30	190
32	189
34	187
36	186
38	184
40	182
45	179
50	175
55	171
60	160
65 +	150

diastole. With increasing heart rates, decreased diastolic filling time, and increased demands of the heart for oxygen (heart rate being one of the major determinants of myocardial oxygen demand), coronary blood flow may become critical, and angina pectoris, congestive failure, or occasionally myocardial infarction may be produced. Furthermore, if the heart muscle contracts poorly and cannot sustain strong contractions at moderate or rapid rates, heart failure may follow.

Heart rate, then, is an immediate response to stress that is effective in maintaining or increasing cardiac output but whose value depends on the patient's age, functional state of the myocardium, and amount of obstructive disease in the coronary arteries.

Dilation

The second reserve mechanism of the heart is *dilation*. With dilation, the muscle cell stretches. The relationship between the cardiac output (the amount of blood the heart pumps in each unit of time) and the length of the heart muscle cell at the end of diastole is expressed in the well known *Starling relationship*, which states that as the end-diastolic fiber length increases, so does the cardiac output (Fig. 14–1).

Like heart rate, however, the usefulness of dilation is self-limiting. There is a point beyond which the stretching of the muscle cell leads not to an increase in cardiac output but to a decrease. This is partly explained by the *Laplace relationship*, which states that the tension in the wall of a chamber such as the left ventricle is related directly to the pressure in that chamber and its radius. Put another way, as the radius of the chamber increases (dilation), so does the wall tension, as long as the pressure in the chamber rises or does not fall.

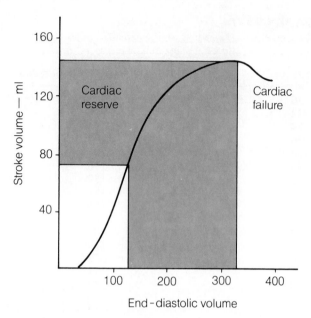

FIGURE 14-1

The Starling curve. As the end-diastolic fiber length increases, so does the cardiac output. At a self-limiting end point, further stretching results in a lessened cardiac output.

Because wall tension is directly related to the demand of the myocardium for oxygen, it is not difficult to see that eventually the radius will dilate to such a degree that the demand of the heart for oxygen cannot be met. In this instance, dilation has advanced to the point where it is no longer providing an increase in cardiac output, and the pump has started to fail.

Hypertrophy

The third reserve mechanism of the heart is the ability of the individual cardiac muscle cells to *hypertrophy*. The process of hypertrophy requires time and is not an acute adjustment to stress. If the stress is applied long enough, however, such as with systemic or pulmonary hypertension or significant stenosis of the aortic or pulmonary valve (pressure loads), the muscle of the chamber pumping against the resistance may hypertrophy to such a degree that it effectively outgrows its blood supply and becomes ischemic. When this happens, hypertrophy ceases to be a useful compensatory mechanism, and the heart's pumping ability decreases. A similar situation may occur with the imposition of a volume load on the pumping ventricle, as occurs with mitral or aortic regurgitation.

Increased Stroke Volume

The fourth reserve mechanism of the heart is to increase its *stroke volume*, the amount of blood that it ejects into the circulation with each systole. It can do this either by increasing the percentage of the end-diastolic volume ejected with each beat (increase the ejection fraction through an increase in contractility) or by increasing the

amount of blood presented to the heart (increased venous return). This is commonly accomplished by the reflexive increase of sympathetic nervous system activity, which increases venous tone. Venous pressure is then raised, and thus venous return to the heart is increased.

Venous return also is increased by elevated body temperature, which shortens the time required for blood to circulate completely through the body; by recumbence, in which case the volume of blood that is held in the legs as a result of gravity largely is returned to the central circulation and presented to the heart; or by taking a deep breath, which increases intrathoracic negativity, thereby "sucking" more blood into the chest. Also, any increase in intravascular volume will increase venous return. By an increase in either ejection fraction (contractility) or venous return (volume), stroke volume and cardiac output will increase. As with other mechanisms of response to stress, increased venous return ("preload," to the physiologist) and increased contractility may not function to increase cardiac output. For example, the myocardium may be so fatigued (depressed contractility) that it cannot respond to further attempts to improve its force of contraction. Similarly, an increase in venous return may cause increased dilation and decrease, rather than improve, cardiac output.

This simplistic review of cardiovascular responses to stress is designed to promote a basic understanding of the topic and to indicate how the responses can be overwhelmed. In addition, it will assist in generating an appreciation for approaching clinical situations, both diagnostic and therapeutic, from a physiological cause-and-effect point of view.

Pathophysiology of Heart Failure

When the normal cardiac reserves for responding to stress are inadequate to meet the metabolic demands of the body, the heart fails to do its job as a pump, and heart failure results. Also, as stated earlier, dysfunction of any of the components of the pump ultimately may result in failure. Heart failure was very simply and appropriately defined in 1933 by Lewis as "a condition in which the heart fails to discharge its contents adequately."[1] This definition is as good today as it was in the 1930s. It is estimated that 10% of the population older than the age of 75 years have some degree of heart failure. The prognosis for heart failure is rather dismal, and those with severe compromise of left ventricular function have a 50% mortality rate at 1 year.

Causes of Failure

Dysrhythmias

Disorders of the cardiac *rhythm* can produce or contribute to failure in several ways.[2] *Bradycardia* allows for increased diastolic filling and myocardial fiber stretch with an associated increase in stroke volume (Starling relationship). Cardiac output therefore is preserved. This is well tolerated in healthy people; resting bradycardia is, in fact, a result of high levels of aerobic physical conditioning. In the diseased heart, however, contractility is decreased, the useful limits of the Starling relationship are exceeded, and cardiac output may be diminished.

With *tachycardia*, diastolic filling time is decreased, myocardial oxygen demand is increased, and the diseased myocardium or the heart with significant CAD may tolerate the burden poorly and fail or develop ischemia, injury, or infarction. Furthermore, frequent premature contractions may decrease the cardiac output, a circumstance that may be poorly tolerated in a patient with marginal pump function.

Valve Malfunction

Valve malfunction can lead to pump failure either by *pressure load* (obstruction to outflow of the pumping chamber, such as valvular aortic stenosis or pulmonary stenosis), or by *volume load* (the valve may be regurgitant as with mitral and aortic insufficiency), which presents an increased volume of blood to the left ventricle.[2]

Valve abnormalities that impose either a pressure load or a volume load on one or more chambers usually are slowly progressive conditions that cause the heart to use its long-term defense mechanisms of dilation and hypertrophy. Both these mechanisms can be overcome, with resultant pump failure.

Less commonly, an acute volume load is imposed on the heart, causing a rapid onset of pump failure. Bacterial endocarditis of the aortic or mitral valves, rupture of a portion of the mitral valve apparatus (papillary muscle or chordae tendineae), or rupture of the interventricular septum is the usual cause. In these cases, initial therapy is designed to support the heart during the period of acute insult so that the long-term compensatory mechanisms can be used. If this is not successful, however, emergency replacement of the abnormal valve or closure of the septal defect is indicated.

Heart Muscle Abnormalities

Abnormalities of the *muscle* that cause ventricular failure include myocardial infarction, ventricular aneurysm, extensive myocardial fibrosis (usually from atherosclerotic coronary heart disease or prolonged hypertension), endocardial fibrosis, primary myocardial disease (cardiomyopathy), or excessive hypertrophy due to pulmonary hypertension, aortic stenosis, or systemic hypertension.

Myocardial Rupture

In acute myocardial infarction, *myocardial rupture* presents as a dramatic and often catastrophic onset of pump failure and is associated with a high mortality. Rupture usually occurs during the first 8 days after infarction, during the period of greatest softening of the damaged myocardium. Fortunately, myocardial rupture is a relatively rare complication of infarction. Rupture of a papillary muscle, of the interventricular septum, or of the free wall of the left ventricle may occur.

Rupture of a Papillary Muscle

There are two papillary muscles in the left ventricle that are thumblike projections of muscle to which the restraining "guide wires" of the mitral valve, the chordae tendineae, are attached. The papillary muscle may be involved in the infarction process and very occasionally may rupture.[2] When it does, there is a sudden loss of restraint of one of the leaflets of the mitral valve, and free mitral regurgitation occurs with each contraction of the left ventricle. This sudden profound pressure and volume load on the left atrium is reflected through the pulmonary veins to the pulmonary vascular bed, and the acute onset of symptoms of pulmonary vascular congestion is noted. This usually is manifested as severe dyspnea and frank pulmonary edema. At the bedside, a loud murmur lasting throughout systole is present. Very often, nothing can be done to save the patient, although occasionally emergency mitral valve replacement can be accomplished successfully.

Rupture of the Interventricular Septum

Sudden heart failure is seen occasionally in acute myocardial infarction as a result of rupture of the interventricular septum. Like rupture of the papillary muscle, septal rupture is uncommon, but when it does appear, it also usually is noted in the first week after damage. Septal rupture is clinically characterized by chest pain, dyspnea, shock, and a rapid onset of evidence of pump failure. There is a loud murmur that lasts throughout systole at the lower left sternal border and often is accompanied by a thrill that one can feel by placing the hand over the precordium at the left sternal border. As with all myocardial ruptures, the prognosis of septal rupture is poor; however, it is occasionally possible to repair these ventricular septal defects by emergency surgery involving cardiopulmonary bypass.

Ruptures of a papillary muscle and the interventricular septum are virtually indistinguishable at the bedside, with both presenting as sudden onset of left ventricular failure, a new murmur, and occasionally a palpable thrill. The location of the infarction is not helpful, and the clinical course in each is rapidly downhill. Emergency cardiac catheterization is the only way to differentiate the two clearly.

Rupture of the Left Ventricle

Mechanical failure of the heart seen in acute myocardial infarction is another relatively rare event and is due to rupture of the free wall of the left ventricle and the spilling of blood into the pericardial cavity. This results in acute compression of the heart or tamponade and the inability of both chambers to fill adequately. There is then very sudden pumping failure with associated shock and death.

Rupture of the free wall may be preceded by or associated with a return of chest pain as the blood dissects through the necrotic myocardial wall. Sudden vascular collapse as occurs with ventricular fibrillation, but with an unchanged rhythm on the electrocardiogram (electromechanical dissociation), suggests rupture of the ventricular free wall. As with rupture of the papillary muscle and interventricular septum, rupture of the free wall of the left ventricle carries with it an extremely poor prognosis.

Responses to Failure

When the heart's normal reserves are overwhelmed and failure occurs, certain physiological responses to the decrease in cardiac output are important. All these responses represent the body's attempt to maintain a normal perfusion of vital organs.

Increased Sympathetic Tone

The primary acute adjustment to heart failure is an increase in sympathetic nervous system influence on the arteries, veins, and heart. This results in increased heart rate, increased venous return to the heart, and increased force of contraction; in addition, sympathetic tone helps maintain a normal blood pressure. The price extracted for this adjustment is an increase in myocardial oxygen demand and oxygen consumption, a request that may be met inadequately in the patient with significant obstructive CAD or poor pump contractility.

As a result of the autonomic nervous changes and other factors, the blood flow to the essential organs, specially the brain and heart, is maintained at the expense of less essential organs such as the skin, gut, and kidneys. With severe congestive heart failure, there is sufficient decrease in blood flow to the skeletal muscles to cause a *metabolic acidosis* (lactic acidosis from hypoxemia) that must be considered when a treatment program is planned.

Sodium and Water Retention

When the kidneys sense a decreased volume of blood presented for filtration, they respond by retaining sodium and water and thereby try to do their part in increasing the central blood volume and venous return. With an increase in circulating blood volume and venous return to the heart, there is an increase in end-diastolic fiber length (dilation) and, within limits, an increase in stroke volume and cardiac output. With a failing heart, however, an increased circulatory volume may be too great a burden for the ventricle, and failure may be worsened.

In some patients with prolonged failure, the remaining heart cells increase the pumping efficiency with hyper-

trophy, and the clinical findings of heart failure may improve or disappear (Fig. 14–2).

Assessment of Heart Failure

Left Ventricular Failure

It is useful to think of the clinical features of heart failure as coming from failure of either the left ventricle, the right ventricle, or both. When the *left ventricle* fails, its inability to discharge its contents adequately results in dilation, increased end-diastolic volume, and increased intraventricular pressure at the end of diastole. This results in the inability of the left atrium to empty its contents into the left ventricle adequately, and pressure in the left atrium rises. This pressure rise is reflected into the pulmonary veins, which bring blood from the lungs to the left atrium. The increased pressure in the pulmonary vessels results in pulmonary vascular congestion, which is the cause of the most specific symptoms of left ventricular failure.

See Display Box 14–1 for a summary of the signs and symptoms of left-sided heart failure.

Pulmonary Vascular Congestion

The symptoms of pulmonary vascular congestion are dyspnea, orthopnea, paroxysmal nocturnal dyspnea, cough, and acute pulmonary edema.

Dyspnea, characterized by rapid, shallow breathing and a sensation of difficulty in obtaining adequate air, is distressing to the patient. Occasionally, a patient may complain of insomnia, restlessness, or weakness, which is caused by the dyspnea.

Orthopnea, the inability to lie flat because of dyspnea, is another common complaint of left ventricular failure related to pulmonary vascular congestion. It is important to determine whether the orthopnea is truly related to heart disease or whether elevating the head to sleep is merely the patient's custom. For example, if the patient states that he sleeps on three pillows, one might hasten to conclude that he is suffering from orthopnea. If, however, when the patient is asked why he sleeps on three pillows, he replies that he does this because he likes to sleep at this elevation and has done so since before he had symptomatic heart disease, the condition does not qualify as orthopnea.

Paroxysmal nocturnal dyspnea (PND) is a well known complaint characterized by the patient's awakening in the middle of the night because of intense shortness of breath. Paroxysmal nocturnal dyspnea is thought to be caused by a shift of fluid from the tissues into the intravascular compartment as a result of recumbence. During the day, the pressure in the veins is high, especially in the dependent portions of the body, due to gravity, increased fluid volume, and increased sympathetic tone. With this increase in hydrostatic pressure, some fluid escapes into the tissue space. With recumbence, the pressure in the dependent

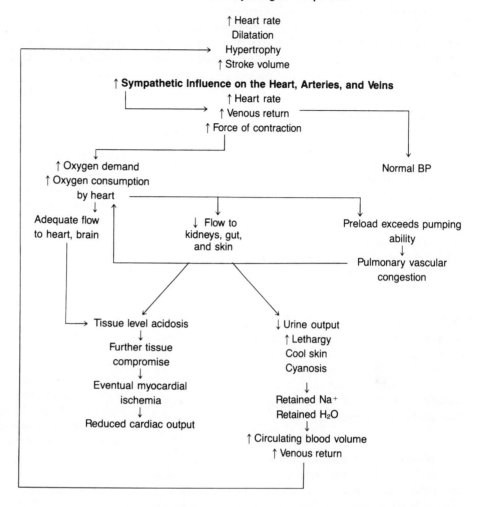

Overwhelmed Physiological Responses

↑ Heart rate
Dilatation
Hypertrophy
↑ Stroke volume

↑ Sympathetic Influence on the Heart, Arteries, and Veins
↑ Heart rate
↑ Venous return
↑ Force of contraction

↑ Oxygen demand
↑ Oxygen consumption
by heart

Normal BP

Adequate flow
to heart, brain

↓ Flow to
kidneys, gut,
and skin

Preload exceeds pumping
ability
↓
Pulmonary vascular
congestion

Tissue level acidosis
↓
Further tissue
compromise
↓
Eventual myocardial
ischemia
↓
Reduced cardiac output

↓ Urine output
↑ Lethargy
Cool skin
Cyanosis
↓
Retained Na+
Retained H₂O
↓
↑ Circulating blood volume
↑ Venous return

FIGURE 14–2
The vicious cycle of heart failure.

DISPLAY BOX 14–1
Signs and Symptoms of Left Ventricular Failure

- Pulmonary vascular congestion
- Dyspnea
- Orthopnea
- Paroxysmal nocturnal dyspnea (PND)
- Irritating cough
- Acute pulmonary edema
- Decreased cardiac output
- Atrial gallop—S₄
- Ventricular gallop—S₃
- Lung crackles
- Dysrhythmias
- Wheezing breath sounds
- Pulsus alternans
- Weight gain
- Cheyne–Stokes respirations
- Radiographic evidence of pulmonary vascular congestion

capillaries is decreased, and fluid is resorbed into the circulation. This increased volume represents an additional amount of blood that is presented to the heart to pump each minute (increased preload) and places an additional burden on an already congested pulmonary vascular bed, with acute onset of dyspnea the resultant symptom. Keep in mind that PND occurs not only at night but also at any time during acute hospitalizations that require bed rest.

An *irritating cough* is one symptom of pulmonary vascular congestion that often is overlooked but that may be a dominant symptom. It may be productive but is usually dry and hacking in character. This symptom is related to congestion of bronchial mucosa and an associated increase in mucus production.

Acute pulmonary edema is the most florid clinical picture associated with pulmonary vascular congestion. It occurs when the pulmonary capillary pressure exceeds the pressure that tends to keep fluid within the vascular channels (approximately 30 mm Hg). At these pressures, there is transduction of fluid into the alveoli, which in turn diminishes the area available for the normal transport of oxygen into and carbon dioxide out of the blood within the pulmonary capillary bed. Acute pulmonary edema is characterized by intense dyspnea, cough, orthopnea, profound anxiety, cyanosis, sweating, noisy respirations, and very often chest pain and a pink, frothy sputum from the mouth. It constitutes a genuine medical emergency and must be managed vigorously and promptly.

Decreased Cardiac Output

In addition to the symptoms that result from pulmonary vascular congestion, left ventricular failure also is associated with nonspecific symptoms that are related to decreased cardiac output. The patient may complain of weakness, fatigability, apathy, lethargy, difficulty in concentrating, memory deficit, or diminished exercise tolerance. These symptoms may be present in chronic low-output states and may dominate the patient's complaints. Unfortunately, these symptoms are nonspecific and often are ascribed to depression, neurosis, or functional complaints. Therefore, these potentially important indicators of deteriorating pump function often are not recognized for their true import, and the patient is either inappropriately reassured or placed on a tranquilizer or mood-elevating preparation. Remember, the presence of the nonspecific symptoms of low cardiac output demands a careful evaluation of the heart as well as the psyche—an examination that will yield the information that will dictate proper management.

Heart Sounds and Crackles

Physical signs associated with left ventricular failure that are easily recognized at the bedside include third and fourth heart sounds (S_3, S_4) and crackles in the lungs.

S_4, or *atrial gallop*, is associated with and follows atrial contraction and is heard best with the bell of the stethoscope very lightly applied at the cardiac apex. The left lateral position may be required to elicit the sound. It is heard just before the first heart sound (S_1) and is not always a definitive sign of congestive failure, but may represent decreased compliance (increased stiffness) of the myocardium. It therefore may be an early, premonitory indication of impending failure. An S_4 is common in patients with acute myocardial infarction and likely does not have prognostic significance, but it may represent incipient failure.

S_3, or *ventricular gallop*, is an important sign of left ventricular failure and in adults almost never is present in the absence of significant heart disease. Most physicians would agree that treatment of congestive failure is indicated with the appearance of this sign.

S_3 is heard in early diastole after the second heart sound (S_2) and is associated with the period of rapid passive ventricular filling. It also is heard best with the bell of the stethoscope applied lightly at the apex, with the patient in the left lateral position, and at the end of expira-

tion (see the section on auscultation in Chapter 12, for further detail).

The *crackles* or fine moist rales most commonly heard at the bases of the lungs posteriorly often are recognized as evidence of left ventricular failure, as indeed they may be. Before these crackles are ascribed to pump failure, the patient must be instructed to cough deeply to open any basilar alveoli that may be compressed as a result of recumbence, inactivity, and compression from the diaphragm beneath. Crackles that fail to clear after cough (post-tussic) need to be evaluated; those that clear after cough probably are clinically unimportant. It is, however, important to note that the patient may have good evidence of left ventricular failure on the basis of a history of symptoms suggesting pulmonary vascular congestion or the finding of S_3 at the apex and yet have quite clear lung fields. It is not appropriate to wait for the appearance of crackles in the lungs before instituting therapy for left ventricular failure.

Dysrhythmias

Because an increase in heart rate is the heart's initial response to stress, sinus tachycardia might be expected and often is found in the examination of a patient with pump failure. Other rhythms associated with pump failure include atrial premature contractions, paroxysmal atrial tachycardia, and ventricular premature beats. Whenever a rhythm abnormality is detected, one must attempt to define the underlying pathophysiological mechanism; therapy then can be properly planned and instituted.

Other Signs

Other signs of left ventricular failure that may be noted in addition to an S_3, crackles in the lungs, and supraventricular rhythms include wheezing breath sounds, pulsus alternans (an alternating greater and lesser volume of the arterial pulse), weight gain, and Cheyne–Stokes respirations. Indeed, patients may awaken at night during respiratory height of a Cheyne–Stokes cycle, a situation that may be interpreted falsely as PND but that may have the same pathophysiological significance. Weight gain resulting from retention of salt and water by the kidneys is a useful sign that the patient may follow at home. Daily weight should be recorded in the morning after voiding and before breakfast.

Radiographic Findings

Radiographic examination of the chest often helps the clinician diagnose heart failure. Careful evaluation of the chest roentgenogram may demonstrate changes in the blood vessels of the lungs that result from an increase in pulmonary venous pressure. Radiographic findings may be present in the absence of crackles, and careful examination of the chest film is necessary if left ventricular failure is suspected.

Right Ventricular Failure

Failure of the *right ventricle* alone often is the result of severe underlying lung disease and such conditions as severe pulmonary hypertension (primary or secondary), stenosis of the pulmonary valve, and a massive pulmonary embolus. The right ventricle tolerates a volume load well, and pure right ventricular failure usually is due to resistance to outflow (pressure load). More commonly, however, right ventricular failure is the result of failure of the left ventricle. In this situation, symptoms and signs of both left and right ventricular failure are present, and the symptoms of left ventricular failure may improve as the right ventricle fails through relief of left ventricular preload and decrease in pulmonary vascular congestion. See Display Box 14–2 for a summary of the signs and symptoms of right ventricular failure.

Low Cardiac Output

In contrast to left ventricular failure, in which specific symptoms usually can be related to a single underlying mechanism—pulmonary vascular congestion—the symptoms of right heart failure are not so specific, and many are related to a low cardiac output. Fatigability, weakness, lethargy, or difficulty in concentrating may be prominent. Heaviness of the limbs (especially the legs), an increase in abdominal girth, inability to wear previously comfortable shoes, and weight gain reflect the ascites and edema associated with right ventricular failure.

In addition, symptoms of the underlying pulmonary disease usually dominate complaints if failure is due to a primary pulmonary problem, usually chronic bronchitis or emphysema. Occasionally, bronchiectasis or restrictive lung disease may be the primary pulmonary problem, but chronic bronchitis and emphysema are by far the most common pulmonary causes of right ventricular failure.

DISPLAY BOX 14–2
Signs and Symptoms of Right Ventricular Failure

- Low cardiac output
- Jugular vein distention
- Dependent edema
- Dysrhythmias
- Right ventricular S_3 and S_4
- Hyperresonance with percussion
- Low immobile diaphragms
- Decreased breath sounds
- Increased anteroposterior chest diameter

Jugular Vein Distention

When the right ventricle decompensates, there is dilation of the chamber, an increase in right ventricular end-diastolic volume and pressure, resistance to filling of the ventricle, and a subsequent rise in right atrial pressure. This increasing pressure is in turn reflected upstream in the venae cavae and can be recognized by an increase in the jugular venous pressure. One can evaluate this best by looking at the veins in the neck and noting the height of the column of blood. With the patient lying in bed and the head of the bed elevated between 30° and 60°, the column of blood in the external jugular veins will be, in the normal person, only a few millimeters above the upper border of the clavicle, if it is seen at all (Fig. 14–3).

When an observation of venous pressure is recorded, the height of the column of blood above the sternal angle and the elevation of the head of the bed should be included. This will then provide a useful basis for comparison of future observations.

Edema

Edema often is considered a reliable sign of heart failure, and, indeed, it often is present when the right ventricle has failed. It is the least reliable sign of right ventricular dysfunction, however. Many people, particularly the elderly, spend much of their time sitting in a chair with the legs dependent. As a result of this body position, the decreased turgor of subcutaneous tissue associated with old age, and perhaps primary venous disease such as varicosities, ankle edema may be produced that reflects these factors rather than right ventricular failure.

When edema does appear related to failure of the right ventricle, it is dependent in location. If the patient is up and about, it will be noted primarily in the ankles and will ascend the legs as failure worsens. When the patient is put to bed, the dependent portion of the body becomes the sacral area, and edema should be looked for there. In addition, other signs of right ventricular failure should be present before the diagnosis is made. Dependent edema alone is inadequate documentation of the status of the right ventricle. With congestion of the liver, this organ may enlarge and become tender, ascites may be present, and jaundice may be noted.

Other Signs

As with left ventricular failure, sinus tachycardia and the other rhythms associated with pump failure may be present. In addition, right ventricular S_3 and S_4 are not uncommon. They are heard best at the lower left sternal border, with the bell of the stethoscope applied lightly to the chest, and can be recognized by an increase in intensity with inspiration. Finally, signs of any underlying cause of right ventricular failure may be present, such as hyperresonance with percussion, low immobile diaphragms, decreased breath sounds, increased anteroposterior chest

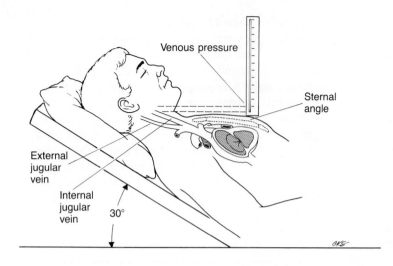

FIGURE 14–3
An assessment of jugular venous pressure. The highest point at which jugular vein pulsations can be seen is noted. The vertical distance between this point and the sternal angle is measured and recorded as centimeters "above or below" the sternal angle.

diameter, and use of the accessory muscles of respiration in patients with severe pulmonary emphysema.

Classification of Heart Failure

Heart failure may be present in varying degrees of severity. In acute myocardial infarction, heart failure has been simply and usefully classified by Killip into four classes: I, no failure; II, mild to moderate failure; III, acute pulmonary edema; and IV, cardiogenic shock.

Early, moderate (Killip class II) failure and chronic failure often are characterized by an S₃, increased heart rate (usually sinus rhythm), and possibly fine post-tussic crackles (rales) at the lung bases. In addition, evidence of pulmonary vascular congestion (often without pulmonary edema) often is seen on the chest roentgenogram, and dysrhythmias may be present: atrial premature contractions, atrial fibrillation, atrial flutter, paroxysmal atrial tachycardia, and junctional rhythms. The patient may be reasonably comfortable at rest or may have symptoms of low cardiac output or pulmonary vascular congestion. Symptoms are increased with activity.

Acute pulmonary edema (Killip class III) is a life-threatening situation characterized by transudation of fluid from the pulmonary capillary bed into the alveolar spaces, with associated extreme dyspnea and anxiety. Immediate care is required if the patient's life is to be saved.

Cardiogenic shock (Killip class IV) is the most ominous pump failure syndrome and is associated with the highest mortality, even with aggressive care. Cardiogenic shock is recognized clinically by:

- a systolic blood pressure less than 80 mm Hg (often it cannot be measured)
- a thready pulse that often is rapid
- pale, cool, and sweaty skin that frequently is cyanotic
- restlessness, confusion, and apathy
- possible alteration from usual mental status
- decreased or absent urine output

These manifestations of shock are a reflection of the profound inadequacy of the heart as a pump and usually reflect a large amount of muscle damage (40% or more of the left ventricular mass).

Some patients with significant, long-standing arterial hypertension will have manifestations of cardiogenic shock at relatively normal pressures. These people require a higher pressure to perfuse vital organs and maintain viability. Knowledge of the preceding blood pressure history is of great importance in recognizing these people. Not all clinical circumstances of cardiogenic shock are associated with an inadequate cardiac output, however. Depending on modifying circumstances, such as fever, the cardiac output occasionally may be normal or even increased.

The failure to decrease coronary care unit mortality below 10% to 20% is due largely to only modest improvement in the management and mortality of severe pump failure syndromes, especially cardiogenic shock. The mortality rate for cardiogenic shock remains at 81%, and more than two-thirds of the cases seen at autopsy document severe stenosis (> 75% of luminal diameter) of all three major coronary vessels, or severe myocardial structural damage.[3]

Killip Classification of Heart Failure

I—No failure
II—Mild to moderate failure
III—Acute pulmonary edema
IV—Cardiogenic shock

Management of Heart Failure

The physiological responses to heart failure form a rational basis for treatment. The goals of the management of congestive heart failure are to reduce the work of the heart, to increase cardiac output and myocardial contractility, and to decrease retention of salt and water.

Goals for Management of Heart Failure

- Reduce work of the heart
- Increase cardiac output and myocardial contractility
- Decrease retention of salt and water

Bed Rest

Because the heart cannot be put to complete rest to heal in the same fashion as a broken bone, the best that can be done is to put the entire patient to rest; thereby, through inactivity, the overall pumping demand on the heart is decreased. *Bed rest* is therefore an important part of the treatment of congestive heart failure, especially in acute and refractory stages.

In addition to decreasing the overall work demands made on the heart, bed rest assists in lowering the work load by decreasing the intravascular volume through a recumbence-induced diuresis. Studies of prolonged bed rest have demonstrated that within 48 to 72 hours of inactivity there is a decrease of plasma volume of 300 ml or more. Although this is not a great volume in terms of the overall intravascular fluid compartment, it does assist in decreasing the volume load that is presented to the failing heart. It therefore assists in decreasing dilation of the heart chambers and establishing a compensated state. This effect results from stimulation of atrial stretch receptors that sense the increased volume of blood returning to the right side of the heart, which would be sequestered in the lower extremities if the patient were upright. These receptors then "turn off" the production of antidiuretic hormone, and a diuresis follows. By decreasing intravascular volume and therefore the amount of blood presented to the heart to pump (preload), compensation of the heart may be enhanced.

Diuretics

In addition to bed rest, *salt* and *water restriction* and *diuretics*, either oral or parenteral, will decrease preload and the work of the heart.

All diuretics, regardless of the route of administration, may cause significant changes in the serum electrolytes, especially potassium and chloride. Therefore, regular determination of serum electrolytes is important in patient follow-up. This is particularly true when the patient also is receiving digitalis because low potassium produced by diuretics predisposes to digitalis toxicity, a life-threatening but avoidable complication. Because of this possibility, potassium supplements customarily are or-

dered when potassium-depleting diuretics are given, especially when digitalis is given as well.

The choice of route of administration of the diuretic is largely a function of the gravity of the clinical situation. Mild to moderate left ventricular failure (manifested by sinus tachycardia, post-tussic rales, and S_3) usually can be managed with oral preparations; however, acute pulmonary edema, a life-threatening situation, demands more drastic approaches, and the parenteral route should be chosen.

Other modifiers of preload and afterload are valuable approaches to the management of acute and chronic failure states. Both pharmacologic and mechanical methods are useful.

Morphine

Morphine is a most useful drug in the treatment of pulmonary edema. It achieves its primary physiological usefulness through a peripheral vasodilating effect, forming a peripheral pool of blood (bloodless phlebotomy) that decreases both venous return and the work of the heart. In addition, morphine allays the great anxiety associated with severe dyspnea and quiets the patient, thereby decreasing the respiratory pump mechanism for increasing venous return. Morphine also decreases arterial blood pressure and resistance, lessening the work of the heart (decreased afterload).

Reduction of Circulating Blood Volume

An even more dramatic method of decreasing preload and the work of the heart is *phlebotomy*, a procedure that is useful in the patient with acute pulmonary edema because it immediately removes a volume of blood from the central circulation, decreases venous return and filling pressure, and provides rather prompt reversal of some basic hemodynamic problems.

Phlebotomy may be bloodless (*rotating tourniquets*), or whole blood may be removed directly from the circulation. Tourniquets are less effective than direct removal of blood.

Although phlebotomy may be helpful in managing acute pulmonary edema, it may be dangerous in the patient who does not have an increased intravascular volume. This situation most commonly occurs in patients with acute myocardial infarction in whom there is extensive muscle damage and rapid onset of pulmonary edema before the kidneys can compensate for a diminished cardiac output by sodium and water retention.

Nitrates and Vasodilator Therapy

The use of *nitrates*, both acutely and chronically, has been advocated in the management of heart failure. By causing peripheral vasodilation, the heart is "unloaded" (decreased afterload), with a subsequent increase in cardiac output, decrease in pulmonary artery wedge pressure (a measurement that reflects the degree of pulmonary vascular congestion and the severity of left ventricular failure), and decrease in myocardial oxygen consumption. This form of therapy has been found useful in mild to moderate failure and acute pulmonary edema failure associated with myocardial infarction, chronic refractory left ventricular failure, and failure associated with severe mitral regurgitation. At present, parenteral vasodilator therapy (intravenous nitroglycerin or sodium nitroprusside) requires accurate hemodynamic monitoring of arterial and pulmonary wedge pressure (arterial cannula and Swan–Ganz catheter) and use of an infusion pump to titrate carefully the dose delivered.

Nitroprusside must be used with care. Long-acting nitrate therapy usually is given with nitroglycerin ointment. Some patients who have received maximal benefit from other forms of therapy for left ventricular failure have been improved substantially by vasodilator treatment. Long-term nitrate therapy not only relieves symptoms but appears to improve the prognosis of heart failure.

Digitalis

Although modification of the work of the heart by decreasing preload and afterload is indicated in heart failure and at times permits avoidance of drugs that increase the force of myocardial contraction, inotropic agents remain important therapeutic tools.

Digitalis is the primary drug for increasing contractility. This inotropic drug has a multiplicity of uses in cardiology and also is potentially one of the most dangerous, a fact recognized in 1785 by William Withering, discoverer of the pharmacologic value and toxicity of digitalis (foxglove): "Foxglove when given in very large and quickly repeated doses occasions sickness, vomiting, purging, confused vision, objects appearing green or yellow, increased secretion of urine with frequent motions to part with it and sometimes inability to retain it; slow pulse even as low as 35 in a minute, cold sweats, convulsions, syncope and death."[4] In the failing heart, digitalis slows the ven-

tricular rate and increases the force of contraction, increasing cardiac efficiency. As cardiac output increases, a greater volume of fluid is presented to the kidneys for filtration and excretion, and intravascular volume decreases.

In early failure with acute myocardial infarction, digitalis may increase the potential amount of damaged myocardium by causing increased contractility and therefore increased myocardial oxygen demand.[5] Treatment of failure in this circumstance probably is best if preload or afterload is decreased through the use of diuretics or nitrates. Patients with more severe heart failure are likely to benefit from long-term digitalis therapy. Maintaining a serum drug level of 1.54 to 2.56 nmol/liter can improve exercise tolerance and quality of life in those with congestive heart failure. Of course, if a significant drop in central aortic pressure occurs, coronary artery perfusion may fall and the area of damage increase. The key lessons here are that any medication has potentially ominous side effects, that a management regimen must be selected with care and with a full understanding of potential adverse effects, and that close patient monitoring is mandatory.

Positive Inotropics

Dopamine, at low doses of 2.5 to 5.0 μg/kg, will stimulate α-adrenergic, β-adrenergic, and dopamine receptors. This results in a release of catecholamines from nerve storage sites, improving contractility and dilating renal, splanchnic, cerebral, and coronary vessels. A small reduction in systemic vascular resistance may be noted. At higher doses (5–10 μg/kg), a positive inotropic (force of contraction), chromotropic (heart rate), and dromotropic (speed of conduction) response occurs. This increases heart rate, cardiac output, and stroke volume. At maximal doses (10–20 μg/kg), vasoconstriction occurs, increasing cardiac workload.

Dobutamine stimulates only β-adrenergic receptors and results in less vasoconstriction. Dosing is similar to that with dopamine, but the synthetic dobutamine will improve stroke volume and cardiac output with less vasoconstriction and tachycardia.

Amrinone will reduce cardiac filling pressures and systemic vascular resistance to improve cardiac output. The clinical trials of amrinone produced variable results, but arterial and venous dilation had a positive inotropic impact. Amrinone is most likely to be used for patients with markedly elevated filling pressures.

Mechanical Measures

Mechanical support of the left ventricle began in 1967 with *intra-aortic balloon counterpulsation* or pumping (IABP).[6] This temporary support enhances coronary blood flow, improves stroke volume, and reduces left ventricular preload and afterload. Chapter 13 fully discusses IABP.

During the 1970s, mechanical support expanded. The use of *extracorporeal membrane oxygenation* (ECMO) emerged. This device replaces cardiac/lung function, resulting in a forward flow of blood and gas exchange.[7] Extracorporeal membrane oxygenation may be used to buy time until definitive treatment such as coronary artery bypass surgery, septal repair, or heart transplantation can occur.

Left ventricular assist devices (LVAD) have been used as "bridge" therapy to maintain life until surgery or transplantation can be performed.[8] These devices provide forward flow to maintain coronary artery and systemic circulation (see Chapter 13).

The application of mechanical support devices is limited to major tertiary medical care systems. The success of IABP has established its use in cardiogenic shock management. The focus of research in the future likely will include expanded applications of ECMO and LVADs.

CASE STUDY

Bob White, a white man, 56 years old, did well in CCU for about 12 hours after the onset of his acute anterior lateral MI. His pain was controllable and his rhythm was NSR at 85. During the night, his nurse noted a steady increase in heart rate. By morning, bibasilar crackles developed. His weight increased by 1.3 kg. He was short of breath and his oxygen was increased from 2 liters per nasal cannula to 6 liters per nasal cannula and 40% via face mask, to keep his pulse oximetry $\geq$ 92%. Lasix was given with poor results (200 ml/2 hours). Mr. White's color had been pale, but now his skin was cool and diaphoretic. An S_3 and S_4 had been present since admission. Bob was frightened and could get comfortable only with the head of his bed elevated 60°. His JVD was elevated.

A Swan–Ganz catheter was placed via a right subclavian approach. Initially his readings were:

PAS/PAD = 42/22 mm Hg
PCWP = 20 mm Hg
C.O. = 3.4 L/minute
C.I. = 1.84 L/minute/BSA
SVR = 1250 dynes/second/cm^5
BP = 90/50 mm Hg
HR = 120/minute

Dobutamine was initiated at 5 µg/kg. After the completion of the Swan–Ganz insertion, Mr. White developed chest pain. This moderate pain radiated down his left arm and was relieved by NTG 1/150 sublingually × 2. Unfortunately, his BP could not withstand the NTG, and fell to 80/50.

It was decided that an IABP would be placed. Using a right femoral approach, the IABP was placed successfully and 1:1 counterpulsation was begun. After 2 hours:

PAS/PAD = 28/16 mm Hg
PCWP = 16 mm Hg
C.O. = 4.32
C.I. = 2.34 L/minute/BSA
SVR = 1080 dynes/second/cm^5
BP = 100/56 mm Hg
HR = 105/minute

A serum potassium was verified as 4.2 and another Lasix 20-mg dose was given, because the bibasilar crackles continued. Within 2 hours, a diuresis of 540 ml occurred.

Although close monitoring and assessment were required, this patient's outcome had been influenced positively by rapid assessment and intervention to reverse left ventricular heart failure.

Nursing Care Plan 14–1 is an example of a standard plan of care for the patient with heart failure.

(*Text continues on page 326*)

Clinical Research

Reedy J, et al: Mechanical cardiopulmonary support for refractory cardiogenic shock. Heart Lung 19:514–523, 1990

Support of 38 patients ranging in age from 10 to 78 years was provided with extracorporeal membrane oxygenation (ECMO) at St. Louis University Medical Center. This group of patients was unresponsive to conventional management and their diagnoses included acute myocardial infarction (12 patients), ischemic disease (15 patients), end-stage cardiomyopathy (7 patients), congenital disease (3 patients), and transplant graft rejection (1 patient). The support with ECMO averaged 28 hours, and 92% experienced hemodynamic stability.

This study concluded with nine patients being discharged (24%) and surviving long term. Based on the data, ECMO may best be applied for 12–24 hours, with a patient younger than 60 years old, having an acute situation requiring surgical intervention, angioplasty, or cardiac transplantation. ECMO can result in an increased survival for selected patients with refractory cardiogenic shock or cardiac arrest.

NURSING CARE PLAN 14–1:
The Patient With Heart Failure

NURSING DIAGNOSIS	OUTCOME CRITERIA/ PATIENT GOALS	NURSING INTERVENTIONS
Decreased cardiac output: related to overwhelmed physiological responses of heart failure; ↑ *rate, dilatation, hypertrophy, or* ↑ *stroke volume.*	• Maintain hemodynamic stability (BP greater than 90/xxx, normal heartrate, CI ≥ 2.2 L/min)	1. Keep patient on bed rest. 2. Assess urine amount and specific gravity routinely, q4h. 3. Measure hemodynamic parameters q2h or prn (PAP, PCWP, CVP). 4. Monitor ECG for rate and rhythm. 5. Assess heart sounds q4h for S_3 or S_4. 6. Assess breath sounds q4h for crackles. 7. Check ABGs and O_2 saturation with oximetric device. 8. Maintain O_2 as ordered. 9. Evaluate patient perceptions of subjective symptoms (SOB, angina, etc.). 10. Maintain IV access. 11. Give diuretics (Lasix) as ordered. 12. Give nitrates/vasodilators (nitroprusside) as ordered. 13. Maintain accurate intake and output measurements. 14. Restrict sodium and water, as ordered.
Decreased cardiac output: related to myocardial muscle damage from an acute infarction, acute structural changes (papillary muscle rupture, septal rupture), or valvular disease.	• Maintain hemodynamic stability (BP greater than 90/xxx, normal HR, CI ≥ 2.2 L/min	1. Keep patient on bed rest. 2. Take vital signs q15m until stable. 3. Monitor ECG for rate and rhythm. 4. Measure hemodynamic parameters q1h (PAP, PCW, CVP) and prn. 5. Assess heart sounds for S_3, S_4, or loud murmurs q4h. 6. Assess lungs for breath sounds and crackles q2h. 7. Administer O_2 to keep arterial saturation greater than 90%. 8. Verify acid–base balance with ABGs, as ordered.

(continued)

NURSING CARE PLAN 14–1: (Continued)
The Patient With Heart Failure

NURSING DIAGNOSIS	OUTCOME CRITERIA/ PATIENT GOALS	NURSING INTERVENTIONS
		9. Record hourly urine outputs, per indwelling catheter.
		10. Maintain IV access.
		11. Administer dopamine, dobutamine, or amrinone, as ordered, for maintaining adequate BP and urine output.
		12. Monitor lab values: ABGs, electrolytes, Hgb, Hct, drug levels.
		13. Administer vasodilators (nitroprusside, nitroglycerin), as ordered.
		14. Follow documentation of chest radiographic results.
		15. Prepare for IABP pumping, as indicated.
		16. Administer antiarrhythmics, as ordered.
Decreased tissued perfusion: related to decreased cardiac output, tissue hypoxemia, acidosis, and possible thrombi or emboli.	• Skin will be warm and dry, patient will show improved mental status.	1. Assess for change in mentation q1h and prn.
		2. Assess for skin color, cyanosis, temperature, and diaphoresis q2h.
		3. Assess urine output and specific gravity q1h.
		4. Assess the quality and presence of distal peripheral pulses q2h.
		5. Assess bowel sounds q4h; place NG if ileus present.
		6. Assess for liver congestion (RUQ pain, increased liver size, tenderness) q4h.
		7. Vital signs q1–4h as indicated.
		8. Position patient for relief of pressure on dependent areas of body.
		9. Assess calf for a + Homan's sign.
		10. Evaluate all subjective symptomatic complaints.
		11. Evaluate lab values (BUN, creatinine, Hgb, Hct, ABG), as ordered.

(continued)

NURSING CARE PLAN 14–1: (Continued)
The Patient With Heart Failure

NURSING DIAGNOSIS	OUTCOME CRITERIA/ PATIENT GOALS	NURSING INTERVENTIONS
		12. Report all abnormal findings to physician.
		13. Maintain the patient on bed rest.
Impaired gas exchange: related to pulmonary congestion, pulmonary hypertension, decreased peripheral perfusion resulting in lactic acidosis and lowered cardiac output.	• Maintain adequate ventilation and oxygenation.	1. Assess work of breathing (rate, rhythm, and depth) q2h.
		2. Assess breath sounds q2h and prn.
		3. Assess cyanosis, if present.
		4. Provide supplemental oxygen, as ordered.
		5. Monitor O_2 saturation with an oximetric device.
		6. Check ABGs as ordered and prn.
		7. Minimize O_2 consumption by providing bed rest.
		8. Correct the acid/base balance with $NaHCO_3$ as ordered.
		9. Assess hemodynamics (PAP, PCWP, CVP) q1h and prn.
		10. Position patient to facilitate gas exchange (elevate the head of the bed).
		11. Prevent atelectasis by TC&DB q2h and prn.
		12. Follow the documentation of chest radiographic results.
		13. Administer diuretics (Lasix) as ordered.
		14. Administer bronchodilators (aminophyline) as ordered.
		15. Administer cardiotonics (digoxin) as ordered.
Fluid volume excess: related to cardiac output reduction, sodium and water retention by the kidneys, hypoperfusion to peripheral tissues and pulmonary hypertension.	• Adequate urine output will be maintained with diuretic therapy (>30 ml/hr).	1. Assess hemodynamic parameters (PAP, PCWP, CVP) q2h and prn.
		2. Assess ECG monitor for rate and rhythm.
		3. Assess BP q1–2h and prn.
		4. Evaluate urine output for amount and specific gravity, q1h.
		5. Assess breath sounds q2h.

(continued)

NURSING CARE PLAN 14–1: *(Continued)*
The Patient With Heart Failure

NURSING DIAGNOSIS	OUTCOME CRITERIA/ PATIENT GOALS	NURSING INTERVENTIONS
		6. Assess JVD q2h or after diuretic therapy.
		7. Assess heart sounds for an S_3 or S_4 q4h.
		8. Evaluate presence and quality of the peripheral pulses q4h.
		9. Maintain an accurate input and output record.
		10. Weigh patient daily.
		11. Maintain fluid and sodium restrictions.
		12. Position patient to facilitate gravity drainage of extremities.
		13. Passive range-of-motion (ROM) exercises to encourage peripheral edema to return to the vascular bed.
		14. Place on airflow bed if the dependent edema is severe.
		15. Evaluate lab values: Na, K, Hgb, Hct.
		16. Administer diuretics, as ordered.
		17. Maintain IV access, but use minimal fluids to keep the line open or use a capped line.
High risk for activity intolerance: related to low cardiac output, inability to meet metabolic needs of skeletal muscle, pulmonary congestion leading to hypoxemia and dyspnea or poor nutrition during a critical illness.	• Patient will show progress in activity without severe symptoms.	1. Maintain patient on bed rest while acutely ill.
		2. Progress patient to sitting in a chair; elevate patient's legs.
		3. Maintain passive ROM while critically ill.
		4. Evaluate vital signs as activity progression occurs.
		5. Use rest periods between times of activity.
		6. Maintain supplementary O_2 as ordered.
		7. During activity assess ECG, dyspnea, cyanosis, work of breathing, respiratory rate, and subjective statements.
		8. Provide diet as ordered (sodium and water restriction will be likely).

(continued)

NURSING CARE PLAN 14–1: (Continued)
The Patient With Heart Failure

NURSING DIAGNOSIS	OUTCOME CRITERIA/ PATIENT GOALS	NURSING INTERVENTIONS
High risk for knowledge deficit: related to disease state, treatments, medications, complications, and lifestyle changes.	• Patient will identify symptoms that warrant medical attention, use rest periods and progress activity to perform ADL, will state name, dose, timing, and purpose of each medication.	1. Begin progressive teaching plan—document the material presented and the patient's response. 2. Include the family/significant others in progressive teaching plan. 3. Use both verbal and written instruction formats. 4. Encourage questions from the patient and family.
	• Patient will attend cardiac rehabilitation classes.	5. Advise patient to begin formal cardiac rehabilitation classes. 6. Plan follow-up care for after discharge. (See sample progressive teaching plan in Chapter 15.)
Anxiety: related to critical illness, fear of death or disfigurement, role changes within social setting, or permanent disability.	• Patient will express anxieties to appropriate resource person.	1. Provide environment that encourages open discussion of emotional issues. 2. Mobilize patient's support system and involve these resources as appropriate. 3. Allow time for patient to express self. 4. Identify possible hospital resources for patient/family support. 5. Encourage open family-to-nurse communications regarding emotional issues. 6. Validate patient and family knowledge base regarding the critical illness. 7. Involve religious support systems as appropriate.

Summary

The general outlook for patients with cardiogenic shock is poor for both the short and the long term. Heart failure, with its accompanying symptoms of low cardiac output or pulmonary vascular congestion or both, is one of the major sources of disability in cardiovascular disease. Its recognition and pathophysiologically based management are of paramount importance if a patient's functional capacity and vocational and community viability are to be optimized and maintained.

REFERENCES

1. Lewis T: Diseases of the Heart. New York, Macmillan, 1933
2. Morris DC, et al: "The Recognition and Treatment of Myo-

cardial Infarction and Its Complications" In Hurst JW, et al (eds): The Heart, Arteries and Veins, pp 1054–1075, 7th ed. New York, McGraw-Hill, 1990

3. Goldberg RJ, et al: Cardiogenic shock after acute myocardial infarction. N Engl J Med 325:1117–1122, 1991

4. Withering W: An Account of the Foxglove and Its Medical Uses, with Practical Remarks on Dropsy and Other Diseases. London, CGJ and J Robinson, 1785

5. Marcus FI, Huang SI: "Digitalis" In Hurst JW, et al (eds): The Heart, Arteries and Veins, pp 1748–1758, 7th ed. New York, McGraw-Hill, 1990

6. Schott KE: Intra-aortic balloon counterpulsation as a therapy for shock. Critical Care Nursing Clinics of North America 2:187–193, 1990

7. Reedy J, et al: Mechanical cardiopulmonary support for refractory cardiogenic shock. Heart Lung 19:514–523, 1990

8. Wampler RK, et al: Treatment of cardiogenic shock with a hemopump left ventricular assist device. Ann Thorac Surg 52:506–513, 1991

BIBLIOGRAPHY

Chatterjee K, Cheitlin M, et al: Cardiology: An Illustrated Text Reference, vols 1 and 2. Philadelphia, JB Lippincott, 1991

Guyton AC: Textbook of Medical Physiology, 8th ed. Philadelphia, WB Saunders, 1991

Porth CM: Pathophysiology: Concepts of Altered Health States. Philadelphia, JB Lippincott, 1990

STUDY QUESTIONS

1. Which of the following mechanisms is *not* one of the reserve mechanisms of the heart?

   a. dilation as described by the Starling relationship
   b. decreased heart rate with increased filling time
   c. hypertrophy—in chronic conditions
   d. stroke volume, which increases the percentage of diastolic volume ejected

2. Pulmonary vascular congestion, dyspnea, and orthopnea may occur in

   a. right heart failure only
   b. left heart failure only
   c. both right and left heart failure
   d. none of the above

3. When physiological responses become overwhelmed as in the vicious cycle of heart failure, all of the following occur *except*

   a. tissue alkalosis and ischemia
   b. increased oxygen consumption by the heart
   c. reduced cardiac output
   d. preload exceeds pumping ability of the heart

4. Which dose of dopamine may be indicated in heart failure?

   a. 2–5 µg/kg
   b. 10–20 µg/kg
   c. > 20 µg/kg
   d. any dose, because dopamine is titrated for the desired effect

CHAPTER 15

Acute Myocardial Infarction

BEHAVIORAL OBJECTIVES

Based on the content in this chapter, the reader should be able to:

1. Describe the continuum of pathophysiological events that occur between angina and acute myocardial infarction (MI).
2. List the three major coronary arteries and the structures supplied by their circulation.

Hudak: Critical Care Nursing:
A Holistic Approach, 6th ed. © 1994
J. B. Lippincott Company.

3. Describe the pathophysiology and anticipated interventions for cardiogenic shock.
4. Describe the content offered in patient/family education while the recovering MI patient remains in the critical care unit.
5. List and describe four complications of an acute MI.

Description

Although the mortality associated with problems of the heart and vessels has decreased by 25% since the 1970s, cardiovascular disease remains the most serious threat to life and health in the United States.[1] For men, the chance of heart disease developing before 60 years of age is 1 in 3; the risk for women is 1 in 10. It has been estimated that 20% of Americans have one or more cardiovascular diseases. Each year, 1,500,000 people have myocardial infarctions (MI), which result in approximately 540,400 deaths. Two-thirds of all cardiovascular deaths are related to arteriosclerosis, and half of those deaths occur within 2 hours of symptom onset and before hospitalization.

As overwhelming as the mortality and morbidity statistics appear, much progress has been made in diagnosis, management, and therapy to combat cardiovascular disease successfully. The mortality rate is declining by 2% per year. Since the Framingham study of risk factors in 1951 and the development of coronary care units in the same decade, the critical care nurse has played a major role in reducing the mortality associated with heart disease.

Sophisticated prehospital care and continuous cardiac monitoring have dramatically decreased the number of deaths caused by dysrhythmias. Following an acute MI, the most frequent cause of death is now left ventricular heart failure. Prognosis after discharge is determined by three factors. The degree of left ventricular dysfunction is the strongest predictor of mortality, followed by the frequency of premature ventricular beats, and evidence of ischemia (either spontaneous or exercise-induced).

The role of the critical care nurse has evolved rapidly. To combat cardiovascular disease, the nurse must have finite assessment skills, intervene quickly, and reevaluate the results of the interventions. Complete discharge planning and "cardiac rehabilitation" programs have enabled patients to return home, maximizing their health status. The role of the nurse, in both acute and nonacute settings, cannot be minimized.

Physiological Principles

Coronary Circulation

Infarct location can affect prognosis. Because the process of an MI begins with coronary artery disease leading to decreased blood flow, it is imperative to understand the functional anatomy of the major coronary arteries.

There are two major coronary arteries, the left and the right.[2] The left main coronary artery has two branches. The left anterior descending (LAD; also called the "widow maker"), passes down the anterior wall toward the apex of the myocardium. It supplies blood flow to two-thirds of the intraventricular septum, most of the apex, and the anterior left ventricle. The left circumflex flows from the left coronary toward the left lateral wall of the left ventricle. The circumflex supplies blood flow to the left atrium, the entire posterior wall, and the posterior one-third of the intraventricular septum (Fig. 15–1).

The right coronary artery (RCA) comes off the aorta on the right side of the pulmonary artery and travels along the right lateral wall to the posterior heart. The RCA supplies the right atrium, right ventricle, sinoatrial (SA) node, atrioventricular (AV) node, posterosuperior intraventricular septum, part of the left atrium, and the posterior and diaphragmatic surface of the left ventricle. Thus, the coronary arteries manage to distribute blood flow to the very active heart tissue.

Seventy-five percent of the population has dominant flow through the RCA; 10% have dominant flow through the LCA; and 5% have an even balance of blood flow. Five percent of hearts have the left ventricle supplied by the LCA, due to a congenitally small RCA. People with left-dominant flow are more likely to succumb to a coronary occlusion. Although infarcts can occur on any wall of the myocardium, the term "myocardial infarction" commonly refers to a left ventricular infarct. The impact of a left ventricular infarct is dramatically symptomatic, and our common diagnostic tools can recognize and locate left

The Coronary Artery Blood Supply

Left Main Coronary Artery
- Left anterior descending supplies
  - Anterior two thirds of ventricular septum
  - Anterior left ventricle
  - Entire apex
  - Most of right and left bundle branches
- Left circumflex supplies
  - 40%–45% of hearts: SA node
  - Left atrium
  - Entire posterior wall

Right Coronary Artery Supplies
- Posterosuperior ventricular septum
- Part of the left atrium
- Right atrium
- 55%–60% of hearts: SA node
- AV node
- Right ventricle
- Posterior left ventricle
- Diaphragmatic left ventricle

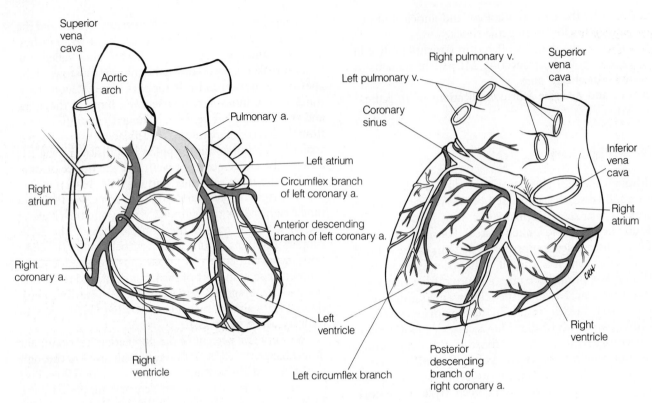

FIGURE 15–1
Coronary circulation. (From Porth CM: Pathophysiology: Concepts of Altered Health States, 3rd ed. Philadelphia, JB Lippincott, 1990)

ventricular damage. As diagnostic skills expand, more attention may be given to infarcts of the other chambers.

Collateral Circulation

Collateral circulation has received much attention. During ischemic attacks, homocoronary anastomosis occurs. The blood flow is unable to pass through the occluded vessel. As pressure builds on the proximal side of the occlusion, flow is redirected and new vessels develop. This collateral circulation allows the vascular pressure to be relatively equal and provides alternate coronary circulation routes, minimizing ischemic potential.

Pathophysiological Principles

Because MI is a "segmental" disease of the myocardium, physiological considerations of global heart disease will not always apply. Rather than an epidemic loss of myocardial function, the MI creates a partial loss, based on location and severity of tissue necrosis.

An MI is the result of coronary artery disease (CAD) with concomitant tissue damage and necrosis. The coronary artery damage may be traced to thrombosis, atherosclerosis, or spasm. The cardiac tissue dependent on blood flow from the diseased artery will become ischemic and necrotic, resulting in an infarct.

Atherosclerosis

For many years, the etiology of "coronary thrombosis," or clot occlusion, of a coronary artery was believed to cause an MI. The thrombosis found on postmortem examination usually resulted in blood flow that was compromised to the extent of causing a full myocardial wall thickness, or "transmural" infarct, and tissue death.

As dissection study continued, it became clear that the final event may have been thrombotic but that the narrowing of the coronary artery had begun by the development of plaque, known as atherosclerosis. The term "atherosclerosis" comes from the Greek word *athere*, which means "porridge" or "gruel." This term seems to describe the gross appearance of the plaque substance.

Atherosclerosis actually is an insidious process, beginning long before symptoms occur. In atherosclerosis, the intima (inner lining) of the artery undergoes focal changes. Muscular arteries, such as the coronaries, carotid, aortic, iliac, femoral, and popliteal arteries, are most susceptible.

Spots develop on the artery's intimal wall. These minor elevations cause a proliferation of intimal cells, and eventually a "cap" of cells is formed. The center of this small cap consists of necrotic intimal cells and cholesterols. As the cap becomes larger, it is known as plaque. Plaque develops best in plasma that is rich in low-density lipoproteins (cholesterol). The inflammatory process causes these cholesterols to gravitate toward disruptions in the otherwise smooth intimal lining. Although the origin of intimal injury resulting in intimal spotting is unclear, cigarette smoking and hypertension are known to aggravate intimal injury.

As the plaque increases in size, platelet adhesion begins. This process can continue to the point of slowing arterial blood flow from a rushing state to merely a trickle by reducing arterial diameter.

Much attention has been given to coronary artery spasm. A blood vessel, narrowed by atherosclerosis, can be occluded if spasm occurs. It is believed that many partial wall thickness infarcts, or nontransmural infarcts, are the result of coronary spasm. Atherosclerotic arteries respond to vasodilator stimuli paradoxically, causing vasoconstriction.[3]

As arterial blood flow is decreased, the myocardial tissue's need for oxygen and nutrients continues. The same work of pumping blood must be accomplished with less available energy and oxygen. The tissue that depends on the blood supply becomes ischemic as it functions with less oxygenated blood. Anaerobic metabolism can provide only 6% of the total energy needed. Glucose uptake by the cells is markedly increased as glycogen and adenosine triphosphate stores are depleted. Potassium rapidly moves out of the myocardial cells during ischemia. An acidotic cellular bath develops, further compromising cellular metabolism.

Myocardial Infarction

If the reduced blood flow is reestablished to normal levels, the ischemic event will terminate. This transient myocardial ischemia is known as "angina." If the ischemia were to continue while myocardial oxygen requirements persevered, the tissue would become necrotic because the energy demands would exceed the oxygenated blood's energy supply. This is an MI.

Necrotic myocardial tissue cannot be revived. Surrounding the dead tissue is a zone of ischemic tissue that has suffered less, remaining viable on severely compromised blood flow. It is a major therapeutic goal to prevent the ischemic concentric rings of tissue from becoming necrotic. If the ischemic rings cannot be saved, the resulting damage is referred to as an "extension" of the acute MI.

Transmural Infarction

As mentioned earlier, infarct size and location have enormous impact on prognosis and survival. Transmural infarcts result in necrosis of all layers of the myocardium.

Because the heart functions as a squeezing pump, systolic efforts to empty the ventricle can be reduced markedly by a segment of the myocardial wall that is dead and nonfunctional. If the area of the transmural infarct is small, the necrotic tissue may be "dyskinetic." As this muscular wall squeezes during systole or relaxes with diastolic filling, dyskinetic tissue does not remain in synchronous motion with the healthy myocardial wall. If the transmural infarct area is larger, the dead tissue may become "akinetic," lacking any motion and therefore interfering with efficient pumping (Fig. 15–2).

During the process of necrosis, the transmural infarct area may weaken. As the rest of the chamber goes through isotonic contraction, the necrotic area may bulge with an aneurysm or even rupture under the effort to create an adequate systolic contraction.

Subendocardial Infarction

Not all infarcts affect the full wall thickness. Subendocardial infarcts are common and involve necrosis of the inner layers of the myocardium. The subendocardial tissue is most vulnerable to ischemia; the outer wall, the epicardium, is the least vulnerable. Because myocardial muscle layers are "wrapped" for efficient squeezing (layers crisscross over each other), a subendocardial infarct will have less impact on wall motion than will a transmural infarct (see Figure 15–2).

Initial Assessment

History

The nursing assessment of a patient with a probable MI must be organized and thorough. It is best to start with the patient's history because this establishes rapport and provides valuable data. A generalized history should be obtained, with emphasis placed on the cardiovascular system.

Historical data that include the presence or absence of "risk factors" should be gathered. The Framingham, Massachusetts study of the late 1940s and early 1950s identified five risk factors for heart disease. During this prospec-

---

Framingham's Risk Factors

- Hypercholesterolemia: >275 mg/dl
- Cigarette smoking: >20/day
- Obesity: >120% of ideal weight
- Hypertension: >160/90
- Sedentary lifestyle

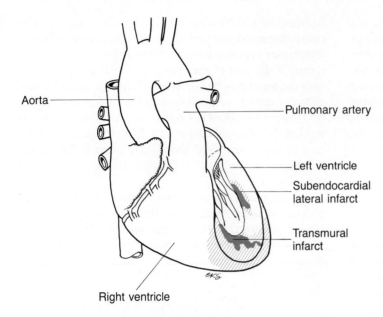

Aorta

Pulmonary artery

Left ventricle

Subendocardial lateral infarct

Transmural infarct

Right ventricle

FIGURE 15–2
Schematic drawing comparing transmural and subendocardial infarctions. Note that the transmural infarct of the inferior/septal wall has a large necrotic area on the interior of the ventricle, which decreases in intensity but increases in size. The subendocardial lateral infarct does not involve all muscle layers and is of less intensity and size.

tive study of a large, random population, several factors were noted to increase a person's propensity for heart disease. The major factors identified were elevated blood cholesterol, cigarette smoking, obesity, hypertension, and sedentary lifestyle.

Other factors may potentiate the development of CAD. These factors relate to the incidence of heart disease, but not the severity of the heart disease[4]:

- family history of heart disease
- type "A" personality (intense ambition, competitive outlook, and fast pace)
- diabetes mellitus or abnormal glucose tolerance test
- male sex
- use of oral contraceptives
- menopause
- high-cholesterol and high-fat diet

The patient's description of the acute event is important. Often, the precipitating events involve cold weather, exercise, heavy meals, stress, emotional events, or Valsalva actions such as a bowel movement. Some people have symptoms at rest, but usually there is an activity involved that increases the metabolic requirements of the body.

Angina

Typically, the pain is precordial. Angina (from a Latin word meaning "squeezing") often presents as a crushing, squeezing, constructing, choking, or burning pain. The sensation is sharp and stabbing, or sore, aching, and dull. The pain may radiate behind the sternum to the left chest, left arm, neck, jaw, or left shoulder. Visceral pain from the myocardium sometimes is poorly localized, and over 100 conditions have been improperly diagnosed as angina.

Commonly, gastric distress, peptic ulcer disease, and gallbladder disease are misdiagnosed as the problem.

Advanced diagnostic skill has enabled practitioners to differentiate types of angina. "Stable angina" is the paroxysmal substernal pain, relieved by rest or nitroglycerin.[5] This transient bout of ischemia presents similarly to the patient each time. The pain can be controlled with nitroglycerin.

More severe than stable angina is "unstable angina," also known as "preinfarction angina" or "crescendo angina." Unstable angina is characterized by more severe or more frequent attacks, occurring with less provocation or at rest. Usually, two nitroglycerin tablets are insufficient to relieve pain. About 16% to 20% of patients with unstable angina will have MI. During an unstable anginal attack, the electrocardiogram (ECG) will reveal significant ST segment depression.

The last category of angina is known as "Prinzmetal's," or "variant," angina. Typically, the pain occurs without precipitating factors because it is due to coronary artery spasm. The ECG will show ST segment elevation (usually seen only with an MI) rather than the ischemic ST depression seen in typical angina.

The pain of an acute MI is similar to anginal pain, but more severe. Although anginal pain may last minutes and be relieved with nitroglycerin, MI pain can last hours and is relieved best with narcotics such as morphine. As many as 25% of patients with acute MI will experience little or no pain.

As the nurse assesses the patient, it is likely that symptoms of a severe autonomic response will be apparent. Patients with cardiac pain (anginal or MI) often are very still. Pallor and diaphoresis often occur. Cyanosis may be present, but the skin often will look gray or washed-out. Vomiting and bradycardia may be present. Syncope is not rare. Some patients will complain of the feeling of "impending doom," and most are very frightened.

It is of value to be able to differentiate between symptoms of right-sided and left-sided heart disease. Right-sided failure (congestive heart failure) presents with edema, distended jugular veins, peripheral venous congestion, an enlarged liver, cyanosis, and crackles. Left-sided heart failure presents with a "shock" picture of gray skin, mottled lower extremities, dyspnea, orthopnea, low blood pressure, and low urine output. Further diagnostic studies often are needed to establish a conclusive etiology.

Diagnostic Studies

Critical care nurses will need to anticipate diagnostic studies required to verify the medical diagnosis. Continuous cardiac monitoring for dysrhythmias and response to treatment will begin on admission. A 12-lead ECG may confirm the presence of heart disease.

Electrocardiogram Findings

On the 12-lead ECG, ischemic but functional myocardial tissue will produce changes in the T wave, causing inversion as the electrical current is directed away from the ischemic tissue.[6] More seriously, ischemic tissue will alter the ST segment, causing ST depression.

With an infarct, the dead myocardium does not conduct electricity and fails to repolarize normally, resulting in ST segment elevation. As the necrosis develops, with healing of the ischemic rings around the necrotic area, Q waves develop. The necrotic area is an electrically inactive scar, but the ischemic zone will reflect T wave changes as ischemia recurs. Initially, with an MI, the ST elevation is accompanied by tall T waves. Hours to days later, the T waves invert. As the MI ages, Q waves remain, and the ST segments return to normal.

The 12-lead ECG also identifies the location of the ischemic or infarcted tissue. By the presence of the specific lead changes, as well as reciprocal changes occurring on the other walls, infarct area and size are determined (Table 15–1 and Figs. 15–3 to 15–5).

Subendocardial infarcts of partial wall thickness are documented by persistent ST depression, T wave inversion with Q waves, or both. The presence or absence of permanent Q waves will not always indicate MI. For example, right ventricular hypertrophy causes Q waves in V5 and V6. Because Q waves are not always abnormal, further diagnostic studies are needed.

Cardiac Enzymes

Traditionally, serial studies of cardiac enzymes are obtained through blood samples drawn every 8 hours for 1 to 2 days. When tissue injury occurs, large proteins escape from inside the cardiac muscle cell and enter the circulation. The enzymes that should be observed are creatine

TABLE 15–1
Specific Electrocardiogram (ECG) Changes for Acute Transmural Myocardial Infarctions

Infarct Area	ECG Changes
Anterior	ST segment elevation in leads V_3–V_4; reciprocal changes (ST depression) in leads II, III, aVF (Fig. 12–3)
Inferior	ST segment elevation in leads II, III, aVF; reciprocal changes (ST depression) in V_1–V_6, I, aVL (Fig. 12–5)
Lateral	ST segment elevation in I, aVL, V_5–V_6 (Fig. 12–4)
Posterior	Reciprocal changes in II, III, aVF; predominant R waves in V_1–V_2
Right ventricle	Mimic inferior wall changes

kinase (CK), lactic dehydrogenase (LDH), and serum glutamic oxaloacetic transaminase (SGOT).[7] False-positive results occur in as many as 15% of patients. Isolated enzymes are available to assist in determining the cardiac origin of CK and LDH (see discussion of serum enzyme studies in Chapter 12).

Other Diagnostic Procedures

If the physician desires further diagnostic data, exercise stress testing can be used to determine functional capacity of the heart under stress in a controlled environment. The blood pressure, heart rate, rhythm, and ischemic ECG changes are monitored during a graded treadmill workout. While the exercise intensity is gradually increased, the left ventricle is observed for dysrhythmias, signs of failure, hypotension, and angina.

Vectorcardiography is a noninvasive measure of electrical axis for speed and direction of conduction and disturbances such as left ventricular and right ventricular hypertrophy and heart blocks. Thallium scintigraphy allows for myocardial imaging after an injection of thallium-201. A "cold spot" occurs in the image corresponding to the area of ischemia.

Invasive diagnostic tests are not without risk, but they provide valuable and accurate data. Coronary angiography (heart catheterization) allows for the direct visualization of the major coronary arteries and direct measurement of left ventricular function. Under the fluoroscope, a catheter is passed through the femoral artery to the aortic arch. The vessel to be studied can be located and a dye injection selectively administered. Coronary artery lesions are visualized, and permanent visual recordings are made.

Pressure readings of all cardiac chambers can be made during a heart catheterization. Radiopaque dye allows the left ventricle to be studied in peak systole and peak diastole. The still films of the functioning ventricle can be

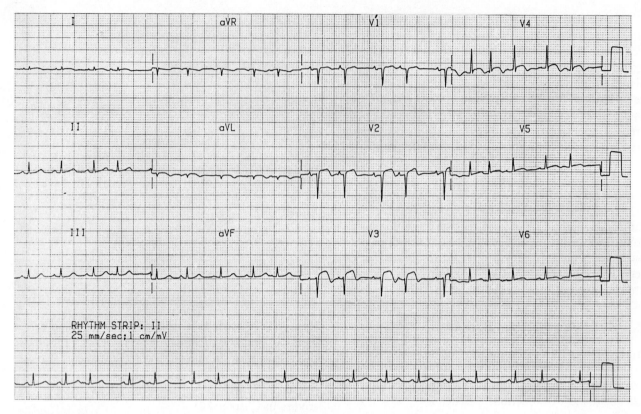

FIGURE 15–3
Acute anterolateral infarct. Note the ST segment elevation in V_2 to V_6, I, and aVL. There are
no reciprocal changes. The rhythm is a sinus tachycardia with premature atrial contractions.

compared with the cardiac cycle (determined by ECG) to determine left ventricular end-diastolic volume, stroke volume, and ejection fraction. A comparison of these three values is helpful in determining the degree of compromise in an infarcted left ventricle (see Chapter 12 for a full discussion of cardiovascular diagnostic techniques).

Often, the findings of atherosclerosis are simultaneously diagnosed and treated during heart catheterization. Percutaneous transluminal coronary artery angioplasty can be performed on vessels with demanding occlusions (see Chapter 13). Plaque in the involved vessel is cleared by expanding a small balloon located on the catheter. Although this plaque lesion may not have created the original infarct, concomitant lesions are not that rare. Therefore, as a diagnostic evaluation of the diseased vessel and myocardial tissue damage is occurring, a new, smaller, but potentially harmful lesion is treated.

Assessment and Management

Reducing Morbidity and Mortality

After the history and diagnostic studies determine the presence of an acute MI, the medical and nursing roles vary. The physician will focus on minimizing complications through preservation of the functional left ventricular wall, limiting ventricular dysrhythmias, controlling

heart failure, and limiting cardiac workload. The nurse's focus will be to control pain, perform an ongoing assessment, report symptoms, and provide patient/family education. Together, the physician and nurse share the common goal of decreasing the inpatient mortality through prevention of further tissue damage.

About 50% of patients with an acute MI die before admission to a hospital. Fifteen percent will die during hospitalization and 10% within a year of discharge.[8] Sudden death appears to result from the fatal triad of ischemia, dysrhythmias, and left ventricular dysfunction. Long-term antiarrhythmic therapy has not produced satisfying statistical reports, with studies describing rhythm disturbances as the etiology of 52% to 74% of all postdischarge deaths.

Anti-ischemic therapy, primarily with β-blockers, has been shown to reduce the risk of death, although the exact mechanism still is conjectural. Control of ischemia with coronary bypass surgery (see Chapter 16) has been successful in cases of LAD lesions or three-vessel disease when the patient presents with stable angina after MI.

Pain

Chest pain can be assessed for location, duration, and the patient's description. It is helpful to have the patient evaluate his or her pain on a scale of 1 to 10, with 10 being the

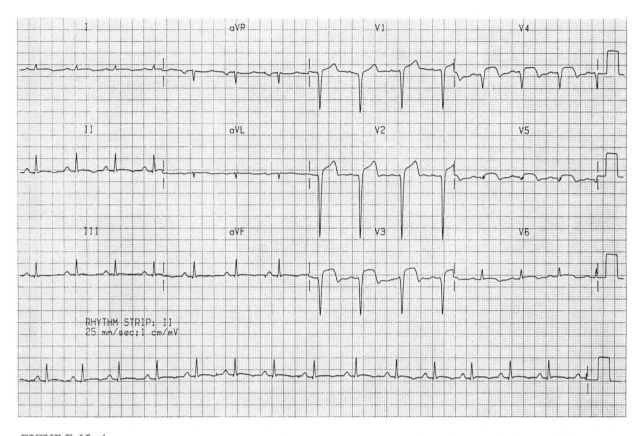

FIGURE 15–4

Acute lateral infarct, with an old inferior infarct that extended into an acute anterior lateral infarct later in the day. Note the elevated ST segments and T wave inversion in V_3 to V_6, I, and II. The rhythm is a normal sinus rhythm. The old inferior infarct presents as residual Q waves in leads II, III, and aVF.

worst. This helps quantitate a subjective experience. Duration and onset factors should be identified. A rhythm strip can be placed in the patient's record. Although ischemic changes are noted best by 12-lead ECG, dysrhythmias may occur during chest pain.

The definitive treatment of ischemic chest pain is administration of an agent in the nitrate group. Nitroglycerin (tablets or continuous infusion) acts on the vascular bed. A relative hypovolemia occurs with a lessened venous return as the result of peripheral pooling of blood. Nitrates act more on veins than on arteries, but selectively dilate the coronary arteries. They cause a significant decrease in the left ventricular filling pressure and a slight increase in cardiac index and stroke volume. Nitroglycerin eases the myocardial workload by decreasing preload. Nitroglycerin tablets can be repeated every 5 minutes until relief is obtained, but long-acting nitrate administration is accomplished best intravenously (Display Box 15–1).

The pain accompanying an MI is treated best with narcotics. Morphine given in small increments of 1 to 2 mg by intravenous (IV) push is the traditional choice. Morphine, a potent vasodilator, decreases preload and provides an analgesic effect. Some patients benefit from the euphoric side effect of morphine, finding that it relaxes and calms them.

Either method of pain relief can result in hypotension.

Again, the patient's pain relief should be assessed on a scale of 1 to 10. The blood pressure should be checked frequently (every 5–10 minutes) until the pain has subsided.

The presence of hypotension (< 100 mm Hg systolic) can indicate impending shock or an adverse response to therapy. Modified Trendelenburg position, with the feet slightly elevated, may help. Some patients with acute MI cannot tolerate having their bed flat, so positions should be changed carefully. Hypotension seen only during chest pain indicates a compromised mechanical pump during ischemia.

Hypertension causes the myocardium to work harder. Convalescing hearts need to have their workload limited. A blood pressure of less than 150 mm Hg systolic is ideal.

After relief of chest pain, the most important therapeutic goal is to maximize the cardiac output while limiting the cardiac workload. This requires a delicate balance of pharmacologic interventions and continuous assessment of the hemodynamic state.

Myocardial Workload

Minimizing the cardiac workload can be accomplished in various ways. β-Adrenergic blockade (eg, propranolol) will decrease heart rate and contractility, and is indicated if

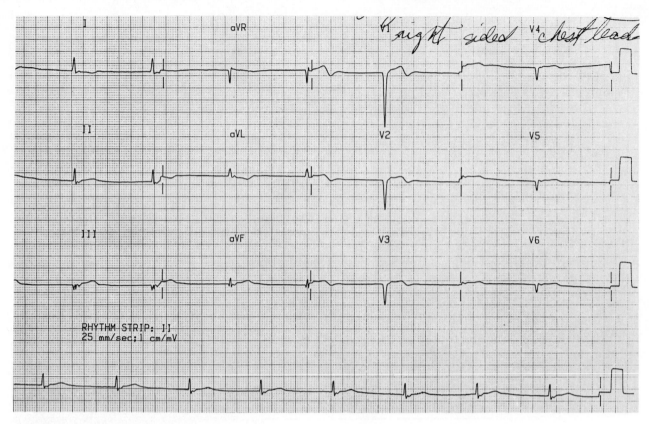

FIGURE 15–5

Acute inferior infarct. The ST segments are elevated in II, III, and aVF. Reciprocal change of ST segment depression is seen in I and aVL. The unusual precordial lead configuration (leads V_1–V_6) occurred because the tracing was done across the right chest, since a transthoracic pacemaker wire was on the left chest. The rhythm is complete heart block, at a rate of less than 50 beats/minute, which was not tolerated by this patient. The patient was stabilized with a temporary pacemaker, and this heart block resolved as the acute infarct evolved.

S_3 develops (heard at the end of rapid ventricular filling) and a gallop rhythm exists, indicating the presence of heart failure. Because propranolol will decrease rate and contractility, the patient should have an adequate heart rate ($\geq$ 55 beats/minute) and blood pressure ($\geq$ 95 mm Hg systolic) and no heart block before the onset of therapy. Use of β-adrenergic blockers will improve mortality and morbidity for acute MI patients.[9]

Calcium antagonists often are used to decrease afterload (the pressures the ventricle must push against to pump blood) and decrease contractility. This substantially reduces the risk of reinfarction or extension of the acute MI. Calcium antagonists also act directly on the coronary arteries, producing vasodilation. Nifedipine is the most effective calcium antagonist. Verapamil and diltiazem provide less direct arterial dilatation but have strong antiarrhythmic qualities, slowing transmission through the SA and AV nodes. Verapamil and diltiazem are effective in terminating supraventricular tachycardias. Calcium channel blockers, used prophylactically, have the best results with postinfarction angina and non-Q wave infarcts (subendocardial MI; Table 15–2).

The use of low-flow oxygen assists in maximizing the oxygen saturation of arterial blood and is very beneficial to the recovering myocardium.

Myocardial work can be limited only through the reduction of energy expenditures by the entire body. Small meals that are easily digestible should be encouraged. Bed rest with a gradual increase in the activities of daily living can help keep the metabolic rate lowered. It is important to keep the environment calm and to reduce stressors during the early stages of recovery. Often, minor tranquilizers are given. Stool softeners are used to prevent Valsalva action during bowel movements.

Accurately recorded intake and output records along with daily weights help the fluid balance assessment. An IV line must be maintained so that emergency drugs can be given if needed.

Anticoagulation Drug Therapy

The use of anticoagulation agents has been controversial. Heparin therapy at one time was standard during the acute phase of MI. Recent studies show that patients who have large anterior MIs with large dyskinetic areas are most at risk for systemic arterial emboli and may benefit from systemic anticoagulation. Minidose heparin (5,000 U given subcutaneously every 12 hours) will effectively prevent venous emboli for patients with heart failure, obesity, edema, or established vascular disease.

Thrombolytic Therapy

Clot dissolution resulting in reperfusion of the thrombosed coronary arteries has, in selected circumstances, become the standard practice for minimizing myocardial infarctions. This widely studied therapy (22 clinical trials, all multi-institutional and many international) has strict patient selection and patient exclusion criteria (Table 15–3). Mortality has been reduced 2% to 18%[10] in studied patients, although the complications limit the application of thrombolytic agents.

Three agents are approved for clinical use: streptokinase, tissue plasminogen activator, and anisoylated plasminogen streptokinase activator. Thrombolytic agents convert plasminogen to an enzyme, plasmin, which actively catalyzes fibrin into fibrin degradation products. Although each agent works slightly differently, the end result is clot lysis (Table 15–4).[11]

Patients presenting within 4 to 6 hours of the onset of symptoms are candidates for thrombolytic therapy. After screening for inclusion–exclusion criteria, the thrombolytic agents will be administered in the emergency department. One ASA (acetylsalicylic acid; aspirin) tablet is given (325 mg) and three peripheral IV sites are established (one line for the thrombolytic agent, one line for other IV drugs, and an 18-gauge line for drawing blood samples). Patients who receive a thrombolytic agent will bleed cutaneously, and safety measures are an important focus for injury prevention.

The patient is moved to the critical care unit where systemic heparinization (5,000-U bolus and continuous infusion to keep partial thromboplastin time [PTT] 2 to 2.5 times normal) and close monitoring occur. Reperfusion rates of 75% to 80%[12] are anticipated. Monitoring will include assessment of chest pain, which should subside, watching for rapid decline of ST segments and early peaking of CK-MB enzymes, and rhythm evaluation. Commonly seen "reperfusion rhythms" (24%–83%) include accelerated idioventricular rhythm (AIVR), malignant ventricular tachycardias, and AV block. Recognition of these rhythms is essential because AIVR usually is well tolerated and therefore untreated. Rhythm disturbances are the most common 70 to 120 minutes after the thrombolytic therapy is initiated. Careful evaluation of blood pressure for hypotension is essential.

Evaluation for complications remains a key nursing intervention. Reocclusion and reinfarction (10%–20%)

TABLE 15–2
Comparison of Calcium Channel Blockers

	Nifedipine	Diltiazem	Verapamil	Amiodipine
Coronary blood flow	↑	↑	↑	↑
Myocardial O₂ demand	↓	↓	↓	↓
Vasodilate periphery	↓ ↓	↓	↓	↓ ↓
Cardiac output	↑	↑ ↓	↑ ↓	↑
Slow AV/SA conduction	No	Yes	Yes	No
Myocardial contractility	↓	↓	↓ ↓	↓

AV, atrioventricular; SA, sinoatrial.

Adapted from Frishman WH, Sonneblick EH: Calcium channel blockers. In Hurst JW, et al (eds): Heart, Arteries and Veins, p 1733. New York, McGraw-Hill, 1990.

TABLE 15–3
*Patient Selection Criteria
for Thrombolytic Therapy*

Inclusion by Symptoms

• Recent onset (<6 hr) of acute MI symptoms
  • Pain; chest pain that may radiate to arm, jaw, neck, or back
  • ECG: evidence of an acute MI, ST segment elevation

Exclusion by History

• Recent major surgery (<10 days)
• Recent trauma (<10 days)
• CVA (within 2 months)
• Recent gastrointestinal or genitourinary bleeding (<10 days)
• Severe hypertension (≥180/110 mm Hg)
• Acute pericarditis
• Subacute bacterial endocarditis
• Recent streptococcal infection (<6 months)
• Pregnancy
• Severe liver dysfunction
• Hemorrhagic ophthalmic disease
• Aortic dissection
• Age over 75 years
• Oral anticoagulant therapy
• Previous SK or APSAC therapy (<1 year)

MI, myocardial infarction; ECG, electrocardiogram; CVA, cerebrovascular accident; SK, streptokinase; APSAC, anisoylated plasminogen streptokinase activator.

From TIMI II: Comparison of invasive and conservative strategies after treatment with IV t-PA in acute MI. N Engl J Med 320:618–627, 1989.

is noted by recurring chest pain, ST segment elevation, and hemodynamic instability. Bleeding may be a major (intracranial hemorrhage, 1%) or a minor (gastrointestinal, genitourinary, or cutaneous, 5%–19%) issue. Hypotension (4.3%–7.2%), embolic cerebrovascular accident (0.4%–2%), and allergic reactions (1%–5%) may be noted.[12]

Anticoagulation with heparin may continue for 24 to 72 hours. Nitroglycerin infusions are initiated to keep the patient pain free and the systolic blood pressure ≥ 90 mm Hg. β-Blocker therapy (oral agents) is indicated if the heart rate (>60/minute) and the blood pressure (≥90/mm Hg systolic) allow.

Further evaluation or interventions may include heart catheterization, enzyme evaluation, PTT evaluation, and other care measures provided to the acute MI patient. Although these patients require close observation, their recovery often is dramatic because the ischemic process is arrested.

Cardiogenic Shock

The previously outlined therapy and assessments allow the nurse to manage the patient with an uncomplicated infarction quite well. Many patients who experience infarcts will have more dramatic symptoms of heart failure, and present in a shock state. When the patient's blood pressure falls below 95 mm Hg systolic or climbs above 150 mm Hg systolic, crackles develop, and urine output decreases, a more aggressive approach is needed. In-hospital mortality rate for cardiogenic shock is 77%.[13]

Clinical Research

Lepley-Frey D: Dysrhythmias and blood pressure changes associated with thrombolysis. Heart Lung 20:335–341, 1991

The purpose of this study was to determine the incidence of reperfusion dysrhythmias and associated hemodynamic changes after the administration of tissue plasminogen activator (t-PA) in the patient with acute myocardial infarction. Before receiving the t-PA, all 41 subjects were not receiving antiarrhythmic drugs and were free of chronic dysrhythmias. Dysrhythmias occurred at a mean time of 98 minutes in 80% (30) of the 41 patients after the start of the infusion. The most frequent dysrhythmia was sinus bradycardia, followed by idioventricular and accelerated idioventricular rhythms, ventricular premature contractions, ventricular tachycardia, and ventricular fibrillation. Within 48 hours of the t-PA infusion, 37 patients had coronary artery angiography, and 30 (81%) had reperfusion. Of these 30 patients, 90% had developed dysrhythmias after the start of the t-PA infusion. Of the remaining seven patients showing no reperfusion, 71% (5) did not have dysrhythmias. Based on the findings that 93% of the patients with dysrhythmias had reperfusion, the author concluded that the absence of dysrhythmias could indicate lack of reperfusion and the development of dysrhythmias could suggest reperfusion. Using this information, the critical care nurse will recognize the need for close monitoring during the 1.5 hours after the start of t-PA infusion and will understand that dysrhythmia occurrence may suggest successful myocardial reperfusion.

TABLE 15–4
Comparison of Approved Thrombolytic Agents

	SK	t-PA	APSAC
Dose	1.5 million units in 60 minutes	6–10 mg bolus initially, 50 mg: first hour 20 mg: second hour 20 mg: third hour (Dose may be varied if weight is ≤65 kg)	30 units in 2–5 min
Half-life	23 min	5 min	90 min
Blood clearance	Hours	30–40 min	4–6 hr
Cost (per treatment)	$390	$2,200	$1,700
Variance in complications		Highest reocclusion rates	Highest allergic rate; highest hypotensive rates

SK, streptokinase; t-PA, tissue plasminogen activator; APSAC, anisoylated plasminogen streptokinase activator. Adapted from Daily EK: Clinical management of patients receiving thrombolytic therapy. Heart Lung 20: 559–565, 1991.

To monitor fluctuations in hemodynamic status adequately, one a thermodilution cardiac output catheter (eg, Swan–Ganz) must be used. Because most MIs involve the left ventricle, measurement of the central venous pressure (CVP) will not reflect changes in left ventricular filling pressures. The pulmonary capillary wedge pressure (PCWP) provides an indirect measurement of left ventricular filling pressures. If the pulmonary artery diastolic pressure is within 1 to 3 mm Hg of the PCWP, this value can be used as well. Optimal filling pressure is below 18 mm Hg, as long as satisfactory systemic flow is maintained (see Chapter 12).

Using the thermodilution technique, cardiac output and index can be determined. A cardiac index (CI) of 2.2 L/minute (cardiac output divided by body surface area) will provide adequate systemic flow. The clinical status can be assessed further by comparing the CI with the PCWP (Table 15–5).

If the clinical picture is one of volume depletion, the patient's PCWP will be less than 18 mm Hg, whereas the CI will be less than 2.2 L/minute/m². Tachycardia, low urine output, and elevated serum sodium and hematocrit may be present. Careful volume replacement with crystalloid IV fluids is indicated. Nitrates and narcotics must be used with care because further systemic lowering of the blood pressure may occur. Although a vasopressor (dopamine or dobutamine) may elevate the systemic pressure, vasopressors are least effective in the setting of volume depletion. Pulmonary congestion will present as a PCWP over 18 mm Hg and a high CI, over 2.2 L/minute/m². This

TABLE 15–5
Hemodynamic Assessment of the Myocardial Infarction

Pulmonary Capillary Wedge Pressure (mm Hg)	Cardiac Index (L/min/m²)	Clinical State	Anticipated Therapy
<18	>2.2	Normal	Reduced metabolic needs
<18	<2.2	Volume depletion	Volume expansion with crystalloids
>18	>2.2	Pulmonary congestion	Diuretics Nitrates
>18	<2.2	Cardiogenic shock	Vasopressors Inotropic agents Afterload reducers IAPB

IAPB, intra-aortic balloon pump.

volume overload state presents with tachycardia, crackles, dyspnea, orthopnea, possible hypoxemia, and diaphoresis. The blood pressure may be elevated in the early stages. Diuretics such as furosemide effectively will reduce intravascular volume. Careful monitoring of serum potassium is needed because diuretic therapy will deplete potassium. Potassium replacement should maintain a serum level of 3.5 mEq/L for the convalescing myocardium.

Diuresis also is obtained through the use of low-dose dopamine or dobutamine (2–5 µg/kg/minute). Dopamine will enhance the systemic blood pressure and increase the renal blood flow, allowing for increased urine formation through normal physiological mechanisms. Dopamine will raise systemic vascular resistance, while dilating renal and mesenteric vascular beds. Dobutamine will minimally alter vascular tone, and actually induce reflexive arterial dilation and decrease systemic vascular resistance. It is important to maintain low dose levels because higher dopamine and dobutamine doses have catecholamine-like effects and will decrease renal blood flow.

Digitalis has been used extensively in the management of congestive failure.[14] Digitalis will decrease heart size and therefore decrease myocardial oxygen consumption (MvO_2). Myocardial oxygen consumption is determined by evaluation of heart rate, contractility, and preload/afterload. Digitalis has a negative chronotropic effect (slows heart rate), a positive inotropic effect (increases contractility), and a negative dromotropic effect (slows electrical impulses). Response to digitalis is delayed in the presence of ischemic myocardium. Although a popular therapy, digitalis can increase infarct size by stimulating MvO_2 if failure is not present.

Cardiogenic shock will present with a PCWP greater than 18 mm Hg and a CI less than 2.2 L/minute/m². The patient will be fatigued and restless and eventually experience drowsiness and stupor. In addition, hypotension of 80 mm Hg systolic or less and oliguria or anuria may ensue. The skin appears gray, mottled, and cool, and diaphoresis often is present. Hypoxemia and acidosis are common.

Shock is accompanied by an intense neurohumoral response. Usually, 40% or more of the left ventricle must be infarcted to cause cardiogenic shock. In an attempt to improve the weakened left ventricle's pumping action, norepinephrine and epinephrine are released. Plasma glucose, free fatty acids, and glucagon are increased as potential energy sources. The MvO_2 increases and lactate acids form as a result of anaerobic metabolism. The catecholamine response causes increased capillary permeability, resulting in interstitial edema and intravascular volume depletion. All the physiological responses to shock increase the MvO_2 while decreasing the myocardial pumping action.

In cardiogenic shock, vasopressors are needed to maintain systemic blood pressures. Dopamine may be used, but often dobutamine is preferred. Dobutamine in small doses of 2 to 5 µg/kg/minute will improve cardiac contractility and decrease afterload and systemic vascular resistance, and it has less of a tachycardic side effect than dopamine. There also is less renal artery vasodilation with dobutamine.

The severe hypotension of cardiogenic shock often is managed with norepinephrine (Levophed, Winthrop Pharmaceuticals, New York, NY). At dosages of 2 to 6 µg/kg/minute, norepinephrine will increase the blood pressure by arterial constriction, which results in an increased peripheral vascular resistance. Although this increases MvO_2, norepinephrine causes direct coronary artery dilation.

Often, vasodilators are added to the therapy to reduce the afterload. Nitroprusside is an effective vasodilator that reduces systemic vascular resistance and therefore enhances stroke volume. The systemic vascular vasodilation can markedly reduce venous return, and it is important to keep diastolic blood pressure at least 60 mm Hg. Having a short half-life of only minutes, nitroprusside can be titrated to the desired effect. Long-term nitroprusside therapy (over 72 hours) may cause thiocyanate or cyanide toxicity, and follow-up therapy often is accomplished with IV nitroglycerin or long-acting nitrates applied topically (Nitro-Bid, Marion Laboratories, Inc., Kansas City, MO).

The maximum support that can be offered to the failing left ventricle is the intra-aortic balloon pump. Occupying 40 ml of space in the proximal aorta, the inflated balloon will, during diastole, displace arterial blood into the coronary arteries and systemic circulation. Coronary artery perfusion is enhanced, and the MvO_2 is lowered. Lactate production is decreased as systemic circulation is augmented. This treatment is as complex as it is successful. It is discussed in depth in Chapter 13.

As in all MIs, the goal of minimizing further tissue necrosis is a goal in cardiogenic shock as well. The challenge to improve MvO_2 while decreasing the work of the ventricle and maintaining systemic circulation is enormous. Modern pharmacologic therapies and treatment modalities require constant bedside assessment and intervention. The role of the critical care nurse in dealing with cardiogenic shock is vital, challenging, and dynamic.

Patient/Family Education

Ongoing patient and family education must begin on admission. A severely compromised, critically ill patient may lack the ability to process and retain new information, but usually is motivated to learn after the life-threatening event. All procedures should be explained in the amount of detail the patient can absorb.

Many successful cardiac rehabilitation programs have been started by nurses who identified the correlation between patient compliance and mortality rates. A brief sample of a progressive teaching plan is found in Display Box 15–2. Cardiac rehabilitation must include physicians,

---

DISPLAY BOX 15–2
Sample Continuum of Patient/Family Educational Goals After Acute MI

When mastery of content is to be expected:	Acute Phase	Before ICU Discharge	At Hospital Discharge
Pathophysiology of heart disease	Can identify angina, using 1–10 scale for reference	Can initiate treatment of angina (rest, NTG, O_2 use)	Knowledgeable about medications, when to seek medical assistance
Environment of hospital	Understands procedures	Asks appropriate questions	Knowledgeable about disease process and therapy
Lifestyle modifications	Complies with activity limitations Complies with dietary limitations	Can state relationship between activity and cardiac work load Begins light activity States risk factors Selects appropriate meals	Can progress activity as tolerated Placement in cardiac rehabilitation program Can state dietary restrictions
Treatment of disease	Accepts medications as ordered	Can identify medications Can identify risk factors	Knowledgeable about medications, dose, timing, action, and side effects Plans for risk factor reduction Begins cardiac rehabilitation program
Emotional adaptation	Accepts sedation to minimize stress	Begins to communicate about lifestyle changes Becomes involved with resolving emotions related to surviving a critical illness	Involves self and loved ones in plans for lifestyle changes Expresses feelings Participates in group recovery program

---

dietitians, physical therapists, and nurses who develop a multidisciplinary team approach to the patient's recovery.

Complications

Special clinical conditions may develop during the convalescence of the patient with an acute infarct. These events, although not entirely predictable, can be managed at the time of occurrence.

Pericarditis

Pericarditis occurs at the 48- to 72-hour postinfarct period with chest pain that may be confused with ischemic pain. This precordial pain intensifies with deep breathing, and a friction rub often can be heard. Some friction rubs are transient, and therefore the absence of such a rub is not conclusive. Anti-inflammatory agents such as aspirin, indomethacin, and corticosteroids, given in usual dosages, can bring dramatic relief.

Ischemic Chest Pain

Recurrent postinfarct chest pain that is ischemic in nature should be treated aggressively. There may be ischemic ECG changes (ST segment depression) and enzyme elevations. Angiography and possible revascularization (coronary artery bypass grafting) should be considered while nitrates are administered. Further progressive loss of myocardial tissue can be minimized and the extension of the infarct aborted with careful hemodynamic assessment for decreasing the MvO_2.

Dysrhythmias

Dysrhythmias often accompany acute infarcts. Often, the dysrhythmia is caused by a failing left ventricle rather than being a direct consequence of conduction system ischemia.

The pulse should be assessed ideally by an apical auscultation and simultaneous radial palpation. Apical–radial pulse assessment will document whether extrasystoles perfuse to the radial artery. It is important to remember that extrasystoles on a rhythm strip may be electrical events without a mechanical response, resulting in a decreased cardiac output.

Dysrhythmias must be treated and minimized in the presence of an acute MI. Ischemic myocardium has a lower fibrillatory threshold, and few ventricular dysrhythmias are considered benign after an infarct. The management of dysrhythmias is considered in detail in Chapter 13, in the discussion of commonly used antiarrhythmic agents.

Supraventricular rhythms may be the result of high left atrial pressures caused by left ventricular failure. Although most rhythm disturbances are manageable with drugs or cardioversion, adequate response to therapy may be delayed until the ventricle heals. Synchronized cardioversion may convert atrial fibrillation, atrial flutter, and nonparoxysmal atrial tachycardias. Paroxysmal atrial tachycardia will respond to verapamil (5–10 mg IV infusion over 10 minutes). Digitalis can be effective but does not work promptly in the ischemic heart. Propranolol often is used if heart failure is not severe.

Many ventricular dysrhythmias will respond to lidocaine therapy. After a bolus loading dose of 1 mg/kg IV push, a continuous infusion of 1 to 4 mg/minute is begun. Lidocaine will decrease the automaticity of the Purkinje fibers and prevent a reentry circuit of tachyarrhythmias by depressing the action potential duration.

Some ventricular dysrhythmias will not respond to lidocaine. The ischemic myocardium may suffer left ventricular failure, hypoxia, hypokalemia, or acidosis, all contributing to a less-than-predictable response. Bretylium, given with a loading dose of 5 mg/kg and followed by a maintenance infusion of 1 to 2 mg/minute is effective therapy for recurrent ventricular tachycardia or fibrillation. Bretylium produces a slow initial response (often 20–25 minutes after the loading bolus), so supportive resuscitative measures should be maintained during this time. Orthostatic hypotension may become a problem during continuous infusion.

Other ventricular antiarrhythmic agents may be used. Procainamide, quinidine, propranolol, and phenytoin sometimes are effective. Overdrive pacing may be indicated. The therapeutic goal of dysrhythmia control is to maintain cardiac output while reducing cardiac workload. This can be assessed by monitoring hemodynamics, blood pressure, urine output, general appearance, and level of consciousness.

Inferior infarctions or occlusion of the RCA will result in conduction disturbances at the AV node for about 10% of the population. Because the inferior wall is small in area and AV node infarcts are rare, these conduction disturbances are transient. Usually Mobitz I (Wenckebach) block will appear and may progress to AV dissociation. If the ventricular rate is too bradycardic to maintain a sufficient blood pressure, transvenous pacing is indicated.

When the lesion is high in the LAD artery, resulting

in an anterior infarct, the development of heart block has serious consequences. The conduction system may be critically damaged at the level of the bundle branches. Multifascicular block occurs, involving two of the three bundles. Mobitz II block (intermittent, nonconducted P waves) may occur, and the cardiac output will fall dramatically. Mortality is high for patients with anterior infarcts with heart block; 70% to 80% will die. Pacemakers are indicated for all anterior infarcts with heart block. Some patients will not respond to pacing if the tissue damage to the left ventricle is extensive.

Patients with inferior wall infarcts should be suspected of also having suffered right ventricular infarcts. This will present as acute congestive failure with hypotension, jugular vein distention, dyspnea, crackles, and an elevated CVP. Management of right ventricular infarcts is critical, because volume support is given to *increase* preload.[15] Usual MI management (decreasing the preload) is deleterious.

Catastrophic Complications

The most catastrophic complications of an infarct are intraventricular septal rupture, papillary muscle dysfunction or rupture, and cardiac rupture. These clinical situations develop rapidly and result in almost immediate physiological deterioration.

Septal Rupture

Intraventricular septal rupture presents as a new, loud, systolic murmur, progressive dyspnea, tachycardia, and pulmonary congestion. Oxygen samples taken from the right atrium, right ventricle, and pulmonary artery will show higher PO_2 in the right ventricle than in the right atrium because the oxygenated left ventricular blood is shunted to the right ventricle. This testing can be accomplished during pulmonary artery catheterization. Urgent cardiac catheterization and surgical correction are needed. The patient can be supported with afterload reducers (nitroprusside) and diuretics until emergency surgery is possible. Some fibrosis of the tissue is needed for suturing and it often is impossible to maintain the patient medically until this occurs.

Papillary Muscle Rupture

Papillary muscle rupture carries a 95% fatality rate. Clinical presentation of sudden-onset valvular failure is similar to that of septal rupture, except that progressive oxygen testing will show equal PO_2 levels in the right atrium, right ventricle, and pulmonary artery. Pulmonary artery pressures will be very high and the waveform will reflect a large

V wave. Emergency surgery is required within hours of the onset of symptoms.

Cardiac Rupture

Cardiac rupture presents with sudden neck vein distention, hypotension, and electromechanical dissociation. This event occurs so suddenly and with such severity that lifesaving efforts are futile.

CASE STUDY

Mrs. Jones, a 62-year-old white woman, was brought to the Emergency Department by a "911" ambulance at 8:30 PM. While unloading groceries at 2:00 PM, she experienced nausea and left chest heaviness. The discomfort subsided when she sat down. During a brief nap, she awoke to intense jaw pain, chest heaviness, and nausea. Mrs. Jones called "911."

Her findings on admission to the ED included: awake, alert, oriented, and cooperative but in a moderate amount of distress. Skin was pale, cool, and diaphoretic. BP 92/40, HR 105-irregular, RR 26 on 2 L/nasal cannula, T 98.0°F, HT 5′4″, WT 60 kg.

The ED staff started a left forearm 20-gauge IV and a right antecubital 18-gauge IV. Her monitor displayed ST segment elevation with frequent PVCs. A lidocaine bolus of 60 mg was given IV push and a lidocaine infusion at 2 mg/minute was started. She rated her chest pain at an "8" on 1–10 scale. An NTG infusion was started and titrated up to 20 mg to relieve her pain to "0." A thorough history revealed no other illness, and hospitalization only for childbirth × 3. She had no allergies to medications or foods.

On physical exam, neurologic findings were normal. Heart exam showed S_1 S_2, no rubs, no murmurs. Peripheral pulses were present but thready. No edema, no increased JVD. Lungs had bilateral basilar crackles. No cyanosis, no clubbing. Respiratory pattern was regular but tachypneic. Abdomen was not tender in spite of nausea, with active bowel sounds. No emesis. GU exam was deferred.

Admission work-up included:

ECG: ST segment elevation II, III, AVF, PR 0.26, QRS 0.06, RR regular except for 4 PVCs/minute, HR 105

LABS: SMA 22, CK-MB, Hg & HCT, WBC, PT, PTT ordered

X-RAY: Portable chest radiograph shows bilateral fluffy infiltrates consistent with CHF, no cardiac enlargement

Mrs. Jones was admitted to CCU with the diagnosis of "Rule out MI." Her status was unchanged except for nausea relief with inapsine, ½ ml IV push. Her VS = BP 98/44, HR 100, 1st degree AV block, no PVCs, RR 26, T 98.0°F.

About 90 minutes after admission, the RN noticed a Wenckebach rhythm. Mrs. Jones was sleeping, but awakened when the RN took her BP. It was 84/40. She stated her pain had returned, and was a "4" on the 1–10 scale. The RN administered morphine sulfate 2 mg, IV push and increased the NTG to 25 μg, with complete relief. A dobutamine infusion was started at 5 μg/kg/minute. Within 30 minutes her BP was 100/48. The

Wenckebach rhythm persisted and the lidocaine infusion was discontinued.

Mrs. Jones' lab work returned within normal limits except for CK = 784, MB (myocardial band) +, K = 3.4. Her diagnosis was confirmed as an acute inferior wall infarction.

Mrs. Jones was anxious but cooperative. With her husband at the bedside, the cardiologist suggested a heart catheterization could be performed safely in 48 hours. It was explained that her delay from initial symptoms to hospitalization precluded the use of thrombolytic therapy. The following orders were written:

Heparin 5,000 units SQ, q12h

Enteric-coated ASA, i qD

KCl 10 mEq/50 ml over 1h × 3 IVPB

Colace i, po bid

Dobutamine 2–5 μg/kg/minute to keep systolic pressure ≥95 mm Hg

Titrate NTG gtt. to relieve pain, keep BP ≥ 95/mm Hg systolic

MSO₄ 2 mg IV push q30 min for pain unrelieved with NTG

Bed rest

O₂ 2–4 LPM, nasal cannula

Low-cholesterol, low-fat diet; start as clear liquids

Weight now and qD

I&O

Cardiac enzymes q8h × 3

ECG q AM × 3

Portable chest radiograph in AM

SMA 22, PTT in AM × 2

Mrs. Jones slept through the night except when awakened for q2h VS and assessments. Her skin was pale, warm, and dry. The nausea subsided. Both the Wenckebach rhythm and the bibasilar crackles persisted.

The AM labs revealed CK = 1136, MB +, K = 4.2. Lasix was given, 20 mg IV push. The 12-lead ECG was unchanged except the rhythm was Wenckebach. By noon, she had diuresed 850 ml and the crackles were diminishing. At approximately 2 PM the Wenckebach rhythm converted to 1st degree AV block. VS: BP 110/54 HR 92, RR 22, T 97.8°F. No rubs or murmurs developed. With her nausea gone, her appetite returned and she remained pain free.

During the afternoon visit with her husband, cardiac rehabilitation began with a booklet, video, and RN explaining heart disease. The Jones' questions were appropriate and demonstrated an understanding of the content presented. Mrs. Jones decided to have the heart cath and plans were made to cover that educational content at 6 PM when her husband returned.

At bedtime the RN noted her lungs were clear, but the heart block was still present. Mrs. Jones slept all night except for q4h VS and assessments. She was NPO for the heart cath. At 8 AM she received her pre-cath Benadryl 50 mg, PO. She went to the cath lab, pain free.

Returning from the cath lab at 11 AM, she was kept flat in bed. A pressure dressing was on the right femoral area and distal

(Text continues on page 348)

NURSING CARE PLAN 15–1:
The Patient With Acute Myocardial Infarction

NURSING DIAGNOSIS	OUTCOME CRITERIA/ PATIENT GOALS	NURSING INTERVENTIONS
Alteration in comfort: chest pain related to angina, MI	• Patient will have relief from chest pain.	1. Administer pain medication (nitrates or narcotics) as ordered. 2. Assess relief of pain (using the scale of 1–10). 3. Instruct the patient to notify staff of further pain. 4. Minimize MvO_2; encourage bed rest; provide quiet environment, easily digestible meals, stool softeners. 5. Obtain 12-lead ECG as ordered. 6. Assess history: onset location, duration description, severity of pain (using the scale of 1–10), radiation, precipitating events. 7. Initiate or maintain IV line and oxygen (2–4 L/min).
Decreased cardiac output: electrical factors affecting rate, rhythm, or conduction	• Maintain a cardiac rhythm with adequate systemic perfusion.	1. Conduct continuous cardiac monitoring in MCL_1 or lead II. 2. Document rhythm strip during every shift and as changes in rhythm occur. 3. Assess BP, apical/radial pulse for extrasystoles, perfusion of extrasystoles. 4. Administer antiarrhythmics, as ordered. 5. Check skin color, temperature. 6. Obtain 12-lead ECG, as ordered.
Decreased cardiac output: mechanical factors relating to preload, afterload, left ventricular failure	• Maintain hemodynamic stability.	1. Assess BP, dyspnea, level of consciousness, hypoxemia, tachypnea, orthopnea, crackles, S_3 ventricular gallop, jugular vein distention, urine output, daily weight, peripheral edema, skin color, and temperature. 2. Maintain IV line, intake and output, oxygen, and bed rest. 3. Assess hemodynamic parameters: PCWP, CO, and CI. 4. Give medication as ordered: diuretics, crystalloid fluids, nitrates, vasopressors, inotropic agents, afterload reducers.

(continued)

NURSING CARE PLAN 15–1: (Continued)
The Patient With Acute Myocardial Infarction

NURSING DIAGNOSIS	OUTCOME CRITERIA/ PATIENT GOALS	NURSING INTERVENTIONS
		5. Assess blood gases.
		6. Monitor cardiac rhythm.
		7. Assess electrolyte balance, especially serum potassium.
		8. Minimize hypoxemia, acidosis, dysrhythmias, pain.
		9. Assess anxiety level of patient and family; instruct and inform at the appropriate level.
		10. If needed, prepare for IAPB.
Knowledge deficit: related to illness and impact on patient's future	• Patient will comply with ADL limitations.	1. Initiate nurse–patient relationship that encourages questioning and uses both formal and informal styles.
		2. Include family in care and teaching.
		3. Begin cardiac rehabilitation education: risk factors, pathophysiology, when to seek medical attention, medications, progressive ADL, diet, sexual activity, returning to work, stress reduction.
	• Patient will ask pertinent questions.	4. Evaluate patient's understanding; document teaching and patient's response on the record.
Anxiety: stress related to fear of illness/ death and critical care environment	• Patient will recognize and express concerns and fears.	1. Explain environment, all procedures, expectations and equipment.
		2. Allow patient free expression.
		3. Maximize patient's control of ADL.
		4. Include family in patient's care.
	• Patient will use effective coping mechanisms.	5. Assess for normal grieving process: anger, denial, depression, acceptance.
		6. Sedate as needed if ordered by physician.
		7. Maximize effective coping styles.
		8. Document patient's emotional response to critical illness.
	• Patient will demonstrate reduction in fear and anxiety.	9. Spend quiet time with patient so that feelings and fears may be explored.

(*continued*)

NURSING CARE PLAN 15–1: (Continued)
The Patient With Acute Myocardial Infarction

NURSING DIAGNOSIS	OUTCOME CRITERIA/ PATIENT GOALS	NURSING INTERVENTIONS
High risk for altered tissue perfusion: thrombolytic therapy impact on myocardial tissue	• Patient will have relief of chest pain.	1. Assess all recurring chest pain: onset, location, duration, description, severity (using scale of 1–10) radiation, precipitating factors. 2. Initiate three peripheral IV sites and O_2 (2–4 L/min). 3. Administer IV NTG, as ordered. 4. Assess pain relief (using 1–10 scale). 5. Instruct patient to inform staff of further pain. 6. Minimize MvO_2 with restful environment.
		7. Obtain 12-lead ECG, as ordered.
	• Maintain a cardiac rhythm with adequate perfusion.	8. Conduct continuous cardiac monitoring in MCL_1 or lead II. 9. Document all changes in rhythm with a rhythm strip. 10. Assess rhythm for AIVR, AV block, or VT. 11. Assess hemodynamic tolerance of all rhythms. 12. Administer antiarrhythmics, as ordered.
	• Patient will have minimal bleeding.	13. Assess neurologic, GU, and GI systems hourly while awake, q2h if asleep. 14. Assess occult blood in all secretions/fluids. 15. Assess PTT q2–4h to be 2–2.5 times normal, or as ordered. 16. Gentle oral care; assess gingival bleeding. 17. Provide safe environment to prevent falls, bruising or injury.
	• Maintain hemodynamic stability.	18. Assess BP, dyspnea, level of consciousness, hypoxemia, tachycardia, tachypnea, orthopnea, crackles, S_3, JVD, urine output, daily weight, edema, skin color, and temperature.

(continued)

NURSING CARE PLAN 15–1: (Continued)
The Patient With Acute Myocardial Infarction

NURSING DIAGNOSIS	OUTCOME CRITERIA/ PATIENT GOALS	NURSING INTERVENTIONS
		19. Assess hemodynamic parameters: PCWP, CO, CI; assess blood gases.
		20. Monitor cardiac rhythm.
	• Patient will not experience an allergic reaction.	21. Assess all complaints of itching/hives.
		22. Administer hydrocortisone 100 mg, IVP, as ordered.
		23. Administer Benadryl, 50 mg IVP, as ordered.
High risk for alteration in comfort: chest pain related to pericarditis	• Patient will have relief from pain.	1. Assess pain: onset, location, duration, description, severity (using scale of 1–10), radiation, precipitating factors.
		2. Determine whether pain increases with deep breathing, presence of friction rub.
		3. Assess rhythm, BP, and heart rate during pain.
		4. Administer anti-inflammatory agents as ordered.
		5. Explain pathology to patient.
		6. Assess pain relief (using scale of 1–10).
High risk for decreased cardiac output: profound shock and heart failure related to acute structural changes (septal rupture, papillary muscle rupture, or cardiac muscle rupture)	• Maintain hemodynamic stability.	1. Assess for sudden onset hypotension, systolic murmur, and pulmonary edema.
		2. Assess hemodynamic parameters: PCWP, cardiac output, CI.
		3. Prepare for IABP support and possible surgery.
		4. Administer afterload reducers and vasopressors as ordered.
		5. Minimize MvO_2: bed rest, supplemental oxygen, NPO, quiet environment.
		6. Monitor cardiac rhythm.
		7. Provide emotional support and appropriate explanations to patient and family.
High risk for anxiety: related to critical illness, fear of death or disfigurement, role changes within social setting or permanent disability	• Patient will express anxieties to appropriate resource person.	1. Provide environment that encourages open discussion of emotional issues.

(continued)

NURSING CARE PLAN 15-1: (Continued)
The Patient With Acute Myocardial Infarction

NURSING DIAGNOSIS	OUTCOME CRITERIA/ PATIENT GOALS	NURSING INTERVENTIONS
		2. Mobilize patient's support system and involve these resources as appropriate.
		3. Allow time for patient to express self.
		4. Identify possible hospital resources for patient/family support.
		5. Encourage open family-to-nurse communications regarding emotional issues.
		6. Validate patient and family knowledge base regarding the critical illness.
		7. Involve religious support systems as appropriate.

circulation to the right leg and VS were assessed q15 minutes. The dobutamine and NTG were slowly weaned off. She was stable. Her preliminary report from the cath lab described a 90% occlusion of the proximal RCA. Surgery was offered as an option.

In her sleep that night, Mrs. Jones converted into a NSR at a rate of 88 beats per minute. While bathing in the morning, Mrs. Jones found that she fatigued easily. This lack of energy frightened her and she described it to the nursing staff as "feeling pooped out." When these data were communicated to the cardiologist, it was suggested that although her strength would return over time, surgical bypass of the right coronary artery surely would improve her fatigue and minimize her potential for heart failure.

Mrs. Jones had been worried about taking a vein from her leg, because this had caused severe pain and scarring for her sister. Once the surgeon consulted and suggested an internal mammary graft, Mrs. Jones agreed to have the bypass performed.

Nursing Care Plan

Critical care nursing began as complex care and assessments were made by nurses specially trained to care for cardiac patients. Although the role of the critical care nurse has evolved enormously, the challenge of caring for patients with acute MI remains. The nurse can no longer "watch" patients but must rapidly assess complex physiological processes and anticipate sophisticated interventions. The declining mortality rate speaks to our success in

meeting the challenge of the patient with an acute MI. After assessment data are gathered, the nurse must design a plan of care that provides for the patient's current needs and anticipates potential problems. The plan of care should be designed in a manner that permits evaluation of the care given by observation of patient outcomes and interventions and by quality assurance assessments of patient records.

Nursing Care Plan 15-1 is a sample standardized plan of care for the patient with an acute MI. This plan would need to be individualized before implementation for a specific patient.

REFERENCES

1. American Heart Association: Textbook of Advanced Cardiac Life Support, 2nd ed, pp 2–3. American Heart Association, Dallas, 1990
2. Healy BP: "Pathology of Coronary Atherosclerosis" In Hurst JW, et al (eds): The Heart, Arteries and Veins, pp 924–926, 7th ed. New York, McGraw-Hill, 1990
3. Shah P: Pathophysiology of unstable angina. Cardiol Clin 9:11–26, 1991
4. Rackley CE, et al: "Multivalvular Disease" In Hurst JW, et al (eds): The Heart, Arteries and Veins, pp 883–885, 7th ed. New York, McGraw-Hill, 1990
5. Lambert CR: Pathophysiology of stable angina pectoris. Cardiol Clin 9:1–10, 1991
6. Castellanos A: "The Resting Electrocardiogram" In Hurst

JW, et al (eds): The Heart, Arteries and Veins, pp 268–273, 7th ed. New York, McGraw-Hill, 1990

7. Sobel BE: "Cardiac Enzymes and Other Macromolecular Markers of Myocardial Injury" In Hurst JW, et al (eds): The Heart, Arteries and Veins, pp 972–974, 7th ed. New York, McGraw-Hill, 1990

8. Waller BF: Pathology of acute MI. Cardiol Clin 6:1–2, 1988

9. Hjalmarson A, Olsson G: Myocardial infarction: Effects of beta blockade. Circulation 84(Suppl):101–107, 1991

10. Kline EM: Clinical controversies surrounding thrombolytic therapy in acute MI. Heart Lung 19:596–601, 1990

11. Cole PL: Thrombolytic therapy: Then and now. Heart Lung 20:543–551, 1991

12. Daily EK: Clinical management of patients receiving thrombolytic therapy. Heart Lung 20:559–565, 1991

13. Goldberg RJ, et al: Cardiogenic shock after acute MI. N Engl J Med 325:1117–1123, 1991

14. Marcus FI, Huang SK: In Hurst JW, et al (eds): The Heart, Arteries and Veins, pp 1746–1758. New York, McGraw-Hill, 1990

15. Finesilver C, Metzler DJ: Right ventricular infarction. Am J Nurs 91(4):32–38, 1991

16. Jugdutt BI: Intravenous nitroglycerin unloading in acute MI. Am J Cardiol 68:520–630, 1991

17. Lepley-Frey D: Dysrhythmias and blood pressure changes associated with thrombolysis. Heart Lung 20:335–341, 1991

18. TIMI II: Comparison of invasive and conservative strategies after treatment with IV t-PA in acute MI. N Engl J Med 320:618–627, 1989

BIBLIOGRAPHY

Chatterjee K, Cheitlin M, et al: Cardiology: An Illustrated Text Reference, vols 1, 2. Philadelphia, JB Lippincott, 1991

Guyton AC: Textbook of Medical Physiology, 8th ed. Philadelphia, WB Saunders, 1991

Porth CM: Pathophysiology: Concepts of Altered Health States, 3rd ed. Philadelphia, JB Lippincott, 1990

STUDY QUESTIONS

1. How was the early diagnosis of acute MI made in Mrs. Jones, the case study patient?

    a. heart catheterization
    b. treadmill and exercise stress testing
    c. chest radiograph
    d. history, physical examination, and ECG

2. Which coronary artery supplies the inferior wall of the left ventricle?

    a. LAD
    b. RCA
    c. circumflex
    d. LAD and part of the circumflex

3. If Mrs. Jones had a Swan–Ganz catheter in place, which readings would you anticipate during her first hospital day?

    a. increased cardiac index and increased wedge pressure
    b. increased cardiac index and decreased wedge pressure
    c. decreased cardiac index and increased wedge pressure
    d. decreased cardiac index and decreased wedge pressure

4. Assessing for the presence of heart failure might include

    1. drawing a CK-MB
    2. auscultating the breath sounds
    3. doing a 12-lead ECG
    4. listening for the presence of a S_3

        a. 1 and 3
        b. 2 and 4
        c. 4 only
        d. all of the above

5. Of the common complications of MI, Mrs. Jones experienced
    1. pain
    2. dysrhythmias
    3. pericarditis
    4. cardiac rupture

        a. 1 only
        b. 2 only
        c. 1 and 2
        d. all of the above

(continued)

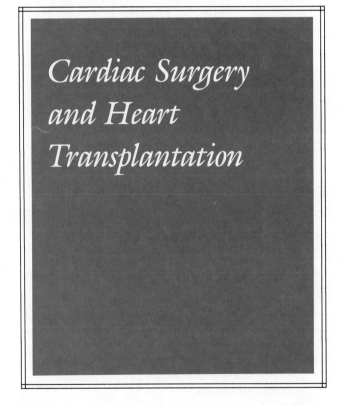

CHAPTER 16

Cardiac Surgery and Heart Transplantation

Hudak: Critical Care Nursing:
A Holistic Approach, 6th ed. © 1994
J. B. Lippincott Company.

351

BEHAVIORAL OBJECTIVES

Based on the content in this chapter, the reader should be able to:

1. Compare and contrast the pathophysiological impacts of stenosis and insufficiency in the mitral and aortic valves.
2. Describe the cardiopulmonary bypass process.
3. Describe five key assessment areas in the early postoperative period.
4. Discuss causes, assessments, and interventions for the hypotensive postoperative cardiac surgery patient.
5. Relate nursing care to the pathophysiological events occurring after cardiac transplantation.

Description

Despite emphasis on modifying and preventing risk factors, cardiovascular disease remains a leading cause of disability and death in the United States. Development of new treatments such as thrombolytic therapy, balloon and laser angioplasty, and atherectomy have improved medical management of cardiac disease. However, surgical intervention is still the treatment of choice for some patients.

Cardiac surgery as we know it today was made possible by the development and practical application of cardiopulmonary bypass by Gibbon in 1953.

This chapter discusses two common situations requiring cardiac surgery (myocardial revascularization and acquired valvular disease) and then discusses in detail the procedure of open heart surgery and subsequent postoperative assessment and nursing care. Finally, heart transplantation and the issues specific to this procedure are discussed.

Coronary Artery Bypass Grafts (CABG)

The first saphenous vein aortocoronary bypass graft was performed in 1964. Since then, the procedure has become an acceptable treatment for coronary artery disease (CAD). Compared to medical treatment, coronary artery bypass grafting (CABG) has proven effective in relieving angina and improving exercise tolerance,[1] and it prolongs life in patients with left main CAD and three-vessel disease with poor left ventricular function.[2] With the introduction of percutaneous transluminal coronary angioplasty (PTCA), however, the indications for CABG are being questioned (see Chapter 13). Currently five prospective randomized trials are in progress comparing PTCA with CABG. One of the largest, the U.S. and Canada Bypass Angioplasty Revascularization Investigation (BARI), is being done by the National Heart, Lung, and Blood Institutes. It will look at 2,400 patients and is due to be completed between 1994 and 1996.

Increased use of PTCA has eliminated many CABG candidates with low operative risk. Patients selected for CABG today are older, have more advanced coronary disease and worse left ventricular function, and many have had previous CABG.[3,4] Postoperatively, their care is more complex.

Saphenous Vein Grafts

Either the saphenous vein or the internal mammary artery (IMA) can be used for CABG. The saphenous vein can be taken from above or below the knee, but vein from below the knee is generally preferred because it is close in diameter to the size of the coronary artery. The vein is removed from an incision made along the inner aspect of the leg.

The obstruction in the coronary artery is bypassed by anastomosing one end of the vein graft to the aorta (proximal anastomosis) and the other end to the coronary artery just past the obstruction (distal anastomosis). Saphenous vein grafts can be *simple*, with an end-to-side anastomosis

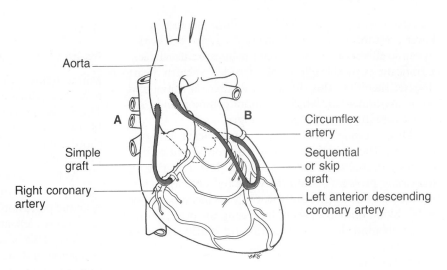

FIGURE 16–1
Aortocoronary bypass grafts using saphenous vein. (**A**) Simple graft from aorta to right coronary artery. (**B**) Sequential graft from aorta to left anterior descending coronary artery to diagonal or circumflex artery.

to the aorta and the coronary artery, or *sequential* (also called *skip*), with an end-to-side anastomosis to the aorta, a side-to-side anastomosis to one coronary artery, and an end-to-side anastomosis to another coronary artery (Fig. 16–1).

Advantages and Disadvantages of Internal Mammary Artery for Myocardial Revascularization

Advantages

- Improved short- and long-term patency rates over saphenous vein grafts
- Diameter close to diameter of coronary arteries
- Aortic anastomosis not required
- IMA retains its nervous system innervation and thus has the ability to adapt size to provide blood flow according to myocardial demands
- No leg incision if only IMA used
- Vascular endothelium adapted to arterial pressure and high flow, resulting in decreased intimal hyperplasia and atherosclerosis

Disadvantages

- Dissection of IMA takes longer, resulting in longer cardiopulmonary bypass time
- Extensive dissection may increase risk of postoperative bleeding
- Pleural space entered, so pleural chest tube required postoperatively
- Postoperative pain may be increased due to entry into pleural space and extensive dissection
- In patients with diabetes mellitus or advanced age, use of bilateral IMAs can increase the risk of infection and sternal nonunion (Pelletier and Carrier, 1991)

Internal Mammary Artery Grafts

The IMA is also used for myocardial revascularization. The IMA is the second branch of the subclavian artery and descends down the anterior chest wall just lateral to the sternum behind the costal cartilage.

IMA grafts have shown a lesser degree of atherosclerosis over time and superior early and late graft patency rates compared with saphenous vein grafts. Ninety percent of IMA grafts were patent 10 years postoperatively, whereas more than 50% of saphenous vein grafts were occluded within 10 years.[5] IMA grafts were also associated with lower long-term morbidity and improved long-term survival.[6] Other advantages and disadvantages of myocardial revascularization using the IMA are shown in the accompanying box.

To isolate the IMA, the pleural space is entered, the IMA is dissected free, and the intercostal artery branches from the IMA are cauterized. The IMA is used as a pedicle graft (ie, the proximal end remains attached to the subclavian artery), and both the left and the right IMA can be used. Because the left IMA is longer and larger than the right, it is usually used to bypass the left anterior descending (LAD) coronary artery. The right IMA is anastomosed to the right coronary artery (RCA) or the circumflex coronary artery (CIRC).

Acquired Valvular Heart Disease

Description

Cardiac valves maintain the unidirectional flow of blood. If structural changes occur as a result of disease, this function is disrupted. Abnormalities can affect the tricuspid, pulmonic, mitral, and aortic valves. Least common are pulmonic and tricuspid valve abnormalities. Pulmonic valve changes usually result from congenital anomalies. Tricuspid valve disease can be caused by endocarditis, rheumatic fever, or left-sided heart failure. Because of the lower pressures on the right side of the heart, the hemodynamic effects of tricuspid abnormalities are usually less significant than the effects of left-sided valvular heart disease; therefore, this discussion focuses on mitral and aortic abnormalities, which are more common and produce profound hemodynamic changes.

Disease causes either stenosis or insufficiency (regurgitation). The stenotic valve has a narrowed orifice that creates a partial obstruction to blood flow, resulting in increasing pressure behind the valve and decreasing forward blood flow. The insufficient valve is incompetent or leaky; blood flows backward, increasing the pressure and volume behind the valve. Stenosis and insufficiency can occur alone or in combination, in the same valve, or in more than one valve.

Assessment and Diagnosis

The diagnosis of valvular disease is suggested by the history, clinical signs and symptoms, physical examination, and auscultation of the characteristic murmur (see p. 144). Diagnosis is confirmed by echocardiography and right and left heart catheterization. Echocardiography shows abnormal movement or thickening of the valve leaflets, valve area, and changes in the chamber size behind the diseased valve. Doppler echo reveals abnormal blood flow patterns. During cardiac catheterization valvular gradients are measured. Normally there is no gradient; however, with stenotic valves a pressure difference develops.

To determine the gradient across the mitral valve, left atrial and left ventricular pressures are measured during diastole. If there is a gradient of more than 15 to 20 mm Hg (ie, left atrial diastolic pressure is 15–20 mm Hg higher than left ventricular diastolic pressure), severe mitral stenosis exists. Valve area is also calculated during cardiac catheterization. The normal mitral valve area is 4 to 6 cm^2. An area less than 1.5 cm^2 signifies critical mitral stenosis, and surgery is indicated.

To determine the gradient across the aortic valve, left ventricular and aortic root pressures are measured during systole. A gradient of more than 50 mm Hg (ie, left ventricular systolic pressure is 50 mm Hg higher than aortic root systolic pressure) is associated with clinically significant aortic stenosis. Normal aortic valve area is 2.6 to 3.5 cm^2. Hemodynamically significant aortic stenosis occurs if the valve area is less than 1 cm^2.

Valvular insufficiency is diagnosed by regurgitation of the contrast medium backward through the incompetent valve. Mitral insufficiency causes the dye to flow from the left ventricle to the left atrium during ventricular systole. Aortic insufficiency produces regurgitation of contrast medium from the aortic root into the left ventricle during ventricular diastole.

Mitral Stenosis
Pathophysiology

Mitral stenosis occurs most frequently as a result of rheumatic heart disease, bacterial endocarditis, or calcification. The disease process causes fusion of the commissures and fibrotic contraction of valve leaflets, commissures, and chordae tendineae. Forward blood flow is impeded as the valve orifice becomes smaller.

As forward flow from the left atrium to the left ventricle decreases, cardiac output drops, creating a decrease in systemic perfusion. Blood backed up behind the stenotic valve causes left atrial dilatation and increased left atrial pressure. This is reflected backward into the pulmonary circulation, and, with prolonged high pressures, fluid moves from the pulmonary capillaries into the interstitial space and eventually the alveoli. Pulmonary hypertension develops, with thickening of the pulmonary arterial walls. If the process is not interrupted, right heart failure develops when the right ventricle is unable to pump against the high pulmonary vascular resistance.

Clinical Manifestations

Patients with mitral stenosis complain of fatigue, tiredness, exertional dyspnea, orthopnea, or even pulmonary edema; they can develop hemoptysis as a result of pulmonary hypertension. Left atrial dilatation causes atrial fibrillation in 40% to 50% of the patients (Fig. 16–2).

Mitral Insufficiency
Pathophysiology of Chronic Insufficiency

Chronic mitral insufficiency can result from rheumatic heart disease (49%), myxomatous degeneration of the mitral valve (40%), myocardial ischemia (4%),[7] or left ventricular dilatation. Rheumatic disease causes valve cusps to become thickened and contracted, preventing valve closure. Myxomatous changes cause enlarged leaflets or stretched or ruptured chordae, which allow the leaflets to balloon backward into the left atrium during ventricular systole. Left ventricular dilatation stretches the mitral valve annulus, pulling the leaflet edges apart so they no longer approximate. Regardless of cause, the result is backward blood flow.

During ventricular systole, some of the left ventricular blood regurgitates into the atrium rather than being ejected through the aortic valve. This decreases the forward cardiac output. Left ventricular hypertrophy occurs in an attempt to improve the cardiac output, but this can actually worsen the regurgitation. Left ventricular volume overload causes left ventricular dilatation. Regurgitant flow into the left atrium causes increased left atrial pressure and dilatation. This volume overload can be reflected backward to the pulmonary circulation; however, pulmonary

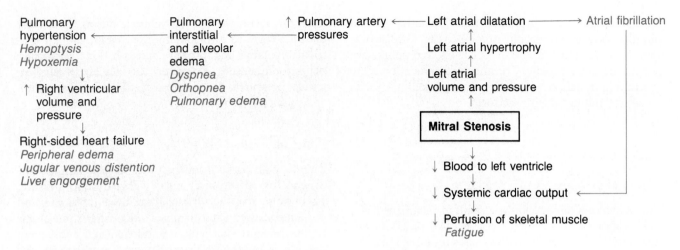

FIGURE 16–2
Hemodynamic and physiological effects of mitral stenosis. The resulting clinical signs and symptoms are noted in color.

and right heart symptoms usually do not occur until late in the disease process.

Clinical Manifestations

Patients with mitral regurgitation commonly complain of fatigue, palpitations, and sometimes shortness of breath (Fig. 16–3).

Pathophysiology of Acute Insufficiency

Endocarditis, chest trauma, or myocardial infarction can result in acute mitral insufficiency. Endocarditis erodes or perforates the valve leaflets or chordae. Trauma can rupture the chordae, and myocardial infarction can cause papillary muscle rupture (see p. 342), allowing blood to flow backward into the left atrium during ventricular systole.

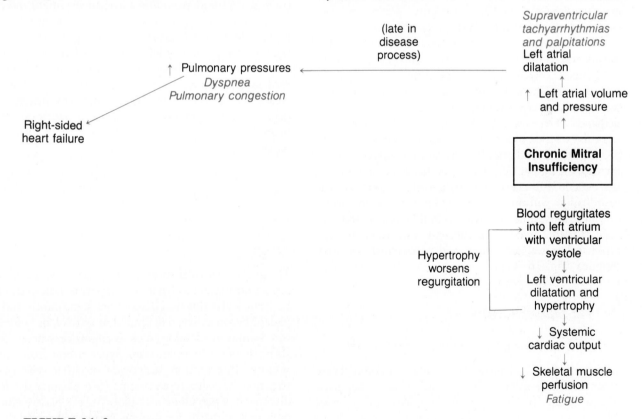

FIGURE 16–3
Hemodynamic and physiological effects of chronic mitral insufficiency. The resulting clinical signs and symptoms are noted in color.

In acute mitral regurgitation, there is insufficient time for dilatation or hypertrophy to compensate. Cardiac output decreases dramatically, shock ensues, and pulmonary edema develops rapidly. Treatment of choice for acute mitral regurgitation with hemodynamic compromise is emergent mitral valve replacement.

Aortic Stenosis

Pathophysiology

Aortic stenosis can develop as a result of rheumatic fever, calcification of a congenital bicuspid valve, or calcific degeneration. The disease process causes fusion of the commissures and fibrous contractures of the cusps, obstructing left ventricular outflow.

Forward cardiac output is diminished, and the left ventricle hypertrophies to maintain the cardiac output. As the stenosis worsens, compensation fails, and volume and pressure overload in the left ventricle cause left ventricular dilatation. Increased left ventricular pressures are reflected backward through the left atrium and pulmonary vasculature.

Clinical Manifestations

Diminished cardiac output in the person with aortic stenosis can lead to two major problems—angina and syncope. Extreme left ventricular hypertrophy increases myocardial oxygen demand at the same time that cardiac output and coronary artery perfusion are decreased, creating ischemic myocardium evidenced by angina. Syncope occurs in the late stages of aortic stenosis when the forward cardiac output cannot increase to meet the body demands of exercise. As the patient with severe aortic stenosis exercises, blood vessels to skeletal muscles dilate to increase the blood supply. The normal response is to increase the cardiac output to meet this demand; however, the patient with aortic stenosis is unable to do so. The vasodilation without a concomitant increase in cardiac output results in insufficient cerebral perfusion and syncope. Patients with aortic stenosis also experience exertional dyspnea, orthopnea, and paroxysmal nocturnal dyspnea (Fig. 16–4).

Aortic Insufficiency

Pathophysiology of Chronic Insufficiency

Rheumatic fever and aneurysm of the ascending aorta are common causes of chronic aortic insufficiency. Rheumatic disease results in thickened and retracted valve cusps, whereas aortic aneurysm causes annular dilatation. Both problems prevent the edges of the valve leaflets from approximating, allowing blood to regurgitate backward from the aorta into the left ventricle during ventricular diastole. Forward cardiac output decreases, and left ventricular volume and pressure increase. Left ventricular hypertrophy ensues. Eventually the increase in left ventricular pressure is reflected backward into the left atrium and pulmonary circulation.

Clinical Manifestations

Patients with aortic insufficiency experience fatigue, low diastolic blood pressure, and a widened pulse pressure. Their pulse may be characterized by a rapid rise and sudden collapse (water-hammer or Corrigan's pulse) due to the forceful ventricular contraction and subsequent diastolic regurgitation from the aortic root into the left ventricle. They may also complain of angina, because aortic insufficiency creates an imbalance between left ventricular myocardial oxygen supply and demand. As left ventricular hypertrophy worsens, the oxygen demand increases, but regurgitant flow from the aortic root during diastole decreases coronary artery perfusion. Angina with aortic insufficiency is less common than with aortic stenosis (Fig. 16–5).

Pathophysiology of Acute Insufficiency

Acute aortic insufficiency can be caused by blunt chest trauma, ruptured ascending aortic aneurysm, or infective endocarditis. The patient with acute aortic insufficiency rapidly develops left heart failure and pulmonary edema because compensatory left ventricular hypertrophy does not have time to develop. In response to the diminished cardiac output, systemic vascular resistance (SVR) increases to maintain the blood pressure. This increases the degree of regurgitation and worsens the situation. Treatment for acute aortic insufficiency is emergent aortic valve replacement.

Management of Valvular Heart Disease

Surgery

The goals of valvular surgery are to relieve symptoms and restore normal hemodynamics. Surgery is indicated before left ventricular function deteriorates significantly and the patient becomes severely limited in activity, or before severe symptoms develop, such as angina or syncope from aortic stenosis or pulmonary hypertension from mitral stenosis. Intervention can consist of either valve reconstruction or valve replacement. (See Chapter 13 for a discussion of percutaneous balloon valvuloplasty, which is indicated primarily for patients considered too high risk for surgery). Because reconstruction is associated with decreased operative mortality and fewer thromboembolic

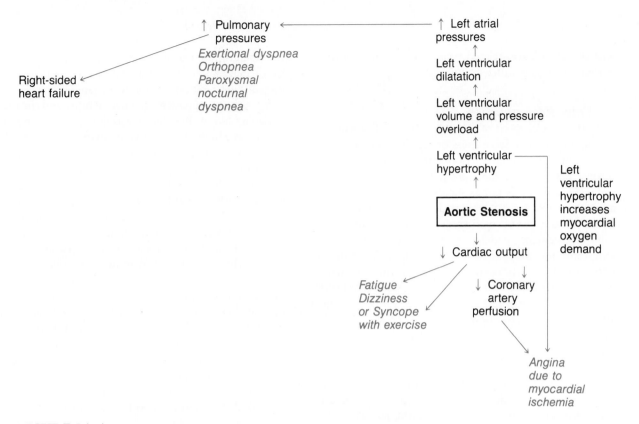

FIGURE 16–4
Hemodynamic and physiological effects of aortic stenosis. The resulting clinical signs and symptoms are noted in color.

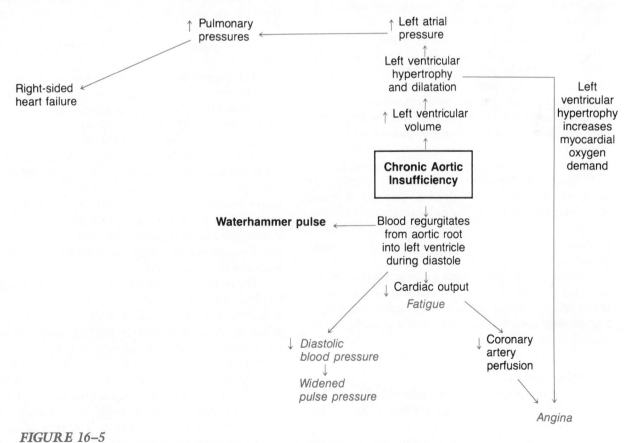

FIGURE 16–5
Hemodynamic and physiological effects of chronic aortic insufficiency. The resulting clinical signs and symptoms are noted in color.

and anticoagulation-related complications than valve replacement, it is gaining popularity.

Valve Reconstruction

With the development of transesophageal echocardiography to assess the effectiveness of repair intraoperatively, the use of valve reconstruction is increasing. Most valve reconstruction procedures are performed on the mitral valve. Although it is not as successful for mitral stenosis, an estimated 90% of valves with degenerative mitral insufficiency could be reconstructed.[8] Compared with mitral valve replacement, reconstruction eliminates the need for long-term anticoagulation; decreases the risks of thromboembolism and endocarditis; decreases the need for reoperation (20% at 10 years);[9] and increases survival (90% at 5 years).[10] For aortic valve disorders, however, most attempts at reconstruction have not been successful because of late insufficiency and restenosis. Aortic valve reconstruction is considered an experimental procedure.[11]

A common reconstruction technique for mitral stenosis is commissurotomy. Although not indicated for patients with severe mitral stenosis, it can be effective for those with moderate stenosis with minimal calcification and regurgitation. During commissurotomy the fused commissures are surgically divided. Calcified tissue is debrided and fused, and shortened chordae are incised. This improves leaflet mobility and increases the mitral valve area, decreasing the degree of stenosis.

Mitral insufficiency can also be treated with reconstruction. If annular dilatation causes the regurgitation, annuloplasty can be performed using sutures or a prosthetic ring (eg, Carpentier-Edwards annuloplasty ring). The ring is sewn around the mitral annulus so that excess annular tissue is drawn up. Suturing and the ring reduce the circumference of the enlarged annulus so that the edges of the leaflets coapt, diminishing regurgitation. If the chordae tendineae are stretched or ruptured, surgical shortening or transposition of chordae to substitute for ruptured chordae can be effective. Redundant mitral leaflets are repaired by resecting a portion of the leaflet, and perforated valve leaflets can be reconstructed by patching. Such repairs are usually supported by an annuloplasty ring.

Reconstruction procedures are more likely to be successful if performed early in the course of the disease, before left ventricular function deteriorates and irreparable damage occurs. If reconstruction cannot be accomplished, valves are replaced.

Valve Replacement

The first valve replacement was performed by Harken and Starr in 1960 with a caged ball prosthesis. Since then, many new valve designs have evolved.

The ideal prosthetic valve would be durable and last for the patient's life. It would have normal hemodynamics with unimpeded, nonturbulent blood flow through a central opening, no transvalvular gradient, and no regurgitation when closed. It would be nonthrombogenic and not damaging to blood components, and it would also be acceptable to the patient in terms of noise and the need for anticoagulation. In other words, it would perform exactly as a normal human valve. Unfortunately, no artificial valve currently meets these criteria, so research continues.

More than 30,000 valves are implanted annually in the United States.[12] Two major types of prosthetic valves are currently available—mechanical and biological. Mechanical valves are made entirely of synthetic materials, whereas biological valves combine synthetic materials with chemically treated biological tissues. Mechanical valves include the caged ball, tilting disc, and bileaflet designs.

The caged ball valve consists of a plastic or metal ball inside of a metal cage attached to a sewing ring. When pressure behind the valve increases, the ball is forced down into the cage, and blood flows around it. When pressure in front of the valve increases, the ball is forced upward against the sewing ring, preventing regurgitant flow. An example of the caged ball valve is the Starr-Edwards.

Hemodynamically, the ball in the cage produces a central obstruction to blood flow, which can result in a small stenotic pressure gradient, and ventricular outflow may be partially obstructed because of the cage's size and high profile. Because of the thrombogenicity of the plastic and metal and the turbulent flow around the ball and through the cage, blood clots can form on or around the valve. Thromboembolism is a common problem, and chronic anticoagulant therapy is essential. Caged ball valves have good long-term durability.

The tilting disc valve is constructed of a disc held in place by struts attached to a sewing ring. When the pressure behind the valve increases, the disc tilts open approximately 60° to 80°, allowing blood to flow around it. When the pressure in front of the valve increases, the disc tilts back flat with the sewing ring to close. Because of its semicentralized flow and lower profile, the tilting disc valve produces less obstruction to blood flow and has better hemodynamic characteristics than the caged ball valve. It has good long-term durability, but the risk of thromboembolism requires long-term anticoagulant therapy. Examples of the tilting disc valve are the Medtronic-Hall and the Omniscience.

The newest type of mechanical prosthesis is the bileaflet tilting disc valve, which consists of two pyrolytic carbon semicircular discs or leaflets hinged to a sewing ring. When the pressure behind the valve increases, the leaflets open perpendicular to the sewing ring, and blood flows through the central opening with minimal obstruction. When pressure in front of the valve increases, the leaflets return to their flat position against the sewing ring, preventing insufficiency. An example of the bileaflet tilting disc valve is the St. Jude Medical. This type of valve has good hemodynamic characteristics and durability, but is thrombogenic and requires long-term anticoagulation.

Biological prostheses, or tissue valves, offer another

alternative for valve replacement. The porcine heterograft is constructed of an excised pig aortic valve preserved in glutaraldehyde and mounted on a frame attached to a sewing ring. Examples of porcine valves are the Hancock and the Carpentier-Edwards.

Biological prostheses provide good hemodynamics except in smaller sizes where obstruction to flow and a gradient can occur. Their main advantage is the lower risk of thromboembolism compared to mechanical valves. Because the majority of thromboembolic events occur during the first 3 months after implant, most patients with biological valves receive anticoagulants during that time only and none subsequently. However, the decision for anticoagulation must be based on the patient's condition. Patients in chronic atrial fibrillation undergoing mitral valve replacement frequently receive long-term anticoagulation therapy even with a biological prosthesis because of stagnant blood flow in the atria, which predisposes to clot formation.

A disadvantage to biological valves is their lack of durability. Valves studied at autopsy have shown structural deterioration beginning as early as 6 years after implant, and their durability is usually considered to be less than 10 years. However, recent studies show less evidence of calcification and structural deterioration when the valves are placed in older patients.[13]

Human aortic homografts are another alternative for biological valve replacement. The cadaver aortic valve is excised and frozen. For implant, it is trimmed to the correct size and sewn into place. Homografts have excellent hemodynamic characteristics and are nonthrombogenic, so anticoagulation is not needed; however, their availability is limited. Long-term durability is currently being studied and appears comparable to that of porcine valves.[14] Structural degeneration may be caused by the immune response of the recipient.[15]

Because no "ideal" prosthetic valve has been developed, advantages and disadvantages must be weighed to choose the appropriate valve for each patient. Mechanical valves offer the benefits of good long-term durability but pose a significant risk of thromboembolism and require long-term anticoagulation. Biological valves decrease the risk of thromboembolism and can obviate the need for long-term anticoagulation; however, their durability is not as good as that of mechanical valves.

Mechanical valves are generally placed in patients whose life expectancy is more than 10 years. Biological valves are indicated for patients who are unable to comply with an anticoagulation regimen, for those in whom a long-term anticoagulation regimen is contraindicated, and for women of childbearing age who plan pregnancy (warfarin crosses the placental barrier). Frequently, older patients receive a bioprosthesis because these valves deteriorate more slowly in older persons, the need for long-term durability of the valve is less, and the risk of anticoagulation may increase with advancing age.

The surgical approach for valve replacement is by the

Advantages and Disadvantages of Prosthetic Cardiac Valves

Mechanical Valves

- Good long-term durability
- Adequate hemodynamics
- High risk of thromboembolism; long-term anti-coagulation required
- Increased risk of bleeding complications

Biological Valves

- Poor long-term durability
- Better hemodynamics than mechanical valves except in small sizes
- No hemolysis
- Low incidence of thromboembolism; anticoagulation may not be required
- Fewer bleeding complications

---

median sternotomy incision, using cardiopulmonary bypass and myocardial preservation techniques. The mitral valve is approached through the left atrium. Rather than excising the native valve, the chordae and papillary muscles are preserved when the prosthetic valve is sutured in place. This helps maintain left ventricular function and ejection fraction.[16] The aortic valve is approached through the ascending aorta. The native aortic valve is excised, the annulus is sized, and the prosthetic valve of correct size is sutured to the annulus. Once the surgery is completed, the patient is transferred to the critical care unit.

Cardiac Surgery

Preoperative Preparation

Preoperative preparation for cardiac surgery has psychological and physiological components. The physiological preparation is similar to that for any preoperative patient. An important aspect of psychological preparation is effective preoperative teaching, which reduces anxiety and physiological responses to stress before and after surgery. An explanation of the surgical procedure and the intraoperative and postoperative experiences should be included. Because the patient is generally not in the critical care unit preoperatively, a tour of the unit helps familiarize the patient and family with the specialized equipment and environment. Seeing a patient who is successfully recovering from cardiac surgery helps instill confidence and allay anxiety. Specific teaching topics related to the patient's stay in the critical care unit are shown in the display box.

Numerous invasive lines are placed in the patient before surgery and are used for monitoring during and

---

DISPLAY BOX 16–1
Preoperative Teaching of the Cardiac Surgery Patient: The Critical Care Unit Experience

1. Equipment, tubes, and lines used in critical care
   a. Cardiac monitor
   b. Arterial line
   c. Thermodilution catheter
   d. IVs and IV infusion pumps
   e. Endotracheal tube and ventilator
      1. Suctioning
      2. Inability to talk
      3. How to communicate when intubated
      4. When extubation can be anticipated
   f. Foley catheter
   g. Chest tubes
   h. Pacing wires
   i. Nasogastric tube
   j. Soft hand restraints

2. Incisions and dressings
   a. Median sternotomy incision
   b. Leg incision (is saphenous vein is used)

3. Patient's immediate postoperative appearance
   a. Skin yellow due to use of Betadine solution in operating room
   b. Skin pale and cool to touch due to hypothermia during surgery
   c. Generalized "puffiness" especially noticeable in neck, face, and hands due to third spacing of fluid given during cardiopulmonary bypass

4. Process of awakening from anesthesia
   a. Patient recovers in the critical care unit; does not go to the postanesthesia care unit
   b. Sensations patient will feel
   c. Noises patient will hear
   d. May be aware or able to hear but unable to respond

5. Discomfort from incision, chest tubes, and endotracheal tube
   a. Amount of discomfort to be expected
   b. When pain might be expected
   c. Relief mechanisms
      a. Positioning/splinting
      b. Medications

6. Postoperative respiratory care
   a. Turning
   b. Effective coughing and deep breathing after extubation
   c. Use of pillow to splint median sternotomy incision
   d. Incentive spirometry
   e. Have patient practice b, c, and d preoperatively

7. Postoperative activity progression

8. Visiting policy in critical care area

---

after surgery. These include a thermodilution catheter, arterial line, and Foley catheter. The patient is intubated, and a nasogastric tube and additional intravenous lines may also be inserted. As long as the hemoglobin is >11 gm/dl, 2 to 3 units of whole blood may be withdrawn from the patient at the beginning of surgery.[17] Plasma volume expanders are given to maintain the patient's volume and produce hemodilution. Infusion of this blood at the end of the procedure decreases the need for banked blood.

Surgical Procedure

Median Sternotomy Incision

The surgical approach most commonly used for myocardial revascularization, valve surgery, or cardiac transplantation is the median sternotomy incision. The sternum is split with a sternal saw from the manubrium to below the xyphoid process. The ribs are spread to expose the anterior mediastinum and pericardium. Once the pericardium is opened and the heart and aorta are exposed, the patient is placed on cardiopulmonary bypass.

Cardiopulmonary Bypass

Because the heart must be still (not beating) and empty during the surgery, a cardiopulmonary bypass machine is used. This machine, also called a pump oxygenator, assumes the job of oxygenating the patient's blood and circulating it throughout the body.

Before implementation of the bypass, the pump tubing is primed with a balanced electrolyte solution; blood is not used. The patient's deoxygenated venous blood is brought to the pump either through one cannula that is placed in the right atrial appendage or by two cannulas, one of which is placed directly in the inferior vena cava and the other directly into the superior vena cava. Another cannula is placed in the ascending aorta to return oxygenated blood to the patient's systemic circulation (Fig. 16–6). Heparin is administered throughout cardiopulmonary bypass to prevent massive extravascular coagulation as the blood circulates through the mechanical parts of the bypass system. After bypass is established, the blood is pumped through the circuit by a series of roller-type pumps which, unlike normal heart function, produce a nonpulsatile flow. Venous blood from the patient flows

1. Patient's deoxygenated blood enters the bypass circuit from the venous cannulas in the superior and inferior vena cavae.
2. Blood is temporarily held in the reservoir.
3. The oxygenator adds oxygen and removes carbon dioxide from the patient's blood.
4. The heat exchanger initially cools, then rewarms the patient's blood.
5. Roller pumps pump the blood through the circuit and back to the patient.
6. Oxygenated blood is returned to the ascending aorta by way of the aortic cannula.

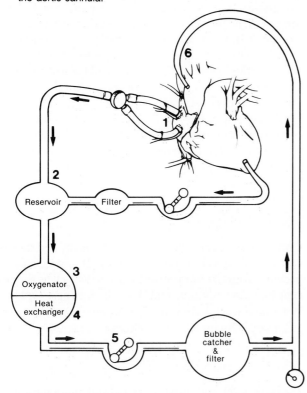

FIGURE 16–6
Flow of blood through the cardiopulmonary bypass circuit. (Adapted from Conahan TJ: Cardiac Anesthesia. Menlo Park, California, Wesley Publishing Co, 1981)

through the venous cannula to the cardiotomy reservoir and then into the oxygenator where exchange of oxygen and carbon dioxide occurs. The blood then travels through the heat exchanger, where it is cooled initially and later rewarmed.

During bypass the patient's core body temperature is lowered to 28° to 32°C to decrease metabolism. For each 1°C drop of body temperature the metabolic demands of the body decrease by 7%. This helps protect the major organ systems from possible ischemic injury and adverse effects of nonpulsatile perfusion during cardiopulmonary bypass.

Oxygenated blood is filtered and returned to the patient's ascending aorta by way of the arterial cannula (see Figure 16–6). Once extracorporeal circulation is established and systemic hypothermia is achieved, the aorta is cross-clamped just above the coronary arteries, and either crystalloid or blood cardioplegia solution is infused into the aortic root. The formula varies, but cardioplegia solution is a balanced electrolyte solution high in potassium. Oxygenated blood from the bypass circuit or oxygenated crystalloid can be added to the cardioplegia solution.

After the aorta is cross-clamped, no blood circulates through the coronary arteries, so the myocardium becomes ischemic. Cold cardioplegia solution at 4°C is infused into the aortic root under pressure. As it circulates through the coronary arteries, the high potassium concentration causes immediate asystole and relaxation, and the cold produces myocardial hypothermia. Asystole and hypothermia both protect against myocardial ischemia by decreasing the metabolic need of myocardial tissue. Oxygen consumption can decrease to less than 5% of normal.[18] The inclusion of blood or oxygenated crystalloid in the cardioplegia solution lessens myocardial ischemia by supplying oxygen. Additional cardioplegia solution is infused into the aortic root every 15 to 30 minutes or whenever cardiac electrical activity recurs.

Because perfusion of cardioplegia solution through occluded or diseased coronary arteries may not produce an even myocardial cooling, inadequately cooled areas risk ischemic damage. Therefore, hypothermia is also applied topically by pouring iced normal saline slush over the heart into the pericardial well. Cardioplegia with concomitant topical hypothermia cools the heart evenly while maintaining the myocardial temperature at 8° to 15°C. Thus, throughout surgery a threefold approach protects the patient against possible detrimental effects: systemic hypothermia, cold cardioplegia, and topical cardiac hypothermia.

After surgery is completed, the heat exchanger rewarms the blood to return the patient's core temperature to 37°C. After air is vented from the heart chambers and the aortic root, the aortic cross-clamp is removed so that blood again perfuses the coronary arteries, warming the myocardium. As perfusion and rewarming continue, a spontaneous cardiac rhythm can resume, ventricular fibrillation can develop (necessitating internal defibrillation), or pacing can be needed to initiate a rhythm. After a reliable rhythm with a rate adequate to maintain the cardiac output and blood pressure is established, total cardiopulmonary bypass is reduced to partial bypass. During partial bypass, some of the patient's blood circulates through the heart and lungs while some continues to circulate through the pump. If adequate arterial pressures are maintained, the patient's heart assumes total responsibility for the cardiac output, and bypass is discontinued. After the heart can maintain an adequate cardiac output, the cannulas are removed from the right atrium and aorta. Heparinization is reversed by the administration of protamine sulfate. If the patient cannot maintain adequate cardiac output during the weaning process, positive inotropic agents or intra-aortic balloon counterpulsation (IABP) can be instituted (see Chapter 13).

Completion of Surgery

If cardiac pacing is thought to be needed postoperatively, temporary pacing electrodes are placed on the epicardial surface of the heart and brought out through the chest wall on either side of the median sternotomy incision. Ventricular pacing electrodes are typically located to the left and atrial wires to the right (Fig. 16–7).

Chest tubes placed in the mediastinum and pericardial space for drainage are brought out through stab wounds just below the median sternotomy. If the pleural space has been entered, pleural tubes are also placed. After adequate hemostasis is obtained, the edges of the sternum are approximated with stainless steel wires, the incision is closed, and dressings are applied.

Assessment and Management of the Postoperative Cardiac Surgical Patient

Immediate Postoperative Period

Patients are transported directly to the critical care unit, where they recover from the anesthesia and where they usually remain for 24 to 48 hours postoperatively. They arrive with numerous lines and tubes attached (Fig. 16–8). Immediate postoperative nursing goals include maintenance of adequate ventilation, oxygenation, and hemodynamic stability. Rapid recognition of and intervention for changes in the patient's condition are imperative, because the person undergoing cardiac surgery is

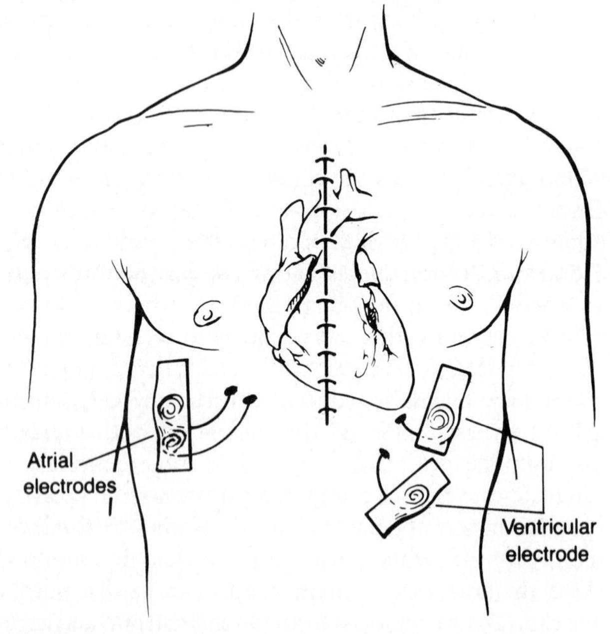

FIGURE 16–7
Temporary epicardial pacing wires: position of atrial and ventricular wires on chest wall. (Adapted from Finkelmeier BA, O'Mara SR: Temporary pacing in the cardiac surgical patient. Crit Care Nurse 4:109, 1984)

often more unstable than other surgical patients because of the effects of cardiopulmonary bypass and cardiac manipulation. Nursing care should be guided by the type of procedure done, the postoperative orders, and the advanced assessment, problem-solving, and technical skills that the critical care nurse possesses.

Ventilation/Oxygenation

The patient is ventilated by a volume ventilator on intermittent mandatory ventilation or assist-control mode (see Chapter 19). In some centers, 5 cm of positive end-expiratory pressure (PEEP) is used to decrease atelectasis and postoperative bleeding. The nurse should auscultate breath sounds immediately to assess for endotracheal tube placement, pneumothorax, and secretions; apply the arterial blood oxygen saturation (SaO_2) monitor; and obtain a chest x-ray and arterial blood gases (ABGs) within the first 15 to 30 minutes after admission. Suction as needed, and intervene as ordered for any abnormalities in the SaO_2 or ABGs.

Cardiac Rhythm

Connect the cardiac monitor, assessing the rate and rhythm, and obtain apical and radial pulses. If a pacemaker is present, assess its capture and sensing, as well as the percent of paced rhythm, and note the settings. Obtain a potassium level within the first 30 minutes, and treat as necessary. Obtain a 12-lead electrocardiogram (ECG).

Hemodynamic Stability

Connect, level, and zero the arterial and pulmonary artery lines. Assess the waveforms and record the values. Obtain thermodilution cardiac output, and administer vasoactive or inotropic medications or volume as needed to maintain the blood pressure and cardiac output (see Chapter 12).

Mixed Venous Oxygen Saturation (SvO_2) Monitoring

Mixed venous oxygen saturation (SvO_2), the amount of oxygen in the blood returning to the right side of the heart, depends on three factors—oxygen supply, oxygen delivery, and oxygen consumption. Oxygen supply (amount of oxygen in the arterial blood) is dependent on the amount of hemoglobin and the oxygen saturation of that hemoglobin (SaO_2). Pulmonary dysfunction or bleeding can decrease the arterial oxygen concentration. Oxygen delivery to the tissues is determined by the cardiac output (CO). The greater the CO, the more oxygen delivered; the lower the CO, the less oxygen delivered. Oxygen consumption (the amount of oxygen used by the tissues) increases if the tissues' metabolic demand increases (eg,

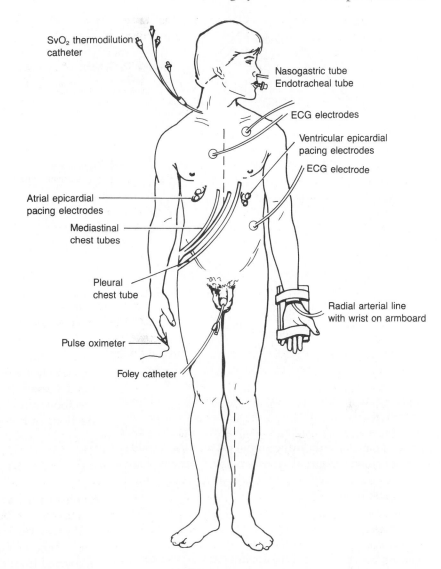

SvO₂ thermodilution catheter

Nasogastric tube
Endotracheal tube

ECG electrodes

Ventricular epicardial pacing electrodes

ECG electrode

Atrial epicardial pacing electrodes

Mediastinal chest tubes

Pleural chest tube

Radial arterial line with wrist on armboard

Pulse oximeter

Foley catheter

FIGURE 16–8
Typical postoperative appearance of a patient after cardiac surgery.

hyperthermia, shivering, and activity) and decreases if metabolic needs decrease (eg, hypothermia, anesthesia, and use of neuromuscular blocking agents). The oxygen left over after tissue use is the SvO_2. Normal SvO_2 ranges from 60% to 80% (Fig. 16–9).

The postoperative cardiac surgical patient with adequate SaO_2, hemoglobin, and CO often has a high SvO_2 initially, because hypothermia and the effects of anesthesia and neuromuscular blockade decrease the tissue demand for oxygen. As rewarming occurs and the patient awakens from anesthesia, tissue demand increases; the SvO_2 decreases but should remain above 60%.

The SvO_2 is intended to reflect the interaction of all aspects of oxygenation rather than a single parameter. It can help in early detection of abnormalities in oxygen supply, delivery, or consumption, and in assessing the effectiveness of interventions such as titration of vasoactive or inotropic drugs or ventilator changes. However, it should never substitute for careful monitoring of each parameter

individually. Noll and Fountain[19] examined the relationship of SvO_2 and CO early after cardiac surgery and found no statistically significant correlation. Measurements of SvO_2 should not be substituted for cardiac output measurements in the open heart surgery patient, even if SaO_2, Hgb, and oxygen consumption remain stable.

Chest Drainage/Bleeding

Connect the chest drainage container to suction (usually 20 cm H_2O), and position the drainage tubes without loops or kinks. Measure and record the amount and character of the drainage initially and then hourly. Assess for chest tube patency by observing for free-flowing drainage or the presence of clots in the tubing. Air leaks are assessed by watching for bubbling in the water seal chamber. If an air leak is present, implement troubleshooting techniques (see Chapter 19). Obtain a hemoglobin and hematocrit within the first 30 minutes.

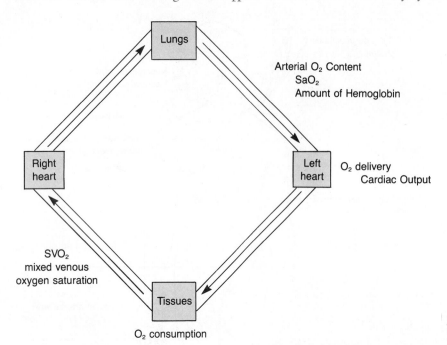

FIGURE 16–9
Factors affecting SVO_2.

Urine Output

Measure and record the urine output initially, and hourly thereafter. Because of hemodilution during cardiopulmonary bypass, an obligatory postoperative diuresis should ensue. Frequently, the urine output exceeds 100 to 200 cc per hour, and the specific gravity is low. Note any cloudiness or pink or red color to the urine, which could indicate hemoglobinuria.

Hypothermia

During rewarming on cardiopulmonary bypass, the patient's core temperature is returned to 37°C. However, as this warmed blood begins to circulate to the periphery, heat transfer to the surrounding tissues causes the core temperature to drop again. Patients frequently enter the critical care unit with a temperature in the 35° to 36°C range. Hypothermia causes peripheral vasoconstriction and a shift of the oxygen-hemoglobin dissociation curve to the left, so less oxygen is released from the hemoglobin to the tissues. See discussion on hypothermia in chapter 29.

Assess the patient's temperature on admission using pulmonary artery or tympanic membrane temperature; these are considered accurate indicators of core temperature.[20] Rectal temperatures do not correlate with core temperature measurements until 8 hours postoperatively,[21] and bladder temperature differs significantly from core temperature with rapid cooling and rewarming.[22] Increase the room temperature, and use radiant heat and blankets to increase core temperature to 37°C. Rewarming by fluid-filled thermal blankets is ineffective until the patient is peripherally vasodilated.[23] Accomplish rewarm-ing slowly to prevent hemodynamic instability due to rapid vasodilation. Avoid shivering, because it increases metabolic rate, oxygen consumption, carbon dioxide production, and myocardial workload.

Neurologic Status

Perform a neurologic assessment, including level of consciousness, pupillary reaction, ability to follow commands, and strength and movement of extremities, initially, hourly, and whenever a change is noticed until the patient is fully recovered from the anesthesia. Generally, patients return to the critical care area unconscious as a result of anesthesia and awaken gradually. Orient and reassure the patient frequently.

Postoperative Complications

Cardiac surgery patients risk developing problems because of their basic disease and the surgical trauma. In addition, the nurse caring for these persons must confront problems caused by cardiopulmonary bypass and intraoperative hypothermia. Because of abnormal blood interface and altered blood flow patterns, cardiopulmonary bypass produces profound physiological effects (Table 16–1) that make the postoperative course and care of the cardiac surgery patient unique and challenging. This discussion focuses on problems encountered early in the postoperative course of both CABG and valve surgery patients while they are in the critical care unit. Nursing Care Plan 16–1 defines the specific nursing interventions.

TABLE 16–1
Effects of Cardiopulmonary Bypass

Causes	Clinical Implications
Increased Capillary Permeability	
Interface between blood and nonphysiological surfaces or bypass circuit leads to • Complement activation that increases capillary permeability; • Platelet activation—platelets secrete vasoactive substances that increase capillary permeability; • Release of other vasoactive substances that increase capillary permeability.	Large amounts of fluid move from the intravascular to the interstitial space during and up to 6 h after cardiopulmonary bypass. Patient becomes edematous.
Hemodilution	
Solution used to prime extracorporeal circuit dilutes patient's blood. Secretion of vasopressin (ADH) is increased. Levels of renin–angiotensin–aldosterone are increased because of nonpulsatile renal perfusion. Total body water is increased.	Decreased blood viscosity improves capillary perfusion during nonpulsatile flow and hypothermia. Hgb and Hct decrease. Levels of coagulation factors are decreased because of dilution. Intravascular colloid osmotic pressure is decreased, contributing to movement of fluid from intravascular to interstitial spaces. Water is retained at collecting tubule of kidney. Aldosterone causes retention of sodium and water at renal tubule. Weight gain occurs.
Alterations in Coagulation	
Procoagulant effects: • Interface between blood and nonendothelial surfaces of bypass circuit activates intrinsic coagulation cascade. • Platelet damage activates intrinsic pathway. Anticoagulant effects: • Interface between blood and nonendothelial surfaces of bypass circuit causes platelets to adhere to tubing and to clump; abnormal platelet function; activation of coagulation cascade, which depletes clotting factors; denaturization of plasma proteins, including coagulation factors. • Coagulation factors decreased as a result of hemodilution. • Heparin and protamine.	Risk of microemboli is increased. Platelet count decreases by 50% to 70% of baseline. Abnormal postoperative bleeding occurs. Possibility of bleeding diathesis exists.
Damage to Blood Cells	
Exposure of blood to nonendothelial surfaces causes mechanical trauma and shear stress. • Platelet damage. • Red blood cell hemolysis. • Leukocyte damage.	Platelet count is decreased. Free hemoglobin and hemoglobinuria are increased. Hct is decreased. Immune response is diminished.
Microembolization	
Emboli from tissue debris, air bubbles, platelet aggregation.	Microemboli to body organs (brain, lungs, kidney) are possible.
Increased Systemic Vascular Resistance (SVR)	
Catecholamine secretion increased when cardiopulmonary bypass initiated. Renin secretion due to nonpulsatile flow to kidney. Hypothermia.	Hypertension is possible. Increased SVR may decrease cardiac output.

(continued)

TABLE 16-1
Effects of Cardiopulmonary Bypass (Continued)

Causes	Clinical Implications
Alteration in Carbohydrate Metabolism	
Insulin release is suppressed.	Postoperative hyperglycemia.
Glycogenolysis is stimulated by increase in catecholamines.	Glucosuria may occur.
Decreased perfusion pressure alters glucose transport across cell membrane.	

Alterations in Fluid and Electrolyte Balance

After cardiopulmonary bypass, total body fluid volume increases as a result of hemodilution, increased vasopressin levels, and nonpulsatile renal perfusion that activates the renin–angiotensin–aldosterone mechanism. Patients can return to the critical care area with a positive fluid balance of 2 to 3 liters or more, and extracellular fluid volume can increase by as much as 20% over preoperative levels. The amount of increase is directly proportional to the amount of time on bypass, and up to 15 lb of body water can be gained. Because of hemodilution, the colloid osmotic pressure of the plasma is decreased.

In addition to fluid retention, capillary permeability is markedly increased because vasoactive substances are released during cardiopulmonary bypass. Increased fluid volume, increased capillary permeability, and decreased plasma colloid osmotic pressure cause large amounts of fluid to move from the intravascular to the interstitial space during and up to 6 hours after surgery. The patient appears edematous (especially the face, neck, and hands) and often develops an intravascular volume deficit.

Intravascular hypovolemia is manifested clinically by decreased central venous pressure (CVP), decreased pulmonary artery diastolic pressure (PAD), and decreased pulmonary capillary wedge pressure (PCWP). If left untreated, low cardiac output and hypotension can occur. Abnormal postoperative bleeding and vasodilation as the body's temperature normalizes can contribute to the hypovolemia.

Initial treatment is aimed at restoring adequate intravascular volume by administering fluids. Colloids (hetastarch or Plasmanate) provide more effective volume expansion than crystalloids because they increase colloid osmotic pressure, drawing interstitial fluid back into the vasculature. Adequacy of fluid administration should be determined by PAD, PCWP, cardiac output, and blood pressure measurements.

Fluid usually shifts back into the vascular space during the first several postoperative days as capillary membrane integrity improves and plasma colloid osmotic pressure

Clinical Research

Ley J, Miller K, Skov P, and Preisig P. Crystalloid versus Colloid Fluid Therapy After Cardiac Surgery. Heart Lung 19:31–40, 1990.

The purpose of this study was to examine the difference between crystalloid and colloid therapy regarding hemodynamics and fluid requirements after cardiac surgery. Twenty-one patients post CABG or valve replacement were randomly assigned to a crystalloid or colloid protocol. The crystalloid group received 0.9% normal saline (NS) at 10 ml/kg/h, and the colloid group received 6% hydroxyethyl starch (hetastarch, HES) at 5 ml/kg/h initially. Both solutions were administered over an 8-hour period and titrated to maintain a cardiac index (CI) greater than 2 L/min/M. The use of HES significantly reduced fluid requirements and produced greater hemodynamic stability than the use of NS. Fluid intake was significantly higher during the 8 hours for the NS group than for the HES group (4655 cc vs. 1918 cc), and the NS group experienced significantly more weight gain in the first 12 hours (2.32 kg vs. 0.26 kg). The HES group exhibited greater hemodynamic stability, with increased systolic BP, CO, and CI after 2 hours of treatment, and after 3 hours, the CI was significantly higher. The HES group also experienced a significantly shorter ICU stay (49.5 h vs. 68.1 h).

normalizes. Renal excretion of excess body fluid results in spontaneous diuresis and weight loss. Fluid and sodium restriction may be ordered until body weight and fluid balance return to normal.

The most common postoperative electrolyte imbalance is an abnormal potassium level. Hypokalemia can result from hemodilution, diuretics, and the effects of aldosterone, which causes potassium secretion into the urine at the distal renal tubule as sodium is retained. Hyperkalemia can occur as a result of large amounts of cardioplegia solution or acute renal failure.

Potassium levels should be checked on admission to ICU, every 2 to 4 hours for the first 8 hours postoperatively, and daily for several days. Based on these laboratory values, potassium supplements should be given as ordered.

Decreased Cardiac Output

Cardiac output (CO) is the product of heart rate (HR) and stroke volume (SV).

$$CO = HR \times SV$$

Preload   Afterload   Contractility

Decreased cardiac output can result from alterations in heart rate, stroke volume, or both. Abnormalities in heart rate are discussed as a separate postoperative problem under "Cardiac Dysrhythmias."

Stroke volume is dependent on preload, afterload, and contractility. An abnormality in one or more of these parameters can cause a decrease in output (see Chapter 12).

Low Preload

Left ventricular preload is the volume of blood in the left ventricle at the end of diastole. It reflects the volume status of the patient and is measured by the PCWP using the thermodilution catheter or by the left atrial mean pressure (LAPM) using a catheter placed directly into the left atrium and brought out through the chest wall at the end of surgery. Normal LAPM is approximately equal to the normal PCWP.

Because postoperative cardiac surgery patients frequently experience intravascular hypovolemia, the assessment of PCWP or LAPM is imperative to optimize cardiac output.

What should be considered "normal" PCWP must be related to the individual patient. For example, normal PCWP usually ranges from 6 to 12 mm Hg. Because of surgical manipulation and cardiopulmonary bypass, the PCWP in patients undergoing cardiac surgery usually must be maintained above 10 mm Hg. If the patient has valve disease, even higher filling pressures may be re-quired. Valvular stenosis or insufficiency causes volume and pressure overload, which in turn cause hypertrophy and dilatation of the chamber behind the valve. Valve replacement corrects the flow obstruction or leak; however, the myocardial changes of hypertrophy and dilatation take months to improve. You can think of it as a balloon that has been left inflated for several weeks. If you let the air out, it has little elastic recoil. To maximize cardiac output, you must increase the filling volume (increase PCWP or LAPM) to stretch this dilated myocardium for optimal contractility (Starling's principle). Clinically, a PCWP of 10 mm Hg is usually the low limit of "normal" for a valve patient, and a PCWP as high as 18 to 20 mm Hg can be considered "normal" and necessary to maintain adequate output. Patients with poor left ventricular function due to a large infarction or left ventricular aneurysm also need a higher PCWP for optimal stretch and contractility according to Starling's principle. If the patient is on PEEP to decrease postoperative bleeding, the PCWP may not truly reflect the left ventricular preload. By increasing intrathoracic pressure, PEEP falsely elevates the PCWP.

Low preload is treated by administering Plasmanate, hetastarch, crystalloids, autotransfusion, or blood (if the hematocrit is low). The goal of fluid replacement is a PCWP or LAPM that produces an adequate output and blood pressure for each patient.

Increased Left Ventricular Afterload

Afterload is the resistance to ejection of blood from the left ventricle and is determined in part by the degree of constriction or dilation of the arterial circulation. It is measured by systemic vascular resistance (SVR), which is calculated by the formula

$$SVR = \frac{MAP - CVP}{CO} \times 20$$

where MAP is mean arterial pressure, CVP is central venous pressure, and CO is cardiac output. Normal values are 800 to 1200 dynes/sec/cm^{-5}.

Afterload can be elevated after cardiac surgery as a result of hypothermia, release of vasoactive substances during bypass, increase in catecholamines, renin, and angiotensin, or a history of hypertension. High afterload increases myocardial workload and oxygen demand and decreases output.

If the cause is hypothermia, warming the patient with blankets and radiant heat, a heating blanket, or a heat lamp can lower the SVR. Care should be taken not to rewarm the patient too quickly, because rapid vasodilation could cause hypotension.

Increased afterload can also be treated by administering vasodilating drugs such as nitroprusside. If the blood pressure seems low to administer nitroprusside, the drug can be started at very low doses. Often the vasodilation produced by a low dose of nitroprusside increases the output enough that there is no change in blood pressure.

Decreased Contractility

Contractility is the ability of the myocardial muscle fibers to shorten independent of preload and afterload. Contractility is measured by left ventricular stroke work index (LVSWI), which is calculated by the formula

$$LVSWI = \frac{(MAP - PAD)SV \times 0.0136}{BSA}$$

where MAP is mean arterial pressure, PAD is pulmonary artery diastolic pressure, SV is stroke volume, and BSA is body surface area.

The normal range for LVSWI is 35 to 85 g/m^2 per beat, but a "normal" postoperative LVSWI in a patient after cardiac surgery can be lower than 35 because of the effects of surgical manipulation of the myocardium, cardiopulmonary bypass, cardioplegia, and ischemia during the aortic cross-clamping. Abnormal decreases in LVSWI can be caused by myocardial infarction, changes in the ventricular muscle as a result of valve disease, or abnormalities of myocardial pH, electrolytes, or oxygenation.

If the underlying cause can be identified, it should be corrected. Positive inotropic medications such as dopamine, dobutamine, or amrinone can also be effective. Because postsurgical depression of myocardial function lasts only 6 to 18 hours postoperatively, attempts to wean these drugs can begin on the first postoperative day.

Alterations in Blood Pressure

After cardiac surgery, it is not unusual for hypotension or hypertension to develop quickly. Nursing interventions should be directed toward anticipating such changes and intervening to prevent them or to rapidly restore the blood pressure to a normotensive range. Generally, the systolic pressure should be kept in the 90 to 150 mm Hg range. These parameters can vary depending on the patient and events in the operating room.

Hypotension

The patient is usually considered hypotensive if the systolic blood pressure is less than 90 mm Hg. In CABG, the saphenous vein grafts can collapse if the perfusion pressure is too low (veins do not have the muscular walls that arteries do), resulting in myocardial ischemia. Inadequate tissue and organ perfusion can result from a systolic blood pressure lower than 90 mm Hg, especially in the previously hypertensive patient.

Hypotension can be caused by decreased intravascular volume, vasodilation as a result of rewarming, poor left ventricular contractility, or dysrhythmias. If the patient is hypovolemic, rapid infusion of volume expanders as ordered by the physician should increase the blood pressure.

If the volume expansion alone does not correct the hypotension, or if the low blood pressure is caused by decreased contractility, a vasopressor drug can be ordered. For example, dopamine started at 2 to 10 µg/kg/min has a primarily β-stimulating effect to increase contractility and blood pressure. If the hypotension is caused by dysrhythmia, interventions are aimed at correcting the dysrhythmia or obtaining a ventricular rate adequate to maintain the output (see discussion of cardiac dysrhythmias on page 168).

Hypertension

Hypertension is particularly dangerous in the postoperative cardiac surgery patient because it can cause rupture or leakage of suture lines and increase bleeding. Postoperative hypertension can result from a history of hypertension, increased levels of catecholamines or renin, hypothermia, or pain. Some patients are hypertensive postoperatively without an obvious cause.

A systolic blood pressure of 150 mm Hg or more is usually considered hypertensive and should be treated. Nitroprusside, a vasodilator, can be titrated to bring the blood pressure into an acceptable range. Sometimes the blood pressure increases when the patient is stimulated by noise or nursing care procedures but returns to normal levels when the patient sleeps. This hypertension can often be controlled by intravenous analgesics or sedatives. Pain may also cause hypertension that can be managed by analgesics.

Unless the patient was hypertensive preoperatively, postoperative hypertension is usually transient, and the nitroprusside dose can be decreased within 24 hours. If this is not possible, oral antihypertensives can be started to facilitate discontinuation of the nitroprusside.

Postoperative Bleeding

Although bleeding from the chest tubes after cardiac surgery is expected, the nurse must differentiate between normal and excessive drainage. Normal chest tube drainage is dark red, thin, serosanguineous, and does not clot in the chest tubes because it is defibrinated. Usually, there is not more than 200 cc of drainage per hour for the first 1 to 2 hours, with the amount decreasing subsequently. The actual amount of drainage is important, but the hourly trend must also be considered. If the drainage amount is excessive initially, but the trend is decreasing, this is less worrisome than a trend of increasing drainage.

Some patients normally bleed more than others. Patients who have had the IMA used for one of the grafts can have increased bleeding initially because of dissection of the chest wall to isolate the IMA. Those undergoing cardiac surgery for a second or third time may also bleed more because of the dissection of scar tissue and adhesions created by previous surgeries.

Arterial Bleeding

Although rare, arterial bleeding is a life-threatening emergency that usually results from rupture or leakage of suture lines at one of three sites: the proximal anastomosis of the vein graft to the aorta, the distal anastomosis of the vein graft to the coronary artery, or the aortic cannulation site where oxygenated blood is returned to the patient during cardiopulmonary bypass.

With an arterial bleed, the chest drainage container fills up with bright red blood within minutes, and the patient becomes hypovolemic and hypotensive extremely rapidly. Lost blood must be replaced as quickly as possible with blood or volume expanders until the chest can be reopened and surgical repair accomplished.

Venous Bleeding

Venous bleeding is more common than arterial bleeding and is caused by surgical problems or coagulopathy. Faulty hemostasis of one or more vessels results in abnormal bleeding. Coagulopathy can have multiple causes. Coagulation factors may be used during cardiopulmonary bypass more quickly than the body can replace them, and they are diluted by the pump primer solution. Thrombocytopenia can be present because of platelet destruction or loss of platelets by adherence to the bypass circuit tubing. Platelets may not work effectively because of damage from cardiopulmonary bypass or preoperative antiplatelet medication (eg, A.S.A.). The fibrinolytic system responsible for clot breakdown can be abnormally activated by surgery, increased levels of catecholamines, or stress.

Heparin "rebound" can also cause postoperative bleeding. After the patient is taken off cardiopulmonary bypass, intravascular heparin is neutralized by protamine. As the body temperature increases and the peripheral circulation improves, nonneutralized heparin shifts or "rebounds" from the interstitial spaces, resulting in a re-anticoagulation.

Treatment of Bleeding

Controlling hypertension, maintaining chest tube patency to prevent cardiac tamponade, and maintaining adequate intravascular volume are essential actions while caring for a bleeding patient. Whether chest tubes should be milked or stripped routinely is controversial. Negative intrathoracic pressures up to −400 cm water can be generated with vigorous stripping. This can entrap intrathoracic tissue in the chest tube drainage holes and increase bleeding. However, if the tubes become occluded, life-threatening cardiac tamponade can develop. More research is needed to determine the effect of chest tube stripping on postoperative bleeding. Gentle milking when clots are evident should be implemented to ensure patency.

To maintain normovolemia, adequate cardiac output, and sufficient blood pressure, the blood loss must be replaced. Autotransfusion of the chest drainage (see Chapter 13) is an excellent way to accomplish this without the risks of heterologous blood transfusion. If the hematocrit is low, fresh whole blood or packed red cells can be given. Usually, transfusion is indicated only if the hematocrit is below 28% to 30% because, as excess volume is excreted, the hematocrit increases. Plasmanate or hetastarch can be given if the hematocrit is adequate.

Treatment is also aimed at decreasing the amount of bleeding and correcting the underlying cause. PEEP of 5 to 10 cm added to the ventilator can decrease venous oozing by increasing intrathoracic pressure. Vital signs must be observed closely if PEEP is used, because the increased intrathoracic pressure can decrease venous return, causing low cardiac output and hypotension.

Laboratory work, including activated clotting time (ACT), prothrombin time (PT), partial thromboplastin time (PTT), fibrinogen, bleeding time, and platelet counts, helps determine appropriate treatment. The ACT, PT, and PTT assess the time required for the patient's blood to clot and are prolonged in the presence of heparin. If the results are abnormally prolonged, heparin "rebound" may be the cause of bleeding, and intravenous protamine can be given.

Bleeding time measures the ability of platelets to adhere to the blood vessel wall and aggregate to form a platelet plug. The bleeding time can be prolonged even when the platelet count is adequate, if platelet function is abnormal.

Thrombocytopenia can also cause abnormal bleeding. Normally, the platelet count drops to 50% to 70% of baseline when cardiopulmonary bypass is initiated. If the postoperative platelet count is less than 50,000/mm^3 or the patient's platelets are not functioning normally, platelet concentrate can be administered. Desmopressin acetate (DDAVP), an analog of vasopressin that lacks vasopressor activity, can also be given. It is thought to increase platelet aggregation.[24] The platelet count usually returns to normal within 24 hours postoperatively as platelets sequestered in the spleen are released to the general circulation.

If the PT, PTT, or fibrinogen is abnormal, fresh frozen plasma (FFP) or cryoprecipitate can be used. FFP is rich in fibrinogen and factors V and VII; cryoprecipitate supplies factors VIII and XIII. These replace clotting factors diminished as a result of cardiopulmonary bypass and hemodilution.

If the bleeding is not stopped by these interventions and the chest tube drainage is more than 400 cc per hour for longer than 3 hours or more than 100 cc per hour for longer than 6 hours, surgical reexploration is indicated.

Early Cardiac Tamponade

Cardiac tamponade can occur if blood accumulates around the heart and compresses the myocardium. This impedes venous return, decreasing both cardiac output and blood pressure. Tamponade is an uncommon complication if the chest tubes are kept patent; however, if it does occur, it is dangerous and must be recognized and treated quickly.

Signs and symptoms include decreasing blood pressure accompanied by rising CVP and PCWP. CVP and PCWP values can become closer to one another (ie, they equalize) as blood surrounding the heart compresses the right and left ventricular chambers. A paradoxical pulse can be present (greater than 10 mm Hg decrease in systolic pressure with inspiration). This can be a clue to tamponade, but paradoxical pulse does not always occur with tamponade after cardiac surgery. Patients with pulmonary disease and those on ventilators can have a decrease in systolic pressure with inspiration when they do not have tamponade. Another clue can be an abrupt decrease in chest tube drainage that has been initially brisk, suggesting an acute chest tube occlusion. Definitive diagnosis is made by chest x-ray, which shows mediastinal widening, or by echocardiography, which demonstrates fluid in the pericardial space.

Treatment for postoperative tamponade includes fluids and vasopressors to maintain the cardiac output and blood pressure until surgical decompression is done. Generally, pericardiocentesis is not used for postoperative cardiac tamponade, because pericardial blood is usually clotted and cannot be aspirated with a needle.

Cardiac Dysrhythmias

Both brady- and tachyarrhythmias are common postoperatively and can decrease cardiac output. They are treated similarly to dysrhythmias occurring in any cardiac patient (see Chapter 13).

Tachyarrhythmias can be dangerous because they compromise cardiac output by decreasing ventricular diastolic filling time. They also decrease coronary artery perfusion and increase myocardial oxygen demand.

Sinus tachycardia can be caused by hypovolemia or side effects of inotropic drugs (especially dopamine). Catecholamine release during surgery, pain, anxiety, or fever may be a contributing factor. Treatment is directed toward correcting the underlying cause.

Premature ventricular contractions (PVCs) are common as a result of surgical trauma and manipulation, electrolyte imbalances (especially hypokalemia), changes in pH and PO_2, and catecholamine release due to pain or anxiety. Occasionally tactile irritation from the thermodilution catheter or mediastinal chest tubes also causes PVCs. Lidocaine should be used to suppress PVCs while the underlying cause is identified and treated. If ventricular tachycardia or ventricular fibrillation develops, treatment with lidocaine or defibrillation according to accepted protocols must be initiated.

Twenty percent to 40% of cardiac surgery patients develop supraventricular tachycardias (SVT),[25] including paroxysmal atrial tachycardia (PAT), atrial fibrillation, and atrial flutter. Most often these arrhythmias develop 24 to 36 hours postoperatively. If the ventricular rate associated with the SVT is rapid, cardiac output can fall. Loss of atrial kick (contribution to cardiac output by atrial contraction) with atrial fibrillation and flutter can contribute to this decrease. If hemodynamic compromise ensues, SVT can be managed by intravenous verapamil, synchronized cardioversion, or several seconds of rapid atrial pacing by the temporary atrial epicardial pacing electrodes. Recent studies indicate that cardiopulmonary bypass can cause hypomagnesemia and that administration of magnesium postoperatively significantly decreases the number of atrial fibrillation episodes.[26]

In postoperative valve patients (especially mitral valve patients), atrial fibrillation is common because of long-standing atrial dilatation and stretching. Many of these patients have had chronic atrial fibrillation preoperatively. If the ventricular response to the fibrillation is controlled, treatment may include digitalization or, in those who are already digitalized, adding quinidine. If the ventricular response is rapid, intravenous verapamil may slow it. Cardioversion is not usually indicated if the fibrillation has been chronic.

Bradyarrhythmias (sinus brady, idiojunctional) and blocks (bundle branch block, second and third degree AV block) occur postoperatively owing to depression of the conduction system cells by cardioplegia or injury to nodes and conduction pathways by surgical manipulation, sutures, or local edema. Valve surgery patients are particularly at risk because of the proximity of the cardiac conduction system to the mitral and aortic valves.

In most patients bradyarrhythmias and blocks resolve as the effects of cardioplegia diminish and the surgical edema subsides. If the cardiac output is decreased as a result of a bradyarrhythmia, AV or ventricular pacing is indicated to maintain an adequate heart rate. Atropine can be used for temporary treatment.

Pulmonary Dysfunction

Cardiac surgery patients are more at risk for developing pulmonary complications than other surgical patients because of the effects of cardiopulmonary bypass. During bypass, pulmonary ventilation is halted or diminished because the oxygenator, not the lungs, oxygenates the blood. This results in pulmonary atelectasis. When the pulmonary circulation is restored, perfusion of nonventilated alveoli occurs, shunting nonoxygenated blood into the systemic circulation. Because of increased capillary permeability, fluid may move into the pulmonary interstitium and alveoli. This hampers gaseous diffusion and can increase secretions. Hypoxemia can develop. Large tidal volumes and PEEP are often used to prevent alveolar collapse, treat atelectasis, and improve oxygenation. Secretions are removed by endotracheal suctioning, and ventilatory status is assessed by SaO_2 monitoring and ABG determination. Patients are usually weaned from the ventilator the evening of surgery or the next morning if extubation criteria are met (see Chapter 19), hemodynamic parameters are stable, and the chest tube drainage is within normal limits. Patients with preexisting pulmonary disease may remain on the ventilator longer.

After extubation, coughing and deep breathing are done every 1 to 2 hours with incentive spirometry every 2 hours. Mobilization should begin as soon as possible. Because the median sternotomy incision and chest tubes cause pain, they can interfere with coughing and deep breathing. Splinting the chest incision with a small pillow and providing pain medications before incentive spirometry and coughing can facilitate pulmonary hygiene.

Renal Failure

Although renal failure is an uncommon complication, cardiac surgery patients are more at risk than others because of cardiopulmonary bypass. Renal blood flow is decreased during bypass, blood cells are damaged, and free hemoglobin is released from red blood cell destruction. Cellular debris and free hemoglobin can damage renal tubules. This risk accelerates with increasing time on bypass and with preexisting renal dysfunction.

Hematuria can occur because of renal filtration of hemoglobin. Maintaining adequate urinary output is imperative to prevent renal tubular damage and obstruction from cellular debris and hemoglobin. Lasix or mannitol can be given to promote urine flow.

Prerenal factors also cause postoperative renal failure. Decreased cardiac output, hypotension, and hypovolemia decrease renal blood flow and should be treated aggressively. Renal dose dopamine can improve renal blood flow.

Neurologic Dysfunction

Postoperative neurologic dysfunction can vary in severity from mild temporary impairments in concentration to periods of agitation and confusion to major cerebrovascular accident or coma. The risk of neurologic complications increases with increasing age, prolonged cardiopulmonary bypass time, preexisting carotid or cerebrovascular disease, and valve disease, especially if atrial fibrillation is present.

Altered cerebral perfusion and microembolization of fat, fibrin, or platelet aggregates during cardiopulmonary bypass, and embolization of clots, particulate matter, or air can all be causes of neurologic sequelae. Atrial clots occur commonly in patients with atrial fibrillation because of sluggish atrial blood flow. When a rhythm is reestablished after bypass, these clots can embolize. During manipulation of diseased valves, calcified material can break loose. Atheromatous plaque in the ascending aorta can also embolize when the aorta is manipulated during cannulation or proximal vein graft anastomosis. Air embolism arising from air trapped in the cardiopulmonary bypass system or from inadequate venting of air from the heart and aortic root can also cause neurologic deficits.

Identifying those at increased risk and assessing neurologic status frequently can facilitate recognition of potential problems early so that intervention can begin. Maintaining adequate cardiac output, blood pressure, and ABGs ensures normal cerebral perfusion and oxygenation.

Wound Infection

Postoperative wound infection can develop in the leg or median sternotomy incision or in chest tube insertion sites. Infection risk is increased by obesity, diabetes mellitus, malnutrition, operative time greater than 6 hours, and more than one surgery in a single admission (eg, reoperation for postoperative bleeding).

An ongoing assessment for signs of wound infection should be conducted. These include erythema, drainage, and temperature elevation that persists more than 72 hours postoperatively. Early temperature elevation as high as 38.9°C during the first 48 hours after surgery is a normal response to cardiopulmonary bypass and usually not a sign of infection.

Wound infection is not an early postoperative problem and is usually not evident until after the patient leaves the critical care unit. However, meticulous care should be taken to prevent infection by keeping incisions clean and dry and changing soiled dressings with aseptic technique.

Postoperative Pain

After cardiac surgery the patient can experience pain resulting from the chest or leg incision, the chest tubes, or rib spreading during surgery. Although pain perception varies from person to person, the median sternotomy incision is usually less painful than a thoracotomy incision, and most people report that the pain is worst the first 3 to 4 days postoperatively. Discomfort from the leg incision often worsens after the patient is ambulatory, especially if leg swelling occurs. Stretching of back and neck muscles as the ribs are spread and immobilization for several hours during surgery can cause back and neck discomfort. Patients having IMA grafting can have increased pain because of more stretching of the intercostal muscles and because of incision into the parietal pleura, which is richly innervated.

Angina after CABG can indicate graft failure; therefore, the nurse must be able to differentiate angina from incisional pain. Typical median sternotomy pain is localized, does not radiate, and can be sharp, dull, aching, or burning. It is often worse with deep breathing, coughing, or movement. Angina is usually precordial or substernal, not well localized, and frequently radiates to arms, neck, or jaw. It is often described as a pressure sensation and is not affected by respiration or movement.

Pain often stimulates the sympathetic nervous system, increasing heart rate and blood pressure, which can be detrimental to the patient's hemodynamics. Discomfort can also result in diminished chest expansion, increased atelectasis, and retention of secretions.

The goals of nursing management should be to provide pain relief, maximize comfort, and alleviate factors that enhance pain perception, such as anxiety and fatigue.

Thrombosis/Embolism after Valve Replacement

The risk of thromboembolism is present in all patients undergoing valve replacement, but it is greatest with a mechanical valve in the mitral position and in patients with atrial fibrillation. Anticoagulation reduces but does not eliminate the risk of these complications, and it increases the risk of significant hemorrhage.

Clots can form on the mechanical valve, obstructing blood flow through it or preventing proper valve closure, which results in regurgitant flow. Hemodynamic deterioration, development of a new murmur, or change in the normal valve sound may suggest these complications.

Infective Endocarditis after Valve Surgery

Patients undergoing valve reconstruction or replacement are at risk for developing valvular endocarditis. Early postoperative endocarditis is usually associated with median sternotomy infection or sepsis from urinary tract infection or invasive lines. Because endocarditis takes time to develop, the critical care nurse's role is primarily prevention. Early removal of the Foley catheter, invasive intravenous lines, and arterial line as well as early recognition and treatment of wound infections can prevent this complication.

Heart Transplantation

Description

The first human-to-human heart transplant was performed by Dr. Christiaan Barnard in 1967; however, because of poor long-term survival, cardiac transplantation remained primarily an experimental procedure. With the 1983 introduction of cyclosporine to treat rejection, heart transplantation has become a therapeutic alternative. In 1990, 1,863 heart transplants were performed in the United States, but the number has reached a plateau because of the unavailability of donors. Internationally, the average 1-year survival rate is 80% to 90% and the 10-year survival is 72%.[27] The goals of cardiac transplantation are to prolong survival in patients with terminal heart disease and to improve functional ability and quality of life.

Indications for Cardiac Transplantation

Transplantation is indicated for end-stage heart disease resulting from cardiomyopathy, severe CAD, valvular heart disease, congenital heart disease, or myocarditis. These conditions must not be manageable by conventional medical or surgical therapy. Those accepted for transplantation are New York Heart Association functional class III or IV and have a life expectancy of less than 6 to 12 months. They must demonstrate emotional and psychosocial stability and a willingness and ability to comply with lifelong immunosuppressive drug therapy.

Contraindications to Cardiac Transplantation

Initially, patients more than 55 years old were not accepted for transplant. Recently, however, favorable outcomes have been achieved in older patients. Therefore, exclusion because of age is based on the person's physiological rather than chronological age.

Patients with insulin-dependent diabetes mellitus were also routinely rejected for transplantation, because

---

Contraindications to Cardiac Transplantation

- **Fixed pulmonary hypertension** with pulmonary vascular resistance >480–640 dynes/sec/cm^{-5} (>6–8 Wood units). Risk of right ventricular failure of donor heart. High pulmonary vascular resistance increases right ventricular afterload. Unlikely that donor heart could acutely increase right ventricular work load to overcome this resistance. (Heterotopic transplant or oversized donor heart may be considered.)
- **Active infection.** Overwhelming infection and increased mortality may occur with immunosuppressive therapy.
- **Malignancy.** Rapid growth and spread of an existing carcinoma may occur with immunosuppressive therapy.
- **Recent unresolved pulmonary infarct.** Increases posttransplant risk of pulmonary infection.
- **Irreversible hepatic or renal dysfunction.** (*If due to cardiac failure and if reversible with improved cardiac output from donor heart, then not a contraindication.*) Increases risk of morbidity. Cyclosporine and azathioprine are toxic to liver and kidneys.
- **Active peptic ulcer disease.** Corticosteroids used for immunosuppression can exacerbate problem.
- **Psychosocial instability or alcohol or drug dependence.** Difficulty complying with lifelong medical regimens and immunosuppressive therapy.
- **Advanced peripheral or cerebral vascular disease.** May increase morbidity. May attenuate benefit of transplant.

corticosteroid immunosuppression can exacerbate the diabetes. Recently this criterion has been relaxed, and many centers consider insulin-dependent diabetics who are free of diabetic retinopathy, neuropathy, nephropathy and vascular disease. Other contraindications to transplantation are described in the accompanying box.

Donor Considerations

When a patient meets the criteria for transplantation, the search for a donor begins. To minimize ventricular myocardial damage, the maximum time the donor heart can be ischemic (ie, the time from aortic cross-clamping during removal from the donor until restoration of coronary artery circulation after implant in the recipient) is 4 to 5 hours. Therefore, distance for transport of the donor organ is limited to a flying radius of about 3 hours.

To ensure relative immunologic compatibility between donor and recipient, Panel Reactive Antibody (PRA) testing is done. The recipient's serum is incubated with a random pool of lymphocytes. If no lymphocyte destruction occurs, the crossmatch is negative, indicating that the recipient has no preformed cytotoxic antibodies and transplantation may proceed. Donor-specific crossmatching is not usually done because of the time limitation. Donor and recipient are also matched by identical ABO blood groups and comparable body size and weight. If a suitable donor is found, the heart is preserved with cold cardioplegia solution, removed, immersed in cold saline solution at 6°C, and transported to the recipient's location.

Surgical Procedure

Orthotopic Transplantation

Orthotopic transplantation is performed most commonly. The recipient's heart is excised, and the donor heart is implanted in its place. A median sternotomy incision is made, cardiopulmonary bypass is initiated, and the recipient's heart is removed by incising the left and right atria, pulmonary artery, and aorta. The atrial septum and posterior and lateral walls of the recipient's atria are left intact, including the areas of the SA node, inferior and superior vena cavae to the right atrium, and pulmonary veins to the left atrium. The remnant atria serve as anchors for the donor heart.

The donor atria are trimmed to preserve the anterior atrial walls, SA node, and internodal conduction pathways. Then anastomoses are made between the recipient and donor left and right atria, the pulmonary arteries, and the aortas. Cardiopulmonary bypass is weaned off, and the donor heart assumes the role of providing the cardiac output (Fig. 16–10).

Heterotopic Transplantation

An infrequently used technique is heterotopic transplantation, or piggyback procedure, in which the recipient's heart is left in place and the donor heart is placed next to it in the right chest. The two hearts are connected in parallel by anastomoses made between the donor and recipient left and right atria, aortas, and pulmonary arteries using a synthetic tube graft. By allowing blood to flow through

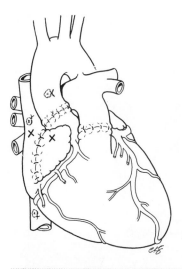

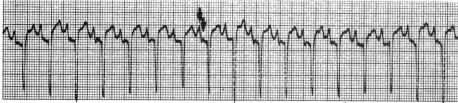

FIGURE 16–10
Orthotopic method of transplantation. Both the donor and the recipient SA nodes are intact (**X**). This results in an ECG tracing as shown. Note the double P wave, at independent rates.

either or both hearts, two functional hearts work together to provide the cardiac output (Fig. 16–11).

Heterotopic transplantation can be used in patients with pulmonary hypertension in whom the donor heart alone would not have a strong enough right ventricle to pump against the increased pulmonary vascular resistance. It can also be used as a lifesaving procedure in urgent cases if the only available donor heart is too small for the size of the recipient. Limitations of heterotopic transplantation include thromboembolism from the native heart with need for anticoagulation, limited space in the chest cavity, and, in ischemic heart disease, ongoing angina and the possibility of ischemia induced arrhythmias in the native heart.

Assessment and Management Posttransplant

Postoperative care of the transplant patient is similar to that for any person undergoing cardiac surgery as discussed previously; however, several major differences present additional nursing challenges. These differences include changes in cardiac rhythm and function caused by denervation of the donor heart and the potential for right ventricular failure. Only the more common orthotopic transplantation is discussed here.

Changes in Cardiac Rhythm and Function

Remnant P Waves

Because the recipient SA node and portions of the recipient atria are left intact, two P waves are usually seen on the ECG. The recipient SA node initiates an impulse that depolarizes the remnant recipient atria; however, this depolarization wave usually does not cross the atrial suture line. The donor SA node initiates the impulse that causes depolarization of the entire donor heart and elicits the QRS complex. Because the two sets of atria beat independently of each other, two different P waves appear on the ECG. Remnant P waves can be identified by their dissociation or lack of relationship to the QRS complexes. They usually occur at a slower rate than the donor P waves, and their rate can speed up or slow down because the remnant P waves are still under autonomic nervous system influence, whereas the donor P waves are denervated. The two sets of atria can also be in different rhythms. For example, the recipient atrial remnants can be in atrial fibrillation while the donor heart is in normal sinus rhythm.

Effects of Denervation

During donor heart removal, the nerve supply is severed, resulting in no autonomic nervous system innervation of the transplanted heart. Because of the loss of vagal influence, the resting sinus rate is higher than normal—usually between 90 and 110 beats per minute—and heart rate

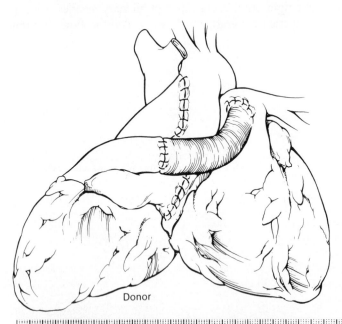

Donor

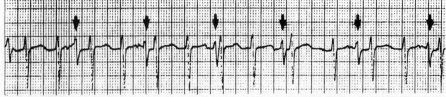

FIGURE 16–11
Heterotopic method of transplantation. The donor heart is anastomosed with a Dacron graft to the recipient's heart. This results in an ECG tracing as shown. Note the "extra" QRS at an independent rate.

variations due to respiration do not occur (see Table 16–2). If a supraventricular tachyarrhythmia develops, Valsalva's maneuver or carotid sinus pressure have no effect, and cardioversion is often required.

Decreased donor SA node automaticity can also occur after transplant as a result of injury to the node during procurement, transport, surgical procedure, or postoperative edema of the atrial suture line. Generally, these problems resolve within 1 to 2 weeks posttransplant, but Isuprel or temporary pacing may be needed to maintain an adequate heart rate. Atropine, which blocks vagal stimulation, is ineffective in treating bradyarrhythmias in the transplanted heart because there is no parasympathetic innervation. If the sinus rate is reduced, junctional rhythms can occur earlier than normal because of the loss of vagal tone.

Normal cardiovascular reflexes are also removed by denervation. In the normal heart, increased body metabolic demands cause direct compensatory stimulation of the heart by the sympathetic nervous system, which immediately increases heart rate, contractility, and cardiac output. Because direct sympathetic nervous system stimulation of the transplanted heart is absent, this response is mediated through release of circulating catecholamines from the adrenal medulla. Therefore, increases in heart rate, contractility, and cardiac output occur much more slowly than normal. With exercise, heart rate and cardiac output increase gradually over 3 to 5 minutes and remain elevated for a longer period of time after exercise. Prolonged warm-up before and cool down after exercise help compensate for these changes.

Orthostatic hypotension can occur because the normal, immediate reflex tachycardia, which compensates for venous pooling with position change, does not occur. When patients begin ambulating, they should be cautioned to change position gradually to prevent orthostatic hypotension.

Because of denervation, the cardiac effects of medications normally mediated by the autonomic nervous system are abnormal. Atropine, which increases heart rate by blocking parasympathetic influence, is ineffective. Instead, pharmacological management of symptomatic bradyarrhythmias is achieved with isoproterenol, because it stimulates myocardial β-receptors directly.

Digitalis preparations are ineffective in decreasing the heart rate or increasing the AV nodal refractory period, because these effects are mediated primarily by the parasympathetic nervous system. Digitalis does increase myocardial contractility by its direct action on myocardial cells. β-Blocking drugs or calcium channel blockers (eg, verapamil) can be used to control supraventricular tachyarrhythmias in the transplanted heart; carotid sinus pressure, Valsalva's maneuver, and digitalis are ineffective.

Finally, denervation prevents transmission of pain impulses from ischemic myocardium to the brain, so the patient does not experience angina. Severe myocardial ischemia or infarction can go unnoticed. For this reason ECG stress testing and annual coronary angiography are

TABLE 16–2
The Denervated Heart

Effects of Denervation	Implications for Nursing
Resting sinus rate is >90 beats/min.	Slower heart rate can indicate sinus node dysfunction.
Change in heart rate in response to metabolic demands is slower than normal.	Do not use tachycardia as a reliable early sign of decreased cardiac output.
	Instruct patient to warm up and cool down during exercise over 20-min period.
Absence of reflex tachycardia in response to position change and pooling of blood in the extremities can cause orthostatic hypotension.	Instruct patient to change position gradually to prevent dizziness or syncope.
Response to medications whose effects are mediated by the autonomic nervous system is altered.	Treat bradyarrhythmias with isoproterenol or pacing rather than atropine.
	Treat supraventricular tachyarrhythmias with β-blockers, Ca⁺ blockers, or cardioversion rather than Valsalva's maneuver, carotid sinus pressure, or digitalis preparations.
	Use isoproterenol, dobutamine, inocor, or epinephrine for inotropic support.
Only mechanism by which heart rate and contractility can increase is through circulating catecholamines.	Use β-blockers with caution.
Transmission of pain impulses from ischemic myocardium is lost.	Patient may have ischemic myocardium but usually does not experience angina.

usually performed. Recently, however, Stark, McGinn, et al.[28] described two orthotopic transplant recipients with documented coronary ischemic events who had chest pain typical of angina pectoris. Banner and Yacoub[29] have also observed orthotopic transplant patients with exertional angina associated with myocardial ischemia. These reports provide evidence that some reinnervation after orthotopic transplant may occur; however, further research is needed in this area.

Potential for Ventricular Failure

Posttransplant ventricular failure, causing decreased cardiac output, occurs for the same reasons as in other cardiac surgical procedures. In addition, global ischemic time may be longer depending on the distance the heart must be transported, and some myocardial depression can be present as a result of positive inotropic support of the donor.

Right ventricular failure is more common after transplant. Often, there is some degree of pulmonary hypertension because of chronic left ventricular failure. Postoperative changes in pH or ABGs can cause pulmonary vascular spasm, compounding the problem. Both pulmonary hypertension and spasm increase the pulmonary vascular resistance, or resistance to ejection of blood by the right ventricle. Normal pulmonary vascular resistance ranges from 37 to 250 dynes/sec/cm^{-5} and is calculated by the formula

$$\text{pulmonary vascular resistance} = \frac{\text{PAM} - \text{PCWP} \times 80}{\text{CO}}$$

where PAM is pulmonary artery mean pressure, PCWP is pulmonary capillary wedge pressure, and CO is cardiac output. The normal right ventricle of the donor heart may be unable to acutely increase its output to overcome a high preexisting pulmonary vascular resistance.

Signs of acute right ventricular failure include elevated CVP and jugular venous distention. Left ventricular cardiac output decreases as the right ventricle is unable to pump enough blood through the lungs.

A good drug for treating ventricular failure in the transplanted heart is isoproterenol. It directly stimulates β_1-receptors of the denervated heart, increasing contractility. It also stimulates β_2-receptors in the lungs, decreasing pulmonary vascular resistance and the right ventricular workload. If isoproterenol is ineffective in decreasing elevated pulmonary vascular resistance, nitroglycerin, nitroprusside, prostacycline, or amrinone[30] may be successful. Other drugs that can increase contractility of the denervated heart are epinephrine, dobutamine, and amrinone.

Complications

Rejection of the Transplanted Heart

The normal immune response that protects the body against invasion by foreign substances has two components—humoral and cellular. Humoral immunity is mediated by B cell lymphocytes that recognize foreign material as antigenic and produce antibodies or immunoglobulins

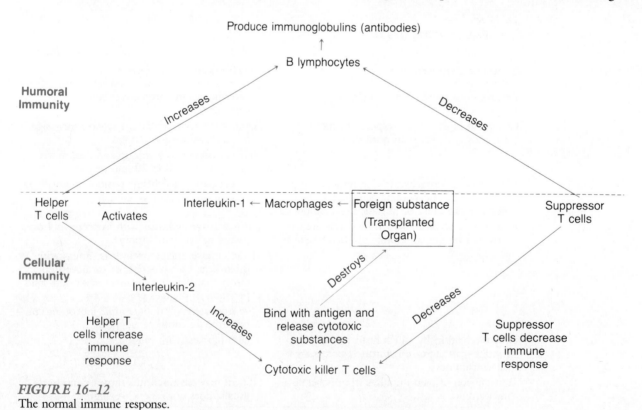

FIGURE 16–12
The normal immune response.

to directly destroy the antigen. Cellular immunity is mediated by T cell lymphocytes, including cytotoxic (or killer), helper, and suppressor T cells. Cytotoxic T cells mature and proliferate as a result of stimulation by interleukin-2 (IL-2) produced by the helper T cells. Cytotoxic T cells directly attack the foreign substance. Helper T cells activated by interleukin-1 (IL-1) from macrophages release IL-2, which increases the cytotoxic response of killer T cells. Helper T cells also interact with the humoral system to increase B cell antibody production. In other words, helper T cells increase the immune response. Suppressor T cells decrease both T cell and B cell activity, so they decrease the immune response (Fig. 16–12). Normally helper and suppressor T cells work in balance. (For a more detailed discussion of immunology see Chapter 47).

Because the transplanted heart is not immunologically identical to the recipient, it acts as an antigen or foreign substance, triggering the immune system to reject it. Cytotoxic T lymphocytes directly attack the donor heart and destroy tissue. Both humoral and cellular immune responses can be responsible for graft rejection.

Rejection can occur at any time, but the risk is highest 10 to 18 days posttransplant, and the earlier and more severe the rejection episode, the worse the prognosis for graft survival. There are three different types of rejection: hyperacute, acute, and chronic.

Hyperacute Rejection

Hyperacute rejection occurs in the operating room immediately after transplant. It is a humoral immune response in which the recipient has preformed antibodies that immediately react against antigens of the donor heart. Coronary arterial damage occurs, resulting in severe thrombosis and graft necrosis. Hyperacute rejection is life-threatening and cannot be reversed. Retransplantation is necessary for patient survival. Hyperacute rejection is uncommon and can usually be prevented by ABO cross-matching and a negative pretransplant PRA.

Acute Rejection

Acute rejection occurs within the first 3 months after transplantation, and most patients experience two or more episodes. This type of rejection is cell mediated and is a major cause of death within the first year after transplantation.

Acute rejection occurs when antigens on the donor heart trigger lymphocytes to mature into helper T cells. The helper T cells increase the production of cytotoxic killer T cells, which bind to the transplanted heart and damage it by secretion of lysosomal enzymes and lymphokines.

Acute rejection is usually clinically asymptomatic in the patient receiving cyclosporine immunosuppression until it is far advanced. Therefore, endomyocardial biopsy is done to diagnose rejection. The biopsy is obtained by passing a cardiac bioptome (a catheter with a scissor at the end) through the right internal jugular vein into the right ventricle under fluoroscopy. Usually three to five samples are taken, because not all areas of the myocardium may be equally affected by the rejection process, and the inflammatory response of cells from previous biopsies can give false results. Biopsy specimens are examined microscopically for evidence of vascular and interstitial lymphocyte infiltration and myocyte damage.

Endomyocardial biopsy is currently the only certain way to diagnose rejection; however, research continues to find less invasive methods. Several methods are available to specifically reverse acute graft rejection diagnosed by endomyocardial biopsy. Steroid pulse is usually tried first. The patient is given methylprednisolone Igm IV bolus for 3 days; then the maintenance steroid dosage is continued.

If the rejection episode fails to respond to an increase in steroids alone, two other medications, antithymocyte globulin (ATG) and Orthoclone OKT3, are available.

ATG is produced by injecting human lymphocytes into rabbits, goats, or horses. These animals produce antibodies that, when given to the transplant recipient, coat the T cells so they can be eliminated by macrophages. Levels of circulating T cells are monitored to determine the dosage.

OKT3 is a monoclonal antibody preparation to human T cells. It reverses acute rejection by blocking the generation and function of T cells. See further discussion on page 384.

Chronic Rejection

Chronic rejection occurs from 3 months to years after transplantation and is mediated by both B and T cells. It is characterized by diffuse, rapidly progressing CAD that causes ischemic myocardial damage and progressive loss of heart function. Five years after transplant, the incidence of severe CAD is 40% to 50%;[31] thus, chronic rejection is a major factor limiting long-term survival. Because the heart is denervated, angina cannot be used as a warning for the development of CAD. Decreased exercise tolerance during stress testing and annual coronary angiography are used for diagnosis. Because the disease is diffuse, CABG cannot adequately revascularize the heart, and retransplantation may be the only definitive treatment.

Treatment of Rejection by Immunosuppression

Immunosuppressive drugs must be taken for the rest of the recipient's life to prevent rejection. Most immunosuppressive regimens use a combination of three drugs—cyclosporine, azathioprine, and prednisone. By combining the three drugs, the doses of each can be reduced so that individual side effects are decreased.

Cyclosporine

Cyclosporine is used to prevent rather than reverse acute rejection. It acts selectively on the immune system, causing

T lymphocytes to become unresponsive to IL-1 so that they do not express receptors for IL-2. This prevents maturation of helper and cytotoxic T cells. Cyclosporine also suppresses humoral immunity to the extent it is dependent on T helper cells.

Because cyclosporine selectively inhibits T cells, T cell-independent humoral immunity remains intact, the bone marrow is not suppressed, and neutrophils remain viable. This selective immunosuppression reduces the risk of infection compared to the broad suppression of other medications. However, any immunosuppression markedly decreases the patient's resistance to infection.

Cyclosporine is given by continuous intravenous infusion until the patient can receive it orally. Doses are determined by daily trough blood levels to find the therapeutic "window" between organ rejection and cyclosporine toxicity. Nephrotoxicity is a common side effect of cyclosporine. Patients with impaired renal function before transplantation are at increased risk for posttransplant cyclosporine-induced renal failure. Blood urea nitrogen (BUN) and creatinine levels should be monitored daily in the immediate posttransplant period, and if nephrotoxicity is developing, the dose of cyclosporine can be reduced.

Hypertension is another side effect of cyclosporine. Usually, it can be controlled with nitroprusside in the early postoperative period. Oral antihypertensives are usually needed for chronic long-term therapy.

Azathioprine

Azathioprine is used with cyclosporine to prevent rejection. It is an antimetabolite that interferes with DNA synthesis in rapidly dividing cells. This prevents rejection by decreasing the body's ability to generate helper and cytotoxic killer T cells.

A major side effect of azathioprine is bone marrow suppression, especially leukopenia and neutropenia, which makes the recipient more susceptible to infection. Generally azathioprine is given in a dosage that does not decrease the leukocyte count below 5,000/mm^3.

Corticosteroids

The third drug in triple drug antirejection therapy is a corticosteroid. Steroids decrease antibody production and inhibit antigen-antibody complex formation. By inhibiting IL-1 and IL-2, they depress the maturation of killer T cells and reduce cell-mediated immunity.

Steroids are used both to prevent rejection and to reverse established rejection. The dose is tapered to a maintenance level, usually within 6 weeks.

Early postoperative side effects of corticosteroids include sodium and water retention, gastrointestinal ulceration, altered glucose metabolism, and psychological changes. Intervention to prevent or minimize these problems is imperative.

New Approaches to Immunosuppression

OKT3

Several alternatives to triple immunotherapy are under investigation. OKT3, a monoclonal antibody against human T cells, is currently given to reverse acute rejection episodes. It is being investigated for induction of immunosuppression immediately after transplant. OKT3 induction can allow reduction of the cyclosporine dosage or discontinuation of long-term steroid therapy,[32] thereby diminishing cyclosporine-induced hypertension and nephrotoxicity[33] or the incidence of steroid-associated complications.

FK 506

FK 506, a new investigational drug, is undergoing clinical trials as a primary immunosuppressant alternative to cyclosporine and as rescue therapy for acute rejection. Made from a soil fungus, it suppresses T helper cell activation and interleukin-2 (IL-2) production. FK 506 and low dose steroids obtain immunosuppression at least comparable, if not superior, to cyclosporine-based triple immunotherapy.[34] Because FK 506 can be used without steroids after the first several weeks, steroid-related complications are decreased. It also produces less hypertension and nephrotoxicity than cyclosporine[35] and appears able to reverse established cardiac rejection refractory to other known forms of therapy.[36]

Infection

Infection is a major cause of morbidity and mortality after transplantation, especially during the first 3 months when high dosages of immunosuppressants allow for growth of nosocomial or opportunistic organisms. Prevention, detection, and early treatment are primary nursing care goals. The extent of isolation needed for the transplant recipient is controversial. Walsh, Guttendorf, et al.[37] compared protective isolation (private room with use of cap, mask, gown, gloves, and strict handwashing) to no isolation (admission to open ward using routine handwashing practices) and found an increase in fungal infections (in the no-isolation group) to be the only statistically significant difference in the incidence of infection between the two groups. Isolation practices vary widely. Lange, Prevost, et al.[38] surveyed heart transplant programs across the United States for their use of infection control measures, including handwashing, mask, gown, gloves, head cover, shoe covers, 3-minute scrub, and admission to private room. Of the 120 centers, 51.6% used maximal precautions (4–8 of these measures), and 48.4% used minimal precautions (1–3 measures). There was no significant correlation between the number of infection control measures and survival rate. However, 98% of the centers admitted transplant recipients to private rooms. Good hand-washing is also imperative.

The lungs are the most common site of infection. To prevent colonization of the respiratory tract, strict aseptic technique should be used in suctioning; the endotracheal tube should be removed as soon as possible, usually within the first 12 to 24 hours posttransplant. Coughing, deep breathing, and incentive spirometry are then implemented, and chest x-rays are assessed daily.

Bacteremia can result from numerous indwelling intravascular lines. Vascular access and monitoring devices should be removed within 24 hours postoperatively, if possible. To prevent urinary tract infection and subsequent bacteremia, the Foley catheter should also be removed within 24 hours.

Wound infections can develop and are more severe than in cardiac surgery patients who are not immunosuppressed. Meticulous aseptic technique should be used in caring for any entry into the skin, and any drainage should be reported immediately and cultured. Chest tubes should be removed 24 hours postoperatively, if possible.

Usually broad spectrum prophylactic antibiotics are given for 48 hours post transplant or until invasive lines and drains are removed. In some centers, patients receiving increased immunosuppression for an episode of acute rejection are given acyclovir as prophylaxis against cytomegalovirus (CMV). Patients seronegative for CMV receive only CMV-negative blood and blood products.

If infection develops in the immunosuppressed patient, the usual signs and symptoms can be absent. A rise in temperature to 37.2°C is significant and should be reported. The leukocyte count should be monitored. Normally, after transplant it is slightly elevated owing to surgery and steroids; however, if elevation persists, a left shift develops, or a rapid elevation occurs after a decline, infection is suggested. If the white blood cell count is low (<5000/mm³), the dosage of azathioprine may need reduction. Early recognition of infection is imperative to prevent morbidity and mortality.

Bleeding

The transplant patient has a greater risk of bleeding than other cardiac surgical patients. The pericardial sac is larger than normal because of stretching to accommodate an enlarged heart. If a smaller, healthy heart is implanted, the pericardial sac becomes a reservoir that can conceal postoperative bleeding, and cardiac tamponade can ensue. Liver congestion from pretransplant heart failure can cause a decrease in coagulation factor production, which can also exacerbate bleeding.

Caring for a cardiac transplant patient is similar to caring for other cardiac surgical patients, with the added dimension of immunosuppression and increased potential for infection. With skilled nursing and medical care, com-plications can be minimized and the recipient can be discharged from the hospital within several weeks and restored to a satisfying life and long-term normal functioning.

CASE STUDY

Mr. C is a 62-year-old man with a history of an anterior MI 2 years ago and hypertension controlled by medication. Preoperatively, he was taking aspirin (325 mg orally q.d.) and had stopped smoking 10 years ago. He has just returned to the ICU after CABG × 3 with an IMA graft to the LAD and saphenous vein graft to the RCA and diagonal.

Mr. C is mechanically ventilated on 50% FIO_2 with 5 cm PEEP. His breath sounds are clear and equal bilaterally, and the SaO_2 is 98%. Neurologically, he is unresponsive with pinpoint pupils. The monitor shows sinus tachycardia at 110 with occasional PVCs. He has atrial and ventricular epicardial pacing wires, but they are not connected to the pacemaker. His BP is 90/60, core temperature 35.9°C, cardiac index (CI) 1.6 L/min/M, PCWP 8 mm Hg, SVR 1,800, LVSWI 25, and SvO_2 55%. The chest tubes have drained 250 cc, and the urine output is 100 cc.

Based on her assessment, the nurse knows that Mr. C's neurologic and respiratory status are as expected immediately postoperatively. His BP is adequate, but the CI and SvO_2 are low. The PCWP of 8 indicates that Mr. C is hypovolemic. The nurse understands that the high SVR, indicating vasoconstriction, is most likely elevated because of the low core temperature and as a compensatory mechanism for hypovolemia. Both the low PAD (preload) and high SVR (afterload) contribute to Mr. C's low CI. His BP is probably low because of hypovolemia. The chest tube drainage of 250 cc is probably normal this early postop, but the trend should be watched.

After his nurse consults with the physician, Mr. C receives 500 cc hetastarch over 30 minutes, autotransfusion of the chest tube drainage, and radiant heat and blankets to increase the core temperature.

Two hours postop, the nurse notes that Mr. C is starting to arouse. He opens his eyes and moves all extremities weakly. His parameters are as follows: BP 170/90, core temp 36.2°C, CI 2.1 L/min/M, PCWP 10, SVR 1600, LVSWI 30, SvO_2 60%, urine output 50 cc per hour, and chest tube drainage 400 cc per hour for the last 2 hours with few clots forming in the tubing. CI, PCWP, and LVSWI have all improved; however, the PCWP is still low for Mr. C, who is on 5 cm PEEP and has a past history of MI. The core temperature, which is increasing slowly, is still low and may still be contributing to the increased SVR. Mr. C's nurse determines that the chest drainage of 800 cc over 2 hours is excessive and Mr. C's BP is now too high. Hypertension is not unexpected, because Mr. C. was hypertensive preoperatively.

After reporting her assessments to Mr. C's physician, the 800 cc of chest drainage are autotransfused rapidly, and a nitroprusside drip is started to control the hypertension. Lowering the BP should also help decrease the bleeding. Mr. C's physician orders an activated clotting time (ACT), bleeding time, and platelet count.

In evaluating the results of the blood work, the nurse recognizes that the ACT is normal, the bleeding time is prolonged, and the platelet count is 105,000/mm³. Because the ACT is

(*Text continues on page 386*)

NURSING CARE PLAN 16–1:
Cardiac Surgery and Heart Transplantation

NURSING DIAGNOSIS	OUTCOME CRITERIA/ PATIENT GOALS	NURSING INTERVENTIONS
Decreased cardiac output: related to changes in left ventricular preload, afterload, and contractility.	• Hemodynamic stability: BP, CO, PCWP, LAPM, SVR, and LVSWI and SvO_2 will be within patient's normal limits.	1. Maintain arterial, thermodilution and LAP lines. 2. Assess hemodynamic parameters, including BP, PCWP, LAPM and SVO_2 continuously, and CO, SVR, LVSWI every 1–2 hours. 3. Administer volume as ordered to optimize PCWP or LAPM. 4. Administer nitroprusside or other vasodilators as ordered to decrease a high SVR. 5. Administer positive inotropic agents as ordered to optimize LVSWI. Posttransplant use isoproterenol. 6. Administer vasopressors as ordered for hypotension <90 mm Hg systolic. 7. Assess core body temperature and if lower than 37°C increase room temperature and apply blankets and radiant heat. Warm slowly to prevent shivering or rapid vasodilation. 8. Maintain normal pH and ABGs.
Decreased cardiac output: related to right ventricular failure, post transplant.	• CVP and pulmonary vascular resistance will be within patient's normal limits.	1. Assess CVP. 2. Calculate pulmonary vascular resistance. 3. Administer isoproterenol or other vasodilator to decrease elevated pulmonary vascular resistance.
Decreased cardiac output: related to acute rejection.	• Rejection will be prevented.	1. Administer immunosuppressive medications, as ordered. 2. Monitor cyclosporine trough levels. 3. Prepare patient for endomyocardial biopsy.
Decreased cardiac output: related to dysrhythmias or conduction disturbances.	• Cardiac rate and rhythm will be adequate to maintain systemic perfusion.	1. Monitor cardiac rate and rhythm continuously. 2. Document rhythm strip every shift and with any change. 3. Assess BP and apical and radial pulse.

(continued)

NURSING CARE PLAN 16–1: *(Continued)*
Cardiac Surgery and Heart Transplantation

NURSING DIAGNOSIS	OUTCOME CRITERIA/ PATIENT GOALS	NURSING INTERVENTIONS
		4. If temporary pacemaker is in use, assess proper functioning including rate, capture, sensing, and settings; maintain electrical safety.
		5. Maintain normal electrolyte levels—especially potassium.
		6. Maintain adequate ABGs.
		7. Administer antiarrhythmics, as ordered.
		8. Relieve anxiety or pain which can aggravate dysrhythmias.
		9. Obtain 12-lead ECG.
Decreased cardiac output: related to dysrhythmias in the denervated heart post transplant.	• Sinus mechanism will be maintained between 90 and 110 beats/min.	1. Administer isoproterenol or use pacemaker as ordered for brady-arrhythmias—not atropine.
		2. Use β-blockers, Ca^+ channel blockers, or cardioversion as ordered for SVT—not vagal maneuvers or digitalis.
Fluid volume deficit: related to increased capillary permeability with fluid shift from intravascular to interstitial space.	• Intravascular volume will be sufficient to maintain adequate cardiac output.	1. Assess BP, CVP, PCWP, LAPM continuously.
		2. Administer crystalloids, colloids, or blood as ordered.
		3. Measure input and output.
		4. Autotransfuse chest tube drainage according to unit protocol.
Fluid volume excess: related to hemo-dilution, increased vasopressin, and aldosterone levels.	• Adequate urine output will be maintained.	1. Assess CVP, PCWP, LAPM continuously.
		2. Assess for peripheral edema.
		3. Measure input and output.
		4. Weigh patient daily.
		5. Administer mannitol, Lasix or other diuretic, as ordered.
		6. Implement fluid restriction, as ordered.
		7. Maintain sodium restriction, as ordered.
Altered tissue perfusion: related to cardiopulmonary bypass, decreased cardiac output, hypotension.	• Systolic BP will be maintain between 90 and 150 mm Hg and SvO_2 between 60% and 80%.	1. Assess BP, hemodynamic parameters, and SvO_2.
	• Peripheral pulses will be palpable.	2. Assess skin and peripheral pulses.
	• Return of preoperative mental status.	3. Implement measures to optimize cardiac output.

(continued)

NURSING CARE PLAN 16–1: (Continued)
Cardiac Surgery and Heart Transplantation

NURSING DIAGNOSIS	OUTCOME CRITERIA/ PATIENT GOALS	NURSING INTERVENTIONS
		4. Administer vasopressors, as ordered.
		5. Assess neurological status including pupillary reaction, level of consciousness, and response to commands initially, hourly, and whenever a change is noted until the patient is fully recovered from anesthesia.
Altered tissue perfusion: related to denervation of the donor heart post transplant.	• Patient will have no episodes of postural hypotension.	1. Instruct patient to change position slowly.
		2. Instruct patient to warm up and cool down over prolonged period with exercise.
Impaired gas exchange: related to cardiopulmonary bypass, anesthesia, poor chest expansion, atelectasis, retained secretions.	• SaO_2 and SvO_2 will remain within normal limits.	1. Assess rate and depth of respiration.
		2. Auscultate breath sounds.
		3. Maintain patent airway and integrity of ET tube and ventilator.
		4. Monitor SaO_2 and SvO_2 continuously.
		5. Obtain chest x-ray.
		6. Obtain ABGs.
		7. Adjust tidal volume, FIO_2 and respiratory rate as ordered to optimize blood gases.
		8. Apply PEEP as ordered to improve oxygenation. Observe for decreased BP and CO as a result of PEEP.
		9. Suction as needed and observe amount, color, and consistency of secretions.
		10. Extubate as ordered when patient is alert and extubation criteria are met.
		11. After extubation: administer oxygen; cough, deep breathe q1–2h initially then q2–4h; assist with incentive spirometry q2h; advance activity as tolerated.
		12. Teach patient how to splint median sternotomy incision.
		13. Administer analgesics to facilitate coughing and incentive spirometry.

(continued)

NURSING CARE PLAN 16–1: (*Continued*)
Cardiac Surgery and Heart Transplantation

NURSING DIAGNOSIS	OUTCOME CRITERIA/ PATIENT GOALS	NURSING INTERVENTIONS
Alterations in comfort: related to ET tube, surgical incisions, chest tubes, rib spreading.	• Patient will verbalize relief from pain, appear comfortable, and be able to rest.	1. Assess character, location, intensity, and duration of pain. 2. Differentiate between pain from the median sternotomy and pain from angina. 3. Position for comfort and provide comfort measures such as back rubs. 4. Teach patient to splint median sternotomy incision. 5. Alleviate factors which enhance pain perception such as fatigue and anxiety. 6. Administer analgesics, as ordered.
High risk for anxiety: related to fear of death, surgery, critical care unit environment, recovery process.	• Anxiety will be reduced; patient will appear relaxed without presence of physiological responses to anxiety.	1. Implement preoperative teaching. 2. Orient patient to time and place while awakening and inform that surgery is completed. 3. Assess anxiety level and physiological responses to anxiety such as increased BP and heart rate. 4. Establish trusting, confident relationship with patient and family. 5. Allow patient and family to verbalize feelings and fears. 6. Reassure patient and identify examples of progress (eg, extubation). 7. Provide opportunity for patient and family to participate in care. 8. Administer sedatives as ordered.
High risk for fluid volume deficit: related to abnormal bleeding.	• Chest tube drainage will be less than 100 cc/h.	1. Assess character, amount, and trend of chest tube drainage hourly. 2. Maintain chest tube patency by milking or stripping as needed. 3. Maintain systolic blood pressure below 150 mm Hg. 4. Autotransfuse chest drainage according to unit protocol. 5. Apply PEEP as ordered. 6. Obtain Hgb and Hct.

(*continued*)

NURSING CARE PLAN 16–1: (Continued)
Cardiac Surgery and Heart Transplantation

NURSING DIAGNOSIS	OUTCOME CRITERIA/ PATIENT GOALS	NURSING INTERVENTIONS
		7. Administer volume expanders or blood as ordered to maintain adequate PCWP or LAPM.
		8. Obtain ACT, PT, PTT, bleeding time, platelet count, and fibrinogen levels as ordered.
		9. Administer protamine, platelets, FFP as ordered.
High risk for decreased cardiac output: related to cardiac tamponade.	• Patient will have no evidence of cardiac tamponade.	1. Assess for decreasing BP and increasing and equalizing CVP and PCWP.
		2. Assess for paradoxical pulse >10 mg Hg.
		3. Assess patency of chest tubes and for abrupt decrease in amount of drainage.
		4. Milk or strip chest tubes to restore patency.
		5. Administer fluids or vasopressors as ordered to maintain CO and BP.
		6. Obtain chest x-ray as ordered.
		7. Anticipate patient's return to OR.
High risk for infection: related to surgical procedure, invasive lines, drainage tubes, hypoventilation, retained secretions, or immunosuppression for post transplant patients.	• Patient will be free from postoperative infections.	1. Assess incisions and all invasive lines and tubes daily for erythema, swelling, and drainage.
		2. Assess temperature q4h.
		3. Discontinue invasive lines and drainage tubes as soon as possible.
		4. Keep incisions clean and dry.
		5. Administer prophylactic antibiotics as ordered.
		6. Assess breath sounds q4h.
		7. Assist patient to cough and use incentive spirometer q2h.
		8. Observe character and consistency of sputum.
		9. Increase activity level as tolerated.
	• The post transplant patient will not develop postoperative infections.	10. Implement private room and meticulous handwashing or protective isolation per unit protocol.

(continued)

NURSING CARE PLAN 16–1: (*Continued*)
Cardiac Surgery and Heart Transplantation

NURSING DIAGNOSIS	OUTCOME CRITERIA/ PATIENT GOALS	NURSING INTERVENTIONS
		11. Report any temperature elevation.
		12. Obtain cultures of wounds, urine, sputum as ordered.
		13. Administer mycostatin oral rinse as ordered.
		14. Monitor cyclosporine and leukocyte levels.
		15. Use strict aseptic technique when caring for all incisions and insertion sites.
High risk for alterations in pattern of urinary elimination: related to hemodilution, cardiopulmonary bypass, decreased cardiac output, renal failure, post transplant cyclosporine nephrotoxicity.	• Urine output will be within acceptable limits.	1. Measure urine output hourly.
		2. Obtain urine specific gravity q4h.
		3. Observe for hematuria.
		4. Maintain adequate cardiac output, BP, and intravascular fluid volume.
		5. Administer mannitol, Lasix or other diuretic as ordered.
		6. Administer renal dose dopamine as ordered.
		7. Assess BUN, creatinine, and cyclosporine trough levels and notify physician if elevated.
High risk for anxiety: related to critical illness, fear of death or disfigurement, role changes within social setting, or permanent disability.	• Patient will be able to express anxieties to appropriate resource person.	1. Provide environment that encourages open discussion of emotional issues.
		2. Mobilize patient's support system and involve these resources as appropriate.
		3. Allow time for patient to express self.
		4. Identify possible hospital resources for patient/family support.
		5. Encourage open family–nurse communications regarding emotional issues.
		6. Validate patient and family knowledge base regarding the critical illness.
		7. Involve religious support systems as appropriate.

normal, his nurse knows that adequate protamine was given to neutralize the heparin. The platelet count of 105,000/mm³ is low but expected at this time because of the effects of cardiopulmonary bypass. Prolonged bleeding time indicates that Mr. C's platelets are not functioning properly. This could be a result of the aspirin he was taking preoperatively and of the cardiopulmonary bypass. The physician orders transfusion of 5 units of platelet concentrate.

Four hours postoperatively, Mr. C is on a nitroprusside drip at 3 µg/kg/min. His BP is 136/85, CI 2.5 L/min/M, PCWP 12, SVR 1,050, LVSWI 32, SaO₂ 62%, core temp 36.8°C, and urine output 75 cc per hour. The chest tube drainage has been 350 cc and 200 cc for the last 2 hours, respectively. Mr. C is responding appropriately to commands and moves all extremities.

Mr. C's hemodynamic profile is normal, and his BP and SVR have decreased as a result of the vasodilating effects of nitroprusside. The chest tube drainage is still high but decreasing hourly, indicating that the bleeding is now under control. The nurse's assessments and interventions were critical in stabilizing Mr. C's condition.

Nursing Care Plan 16–1 outlines the nursing care for the patient after cardiac surgery or heart transplantation.

Summary

Cardiac surgery—from bypass grafting to valve reconstruction or replacement to transplantation—is one component of a multitude of approaches to the treatment of cardiovascular disease. It offers a unique challenge to the critical care nurse to integrate theoretical knowledge, assessment skills, and problem-solving ability to provide optimal nursing care.

REFERENCES

1. Hammermeister K, Morrison D: Coronary bypass surgery for stable angina and unstable angina pectoris. Cardiol Clin 9:135–155, 1991
2. Nawasokwa O, Koss J, Friedman G, Grunwald A, Bodenheimer M: Bypass surgery for chronic stable angina: Predictors of survival and strategy for patient selection. Ann Intern Med 114:1035–1049, 1991
3. King S, Ivanhoe R: Has multivessel angioplasty displaced surgical revascularization? Cardiovasc Clin 21:123–127, 1991
4. Bass L: Essentials of Cardiovascular Nursing, pp 217–240. Maryland, Aspen Publishers, 1991
5. Bourassa M: Long term clinical results after CABG surgery. Cardiovasc Clin 21:101–121, 1991
6. Hall R: Coronary artery bypass in perspective. Tex Heart Inst J 16:127–130, 1989
7. Cosgrove D: Surgery for degenerative mitral valve disease. Semin Thorac Cardiovasc Surg 1:183–193, 1989
8. Cosgrove D: Surgery for degenerative mitral valve disease. Semin Thorac Cardiovasc Surg 1:183–193, 1989
9. Livesay J, Talledo O: Current preference for mitral valve reconstruction. Tex Heart Inst J 18:87–92, 1991
10. Loop F: Long term results of mitral valve repair. Semin Thorac Cardiovasc Surg 1:203–210, 1989
11. Crumbley A, Crawford F: Long term results of aortic valve replacement. Cardiol Clin 9:353–380, 1991
12. Wernly J, Crawford M: Choosing a prosthetic heart valve. Cardiol Clin 9:329–338, 1991
13. Crumbley A, Crawford F: Long term results of aortic valve replacement. Cardiol Clin 9:353–380, 1991
14. Grunkmeier G, Rahimtoola S: Artificial heart valves. Annu Rev Med 41:251–263, 1990
15. Crumbley A, Crawford F: Long term results of aortic valve replacement. Cardiol Clin 9:353–380, 1991
16. Assey M, Spann J: Indications for heart valve replacement. Clin Cardiol 13:81–88, 1990
17. Goodnough L, Johnston M, Ramsey G, Sayers M, Eisenstadt R, Anderson K, Rutman R, Silberstein L: Guidelines for transfusion support in patients undergoing coronary artery bypass grafting. Ann Thorac Surg 50:675–683, 1990
18. Noll M, Fountain R: The relationship between mixed venous oxygen saturation and cardiac output in mechanically ventilated coronary artery bypass graft patients. Prog Cardiovasc Nurs 5:34–40, 1990
19. Osguthorpe S, Tidwell S, Ryan W, Paull D, Smith T: Evaluation of the patient having cardiac surgery in the postoperative rewarming period. Heart Lung 19:570–573, 1990
20. Finke C: Measurement of the thermoregulatory response: A review. Focus Crit Care 18:408–412, 1991
21. Howie J: Hypothermia and rewarming after cardiac operation. Focus Crit Care 18:414–418, 1991
22. Finke C: Measurement of the thermoregulatory response: A review. Focus Crit Care 18:408–412, 1991
23. Howie J: Hypothermia and rewarming after cardiac operation. Focus Crit Care 18:414–418, 1991
24. Pelletier L, Carrier M: Early postoperative care and complications. Cardiovasc Clin 21:3–24, 1991
25. Crosby L, Woll K, Wood K, Pifalo W: Effect of activity on supraventricular arrhythmias after coronary artery bypass surgery. Heart Lung 19:666–670, 1990
26. Fanning W, Thomas C, Roach A, Tomichek R, Alford W, Stoney W: Prophylaxis of atrial fibrillation with magnesium sulfate after coronary artery bypass grafting. Ann Thorac Surg 52:529–533, 1991
27. Dec G, Semigran M, Vlahakes G: Cardiac transplantation: Current indications and limitations. Transplant Proc 24: 2095–2106, 1991
28. Stark R, McGinn A, Wilson R: Chest pain in cardiac transplant recipients. New Engl J Med 324:1791–1794, 1991
29. Banner N, Yacoub N: Physiology of the orthotopic cardiac transplant recipient. Semin Thorac Cardiovasc Surg 2:259–270, 1990
30. Deeb G, Bolling S: Role of amrinone in potential heart transplant patients with pulmonary hypertension. J Cardiothorac Vasc Anesth 8:33–37, 1989
31. Smith S: Tissue and Organ Transplantation. St. Louis, Mosby Year Book, 1991

32. O'Connell J, Renlund D: Diagnosis and treatment of cardiac allograft rejection. Cardiovasc Clin 20:147–162, 1990
33. Pezze J, Whitman K: Orthoclone OKT3: An overview of the monoclonal antibody and nursing considerations it presents. Crit Care Nurse 11:98–107, 1991
34. Armitage J, Kormos R, Fung J, Lavee J, Fricker F, Griffith B, Stuart R, Marrone G, Hardesty R, Todo S, Tzakis A, Starzl T: Preliminary experience with FK506 in thoracic transplantation. Transplantation 52:164–167, 1991
35. Starzl T, Fung J, Todo S, Tzakis A: Notes on FK506. Transplant Proc 23:2178–2179, 1991
36. Armitage J, Kormos R, Fung J, Lavee J, Fricker F, Griffith B, Stuart R, Marrone G, Hardesty R, Todo S, Tzakis A, Starzl T: Preliminary experience with FK506 in thoracic transplantation. Transplantation 52:164–167, 1991
37. Walsh T, Guttendorf J, et al: Value of protective isolation procedures in cardiac allograft recipients. Ann Thorac Surg 47:539–545, 1989
38. Lange S, Prevost S, Lewis P, Fadol A: Infection control practices in cardiac transplant recipients. Heart Lung 21:101–105, 1992

BIBLIOGRAPHY

Ahrens T: SvO$_2$ monitoring: Is it being used appropriately? Crit Care Nurse 10:70–72, 1990
Allen J: Physical and psychosocial outcomes after coronary artery bypass graft surgery: Review of the literature. Heart Lung 19:49–54, 1990
Farrel T, Camm A: Action of drugs on the denervated heart. Semin Thorac Cardiovasc Surg 2:279–289, 1990
Gallo J, Todd B: Mediastinitis after cardiac surgery. Crit Care Nurse 10:64–68, 1990
Imperial F, Cordova-Manigbas L, Ward C: Cardiac transplantation. Crit Care Nurs Clin North Am 1:399–415, 1989
Ledoux D: Management of heart failure in cardiac surgical patients: Amrinone and other pharmacologic agents. Prog Cardiovasc Nurs 5:78–83, 1990
Ley J, Miller K, Skov P, Preisig P: Crystalloid versus colloid fluid therapy after cardiac surgery. Heart Lung 19:31–40, 1990
Martin E, Harris A, Johnson N, Lester L, Nelles S, Patton S, Walton M: Autotransfusion systems. Crit Care Nurse 9:65–73, 1989
Shaefer M, Williams L: Nursing implications of immunosuppression in transplantation. Nurs Clin North Am 26:291–315, 1991
Stradtman J, Ballenger M: Nursing implications in sternal and mediastinal infections after open heart surgery. Focus Crit Care 16:178–183, 1989
Tennant D, Evans M: Minimizing blood usage after open heart surgery. Focus Crit Care 17:308–312, 1990
Vargo R, Whitman G: Complications after cardiac transplantation. Crit Care Nurs Clin North Am 1:741–752, 1989
Vaska P: OKT3 monoclonal antibody in cardiac transplant patients. Dimens Crit Care Nurs 10:126–132, 1991

STUDY QUESTIONS

1. Effects of cardiopulmonary bypass include all of the following *except*

   a. damage to RBCs
   b. hemodilution
   c. decreased capillary permeability
   d. changes in coagulation

2. Compared with mechanical valves, biological valves

   a. require lifelong anticoagulation
   b. have poor durability
   c. are the valve of choice for patients under 50 years old
   d. have a higher incidence of thromboembolism

3. Postoperative bleeding in the cardiac surgery patient can be treated by

   a. protamine
   b. PEEP
   c. autotransfusion
   d. all of the above

4. Interventions for decreased cardiac index caused by increased afterload soon after cardiac surgery include

   a. autotransfusion
   b. dopamine drip
   c. volume expansion with hetastarch
   d. blankets and radiant heat

5. If the cardiac transplant recipient develops bradycardia, which treatment should *not* be used?

   a. atropine
   b. isoproterenol
   c. pacemaker
   d. epinephrine

6. In the cardiac transplant recipient, acute rejection is diagnosed by

   a. ECG changes
   b. cardiac catheterization
   c. endomyocardial biopsy
   d. cyclosporine levels

UNIT II

*Respiratory
System*

CHAPTER 17

Anatomy and Physiology of the Respiratory System

BEHAVIORAL OBJECTIVES

Based on the content in this chapter, the reader should be able to:

1. Explain the components of total lung capacity.
2. Describe the mechanics of respiration.
3. Define lung compliance.
4. Compare and contrast perfect ventilation and perfusion with decreased ventilation and perfusion.
5. Outline the process of gas diffusion through the alveoli and into the blood and tissues.
6. State the importance of oxygen saturation in assessing the effectiveness of respiration.
7. Describe the key features of the oxygen dissociation curve.
8. List two brain stem centers that regulate respiration.
9. Describe the compensatory mechanisms that control respiration.

Hudak: Critical Care Nursing:
A Holistic Approach, 6th ed. © 1994
J. B. Lippincott Company.

Description

Oxygen is required for the complete catabolism of chemicals that occurs in the production of cellular energy. Although some energy can be stored, cells differ in the amount of energy they can store. Neurons, for example, are thought to have less capacity to store energy than skeletal muscle cells. Also, the amount of energy stored can fuel cell activities for only a short time. These facts partially account for the limited time available in which cardiopulmonary resuscitation can be initiated successfully.

Catabolic energy-producing reactions produce carbon dioxide. High levels of this waste product can seriously impair cell function. Therefore, there is a critical need for providing oxygen to body cells and at the same time removing carbon dioxide from the body. Strictly defined, *respiration* is the exchange and transport of oxygen and carbon dioxide between cells (of the body) and the external environment (atmosphere).

Accomplishing this in vertebrates (including humans) involves both the respiratory and the cardiovascular systems: the former to provide exchange of these gases between atmosphere and blood, and the latter to transport these gases to and from the cells of the body. At times it is difficult to establish priorities between these two systems; it is better to consider them as being equally critical to the dynamic stability of the human body.

In this chapter, we examine four general areas of respiration in the following order:

1. Pulmonary ventilation—the actual flow of air in and out between the atmosphere and the alveoli of the lung.
2. Pulmonary circulation—the flow of mixed venous blood through the lungs.
3. Gas transportation between the alveoli and the cells.
4. Regulation of ventilation by control mechanisms of the body with regard to rate, rhythm, and depth.

Ventilation

Lung Volumes

The flow of air in and out of the lungs provides tangible measures of lung volumes. Although referred to as "pulmonary function" measures, in reality these volumes represent *pulmonary anatomy* measures. In the evaluation of ventilation, structure or anatomy often determines functionality.

Ventilatory Function Tests

Ventilatory or pulmonary function tests measure the ability of the chest and lungs to move air into and out of the alveoli. These measurements are influenced by exercise and disease. Age, sex, body size, and posture are other variables that are taken into consideration when the test results are interpreted.

Volume Measurements

Volume measurements show the amount of air contained in the lungs during various parts of the respiratory cycle (Fig. 17–1). Each *volume* is not divisible into smaller parts, because it represents a basic unit.[1]

- *Tidal volume* (VT) is the volume of air moved in and out with each normal respiration. It measures about 500 ml in normal young males.
- *Inspiratory reserve volume* (IRV) represents the amount of air one can forcibly inhale after a normal tidal inspiration. IRV is usually about 3,000 ml.
- *Expiratory reserve volume* (ERV) is the volume of air one can forcibly exhale after a normal tidal exhalation. ERV is usually about 1,100 ml.
- *Residual volume* (RV) is the volume of air remaining after forced expiration. This volume can be measured only by indirect spirometry, whereas the others can be measured directly.

Capacity Measurements

Capacity measurements quantify a part of the pulmonary cycle. They are measured as a combination of the previous volumes.

- *Inspiratory capacity* (IC) is the amount of air that can be inhaled forcibly when starting from a normal expiratory level. It is equal to the VT plus the IRV and is about 3,500 ml.
- *Functional residual capacity* (FRC) is the amount of air remaining at the end of normal expiration. It is the sum of the ERV and the RV and is about 2,300 ml.
- *Vital capacity* (VC) is the maximal amount of air that can be forcibly expired after a forced maximal inspiration. It is the sum of the IRV, VT, and ERV. This volume is about 4,600 ml in a normal male.
- *Total lung capacity* (TLC) is equal to the volume to which the lungs can be expanded with greatest inspiratory effort. The volume of the capacity is about 5,800 ml.

Dynamic Measurements

The following measurements, called dynamic measurements, provide data about airway resistance and the energy expended in breathing (work of breathing).

- *Respiratory rate or frequency* (f) is the number of breaths per minute. At rest, f equals about 15.
- *Minute volume,* sometimes called minute ventilation

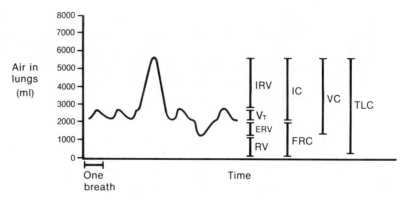

FIGURE 17–1
Volume and capacity measurements. Two resting respiratory cycles illustrate tidal volume (V_T) followed by a forced inspiration showing inspiratory reserve volume (*IRV*). One resting cycle followed by forced expiration shows expiratory reserve volume (*ERV*), followed by one resting cycle. Residual capacity (*RC*) is shown as approximately 1200 ml. Inspiratory capacity (*IC*), functional residual capacity (*FRC*), vital capacity (*VC*), and total lung capacity (*TLC*) are shown as the sum of their respective volumes.

(V_E), is the volume of air inhaled and exhaled per minute. It is calculated by multiplying V_T by f. At rest V_E equals approximately 7,500 ml/min.

• *Dead space* (V_D) is the part of the V_T that does not participate in alveolar gas exchange. V_D (measured in ml) comprises the air contained in the airways (anatomical dead space) plus the volume of alveolar air that is not involved in gas exchange (physiological dead space; eg, air in an unperfused alveolus due to pulmonary embolism or, more commonly, air in underperfused alveoli).

Adult anatomical dead space is usually equal to the body weight in pounds (eg, 140 ml in a 140-lb person). In the healthy person, V_D is composed only of anatomical dead space. Physiological dead space occurs in certain disease states.

One obtains V_D by subtracting the partial pressure of arterial carbon dioxide ($PaCO_2$) from the partial pressure of the carbon dioxide of alveolar air ($PaCO_2$). The normal value of V_D in healthy adults is typically less than 40% of the V_T. This value of the V_D/V_T ratio is used to follow the effectiveness of mechanical ventilation.

• *Alveolar ventilation*, the complement of V_D, is expressed as the *volume of tidal air that is involved in alveolar gas exchange*. This volume is represented as volume per minute by the symbol V_A. V_A indicates effective ventilation. It is more relevant to the blood gas values than either V_D or V_T because these last two measures include physiological dead space. V_A is calculated by subtracting V_D from V_T and multiplying the result by the respiratory rate per minute:

$$V_A = (V_T - V_D) \times f$$

About 2,300 ml of air (FRC) remains in the lung at the end of expiration. Each new breath introduces about 350 ml of air into the alveoli. The ratio of new alveoli air to total volume of air remaining in the lungs is

$$\frac{350 \text{ ml}}{2,300 \text{ ml}}$$

Therefore, new air is only about one-seventh of the total volume contained within the lungs. The normal V_A is 5,250 ml/min (350 ml/breath × 15 breaths/min = 5,250 ml/min).

A normal breath (V_T) can replace 7,500 ml of air per minute (500 ml/breath × 15 breaths/min = 7,500 ml/min), requiring a time of .008 sec/ml:

$$\left(\frac{1 \text{ min}}{7500 \text{ ml}} \times \frac{60 \text{ sec}}{1 \text{ min}} = .008 \text{ sec/ml} \right)$$

Therefore, the FRC of the lungs can be completely replaced in 18.4 seconds (2,300 ml × .008 sec/ml = 18.4 sec), if there is uniform air diffusion. This slow turnover rate prevents rapid fluctuations of gas concentrations in the alveoli with each breath.

Mechanics of Ventilation

Air flows from a region of higher pressure to a region of lower pressure. Therefore, when there is no airflow in or out of the lungs, alveolar and atmospheric pressure have equilibrated. To initiate a breath, airflow into the lungs must be precipitated by a drop in pressure within the alveoli. This involves a complex process of multiple variables, referred to as the *mechanics of ventilation*, and includes the properties of elasticity, compliance, pressure, and gravity.

Elastic Recoil

Elasticity is the return of the original shape of matter after alteration by an outside force.[2] The lungs and the chest are elastic, requiring energy to move but quickly returning to their original shape when the energy is not actively applied.

The downward and upward movement of the diaphragm, which lengthens and shortens the chest cavity, combined with the elevation and depression of the ribs, which increases and decreases the anteroposterior diameter of the cavity, causes the expansion and contraction of the lungs. It is estimated that about 70% of the expansion and contraction of the lungs is accomplished by the change in anteroposterior measurement and about 30% is achieved by the change in length due to movement of the diaphragm.

The lungs—two air-filled spongy structures—are attached to the body only at the pulmonary ligament at the mediastinum. The three lobes of the right lung and the two lobes of the left lung have no other attachment. However, the membrane lining the intrapleural space constantly absorbs fluid or gas that enters this area, thereby creating a partial vacuum. This vacuum holds the visceral pleura of the lungs tightly against the parietal pleura of the chest wall. The parietal (lining the chest wall) and visceral (covering the lung tissue) pleurae slide over each other with each inspiration and expiration, lubricated by the few millimeters of tissue fluid-containing proteins in the intrapleural space.

During inspiration, the diaphragm and intercostal muscles contract, increasing the volume of the chest cavity. The lungs are expanded, and the pressure within the alveolar sacs, the intra-alveolar pressure, becomes slightly negative (-3 mm Hg) with regard to the atmosphere. This slightly negative pressure sucks air into the alveolar sacs through the respiratory passage.

After inspiration, the muscles used for inspiration relax, and the chest cavity returns to its resting position. With this decrease in chest size and resultant compression of the lungs, the intra-alveolar pressure builds to about $+3$ mm Hg and forces air out of the respiratory passages. During maximum respiratory efforts, the intra-alveolar pressure can vary from -80 mm Hg during inspiration to $+100$ mm Hg during expiration. One respiratory cycle consists of one inhalation and one exhalation. At rest, inhalation normally requires about 1 second, which is less than that required for exhalation. Exhalation lasts about 2 seconds.

The lungs continually tend to collapse. Two factors are responsible for this phenomenon. First, the many elastic fibers contained within the lung tissue itself are constantly attempting to shorten. The second and more important factor is the high surface tension of the fluid lining the alveoli. If surface tension is high, the moist interior surfaces of an alveolus are difficult to separate from one another. This increases the energy required to open and fill the alveolus with air during inspiration. If surface tension is low, the alveoli walls more easily separate, making alveolar filling during inspiration less effortful. A lipoprotein substance called surfactant, which is constantly secreted by the epithelial alveolar lining, decreases the surface tension of the fluids of the respiratory passages 7- to 14-fold.[3] The inability to secrete surfactant in the newborn is called *hyaline membrane disease* or *respiratory distress syndrome*.

Compliance

It is evident from the preceding discussion that both the lungs and the thorax itself have elastic characteristics and thus exhibit expansibility. This expansibility is called *compliance* and is a measure of the elasticity of the lungs. Compliance is expressed as the volume increase in the lung for each unit increase in intra-alveolar pressure.

$$\text{compliance} = \frac{\text{change in lung volume (liters)}}{\text{change in lung pressure (cm } H_2O)}$$

Normal total pulmonary compliance, that is, both lungs and thorax, is 0.13 L/cm water pressure. In other words, every time alveolar pressure is increased by an amount necessary to raise a column of water 1 cm in height, the lungs expand 130 ml in volume.

Because inspiration requires muscle contraction, it is an active process requiring energy. Energy is also required to overcome two other factors that tend to prevent expansion of the lungs: (1) nonelastic tissue resistance; and (2) airway resistance, meaning that energy is required to rearrange the large molecules of viscous tissues of the lung itself so that they slip past one another during respiratory movements. Under normal conditions, exhalation is a passive process that requires no energy. The lungs, with the chest wall, simply recoil to their original position.

A normal person at rest expends less than 6% of his total bodily oxygen consumption on the work of breathing. This percentage increases as the airway diameters decrease or compliance decreases.

Conditions or situations that destroy lung tissue, cause it to become fibrotic, produce pulmonary edema, block alveoli, or in any way impede lung expansion and expansibility of the thoracic cage are reducing pulmonary compliance. If compliance is reduced, it is more difficult to

---

DISPLAY BOX 17–1
Common Measures of Airway Diameters

Common measures of airway diameters are the forced expiratory volume (FEV), the forced vital capacity (FVC), and the maximal midexpiratory flow (MMEF). FEV is the volume of air exhaled in a given time period—usually during the first second of the FVC (FEV_1). FVC measures the amount of air in a forceful maximal expiration. Normally it is approximately the same as the VC. MMEF is the volume of air that is exhaled during the midpoint record of the FVC. This also may be termed FVC_{50}—FVC_{25}.

The FEV is expressed in terms of the FVC or the VC. Normally, the FEV_1 is about 80% of a VC. In obstructive disorders such as chronic bronchitis or emphysema, this FEV_1 is a smaller percentage of the VC (or FVC).

expand the lungs for inspiration. (If compliance is increased, it is easier to expand lung tissue.) In the presence of tissue edema, the lungs lose many of their elastic qualities, and increased viscosity of the tissues and fluids increases the nonelastic resistance. The work of breathing is increased, and the energy expended to accomplish the task is also greatly increased. Energy can be required for exhalation if elasticity is lost (emphysema) or air passages are obstructed (asthma).

Pressure

The air that is taken into the respiratory passages is a mixture of primarily nitrogen and oxygen (99.5%) and a small amount of carbon dioxide and water vapor (0.5%). The molecules of the various gases behave as they do in solution and exhibit brownian movement. Therefore, a mixture of gases such as air has all molecular species evenly distributed throughout the given volume. Because of this constant molecular bombardment, the volume of gases exerts pressure against the walls of the container. This pressure can be defined as the force with which a gas or mixture of gases attempts to move from the confines of the present environment. Therefore, each of the components of a mixture such as air accounts for part of the total pressure of the entire mixture. Consequently, if we take 100 volumes of air and place them in a container under 1 atmosphere of pressure (760 mm Hg), by analysis we would find that nitrogen constitutes 79 of the 100 volumes and oxygen accounts for 21 volumes, or 79% and 21% concentration, respectively.

Both these gases are contained at 760 mm Hg pressure in this container. If we now take the same volume of nitrogen and move it to a container of the same volume and allow it to expand until it completely fills all of the volume (100%), we observe that the pressure in the second container drops from 760 to 600 mm Hg. If we do the same thing with the 21 volumes of oxygen and allow them to expand to 100% of the volume, we observe that the pressure in the third container drops from 760 to 160 mm Hg. We conclude then that in the original container the *part* of the total pressure due to nitrogen was 600 mm Hg and the *part* due to oxygen was 160 mm Hg. This pressure of nitrogen is called the *partial pressure* of nitrogen (PN_2) and that of oxygen the *partial pressure* of oxygen (PO_2).

The partial pressure of a gas in a given volume is the force it exerts against the walls of the container. If the walls of the container are permeable, like the pulmonary membrane, the penetrating or diffusing power of a gas is directly proportional to its partial pressure.

It is extremely important to point out that atmospheric air differs from alveolar air in partial pressures of the components. The comparative concentrations of each are shown in Table 17–1.

The difference between atmospheric air and alveolar

TABLE 17–1
Comparison of Gases in Atmospheric and Alveolar Air

Gas	Atmospheric Air (%)	Alveolar Air (%)
N_2	78.62	74.90
O_2	20.84	13.60
CO_2	0.04	5.30
H_2O vapor	0.50	6.20
	100.00	100.00

air is in the increased concentration of carbon dioxide and water in alveolar air. There are two reasons for these differences. First, the air is humidified as it is inspired by the moisture of the epithelial lining of the respiratory tract. At normal body temperature, water vapor has a partial pressure of 47 mm Hg and mixes with and dilutes the other gases, decreasing their partial pressures. Second, molecules in a given volume of gas behave like molecules in a solution and diffuse from an area of high concentration to one of lower concentration.

Gravity

In an erect adult, the force of gravity increases the intrapleural pressure (and therefore the intra-alveolar pressure) at the base of the lungs. Consequently, more air exchange occurs in the upper regions of the lungs than at the bases. Similarly, in any other body position, gravitational forces increase the amount of effort required to ventilate dependent portions of the lungs. This causes a shift in ventilation wherein ventilation of these portions is decreased and ventilation of other, less dependent areas is increased.

Perfusion

The pulmonary circulation provides mixed venous blood exiting the right ventricle of the heart a chance to exchange gas before returning to the left atrium. The pulmonary circulation is unique and differs from other organ specific circulatory beds.

Anatomically, the pulmonary vascular bed has no thick walled muscular vasculature similar to arterioles. This results in a very distensible vascular bed with low resistance to flow. Although the pulmonary circulation receives the same volume of blood as the systemic system, the pulmonary vascular resistance (PVR) is one-sixth the systemic vascular resistance.[4]

If systemic pressures rise, PVR decreases. Using recruitment, previously low or non-perfused pulmonary vessels are opened and low perfused vessels are dilated.

Most of the PVR, at least 50%, is believed to be generated at the level of the capillaries. The size of the capillaries can be influenced by the nearby intra-alveolar pressures. The capillaries not near alveolar surfaces are subject to pressure generated by motion in the connective tissue of the lung. Chemical stimulation (by catecholamines, histamine, angiotensin II, and prostaglandins) results in vasoconstriction. For unknown reasons, hypoxia increases PVR.

A major force in perfusion distribution in the lung is gravity. Low pressures systems, like the pulmonary vasculature, are subject to hydrostatic pressure created by gravity. In an upright position, the dependent base of the lung distends the vasculature, offering very low PVR. The apex vasculature has little perfusion and higher PVR as constriction occurs.

Ventilation–Perfusion

Maximal efficiency in the exchange of gases between blood and alveolus results when ventilation (movement of air in alveoli = $\dot{V}$) and perfusion (movement of blood around alveoli = $\dot{Q}$) correspond equally (Fig. 17–2A). In other words, if an acinus (group of alveoli—the basic unit of respiration) is less ventilated, it needs less perfusion; if it is more ventilated, perfusion must be increased. Ventilation would be, in effect, wasted on an unperfused unit. Similarly, perfusion would be wasted on an unventilated unit. Two reflexes operate normally to facilitate such matching of ventilation and perfusion.

One reflex adjusts perfusion to ventilation (see Figure 17–2B). Here, a low concentration of alveolar oxygen (PaO_2) causes a lowered PaO_2, which, in turn, triggers vasoconstriction of nearby pulmonary arterioles. This effectively *shunts* blood away from an underventilated area. The other reflex adjusts ventilation to perfusion (see Figure 17–2C). If perfusion through an area is impeded (eg, by an embolus plugging the vessel), it results in a local decrease in $PACO_2$. This causes a decrease in $PACO_2$, which, in turn, causes a constriction of the bronchioles and smaller bronchi in the underperfused area. Therefore, the underperfused area is not ventilated as much as before. These reflexes keep the ventilation ($\dot{V} = 4$ L/min) to perfusion ($\dot{Q} = 5$ L/min) ratio at 4 : 5. Thus, the $\dot{V}/\dot{Q}$ ratio is 0.8 under normal circumstances. A high $\dot{V}/\dot{Q}$ ratio indicates ventilation exceeds perfusion; a low $\dot{V}/\dot{Q}$ ratio is reflective of perfusion exceeding ventilation.[5] The lungs react regionally; the $\dot{V}/\dot{Q}$ ratio is 3.0 at the apex and 0.6 at the base, simultaneously.

$\dot{V}/\dot{Q}$ mismatch occurs in many respiratory disorders. If ventilation is in excess of perfusion (eg, after pulmonary embolism), the disorder is described as *dead space-producing* (with a $\dot{V}/\dot{Q} > 0.8$). If perfusion exceeds ventilation (eg, after alveolar atelectasis or collapse), the disorder is *shunt-producing* (with a $\dot{V}/\dot{Q} < 0.8$).

Gas Transportation

Pulmonary Membrane

The pulmonary membrane is composed of all the surfaces in the respiratory wall that are thin enough to permit the exchange of gases between the lungs and the blood. The total area of this membrane in the average normal adult male is about 60 m^2, or about the size of a moderate-sized classroom. It is 0.2 to 0.4 μ thick, or less than the thickness of the average red blood cell. These two outstanding features combine to allow large quantities of gases to diffuse across the pulmonary membrane in a very short period of time.

Diffusion

The factors that govern the rate of diffusion of the gases through the pulmonary membrane are as follows:

- The greater the pressure difference across the membrane, the faster the rate of diffusion.
- The larger the area of the pulmonary membrane, the larger the quantity of gas that can diffuse across the membrane in a given period.
- The thinner the membrane, the more rapid the diffusion of gases through it to the compartment on the opposite side.
- The diffusion coefficient is directly proportional to the solubility of the gas in the fluid of the pulmonary membrane and inversely proportional to molecular size. Therefore, small molecules that are highly soluble diffuse more rapidly than do large molecular gases that are less soluble.

The diffusion coefficients are:

- Oxygen   1
- Carbon dioxide   20.3
- Nitrogen   0.53

The coefficients indicate that CO_2 is the most soluble and N_2 the least soluble of these three gases. They are very similar to one another with regard to molecular size but have quite different solubilities in the fluids of the pulmonary membrane. These differences account for the difference in the rate of diffusion of the gases through the pulmonary membrane.

Tissue Oxygen and Carbon Dioxide

As oxygen diffuses from the lungs to the blood, a small portion of it becomes dissolved in the plasma and cell fluids, but more than 60 times as much combines immediately with hemoglobin. At a PAO_2 of 100 mm Hg, almost 96% of all hemoglobin molecules have combined

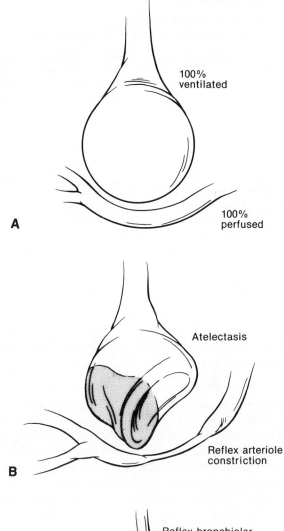

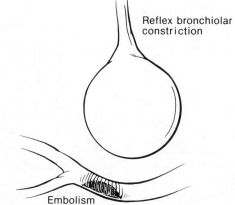

FIGURE 17–2
(**A**) A fully ventilated alveolus with a fully perfused vasculature illustrates the ratio $\dot{V}/\dot{Q} = 1$, where $\dot{V}$ is ventilation and $\dot{Q}$ is perfusion of vascular bed. (**B**) A partially collapsed and filled alveolus with reflex constriction of vasculature illustrates $\downarrow \dot{V} \rightarrow \downarrow PAO_2 \rightarrow \downarrow \dot{Q}$ (**C**) A nearly blocked vasculature with reflex bronchiolar constriction illustrates $\downarrow \dot{Q} \rightarrow \downarrow PACO_2 \rightarrow \downarrow \dot{V}$.

with oxygen. This percentage represents the *saturation* of hemoglobin. Saturation is important because it reflects the oxygen available to tissues more accurately than the PAO_2. It is the oxygen carried on hemoglobin molecules that tissues can access, not the oxygen dissolved in the blood. Hemoglobin carries oxygen to the tissues. Here the oxygen is used by the cells, and carbon dioxide is formed.

As the carbon dioxide diffuses into the interstitial fluids, about 5% is dissolved in the blood, and the remain-

der diffuses into the red blood cells where one of two things occurs:

- Carbon dioxide combines with water to form carbonic acid and then reacts with the acid–base buffer and is transported as the bicarbonate ion.
- A small portion of the carbon dioxide combines with hemoglobin at a different bonding site from that of oxygen and is transported as carbaminohemoglobin.

TABLE 17–2
Relative Partial Pressures

Gas	Atmospheric Air	Alveolar Air	Venous Blood	Arterial Blood
PO_2	159	104	40	100
PCO_2	0.15	40	45	40
PN_2	597	569	569	569

Nitrogen diffuses from the alveolus into the blood. Because there is no carrier mechanism and under standard conditions nitrogen has only slight solubility in tissue fluid, it quickly establishes an equilibrium state on either side of the membrane and therefore is essentially inert.

The relative partial pressure (mm Hg) in the various compartments is summarized in Table 17–2.

It can readily be seen that concentration gradients are established that then foster the diffusion of these gases in the direction that is physiologically advantageous.

Figure 17–3 summarizes the events of gaseous diffusion through the pulmonary membrane and transport to and from the tissues.

Oxyhemoglobin Dissociation Curve

The influence of PaO_2 (the arterial level of oxygen) on saturation, or the attachment of oxygen to hemoglobin, is not a straight-line function. In other words, the relation is not directly proportioned on a 1 : 1 basis. The relations involved are shown in Figure 17–4. The upper right-hand corner illustrates conditions in arterial blood when the normal PaO_2 is at about 100 mm Hg. Then, as the blood circulates through the capillaries, losing oxygen to the interstitial fluid, the curve falls until the PO_2 of venous fluid (40 mm Hg) is reached. At a PO_2 of 40, hemoglobin molecules are still about 70% to 75% saturated with oxygen. This provides a reserve supply of oxygen that can be provided to the tissues in cases of emergency or strenuous exercise. Only about 25% to 30% of the arterial oxygen supply is used to meet tissue needs.

Due to the relations represented by this curve, oxygen can be applied to the tissues even if the PaO_2 is less than 100 (hypoxemia or high-altitude living). Indeed, hemoglobin is approximately 95% saturated at a PaO_2 of 80 mm Hg.

Several factors influence the saturation. Clinically important are the pH, PCO_2, and temperature. These factors exert a Bohr effect on the oxyhemoglobin dissociation curve, shifting it to the right or left (Fig. 17–5). A shift to the right means a decrease in the affinity of hemoglobin for oxygen. This means that less oxygen can be picked up in the lungs but that oxygen is more readily given up to the tissues in the capillaries. Acidity, hypercarbia, and elevation in temperature all lead to a shift to the right. A shift to the left increases the affinity of hemoglobin for oxygen. More oxygen can be picked up in the lungs, but oxygen is less readily released in the capillaries. This could cause tissue hypoxia even with an adequate PaO_2. A fall in PCO_2, seen often in mechanical hyperventilation, has the greatest clinical potential for producing such a condition. Other factors that lead to a shift to the left are alkalinity and hypothermia.

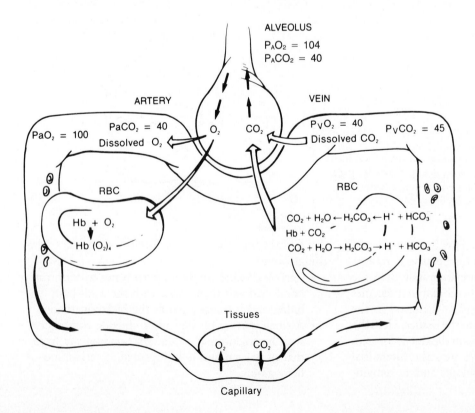

FIGURE 17–3
Movement and partial pressures of oxygen and carbon dioxide, from alveolar air, to arterial blood, to capillary exchange, to venous blood, back to alveolar air. Note the reversibility of the Henderson–Hasselbalch equation, from capillary blood to venous blood at the alveolus.

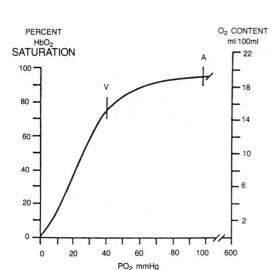

FIGURE 17–4

Normal oxyhemoglobin dissociation curve. Point A illustrates the relationship between the partial pressure of oxygen (PO_2) and the percentage of oxyhemoglobin saturation (HbO_2) in the lungs. Point V illustrates this same relationship in venous blood returning from the tissues. (Smith JJ, Kampine JP: Circulatory Physiology—The Essentials. Baltimore: Williams & Wilkins, 1980)

Regulation of Respiration

Brain Stem Centers and the Respiratory Cycle

Unlike the heart, the lungs have no spontaneous rhythm. Ventilations depend on rhythmic operation of brain stem centers and intact pathways from there to the respiratory muscles. There are two centers in the medulla: (1) a center that stimulates inspiration by diaphragmatic contraction (by way of phrenic nerves); and (2) another center that innervates both inspiratory and expiratory intercostal and accessory muscles.

Note that the phrenic and the intercostal nerves exit the spinal cord at C6, whereas motor nerves that supply accessory muscles exit higher. This has implications for respiratory drive and efficacy in those persons with spinal cord injury.

The pons also contains two centers included in respiration. One is called the pneumotaxic center. The other, the apneustic center, produces sustained inspiration if stimulated. Voluntary control and involuntary control are further established by descending fibers from other brain centers. (These facilitate the alterations in respiration seen, for example, during swallowing, coughing, yawning, and willed action.)

In breathing at rest, the following sequence is thought to occur. The neurons innervating the inspiratory muscles fire bursts of impulses to these muscles, leading to inspiration. These neurons also stimulate the pneumotaxic center. This center, in turn, fires inhibitory impulses back to the inspiratory neurons, causing a halt in inspiration. Expiration follows passively. After expiration, the inspiratory neurons are again stimulated to fire automatically. During exercise or other occasions when more vigorous ventilation occurs, the expiratory neurons of the medulla are postulated to participate in this sequence, causing active exhalation. A more comprehensive picture of the breathing process awaits further data.

Adjustments to the Respiratory Cycle

Respiratory centers in the medulla and pons and specialized sensory tissues in the aorta and carotids, called the aortic and carotid bodies, adjust respiratory rates and

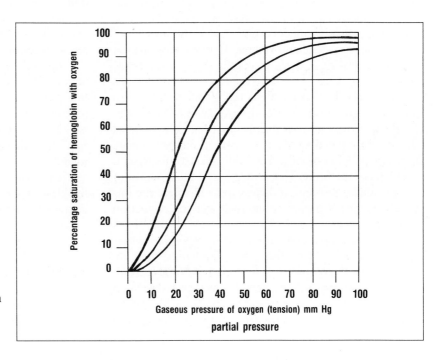

FIGURE 17–5

Right and left shifts of the oxyhemoglobin dissociation curve. (Carpenter KD: "Oxygen Transport in the Blood," Critical Care Nurse Oct: 20–33, 1991)

TABLE 17–3
Peripheral Receptors and Their Regulatory Effect in Ventilation

Peripheral Receptor	Stimulus	Response
Pulmonary stretch receptors (Hering–Breuer reflex)	Lung distention	Vagal stimulus to medulla causing increased expiratory time, leading to slowed rate
Irritant receptors in upper airways	Antigens such as pollen, histamine, and cold air	Vagal stimulus to bronchioles, causing bronchiolar constriction; important in asthma
Juxtacapillary receptors in alveolar walls	Pulmonary capillary distention, inhaled antigens such as anesthetics	Vagal stimulus to medulla, causing increased rate and decreased depth; may lead to apnea
Gamma system receptors in intercostals and diaphragm	Muscle stretch	Increased stretch leads to increased contraction
Gamma receptors in joints and muscles	Muscle stretch	Afferent stimuli to medulla, causing increased rate and depth; important in exercise
Receptors in nose, nasopharynx, larynx	Antigens or mechanical irritants	Sneezing, coughing, laryngeal spasm, bronchoconstriction; important in airway defense

volumes. Changes in PO_2, PCO_2, and pH stimulate all these areas.

The Henderson–Hasselbalch equation shows that carbon dioxide in the blood dissociates into carbonic acid, and then into hydrogen ion and bicarbonate. Hydrogen ion is a strong acid. Practitioners may find it most useful to think of carbon dioxide as an acid, regulated rapidly by the respiratory system.

If the blood carbon dioxide level rises (hypercapnia), the blood pH drops to acidic levels. Because carbon dioxide diffuses rapidly in fluids, it crosses to cerebrospinal fluid (CSF) also, and the CSF pH drops. Central chemoreceptors located in the medulla respond to the low pH by increasing, through medullary stimuli to the muscles of inspiration, both rate and volume. Cerebral vasodilation also occurs during acidosis, increasing the carbon dioxide supply to the CSF.

Low blood pH is most commonly due to hypercapnia, although blood pH can drop because of lactic acid production during anaerobic metabolism, or with renal disease causing hydrogen ion, potassium, and bicarbonate imbalances. A low blood pH is rapidly toxic to all chemical reactions of the body. This principle and the strength of the medullary response to hypercapnia illustrate the importance of carbon dioxide and hydrogen ion regulation to life processes.

Although aortic and carotid bodies respond to hypercapnia and low pH by increasing ventilation, their response is weak compared to medullary actions. Instead, these bodies respond strongly to hypoxia (decreased PO_2). Hypoxia stimulates the carotid bodies, which signal the carotid sinus nerve. This nerve causes the medulla to increase ventilatory rate and depth. The aortic bodies respond somewhat more weakly than the carotid bodies, but in the same way. Low PO_2 stimulates the aortic bodies, which activate the vagus nerve, leading to the medullary increase in ventilation.

For persons with chronically high levels of carbon dioxide, the hypercapnic drive to adjust carbon dioxide can be lost due to accommodation. In such persons, changes in PO_2, and the response of the carotid and aortic bodies, can provide the only stimulus to adjust ventilation. In persons with chronically high PCO_2 and low PO_2, the medulla is depressed by hypercarbia. Therefore, the only stimulus for respirations is hypoxia. Administering oxygen to long-term hypercapnic and hypoxic patients can result in respiratory standstill or apnea.

Table 17–3 shows peripheral receptors and their regulatory effects on ventilation. Normally, peripheral receptors play a minor role in ventilation. Emotional stimuli commonly increase ventilation. Ventilatory rate and depth have been shown to increase before exercise, leading to the hypothesis that cognition of impending exercise affects the medulla.

The compensatory mechanisms discussed in this chapter illustrate the rapidity of the respiratory response to alterations in blood chemistry.

REFERENCES

1. Bates D, et al.: Respiratory Function in Disease, pp. 23–47. Philadelphia: WB Saunders, 1989

2. Bates D, et al.: Respiratory Function in Disease, pp. 23–47. Philadelphia: WB Saunders, 1989
3. Holm B, Notter R (eds): Surfactant Replacement Therapy, pp 273–304. New York: Alan R Liss, 1989
4. Bates D, et al: Respiratory Function in Disease, pp. 23–47. Philadelphia: WB Saunders, 1989
5. Ahrens T: Blood gas analysis of intrapulmonary shunting and dead space. Crit Care Nurs Clin North Am, 1(4): 641–648, 1989

BIBLIOGRAPHY

Guyton AC: Textbook of Medical Physiology, 8th ed. Philadelphia, WB Saunders, 1991
Hole JW Jr: Essentials of Human Anatomy and Physiology, 4th ed. Dubuque, Iowa, WC Brown, 1992
Shapiro B, et al: Clinical Application of Respiratory Care. Chicago, Yearbook Medical Publishers, 1990
Shoemaker W, et al: Textbook of Critical Care. Philadelphia, WB Saunders, 1989

STUDY QUESTIONS

1. Which of the following has an impact on lung compliance?

   a. resting tidal volume
   b. decreased pulmonary artery perfusion
   c. oxygen consumption
   d. brain centers in the medulla

2. Which of the following statements about pulmonary perfusion is *not* true?

   a. pulmonary vascular resistance is one-sixth the systemic vascular resistance
   b. gravity is a major force in pulmonary perfusion distribution
   c. pulmonary vascular resistance rises if the systemic vascular resistance rises
   d. there is normally a mismatch of ventilation and perfusion within the lung

3. The oxygen dissociation curve describes several factors that shift the curve to the right, decreasing the oxygen affinity for hemoglobin. These factors are

   a. tidal volume, functional residual volume, and anatomic dead space
   b. pH, PCO_2, and temperature
   c. alveolar perfusion and diffusion gradients
   d. alterations in barometric pressure

4. The aortic and carotid bodies respond to hypercapnia by

   a. vasodilation of the pulmonary vasculature
   b. vasoconstriction of the pulmonary vasculature
   c. decreasing respiratory rate and depth
   d. increasing respiratory rate and depth

CHAPTER 18

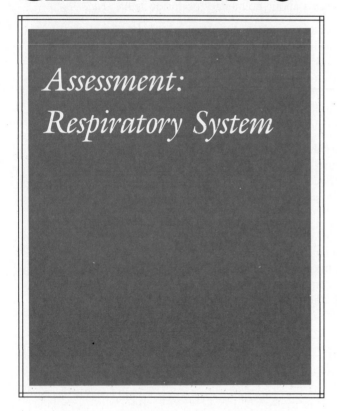

Assessment: Respiratory System

BEHAVIORAL OBJECTIVES

Based on the content in this chapter, the reader should be able to:

1. List five questions to use while gathering history data.
2. Describe four procedures and possible pertinent findings used in respiratory physical examination.

Hudak: Critical Care Nursing:
A Holistic Approach, 6th ed. © 1994
J. B. Lippincott Company.

3. Compare and contrast mixed venous and arterial samples for oxygen, carbon dioxide, pH and oxygen saturation.
4. List the normal values for arterial blood gases.
5. Describe the procedure for obtaining ABGs.
6. Given an example, perform a basic analysis of acid–base interpretation.

Description

Nurses contribute significantly to the care of patients with respiratory problems by taking an illness-specific history and performing a chest physical examination. This assessment allows the nurse an opportunity to establish a base line of information and provides a framework for detection of some of the rapid changes in the patient's condition. Assessments are valuable if made before and after interventions that are likely to alter or improve respiratory status. Because the nurse is with the patient more frequently, it is often the nurse who detects the patient's changing condition rather than the physician, who visits the patient only once or twice a day and who, even with the information provided by daily chest roentgenograms, is less likely to be alert to immediate changes in the status of the patient.

History

The patient history should start with information about the present illness. Often, if the patient is very ill, a relative or friend provides more information.

If dyspnea is present, information about the onset of symptoms is important. Ask whether it occurs only with exertion or only if the patient is lying flat (therefore requiring the patient to sit up, as is seen more commonly in heart failure) and whether it awakens the patient at night (paroxysmal nocturnal dyspnea). Paroxysmal nocturnal dyspnea and orthopnea often signify heart failure but can be seen in severe dyspnea of any cause. The entire course of dyspnea should be described, including exacerbating factors, length of episodes, and relief measures attempted thus far.

Often the dyspnea seen with lung disease is associated with an anterior chest discomfort that must be distinguished from angina. If chest pain is present, one should determine whether there is more than one type of pain. For each type of chest pain, one should determine duration; related factors such as exertion (which usually is seen with cardiac pain), position, or eating habits; whether pain is worsened by breathing or movement (eg, in pleurisy); and what relief measures have been used (eg, rest, nitroglycerin, antacids, or belching).

Illness within the respiratory system often results in the production, or a change in the production, of sputum.[1]

The nurse can ask how much sputum is produced in 24 hours, giving the patient a frame of reference (eg, a tablespoonful or one-half cup). The color of the sputum provides important information about infection. Yellow, green, or brown sputum usually signifies bacterial infection, but clear or white sputum usually indicates absence of bacterial infection. The color usually comes from white blood cells in the sputum. However, yellow color can occur if there are many eosinophils in the sputum, thereby signifying allergy rather than infection. An increase in either the color or the amount of sputum often means infection. Sometimes in infections, the patient is unable to cough up the sputum; a decrease in sputum production associated with worsening hypoxemia and a silent chest can signify bronchiolitis. Usually, though, cough without sputum production means that bacterial infection is not present. One must try to determine whether mucus production comes from the nose or sinuses as postnasal drainage or whether the mucus originates in the chest.

It is important for one to ask whether there has been blood in the sputum; sometimes the patient is afraid to mention it. The amount of blood should be evaluated—from streaks or specks, to blood-colored mucus, to pure blood (bright red or dark). One should also determine whether the blood is associated with sputum production, as it often is in bronchitis and pneumonia, or whether it occurs alone, as is often the case in a pulmonary embolus.

It is important to gather data on the past health history as well.[2] This data should include environmental exposure and risk factors, past medical history, and family history. The patient's use of tobacco should be quantified by amount and how long the patient has smoked or did smoke.

Especially in elderly people, it is important to determine whether regurgitation and aspiration of gastric contents, often occurring at night, cause symptoms of cough, wheeze, or dyspnea.

Physical Examination

Sometimes a chest examination by the nurse is the quickest and most reliable assessment of the situation. Physical diagnosis of the chest includes four procedures:

- inspection, or looking at the patient
- palpation, or feeling the patient
- percussion, or thumping on the patient
- auscultation, or listening to the patient's chest with a stethoscope.

Inspection

Inspection of the patient involves checking for the presence or absence of several factors.

Cyanosis is one of the factors in which we are most

interested. Cyanosis is notoriously hard to detect if the patient is anemic, and the patient who is polycythemic can have cyanosis in the extremities even if oxygen tension is normal.

We generally differentiate between *peripheral* and *central* cyanosis. Peripheral cyanosis occurs in the extremities or on the tip of the nose or ears, even with normal oxygen tensions, if there is diminished blood flow to these areas, particularly if they are cold or dependent. Central cyanosis, as observed on the tongue or lips, has a much greater significance; it means the patient actually has a low oxygen tension.

Labored breathing is an obvious sign to check; we are particularly interested in knowing whether the patient is using the accessory muscles of respiration. The presence of staccato speech may be observed. This is a speech pattern interrupted by breaths of air. Sometimes, the number of words a patient can say before having to gasp for another breath is a good measure of the amount of labored breathing.

An increase in the anteroposterior (AP) diameter of the chest (ie, an increase in the size of the chest from front to back) also is checked. This often is caused by overexpansion of the lungs from obstructive pulmonary disease, but an increase in AP diameter also can be present in a patient who has kyphosis (forward curvature of the spine).

Chest deformities and scars are important in helping us determine the reason for respiratory distress. For instance, a scar may be our first indication that the patient has had part of his lung removed. A chest deformity such as kyphoscoliosis can indicate why the patient has respiratory distress.

The patient's posture also must be observed, because patients with obstructive pulmonary disease often sit and prop themselves up on outstretched arms or lean forward with their elbows on a desk in an effort to elevate their clavicles and thereby gain a slightly greater ability to expand their chests.

The position of the trachea is also important to observe. Is the trachea in the midline as it should be, or is it deviated to one side or the other? A pleural effusion or a tension pneumothorax usually deviates the trachea away from the diseased side. With atelectasis, however, the trachea often is pulled toward the diseased side.

The respiratory rate is an important parameter to follow; it should be counted over at least a 15-second period rather than merely estimated. Often, the respiratory rate is recorded as 20 breaths per minute, which frequently means that the rate was estimated instead of counted.

The depth of respiration is often as meaningful as the respiratory rate. For instance, if a patient were breathing 40 times per minute, one might think severe respiratory problems could be present, but if breaths were quite deep at that rate, it might mean the patient had Kussmaul respirations due to diabetic acidosis or other acidosis. However, if the respirations were shallow at a rate of 40 times per minute, it might indicate severe respiratory dis-

tress from obstructive lung disease, restrictive lung disease, or other pulmonary problems.

The duration of inspiration versus the duration of expiration is important in determining whether there is airway obstruction. In patients with any of the obstructive lung diseases, expiration is prolonged, more than 1½ times as long as inspiration.

Observation of *general chest expansion* is an integral part of examining a patient. Normally, we expect about a 3-inch expansion from maximal expiration to maximal inspiration. Motion of the abdomen in breathing efforts (normal in men more than women) may be observed. Ankylosing spondylitis, or Marie-Strümpell arthritis, is one condition in which general chest expansion is limited. Compare the expansion of the upper chest with that of the lower chest and observe movement of the diaphragm to determine whether the patient with obstructive pulmonary disease is concentrating on expanding the lower chest and using the diaphragm properly. Look at the expansion of one side of the chest versus the other side, realizing that atelectasis, especially that caused by a mucous plug, can cause unilateral diminished chest expansion.

A pulmonary embolus, pneumonia, pleural effusion, pneumothorax, or any other cause of chest pain, such as fractured ribs, can lead to diminished chest expansion. An endotracheal or nasotracheal tube inserted too far, so that it extends beyond the trachea into one of the main stem bronchi (usually the right), is a serious and frequent cause of diminished expansion of one side of the chest. If the tube slips into the right main stem bronchus, the left lung is not expanded, and the patient usually develops hypoxemia and atelectasis on the left side. Fortunately, the nurse who is aware of this potential problem usually recognizes it.

If present, *intercostal retractions* (ie, sucking in of the muscles and skin between the ribs during inspiration) usually mean that the patient is making a larger effort at inspiration than normal. Usually this signifies that the lungs are less compliant (stiffer) than usual. Use of accessory muscles, as seen by lifting of the shoulders, indicates an increased work of breathing.

The effectiveness and frequency of a patient's cough are important to notice, as are sputum characteristics such as amount, color, and consistency.

Palpation

Palpation of the chest is done with the heel of the hand flat against the patient's chest. Often, we are determining whether tactile fremitus is present. We do this by asking the patient to say, "Ninety-nine." Normally, if a patient follows these instructions, a vibration is felt on the outside of the chest by the examiner's hand. This is similar to the vibration one feels after putting a hand on the chest of a cat when the cat is purring. In normal patients, tactile fremitus is present. It can be diminished or absent if there is something that comes between the patient's lung and the hand on the chest wall. For instance, if there is a pleural effusion, thickened pleura, or pneumothorax, either it is impossible to feel this vibration or the vibration is diminished. If the patient has atelectasis due to an occluded airway, the vibration also cannot be felt. Tactile fremitus is slightly increased in conditions of consolidation, but detection of this slight increase can be difficult. Just by palpating over the patient's chest with quiet breathing, one can sometimes feel palpable rhonchi that are due to mucus moving in large airways.

Percussion

In percussing a patient's chest, one must use a finger that is pressed flat against the chest; this finger is struck over the knuckle by the end of a finger from the dominant hand. Normally, the chest has a resonant or hollow percussion note. In diseases in which there is increased air in the chest or lungs, such as pneumothorax and emphysema, there can be hyperresonant (even more drumlike) percussion notes. Hyperresonant percussion notes, however, are sometimes hard to detect. More important is a dull or flat percussion note such as is heard if one percusses over a part of the body that contains no air. A dull or flat percussion note is heard if the lung underneath the examining hand has atelectasis, pneumonia, pleural effusion, thickened pleura, or a mass lesion. A dull or flat percussion note also is heard if one is percussing over the heart.

Auscultation

In auscultation, one generally uses the diaphragm of the stethoscope and presses this firmly against the chest wall. It is important for one to listen to the intensity or loudness of breath sounds and to realize that normally there is a fourfold increase in loudness of breath sounds when a patient takes a maximum deep breath as opposed to quiet breathing. The intensity of the breath sounds can be diminished due to decreased airflow through the airways or to increased insulation between the lungs and the stethoscope. In airway obstruction, such as chronic obstructive pulmonary disease (COPD) or atelectasis, the breath sound intensity is diminished. With shallow breathing, there is diminished air movement through the airways, and the breath sounds also are not as loud. With restricted movement of the thorax or diaphragm, there can be diminished breath sounds in the area of restricted movement. In pleural thickening, pleural effusion, pneumothorax, and obesity there is an abnormal substance (fibrous tissue, fluid, air, or fat) between the stethoscope and the underlying lung; this substance insulates the breath sounds from the stethoscope, making the breath sounds seem less loud.

Generally, there are three types of sounds that are heard in the normal chest[3]:

- vesicular breath sounds, which are heard in the periphery of the normal lung;
- bronchial breath sounds, which are heard over the trachea;
- bronchovesicular breath sounds, which are heard in most areas of the lung near the major airways.

Bronchial breath sounds are high-pitched, seem to be close to the ear, are loud, and include a pause between inspiration and expiration. *Vesicular breath sounds* are of lower pitch, having a rustling quality, and include no noticeable pause between inspiration and expiration. *Bronchovesicular breath sounds* represent a sound halfway between the other two types of breath sounds.

Bronchial breath sounds, in addition to being heard over the trachea of the normal person, are also heard in any situation in which there is consolidation—for instance, pneumonia. Bronchial breath sounds are also heard above a pleural effusion in which the normal lung is compressed. Wherever there is bronchial breathing, there also may be two other associated changes: (1) E to A changes, and (2) whispered pectoriloquy.

An *E to A change* merely means that if one listens with a stethoscope and the patient says "E," what one hears is actually an A sound rather than an E sound. This occurs if there is consolidation.

Whispered pectoriloquy is the presence of a loud volume as heard through the stethoscope when the patient whispers. For bronchial breathing and these two associated changes to be present, there must be either (1) an open airway and compressed alveoli, or (2) alveoli in which the air has been replaced by fluid.

Other sounds heard with auscultation include crackles, wheezes, and rubs. *Crackles* are light, continuous sounds created as small airways are reopened or reinflated during end-inspiration. Crackles occur in pneumonia, congestive heart failure, and pulmonary fibrosis. Both inspiratory and expiratory crackles may be auscultated in bronchiectasis. Loud crackles can be heard in pulmonary edema and in moribund patients. Often loud crackles are audible without a stethoscope because they are generated in the large airways.

Extra sounds such as wheezing mean there is airway narrowing. This can be caused by asthma, foreign bodies, mucus in the airways, stenosis, and so forth. If the wheeze is heard only in expiration, it is called a *wheeze;* if the wheezing sound occurs in both inspiration and expiration, it is usually due to retained secretions.

A *friction rub* is heard if there is pleural disease such as a pulmonary embolus, peripheral pneumonia, or pleurisy, and it is often difficult to distinguish from a rhonchus. If the abnormal noise clears after the patient coughs, it usually means that it was a rhonchus rather than a friction rub.

Certainly, critical care nurses and respiratory thera-

TABLE 18–1
Checklist of Abnormal Respiratory Findings

Bronchitis

Increased respiratory rate (occasional)
Use of accessory muscles (occasional)
Intercostal retraction (occasional)
Prolonged expiratory phase (frequent)
Increased AP diameter of the chest (frequent)
Decreased motion of the diaphragm (frequent)
Decreased intensity of breath sounds
Crackles
Wheezes (frequent)
Crackles and wheezes clear after cough (frequent)

Pneumothorax

Increased respiratory rate
Trachea deviated to side of pneumothorax
Cyanosis (occasional)
Decreased movement of chest on side of pneumothorax (splinting)
Hyperresonance (unreliable sign)
Decreased breath sounds
Decreased tactile fremitus and decreased vocal fremitus (the most reliable signs)

Emphysema

Increased respiratory rate (frequent)
Use of accessory muscles (neck)

Atelectasis

Increased respiratory rate
Increased pulse
Cyanosis (frequent)
Trachea deviated to side of atelectasis
Decreased chest expansion on side of atelectasis (splinting)
Decreased fremitus (tactile and vocal)
Dull or flat percussion note
Decreased breath sounds
Rales (occasional)

Pleural Effusion

Increase in respiratory rate (occasional)
Trachea deviated away from side of effusion
Decreased fremitus (tactile and vocal)
Decreased breath sounds
Above effusion
  Bronchial breathing ⎫
  E to A changes ⎬ due to compressed lungs with open airway
  Whispered pectoriloquy ⎭
Friction rub—after fluid is removed and visceral pleura rubs against parietal pleura

Large Mass Lesion (tumor)

Dullness over tumor
Fine rales (frequent)
Decreased breath sounds if airway is occluded

Intercostal retractions
Propped up on outstretched arms
Prolonged expiratory phase
Increased AP diameter
Decreased chest expansion
Decreased motion of diaphragm
Hyperresonance to percussion
Decreased intensity (loudness) of breath sounds
Little or no increase in loudness of breath sounds with deep breath
Crackles (frequent)
Wheeze (occasional)

Pneumonia

Increased respiratory rate
Cyanosis (occasional)
Decreased expansion (splinting) (frequent)
Increased fremitus (tactile and vocal)
Palpable rhonchi—usually are removed by coughing or suctioning (occasional)
Dullness to percussion
Bronchial breathing, whispered pectoriloquy, and E to A changes (usual if consolidation is extensive)
Crackles—usually clear with cough or suctioning (occasional)
Pleural friction rub (occasional)
Bronchial breathing, E to A changes, and whispered pectoriloquy if airway is open
Pleural friction rub (occasional)

Subcutaneous Emphysema

Crackling sounds that come from air outside the chest in the soft tissue

Pulmonary Edema (congestive heart failure)

Increased respiratory rate
Cyanosis (frequent)
Use of accessory muscles (usual)
Apprehension
Sitting upright (frequent)
Increased fremitus (due to interstitial edema)
Dull percussion note (due to interstitial edema)
Bronchovesicular sounds (due to interstitial edema, often obscured later by rales)
Crackles that increase in amount, volume, and auscultated area (occasional)
Wheezing (occasional)

Pulmonary Interstitial Fibrosis

Increased respiratory rate (frequent)
Intercostal retractions
Cyanosis (late)
Crackles
Bronchovesicular breathing (occasional)

Assessment: Respiratory System 407

pists should learn to participate in chest physical diagnosis so that they can detect changes in the patient's condition as soon as they occur, rather than waiting for the physician's visit once or twice a day or depending on a daily chest film. Table 18–1 is a checklist of abnormal respiratory findings in some common pulmonary disorders.

Diagnostic Tests

Mixed Venous Blood Sampling

Blood obtained from a vein in an extremity gives information mostly about that extremity and can be quite misleading if the metabolism in the extremity differs from the metabolism of the body as a whole, as it often does. This difference is accentuated if the extremity is cold or underperfused as in a patient in shock, if the patient has done local exercise with the extremity such as opening and closing the fist, if there is local infection in the extremity, and so forth.

Sometimes blood is sampled through a central venous line (CVP catheter) in hope of getting mixed venous blood, but even in the superior vena cava or right atrium, where a CVP catheter ends, there is usually incomplete mixing of venous blood from various parts of the body. For complete mixing of the blood, one would have to obtain a blood sample from the pulmonary artery, through a Swan-Ganz catheter, for example; even then one would not get information about how well the lungs are oxygenating the blood.

Oxygen measurements of mixed venous blood indicate whether the tissues are being oxygenated but cannot separate the contribution of the heart from that of the lungs. Normal mixed venous oxygen saturation is 70% to 75%.[4] If the mixed venous blood oxygen is low, it means that either heart or lungs, or both, is at fault. Such a reading can indicate one of two conditions: (1) the lungs have not oxygenated the arterial blood well and, because the tissues extract their usual amount of oxygen from arterial blood, the resulting venous blood has a low oxygen concentration; or (2) the heart is not circulating the blood well, it is taking blood a long time to circulate through the tissues, and the tissues, therefore, must extract more than the usual amount of oxygen from each cardiac cycle because the blood is flowing slowly; this produces a low venous oxygen concentration. See Display Box 18–1.

If it is known that the arterial oxygen concentration is normal (indicating that the lungs are doing their job) but the mixed venous oxygen concentration is low, then one can infer that the heart and circulation are failing. Mixed venous oxygen saturation of 40% to 60% is often found with heart failure, and values less than 40% indicate profound shock.

One advantage of using mixed venous blood instead

Normal Blood Gas Values

	Arterial Blood	Mixed Venous Blood
pH	7.40 (7.35–7.45)	7.38 (7.33–7.43)
PO_2	80–100 mm Hg	35–49 mm Hg
O_2 sat	95% or greater	70%–75%
PCO_2	35–45 mm Hg	41–51 mm Hg
HCO_3^-	22–26 mEq/L	24–28 mEq/L
Base excess (BE)	−2 to +2	0 to +4

---

of arterial blood is that if the oxygen concentration in mixed venous blood is normal, one can infer that the tissues are receiving enough oxygen—usually this means that both ventilation and circulation are adequate. Therefore, if the mixed venous oxygen saturation is monitored and is found to be normal, it ensures both normal oxygenation of blood by the lungs and normal or near normal cardiac function. If the oxygen saturation is low, one should measure arterial oxygen saturation and cardiac output. However, as long as the mixed venous oxygen saturation is normal, one can infer that both the arterial oxygen saturation and the cardiac output are normal. Therefore, these two determinants of the mixed venous oxygen saturation do not have to be measured so frequently as long as the mixed venous oxygen saturation remains normal.

The development of a pulmonary artery flotation catheter that allows continuous monitoring of oxygen saturation ($S\bar{v}O_2$ monitoring) with an oximeter built into its tip provides ongoing assessment of oxygen supply/demand imbalances.[5] Even if the exact mixed venous oxygen saturation measured by this catheter is not completely accu-

---

DISPLAY BOX 18–2
Causes of Low Mixed Venous Oxygen Saturation

- Low arterial saturation due to abnormal lung function, but normal cardiac function
- Normal oxygen saturation and decreased cardiac function (slower blood flow) allowing more tissue extraction of oxygen (increased arteriovenous oxygen difference)
- Combination of the two

rate, certainly the trends recorded are just as useful. Alternatively, one can draw blood from the pulmonary artery through a regular Swan-Ganz catheter, measure the PO_2 or oxygen saturation or both on a blood gas analyzer or oximeter or both, and use the information in the same way.

Finally, there is another rare cause of arterial hypoxemia that is due to a combination of heart and lung failure. Low mixed venous oxygen saturation resulting from decreased cardiac function can occasionally lead to a low arterial oxygen saturation if the lungs cannot raise the oxygen saturation to normal as the markedly desaturated blood traverses the lungs. This is seen only if there is significant shunting of blood in the lungs away from ventilated alveoli. In this case, a decrease in cardiac output in a patient with a large pulmonary shunt can lead to a reduction in arterial PO_2 without any change in the severity of the patient's lung disease. This cause of arterial hypoxemia—low cardiac output and large pulmonary shunt—is uncommon but important to remember.

Noninvasive Measurement of PO_2 and PCO_2

Through oximetry, light-emitting and light-receiving sensors quantitate the amount of light absorbed by oxygenated/deoxygenated hemoglobin in arterial blood. Usually, the sensors are in a clip placed on a finger or ear lobe. The equipment should have a method to evaluate the arterial waveform (an actual waveform or bar code) to eliminate inaccurate data caused by vasoconstriction, low blood volume, shock or any impairment to peripheral circulation.[6] Ear and finger oximetry are frequently substituted for arterial blood gas measurements in the circumstance in which one is most interested in the PO_2 and oxygen saturation and for use in titrating the oxygen up to a specified saturation. Occasionally, ear oximetry or finger oximetry measurements require confirmation with blood gas determinations.

Measurement of end-tidal PCO_2 is limited to patients with an artificial airway present. Actual measurements of exhaled gas allow for an estimation of arterial PCO_2. This method of measurement requires expensive monitoring sets and frequent recalibration. Further development of this technique will bring a wider application of end-tidal PCO_2 monitoring to the bedside.

Arterial Blood Gas Analysis

To definitively determine the scope of pulmonary gas exchange, a direct measure of values is obtained by arterial blood sampling. Arterial blood gases (ABGs) allow for measurement of pH (and therefore acid–base balance), oxygenation, carbon dioxide levels, bicarbonate levels,

oxygen saturation, and base excess or deficit. ABG analysis is indicated to assess the nature, course, and severity of metabolic and respiratory disorders. The procedure requires some skill but, done properly, has little risk. Complications, occurring 0.58% of the time, include vasovagal episodes, localized pain, and small hematomas.[7]

Measuring pH in the Blood

The pH is the negative logarithm of the hydrogen ion concentration, and therefore of the acidity or alkalinity of the blood.[8] A normal pH is 7.35 to 7.45. As hydrogen ions accumulate, the pH drops, resulting in acidemia (acidotic state of the blood). A decrease in hydrogen ions results in an elevation of the pH and alkalemia (an alkalotic state of the blood).

Conditions leading to acidemia or alkalemia are influenced by a multitude of physiologic processes. Some of these processes include respiratory and renal function, tissue oxygenation, circulation, substance ingestion, and electrolyte loss from the gastrointestinal tract (because of vomiting or diarrhea). The identification of a pH variance should lead to the investigation of possible contributing factors.

Measuring Oxygen in the Blood

There are three ways to measure oxygen in blood:

- oxygen content, which is the number of milliliters of oxygen carried by 100 ml of blood;
- the PO_2, or pressure exerted by oxygen dissolved in the plasma;
- the oxygen saturation of hemoglobin, which is a measure of the percentage of oxygen that hemoglobin is carrying related to the total amount the hemoglobin could carry, or

$$O_2 \text{ sat} = \frac{\text{amount of oxygen that hemoglobin is carrying}}{\text{maximal amount of oxygen that hemoglobin can carry}} \times 100$$

The first of these methods is the easiest to understand but the most difficult to measure, so it is not used routinely. The last two methods, which are used routinely, are more understandable if compared with the first method (Table 18–2).

The majority of oxygen carried by the blood is carried by hemoglobin, and a very small amount is dissolved in plasma. The percentage saturation of hemoglobin with oxygen, then, gives a close estimate of the total amount of oxygen carried in blood.

The PO_2 measurement, however, tells only of the pressure exerted by the small amount of oxygen that is dissolved in plasma.

PO_2 is widely used, and it is valuable because PO_2

TABLE 18–2
How Oxygen is Carried in Blood

Dissolved in plasma:	0.3 ml/100 ml blood (reflected by PO_2 90 mg Hg)
Combined with Hgb:	19.4 ml/100 ml blood (reflected by O_2 sat Hgb 97%)
Total in whole blood:	19.7 ml/100 ml blood

(pressure of oxygen dissolved in plasma) and oxygen saturation of hemoglobin (which is closely related to the total oxygen content of whole blood) are related to each other in a definite fashion, and the relation is documented in the *oxyhemoglobin dissociation curve* (see Chapter 17). If the PO_2 in plasma is high, hemoglobin carries much oxygen. If the PO_2 is low, hemoglobin carries less oxygen. Once this relation is known, PO_2 is just as valuable as a measurement of total O_2 content or the percentage of oxygen that hemoglobin is carrying.

Oxygen Content

Oxygen content refers to the total amount of oxygen that is present in blood in any form. Oxygen is carried in blood in only two ways: (1) dissolved in the plasma, and (2) combined with hemoglobin. By far the larger amount of oxygen is carried in combination with hemoglobin, and a very small amount is dissolved in plasma. Oxygen is not very soluble in plasma or water, so only a very small amount can dissolve in plasma. Oxygen content and oxygen saturation of hemoglobin are indicators of the *amount* of oxygen in blood and in the red blood cells, respectively. Normal O_2 content is 19.7 ml O_2 per 100 ml of whole blood.

PO₂ Measurement

The oxygen that is combined with hemoglobin exerts no pressure, but the oxygen that is dissolved in plasma exerts a pressure or tension that can be readily measured and is known as PO_2. The oxyhemoglobin dissociation curve defines the relation between the pressure exerted by dissolved oxygen and the amount of oxygen carried by hemoglobin. It should be made quite clear, though, *that PO_2 is a measure of the pressure or tension exerted by dissolved oxygen and that PO_2 is not a measure of the amount of oxygen in blood.*

Partial Pressure and Barometric Pressure

An explanation of PO_2 must start with an explanation of barometric pressure. Barometric pressure can be thought of as the weight of the atmosphere or the pressure exerted by the atmosphere. At sea level, barometric pressure is 760 mm Hg. We are not conscious of the weight or pressure exerted on us by the atmosphere, partly because the atmosphere is made up of gases. If we dive into water, we are much more aware of the weight or pressure exerted on us

by the water, and this pressure increases as we dive deeper because there is progressively more water above us. Just as in water, the deeper we are in the atmosphere, the higher the barometric pressure. At the top of Pike's Peak (elevation 14,110 feet above sea level) we are near the top of the atmosphere and the barometric pressure is lower—425 mm Hg. Denver (elevation 5,280 feet above sea level) and other cities at similar elevations are between these two extremes. The average barometric pressure in Denver is 625 mm Hg. Of course, as weather fronts approach, the barometric pressure can fluctuate slightly even though the elevation is constant. With high-pressure weather fronts, the barometric pressure can increase by 5 to 10 mm Hg, and with low-pressure fronts the barometric pressure can fall by 5 to 10 mm Hg. In blood gas laboratories, a barometer is necessary for determining the barometric pressure each day.

If one takes a bottle in which a vacuum has been created, inverts this bottle in a pan of water, then removes the cork from the bottle, the water in the pan rises in the bottle (Fig. 18–1). The force that makes the water rise in the bottle is the difference between the barometric pressure exerted on the pan and the absence of barometric pressure in the vacuum bottle.

If we substitute a long tube for the bottle, create a vacuum in the tube, and invert the tube in a container of mercury instead of a pan of water, we have a barometer. Because the vacuum in the tube remains constant, the only factor influencing how high the mercury rises in the tube is the barometric pressure (or weight of the atmosphere) pressing down on the mercury in the container.

Table 18–3 is a simplified explanation of why the arterial PO_2 in Denver is about 72 mm Hg and at sea level about 95 mm Hg.

It should be pointed out that the percentage of oxygen in the atmosphere is 21% (actually 20.93%) everywhere in the atmosphere and that changes in PO_2 with altitude are due to changes in barometric pressure and not to changes in percentage of oxygen present.

Oxygen Saturation of Hemoglobin

Each gram of hemoglobin can carry a maximum of 1.34 ml of oxygen. The percentage of saturation of hemoglobin is defined as the amount of oxygen that hemoglobin *is* carrying compared with the amount of oxygen that hemoglobin *can* carry, expressed as a percentage:

$$\text{Percent } O_2 \text{ saturation of Hgb} = \frac{\text{Amount } O_2 \text{ Hgb is carrying}}{\text{Amount } O_2 \text{ Hgb can carry}} \times 100$$

Because the amount of oxygen that hemoglobin can carry is a constant 1.34 ml/g,

$$1.34 \text{ ml} \times \text{g Hgb} \times \% \text{ saturation Hgb} = \text{No. of ml } O_2 \text{ that Hgb is carrying}$$

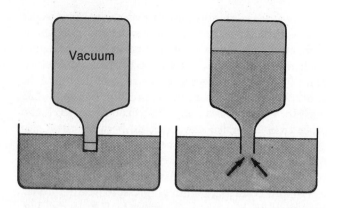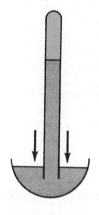

FIGURE 18–1
Effects of barometric pressure.

(It should be noted that there are rare, abnormal types of hemoglobin that cannot carry 1.34 ml of oxygen per gram. There also are rare situations in which normal hemoglobin has been poisoned so that it cannot carry 1.34 ml of oxygen per gram—eg, with sulfhemoglobin or methemoglobin.)

In 100 ml of blood
$$\begin{cases} 1 \text{ g Hgb can carry } 1.34 \text{ ml } O_2 \\ 15 \text{ g Hgb can carry } 15 \times 1.34 \text{ ml } O_2 \end{cases}$$

In Denver, the normal oxygen saturation of hemoglobin in arterial blood is 93% (ie, hemoglobin is carrying 93% of the total amount of oxygen it can carry). Ninety-three percent of 20.1 ml equals 18.7 ml of oxygen carried by hemoglobin in Denver. At sea level, arterial oxygen saturation of hemoglobin is 97%, so hemoglobin is carrying 97% of 20.1 ml, or 19.4 ml of oxygen.

The major factor that determines how much oxygen hemoglobin is carrying is the PO_2 to which the hemoglobin is exposed. At high PO_2, hemoglobin carries more

oxygen; at low PO_2 hemoglobin, carries less oxygen. The exact relation between the amount of oxygen that hemoglobin is carrying and the PO_2 is described by the oxyhemoglobin dissociation curve.

A–a Oxygen Gradient, a/A Ratio, and Fraction of Inspired Oxygen (FIO_2). One should always relate the oxygen content of blood to the FIO_2. For instance, an oxygen saturation of hemoglobin of 96% is normal if the patient is breathing room air, which has an FIO_2 of 21, but is quite abnormal if the FIO_2 is 40. It is useful to calculate the A–a oxygen gradient and a/A ratio for every blood gas. However, much the same information can be obtained if one compares the arterial PO_2 or oxygen saturation with the FIO_2 that the patient is receiving and also looks at the PCO_2 to see the amount of ventilation required to produce the PO_2. The capital "A" is used to designate the alveolus, and the lower-case "a" is used to designate the artery.

The A–a oxygen gradient is the difference between PO_2 in alveolar air and PO_2 in arterial blood. PO_2 is always higher in the alveolus. One calculates the alveolar PO_2 by

TABLE 18–3
Comparison of PO_2 at Sea Level with PO_2 above Sea Level (>5,000 ft)

At Sea Level	At Denver	Remarks
760	630 mm Hg	Average barometric pressure
−47	−47 mm Hg	Water vapor pressure at body temperature (subtracted because in the body this pressure is exerted by water vapor)
713	583 mm Hg	Corrected barometric pressure (in body or completely humidified air at body temperature)
×21%	×21%	Percent of O_2 in the atmosphere
150 mm Hg	123 mm Hg	PO_2 in air that is completely humidified
−40	−36	PCO_2—pressure exerted by CO_2 in alveolus
110 mm Hg	87 mm Hg	PO_2 in alveolus
−5 mm Hg	−5 mm Hg	Gradient for diffusion of O_2 from alveolus into capillary
105 mm Hg	82 mm Hg	PO_2 in capillary blood in lungs
−10 mm Hg	−10 mm Hg	Due to venous shunting
95 mm Hg	72 mm Hg	PO_2 in arterial blood

making several assumptions, and although the result may not be precise, it is accurate enough to be quite useful clinically. One can estimate the alveolar PO_2 at the bedside by

- subtracting the water vapor pressure from barometric pressure;
- multiplying the resulting pressure by the patient's FIO_2;
- subtracting from this $1\frac{1}{4}$ times the patient's arterial PCO_2.

These calculations give the alveolar PO_2. If the arterial PO_2 is subtracted from the alveolar PO_2, the A–a oxygen gradient has been calculated. Frequently, a computer is used to calculate a/A ratios and A–a gradients.

The A–a oxygen gradient is most useful for patients breathing room air, because normal values are well established. An example of the usefulness of the A–a oxygen gradient is in a patient suspected of having a pulmonary embolus, for which arterial hypoxemia is often used as a screening test. However, hyperventilation (which is common in patients with pulmonary emboli) can raise the arterial PO_2 into the normal range. The A–a oxygen gradient remains abnormal and suggests pulmonary embolus even if the PO_2 is normal. For example, a patient at sea level breathing room air with a PO_2 of 85 and PCO_2 of 20 still has a widened A–a gradient of 40 (normal value is less than 20), suggesting pulmonary embolus. The normal range for A–a oxygen gradient increases with age. In young people, the A–a oxygen gradient can normally be as high as 15 mm Hg, whereas in elderly people it can normally be as high as 27 mm Hg. Often, a range of less than 20 is used to encompass all age groups.

The a/A ratio is the percentage of alveolar PO_2 that arterial PO_2 represents. In the preceding example and in Figure 18–2, the a/A ratio is as follows:

$$\frac{\text{Patient's measured arterial } PO_2}{\text{Patient's calculated alveolar } PO_2}$$

$$\frac{90}{100} = 0.9$$

The normal a/A ratio is greater than 0.75.

Abnormal A–a oxygen gradients and a/A ratios are seen in patients with right-to-left shunting, ventilation/perfusion mismatching, and diffusion abnormalities. In patients who are receiving oxygen, the a/A ratio is more useful than the A–a gradient, because the A–a gradient increases as the patient's FIO_2 increases. The a/A ratio does not vary as the FIO_2 is changed. In patients on ventilators, one can change the FIO_2 and still look at the a/A ratio to determine whether oxygen transfer is improving or worsening.

As shown in Table 18–4, the normal values for oxygen in arterial blood in Denver or any other place above sea level are lower than those at sea level, because there is progressively lower PO_2 in the ambient air as one ascends.

$$PAO_2 \quad \text{minus} \quad PaO_2 = \text{A} - \text{a Oxygen Gradient}$$

$$\left(\begin{matrix}\text{Barometric}\\ \text{pressure}\end{matrix}\right) - \left(\begin{matrix}\text{Water vapor}\\ \text{pressure}\end{matrix}\right) \times \left(\begin{matrix}\text{Patient's}\\ FIO_2\end{matrix}\right) - (1\tfrac{1}{4}) \times \left(\begin{matrix}\text{Patient's}\\ \text{Arterial}\\ PCO_2\end{matrix}\right) - \begin{matrix}\text{Patient's}\\ \text{Arterial}\\ PO_2\end{matrix} = \begin{matrix}\text{A} - \text{a Oxygen}\\ \text{Gradient}\end{matrix}$$

Example: In a patient at sea level, breathing room air (FIO_2) with PO_2 of 90 and PCO_2 of 40, this is how the A – oxygen gradient is easily calculated:

$$(760 - 47) \times (.21) - (1\tfrac{1}{4}) \times (40) \quad - \quad 90 \quad =$$

$$(713 \times .21) - 50 \quad - \quad 90 \quad =$$

$$150 - 50 \quad - \quad 90 \quad =$$

$$100 \quad - \quad 90 \quad = \quad 10$$

FIGURE 18–2
A–a oxygen gradient: difference between PO_2 in alveolus and PO_2 in arterial blood.

DISPLAY BOX 18–3
*Determinants of a/A Ratios
and A–a Oxygen Gradients*

- Right-to-left shunts
- Diffusion abnormalities
- Ventilation/perfusion mismatching

Measuring Carbon Dioxide in the Blood

The PCO_2 refers to the pressure or tension exerted by dissolved CO_2 gas in the blood. The PCO_2 is influenced *only* by respiratory causes. Although this is an oversimplification, remember that PCO_2 *is influenced only by the lungs.*

Carbon dioxide is present only in very tiny amounts in the air we breathe. It comes directly from foods we eat. As a result of metabolism for the production of energy, foods are converted by the body tissues to water and CO_2 gas. If the pressure of CO_2 in the cells exceeds 45 mm Hg (the normal arterial value is 35–45 mm Hg), the CO_2 spills over from the cells into the plasma. In plasma, CO_2 can combine with H_2O to form H_2CO_3 (carbonic acid), but there is actually 800 times as much CO_2 in the form of dissolved gas in plasma as is converted to H_2CO_3.

CO_2 gas should be considered an acid substance, because if it combines with water, an acid is formed—carbonic acid, H_2CO_3.

H_2CO_3 dissociates into hydrogen ion, H^+, and bicarbonate, HCO_3^-. Much of the H^+ forms a loose association with the plasma proteins (ie, it is buffered), thereby reducing the amount of free H^+.

The body has to get rid of the waste product, CO_2, and can do so in two ways:

- The less important way is conversion of the CO_2 gas to carbonic acid, H_2CO_3, which dissociates into H^+ and HCO_3^-. The H^+ is excreted by the kidneys, mainly in the form of NH_4^+.
- A much more important way is expulsion of the CO_2 by lungs.

Getting rid of CO_2 gas, then, is one of the main functions of the lungs, and a very important relation exists between the amount of ventilation and the amount of PCO_2 in blood. If the PCO_2 in blood (ie, the dissolved CO_2 gas in blood) is too high, it means that the lungs are not providing enough ventilation. This is called *hypoventilation.* One can therefore detect hypoventilation by finding high levels of PCO_2 in the blood. If the PCO_2 is too low, there is excessive ventilation by the lungs, or *hyperventilation,* and if the PCO_2 is normal, there is exactly the right amount of ventilation.

PCO_2 is much more important than PO_2 in the determination of whether there is normal ventilation, hyperventilation, or hypoventilation, because there are other factors (eg, shunting and diffusion abnormalities) that lower the PO_2 without reducing ventilation.

Measuring Bicarbonate and Base Excess

The term *base excess* refers principally to bicarbonate but also to the other bases in blood (mainly plasma proteins and hemoglobin). Bicarbonate and base excess are influenced *only* by nonrespiratory causes, not by respiratory causes. Again, this is a simplification, but a very important fact to remember—*bicarbonate and base excess are influenced only by nonrespiratory processes.*

TABLE 18–4
Oxygen Values Above Sea Level vs. Sea Level

	Denver	Sea Level
Arterial Blood O_2		
Oxygen content	18.9 ml O_2/100 ml of blood	19.7 ml O_2/100 ml of blood
PO_2	70 mm Hg (range 65–75)	>80 mm Hg
O_2 saturation of Hgb	93% (range 92%–94%)	≥95%
Mixed Venous Blood O_2		
Oxygen content	14–16 ml O_2/100 ml of blood	14–16 ml O_2/100 ml of blood
PO_2	35–49 mm Hg	35–49 mm Hg
O_2 saturation of Hgb	70–75%	70–75%
Ratios and Gradients		
a/A ratio	>.75	>.75
A–a oxygen gradient	<20	<20

DISPLAY BOX 18–4
PCO₂, The Respiratory Parameter

PCO_2 = pressure (tension) of dissolved CO_2 gas in blood; influenced only by respiratory causes

$$Food \xrightarrow[\text{by body}]{\text{converted}} H_2O + CO_2 + energy$$

$$CO_2 + H_2O \rightleftharpoons H_2CO_3 \rightleftharpoons HCO_3^- + H^+$$
Normal PCO_2 = normal ventilation
High PCO_2 = hypoventilation
Low PCO_2 = hyperventilation

DISPLAY BOX 18–5
Normal Arterial Blood Gas Values

pH	7.35–7.45
PO_2	80–100 mm Hg
O_2 Sat	≥95%
PCO_2	35–45 mm Hg
HCO_3^-	22–26 mEq/L
BE	−2 to +2

For our purposes we can define a *metabolic process* as anything other than respiratory causes that affects the patient's acid–base status. Examples of common metabolic (nonrespiratory) processes are diabetic acidosis and uremia.

Normally, HCO_3^- is 22 to 26 mEq/L and the base excess is −2 to +2. If a nonrespiratory process leads to the accumulation of acids in the body or to loss of bicarbonate, bicarbonate values drop below the normal range, and base excess values become negative. However, if a nonrespiratory process causes loss of acid or accumulation of excess bicarbonate, bicarbonate values rise above normal, and base excess values become positive. Base excess can be thought of as representing an excess of bicarbonate or other base. Bicarbonate, then, is base or, in other words, an alkaline substance.

Procedure for Obtaining ABGs

Refined techniques for electrode measurement of arterial blood gases have allowed for rapid laboratory analysis of acid–base imbalances. In the 1960s, ABG specimens were obtained only by physicians. Since the 1970s nurses have been safely obtaining arterial specimens.[9]

The procedure, although basically standardized nationally, varies slightly among institutions. Arterial puncture is considered an advanced skill taught to all critical care nurses. Table 18–5 describes the basic technique, but each nurse should check for any institutional variation.

Do not change the patient's oxygen supplements just before obtaining a sample. Changes to the oxygen delivery systems can require 15 minutes for adaptation. The exception to this rule is during resuscitative efforts.

Recent developments in gas analysis equipment have brought ABG analyzers into the ICU. Nurses involved with this equipment require extra training and must be familiar with all quality control measures involved in the equipment calibration.

Interpretation of Results

Blood Gas Analysis

Normal Values

Normal values for blood gases are listed in Display Box 18–5. Notice that only two measurements, PO_2 and PCO_2, are actually measurements of gases. However, all of these values should be determined in blood gas analyses. It is imperative that a measure of the nonrespiratory (metabolic) component be included, and actual HCO_3^- and base excess are the most useful.

Older persons have values for PO_2 and oxygen saturation near the lower part of the normal range, and younger people tend to have high normal values.

The main emphasis in this discussion is on acid–base interpretation. An acid is any substance that can donate a hydrogen ion, H^+, which can be thought of as the most important part of an acid.

Many substances may include H^+ in their chemical structure, but some cannot donate the H^+ because it is

DISPLAY BOX 18–6
Definitions

Acid: A substance that can donate hydrogen ions, H^+. Example:

$$H_2CO_3 \longrightarrow H^+ + HCO_3^-$$
(acid)

Base: A substance that can accept hydrogen ions, H^+. All bases are alkaline substances. Example:

$$HCO_3^- + H^+ \longrightarrow H_2CO_3$$
(base)

TABLE 18–5
Procedure for Drawing Blood for Arterial Blood Gas Analysis

A. Equipment

1. 5- or 10-ml glass syringe or plastic syringe with vented plunger
2. 10-ml bottle of heparin, 1000 units/ml (multi-dose)
3. No. 22 needle or no. 25 disposable needle (short bevel)
4. Rubber airtight cap
5. Alcohol swab
6. Container of ice (emesis basin or plastic bag)
7. Request slip on which to write patient's clinical status, etc., including
   a. Name, date, time
   b. Whether receiving O_2, and if so show how much and by what route
   c. Temperature

B. Technique

1. Radial artery is generally preferred, although brachial may be used.
2. If a radial approach is used, perform an Allen's test. Simultaneously occlude the radial and ulnar arterial flow. The hand will blanch to pale. Release the ulnar artery flow. A positive Allen's test will return the hand to pink. This ensures arterial flow if the radial artery is no longer patent.
3. Wrist is hyperextended and arm is externally rotated.
   a. Very important to have wrist hyperextended—usually a folded towel under the wrist accomplishes this.
   b. For brachial artery puncture, elbow is hyperextended after placing elbow on towels.
4. 1 ml of heparin is aspirated into the syringe, barrel of the syringe is wet with heparin, and then excess heparin is discarded through the needle, with care taken so that the hub of the needle is left full of heparin and there are no bubbles.
5. Brachial or radial artery is located by palpation with index and long fingers, and point of maximum impulse is found. Clean the site with alcohol.
6. Needle is slowly inserted into the area of maximal pulsation. This is easiest with the syringe and needle approximately 45–90° to the skin.
7. Often the needle goes completely through both sides of the artery and only when the needle is slowly withdrawn does the blood gush up into the syringe.

8. The only certain indication that arterial blood is obtained is pumping of the blood up into the syringe under its own power.
   a. If one has to aspirate blood by pulling on the plunger of syringe—as is sometimes required with a tighter fitting plastic syringe—it is impossible to be positive that blood is arterial. *The blood gas results do not allow one to determine whether blood is arterial or venous.*
9. After 5 ml of blood are obtained, the needle is withdrawn and the assistant puts constant pressure on site of arterial puncture for at least 5 min (10 min if patient is anticoagulated).
10. Any air bubbles should be squirted out of the syringe. Remove the needle and place airtight rubber stopper on syringe. Roll the syringe between palms to mix the heparin.
11. The syringe is labeled and immediately placed into ice or ice water, then taken to the laboratory.
12. Note:
    a. If O_2 saturation is also measured, this provides a cross-check for accuracy of the PO_2 (use PO_2 and pH to calculate O_2 saturation on blood gas slide rule and see whether this calculated O_2 saturation agrees with the measured O_2 saturation plus carboxyhemoglobin (calculated O_2 saturation = measured O_2 saturation + carboxyhemoglobin).
    b. If CO_2 content is also measured, this provides a cross-check for accuracy of PCO_2. (Use PCO_2 and pH to calculate CO_2 content on blood gas slide rule and see whether this calculated CO_2 content agrees with the measured CO_2 content.)
    c. Another way to ensure accuracy is to run the tests in duplicate on two different blood gas analyzers. If there is a discrepancy in the two determinations, the test must be run a third time.
    d. The technician performing analysis should report any suspicion that results are not reliable. For instance:
       1) If syringe comes with air bubbles in it.
       2) If calculated O_2 saturation and measured O_2 saturation do not agree.
       3) If calculated CO_2 content and measured CO_2 content do not agree.

---

too tightly bound. Only those substances that can give up their H^+ are acids.

Bases are substances that can accept or combine with H^+. The terms *base* and *alkali* are used interchangeably.

The pH measurement is the only way to determine whether the body is too acid or too alkaline. Low pH numbers (below 7.35) indicate an acid state, and high pH numbers (above 7.45) indicate an alkaline state.

If the number is lower than 7.35, there is acidemia, and if it is higher than 7.45, alkalemia is present. Acid*emia*

refers to a condition in which the *blood* is too acid. Acid*osis* refers to the *process* in the patient that causes the acidemia. The adjective for the process is acid*otic.* Alkal*osis* refers to the *process* in the patient that causes the alkal*emia,* and the adjective for this process is alkal*otic.*

This much attention has been given to defining the terms because there can be more than one process occurring in a patient at the same time. For instance, if both an acidosis and an alkalosis are occurring at once, the pH indicates which is the stronger of the two processes. The

---

DISPLAY BOX 18–7
Acid–Base Terms

---

pH measurements: Only way to tell if body is too acid or too alkaline
  Acidemia: Acid condition of the blood—pH <7.35
  Alkalemia: Alkaline condition of the blood—pH >7.45
  Acidosis: Process causing acidemia
  Alkalosis: Process causing alkalemia

---

pH is below 7.35 if the acidosis is the stronger, above 7.45 if the alkalosis is the stronger, and between 7.35 and 7.45 if the acidosis and alkalosis are of almost equal strength. The pH value of blood represents an average of the acidoses and alkaloses that are occurring.

Respiratory Parameter: PCO_2

As seen in Table 18–6, there are only two abnormal conditions associated with abnormalities in PCO_2: respiratory acidosis (high PCO_2) and respiratory alkalosis (low PCO_2). See Display Box 18–8.

Respiratory Acidosis

The term *respiratory acidosis* means elevated PCO_2 due to hypoventilation. The causes of respiratory acidosis (high PCO_2) are listed in Display Box 18–9.

It should be noted that *respiratory* acidosis can occur even with normal lungs if the respiratory center is depressed.

Respiratory Alkalosis

The term *respiratory alkalosis* means low PCO_2 due to hyperventilation. The causes are hypoxia, congestive heart failure, anxiety, pulmonary emboli, pulmonary fibrosis, pregnancy, hyperventilation with mechanical ventilator, gram-negative septicemia, hepatic insufficiency, brain injury, salicylates, fever, asthma, and severe anemia. In gram-negative septicemia, the hyperventilation can precede

TABLE 18–6
Respiratory Abnormalities

Parameter	Condition	Mechanism
↑ PCO_2	Respiratory acidosis	Decreased elimination by lungs of CO_2 gas (hypoventilation)
↓ PCO_2	Respiratory alkalosis	Increased elimination by lungs of CO_2 gas (hyperventilation)

DISPLAY BOX 18–8
Signs and Symptoms of Acid–Base Disorders

Acid–Base Disorder	Signs & Symptoms
Respiratory Acidosis	Signs of CO_2 narcosis: headache, lethargy, drowsiness, coma, increased heart rate, hypertension, sweating, decreased responsiveness, tremulousness/asterixis, papilledema, dyspnea (may or may not be present)
Respiratory Alkalosis	Vague symptoms: dizziness, numbness, tingling (parasthesia) of the extremities, muscle cramps, tetany, seizures, increases in deep tendon reflexes, arrhythmias, hyperventilation
Metabolic Acidosis	Kussmaul breathing, Hypotension, Lethargy, Nausea and vomiting
Metabolic Alkalosis	Nonspecific: hyperactive reflexes, tetany, hypertension, muscle cramps, weakness

---

other evidence of septicemia. In patients with congestive heart failure, pneumonia, asthma, pulmonary emboli, and pulmonary fibrosis, the hyperventilation (respiratory alkalosis) continues even if the hypoxia is corrected; thus, hypoxia is not the only cause in these conditions.

Nonrespiratory (Metabolic) Parameters: HCO_3^- and Base Excess

As seen in Table 18–7, there are only two abnormal conditions associated with abnormalities in HCO_3^- or base excess: metabolic alkalosis and metabolic acidosis. See Display Box 18–8.

DISPLAY BOX 18–9
Causes of Respiratory Acidosis (↑ PCO_2)

- Obstructive lung disease
- Oversedation and other causes of reduced function of the respiratory center (even with normal lungs)
- Neuromuscular disorders
- Hypoventilation with mechanical ventilator
- Other causes of hypoventilation: pain, chest wall deformities, etc.

DISPLAY BOX 18–10
Causes of Respiratory Alkalosis (↓ PCO_2)

Hypoxia
Nervousness and anxiety
Pulmonary embolus, fibrosis, etc.
Pregnancy
Hyperventilation with mechanical ventilator
Brain injury
Salicylates
Fever
Gram-negative septicemia
Hepatic insufficiency
Congestive heart failure
Asthma
Severe anemia

Metabolic Alkalosis

The *causes* of metabolic alkalosis (increased HCO_3^- and base excess) are (1) loss of acid-containing fluid from the upper gastrointestinal tract, as by nasogastric suction or vomiting (this loss of acid from the stomach leaves the body with a relative excess of alkali); (2) rapid correction of chronic hypercapnia (it takes the body several days to correct its compensation for hypercapnia—accumulation of excess HCO_3^-—after the hypercapnia is suddenly relieved); (3) diuretic therapy with mercurial diuretics, ethacrynic acid, furosemide, or thiazide diuretics; (4) Cushing's disease; (5) treatment with corticosteroids (ie, prednisone or cortisone); (6) hyperaldosteronism; (7) severe potassium depletion; (8) excessive ingestion of licorice; (9) Bartter's syndrome; (10) alkali administration; and (11) nonparathyroid hypercalcemia.[10]

A rare cause of nonrespiratory alkalosis, which unfortunately is not reflected by an elevated bicarbonate in the blood, is the intravenous infusion of phenytoin (Dilatin), which has a very alkaline pH. Infusion of this alkaline substance causes a short-lived alkalemia not associated with elevated HCO_3^-. Any condition that is associated with a reduction in blood volume (eg, the preceding examples 1 and 3) is said to cause a contraction alkalosis because of a contraction of blood or plasma volume.

Hypokalemia and Hypochloremia. The first three causes of alkalosis listed—fluid losses from the stomach, rapid correction of chronic hypercapnia, and diuretic therapy—will all show correction of the alkalosis in response to administration of sodium chloride. Treatment with potassium chloride may be more reasonable if the potassium is low or if one is trying to prevent accumulation of salt and water. Treatment with two other diuretics, spironolactone (Aldactone) and triamterene (Dyrenium), does not cause metabolic alkalosis. With causes 4 through 9 in the accompanying list, the metabolic alkalosis cannot be corrected by administration of sodium chloride. With the last two causes listed, the response of sodium chloride is variable.

The following is an explanation of the relation between hypokalemia (low K^+), hypochloremia (low Cl^-), and metabolic alkalosis. Normally, in the kidney, sodium (Na^+) and chloride (Cl^-) pass from the blood into the urine at the glomerulus. Further along, this Na^+, which is in the urine, must be reabsorbed from the urine into the kidney tubule cells and then into the blood.

Because Na^+ has a positive charge ($+$), if it is reabsorbed into the cells it must do one of two things:

TABLE 18–7
Metabolic Abnormalities

Parameter	Condition	Mechanism
↑ HCO_3^- or ↑ BE	Nonrespiratory (metabolic) alkalosis	1. Nonvolatile acid is lost; or 2. HCO_3^- is gained
↓ HCO_3^- or ↓ BE	Nonrespiratory (metabolic) acidosis	1. Nonvolatile acid is added (using up HCO_3^-); or 2. HCO_3^- is lost

- It can be reabsorbed with something that has a negative charge (−), such as Cl^-:

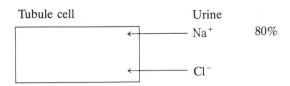

- It can enter the tubule cell in exchange for something else that has a positive charge, such as K^+ or H^+ (which passes from the tubule cell to the urine):

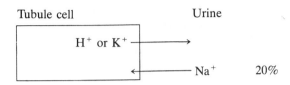

Normally, 80% of the Na^+ is reabsorbed in company with Cl^-, and 20% is exchanged for K^+ or H^+ (Fig. 18–3).

If there is hypochloremia ($\downarrow Cl^-$), the amount of Na^+ that is reabsorbed in the company of Cl^- is reduced, and more Na^+ must be exchanged for K^+ or H^+. If Na^+ is exchanged for K^+ and H^+, the loss of H^+ represents a loss of acid, leaving the patient alkalotic—therefore this is a hypochloremic alkalosis.

If Na^+ is exchanged for K^+ or H^+, only a small amount of K^+ is available; after this is used up, the patient becomes hypokalemic, and H^+ is lost. The loss of H^+ is a

---

DISPLAY BOX 18–11
Causes of Metabolic (Nonrespiratory) Alkalosis ($\uparrow HCO_3^-$)

Fluid losses from upper GI tract—vomiting or nasogastric tube causing loss of acid
Rapid correction of chronic hypercapnia
Diuretic therapy—mercurial, ethacrynic acid (Edecrin), furosemide (Lasix), thiazides
Cushing's disease
Therapy with corticosteroids (prednisone, cortisone, etc)
Hyperaldosteronism
Severe potassium depletion
Excessive ingestion of licorice
Bartter's syndrome
Alkali administration
Nonparathyroid hypercalcemia

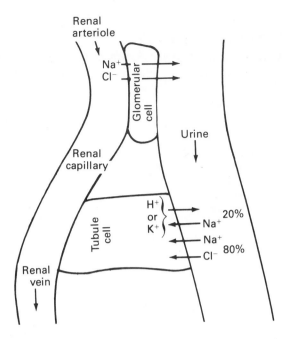

FIGURE 18–3
Process by which low Cl^- and low K^+ can cause metabolic alkalosis.

loss of acid, leaving the patient with an alkalosis—hypokalemic alkalosis.

Metabolic Acidosis

Substances that have a negative charge are attracted to an anode and are called *anions*. The anions that are normally measured (specified) are HCO_3^- and Cl^-. The anions that are not regularly measured but are normally present in blood are called *unspecified* or *unmeasured* anions. They are phosphates, sulfates, creatinates, and proteinates.

The causes of nonrespiratory (metabolic) acidosis (low HCO_3^- and low base excess) can be divided into those causes in which there is an increase in the unspecified anions and those causes in which bicarbonate has been lost and there is no such increase in unspecified anions. (See Display Box 18–12.)

An increase in unspecified anions can be due to accumulation of phosphates, sulfates, and creatinates, as seen in renal failure, or the accumulation of an unusual negatively charged substance such as lactic acid or ketoacids. Often, the unspecified anions are referred to as the *anion gap*. This is obtained by subtracting the sum of HCO_3^- and Cl^- concentration from Na^+ concentration. The normal value is 12 ± 3; if one finds a difference greater than 15, there is said to be an increase in unspecified anions (increased anion gap). Conditions causing this are diabetic ketoacidosis, alcoholic ketoacidosis, poisonings (salicylate, ethylene glycol, methyl alcohol, paraldehyde), lactic acidosis, and renal failure. In these cases, there is accumulation of or ingestion of an unusual acid.

DISPLAY BOX 18–12
Causes of Metabolic Acidosis (↓ HCO_3^- and ↓ BE)

Anion Gap:
With Increase in Unspecified Anions
    Diabetic ketoacidosis
    Starvation ketoacidosis
    Alcoholic ketoacidosis
    Poisonings
      Salicylate
      Ethylene glycol
      Methyl alcohol
      Paraldehyde (rarely)
    Lactic acidosis
    Renal failure

Non-anion Gap:
Without Increase in Unspecified Anions
    Diarrhea
    Drainage of pancreatic juice
    Ureterosigmoidostomy
    Obstructed ileal loop
    Therapy with acetazolamide (Diamox)
    Therapy with ammonium chloride
      (NH_4Cl)
    Renal tubular acidosis
    Intravenous hyperalimentation (rarely)
    Dilutional acidosis

Conditions that cause a metabolic acidosis *without an increase in unmeasured anions* are associated with a high serum chloride. These conditions are diarrhea, drainage of pancreatic juice, ureterosigmoidostomy, obstructed ileal loop, treatment with acetazolamide (Diamox), renal tubular acidosis, treatment with ammonium chloride or arginine hydrochloride, and intravenous hyperalimentation. In most of these latter conditions, there is a deficit of bicarbonate, leaving relatively too much acid.

In all the anion gap conditions, there is an accumulation of an abnormal acid substance in blood, which then reacts with and uses up some of the usual amount of bicarbonate, leaving the patient with reduced levels of bicarbonate and reduced base excess.

One of the most important causes of metabolic acidosis is *lactic acidosis*. Whenever body tissues do not have enough oxygen, they lose their ability to metabolize lactic acid, which then accumulates in the blood. This lactic acid then combines with some of the normal amount of bicarbonate, using up the bicarbonate.

Cardiac arrest is a classic example of lactic acidosis. Other conditions that can be associated with lactic acidosis are shock, severe heart failure, and severe hypoxemia. Tissue hypoxia, seen in all these conditions, leads to the lactate production.

If a patient has a metabolic acidosis with an anion gap of greater than 15, the nurse can ask the laboratory technician to measure whichever unspecified anion might be elevated; for example, if the patient is an uncontrolled diabetic, ketoacids should be measured; if the patient is in shock, lactic acid should be measured.

CO_2 Content

PCO_2 is a respiratory parameter, a gas, and an acid, and it is regulated by the lungs. HCO_3^- and base excess are both nonrespiratory parameters occurring in solution; they are bases (alkaline substances), and they are regulated mainly by the kidneys (not by the lungs). To summarize:

PCO_2—Respiratory Parameter

Gas

Acid

Regulated by the lungs

HCO_3^- or Base Excess—Nonrespiratory Parameter

Solution

Base

Regulated mainly by the kidneys

Where does the CO_2 content fit in this scheme? Determination of electrolytes consists of Na^+, K^+, Cl^-, and CO_2. In this case CO_2 is an abbreviation for CO_2 content, which is composed mainly of bicarbonate; if the term *CO_2 content* were used, it would improve understanding. Note that in conversation CO_2 is sometimes used to mean CO_2 content (mainly bicarbonate) and sometimes to mean CO_2 gas. This double use of the term CO_2 is one of the main difficulties in understanding acid–base problems. One should use the terms *CO_2 content* and *CO_2 gas* to avoid confusion. Better yet, some hospitals are reporting HCO_3^- in place of CO_2 content if electrolytes are ordered.

Display Box 18–13 shows that CO_2 content is mainly bicarbonate (HCO_3^-) and, to a lesser extent, dissolved CO_2 gas. The normal value of CO_2 content, 25.2 mEq/L, consists of 24 mEq/L of HCO_3^- and 1.2 mEq/L of dissolved CO_2 gas. The 1.2 mEq/L of dissolved CO_2 gas is expressed in different terminology: PCO_2 of 40 mm Hg equals 1.2 mEq/L. For changing mm Hg to mEq/L, the conversion factor is 0.03, so 40 mm Hg × 0.03 = 1.2 mEq/L.

HCO_3^-/CO_2 Ratio. In Display Box 18–13, the ratio of HCO_3^- to PCO_2 is 24 : 1.2, or 20 : 1. The body

---

DISPLAY BOX 18–13
CO$_2$ Content

HCO$_3^-$	24	mEq/L
Dissolved CO$_2$ gas	1.2 mEq/L	= 40 mm Hg PCO$_2$
CO$_2$ content	25.2 mEq/L	

---

always tries to keep this ratio of HCO$_3^-$ to PCO$_2$ stable at 20:1. That is, the ratio of alkali (HCO$_3^-$) to acid (PCO$_2$) is normally 20:1. As long the ratio remains 20:1, the pH remains normal. If bicarbonate (HCO$_3^-$) or base excess increases, there is alkalosis, causing the pH to rise. If HCO$_3^-$ or base excess falls, there is acidosis, and the pH falls. If the pH change is due mainly to change in bicarbonate (or base excess), it is said to be due to nonrespiratory (metabolic) causes.

Just the opposite happens with PCO$_2$, which, remember, is an acid substance. If the PCO$_2$ rises, there is an acidosis, causing the pH to fall. If the PCO$_2$ falls, there is an alkalosis, and the pH rises. *If the pH change is due mainly to changes in PCO$_2$, it is said to be due to respiratory causes.*

As seen in Display Box 18–14, acid–base abnormalities can be separated into just four categories for easier understanding. First, they are divided by pH into either alkalemia or acidemia. Next, they are subdivided into either nonrespiratory (metabolic) or respiratory causes. This is the procedure used in interpreting acid–base abnormalities.

pH Factor

pH and Alkalemia. If pH is high, there is an alkalemia. There are two types of alkalemia.

- In *nonrespiratory alkalemia*, the primary abnormality is an increase in bicarbonate. An example

of this is overingestion of bicarbonate or baking soda.
- In *respiratory alkalemia*, the primary abnormality is hyperventilation with loss of CO$_2$ gas. CO$_2$ gas is an acid substance; if it is lost (due to hyperventilation), an alkalosis occurs. An example is a hyperventilation attack in a nervous person.

pH and Acidemia. If the pH is low, there is an acidemia, of which there are just two types.

- In *nonrespiratory acidemia*, the primary abnormality is loss of HCO$_3^-$, usually due to reaction with excessive metabolic acids. An example is diabetic acidosis in which ketoacids accumulate; these acids then react with the normal amount of HCO$_3^-$, using up HCO$_3^-$ and leaving HCO$_3^-$ and base excess levels low.
- In *respiratory acidemia*, there is an accumulation of CO$_2$ gas (high PCO$_2$), an acid substance. An example is a patient with acute respiratory failure who *hypo*ventilates because his airways are obstructed by mucus. In respiratory acidosis there is an accumulation of volatile acid (CO$_2$ gas), but in nonrespiratory acidosis the acids that accumulate are not gases.

pH and Combined Acidosis/Alkalosis. There can be more than one primary acid–base disturbance occurring at the same time. Occasionally, two disturbances are of equal magnitude, and if one is an acidosis and the other an alkalosis, they balance each other and the pH remains normal. Or there can be several acidoses, for instance, occurring at the same time, all adding their effects to make the pH more acidemic than one alone would.

pH Compensation and Correction. There are two ways in which an abnormal pH can be returned toward normal: compensation and correction (Display Box 18–15).

In *compensation*, the system not primarily affected is responsible for returning the pH toward normal. For example, if there is respiratory acidosis (high PCO$_2$) the

---

DISPLAY BOX 18–14
Causes of Alkalemia and Acidemia

Types		Primary Abnormality
Alkalemia (high pH)	Nonrespiratory (metabolic)	↑ HCO$_3^-$
	Respiratory	↓ PCO$_2$
Acidemia (low pH)	Nonrespiratory (metabolic)	↓ HCO$_3^-$
	Respiratory	↑ PCO$_2$

DISPLAY BOX 18–15
Compensation Versus Correction of Acid–Base Abnormalities

In both: Abnormal pH is returned toward normal.

Compensation: Abnormal pH is returned toward normal *by altering the component not primarily affected;* that is, if PCO$_2$ is high, HCO$_3^-$ is retained to compensate.

Correction: Abnormal pH is returned toward normal *by altering the component primarily affected;* that is, if PCO$_2$ is high, PCO$_2$ is lowered, correcting the abnormality.

kidneys *compensate* by retaining bicarbonate to return the ratio between HCO_3^- and PCO_2 to 20:1; when the ratio is 20:1, the pH is normal.

Compensation is complete only in chronic respiratory alkalosis. In the other acid–base disorders, the pH is returned almost but not completely to normal, because the compensation is not complete.

In *correction*, the system primarily affected is repaired, returning the pH toward normal. For example, if there is respiratory acidosis (high PCO_2) vigorous bronchial hygiene and bronchodilators can improve ventilation and lower PCO_2, returning the pH toward normal.

In most cases, physicians, nurses, and paramedics are more interested in correcting the abnormality than in helping the body compensate. In both compensation and correction, the pH is returned toward normal. The body tries hard to maintain a normal pH because the various enzyme systems in all organs function correctly only if the pH is normal. According to newer terminology, *acute* respiratory acidosis means *uncompensated; chronic* respiratory acidosis means *compensated*.

Compensatory Mechanisms for Acid–Base Abnormalities

The body compensates for the various acid–base abnormalities by trying to return the ratio between HCO_3^- and PCO_2 to 20:1—for if this ratio is 20:1, the pH is normal. If the primary process is respiratory, the compensating system is metabolic, and vice versa. If the lungs compensate for a nonrespiratory abnormality, compensation occurs in hours, but the kidneys take 2 to 4 days to compensate for a respiratory abnormality.

Remember, the PCO_2 in mm Hg must be converted to mEq/L by multiplying it by 0.03 before trying it in the 20:1 ratio; for example, PCO_2 of 40 mm Hg $\times$ 0.03 = 1.2 mEq/L.

In *primary respiratory acidosis*, characterized by elevated levels of PCO_2 (an acid), the system at fault is the respiratory system, and compensation occurs through metabolic process. To compensate, the kidneys excrete more acid and less HCO_3^-, thus allowing levels of HCO_3^- to rise, returning the ratio of HCO_3^- to PCO_2 toward 20:1, and therefore returning pH toward normal (Table 18–8).

If the PCO_2 is high (respiratory acidosis) but the pH is normal, it means that the kidneys have had time to retain HCO_3^- to compensate for the elevated PCO_2 and that the process is not acute (has been present at least a few days to give the kidneys time to compensate). Usually, the body does not fully compensate for respiratory acidosis.

In *primary respiratory alkalosis*, characterized by low PCO_2, compensation occurs through metabolic means. The kidneys compensate by excreting HCO_3^-, thus returning the ratio of HCO_3^- to PCO_2 back toward 20:1; this compensation by the kidneys takes 2 to 3 days.

Of the four acid–base abnormalities, it is only in compensation for respiratory alkalosis that the body is able to return the ratio to 20:1 and return pH entirely to normal.

In *primary metabolic acidosis*, the major abnormality is low HCO_3^- (or low base excess). In most cases excess acids, such as ketoacids in diabetic ketoacidosis, have reacted with the normal amounts of HCO_3^-, using up some of the HCO_3^- and leaving a low level of HCO_3^-. The body compensates by hyperventilating, thus lowering the PCO_2 so that the ratio of HCO_3^- to PCO_2 returns toward 20:1. Because the compensating system is the lungs, compensation can occur in hours. However, if the metabolic acidosis is severe, the lungs may not be able to blow off enough CO_2 gas to compensate fully. Actually, in metabolic acidosis the body never compensates fully (never gets the ratio back to 20:1 or the pH back to 7.40).

In *metabolic alkalosis* (ie, presence of excess HCO_3^-), the body compensates with the respiratory system by hypoventilating so that PCO_2 rises and the ratio of HCO_3^- to PCO_2 is returned toward the normal of 20:1, therefore returning the pH to normal. The body is usually unable to compensate completely for metabolic alkalosis.

In this instance, respiratory compensation is by hypoventilation, and this occurs over one or several hours. Hypoventilation allows PCO_2 to rise only to a maximum of 50 to 60 mm Hg before other stimuli of ventilation, such as hypoxia, take over to prevent further hypoventilation.

In compensating for one abnormality, high HCO_3^-, the body creates another abnormality, high PCO_2, but in doing so brings the ratio between HCO_3^- and PCO_2 to 20:1, allowing the pH to return to normal in spite of two abnormalities. These two abnormalities balance each other.

ABG Data Analysis Applied to Clinical Practice

Oxygen Transport to the Tissues

The amount of oxygen that is transported to the tissues is more important than the PO_2. The PO_2 is a measure of intensity or pressure due to oxygen, and oxygen content is a measure of amount of oxygen.

$$O_2 \text{ transport to the tissues} = \text{arterial } O_2 \text{ content} \times \text{cardiac output}$$

The oxygen transported to the tissues depends on (1) the amount of oxygen in arterial blood (arterial oxygen content), and (2) the ability of the heart to pump this blood containing oxygen around to the tissues.

The arterial oxygen content depends in turn on (1) how well the lungs are able to get oxygen from air into the blood, and (2) a normal amount of functioning hemoglobin to carry the oxygen.

Assessment: Respiratory System 421

TABLE 18–8
Compensation for Acidosis and Alkalosis

Parameter	Normal	Abnormal* (Uncompensated)	Compensated
Respiratory Acidosis			
HCO₃⁻ mEq/L	24	24	36
PCO₂ mEq/L	1.2	1.8	1.8
PCO₂ mm HG	40	60	60
ratio	20:1	13:1	20:1
pH	7.40	7.23	7.40
Respiratory Alkalosis			
BE	0	+2.5	−5
HCO₃⁻ mEq/L	24	24	18
PCO₂ mEq/L	1.2	0.9	0.9
PCO₂ mm Hg	40	30	30
ratio	20:1	27:1	20:1
pH	7.40	7.52	7.40
Metabolic Acidosis			
BE	0	−17	−10
HCO₃⁻ mEq/L	24	12	12
PCO₂ mEq/L	1.2	1.2	0.6
PCO₂ mm Hg	40	40	20
ratio	20:1	10:1	20:1
pH	7.40	7.11	7.40
Metabolic Alkalosis			
BE	0	+13	+9
HCO₃⁻ mEq/L	24	36	36
PCO₂ mEq/L	1.2	1.2	1.8
PCO₂ mm Hg	40	40	60
ratio	20:1	30:1	20:1
pH	7.40	7.57	7.40

*The primary abnormality is in the enclosed box.

In summary, oxygenation of the tissue depends on the following:

1. Arterial O₂ content, which depends on
   a. lung's ability to get O₂ into blood
   b. ability of hemoglobin to hold enough O₂
2. Cardiac output (circulation)

Tissue Hypoxia

There are varied pulmonary and nonpulmonary causes for tissue hypoxia, which results from insufficient oxygenation.[11] Four pulmonary reasons can be listed to explain why arterial blood may not be carrying the normal amount of oxygen.

1. Alveolar hypoventilation: associated with high PCO₂.

2. Diffusion defect (at alveolar–capillary level): associated with low or normal PCO₂.
3. Right-to-left shunt (in lung or heart): associated with low or normal PCO₂.
4. Mismatching of ventilation and blood flow in the lungs: associated with low or normal PCO₂. (Blood goes by alveoli that are poorly ventilated. This blood, as it passes through the lungs, picks up little oxygen. This poorly oxygenated blood then returns to the heart and is pumped out through the arteries to the body, thus causing arterial blood to have less than the normal amount of oxygen; see Chapter 17.)

The nonpulmonary causes of tissue hypoxia are (1) reduced blood flow to the tissues (reduced cardiac output); (2) anemia—not enough hemoglobin to carry oxygen; (3) nonfunctioning hemoglobin—enough hemoglobin, but hemoglobin that exists cannot carry oxygen because it has been "poisoned"; and (4) right-to-left cardiac shunts—most frequently seen in cyanotic congenital heart disease.

1. *Reduced blood flow* to the tissues (reduced cardiac output) can be caused by
    a. myocardial infarction
    b. abnormal cardiac rhythm
    c. reduced cardiac function from other causes (eg, congestive heart failure, valvular heart lesion)
    d. hypovolemia (intimately related to anemia)
2. *Anemia*: One gram of hemoglobin carries 1.34 ml O_2, and normally there are 15 g Hgb to carry 15 × 1.34 ml O_2, or 20.1 ml O_2. If there is anemia such that only 7.5 g Hgb are present, 7.5 × 1.34 ml O_2 = 10 ml O_2 are all that can be carried. If anemia is milder (between 7.5 and 15 g Hgb), more O_2 can be carried; if anemia is more severe (less than 7.5 g Hgb), even less O_2 can be carried. Usually the body compensates for anemia by tachycardia, which circulates the blood faster.
3. *Nonfunctioning hemoglobin*: A few rare conditions exist in which there is a normal amount of hemoglobin, but even this normal amount cannot function because it has been poisoned. Some examples of this are:
    a. carbon monoxide poisoning
    b. methemoglobinemia
    c. sulfhemoglobinemia
    In each of these situations, something (eg, carbon monoxide) has combined with hemoglobin, making it hard for oxygen to combine with and be carried by this hemoglobin.
4. In *right-to-left cardiac shunts*, oxygen gets through the lungs normally into the bloodstream, there is enough functioning hemoglobin to carry the oxygen, and the heart is strong enough to circulate the oxygenated blood. However, some venous blood that never passes through the lungs to get oxygenated is *shunted* into the systemic arterial system, and the combination of oxygenated blood plus venous unoxygenated blood is carried through the arteries to the tissues, supplying them with less oxygen than they need.

Compensatory Mechanisms

The patient who is hypoxemic compensates for hypoxia in the following ways:

- tachypnea (rapid breathing);
- tachycardia (rapid heartbeat);
- erythrocytosis (high hemoglobin and hematocrit).

The tachypnea and tachycardia represent extra energy expenditure by the patient. Erythrocytosis simply means increased production of red blood cells by the hypoxic patient's bone marrow in an attempt to get more oxygen to the tissues. If the fault is lack of enough red blood cells, this can be remedied. However, if the fault is in getting enough oxygen through the lungs, increasing the number of red blood cells helps little or not at all. The hypoxemic patient tries all these means of compensating for hypoxemia, and often all of them together are inadequate.

Hypoxia often leads to pulmonary hypertension (high blood pressure in the arteries of the lungs), and this can lead to strain or failure of the right side of the heart.[12]

pH As a Determinant

We first look at the pH to see which side of 7.40 it is on. Even though it is in normal range, pH is usually either above or below 7.40. If the pH is above 7.40, the primary process is probably alkalosis, and if below 7.40, the primary process is probably acidosis. For example:

pH	7.42
PCO_2	52 mm Hg—respiratory acidosis
HCO_3^-	33 mEq/L—metabolic alkalosis

Which is the primary process, respiratory acidosis or metabolic alkalosis? If one consults Figure 18–4, one finds that these numbers can be interpreted in either of two ways, for they fit into two 95% confidence bands—that is, those for chronic (fully compensated) metabolic alkalosis and chronic (fully compensated) respiratory acidosis. How-

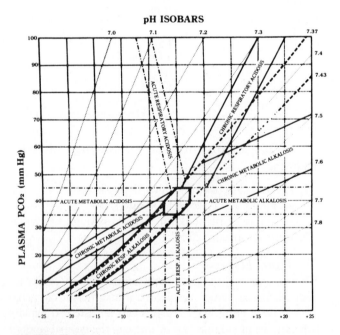

FIGURE 18–4
Ninety-five percent confidence limits of respiratory or metabolic compensation.

ever, following our rule, we see that the pH, although normal, is tending toward alkalemia. Therefore, the primary process is probably alkalosis, and this is a metabolic alkalosis with nearly complete compensation. Often, it is clinically obvious which is the primary abnormality, but sometimes this is not the case.

It must be pointed out that there can be more than one *primary* acid–base abnormality. For example, if there is both a respiratory and a nonrespiratory acid–base abnormality, instead of one compensating for the other, both can be acidoses or both alkaloses, in which case the pH deviates more from normal than if either of the abnormalities were present alone. Here is an example of blood gases to interpret:

Example 1

pH	7.24
PCO₂	38 mm Hg
HCO₃⁻	15.5 mEq/L
BE	−11

Coronary care nurses deciphering a dysrhythmia are taught to first find the P wave; in trying to interpret an acid–base abnormality, one must look first at the pH to determine whether there is an alkalemia or an acidemia. Here we have an acidemia because the pH is low.

Next, look at the PCO₂ to see whether there is a respiratory abnormality. Here there is no abnormality; the PCO₂ is normal.

Next, look at either HCO₃⁻ or base excess to determine whether there is a metabolic abnormality. The HCO₃⁻ and the base excess are low, indicating a metabolic acidosis. We have an acidemia caused by a metabolic acidosis.

Consulting Figure 18–4, one sees that the example falls in the area labeled acute (uncompensated) metabolic acidosis.

Next is a tougher example:

Example 2

pH	7.20
PCO₂	55 mm Hg
HCO₃⁻	20.5 mEq/L
BE	−8

First, look at the pH to see whether there is an alkalemia or an acidemia. Here the pH is low, indicating an acidemia.

Does the PCO₂ indicate a respiratory abnormality? Yes, PCO₂ is high, indicating respiratory acidosis.

Does the HCO₃⁻ or BE indicate a nonrespiratory abnormality? Yes, HCO₃⁻ and BE are low, indicating nonrespiratory (metabolic) acidosis.

Therefore, this is an acidemia caused by combined respiratory and metabolic acidoses.

Consulting Figure 18–4, one sees that this example falls in the area between acute metabolic acidosis and acute respiratory acidosis, indicating that both are occurring.

The Nomogram

The foregoing is all that is necessary to solve most acid–base problems. Some experts feel that the use of confidence limits is a big help or even a necessity in solving acid–base problems. This concept is briefly discussed here and can help explain some of the intricacies of acid–base problems. The use of a nomogram is also presented.

Some of the statements made in the preceding sections are true most of the time but not all of the time. For instance, according to the equation $CO_2 + H_2O \rightleftharpoons HCO_3^- + H^+$, elevations of PCO_2 raise the $HCO_3s]^-$ solely because of the chemical reaction. Several days later, the HCO_3^- is elevated further because the kidneys excrete less HCO_3^- in an effort to compensate.

Ninety-five percent confidence limits have been compiled so that if, for example, the primary problem is chronic respiratory acidosis (fully compensated respiratory acidosis), one can look up the level of HCO_3^- that would be expected in 95% of the cases of chronic respiratory acidosis.

In the nomogram, base excess values are plotted on the horizontal axis and PCO_2 values are plotted on the vertical axis; pH isobars are the sweeping lines of small dots. Cohen, the author who produced this figure, prefers the narrow range of 7.37 to 7.43 for the normal pH range instead of 7.35 to 7.45. Cohen plotted 95% confidence bands for the acute and chronic (uncompensated and compensated) forms of each of the four basic acid–base disturbances. If one knows any two of the three parameters (pH, PCO_2, BE), one can calculate the third and also name the process and determine whether it is acute, chronic, or somewhere in between. Without using the 95% confidence limits or consulting the nomogram, one could occasionally miss the less obvious part of a combined acid–base problem.

Computer Interpretation

Based on the information shown in Figure 18–4, a computer program for acid–base interpretation has been developed. Computer interpretation of acid–base disorders, if combined with calculation of A–a gradients and a/A ratios, and particularly if severely abnormal values are "flagged," is an extremely useful tool in alerting all members of the health care team that immediate action must be taken. The interpretive statements, combined with the printing of severely abnormal values in bold print, clearly indicate to the nurse or therapist that the physician must be called immediately to initiate corrective action. In some institutions, computer-generated reports have given the nurse and therapist the impetus and authority to notify the physician and to see that corrective action is taken.

Management of Hypoxemia

Oxygen Therapy

If oxygen is administered to the patient to treat hypoxemia, tachypnea and tachycardia do not occur, there is no erythrocytosis, and pulmonary hypertension may go away. Complete compensation is possible with oxygen treatment, but sometimes patient compensation is not complete.

It can be seen that supplemental oxygen is rational treatment for the patient with hypoxemia, but long-term continuous oxygen is usually reserved for the patient who, when completely stable, has an oxygen saturation below 85% and who also has one or more of the following:

- right heart failure difficult to manage with digitalis and diuretics
- significant secondary erythrocytosis
- a progressive downhill course with weight loss, progressive muscle wasting, or decreased mental function.

Often such a patient responds to nocturnal oxygen (oxygen for 8 hours at night). If the patient is living at a high altitude, a move to a lower altitude can make supplemental oxygen unnecessary.

Possible CO_2 Retention. Oxygen treatment can lead to CO_2 retention if the oxygen is not carefully controlled.

There are two major reflex stimuli to breathing:

- CO_2 retention (hypercapnic stimulus to breathe), and
- low PO_2 (hypoxic stimulus to breathe).

Small elevations of PCO_2 are a major stimulus to breathing. Increasing the PCO_2 by 4 mm Hg can cause a 100% increase in ventilation. Large elevations in PCO_2 reduce the amount of ventilation by reducing all brain functions including function of the respiratory center.

In patients with large elevation of PCO_2, hypoxemia can be the most important stimulus to breathing. If a patient who no longer has a hypercapnic stimulus to breathing is treated with oxygen, thereby eliminating the hypoxic stimulus to breathe, he or she may breathe even less, significantly worsening the condition. It has become apparent that administration of a controlled amount of oxygen (just enough to raise the PaO_2 to approximately 60 mm Hg) allows the patient to benefit from the oxygen and usually does not reduce ventilation.

It should be clear that oxygen therapy, although often given in a haphazard fashion, requires just as much understanding and precision in dosage as any other form of drug therapy.

Oxygen supplementation can be employed by mask, cannula, tent (pediatrics), or mechanical ventilation. (See Chapter 19.)

Management of Acid–Base Abnormalities

It is important to realize that the body's compensation is only an effort to return the pH toward normal, and the primary abnormality is not corrected. The medical team's definitive treatment is aimed at correcting the primary abnormality.

Metabolic alkalosis (excess HCO_3^-) is treated by getting rid of excess HCO_3^- rather than just allowing PCO_2 to rise and normalize the ratio. Excess HCO_3^- can be corrected by giving the patient acetazolamide (Diamox) to make the kidneys excrete more HCO_3^- or, more commonly, by giving KCl to allow the kidneys to excrete K^+ and Cl^- rather than acids. Sometimes ammonium chloride (NH_4Cl), arginine hydrochloride, or even dilute hydrochloric acid (HCl) is given to react with the excessive HCO_3^-, thereby correcting the metabolic alkalosis.

Respiratory alkalosis (low PCO_2) is treated by having the patient stop hyperventilating. This can be accomplished with sedation.

Metabolic acidosis, in which excess acids have used up HCO_3^- or HCO_3^- has been lost, is treated by supplying HCO_3^- in the form of sodium bicarbonate ($NaHCO_3^-$) orally or intravenously while also treating the cause of acid accumulation or HCO_3^- loss. Multiplying the body weight (in kg) by the deficiency of HCO_3^- (in mEq/L) by 0.3 gives a rough guide to the amount of $NaHCO_3^-$ (in mEq) that should be administered. A 60-kg patient with an HCO_3^- of 4 would be given 360 mEq $NaHCO_3^-$, or

$$24 - 4 = 20 \times .3 \times 60 = 360$$

Administration of large doses of $NaHCO_3^-$ can give the patient a large osmotic load, which can be more detrimental than the acidemia and result in severe alkalosis. Therefore, metabolic acidosis is not usually treated with $NaHCO_3^-$ unless the pH is below 7.25.

Respiratory acidosis (high PCO_2) is treated by increasing ventilation, enabling the lungs to expel CO_2. Although *overtreatment* can occur, *overcompensation* by the body usually does not occur. In fact, complete compensation seldom occurs, so that instead of the ratio returning to 20:1, it returns to almost 20:1, and instead of the pH returning to 7.40, it returns almost to that point.

Summary

The essential need for patients to be comfortable with their breathing makes respiratory assessment a high priority for all critically ill patients. This assessment requires a multitude of data. Each component—the respiratory history, the physical examination, and the diagnostic tests—contributes valuable information. The integration of this data into an action plan and management decisions gives the nurse a framework for the care provided.

REFERENCES

1. Swartz M: Textbook of Physical Diagnosis, pp 214–217. Philadelphia, WB Saunders, 1989
2. Brenner M, Welliver J: Pulmonary and acid–base assessment. Nurs Clin North Am 25:761–770
3. Bates B: A Guide to Physical Examination and History Taking, pp 249–251. New York, JB Lippincott, 1991
4. Voyce S, et al: Pulmonary artery catheters, p 62. In Rippe J, et al: Intensive Care Medicine. Boston: Little, Brown & Co, 1991
5. Mims B: Physiologic rationale of S$\bar{v}$O$_2$ Monitoring. Crit Care Nurs Clin North Am 1:619–627, 1989
6. Ehrhardt B, Graham M: Pulse oximetry: An easy way to check oxygenation. Nursing '90, pp 50–54, March, 1990
7. Irwin R: Arterial puncture of blood gas analysis. In Rippe J, et al: Intensive Care Medicine, pp 155–159. Boston, Little, Brown & Co, 1991
8. Brenner M, Welliver J: Pulmonary and acid–base assessment. Nurs Clin North Am 25:761–770
9. Irwin R: Arterial puncture of blood gas analysis. In Rippe J, et al: Intensive Care Medicine, pp 155–159. Boston, Little, Brown & Co, 1991
10. Irwin R: Physiologic approach to managing respiratory failure, pp 449–454. In Rippe J et al: Intensive Care Medicine. Boston, Little, Brown & Co, 1991
11. Bates D: Respiratory Function in Disease, p 191. Philadelphia, WB Saunders, 1989
12. Irwin R: Physiologic approach to managing respiratory failure, pp 449–454. In Rippe J et al: Intensive Care Medicine. Boston, Little, Brown & Co, 1991

BIBLIOGRAPHY

Ahrens T: Blood gas assessment of intrapulmonary shunting and deadspace. Crit Care Nurs Clin North Am 1:641–648, 1989

Clark J, Votteri B, Ariagno R, Cheung P, et al: Noninvasive assessment of blood gases. Am Rev Respir Dis 145:220–232, 1992

Hurray, J, Saver, C: Arterial blood gas interpretation: Improving perioperative skills. AORN J 55:180–185, 1992

STUDY QUESTIONS

1. Normal breath sounds that are heard over the periphery of the lung are called

   a. bronchial breath sounds
   b. bronchovesicular breath sounds
   c. vesicular breath sounds
   d. loud crackles

2. Mixed venous blood has an oxygen saturation that is

   a. 70% to 75%, which is lower than arterial blood
   b. 80% to 90%, which is lower than arterial blood
   c. 30% to 40%, which is lower than arterial blood
   d. 95% or greater, which is the same as arterial blood

3. This ABG analysis indicates which of the following conditions?

pH	7.31
PCO$_2$	48
PO$_2$	86
HCO$_3^-$	24
BE	−2

   a. respiratory alkalosis
   b. metabolic alkalosis
   c. metabolic acidosis
   d. respiratory acidosis

4. All of the following are symptoms of hypoxia except

   a. confusion and delirium
   b. sweating
   c. tachycardia
   d. vasodilatation

5. The primary abnormality in respiratory alkalosis is

   a. decreased PCO_2
   b. increased PCO_2
   c. decreased HCO_3^-
   d. increased HCO_3^-

6. Compared with a patient at sea level, the PO_2 of a patient at approximately 5,000 feet above sea level is

   a. increased
   b. decreased
   c. the same
   d. unaffected

Bronchial Hygiene

BEHAVIORAL OBJECTIVES

Based on the content in this section, the reader should be able to:

1. Outline a bronchial hygiene plan of care for a specific patient.
2. List and describe the advantages and disadvantages of intermittent positive pressure breathing (IPPB).
3. Describe advantageous positions for postural drainage of any lung field.

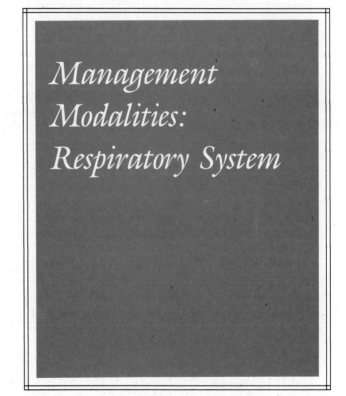

CHAPTER 19

Management Modalities: Respiratory System

Hudak: Critical Care Nursing:
A Holistic Approach, 6th ed. © 1994
J. B. Lippincott Company.

Description

Bronchial hygiene consists of any one or a combination of the following measures: inhaled bronchodilator therapy, aerosol therapy, deep-breathing maneuvers, coughing, and postural drainage. The therapeutic goals of bronchial hygiene are removal of secretions, improved ventilation, and oxygenation. Specific bronchial hygiene depends on existing pulmonary dysfunction.

The need for and the effectiveness of various modalities of bronchial hygiene must be assessed frequently. The evaluation process should be based on physical assessment, chest radiograph, measurement of arterial blood gases (ABGs), and additional sources of information as indicated.

The following discussion is not intended as a specific instructional guide for bronchial hygiene. Techniques of delivery of bronchial hygiene are paramount in the prevention and treatment of pulmonary complications (eg, retained pulmonary secretions in a chronic bronchitic who subsequently develops pneumonia). The nurse should integrate knowledge of normal airway anatomy and lung function as the techniques for the delivery of bronchial hygiene are developed. The nurse should concentrate on the primary phases of lung function that most techniques of bronchial hygiene aim to improve, namely, ventilation and diffusion (Fig. 19–1).

Effective Cough and Deep Breathing

An effective cough is a necessary prerequisite to clear secretions. The objectives of deep breathing and coughing are to promote lung expansion, mobilize secretions, and prevent the side effects of retained secretions (pneumonia, atelectasis, and fever).

Ideally, the patient is positioned upright on the edge of the bed or chair with the feet supported. He or she is instructed to take a slow, deep breath, hold it for at least 3 seconds, and exhale slowly. If secretions are auscultated, then a cough is initiated on maximum inspiration.

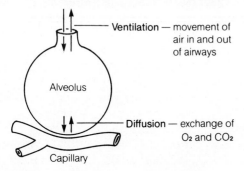

FIGURE 19–1
Primary lung functions: ventilation and diffusion.

There are incentive spirometers that encourage and quantify deep breathing by giving immediate visual feedback to the patient. Flow incentive spirometers consist of plastic chambers with freely moving ping-pong balls. The patient inhales through the mouthpiece of the spirometer to elevate the balls and keep them elevated for as long as possible. With this type of device, the inhaled volume is unknown. Volume incentive spirometers use the same method, but the amount of inspired volume is measured and presented in visual feedback to the patient.

Chest Physiotherapy

Chest physiotherapy consists of postural drainage, chest percussion, and chest vibration. Usually all three methods are used in sequence in different lung drainage positions followed by deep breathing and coughing.

Standard postural drainage positions are based on the anatomy of the lung segments (Fig. 19–2). The lung segments in the apices are above the level of the bronchi they drain into. The correct position to drain these segments is a semi-reclining position with the head up. In contrast, the bases of the lungs are below the level of the bronchi they drain into. To drain these segments, place the patient in the prone position with the hips higher than the head. To drain the right middle lobe and the lingula, place the patient in the supine position or on either side.

Chest percussion involves striking the chest wall with your hands. To percuss the chest, the hands are formed into a cupped shape by flexing the fingers and placing the thumb tightly against the index finger. Percussing the chest wall mechanically dislodges secretions.

The patient's position depends on the segment of lung to be percussed. A towel or pillow case is draped over the area to be percussed, and percussion is performed for 3 to 5 minutes per position. Never percuss over the spine, over the sternum, or below the thoracic cage. If performed correctly, percussion does not hurt the patient or redden the skin.

A clapping sound (as opposed to slapping) indicates correct hand position. Gallon[1] found that if percussion was included in the treatment regimen, the rate of sputum production was significantly greater.

Vibration increases the velocity and turbulence of exhaled air to loosen secretions. This technique is accomplished by placing your hands side by side with fingers extended over the chest area. After the patient inhales deeply, he or she slowly exhales. During exhalation, the chest is vibrated by quickly contracting and relaxing the muscles of your arms and shoulders. Vibration is used instead of percussion if the chest wall is extremely painful.

Stiller et al[2] found that patients treated with positioning, vibration, hyperinflation, and suctioning had a significantly higher resolution of their atelectasis than patients treated with suctioning and hyperinflation alone. Other studies[3] concluded that chest physiotherapy in medical

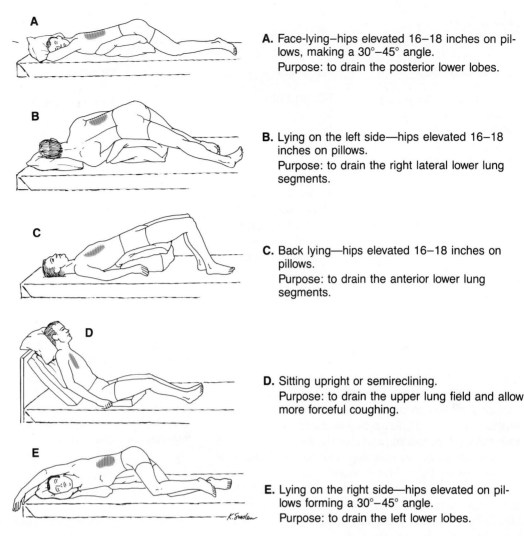

A. Face-lying–hips elevated 16–18 inches on pillows, making a 30°–45° angle.
Purpose: to drain the posterior lower lobes.

B. Lying on the left side—hips elevated 16–18 inches on pillows.
Purpose: to drain the right lateral lower lung segments.

C. Back lying—hips elevated 16–18 inches on pillows.
Purpose: to drain the anterior lower lung segments.

D. Sitting upright or semireclining.
Purpose: to drain the upper lung field and allow more forceful coughing.

E. Lying on the right side—hips elevated on pillows forming a 30°–45° angle.
Purpose: to drain the left lower lobes.

FIGURE 19–2
Positions used in lung drainage.

patients has consistently shown benefit only in patients who produce large amount of sputum. Among surgical patients, the only procedure that clearly reduces the incidence of postoperative pulmonary complications is repeated deep-breathing maneuvers.

Postural drainage is therapeutic positioning of the patient to enable pulmonary secretions to drain by gravity into the major bronchi and trachea. Once drained, these secretions are then expectorated. The position in which the patient is placed depends on which lung segment is involved. The segment to be drained is placed uppermost, with the mainstem bronchus as vertical as possible. The patient must be monitored carefully in the head down position for aspiration, dyspnea, or arrhythmias.

Special Considerations

Nursing personnel may not be trained to administer manual percussion and vibration. In addition, if the patient requires treatment at home, the family may not be available or able to perform chest physiotherapy. In this case, mechanical percussors are available that require very little instruction to use.

In the critical care setting, it may not be feasible to position the patient in all of the depicted lung drainage positions. For patients who cannot tolerate chest physiotherapy (Table 19–1), turning the patient every 2 hours aids in draining the lungs and prevents stagnation of secretions.

Patients with unilateral disease are positioned with the good lung down. Placed in this position, the good lung is better ventilated and perfused. Positioning the "bad" lung down is likely to cause hypoxemia with ventilation/perfusion mismatching and shunting. However, if the "bad" lung has a lung abscess, the preferred position is down. If an abscessed lung is in a gravity dependent position, its purulent contents can drain into the opposite lung. The healthy lung would then be contaminated by the abscessed lung, and gas exchange would most likely be affected.

TABLE 19–1
Contraindications for Chest Physiotherapy

Postural Drainage	Percussion	Vibration
Increased intracranial pressure	Fractured ribs	Same as percussion
Immediately after meals	Traumatic chest injury	
Inability to cough	Pulmonary hemorrhage or embolus	
Acute heart disease	Mastectomy	
Intravascular bleeds	Orthopedic appliances	
	Pneumothorax	
	Metastatic lesion of ribs	
	Osteoporosis	
	Cervical cord trauma	
	Unstable fractures	
	Abdominal trauma	
	Hiatal hernia	
	Obesity	

Bronchodilator Aerosol Therapy

The goals of bronchodilator therapy are to relax the airways, mobilize secretions, and reduce mucosal edema. Various methods to deliver bronchodilator therapy are available (Fig. 19–3). Regardless of the mode of delivery, assessment before, during, and after the therapy is essential.

Assessment before and after treatment includes bedside spirometry (V_T), breath sounds, pulse, and respiratory rate. The last two commonly increase during bronchodilator therapy and can remain elevated up to 1½ hours after treatment. ABG measurement can be indicated but does not take the place of the other assessments. Objective evaluation is crucial, but *subjective* information is also valuable. How does the patient feel? Is breathing better than before the treatment? Can the patient feel movement of air or medication in the lower part of the lungs? How long does the effectiveness of the treatments last? What, if any, are the side effects (eg, jitteriness, palpitations, inability to concentrate, increased heart rate), and how long do these symptoms last?

Inhaled Moisture

The primary purposes of inhaled moisture are hydration of normal mucociliary clearance mechanisms and liquefaction of secretions. Adequate systemic hydration is essential to obtaining optimal results of inhaled moisture.

The most important aspect of inhaled moisture therapy is active deep breathing by the patient, followed by brief breath-holding to allow deposition of aerosolized particles, and then slow, complete exhalation. One must also remember the importance of helping the patient assume the most effective position (being cognizant of any factors such as unstable vertebral fractures that might be

contraindications) to maximize ventilation and, therefore, depth of deposition of aerosolized particles.

Potential hazards include bronchospasm in patients with hyperreactive airways and infection from contaminated equipment. The ultimate success of inhaled moisture therapy depends on clearance of secretions with forceful, rigorous coughing.

Intermittent Positive Pressure Breathing (IPPB)

IPPB is used to improve alveolar ventilation and increase lung expansion. The primary indication is an inability on the part of the patient to generate inspirations of 15 to 20 ml/kg. Patients with restrictive disease or muscle fatigue benefit from IPPB therapy. See Table 19–2.

Successful IPPB treatments are determined by the patient's position, ventilatory pattern, and ability to cooperate and follow instructions.

An adequate ventilatory pattern during an IPPB treatment consists of a deep inspiration aimed at increasing normal tidal volume (V_T) by two to three times. The patient is then instructed to hold his or her breath briefly to provide greater depth and deposition of aerosolized medication, water, or saline. Exhalation should take twice as long as inspiration, resulting in complete exhalation.

If IPPB is indicated, the nurse must be aware of the importance of placing the patient in the most effective position (one that is not contraindicated by any underlying condition, such as unstable vertebral fractures) to facilitate maximal ventilation. The nurse should remain to guide the patient through the treatment.

The role of IPPB in respiratory care has diminished. More cost effective and simpler methods for aerosol medication administration, lung expansion, and secretion clearance have replaced this technique.

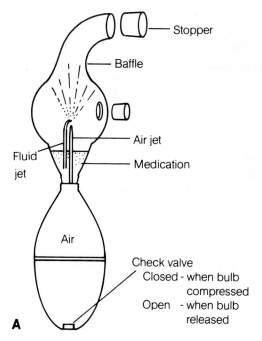

A

Hand-powered nebulizer

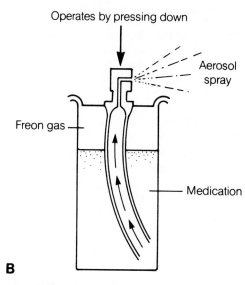

B

Pressurized aerosol cartridge

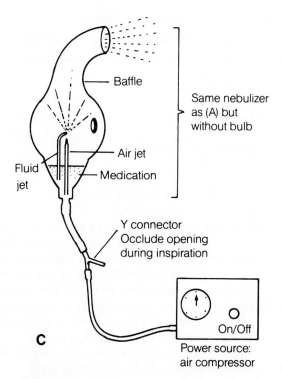

C

Compressor-driven nebulizer

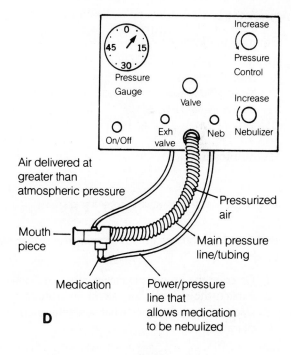

D

IPPB

FIGURE 19–3
Common devices for inhaled bronchodilator delivery.

TABLE 19–2
IPPB (Intermittent Positive Pressure Breathing)

Indications	Contraindications
Reduced vital capacity	Pneumothorax
Failure of simpler methods such as postural drainage and coughing, deep breathing and coughing, incentive spirometry, and hydration to expel secretions	Bullous emphysema
	Increased intracranial pressure
	Tracheoesophageal fistula
	Bronchopleural fistula
Restrictive disorders (ascites, interstitial disease, kyphoscoliosis)	Hypovolemia
Pulmonary edema	Increased dyspnea during treatment
Neuromuscular deficits	Hemoptysis
Sputum induction for tests	Immediately after lung resection; pneumonectomy
Medication delivery (especially in patients with severe hand deformities)	Active pulmonary TB
	Gastric reflux condition (tube feedings or meals within the last hour)

Artificial Airways

Behavioral Objectives

Description

Equipment Features

Airways
    Oral Pharyngeal
    Nasal Pharyngeal
    Endotracheal Tubes

Suctioning Procedure

Humidification

BEHAVIORAL OBJECTIVES

Based on the content in this section, the reader should be able to:

1. Describe the proper placement of an artificial airway.
2. Explain the rationale for care of an artificial airway.
3. Use proper techniques when suctioning an artificial airway.

Description

Rigorous bronchial hygiene and carefully monitored oxygen therapy can eliminate the need for an artificial airway or ventilatory support. If these measures fail to provide adequate oxygenation and removal of carbon dioxide, an artificial airway and ventilatory support become mandatory. Artificial airways have a fourfold purpose:

establishment of an airway

protection of the airway, with the cuff inflated

provision of continuous ventilatory assistance

facilitation of airway clearance.

Knowledgeable, aggressive nursing care is required for maintaining airway patency as well as maximizing therapeutic effects and minimizing damage to the patient's natural airway.

Equipment Features

The selection of the appropriate artificial airway is most important. Any artificial airway increases airway resistance; therefore, it is essential that the largest tube possible be used for intubation. The cuff on the endotracheal or tracheostomy tube must be of low compliance (soft) so that barotrauma to the trachea, vocal cords, and subglottic area is minimized. The competency of the cuff must be established before intubation. Approximately 10 cc of air is injected into the cuff before use. Figure 19–4 illustrates some frequently used artificial airways.

Airways

Oral Pharyngeal

If a patient becomes unconscious or is sedated and lying supine, the innervation of the genioglossal muscle is decreased, causing the tongue to occlude the airway. An oral or nasal pharyngeal airway maintains the air passage.

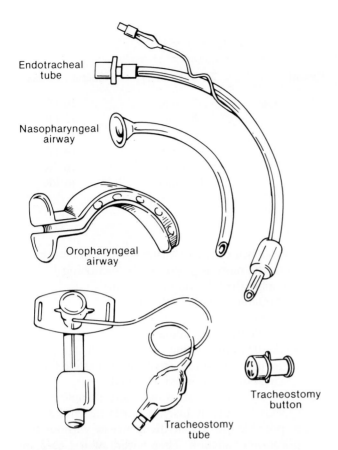

FIGURE 19–4
Five frequently used artificial airways.

Never attempt to place an oral pharyngeal airway in a conscious patient, because it stimulates the gag reflex and can cause vomiting and aspiration. Before placing an artificial airway, always make sure any possible obstruction is cleared. To insert an oral pharyngeal airway, three steps should be followed:

1. Gently open the patient's mouth using a crossed finger technique or a modified jaw thrust.
2. Hold the tongue down with a depressor and guide the airway over the back of the tongue. An optional method is to position the tip of the airway toward the roof of the mouth and gently advance the airway by rotating it 180 degrees.
3. After it is in place, tape the airway with two strips of tape across the top and bottom. Make sure there are no pressure points under the airway on the patient's mouth and that there is enough room for suctioning.

Nasal Pharyngeal

The nasal pharyngeal airway is a flexible tube that is inserted nasally past the base of the tongue to maintain airway patency. Patients with apneic sleep disorders can be taught to insert a nasal pharyngeal airway before bedtime.

To insert a nasal pharyngeal airway the following steps are used:

1. Determine and select the correct tube length by measuring from the tip of the nose to the earlobe. Use a tube with the largest outer diameter that will fit the patient's nostril.
2. Lubricate the tube with water or a soluble jelly.
3. Reassure patient and familiarize him or her with the procedure.
4. Insert the airway into the nostril up to the end of the nasal trumpet.
5. Have the patient exhale with the mouth closed. If the tube is in the correct position, air can be felt exiting from the tube opening. Open the patient's mouth, depress the tongue, and look for the tube's tip just behind the uvula.

To remove the pharyngeal airway, suction the oropharynx and gently remove the airway. The nasal airway may have to be gently rotated to withdraw it from the nares.

Endotracheal Tubes

An ET tube (endotracheal tube) is inserted if the patient needs ventilation or protection of the airway from aspiration. The equipment listed in Table 19–3 is assembled before intubation. Tracheal intubation must be performed by rigorously credentialed personnel to reduce the incidence of complications (Table 19–4).

Position the patient on his or her back with a small blanket under the shoulder blades. This hyperextends the neck and opens the airway. Before insertion, inject air into the endotracheal cuff to ensure the cuff is intact. Deflate the cuff. Confirm that the suction is properly working. Insert the stylet into the endotracheal tube, making sure the tip does not protrude beyond the tube. Lubricate the tube and assist the physician with the insertion. Once placed, inflate the cuff and auscultate the chest bilaterally for equal breath sounds. Insert a bite block or oral airway and secure with tape. Immediately obtain an portable chest x-ray to confirm proper tube placement.

TABLE 19–3
Tracheal Intubation Equipment

Laryngoscope with blades and intact bulb
Suction setup
Correct size endotracheal tube
Stylet
Lubricating jelly (water soluble)
Syringe for cuff inflation
Adhesive tape
4 × 4 gauze dressing
Magill forceps
Tongue blade

TABLE 19–4
Complications of Tracheal Intubation

Trauma
Nosocomial infection
Mechanical problems
Displacement of Tube:
• right mainstem intubation
• gastric intubation
Aspiration
Physiologic problems (tracheal necrosis)
Laryngeal damage and necrosis

TABLE 19–6
Endotracheal Tube Sizes

Patient	ET Tube Size	Suction Catheter
Adult Female	7.0 mm	10 FR
	8.0 mm	12 FR
	8.5 mm	14 FR
Adult Male	8.5 mm	14 FR
	9.0 mm	16 FR
	10.0 mm	18 FR

Endotracheal tubes can be inserted nasally or orally. See Table 19–5 for advantages and disadvantages and Table 19–6 for suggested sizes.

Suctioning Procedure

The presence of an artificial tube prevents the patient from coughing, which is the normal clearing mechanism. It also increases production of secretions because of the presence of a foreign object. Suctioning therefore becomes paramount in removal of secretions and maintenance of patency. The need for suctioning is determined by visual observation of secretions and, more importantly, by chest auscultation for determination of the presence of secretions or mucous plugs in major airways. The following suctioning procedure is recommended:

1. Hyperoxygenate the patient with 100% oxygen, using a bag or the ventilator. (This can be done while the nurse is preparing for suctioning.)
2. Assemble the following equipment:
   a. Atraumatic sterile catheter
   b. Glove
   c. Sterile irrigation container
   d. Sterile normal saline
   e. Syringe containing sterile normal saline for tracheal irrigation when indicated.
3. After the first two steps have been completed, quickly but gently insert a sterile catheter as far as possible into the artificial airway without application of suction. Then withdraw it 1 to 2 cm and apply intermittent suction while rotating and removing the catheter. The aspiration should not exceed 8 to 10 seconds. Prolonged aspiration can lead to severe hypoxemia, changes in pulmonary pressure and volume, and ultimately cardiac arrest.
4. Reestablish ventilatory assistance, allowing the pa-

TABLE 19–5
Airway Placement

Type	Advantages	Disadvantages
Nasal endotracheal	Patient comfort	Can kink and obstruct the airway
	Prevents tube obstruction from biting	Predisposes to nasal or sinus infection
	Easily anchored	Tube and cuff can cause tracheal damage
		High risk for shearing off nasal polyps in asthmatics
Oral endotracheal	Less trauma during intubation than nasally	Predisposes to mouth sores
	Permits use of a larger ET tube	Uncomfortable for patient
		Easily obstructed if not used with bite block
		Tube and cuff can cause tracheal damage
		Complicates effective oral hygiene
		Difficult to secure

Clinical Research

Czarnik R et al: Differential effects of continuous versus intermittent suction on tracheal tissue. Heart Lung 20(2):144–151, 1991

An animal subject study was performed to determine the difference in tracheal damage from the employment of continuous versus intermittent negative pressure endotracheal suctioning. Fifteen dogs were intubated and randomly assigned to receive either continuous or intermittent suctioning with a 14 F catheter. Both groups received 16 catheter passes, 15 minutes apart, over a four-hour period. The continuous suction was applied for 10 seconds during each catheter pass. The intermittent suction was applied 2 seconds with suction, 1 second without suction, for a total of 10 seconds during each catheter pass. The suction pressure was 200 mm Hg. Both groups studied had simple damage, ulceration, and ulceration with necrosis. The study concluded that both continuous and intermittent application of negative pressure during suctioning results in tracheal tissue damage.

---

tient to receive three to five breaths before the procedure is repeated.

It should be noted that patients not on ventilators also need to be hyperoxygenated. The patient should be instructed to take deep breaths while connected to a 100% oxygen source. Patients incapable of taking a deep breath should be assisted by a positive pressure device.

If secretions are tenacious, 3 to 5 ml of sterile normal saline may be injected into the artificial airway. Secretions should be monitored for amount, consistency, odor, and color, and the observations recorded. Changes in any of these characteristics can necessitate changes in therapy. Laboratory analysis of secretions must be performed based on patient assessment and response to existing therapy.

Humidification

An artificial airway excludes normal physiological airway humidification. Therefore, artificial humidification is essential to maintenance of airway patency and clearance of secretions. Determination of adequate airway humidification is based on the consistency and amount of secretions as well as condensation visible in the oxygen tubing leading to the patient. The humidification devices attached to oxygen therapy equipment often become media for bacterial growth. Appropriate care should therefore be taken in the maintenance of all oxygen therapy equipment. Policies should be established to monitor, by culture, the presence of organisms.

Chest Tubes

Behavioral Objectives

Physiological Principles

Chest Anatomy

Pleural Pressures

Equipment Features

Chest Tubes

Drainage Systems
    One-Bottle System
    Two-Bottle System
    Three-Bottle System
    Disposable Drainage Units
    Emerson Pleural Suction Pump

Indications for Chest Tube Placement

Procedure

Chest Tube Insertion

Chest Tube Removal

Assessment and Management

Positioning

Maintaining System Patency

Drainage Monitoring

Water Seal Monitoring

Complications

Dislodgement of Chest Tube

Based on the content in this section, the reader should be able to:

1. Describe the process by which intrapleural negative pressure is generated.
2. List several indications for chest tube placement.
3. Compare and contrast the one-, two-, and three-bottle chest tube drainage systems.
4. Discuss the nursing interventions necessary to prevent complications in a patient with a chest tube drainage system.
5. Describe the nursing actions required to maintain chest tube patency.
6. State three potential complications of chest tube stripping.

Physiological Principles

A short review of chest anatomy and pleural pressures is provided here for understanding of chest tubes and drainage systems.

Chest Anatomy

The chest consists of three compartments: the mediastinum, a right pleural cavity, and a left pleural cavity.

Each pleural cavity is lined with a thin, slippery membrane called the parietal pleura. A similar membrane covers the lung and is called the visceral pleura. A thin layer of fluid with a total volume of 5 to 15 ml acts as a lubricant between the visceral and parietal pleurae, allowing them to slide smoothly over each other during breathing.

Because the two pleurae lie in contact with each other, the pleural space is a "potential" space only. If the area between these membranes becomes an actual space, the lung collapses.

Pleural Pressures

The lung is supported within the chest cavity by intrapleural negative pressure. This negative pressure is created by two opposing forces. The first is the tendency of the chest wall to spring upward and outward. The second is the tendency of the elastic alveolar tissue to contract.

An analogy is two microscopic slides held together by a drop of water placed between them. One is not able to pull the slides apart because of the surface tension of the fluid.

Compare the lung to the two slides. One slide is the visceral pleura; the other is the parietal pleura. The drop of water is pleural fluid. As in the analogy of the slides, the opposing forces attempt to pull the pleurae in different directions. A negative pressure is generated which holds the lung tightly to the chest wall, preventing lung collapse. During inspiration, the intrapleural pressures become more negative. On expiration, the pressures become less negative (Table 19–7).

All gases move from an area of higher pressure to an area of lower pressure. During inspiration, the chest cavity enlarges through diaphragmatic contraction. This increases lung space and causes intrapleural pressure to fall below atmospheric pressure. Air flows from the relatively high atmospheric pressure into the area of low pressure in the lungs.

During expiration, this process is reversed. The diaphragm recoils, decreasing the space in the chest cavity and compressing the lungs. Intrapleural pressure is now higher than atmospheric pressure, causing air to move out of the lungs.

After the respiratory muscles relax, the pressure between the outside air and the lungs is equalized (760 mm Hg at sea level). Because the pressure is equalized, there is no air movement.

Equipment Features

Chest Tubes

Most chest tubes are multifenestrated, transparent tubes with distance and radiopaque markers. This enables the physician to visualize the tube on chest x-ray and position it correctly in the pleural space.

Chest tubes are categorized as pleural or mediastinal, depending on the location of the tube's tip. Patients can have more than one tube in different locations depending on the purposes of the tubes. *All chest tubes are treated as intrapleural tubes for patient safety.*

Larger tubes (20–36 French) are used to drain blood or thick pleural drainage. Smaller tubes (16–20 French) are used to remove air.

Drainage Systems

The chest tube acts as a drain for air or fluid. To reestablish intrapleural negative pressure, a seal for the chest tube that prevents outside air from entering the system is required.

TABLE 19–7
The Effect of Breathing on Intrapleural Pressure

Ventilation Cycle	Intrapleural Pressures
At rest	-5 cm H_2O
Inspiration	-6 to -12 cm H_2O
Expiration	-4 to -8 cm H_2O

The simplest way to accomplish this is to use an underwater system of drainage.

A review of the one-, two-, and three-bottle systems can provide a basis for understanding all commercially available products. Each system has advantages and disadvantages (Table 19–8). Knowledge of these systems enables the nurse to safely manage the most complex chest tube drainage setup.

One-Bottle System

The simplest chest drainage system is the one-bottle system (Fig. 19–5). This system consists of a bottle with a sealed cap. The cap has two openings. One is for an air vent, and the other allows a tube to pass through which extends almost to the bottom of the bottle.

Sterile water is poured into the bottle until the tip of the rigid tube is submerged 2 cm. This creates a water seal by closing the system to outside air. A fluid level higher than 2 cm of water can make breathing more difficult because the patient has a longer column of fluid to move during respiration. More positive pressure is then required to drive drainage out through the water seal.

The top of the tube is connected to about 6 feet of latex rubber that is in turn attached to the open end of the patient's chest tube. The vent in the bottle stays open to allow air from the pleural space to escape. This prevents pressure from building up in the pleural space. Except for the vented cap, the entire drainage system from the chest tube insertion site to the bottle must be airtight.

The fluid level in the water seal fluctuates during respiration. During inspiration, pleural pressures become more negative, causing the fluid level in the submerged tube to rise. During expiration, pleural pressures become more positive, causing the fluid level to descend.

If the patient is being mechanically ventilated, this

TABLE 19–8
Chest Tube Drainage Systems

System	Advantages	Disadvantages
One-Bottle	Simple configuration Easy to ambulate patient	As chest drainage fills up the bottle, more force is needed to allow pleural air and liquid to exit the chest into the bottle A mixture of drained blood and air creates a frothy mixture in the bottle that limits precise measurement of drainage To drain, pleural pressures must be higher than bottle pressures
Two-Bottle	Keeps the water seal at a constant level Allows better observation and measurement of drainage	Adds dead space to the drainage system that has the potential to be drawn into the pleural space To drain, pleural pressures must be higher than bottle pressures Has limitations on excessive air flow capacity in presence of a pleural leak
Three-Bottle	Safest system to regulate suction	More complex, more room for error in the set up and in maintenance
Disposable Units Water seal	Plastic and do not break as easily as bottles	Cost Loss of water seal and accuracy of drainage measurement if unit is tipped over
Flutter valve	Ideal for transport since water seal is maintained if unit tips over One less chamber to fill No problems with evaporation of water Decreased noise level	Cost Valve device doesn't provide visual information on intrapleural pressures because of absence of water fluctuations in the water seal chamber
Screw-valve	Same as above	Same as above Narrow valve limits the amount of volume it can handle; inefficient for large pleural air leaks
Calibrated spring mechanism	Same as above Able to handle large volumes	Cost

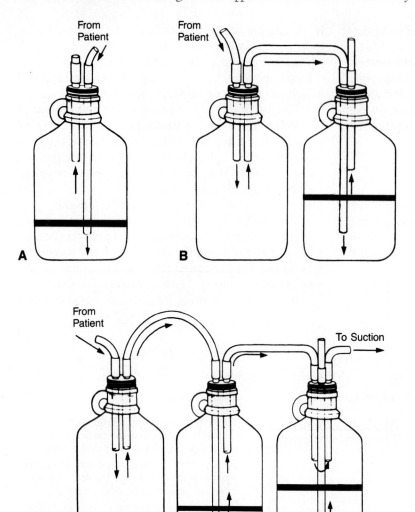

FIGURE 19–5
(**A**) One-bottle system underwater seal drainage.
(**B**) Two-bottle system underwater seal drainage.
(**C**) Underwater seal drainage with suction.

process is reversed. Bubbling should only be seen in the underwater seal chamber during expiration as air and fluid drain from the pleural cavity. Constant bubbling indicates either an air leak in the system or a bronchopleural fistula. This is discussed further under Nursing Management.

Two-Bottle System

In a two-bottle system (see Figure 19–5), the first bottle is the collection receptacle, and the second bottle serves as the water seal. In a two-bottle system, suction can be applied to the underwater seal bottle by connecting it to the air vent.

Three-Bottle System

In the three-bottle system, a suction control bottle is added to the two-bottle system (see Figure 19–5). This is the safest way to regulate the amount of suction. The third bottle is configured similar to the underwater seal bottle.

In this system, it is the depth of the submerged tube in the third bottle and **not the amount of wall suction** that determines the amount of suction applied to the chest tube. The amount of wall suction applied to the third bottle should be sufficient to create a gentle rolling bubble in the bottle. Vigorous bubbling results in water loss, changing suction pressure and increasing the noise level in the patient's unit.

To check for chest tube patency and respiratory cycle fluctuations, the suction must be momentarily disconnected.

Disposable Drainage Units

Disposable chest tube drainage systems mirror, in physiological principles, the bottle setups described above (Fig. 19–6). Some of the brand names include Pleur-evac (Deknatal Division, Fall River, MA), Atrium Compact (Atrium Medical Corp., Hollis, NH), ConMed Pleura-Gard (Con Med Corp., Utica, NY), Emerson 550 (Emerson Co., Cambridge, MA), and the Thora-Klex (Davol

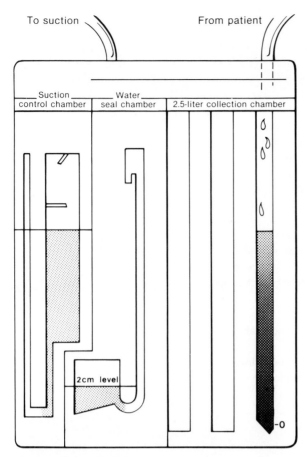

To suction   From patient

Suction
control chamber | Water
seal chamber | 2.5-liter collection chamber

2cm level

-0

FIGURE 19–6
Disposable chest tube drainage system.

Inc., Cranston, RI). The primary differences between them are the methods by which the chest tube drainage systems achieve a pleural seal.

Emerson Pleural Suction Pump

A suction pump commonly used instead of wall suction is the Emerson Pleural Suction Pump. It can be set up using a two- or three-bottle system. In contrast to the wall unit, the pressure control knob on the front of the pump controls the suction generated. The amount of pressure is registered on the suction dial.

Indications for Chest Tube Placement

If injury, surgery, or any disruption in the integrity of the lungs and chest cavity occurs, placement of a chest tube is warranted (Table 19–9). The chest tube is a drain. Its purposes are to remove air, fluid, or blood from the pleural space, to restore negative pressure to the pleural space, to re-expand a collapsed or partially collapsed lung, and to prevent reflux of drainage back into the chest.

Procedure

Chest Tube Insertion

Chest tube insertion can be accomplished in the operating room, in the emergency room, or at the bedside (Display Box 19–1).

Placement is based on the principle that, because of their different densities and weights, air rises and liquid sinks. The insertion site for air removal is near the second intercostal space along the midclavicular line. The insertion site for liquid drainage is near the fifth or sixth intercostal space on the midaxillary line. After heart surgery, placement can be in the mediastinum to drain blood from in front of and beneath the heart.

The nurse is responsible for explaining the procedure and physically preparing the patient. Patients are more likely to experience a favorable outcome if the nurse takes a few minutes to assure and outline in lay terms what is going to be done and why. A description of the sensations the patient will experience is helpful. Administer any analgesics that have been ordered. Position the patient in Fowler's or semi-Fowler's position.

After the skin has been cleaned and anesthetized, the physician makes a small skin incision. A forceps is used to penetrate the pleural space (Fig. 19–7). The tract made by the forceps is then dilated with a finger. The proximal end of the tube is clamped with the forceps and then inserted into the pleural space. If the placement is difficult, a metal trocar can be used to penetrate the chest wall, leaving the tube in place and removing the trocar.

After insertion, the external end of the tube is connected to a chest drainage unit (see Table 19–8). To prevent the tube from dislodging, the skin around the tube is sutured. The ends of the suture are wrapped around the tube and tied off.

Bacteriostatic ointment or petroleum gauze can be applied to the incisional site. Petroleum gauze is preferred because it prevents air leaks; however, it also has the poten-

---

DISPLAY BOX 19–1
Equipment for Chest Tube Insertion

Chest tube tray or thoracotomy tray
Chest tube
1% lidocaine
Antiseptic (povidone-iodine)
Sterile gloves
Large hemostats
Suture material (2–O silk)
Cutting needle
Bacteriostatic ointment or petroleum gauze
Wound dressing materials

TABLE 19–9
Indication for Chest Tube Placement

Indication	Cause
Hemothorax	Chest trauma
	Neoplasms
	Pleural tears
	Excessive anticoagulation
	Post thoracic surgery
Pneumothorax	
Spontaneous: >20%	Bleb rupture
Symptomatic patient	
Presence of lung disease	
Tension	Mechanical ventilation
	Penetrating puncture wound
	Prolonged clamping of chest tubes
	Lack of seal in chest tube drainage system
Bronchopleural fistula	Tissue damage
	Tumor
	Aspiration of toxic chemicals
Pleural Effusion	Neoplasms
Complicated parapneumonia:	Serious cardiopulmonary disease
Gross pus (empyema)	Inflammatory conditions
Gram-positive stain or bacterial culture	
Glucose <40 mg/dl	
pH <7.0	
pH 7.0–7.2 and LDH >1000 IU/L	
Chylothorax	Trauma
	Malignancy
	Congenital abnormalities

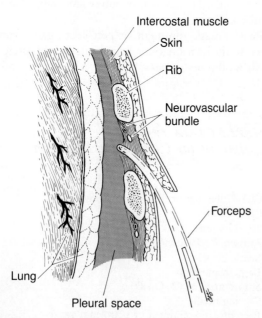

FIGURE 19–7
Forceps penetrates the pleural space to create a track for the chest tube.

tial to macerate the skin and predispose the site to infection. A gauze 4 × 4 with a split is positioned over the tube and taped occlusively to the chest. The tube is taped to the chest to prevent traction on the tube and sutures if the patient moves.

A post-insertion chest x-ray is always ordered to confirm proper positioning.

The lungs are auscultated and the condition of the tissue around the insertion site is evaluated for the presence of subcutaneous air. This assessment provides a baseline for determining improvement or worsening of the patient's condition.

Chest Tube Removal

Opinions differ regarding how chest tubes should be removed. Many thoracic surgeons prefer to clamp the chest tube 12 to 24 hours before removal. This identifies persistent air leaks or reaccumulation of fluid on repeat chest x-ray.

Some patients report that being told the chest tube was to be pulled was sufficient preparation. Premedication before removal alleviated discomfort and pain according to some, and had no effect according to others.

- One day after cessation of air leak
- Drainage of <50–100 cc of fluid per day
- 1–3 days post cardiac surgery
- 2–6 days post thoracic surgery
- Obliteration of empyema cavity
- Serosanguinous drainage from around the chest tube insertion site

The patient is placed in a Fowler's or semi-Fowler's position. The dressing over the insertion site is removed and the area is cleaned. The suture is clipped. The tube is removed in one quick movement at peak inspiration or during expiration. Immediately, the mattress suture is tied to close the incisional area.

The most commonly described patient sensations are burning, followed by pain, pulling, and pressure.[4] The symptoms are generally characterized as intense but of short duration.

Immediately after removal, lung fields are auscultated and a dressing is applied over the site. A chest x-ray is obtained 12 to 24 hours later to assess the presence of residual air or fluid.

Assessment and Management

Vigilant and expert nursing care can prevent serious complications in a patient with a chest tube and drainage system.

Positioning

The ideal position for a patient with a chest tube is semi-Fowler's. To enhance air and fluid evacuation, turn the patient every two hours.

Show the patient how to support the chest wall near the tube insertion site. Encourage coughing, deep breathing, and ambulation. Administration of pain medication before these exercises decreases pain and enhances lung expansion.

Maintaining System Patency

The most serious complication of a chest tube is a tension pneumothorax. If untreated, it is life-threatening. A tension pneumothorax occurs if air enters the pleural space during inspiration but cannot exit during expiration. This process develops if there is any obstruction in the chest tube drainage system. As more air is trapped in the pleural

space, pressure increases until the lung collapses and all soft tissues in the chest are compressed (see Display Box 19–3). The routine practice of clamping chest tubes predisposes patients to this complication. Clamping of chest tubes is recommended in only two situations. One is to locate the source of an air leak if bubbling occurs in the water seal chamber. The second is done momentarily when replacing the chest tube drainage unit. Padded forceps must be used for clamping to avoid cutting the vinyl chest tube.

Nursing care is directed at maintaining patency and proper functioning of the chest tube drainage system. Lift the latex tubing frequently to drain the fluid into the collection container. Coil the latex tubing loosely on the bed to prevent kinks and pooling of blood in a dependent loop hanging on the floor. Never raise the chest tube drainage system above the chest or the drainage will back up into the chest. Check the chest tube drainage system at frequent intervals for drainage and water seal integrity.

Drainage Monitoring

Note the color, consistency, and amount of drainage. Use a pen to mark the level on the drainage system at the end of the shift and at prescribed time intervals. Be alert to sudden changes in the amount of drainage. A sudden increase indicates hemorrhage or sudden patency of a previously obstructed tube. A sudden decrease indicates chest tube obstruction or failure of the chest tube or drainage system.

To reestablish chest tube patency, the following nursing actions are recommended:[5]

1. Attempt to alleviate the obstruction by repositioning the patient.
2. If the clot is visible, straighten the tubing between the chest and drainage unit and raise the tube to enhance the effect of gravity.

- Tachycardia
- Tachypnea
- Agitation
- Diaphoresis
- Midline tracheal shift
- Muffled heart tones
- Absent breath sounds over affected lung
- Hyper-resonance to percussion over affected lung
- Hypotension
- Cardiac arrest
- High pressure alarms (if mechanically ventilated)

3. Squeeze and release the tubing alternately to gently move the clot toward the drainage receptacle.
4. If the chest tube continues to remain blocked, stripping the chest tube is recommended. Routine chest tube stripping without evaluating the patient's situation is controversial and risky (Table 19–10).

Water Seal Monitoring

Monitoring the water seal of the chest tube drainage system is as important as observing the drainage. Visually check to ensure the water seal chambers are filled to the 2 cm water line. If suction is applied, ensure the water line in the suction chamber is at the ordered level. If an Emerson Pleural Suction Pump is used, check the suction gauge. Never occlude an air vent opening.

Observe the underwater seal for respiratory fluctuations. The absence of fluctuations can indicate that the lung is re-expanded or that there is an obstruction in the system. Continuous vigorous bubbling in the water seal without suction can indicate the tube has been displaced or disconnected. Check the entire system for disconnections and inspect the chest tube to see if it is displaced outside the chest.

Bubbling that occurs 24 hours after chest tube insertion in conjunction with a resolved pneumothorax indicates the presence of a bronchopleural fistula. This usually

TABLE 19–10
Potential Complications of Chest Tube Stripping

Generation of excessive negative pressures causing aspiration of lung tissue into eyelets of chest tube
Rupture of alveoli
Persistent pleural leak
Disrupted suture lines
Acute myocardial ischemia
Increase in pulmonary wedge pressure
Increase in venous return to the right heart
Shift in the ventricular septum to the left
Right ventricular interference with left ventricular function
Impedance to left ventricular ejection

occurs in the setting of mechanical ventilation at high tidal volumes and pressures.

Complications

Dislodgement of Chest Tube

If the chest tube falls out or is accidentally pulled out, quickly seal off the insertion site to prevent air from entering the pleural cavity.

Pharmacologic Agents

Behavioral Objectives

Description

Bronchodilators

Anticholinergic Drugs

Asthma Prophylactic Drugs

Anti-Inflammatory Corticosteroid

Oxygen

Antibiotics

BEHAVIORAL OBJECTIVES

Based on the content in this section, the reader should be able to:

1. Name two specific drugs and their mechanisms of action for each category: bronchodilators and anticholinergic drugs.
2. Describe the rationale for categorizing oxygen as a drug.

Description

The distinguishing feature of a group of diseases affecting the lower respiratory tract is spasm of the bronchial smooth muscle. Flow of air through the airways can fluctuate significantly within short periods secondary to an increased responsiveness to various stimuli (eg, noxious fumes and gases, air pollutants, animal dander, extreme cold, and exercise). Bronchospasm is an important component of reversible obstructive airway disease (asthma) and chronic bronchitis. In addition, bronchospasm is frequently associated with viral infections.

A basic understanding of pulmonary drugs and their sites of action (Table 19–11) and of specific pharmacologic agents with knowledge of action, dosage, and side effects (Table 19–12) is crucial for the delivery of safe pharmacologic support and meticulous assessment for drug effectiveness and side effects. Because a full discussion of the multiple pharmacologic agents is beyond the scope of this book, the reader should consult a current pharmacology text for added information.

Bronchodilators

The choice of specific bronchodilator therapy depends on the physician's bias, drug availability, cost, the patient's tolerance, and the patient's compliance. Table 19–12 illustrates pulmonary drugs commonly used at this time, along with actions, dosages, and side effects. Therefore, only major points for emphasis are discussed here.

(*Text continues on page 446*)

TABLE 19–11
Sites of Action of Pulmonary Drugs

1. Receptors of Smooth Muscle—Airways

Smooth Muscle ————

Airway ——————

β ———————— Beta Receptors—Relaxation

α ———————— Alpha Receptors—Contraction

× ———————— Cholinergic Receptors
(ie, Vagus Nerve)—Contraction

2. Cellular Metabolism

	Adenyl cyclase		Phosphodiesterase
Adenosine triphosphate (ATP)	Cyclic AMP (active form)		Cyclic AMP (inactive form)
(Adenyl cyclase is stimulated in the presence of sympathomimetic drugs.)	(Results in specialized cellular function; ie, smooth muscle relaxation.)		(Phosphodiesterase is decreased in the presence of methylxanthines.)

Cyclic AMP is one of the intermediaries of cellular metabolism in the sequence of energy production. It is present in almost all cell membranes and is influenced by a variety of agents, such as hormones and drugs.

3. Mast Cells

———————— Mast Cell

———————— Histamine-Containing Granules

Mast cells with histamine-containing granules are abundant in allergic asthmatics.

TABLE 19–12
Action, Dosage, and Side Effects of Pulmonary Drugs

Pulmonary Drugs	Action	Dosage	Side Effects
1. Broncholidilators			
Methylxanthines	↓ phosphodiesterase with ↑ cyclic AMP (active form)	IV: loading—5 mg/kg; maintenance—0.9 mg/kg PO: aminophylline—1200 mg/24 hr; oxtriphylline (Choledyl)—1600 mg/24 hr NB: Dosages adjusted to maintain serum theophylline levels 10–20 µg/ml	Nausea Vomiting Nervousness Dysrhythmias Seizures

Theophylline—Dosage increased by 50% for smokers who can tolerate the drug if effect is less than optimal.
Dosage decreased by 50% for patients with liver failure, heart failure, hypoxemia, and shock.

Pulmonary Drugs	Action	Dosage	Side Effects
Sympathomimetics	β-Stimulants		Relatively few side effects with recommended dosages
Isoetharine (Bronkosol)	Stimulates adenyl cyclase with ↑ cyclic AMP (active form)	Delivered by nebulizer—either hand-powered or IPPB 0.5 ml with sterile water or normal saline (1:3 conc.) q4h	Tachycardia Palpitations Nausea Headache Changes in blood pressure Nervousness
Terbutaline (Brethine)	Stimulates adenyl cyclase with ↑ cyclic AMP (active form)	5 mg PO q8h; 0.25 mg SC not to exceed 0.5 mg q4h	↑ Heart rate Nervousness Tremor Palpitations Dizziness (Usually transient effects and do not require treatment)
Metaproterenol (Alupent, Metaprel)	Stimulates adenyl cyclase with ↑ cyclic AMP (active form)	Metered dose device: 0.65 mg/metered dose; 20 mg PO tid	Tachycardia Hypertension Palpitations Nervousness Tremor Nausea and vomiting
Albuterol (Salbutamol, Proventyl)	Same as for metaproterenol	Metered dose device: 1–2 inhalations q4–6h Oral: 2–4 mg q6–8h	Mainly fine finger tremors
Bitolterol (Tornolate)	Same as for metaproterenol	Metered dose: 370 mg/puff 2 puffs q4–6h	Derivative of metaproterenol See metaproterenol
Fenoterol (Berota)	Same as for metaproterenol	7.5 mg PO bid/tid and corresponding aerosol dose: 400 mg	
Epinephrine	Same as for metaproterenol	0.2–0.5 mg of 1:1000 solution SC q2h as necessary. Severe attacks: doses may be repeated every 20 min for maximum of three doses	Anxiety Tremors Palpitations Tachycardia Hirsutism (Contraindicated in hypertension, hyperthyroidism, ischemic heart disease, and cerebrovascular insufficiency)

(continued)

TABLE 19–12
Action, Dosage, and Side Effects of Pulmonary Drugs (Continued)

Pulmonary Drugs	Action	Dosage	Side Effects
Summary of Potential Systemic Effects of Sympathomimetics			
Neurological—	Tremulousness, agitation, anxiety, insomnia, dizziness, faintness		
Ophthalmic—	Glaucoma		
Cardiovascular—	Tachycardia, palpitations, dysrhythmias, alterations in blood pressure, angina, vasodilation or vasoconstriction, myocardial necrosis		
Respiratory—	Tracheal and/or bronchial irritation, bronchospasm (paradoxical response), blood gases—decreased PaO_2		
Metabolic—	Hyperglycemia, hyperthyroidism		
Gastrointestinal—	Nausea, vomiting, dry mouth, gagging		
Genitourinary—	Urinary retention—primarily in men with prostate hypertrophy		
Interaction with other drugs—	Insulin, oral hypoglycemic agents, monoamine oxidase inhibitors, general anesthetics, hypotensive agents, thyroid hormone		
2. Steroids	Stimulate adenylate cyclase with ↑ cyclic 3′, 5′-AMP; may facilitate use of β-stimulants; anti-inflammatory action		
Prednisone		Variable; eg, 40–60 mg PO initially and decreasing according to PFT and eosinophil counts (in patients with ↑ Eos 2° to allergin-mediated responses)	Formation of glucose from body protein → ↑ blood sugar; Depletion of bone calcium—osteoporosis; Increase in fat production; Impairment of immunologic response; Reduction of inflammatory response; Increase in gastric acidity; Elevation of blood pressure; Acne
Methylprednisolone (Solu-Medrol)		Variable; eg, 100 mg IV and repeat with one fourth original dose q6h	Same as for prednisone
Beclomethasone (Vanceril)	Virtually same as for other steroids except it is an inhaled preparation with a high topical effect on the airways and low systemic activity	Inhalation device; 2 inhalations (100 μg) qid	Oral candidiasis; Mild oropharyngeal symptoms—discomfort and dryness of throat
3. Cromolyn Sodium (Aarane, Intal)	Prophylactic bronchospasmolytic in allergic asthma; *not* useful in acute bronchospasm; probably strengthens mast cell membrane, preventing release of histamine and therefore decreases bronchospasm in the allergic asthmatic	1 capsule via inhaler device qid	Maculopapular rash; Urticaria; Cough and/or bronchospasm
4. Anticholinergics Atropine sulfate	Parasympathetic antagonist	5 mg of solution	Tachycardia; Dry mouth

Theophylline, a member of the xanthine family, is the most useful bronchodilator for moderate to severe bronchospasm, and it increases diaphragmatic contractibility.[6] It is a safe and effective drug that one can monitor relatively easily by obtaining serum theophylline levels, which are usually between 10 and 20 µg/ml. The incidence of drug toxicity increases at levels greater than 20 µg/ml. Many physicians consider theophylline to be the "first-line" bronchodilator of choice, and it is the first bronchodilator the patient receives. If, after therapeutic levels have been achieved, the patient continues to be symptomatic, a second bronchodilator—an adrenergic agent—can be added.

The adrenergic bronchodilators are those drugs that mimic the sympathetic nervous system (are sympathomimetic) and are relatively short-acting because they are readily metabolized.[7] The choice of a specific agent depends on the preferred route of administration (ie, oral or inhaled), the rapidity of onset, the length of action, and prevalence and type of side effects. These drugs include metaproterenol, isoetharine, isoproterenol, albuterol, and terbutaline. Multiple trials may be needed to evaluate the maximal effectiveness of a timed-release preparation such as Slo-Phyllin or Theolair versus Bronkodyl. If possible, patients should participate in drug selection and schedule. This improves compliance with drug therapy and, ultimately, quality of life.

Anticholinergic Drugs

Atropine sulfate is an agent that has been used for many years preoperatively for drying oral secretions, and many physicians believe that such an agent is contraindicated in patients with lung disease who have excessive secretion production. The parasympathetic action of atropine is effective in blocking neurotransmission by acetylcholine to smooth muscle. This agent can exert significant bronchodilator effect after inhalation while avoiding the drying effect of large systemic doses.

Asthma Prophylactic Drugs

Cromolyn sodium can be used in asthmatic patients whose symptoms are not controlled adequately by bronchodilators. A trial of 1 month is preceded and followed by pulmonary function testing to document response. If an appropriate response cannot be demonstrated, the drug is discontinued. The desired effects of cromolyn are to reduce severity of asthma attacks and to enhance effects of concomitantly administered bronchodilator and steroid therapy. As a result of the latter, one can anticipate a reduction of bronchodilator and steroid dosage.

Anti-Inflammatory Corticosteroid

Steroids apparently stimulate adenyl cyclase with a resultant increase of cyclic 3′,5′-AMP. They can facilitate the action of β-stimulants. They also are anti-inflammatory agents. One must keep in mind that steroid side effects can occur with as little as 10 mg of prednisone per day. The inhaled form of corticosteroid, beclomethasone dipropionate (Beclovent or Vanceril inhaler), can be used either for those patients who require 20 mg or less daily to control asthmatic symptoms or for those who require high-dose steroids. Beclomethasone supplementation can enable the physician to decrease the oral steroid dosage in the latter group. Regardless of whether the patient is transferred totally to inhaled steroids or to a combination of both oral and inhaled steroids, caution must be exercised.[8] Decrement of oral dosage should be very small (eg, 2–3 mg). Pulmonary functions should be monitored carefully. Stressful situations such as exacerbation of severe asthma, trauma, or surgery may warrant a short course of systemic steroids in full therapeutic dosage.

Oxygen

Oxygen is one of the most commonly used forms of medical therapy. Factors that determine tissue oxygenation include (1) alveolar oxygen concentration; (2) diffusion of gases (oxygen) at the alveocapillary membran; (3) ventilation-perfusion ($\dot{V}D/\dot{Q}D$) relations within the lung; (4) the amount and carrying capacity of hemoglobin; and (5) cardiac output.

Therapeutic oxygen is potentially harmful. The dosage of oxygen must be prescribed precisely in terms of percent concentration in the inspired air (eg, FIO_2 0.5, 50% oxygen concentration) or in liters per minute. In most clinical settings, a PaO_2 less than 60 mm Hg is the degree of hypoxemia that indicates a need for supplemental O_2. The goal of this therapy is to raise the PaO_2, with a subsequent reduction of hypoxic vasoconstriction of the pulmonary vascular bed and pulmonary artery pressure and, it is hoped, improvement in right ventricular function and tissue delivery of oxygen.

The critical care nurse must become knowledgeable in the techniques and rationale for the various oxygen delivery devices, even though respiratory therapists may be responsible for oxygen therapy, because they may not have adequate staff to provide constant ICU coverage if they have other responsibilities as well. The nurse should develop the habit of checking this equipment and assessing the patient. What are the blood gases? Is the patient demonstrating signs and symptoms of hypoxemia—tachycardia, tachypnea, diaphoresis, and confusion or behavioral change?

Antibiotics

Ideally, pneumonia is treated with specific antibiotic therapy designed to definitively destroy the cultured microorganism. In reality, less than 20% of infected patients have definitive cultures.[9] Therefore, broad-spectrum antibiotics or combination therapy of double or triple antibiotics are usually employed. Often, nosocomial infections involve more than one organism. The critically ill patient is at increased risk due to mechanical ventilation systems, decreased immune responses, use of steroids, debilitated general health, and cross-infection by health care workers.

Current antibiotic therapy commonly used for the treatment of pneumococcal, staphylococcal, and *Klebsiella* pneumonia and of *Haemophilus* influenza is summarized in Table 19–13. The reader is encouraged to review the subject in a current pharmacology text. Pneumonia with or without preexisting lung disease can be a serious complication. Side effects from potent antibiotic therapy can significantly complicate the situation with such problems as renal and hepatic complications and ototoxicity.

TABLE 19–13
Antibiotic Therapy in Pulmonary Disease*

Pulmonary Complication	Antibiotic	Dosage
Pneumococcal pneumonia with or without COPD	Penicillin	600,000 U procaine penicillin IM q12h (a blood level of 0.02 mg/ml 12 h after start of drug is adequate to kill organism) or IV prep: aqueous penicillin G 300,000–600,000 U IV q3–4h
	Penicillin V	250 mg orally q6h
	Cefazolin	500 mg IM or IV q8h
	Cephalexin	500 mg orally q6h
Staphylococcus pneumonia (production of enzymes that destroy lung tissue)	Antistaphylococcal agents Nafcillin Methicillin Cloxacillin Penicillin	1–2 g IV q4–6h
Klebsiella pneumonia (gram-negative): a very severe pneumonia with high mortality; seen more commonly in chronic/debilitated states[†]	Cephalosporin (Cefazolin)	1 g IM or IV q4–6h
	Gentamicin	Dosage is related to renal function (ie, creatinine clearance); commonly, 3–6 mg/kg/24 h. Aim to achieve a trough blood level not less than 1.5 mg/ml and a peak level not over 10 mg/ml
Pseudomonas pneumonia (gram-negative)[†]	Tobramycin	3–5 mg/kg/24 h, producing blood levels of 2.5 mg/ml in presence of normal renal function
	Gentamicin	3–5 mg/kg/24 h (see *Klebsiella* pneumonia, above)
Haemophilus influenza	Ampicillin	2.0–6.0 g/24 h, increasing to 8–12 g/24 h for serious infections
	Chloramphenicol	3.0–4.0 g/24 h PO (50–100 mg/kg/24 h)

* A complete discussion of antibiotic therapy related to pulmonary disease and/or complications is beyond the scope of this chapter.
† Antibiotic treatment of gram-negative bacterial pneumonias frequently consists of aminoglycoside and a second drug (ie, a cephalosporin). The rationale is based on poor penetration into bronchial secretions by aminoglycosides; in addition, antibiotic resistance occurs frequently with the latter.

Ventilatory Support

BEHAVIORAL OBJECTIVES

Based on the content in this section, the reader should be able to:

1. Define respiratory failure.
2. Identify three events affecting different body systems that can lead to respiratory failure.
3. Discuss five indications for mechanical ventilation.
4. Compare and contrast the function of a manual resuscitator bag and a mechanical ventilator.
5. Discuss three different modes of mechanical ventilation.
6. Discuss three different types of mechanical ventilators.
7. Explain the physiological impact of mechanical ventilation.
8. Discuss four nursing interventions necessary for care of a patient on a ventilator.
9. Given a set of ABG values, barometric pressure, water pressure, and target PaO_2, calculate the ventilator FIO_2 setting.
10. Describe potential complications of mechanical ventilators.

11. List three criteria for weaning a patient from a ventilator.
12. Outline five clinical signs that warrant evaluation and possible discontinuation of weaning.
13. Differentiate between short-term and long-term weaning procedures.
14. Discuss four nursing interventions necessary if weaning a patient from a ventilator.

Description

Once a patient has been intubated and resuscitated successfully, the commitment to mechanical ventilation has been made. This commitment poses a financial and psychological burden on the patient and family. Because mortality is reduced very little, every effort and consideration must be given to avoid mechanical ventilation.

Two approaches that can eliminate the need for mechanical ventilation are

* identification of high-risk patients;
* institution of appropriate measures to forestall or prevent respiratory failure.

Patients are predisposed to developing respiratory failure if any of the systems involved in respiration are compromised or overwhelmed (Table 19–14). The degree of risk for developing respiratory failure depends on the patient's ability to move air, secretions, and blood. Inability to do the latter is reflected clinically as pulmonary edema due to poor cardiac output.

Physiological Principles

Effects of Mechanical Ventilation

To understand the effects of mechanical ventilation, the reader is encouraged to review the physiology of normal respirations and lung compliance as discussed in Chapter 17.

In mechanical ventilation, the relation between pressures in inspiration and expiration is *reversed*. The ventilator delivers air by virtually pumping it into the patient; therefore, pressures during inspiration are positive. The positive pressures pumped into the lungs result in increased intrathoracic pressures and decreased venous return during inspiration. With the institution of positive end-expiratory pressure (PEEP), even greater pressures are generated during inspiration. During expiration, pressures decrease to PEEP level and continue positive throughout expiration. Most patients compensate by increasing peripheral venous tone. If conditions of decreased sympathetic responses (eg, hypovolemia, drugs, old age) are present, hypotension develops. In addition, a large V_T, greater than 10 to 12 ml/kg, which generates pressures

TABLE 19–14
Body Systems and Possible Events Leading to Respiratory Failure

Systems	Events
1. Nervous system	Head trauma
Brain stem	Poliomyelitis
Spinal cord and nerves	Cervical (C1–C6) fractures
	Overdose
2. Muscular system	Myasthenia gravis
Primary—diaphragm	Guillain–Barré
Secondary—respiratory	
3. Skeletal system	Flail chest
Thorax	Kyphoscoliosis
4. Respiratory system	Obstruction
Airways	Laryngeal edema
	Bronchitis
	Asthma
Alveoli	Emphysema
	Pneumonia
	Fibrosis
Pulmonary circulation	Pulmonary embolus
5. Cardiovascular system	Congestive heart failure
	Fluid overload
	Cardiac surgery
	Myocardial infarction
6. Gastrointestinal system	Aspiration
7. Hematological system	Disseminated intravascular coagulation
8. Genitourinary system	Renal failure

greater than 40 cm H_2O, can not only influence the cardiac output but also increase the risk of pneumothorax.

The movement of air through the airways creates friction and turbulence. The more flow, the more friction. If the airway is narrowed, the friction increases even more. Therefore, with spontaneously generated inspiration, more negative pressure must be generated for a given flow of air to occur. With mechanical ventilation, more positive pressure is needed to deliver air through the narrowed airway. This is one of the reasons for a high mortality rate in patients with status asthmaticus requiring mechanical ventilation.

Compliance

In terms of its compliance, the lung is frequently compared with a balloon. Initially it is hard to inflate, until it is stretched. After repeated inflations, the elasticity is lost, and the balloon becomes very easy to blow up.

As the volume of gas is delivered to a patient on a mechanical ventilator, the respirator pressure gauge slowly rises from zero to maximum inspiratory pressure (MIP). The rise in pressure is caused by resistance to flow or resistance to lung and chest wall inflation (see Display Box

---

DISPLAY BOX 19-4
Factors Influencing Maximum Inspiratory Pressure

Flow Resistance

Peak flow
Size of airways
Airway obstructions
External obstructions (ie, kinked ventilator tubing or water in the tubing)

Lung Resistance

Chest size
Volume of air
Elasticity of lung

Chest Wall Resistance

Chest wall deformities
Position of patient
External compression of chest wall or diaphragm (ie, distended abdomen)

19-4). A graph of pressure over time, depicting inspiration, would look like that shown in Figure 19-8.

Dynamic pressures and MIP can give an indication of flow properties of the airways.

Static Pressure. One of the measurements used to obtain compliance is static pressure (SP). SP is obtained by kinking the exhalation valve line when the patient is in maximum inspiration. This holds the volume of delivered air in the patient's chest by preventing exhalation. The pressure recorded at this moment is SP and reflects the force necessary to deliver the preset volume of air to the patient and hold the airways open. Graphically, it would appear as in Figure 19-9. Dividing the V_T by the SP yields compliance.

Equipment Features

Oxygen Delivery Systems

If external or internal respiration is impaired, supplemental oxygen is vital to maintain the patient's cellular function. Oxygen therapy corrects hypoxemia, decreases the

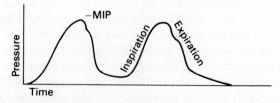

FIGURE 19-8
Graph depicting maximum inspiratory pressure (MIP).

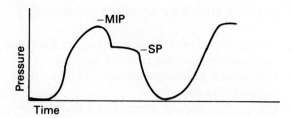

FIGURE 19-9
Graph depicting static pressure (*SP*); *MIP*, maximum inspiratory pressure.

work of breathing, and decreases myocardial work. Oxygen delivery systems are traditionally divided into high-flow and low-flow systems (see Display Box 19-5).

Low-flow oxygen devices work by supplying oxygen at flow rates less than the patient's inspiratory volume. The rest of the volume is pulled from room air. Because of this oxygen and room air mixing, the actual FIO_2 delivered to the patient is unknown. Low-flow oxygen devices are suitable for stable patients with normal respiratory patterns, rates, and ventilation volumes.

High-flow oxygen devices supply flow rates high enough to accommodate two to three times the patient's inspiratory volume. These devices are suitable for patients with shallow breathing patterns and COPD patients who have a hypoxic ventilatory drive. The latter patients are very "sensitive" to oxygen in that a small increment increases their PaO_2 and, at the same time, dramatically increases their $PaCO_2$. In other words, once their hypoxic drive is satisfied, they literally stop breathing.

The approach to oxygen therapy is usually dictated by the physician, the nursing staff, and the respiratory staff's skill and familiarity with the oxygen equipment (Table 19-15).

If lower concentrations of oxygen are needed, the system selected is usually the **nasal cannula**. The cannula can even be used with mouth breathers, because movement of air through the oropharynx creates the Bernoulli effect, pulling oxygen from the nasopharynx. The exact

---

DISPLAY BOX 19-5
Oxygen Delivery Devices

Low-flow	Nasal cannula
	Simple mask
	Rebreather
	Non-rebreather
High-flow	Venturi mask
	Aerosol mask
	Tracheostomy collar
	T-piece
	Face tent

TABLE 19–15
Basic Oxygen Delivery Systems

Method	Rate of Flow (L/min)	Estimated Oxygen Delivered (%)	Features
 Cannula (nasal prongs)	1 2 3 4 5 6	23–24 24–28 28–32 32–36 40 max 44	Convenient Comfortable Nasal passages must be patent Can be used in mouth breathers Exact O_2% depends on patient's minute ventilation >6 L/min dries mucous membranes Allows talking, eating
 Catheter	Same as cannula		Less comfortable May cause abdominal distention in adults >6 L/min dries mucous membranes Not recommended for adults
 Simple mask	5 6 8	40 45–50 55–60	Confining Does not allow eating, coughing Tight face seal necessary Must have >5 L/min to flush CO_2 from mask
 Partial rebreather	6 8 10 12 15	35 40–50 60 60 60	Confining Tight seal is necessary Does not allow eating or coughing Bag may twist or kink

(*continued*)

TABLE 19–15
Basic Oxygen Delivery Systems (Continued)

Method	Rate of Flow (L/min)	Estimated Oxygen Delivered (%)	Features
Non-rebreather	6	55–60	Same as partial
	8	60–80	Never let bag totally deflate
	10	80–90	All rubber diaphragms must be in place and not stick
	12	90	
	15	90	
Venturi mask Jet adapter	*Color** Blue: 4 Yellow: 4–6 White: 6–8 Green: 8–10 Pink: 8–12 Orange: 12	24 28 31 35 40 50	Delivers exact O_2 concentration despite patient's minute ventilation Confining Must fit tightly Doesn't allow for coughing or eating If humidity is added, use compressed air so as to not alter O_2 concentration
T-tube	O_2 is dialed in on humidifier Flow should be high enough to cover patient's minute ventilation		Allows humidity for ET or trach tube Empty condensation in tubing Mist should be visible on exhalation end
Face tent	Same as T-tube		Provides humidity for patients in the recovery room or after extubation Substitutes for face mask if patient finds mask too confining Impractical for long term use

(continued)

TABLE 19–15
Basic Oxygen Delivery Systems (Continued)

Method	Rate of Flow (L/min)	Estimated Oxygen Delivered (%)	Features
 Trach collar	Same as T-tube		Provides humidity to patients with tracheostomies Swivel adapter prevents jarring of the trach tube Frontal port permits suctioning without removing mask Condensation in the collar can drain into the patient's trach tube Secretions and crusts around the stoma can cause irritation and infection

＊Colors refer to Inspiron venturi ports, which are designed to deliver a factory-established percentage of O_2 when set at the specified rate of liter flow.

concentration of oxygen depends on the patient's V_T. If the patient hypoventilates, the oxygen concentration increases in the upper airway. In contrast, if hyperventilation occurs, the concentration of oxygen decreases owing to large amounts of room air diluting the oxygen delivered.

If the oxygen concentration must be constant, the system used is the **Venturi mask**. It delivers an exact percentage of oxygen regardless of a patient's V_T. Patients with COPD who primarily depend on the hypoxic drive to breathe require oxygen delivery by the Venturi system. They can be detected through serial ABG monitoring, which reveals large increases in $PaCO_2$ with small increases in oxygen flow.

As the need for higher concentrations of oxygen occurs, the nasal cannula is replaced by a **mask system**. A simple mask delivers the lowest concentrations of oxygen, and a non-rebreather the highest. If a patient's PaO_2 cannot be maintained using the non-rebreather, respiratory failure with the need for intubation and mechanical ventilation is imminent.

Manual Resuscitator

Before discussing the more sophisticated mechanical ventilators, a brief note about a simple, man-powered model is necessary. Frequently overlooked is the nurse's first important line of defense for acute respiratory failure (ARF)—the manual resuscitator. Common resuscitation bags without reservoirs deliver 0.33 to 0.38 concentrations of oxygen. During artificial resuscitation, hyperinflation before suctioning, or "bagging" of any mechanically ventilated patient, resuscitation bags with reservoirs must be used to deliver 0.74 to 1.0 concentrations of oxygen. It is recommended that corrugated tubes not be used as reservoirs for ventilating bags. A 2.5 L bag with an oxygen flow rate of 15 L/min has been shown to consistently deliver .95 to 1.00 concentrations of oxygen. Use of the 2.5 L reservoir

bag also provides visual assurance that the oxygen lines are intact and the bag is receiving supplemental oxygen. A corrugated tube reservoir varies according to the ventilatory rate, the volume delivered, and the filling time of the bag. If the 2.5 L reservoir bag is not available, a demand valve activated at -3 cm H_2O pressure is an adequate replacement.

Knowledge of the bag, along with skill in using it, is vital. The function of this simple ventilator can be compared with that of the more sophisticated models. With the manual resuscitator

- the *force* of squeezing the bag determines *tidal volume* (V_T) delivered to the patient;
- the *number* of hand squeezes per minute determines the *rate;*
- both the *force* and *rate* at which the nurse squeezes the bag determine the *peak flow.*

While the bag is being used, one must carefully observe the patient's chest to determine whether the bag is performing properly and whether any gastric distention is developing. In addition, the ease or resistance encountered can roughly indicate lung compliance. If a patient becomes progressively harder to "bag," an increase in secretions, hemothorax, pneumothorax, or worsening bronchospasms must be considered.

The following criteria are suggested for selection of a resuscitation bag:

1. The ability of the bag to deliver 100% oxygen in acute situations. (In nonacute maintenance situations, less oxygen concentration is acceptable.)
2. The need for the face mask, if used, to be transparent to enable the nurse to see any vomitus or blood that would create a potential for aspiration.
3. A valve system that functions without jamming in acute situations.
4. The cleaning and recycling endurance of the bag.

Mechanical Ventilators

Most of today's ventilators can be divided into two categories—*volume-cycled* and *pressure-cycled*. Realistically, the type selected depends on the models present in the hospital and the familiarity of the physicians with each type (see Display Box 19–6). Regardless of which type or model is used, the ventilator's function and limitations must be intimately known. A mechanical device used to sustain life is only as good as its design and the medical team using it.

The goal of mechanical ventilation is to maintain an alveolar ventilation appropriate for the patient's metabolic needs and to correct hypoxemia and maximize oxygen transport. The following discussion of ventilators is in order of evolution and use.

Negative Pressure Ventilator

The early negative pressure ventilators were known as "iron lungs." The patient's body was encased in an iron cylinder and negative pressures were generated to enlarge the thoracic cage. Recently, intermittent short-term negative pressure ventilation (INPV) has been used in COPD to correct severe hypercapnic respiratory failure by improving diaphragmatic function. Sauret[10] used INPV in selected cases and prevented the need for more aggressive intubation and ventilatory support.

This ventilator is mobile and fits like a tortoise shell, forming a seal over the chest with a hose connecting the shell to a negative pressure generator. The thoracic cage is literally "sucked up" to initiate inspiration, which is preset manually with a trigger. Negative pressure ventilators are advantageous in that they mimic normal respiration. However, their use is restricted because of their limitations on positioning and movement as well as on large or small body torsos.

Positive Pressure Ventilator

Pressure-Cycled. The pressure-cycled ventilator works on the basic principle that once a *preset pressure* is reached, inspiration is terminated. At this pressure point, the inspiratory valve closes and exhalation occurs passively. Ultimately this means that if a patient's lung compliance or resistance to flow changes, the *volume* of air delivered *varies*.

Clinically, as a patient's lungs become stiffer (less compliant), the volume of air delivered to the patient drops—sometimes drastically. Consequently, to ensure adequate minute ventilation and to detect any changes in lung compliance and resistance, one must frequently monitor inspiratory pressure, rate, and *exhaled* VT. In a patient whose pulmonary status is unstable, the use of a pressure ventilator is not recommended. However, in a very stable patient with compliant lungs, pressure ventilators are adequate and can also be used as a weaning tool in selected patients.

Time-Cycled. The time-cycled ventilator works on the basic principle that once a *preset time* is finished, inspiration is terminated. Expiratory time is determined by inspiratory time and rate (number of breaths per minute). Normal I:E (inspiratory-expiratory) ratio is 1:2.

Volume-Cycled. The volume ventilator is the most frequently used type in critical care settings. The basic principle of this ventilator is that once a *designated volume* of air is delivered to the patient, inspiration is terminated. A piston or bellows pushes a predetermined volume (VT) into the patient's lungs at a set rate. The advantage of a volume ventilator is that despite a change in patient lung compliance, a consistent VT is delivered.

High Frequency Ventilator

Because of the complications associated with positive pressure ventilation, other methods that may be more physiologically compatible are being investigated. The technique of high-frequency ventilation (HFV) is one such method. At present, it is still considered experimental. The exact mechanism by which HFV sustains life remains unclear, but it accomplishes oxygenation by the diffusion of oxygen and carbon dioxide from high to low gradients

---

DISPLAY BOX 19–6
Examples of Mechanical Ventilators

Negative Pressure

Pulmo-Wrap

Pressure-Cycled

Bennett PR-1
Bennett PR-2
Bird
Monaghan 225, 300

Time-Cycled

Baby Bird
Air shields electric ventilator
Monaghan 225
Bennett PR-2

Volume-Cycled

Emerson
Puritan-Bennett MA-1, MA-2
Ohio 550, 560
Scarle 801
Gill 1
Engstrom
Siemens
Bear I, II, 5
Veolar

of concentration. This diffusion movement is increased if the kinetic energy of the gas molecules is increased. (A patient experiencing HFV is somewhat analogous to a panting dog—the dog moves small volumes of air at a very fast rate.)

Basically, three different methods of delivering HFV can be identified (see Display Box 19–7). All involve ventilation at frequencies greater than 240 breaths per minute and use V_T less than or equal to dead space (V_D). Because the range of machines that deliver HFV is so varied, the resulting clinical research data are difficult to interpret. Used clinically, HFV has been found to maintain adequate oxygenation in patients with normal lungs. In patients with diseased lungs, adequate oxygenation is maintained, but PEEP requirements are not reduced. In some cases, the elimination of carbon dioxide has been a problem. Clinical trials have been limited to patients with bronchopleural fistulas, patients with tracheoesophageal fistulas, adult respiratory distress syndrome (ARDS) patients on whom conventional ventilation fails, patients undergoing bronchoscopy or laryngoscopy procedures, and patients clinically deteriorating from acute respiratory failure. Animal studies indicate that HFV can be used without a balloon cuff as long as PEEP is not required.

Because HFV is more compatible physiologically, it does result in more efficient cardiac performance and oxygen transport than other traditional methods. Patients tend to require less analgesia and sedation because of a reduced tendency to fight the ventilator.

Today's Generation of Mechanical Ventilator

Ventilators today have become very complex, incorporating every known cycling mode, pressure wave, and monitoring feature. The most technologically advanced ventilator has a computer and a microprocessor system. Pulse oximetry and end-tidal CO_2 sensors have also been added to the latest generation of ventilators. They provide visual feedback to the respiratory care team as to what the ventilator is doing. The more complex the ventilator, the higher the cost and the greater the margin for error. These ventilators are most appropriate for the patient with high minute ventilation requirements that frequently outstrip the conventional ventilators.

All types of mechanical ventilation require attention to patient care, and careful monitoring by the nurse is still the essence of therapy.

Ventilator Controls

Most ventilators have dials that are similar in function regardless of terminology. Understanding the function of each dial enables the nurse to meet the changing needs of the patient committed to mechanical ventilation.

DISPLAY BOX 19–7
Methods of Delivering High-Frequency Ventilation

High-Frequency Positive Pressure Ventilation (HFPPV)

Positive pressure ventilator
Rates 60–110/min
Uses a small cannula
IE ratios 1:6–1:2

High-Frequency Oscillation (HFO)

Rates 400–2400/min
Primarily used with neonates

High-Frequency Jet Ventilation (HFJV)

Uses pressure jets
Rates 110–400/min
Primarily used with adults

Fraction of Inspired Oxygen (FiO_2)

Most models enable the nurse to directly dial-in oxygen percentage, FiO_2. However, the nurse must not assume that because 100% is dialed-in, the patient is receiving 100%. If a patient requires 50% or higher FiO_2 concentrations, the ventilator needs to be checked frequently for accuracy with an oxygen analyzer. The newer models of volume ventilators, such as the MA-2 (Puritan-Bennet Ventilator Division, Carlsbad, CA) and Bear, have oxygen analyzers in circuit, with constant digital readouts of oxygen concentrations. However, the older models, such as the MA-1 (Monaghan Medical Corp., Plattsburgh, NY) and Monaghan, do not have oxygen analyzers in circuit. Indeed, as long as 50 psi (pounds per square inch) of compressed air is connected, the ventilator will function.

Respiratory Rate

The number of breaths per minute delivered to the patient can be directly dialed-in. In some models, the numbers are marked, whereas in models such as the Monaghan the rate is timed for a full minute with a watch, and the dial is set accordingly. Again, the nurse must not assume, just because the ventilator is set at a specified number of breaths per minute, that this is what is being delivered. Double-check the functioning of the ventilator with a watch that has a second hand. The possibility of mechanical failure is always present.

In the pressure ventilator, the inspiratory time flow-rate control determines the duration of inspiration by regulating the velocity of gas flow. The higher the flow rate, the faster peak airway pressure is reached and the shorter the inspiration. The lower the flow rate, the longer the inspiration. A high flow rate produces turbulence, shallow inspirations, and uneven distribution of volume.

Tidal Volume

In the volume ventilator, a dial or crank is turned to the number of cubic centimeters of air to be delivered with each breath. Again, in the pressure ventilator, manipulation of the inspiratory time flow-rate control determines the magnitude of inspiration. A low flow rate increases V_T and produces better alveolar ventilation than a high flow rate. Use of a Wright respirometer to measure exhaled air checks that the V_T dialed-in is being delivered (Fig. 19–10).

Peak Flow

This is the velocity of air flow per unit of time and is expressed as liters per minute. On the volume ventilator, this is a separate knob. In the pressure ventilator, this is manipulated, again, with the inspiratory time flow-rate control.

Installation of a demand valve in the newer volume ventilators enables a patient to receive the flow of air as demanded. The older models dump the air at the set rate (peak flow) that is dialed-in. The demand valve, besides decreasing airway turbulence, enhances patient comfort.

Pressure Limit

On the volume-cycled ventilators, this knob limits the highest pressure allowed in the ventilator circuit. Once the high pressure limit is reached, inspiration is terminated. Therefore, if the pressure limit is being constantly reached, the designated V_T is not being delivered to the patient. The cause of this can be coughing, accumulation of secre-

tions, kinked ventilator tubing, pneumothorax, decreasing compliance, or simply a pressure limit set too low.

Positive End-Expiratory Pressure (PEEP)

The PEEP knob adjusts the pressure that is maintained in the lungs at the end of expiration. If an intermittent mandatory ventilation (IMV) model is used, this knob may be labeled continuous positive airway pressure (CPAP). CPAP indicates that spontaneous breathing through the ventilator circuit is occurring (non-IMV breaths) and that at the end of these breaths, positive airway pressure is being maintained. PEEP can be visualized on the respiratory pressure gauge. Instead of returning to zero at the end of expiration, the pressure needle drops to PEEP level.

In the newer ventilators, PEEP is built-in. The process by which one obtains PEEP on these ventilators is by keeping the exhalation valve inflated throughout the expiratory phase with a pressure equal to the amount of desired PEEP.

Several other devices can be used to apply PEEP externally on a ventilator or T-piece. They range from spring-loaded diaphragms and plastic cylinder ball valves to a container of water. These devices are applied on the exhalation port of the ventilator circuit. If water is used, for each 1 cm of exhalation tubing extending into the water, 1 cm of PEEP is generated.

Sensitivity

This knob controls the amount of patient effort needed to initiate an inspiration, as expressed by negative inspiratory pull required. Increasing the sensitivity decreases the amount of work the patient must do to initiate a ventilatory breath. Likewise, decreasing the sensitivity increases the amount of negative pressure that the patient needs to initiate inspiration and increases the work of breathing. In some models, sensitivity can be totally dialed-out so that the ventilator is controlling the patient.

Sigh

To understand the function of this knob, some history of initial attempts at mechanical ventilation must be reviewed. Because normal breathing consists of V_T at 5 ml/kg of body weight, patients were initially ventilated at these volumes. However, subsequent studies on dogs showed that atelectasis developed. On further observation of normal breathing, it was noted that persons automatically deepened their V_T two to four times an hour. In an attempt to mimic normal breathing, a sigh mode was incorporated on the ventilators. A sigh mode delivers a bigger breath to patients at a designated volume and rate per hour. Presently, mechanical ventilation is performed at twice normal V_T; with this practice, the need for sighs has been negated except in special cases such as refractive

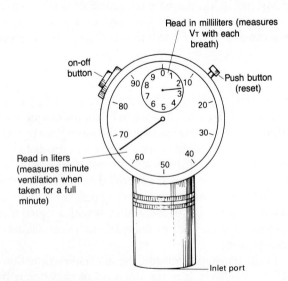

FIGURE 19–10
Wright respirometer—newer model.

atelectasis. With new research on suctioning techniques, use of the sigh mode in conjunction with .100 O_2 is recommended for postsuctioning hyperinflation.

Ventilatory Modes

Several different modes of ventilatory control can be found on ventilators. These modes can be separate dials, or they can be incorporated in the function of another knob such as sensitivity. Some of these modes are *assist, control, assist–control, IMV*, and pressure support (Fig. 19–11).

In the *assist mode*, only the breaths triggered by the patient are delivered at the designated V_T. In this mode, the patient *must* have a drive to breathe. If the patient is unable to trigger a breath, air is not delivered.

In the *control mode*, the ventilator controls the patient. Breaths delivered to the patient are at the rate and volume dialed-in on the ventilator, regardless of the patient's attempts to initiate an inspiration. If the patient is not unconscious or paralyzed, this mode can provoke high anxiety and discomfort.

The *assist–control mode* incorporates the preceding two modes. A basic rate can be set. If the patient wishes to breathe faster, he or she can trigger the ventilator (providing the sensitivity allows). If the patient's drive to breathe is negated, the ventilator "kicks in" at the preset rate. This ensures that the patient never stops breathing while on the ventilator. In the assist–control mode, all breaths—whether triggered by the patient or delivered at a set rate—are at the same V_T. Because of this, hyperventilation (reflected in ABGs as a respiratory alkalosis) can occur.

The *IMV mode* allows intermittent mandatory ventilation. As in the control mode, the rate and V_T are preset. If the patient wishes to breathe above this rate, he or she may. However, unlike the assist–control mode, any breaths taken above the set rate are spontaneous breaths taken through the ventilator circuit. The V_T of these breaths can vary drastically from the V_T set on the ventilator because they are determined by the patient's ability to generate negative pressure in the chest. V_T can vary from 0 to 1 liter.

To understand IMV, one must review the basic functioning of the ventilator. Instantaneously, as the ventilator delivers a preset volume to the patient, a burst of air inflates a balloon in the exhalation port, forcing the air in only one direction—into the patient. After inspiration is terminated, the balloon deflates and air rushes into the area of least resistance—out the exhalation port. This occurs with every ventilator cycle in assist, control, and assist–control modes.

However, if the IMV mode is used, the balloon is inflated *only* during the *mandatory cycles*. The rate and V_T are dialed-in for only the IMV breaths. As the patient triggers above this rate, the balloon is not inflated. These are non-IMV breaths. Because the balloon is not inflated

during these breaths, the ventilator bellows "dump" and air is delivered to the area of least resistance. If the patient generates negative pressure in the chest, some or all of the V_T dumped can be delivered to the patient. If the patient is unable to generate adequate negative pressure, all of the V_T dumped rushes out the exhalation port with none reaching the patient.

Because of this, accurate monitoring of *inspired* V_T must be done. On the newer ventilators, this is accomplished by a continuous digital readout of inspired V_T with alarms set accordingly. On the older models, such as the Monaghan, there are no such monitoring systems. The nurse or respiratory therapist *is* the *alarm system*. With these ventilators, Wright respirometers must be placed in line of the ventilator circuit, between the patient and the exhalation port (Fig. 19–12). A total minute ventilation (MV) is calculated. From this, one subtracts the IMV MV to obtain the patient's MV.

$$\frac{\begin{array}{r} \text{Total MV} \\ - \text{IMV} \end{array}}{\text{Patient's MV}}$$

For example: the total MV, as measured in-line on the Wright respirometer, is 10 liters, and the ventilator is set for an IMV rate of 8 and V_T of 800. The following calculations produce the amount of patient's contribution to ventilation:

Total MV	10	liters
− IMV MV	6.4	liters ($V_T \times$ rate)
Patient's MV	3.6	liters

If the patient fatigues and drops the contribution to less than 3.6 liters, an ABG must be obtained to evaluate the $PaCO_2$. If the IMV rate is set very low and the patient fatigues, MV is reduced drastically. Because of this, the $PaCO_2$ elevates rapidly and the patient can have an arrest—on a mechanical ventilator. Use of IMV as a weaning tool is discussed in the next section.

In selecting a patient for IMV, compliance and respiratory reserve must be evaluated. If compliance and reserve are both low and IMV is instituted, the work of breathing increases dramatically. The controversy continues concerning the use of IMV. Does it re-train by building endurance in respiratory muscles or induce long-term fatigue resulting in weaning failures?

In the IMV mode, the mandatory breaths are delivered at a set rate regardless of whether the patient is in inspiration or expiration. Some ventilators have the IMV mode synchronized (SIMV) so that the mandatory breaths are delivered in synchrony with patient triggering.

The IMV mode is desirable for use in the patient with a high ventilatory drive who "fights the ventilator." In the assist–control mode, this type of patient can trigger the ventilator, developing a severe respiratory alkalosis. Insti-

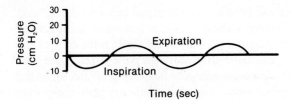

Spontaneous Breathing

Patient has full work of breathing: determining rate, V_T, and rhythm.

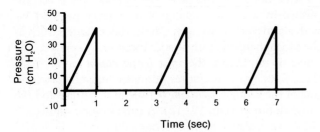

Controlled Ventilation

Patient has no work breathing: ventilator will rhythmically deliver V_T at preset rate.

Assist-Control

Patient has minimal work of breathing during initial expansion of chest, then ventilator will deliver preset V_T.

Intermittent Mandatory Ventilation (IMV)

Patient has a variable work of breathing: the mandatory ventilated breaths occur at a preset rate and V_T, but the patient may take spontaneous breaths between the machine-delivered breaths.

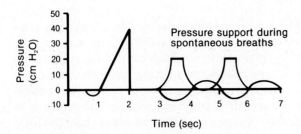

IMV with Pressure Support (12 cm H_2O)

Patient has low-to-moderate work of breathing: the spontaneous breaths are supported with a preset pressure assistance.

FIGURE 19–11
Comparison of ventilatory modes.

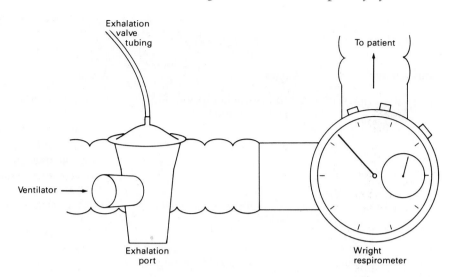

FIGURE 19–12
Wright respirometer in-line circuit is
used to determine MV.

tuting IMV decreases the patient's total minute ventilation, satisfies the need to control the respiratory rate, and
decreases sedation requirements. IMV is also the most
efficient mode to minimize mean thoracic pressure, ventilator complications, and hemodynamic compromise (see
Figure 19–11).

Pressure Support Ventilation (PSV)

The pressure support mode augments or assists spontaneous breathing efforts up to a point where the preset
pressure is reached. This concept is similar to the IPPB
devices used to deliver bronchodilators to nonventilated
patients. It is now incorporated in some of the new ventilators. Pressure support is used at low pressure levels (5–10
cm H_2O) to aid the patient in breathing during the spontaneous breaths in the IMV mode. Specific uses of pressure support are to promote patient comfort, to decrease
the work of breathing necessary to overcome the resistance of the endotracheal tube, and for weaning. Endotracheal tube resistance can be related to the effort needed
in breathing through a straw if one is submerged under
water. The smaller the straw, the larger the effort to move
air from the atmosphere into the lungs. Pressure support
reduces this work. As a weaning tool, pressure support is
thought to increase the endurance of the respiratory muscles by decreasing the physical work and oxygen demands
during spontaneous breathing. According to Petty,[11] PSV
probably offers no advantages to weaning.

Airway Pressure Release Ventilation (APRV)

This mode allows a patient during spontaneous breathing
to exhale at a lower volume than provided by the ventilator. APRV is similar to continuous positive airway pressure (CPAP) except that the end-expiratory pressure is
periodically released and then re-applied in the next breath.

The purpose of this mode is to allow the patient's breaths to
be assisted without increasing inspiratory airway pressures.

Inverse Ratio Ventilation (IRV)

Most ventilators operate with a short inspiratory time and
a long expiratory time; this promotes venous return and
allows time for air to exit out of the lungs. IRV reverses
this ratio so that inspiratory time is much longer than
expiratory time. With this inverse ratio, intrathoracic pressure is often higher.

Indications for Ventilatory Support

Respiratory Failure

Respiratory failure is defined as an inability to maintain an
adequate pH, $PaCO_2$, and PaO_2. *Adequate* means a pH
greater than 7.25, a $PaCO_2$ less than 50 mm Hg, and a
PaO_2 greater than 50 mm Hg with the patient on oxygen.
If the ABGs deteriorate and the patient fatigues, mechanical ventilatory support is indicated (Table 19–16).

Many times, it is the nurse who initially recognizes
the onset of respiratory failure. Simple bedside monitoring can alert the nurse to signs of patient decompensation.
Two simple, noninvasive, and inexpensive indicators that
can be used are respiratory rate and vital capacity.

Normal respiratory rate (RR) is 16 to 20 breaths per
minute. If the rate increases to 25 breaths per minute, the
patient's status must be evaluated and appropriate measures instituted—namely, suctioning, postural drainage,
and chest physiotherapy. Once RR reaches 40/min or
more, the "work of breathing" to maintain less than acceptable blood gas values is high. Eventually, exhaustion
occurs, and ventilatory assistance is required. This process

TABLE 19–16
Indications for Mechanical Ventilation

Parameters	Values	Action
Respiratory rate	<10 breaths/min (diminished drive to breathe)	Evaluate patient and eliminate cause
	16–20 breaths/min	Normal
	28–40 breaths/min	Evaluate patient and institute appropriate measures
	>40 breaths/min	Consider elective intubation/ventilation
Vital capacity	<10–20 ml/kg (poor ventilatory reserve)	Watch for signs of respiratory failure
		Prepare to initiate ventilatory support
Inspiratory pressures	<20 cm water or decreasing trend	
Arterial blood gases		
pH	<7.25	Evaluate in combination with rising $PaCO_2$
$PaCO_2$	>50 mm Hg	Evaluate in combination with decreasing pH
PaO_2	<50 mm Hg while on O_2	Evaluate in combination with the pH and $PaCO_2$
A – a gradient Shunt	≥300 mm Hg	
	≥25–30	
Chest auscultation	Diminished or no breath sounds	Deliver 100% O_2
		Prepare ventilatory support
Heart rate and rhythm	Pulse over 120, dysrhythmias	Monitor for dysrhythmias
Activity	Extreme fatigue, lessened activity tolerance	Evaluate with above and take appropriate measures
Mental status	Confusion, delirium, somnolence	Monitor for hypoxic seizure activity
Physical observation	Use of accessory muscles, fatiguing, extreme work of breathing	Prepare for ventilatory support

can occur over hours or minutes, depending on the patient's respiratory reserve (see Table 19–16).

Vital capacity (VC), the second parameter, is a measure of ventilation. Using a simple bedside spirometer, the patient is asked to take a deep breath and exhale through the spirometer until the lungs are completely emptied. If VC is less than 10 to 20 ml/kg, respiratory reserve is minimal. Serial monitoring of this parameter is more meaningful than a one-spot check. A good clinical example is a patient with a cervical spine injury. Serial monitoring of VC can show the progression of ascending edema and dictate elective rather than crisis intubation and resuscitation.

In summary, identification of high-risk patients, serial monitoring and evaluation of progressive respiratory status, and institution of appropriate measures can forestall or negate the need for mechanical ventilation.

Procedure

Before placing a patient on a ventilator, attach the ventilator to a test lung to adjust the settings to the standard guidelines.

Standard Settings

Fraction of inspired oxygen (FIO_2)	100%
Tidal volume (V_T)	10–15 ml/kg body weight
Respiratory rate (RR)	10–15 breaths/min
Inspiratory flow	40–60 L/sec
Sensitivity	– 2 cm H_2O
Sigh rate (optional)	1–2/min, V_T 20 ml/kg
Positive end-expiratory pressure (PEEP)	0–5 cm

Settings for the patient are determined by the goals of the therapy, and changes of the settings are determined by the patient's response as reflected in ABGs.

Fraction of Inspired Oxygen (FIO_2)

Initially, the patient without a previous blood gas level available is placed on 100% (.100) oxygen. Several calculations determine subsequent ventilator changes in oxygen delivery and evaluate the imbalance between pulmonary perfusion and ventilation. With the alveolar air equation (Fig. 19–13), an oxygen change on the ventilator can be calculated using a target PaO_2. Experienced practitioners usually are able to manipulate ventilator oxygen concentrations without using the lengthy calculation, but to the inexperienced nurse or therapist, this calculation is necessary for safety. To determine the amount of blood that has bypassed the lungs and not picked up oxygen, the a/A ratio and the A–a gradient are calculations that reveal intrapulmonary shunting. Of the two, the a/A ratio depicts a more accurate pulmonary status because it uses the difference in FIO_2 concentrations.

Respiratory Rate and Tidal Volume

$RR \times V_T = MV$. In turn, MV determines alveolar ventilation. These two parameters are adjusted according to the $PaCO_2$. Increasing MV decreases $PaCO_2$; conversely, decreasing MV increases $PaCO_2$. There are special cases, however, in which hypoventilation or hyperventilation is desired. For example, in a head injury, the neurosurgeon may wish a respiratory alkalosis to occur to promote cerebral vasoconstriction. In this case, the V_T and RR are increased to achieve the desired alkalotic pH by $PaCO_2$ manipulation. In contrast, COPD patients whose baseline ABGs consist of elevated carbon dioxide need to be mechanically hypoventilated at their baseline $PaCO_2$. These patients usually have a large acid load, and lowering their carbon dioxide levels rapidly can result in seizures. Patients with restrictive diseases need careful monitoring of their blood gases because they may need lower V_T and higher RR.

Peak Flow

If MV is high, peak flow may need to be increased to provide time for exhalation before a new inhalation is triggered. However, remember that increasing peak flow increases turbulence, which is reflected in increasing airway pressures.

Positive End-Expiratory Pressure (PEEP)

PEEP is used for patients who require FIO_2 levels greater than .50 for more than several hours to achieve adequate arterial oxygen levels. Most often this is the patient who develops acute respiratory distress syndrome (ARDS) with refractive hypoxia. In this case, despite greater concentrations of oxygen administration, the PaO_2 deteriorates rapidly. Currently, PEEP is also being used to control postoperative bleeding in patients who have undergone coronary artery surgery. PEEP is thought to exert a tamponade effect on the area of bleeding. In controlled clinical trials, however, no effect on mediastinal bleeding could be established. Although this is a common practice, the scientific basis for it is non-existent.[12]

Calculating Alveolar Air

P_AO_2 = partial pressure of O_2 in alveolus
PaO_2 = partial pressure of O_2 in arteries
PIO_2 = partial pressure of inspired O_2
P_ACO_2 = partial pressure of CO_2 in alveolus
$PaCO_2$ = partial pressure of CO_2 in arteries
(P_ACO_2 = the patient's $PaCO_2$)
R = respiratory quotient = 1 on O_2 = 0.8

    on room air and reflects $\dfrac{CO_2\ production}{O_2\ consumption}$

Pb = barometric pressure
P_{H_2O} = water pressure
FIO_2 = fraction of inspired oxygen

Alveolar Air Equation: $P_AO_2 = PIO_2 - \dfrac{PaCO_2}{R}$

STEP 1: $PIO_2 = FIO_2 (Pb - P_{H_2O})$

STEP 2: Substituting the following given values,

    aPb of 647 mm Hg
    P_{H_2O} of 47 mm Hg

and a patient on .100 O_2 with a $PaCO_2$ of 40 mm Hg, the equation would read:

$$P_AO_2 = 1.00(647 - 47) - \frac{40}{1}$$
$$= 1.00(600) - 40$$
$$= 600 - 40$$
$$= 560\ mm\ Hg$$

STEP 3: Blood gases are drawn on 100% FIO_2 with the following results:

$pH = 7.40$
$PaO_2 = 300$ mm Hg
$PaCO_2 = 40$ mm Hg

STEP 4: To calculate *target* PaO_2, set PaO_2 and P_AO_2 in ratio form.
Because normal PaO_2 in Denver is 65 to 75 mm Hg, target PaO_2 would be 75 mm Hg.

(Equation) $\dfrac{P_AO_2}{PaO_2} = \dfrac{560}{300} = \dfrac{x}{75}$
(Blood gas)

x = the P_AO_2 to give a target PaO_2 of 75 mm Hg

$(560)\ 75 = 300x$

$\dfrac{(560)\ 75}{300} = x$

$140 = x$

From these calculations, to have a PaO_2 of 75 mm Hg, a P_AO_2 of 140 is needed.

STEP 5: Now to find the FIO_2 that gives a P_AO_2 of 140, substitute the values into the alveolar air equation. (Assume everything else stays constant.)

$$140 = x\ (647 - 47) - \frac{40}{1}$$
$$x = target\ FIO_2$$
$$140 = x\ (600) - 40$$
$$180 = 600x$$
$$.30 = x$$

STEP 6: Therefore, for a target PaO_2 of 75 mm Hg, the FIO_2 on the ventilator can be reduced to .30.

FIGURE 19–13
Calculating alveolar air.

In patients who require greater than 50% oxygen concentrations for prolonged periods, the risk of oxygen toxicity increases. Because oxygen toxicity is time–dose related, PEEP is instituted to decrease the need for high FIO_2 concentrations. It is important to weigh the risk of PEEP against the risk of oxygen concentrations. The physiological effects of PEEP on cardiac output and tissue oxygenation must be monitored through the use of mixed venous and arterial blood gases. (See Chapter 18).

In the patient who does not have adequate circulating blood volume, institution of PEEP decreases blood return to the heart, decreases cardiac output, and decreases oxygen to the tissues. With an increase in PEEP, arterial oxygenation may improve, but if mixed venous oxygenation worsens, PEEP is not therapeutic. If hypotension or decreased cardiac output results from PEEP application, restoring circulating volume usually corrects the hypotension.

To evaluate whether the effects of PEEP are beneficial, monitoring of arterial and mixed venous blood gases, hemodynamic pressures to include cardiac output, compliance, and blood pressure is necessary. Baseline values are obtained before changes in PEEP. PEEP is usually increased in increments of 2.5 to 5 cm of water pressure. The patient is monitored for adverse effects such as hypotension, dysrhythmias, and increased intracranial pressure. If these occur, the PEEP is removed. If PEEP is tolerated, the patient is stabilized on the new PEEP settings for approximately 15 minutes. The monitored parameters are then repeated. Because the goal of PEEP therapy is to increase oxygen delivery to the tissues, a calculation using the following formula can determine its effectiveness:

$$O_2 \text{ delivery} = CO\ [1.34(Hgb)(SaO_2) + 0.003\ PaO_2]$$

where Hgb is hemoglobin concentration, SaO_2 is arterial oxygenation saturation, and PaO_2 is arterial oxygen pressure.

During the PEEP trials, compliance is calculated and monitored. If compliance falls, the risk of pneumothorax or barotrauma must be weighed against the improvement in oxygenation.

Reduction in PEEP is considered if the patient has a PaO_2 of 80 to 100 mm Hg on an FIO_2 of .50 or less and is hemodynamically stable, and the underlying illness is stable or improving. A similar process is followed in reducing PEEP as in adding PEEP. In addition, monitoring of ear or finger oximetry is recommended. If the saturation falls dramatically in the first 3 minutes, the PEEP levels are returned to the previous settings. If oxygenation is maintained at an adequate level, PEEP is reduced, monitoring the parameters discussed above at 1-, 6-, and 12-hour intervals.

PEEP holds the alveoli open by maintaining a pressure greater than atmospheric pressure in the alveoli at the end of expiration. This end-expiratory pressure increases functional residual capacity (FRC) by reinflating collapsed alveoli, keeping the alveoli open, and decreasing the pressure needed to ventilate them. In addition, there is some evidence that keeping the alveoli open enhances surfactant regeneration. If a patient requires high levels of PEEP for a prolonged period, decreasing PEEP must be done slowly. Within 4 hours after PEEP is decreased, airways can start to collapse again owing to hypoxia.

Hemodynamic measurements (PCWP, PAD, PAS) are taken at end-expiration with the patient on PEEP. It is no longer necessary to discontinue PEEP by removing the patient from the ventilator, because it takes a significant amount of time for the effects of PEEP to become reestablished. Hemodynamic measurements can be inaccurate indicators of oxygen delivery to the tissues if a patient is on PEEP and the position of the catheter is not below the left atrium. The position of the catheter should be verified on a lateral chest x-ray. If the catheter tip is lodged within 1 cm of or above the left atrium, the catheter does not reflect accurate left atrial pressures if PEEP is used and left atrial pressures are low.

Sensitivity

One can set sensitivity in some machines by turning the knob (increasing sensitivity) to the point that the ventilator "chatters." Chatter comes from the sound of the ventilator constantly dumping. The dial is then slowly decreased to the point at which the chattering stops. At this point, the ventilator can be triggered whenever -2 cm negative pressure is generated.

Some physicians prefer to have the patient trigger the ventilator. Keeping the patient in control of the ventilator enables him or her to adjust the MV as needed. This is also of benefit to the patient being weaned from the ventilator. In contrast, some physicians prefer to paralyze, anesthetize, dial-out the sensitivity, or increase MV so the patient does not initiate respiration on the ventilator. They prefer to rest the patient while the ventilator does the work of breathing. In the latter case, psychological support must be provided if the patient is alert and awake.

Addition of PEEP can change the sensitivity on a ventilator. For example, if the machine is set so that generation of -2 cm initiates respiration, the patient triggers the ventilator by "sucking" the dial from zero to -2. If 10 cm of PEEP is added, the ventilator is still triggered at -2 cm. However, now the patient must suck the needle from 10 to -2 (-12 cm pressure) to initiate a breath. This increases the patient's work of breathing. Because of this increased work, the patient may stop triggering the machine, decreasing the MV. To correct this, the sensitivity is increased so that inspiration is initiated at 8 cm of pressure. Thus, when the patient sucks the needle from 10 cm to 8 (-2 cm), the work of breathing is decreased to the initial level. If PEEP is decreased to levels less than 8 cm, sensitivity must also be decreased or oversensitivity occurs, resulting in a severe respiratory alkalosis from mechanical hyperventilation (Fig. 19–14).

Dead Space

Dead space is a term designating the addition of tubing between the patient and the exhalation valve. In essence, the patient is rebreathing his exhaled CO_2. Indication for additional dead space is a respiratory alkalosis not mechanically correctable through manipulation of RR and V_T. Clinically, for some physiological reason, the patient is hyperventilating. This type of high ventilatory output failure is often seen in adult respiratory distress syndrome (ARDS). Because it is desirable to correct this alkalosis by correcting the primary ABG abnormality (decreased $PaCO_2$), dead space is sometimes added.

An MV must be calculated before and after addition of dead space. Some patients appear very sensitive to $PaCO_2$ levels. If 5 inches of dead space is added, they can increase their MV so that the effect on the $PaCO_2$ values is negligible, and continued addition of many inches of dead space can force the patient into agonal breathing. If this does occur, simply switching to the IMV mode of ventilation correct the respiratory alkalosis.

There is no set formula for calculating inches of dead space for rises in $PaCO_2$. This is a trial-and-error process. Because 5 inches constitutes a negligible amount, 10 inches is usually applied initially.

It must be stressed that *mechanical manipulation of $PaCO_2$ must be based on pH values.* In other words, if a patient is in metabolic acidosis and the $PaCO_2$ is low because of this, dead space is not indicated. Additional dead space at this time would force the patient into a more severe acidosis.

Lastly, because the partial pressures of CO_2 and O_2 largely determine the total pressure of inhaled gas on a ventilator, increasing the $PaCO_2$ can slightly lower the oxygen values. Since the advent of IMV, dead space is used only in selected cases.

Alarm Systems

Mechanical ventilators are used to support life. Alarm systems are necessary to warn the nurse of developing problems. Alarm systems can be categorized according to volume versus pressure and high versus low. Low-pressure alarms warn of disconnection from the patient. High-pressure alarms warn of rising pressures. Low-volume

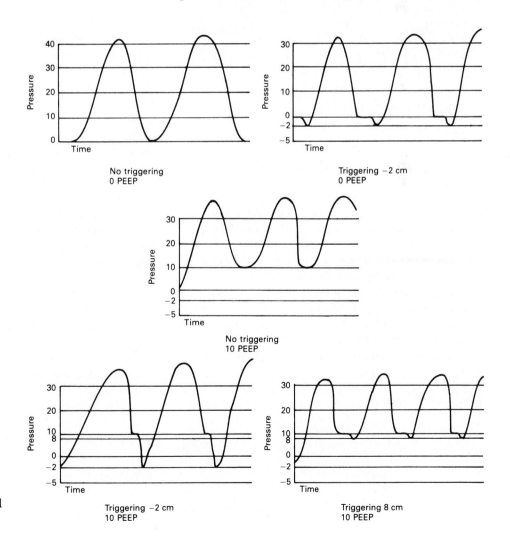

FIGURE 19–14
Respiratory wave forms with different settings of PEEP and triggering.

alarms warn of leaks. Electrical failure alarms are a *must* for all ventilators.

A nurse or respiratory therapist *must* respond to every ventilator alarm. Alarms must never be ignored, disarmed, or placed on "standby." Some trouble-shooting guidelines are presented in Table 19–22.

Humidification and Temperature

Mechanical ventilation bypasses the upper airway, thus negating the body's protective mechanism for humidification and warming. These two processes must be added—a humidifier with a temperature control. All air delivered by the ventilator passes through the water in the humidifier, being warmed and saturated. Because of this, no insensible water loss occurs; such loss is usually 300 to 500 ml/24 h. In most instances, the temperature of the air is about body temperature. In some rare instances (severe hypothermia), the air temperature can be increased. Caution is advised because prolonged, high, inhaled temperatures can cause tracheal burns. Contrary to a dangerous myth, a dry humidifier does *not* decrease pulmonary edema! It only contributes to drying the airway, with resultant mucous plugging and an inability to suction out secretions.

As the air is passed through the ventilator to the patient, large droplets are rained out in the corrugated hose. This moisture is considered contaminated and must be drained into a receptacle and not back into the sterile humidifier. If the water is allowed to build up, resistance is developed in circuit and PEEP is generated. In addition, if left unchecked, the water can be aspirated by the patient. Attention to this is a primary nursing responsibility.

Assessment and Management

The patient who needs ventilatory support also needs primary nursing care (Nursing Care Plan 19–1: The Mechanically Ventilated Patient). Critical care units, mechanical ventilators, and intubation naturally evoke psychological stress. Communications are frustrating and anxiety-producing because the intubated patient is not able to speak. Each patient must be told that the tube prevents talking and that nothing is wrong with the voice. Perhaps the patient can write or use sign language to indicate messages, and the nurse can be more aware of nonverbal communications and body language.

Airway Care

Airway care consists of adequate humidification, measures to mobilize secretions, position changes, and suctioning. Humidification and warming (discussed previously) are accomplished by mechanical additions to the ventilator to prevent airway obstruction from dry secretions and mucous plugs. Mobilizing of secretions through chest physiotherapy and position changes is discussed earlier in this chapter.

Suctioning is done only if necessary, because it exposes the patient to risks such as hypoxemia, atelectasis, infection, and aspiration. Suctioning is done if rhonchi are auscultated or secretions are heard during respiration. A rise in ventilator peak inspiratory pressures can signify plugging or narrowing of the airways by secretions, also indicating a need for suctioning. Pertinent points of suctioning a patient on a ventilator are reviewed here.

Before suctioning, obtain baseline values for vital signs, rhythm, and lung sounds. Check the suction pressure; it should not exceed 100 to 120 mm Hg. The size of the suction catheter should not exceed more than one-half the diameter of the endotracheal tube. Hyperoxygenation with 100% oxygen and hyperinflation at one and one-half the VT for four to five breaths before and after each suctioning period help prevent hypoxemia during suctioning. Hyperinflation and hyperoxygenation are accomplished through the use of a manual resuscitator or resetting the ventilator settings to .100 and using the sigh mode. See Table 19–17. The new ventilators have oxygen suctioning buttons that deliver .100 oxygen for a preset period and automatically return to the previous set level.

After hyperoxygenation and hyperinflation, insert the suction catheter with the suction port open until resistance is met. This indicates the catheter is at the level of the carina. On contact, the cough reflex is usually stimulated. Withdraw the catheter a few centimeters before applying suction. This maneuver prevents atelectasis if you have inadvertently entered a small airway. As you withdraw the catheter, rotate it and intermittently occlude the suction port. This prevents pulling the tracheal mucosa from the tracheal wall with the suction catheter. From the time you enter the patient's airway, you should hold your breath; if you are not finished by the time *you* are out of breath, you have suctioned too long and exposed the patient to hypoxemia and dysrhythmias. Suctioning periods must not be longer than 10 seconds. Allow the patient to rest for short periods between suctioning episodes. Continue to monitor the patient for premature ventricular contractions (PVCs), an increase in heart rate, or a decrease in heart rate. The former are indications of hypoxemia; the latter are indications of vagal stimulation by the AV node. After the suctioning is complete, reassess the patient. If the patient is maintained on PEEP pressures, the use of an adapter with a small slit enables suctioning without loss of pressures.

Endotracheal Tube Care

All endotracheal tubes must be anchored securely to prevent tube movement. If taping obscures skin areas, septum or lip necrosis can occur. Because oral hygiene is given

TABLE 19-17
Hyperinflation and Hyperoxygenation Prior to Suctioning

Method	Advantages	Disadvantages
Manual resuscitator bag	Ability to feel lung compliance Ability to vary flows and volumes to remove mucous plugs	Requires ventilator disconnection which affects oxygen saturation and PEEP levels Inconsistent delivery of volumes and oxygen Generates unknown airway pressures
Ventilator	Maintenance of PEEP levels Fewer effects on hemodynamics	Easy to forget to return setting to previous level Requires a "washout period" for oxygen to reach 100% delivered

every day, it is an opportune time to inspect the skin, nose, and mouth for tissue breakdown. Placement of an oral bite block prevents the patient from biting on the tube or displacing the tube with his or her tongue. The use of a swivel connector (connecting the tube to the ventilator circuit), along with anchoring a large loop of tubing to the bed, facilitates patient movement without tube movement.

If the patient is going to require tracheal intubation and ventilation in excess of 21 days, an early conversion to tracheostomy should be considered.[13] Daily assessment is required, and once the decision to convert to tracheotomy is made, it should be done without delay (Table 19–18).

Tube Cuff Pressures

Tube cuff pressures are monitored every shift to prevent overdistention and excess pressure on the tracheal wall. If a patient is on the ventilator, the best pressure is the lowest possible pressure without having a leak of VT. Physiologically, arterial circulation to the tracheal wall is obliterated by pressures of about 30 mm Hg. If a cuff leak is suspected because of a discrepancy in actual versus measured VT, auscultation at the neck for air turbulence can determine whether the seal is adequate (Fig. 19–15).

One method used to inflate a cuff is called the minimal occluding volume (MOV). The same equipment is used. Air is injected slowly during ventilator inspiration. During this time, auscultate over the trachea. When the harsh "rhonchi" sound is no longer audible or prescribed ventilator VT is being delivered, the MOV has been reached, and the tube cuff is occluding the airway without excessive pressure on the trachea. Do not add extra air.

An alternate method is called the minimal leak technique. The same procedure as the MOV described above is used; however, instead of slowly inflating, a very minute amount of air is withdrawn through the syringe until a harsh rumbling sound is auscultated. Deflation is to be done after suctioning the trachea and oropharynx and on ventilator inspiration. Secretions pooled above the cuff are driven up into the mouth and not aspirated.

Gastrointestinal Care

Recent studies indicate that maintaining the natural gastric acid barrier in the stomach plays a major role in decreasing incidence and mortality from nosocomial pneumonia.[14] Intubated patients have a tenfold increase in nosocomial pneumonia. It is the second most common

TABLE 19–18
Early Conversion From ET Tube to Tracheostomy Tube

Advantages	Disadvantages
Prevents further injury from ET tube	Cost of procedure
Increases patient comfort and psychological well-being	Risk of bleeding
Facilitates suctioning and mouth care	Risk of dislodging tube into SQ tissues
More secure artificial airway	Scar and/or disfigurement
Facilitates ambulation and allows for transfer to non-acute setting	
Permits verbal communication	
Facilitates oral nourishment	

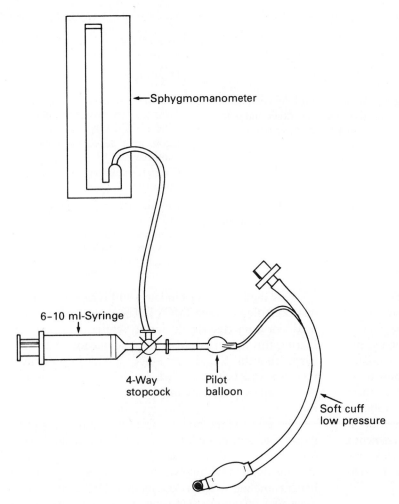

← Sphygmomanometer

6-10 ml-Syringe

4-Way stopcock

Pilot balloon

Soft cuff low pressure

FIGURE 19–15
Monitoring cuff pressures.

1. The pilot balloon tubing is attached to a syringe and mercury manometer by a four-way stopcock.
2. The stopcock is tuned off to the patient.
3. Air pressure is added to the system by compressing the syringe until the mercury manometer reads 20 mm Hg.
4. The stopcock is then turned on to the patient, manometer, and syringe. Pressure can be increased or decreased by manipulation of the syringe.
5. After the pressure is set, preferably at 20 or less at the end of ventilator inspiration, the stopcock is closed to the pilot balloon and the manometer.
6. The pressures are then recorded on the ventilator flowsheet.

hospital acquired infection and the leading cause of death from nosocomial infections. Factors that lead to nosocomial pneumonia are oropharyngeal colonization, gastric colonization, aspiration, and compromised lung defenses.

The widespread use of antacids or H₂ (or histamine H₂ blockers) type blockers to guard against stress bleeding in mechanically ventilated patients can increase colonization of the upper GI tract owing to decreased gastric acidity and predispose the patient to nosocomial infections. Two recently developed approaches are selective decontamination of the GI tract with topical antimicrobial substances[15] and stress ulcer prophylaxis that does not alter the pH of the stomach.[16] Kappstein et al[17] compared the use of sucralfate (a cytoprotective substance) with cimetidine and found a decreased incidence in mortality in the sucralfate group versus the cimetidine group.

Nutritional Support

Nutritional support of ventilated patients should be instituted early. Current research verifies that the many side effects of clinical starvation can lead to pulmonary complications and death, as listed below and in Display Box 19–8.

Respiratory Muscles

Respiratory muscles, like all other body muscles, need energy to work. If energy needs are not met, muscle fatigue occurs. Muscle fatigue leads to discoordination of respiratory muscles and a decrease in VT. Hypomagnesemia and hypophosphatemia have been implicated in muscle fatigue caused by depleted levels of ATP.

DISPLAY BOX 19–8
Results of Clinical Starvation

Atrophy of respiratory muscles
Decreased protein
Decreased albumin
Decreased cell-mediated immunity
Decreased surfactant production
Decreased replication of respiratory epithelium
Intracellular depletion of ATP
Impaired cellular oxygenation
Central respiratory depression

With prolonged starvation the body cannibalizes the intercostal and diaphragmatic muscles for energy. In addition, the respiratory muscles of a patient on long-term ventilation atrophy from inactivity and passive movement by the ventilator. If clinical starvation is not corrected, weaning may be impossible.

Starvation has also been linked to emphysematous changes. In starvation, protein synthesis is decreased, which in turn adversely affects lung tissue elasticity and surfactant production. The potential for pulmonary infection is increased because the normal bacterial clearance mechanisms and immunologic competence are impaired.

Central Nervous System

Normally, hypoxia or hypercapnia stimulates an increase in the rate and depth of breathing. Starvation for 20 days in a normal person weakens this response. If a patient on a ventilator has been on a long period of fast, the normal stimulus to breathe from hypoxia and hypercapnia is blunted. Coupled with respiratory muscle dysfunction and lack of energy, this can make weaning. After starvation is corrected, the response is normalized. This response can also be acquired as the result of long-term residence at high altitudes or can be inherited.

Nutritional Replacement

If the gastrointestinal tract is intact, nutrition can be provided by a feeding tube. Many chronically ill patients, such as those with COPD, have long-standing protein/caloric malnutrition. The concentration is initially diluted, and the rate of administration is slow. The patient is observed for side effects such as diarrhea or hyperosmolar dehydration. Blood sugar determinations and urinalyses for sugar and acetone are done. If the patient tolerates the tube feedings, first the rate and then the concentration are increased.

If tube feedings cannot be tolerated, parenteral hyperalimentation is considered. (See Chapter 35.) If used, one must observe strict aseptic technique to minimize the risk of infection.[18] Basic caloric requirements are usually increased by 25% for hospital activity and stress associated with treatment. Large glucose loads increase carbon dioxide production and can precipitate respiratory failure in a compromised patient. High amino acid infusion also increases oxygen consumption. All ventilator patients who require long-term ventilation need 2,000 to 2,500 calories per day. On the day the patient is to be weaned, the caloric intake is decreased to approximately 1,000 calories and glucose intake limited. This mobilizes fat and produces decreased carbon dioxide levels in the blood.

Eye Care

Eye care in the ventilator patient is an important part of nursing care. Frequent assessment and instillation of ophthalmic ointment or drops decreases corneal drying. If the blink reflex is lost, the lids must be taped to prevent corneal abrasions, drying and inadvertent trauma. Scleral edema can occur in the ventilated patient if the venous pressure is raised, decreasing drainage of blood from the ocular tissues. Raising the head of the bed and proper taping of the ET tube can prevent or reduce scleral edema.[19]

Psychological Care

The ventilated patient is subjected to extreme physical and emotional stress in the critical care environment. Sleep deprivation and sensory overstimulation occur daily in a repetitive cycle. Treatments can often seem dehumanizing. In many cases, the prognosis is poor, and the possibility of death is ever present. Feelings of helplessness and lack of control can be overwhelming. The patient may

---

Clinical Research

Smith C et al: Diarrhea associated with tube feeding in mechanical ventilated critically ill patients. Nursing Res 39(3):148–152, 1990

Nutritional support of patients receiving mechanical ventilation is often accomplished with tube feedings. Of 73 ventilated and tube-fed patients, 63% had diarrhea. Incidence of diarrhea with tube feedings was higher among ventilated patients than among non-ventilated patients. Use of antibiotics and serum albumin levels were not statistically significant factors. Higher rates of infusion, greater tube feeding osmolality, and changes in tube feeding products were predictors of diarrhea. The duration of diarrhea could be predicted within the first 5 days of tube feeding. Diarrhea was associated with the use of higher osmolalty products and an infusion rate 10 cc/hour higher than in subjects without diarrhea. Nurses caring for ventilated patients with diarrhea should plan for increased need for skin care, emotional support, and close observation of fluid and electrolyte balances.

attempt to gain some element of environmental control through complaining or constant demanding. If coping mechanisms are incapable of dealing with stress, the patient may totally withdraw, exhibiting depression, apathy and lack of emotional involvement.

If a patient has been struggling for years to breathe, assisted ventilation can precipitate a psychological dependence. It seems logical that if, for the first time in years, a patient is receiving enough oxygen to meet metabolic needs and does not have to struggle for air, she or he would be reluctant to give up this feeling of normalcy and comfort. In this situation, weaning can become even more stressful for staff and patient. In fact, the patient may never wean because the staff is reluctant to "torture" the patient during the weaning process.

This is a stressful time for the family of a patient in the critical care unit. They must deal with a strange environment, a critically ill loved one, and the financial strain imposed by the illness. As soon as possible, the family should be familiarized with the physical surroundings, informed of visiting hours, and given progress reports on the condition of the patient. If the patient is critical, visiting hours should be made flexible until the patient stabilizes. Each member of the health care team should be aware of the established guidelines for family involvement in patient care.

Complications of Mechanical Ventilation

The patient on a mechanical ventilator requires observant, skillful, and *repetitive* nursing care. Complications that can occur with this therapy can be minimized—*prevention* is the key (see Display Box 19–9).

Airway Complications

Aspiration can occur before, during, or after intubation. One can minimize the risk of aspiration after intubation by securing the tube, maintaining an inflated cuff, and continuing adequate tube or oral suctioning. If resuscitation was prolonged and gastric distention occurred, the airway must be secured before passing a nasogastric tube for stomach decompression. If aspiration does occur, the potential for the development of ARDS increases.

Most ventilator patients need to have both hands restrained, because self-extubation with aspiration is an ever present complication. In addition, self-extubation with an inflated cuff can result in vocal cord damage.

The procedure of intubation itself is a high risk. Examples of intubation complications include:

- prolonged and complicated intubation → increased hypoxia and tracheal trauma;

> ### DISPLAY BOX 19–9
> #### Complications of Mechanical Ventilation
>
> **Airway**
>
> Aspiration
> Decreased clearance of secretions
> Predisposition to infection
>
> **Endotracheal Tube**
>
> Tube kinked
> Tube plugged
> Rupture of pyriform sinus
> Tracheal stenosis
> Tracheal malacia
> Right main stem intubation
> Cuff failure
> Sinusitis
> Otitis media
> Laryngeal edema
>
> **Mechanical**
>
> Ventilator malfunction
> Hypoventilation
> Hyperventilation
> Tension pneumothorax
>
> **Physiological**
>
> Water and NaCl retention
> Left ventricular dysfunction → hypotension
> Stress ulcers
> Paralytic ileus
> Gastric distention
> Starvation

- main stem intubation (usually right) → unequal ventilation, increasing the mortality rate;
- intubation of pyriform sinus (rare) → pharyngeal abscess.

Pseudomonas pneumonia frequently develops in cases of prolonged intubation and is always a potential possibility from contaminated equipment.

Endotracheal Tube Problems

If the tube is placed nasotracheally, a severe sinus infection can develop. Alternatively, because of the position of the tube in the pharynx, the orifice to the inner ear can become occluded, resulting in a severe otitis media. Whenever a patient complains of ear or sinus pain or develops a fever of unknown etiology, the sinuses and ears must be checked for possible sources of infection.

Some degree of tracheal damage results from prolonged intubation. Tracheal stenosis and malacia can be minimized if cuff pressures are minimized. Arterial circulation is occluded at cuff pressures of about 30 mm Hg. A decreased incidence of both stenosis and malacia has been reported when cuff pressures are kept at about 20 mm Hg. If laryngeal edema is present, life-threatening postextubation stridor can occur.

Mechanical Problems

Ventilator malfunction is a potentially serious problem. Every 2 to 4 hours ventilator checks are done by nursing or respiratory staff. Inadequate V_T is caused by leaks in the circuit or cuff, disconnected tubing or ventilator, or obstruction to flow. The latter is caused by kinked tubing, retained secretions, severe bronchospasms, coughing spasms, or biting on the endotracheal tube (see Table 19–22).

Iatrogenically induced complications include mechanical overventilation causing respiratory alkalosis and mechanical underventilation causing respiratory acidosis or hypoxemia. ABG studies determine the effectiveness of mechanical ventilation. Note, however, that COPD patients are ventilated at *their normal ABG values*, which can involve high carbon dioxide levels.

Barotrauma

Mechanical ventilation involves "pumping" air into the chest, creating positive pressures during inspiration. If PEEP is added, the pressures are increased and continued throughout expiration. These positive pressures can rupture an alveolus or emphysematous bleb. Air then enters the pleural space, creating a tension pneumothorax—an emergency situation. The patient can suddenly develop extreme dyspnea and complain of pain on the affected side. Ventilator pressures depict a sharp increase on the gauge, with the high pressure alarms sounding. On auscultation, the breath sounds on the affected side are decreased or absent. Observation of the patient may reveal a tracheal deviation. Probably the most prominent sign is the resultant hypotension and bradycardia that deteriorates into a cardiac arrest without timely medical intervention. Until the physician is available to decompress the chest with a needle, the nursing intervention is to remove the patient from the positive pressure source and ventilate by the manual resuscitator, providing the patient with small rapid breaths.

Decreased Cardiac Output

Decreased cardiac output reflected by hypotension when a patient is initially committed to a ventilator is attributed to lack of sympathetic tone and decreased venous return. In addition to hypotension, other signs and symptoms can include unexplained restlessness, decreased levels of consciousness, decreased urine output, weak peripheral pulses, slow capillary refill, pallor, fatigue, and chest pain. Hypotension is usually corrected by increasing fluids to correct the hypovolemia.

Positive Water Balance

The decreased venous return to the heart is sensed by the vagal stretch receptors located in the right atrium. This sensed hypovolemia stimulates the release of antidiuretic hormone from the posterior pituitary. The decreased cardiac output leading to decreased urine output compounds the problem by stimulating the renin–angiotensin–aldosterone response. The patient who is mechanically ventilated, hemodynamically unstable, and requiring large amounts of fluid resuscitation can experience extensive edema, including scleral and facial edema.

Weaning from Mechanical Ventilation

From the time the patient is placed on mechanical ventilation, the goal of weaning is present. The process to achieve this goal includes:

- correction of the cause of respiratory failure;
- maintenance of muscle strength;
- proper nutrition;
- psychological preparation.

Each of these phases is as important as the others for a successful discontinuance of ventilatory support.

Each patient is evaluated daily for the possibility of weaning. Generally, patients are categorized as:

- short-term ventilation recipients experiencing uncomplicated extubation;
- long-term ventilation recipients requiring prolonged weaning time.

The former usually require only a short trial of 20 minutes before extubation; the latter require a tedious 3 to 4 weeks of weaning associated with numerous problems.

The criteria listed in Table 19–19 are suggested for assessing the patient's potential to be weaned. All criteria must be evaluated within the context of the patient's disease process and capabilities.

Short-Term Weaning

Before any weaning is initiated, proper preparation of the patient is necessary. All patient resources must be mobilized. Patients ventilated for 24 to 48 hours meet the

TABLE 19–19
Criteria for Weaning

Weaning Tests

Vital Capacity (VC): 10–15 cc/kg
Tidal Volume (V_T): 4–5 cc/kg
*Minute Ventilation (MV):** 6–10 liters
Maximum Voluntary Ventilation (MVV)†: Double the MV
Inspiratory Force‡: 20 cm H_2O or greater
Compliance: −20 ml/cm H_2O or greater
RR: <20/min

Ventilator Settings

FIO_2: <.50
PEEP: 0
V_T: Average for the patient

ABGs

$PaCO_2$: Normal for the patient
$P(A−a)O_2$: >200–300 mm Hg (100% FIO_2)
PaO_2: 60–mid 70 or normal for patient
pH: Normal with all electrolyte imbalances corrected

Endotracheal Tube

Position: Above the carina on x-ray
Size: 8.5 mm diameter or greater
Tracheostomy: For long-term weans

Nutrition

Daily calories: 2000–2500/day
Day of wean: 1000 with limited glucose intake
Time: At least 1 h after a meal

Airway

Secretions: Antibiotics if change in color; suctioned well and rested
Bronchospasms: Controlled with β-adrenergics, theophyllines, or steroids
Position: Up in chair, semi-Fowler's, or positioned for maximizing air exchange or diaphragm movement

Drugs

Sedating agents: Stopped more than 24 h
Paralyzing agents: Stopped more than 24 h

Emotional

"Psyched up" for the wean

Physical

Stable; no new acute process; rested

---

* Minute Ventilation. If MV is higher than 20 liters, the work of breathing is high. The patient may well wean, but after a couple of hours may fatigue and need to be reintubated. When MV is less than 6 liters, hypoventilation will occur. The etiology for hypoventilation needs to be investigated because often the cause is sedation.
† Maximum Voluntary Ventilation (MVV) is obtained by having the patient breathe as hard and as fast as possible for 15 sec. Multiply this by 4 and the answer is total MVV for 1 min. MVV is an objective measurement of the patient's ventilatory reserve. If the patient's work of breathing postextubation is increased and ventilatory reserve is low, reintubation may be needed.
‡ Inspiratory Pressure. Inspiratory pressure gives an indication of inspiratory muscle strength. A pressure less than −20 ml/cm H_2O pressure indicates muscle weakness. The work of breathing will be very costly and fatigue will result.

---

criteria for short-term weaning, provided that the initial cause necessitating ventilation is corrected.

Procedure

Standard steps in weaning are as follows:

1. Start weaning in the morning, not at night when the patient is tired.
2. Explain the procedure to the patient.
3. Suction.
4. Obtain spontaneous parameters.
5. Administer bronchodilators if ordered.
6. Suction.
7. Rest the patient for 15 to 20 minutes.
8. Elevate the head of the bed.
9. Stay with the patient; support, reassure, and evaluate the patient's response to weaning.

Methods

T-Piece. If weaning by **T**-piece is selected, the following procedure is recommended. Collect all physiological data (Table 19–20). Connect the **T**-piece set at the desired FIO_2 to the patient. Usually, 20 to 30 minutes on a **T**-piece is sufficient to evaluate the potential for extubation. Continue to collect physiological data every 5 to 10 minutes or as needed. At the end of 30 minutes, collect ABGs and evaluate the patient for signs of fatigue. If the criteria for weaning are met at this time, extubation is warranted. Extubation should not be done unless some-

TABLE 19–20
Assessment Criteria That May Terminate Weaning From Mechanical Ventilation

Physiological Data

Pulse: Increase or decrease of 20 beats/min or more
Blood pressure: Systolic increase or decrease of 20 mm Hg
Respiratory rate: Change of 10 breaths/min; respiratory rate >25 breaths/min or <8 breaths/min

Psychological/Subjective Data

Dyspnea
Panic
Pain
Fatigue

Objective Observations

Dysrhythmias: PVCs >4/min
Increased accessory muscle use
Increased intercostal retractions
Increased flaring of nostrils
Erratic breathing pattern (paradoxical breathing, increased restlessness, increased drowsiness)
ABGs deteriorating: Increased $PaCO_2$ resulting in pH < 7.35 or oxygen desaturation via oximetry

one qualified to reintubate is present. Post-extubation stridor is sudden and can be fatal. Use of inhaled racemic epinephrine can be tried to constrict capillaries topically and to decrease edema.

Intermittent Mandatory Ventilation. Short-term weaning by IMV is as effective as T-piece weaning. IMV can involve more time, because each incremental rate decrease must be followed by a blood gas determination. The steps outlined for T-piece weaning apply to IMV. The IMV rate is usually decreased by increments of two until a rate of two or zero is reached. At this point, the patient can be evaluated by the weaning criteria to determine the potential for extubation.

Weaning by any method should be terminated if any of the termination criteria are seen. Determination of ABGs and VC before termination can provide data on which to base further weaning plans.

CASE STUDY

A 69-year-old man weighing 67 kg was admitted to the Post Anesthesia Care Unit after coronary artery bypass. Initially he was placed on

IMV	10
FIO_2	100%
PEEP	5 cm
VT	800 cc

Subsequent ABGs revealed

pH	7.38
PaO_2	520
$PaCO_2$	38

The oxygen was reduced to 60%, then 40%, and ABGs documented a normal oxygen level. The patient continued hemodynamically stable throughout the evening and was treated only with renal dose dopamine and two units of 5% albumin. At 11:00 PM he awoke, made no effort to initiate ventilations, and drifted back to sleep immediately.

At 6:00 AM the patient was easily arousable, physiologically stable, and initiating an occasional breath. The IMV rate was decreased by increments of two until a rate of two was reached. Spontaneous parameters at this time revealed

VT	400 cc
VC	1,000 cc
VE	4.8 liters
Respiratory rate	12/min
MIF	−50 cm H_2O

ABGs continued to be normal. The patient was alert and communicated to the staff his desire to have the tube removed. After evaluation of the patient's clinical status and all available data, extubation was carried out. Postextubation blood gases were normal. The patient was awake and continued to present a good clinical picture. This patient demonstrates a short-term, easy, and safe wean from the ventilator.

Long-Term Weaning

Once a patient is ventilated for more than 30 days, discontinuing ventilation is more difficult. The same principles that apply to short-term ventilation apply to long-term ventilation (see Table 19–19). The process is more prolonged, often taking weeks, and the criteria applied must be adjusted to chronic disease process.

Procedure

After the decision is made to begin weaning, a team approach is necessary. The team should include the physician, nursing staff, respiratory therapist, physical therapist, nutritional therapist, and psychologist. A care plan is devised that includes daily exercise, walking, and wheelchair trips outside the critical care unit. The weaning process is reviewed at this time, short-term goals are formulated, and misgivings that can hinder the weaning process are expressed. Any manipulative behavior on the part of the patient is addressed at this time, and a systematic approach to the problem is defined. A designated primary nurse should coordinate and evaluate the weaning process daily.

After the plan of care is decided, the primary nurse discusses the plan with the patient and family. If the patient wishes to set personal goals, they should be incorporated. At this time, the patient should be informed of the consequences of not being able to wean from the ventilator.

Methods

T-Piece. If the T-piece is selected as the method of weaning, a schedule of time on the ventilator and time on the T-piece is prepared. The number of minutes on the T-piece is totalled every 24 hours. The goal is to increase the time off the ventilator until the patient is able to tolerate 48 hours off the ventilator. The best way to provide ventilation (rest periods) during the wean is by assist–control mode or IMV at high rates. IMV at low rates may not provide sufficient rest for the respiratory muscles, resulting in a weaning failure because of fatigue. If the T-piece is chosen as the weaning tool, the following schedule is suggested:

1. Initially, wean only during the day.
2. Obtain serial ABGs and other physiological parameters.
3. Start with 5-minute weaning periods per hour.
4. Gradually increase the 5-minute weans further into the day.
5. Stress patient, but do not overfatigue.
6. Increase weaning periods to 10 min/hour.
7. Increase weaning periods by 5-minute increments until 30 min/hour is attained.

8. Increase rest periods to 1 hour after weaning periods of 30 minutes are achieved.
9. Decrease VT on the respirator by 50 cc/day.
10. After 8-hour weaning periods are attained, extend weaning into late night and early morning.
11. Continue 1-hour rests between weaning periods.
12. Wean through the night—*slowly;* this is the crucial period.
13. Wean accomplished.

During this prolonged weaning process, a record is maintained by the primary nurse and the patient as to the total number of hours accomplished off the ventilator each day. An additional record with ABG values and spontaneous parameters is also maintained. These records ensure that the patient is actually increasing the time off the ventilator and provide positive feedback for the patient and staff.

Usually, this process is not as progressive and uncomplicated as described. Many delays and setbacks occur. Weekly nursing care sessions provide staff support, redefine goals, and address new nursing diagnoses.

Intermittent Mandatory Ventilation. The preparations for IMV are the same as those described previously. The IMV rate is decreased slowly. Theoretically, this provides the patient time to exercise the muscles of respiration, although there are no clinical data to support this theory. Skillful evaluation by the team for hypoventilation and hypercapnia due to fatigue is essential. VT also can be slowly decreased as the weaning progresses. Monitoring is done with serial ABGs and with the patient's contributory minute ventilation.

Table 19–21 outlines some equipment and techniques that can prove useful in the weaning process.

Continuous Positive Airway Pressure (CPAP). The use of CPAP at 5 cm H_2O or less in weaning continues to be controversial. However, it can be beneficial to those patients with unstable airways and large alveolar-to-arterial PO_2 gradients that result in early alveolar collapse. Because of this, the patient with ARDS can benefit from PEEP or CPAP during weaning.

Pressure Support Ventilation (PSV). Pressure support is a new weaning and ventilation method. The use of pressure support is thought to increase endurance and retrain the respiratory muscles to breathe. One way to wean with PSV is to start with a pressure level that produces a desired VT. The pressure is then reduced in small increments provided the VT continues adequate. Another weaning method is to combine the use of PSV with IMV. The IMV rate is reduced (as described earlier) while the patient's spontaneous breaths are augmented with PSV at low levels.

Regardless of the weaning method selected, the approach must be consistent, team based, and evaluated daily. Setbacks during the wean are common. The goal is a successful wean with the return of the patient to a life free from mechanical ventilation.

TABLE 19–21
Adjuncts to Weaning

Fenestrated Trach*
- Provides for communication during weaning periods

Kirshner Button
- Provides for communication during weaning periods
- Less resistance to breathing and coughing up secretions than with the fenestrated trach

Large ET Tubes (>8.5 mm)
- Small-diameter endotracheal tubes increase resistance to breathing, thereby increasing work of breathing

Postural Drainage and Percussion
- Aids in removal of secretions

Exercise
- Provides increased stimulation to breathing
- Increases and changes environmental stimuli

Nutrition
- Provides energy for breathing
- Maintains protein balance
- Aids in resistance to infection

IPPB
- Provides periods of hyperinflation and rest during weaning periods
- May maintain patient when weaned

Pulse Oximetry
- Provides noninvasive monitoring of O_2 saturation

* The fenestrated trach tube has an opening in the outer cannula but not the inner cannula. With the inner cannula in place and the cuff inflated, the patient is easily mechanically ventilated. During the weaning process, the inner cannula is removed, the cuff deflated, the outer cannula capped, and supplemental oxygen supplied via nasal cannula. This system permits air to pass from the patient's nares through the hole in the outer cannula (fenestration in the trach tube) and past the vocal cords, allowing verbal communication on the part of the patient.

Troubleshooting

Table 19–22 outlines some of the common problems encountered with mechanical ventilators, suggests possible causes of each problem, and recommends actions to alleviate the problem.

Nursing Care Plan

After the initial crisis is over, a nursing care plan for a coordinated approach to the patient should be developed. Inherent in the plan is the opportunity for the patient to gain some control over the environment and the activities of daily living. A plan must include ways to minimize the work of breathing, periods of rest, and ways to decrease

(*Text continues on page 478*)

NURSING CARE PLAN 19–1:
The Mechanically Ventilated Patient

NURSING DIAGNOSIS	OUTCOME CRITERIA/ PATIENT GOALS	NURSING INTERVENTIONS
Ineffective airway clearance: related to intubation, ventilation, disease process, debilitated state, and fatigue.	• Patient airway will be maintained.	1. Auscultate breath sounds q2–4h and prn.
		2. Suction only when rhonchi are auscultated (suction pressures should not exceed 100–120 mm Hg). Hyperoxygenate with 4–5 breaths of 100% O_2 and hyperinflate with $1\frac{1}{2}$ times the V_T using a manual resuscitation bag or ventilator. Auscultate breath sounds after suctioning.
		3. Monitor ventilator humidifier and temperature (95–100° F).
		4. Monitor hydration status of patient to prevent viscous secretions.
		5. Monitor dynamic ventilator pressures for sudden increases indicating plugging of airways.
		6. Administer saline lavage as indicated for removal of thick secretions.
		7. Administer chest physiotherapy as indicated with frequent changes in position.
		8. Administer bronchodilator drugs, as ordered, and evaluate their effectiveness on bronchospasms.
		9. Turn and position to facilitate gravity drainage of secretions.
Impaired gas exchange: related to retained secretions, disease process, or improper ventilator settings.	• Arterial blood gases will be within normal range for the patient.	1. Obtain ABGs 10–30 min after ventilator changes occur.
		2. Monitor ABGs or oximetry during periods of weaning.
		3. Assess whether certain positions cause decreased PaO_2 or precipitate respiratory discomfort.
		4. Monitor for signs and symptoms of hypoxia and hypercapnia.
Ineffective breathing pattern: related to fatigue, improper ventilator settings, increased secretions, or endotracheal tube obstruction.	• Patient will maintain an effective breathing pattern.	1. Perform ventilator checks by qualified nursing personnel or respiratory personnel q1–2h.
		2. Evaluate all alarms and determine cause, stat.

(continued)

NURSING CARE PLAN 19–1: *(Continued)*
The Mechanically Ventilated Patient

NURSING DIAGNOSIS	OUTCOME CRITERIA/ PATIENT GOALS	NURSING INTERVENTIONS
		3. Maintain a manual resuscitator at the bedside at all times.
		4. Monitor tubing for disconnect, kinking, leaks, or obstruction.
		5. Evaluate cuff pressure/leaks.
		6. Insert a bite block or oral airway to prevent biting on the tube.
		7. Secure endotracheal tube with holder or adhesive tape. Check for breath sounds bilaterally after loosening or changing the tape. Note position at lips in reference to cm markings on the tube.
		8. Position patient to prevent occlusion or dislodging of the tube.
		9. Restrain patient to prevent self-extubation, as per unit protocol.
		10. Evaluate proper positioning of endotracheal tube by x-ray placement and bilateral auscultation.
Altered nutrition, less than body requirements: related to critical illness, increased metabolic needs, lack of ability to consume foods orally.	• Patient will maintain body weight and approach normal weight.	1. Weigh patient daily.
		2. Maintain high caloric intake by tube feedings, total parenteral nutrition, and intralipids. Avoid high carbohydrate loads which can elevate $PaCO_2$ levels during weaning.
		3. Once trached, evaluate and initiate oral feeding as patient tolerates.
Impaired verbal communication: related to endotracheal tube placement.	• Maintain communication by alternate methods.	1. Explain environment, all procedures, expectations, and equipment.
		2. Keep call bell by patient at all times.
		3. Provide notepad and pencil, slate, letter or picture board for communication. Ask "yes" or "no" questions.
		4. Reassure patient that voice will return once the endotracheal tube is removed.

(continued)

NURSING CARE PLAN 19–1: (Continued)
The Mechanically Ventilated Patient

NURSING DIAGNOSIS	OUTCOME CRITERIA/ PATIENT GOALS	NURSING INTERVENTIONS
		5. Anticipate and support patient during periods of anxiety and frustration.
		6. Remain with patient during process of weaning from ventilator.
Anxiety: related to fear of illness/death and critical care environment; patient and family.	• Patient will use effective coping mechanisms.	1. Maximize patient's control of ADL.
		2. Include family in care.
		3. Sedate as needed if ordered by physician.
		4. Maximize effective coping styles.
		5. Document patient's emotional response to critical illness.
		6. Monitor for signs of ICU psychosis.
		7. Collaborate with physician in providing prognosis and realistic information at patient's level of understanding.
		8. Provide for periods of uninterrupted sleep.
Pain: related to mechanical ventilation, endotracheal tube placement.	• Pain will be relieved or controlled.	1. Maintain tubing position to prevent pulling or jarring of the endotracheal tube.
		2. Adjust ventilator flow rates for comfort.
		3. Adjust ventilator sensitivity to decrease patient's effort to initiate breathing.
		4. Position patient with head of bed up unless contraindicated. Change position q2h.
		5. Administer analgesic medications as ordered.
High risk for injury: related to mechanical ventilation, endotracheal tube, anxiety, stress.	• Patient will be free from injury during mechanical ventilation.	1. Monitor ventilator for sharp increases on pressure gauge.
		2. Observe for signs and symptoms of barotrauma.
		3. Monitor cuff pressures q2–4h; maintain cuff pressures 20 mm Hg.
		4. Restrain patient to prevent self-extubation.

(continued)

NURSING CARE PLAN 19–1: (Continued)
The Mechanically Ventilated Patient

NURSING DIAGNOSIS	OUTCOME CRITERIA/ PATIENT GOALS	NURSING INTERVENTIONS
		5. Remove NG ASAP or replace with small feeding tube.
		6. Position ventilator tubing to prevent traction on endotracheal tube.
		7. Assess endotracheal tube length and document Q shift (ie, "22 cm at tip").
	• Patient will not develop stress gastric ulcers.	8. Administer antacids and H_2 gastric blockers, as ordered.
		9. Sedate patient, as needed.
		10. Monitor patient for abdominal distension, pH of NG aspirate, Hgb and Hct, auscultate bowel sounds, and check stool for occult blood.
High risk for alterations in tissue perfusion: related to positive pressure ventilation, PEEP, hypotension.	• Maintain stable hemodynamics and mentation.	1. Monitor vital signs, PAPs, PCWP, peripheral perfusion, LOC, and input and output.
		2. Perform measurements of hemodynamics with each change in PEEP setting.
		3. Draw mixed venous gases 20 min after each PEEP setting change, as ordered.
		4. Hyperoxygenate/hyperventilate prior to suctioning.
High risk for high risk of infection: related endotrachael tube placement debilitated state.	• Patient will not acquire a nosocomial infection.	1. Evaluate color, amount, consistency, and odor of sputum with each suctioning.
		2. Collect specimens for culture and sensitivity, as indicated.
		3. Maintain sterile technique when suctioning.
		4. Change ventilator tubing q24–72h.
		5. Perform oral hygiene every shift.
		6. Monitor vital signs for indications of infection.
		7. Palpate sinuses and visually inspect the tympanic membrane for fevers of unknown origin.

(continued)

NURSING CARE PLAN 19–1: (Continued)
The Mechanically Ventilated Patient

NURSING DIAGNOSIS	OUTCOME CRITERIA/ PATIENT GOALS	NURSING INTERVENTIONS
		8. Drain condensed water in ventilator tubing externally away from airway and humidifier reservoir.
		9. Wash hands frequently.
		10. Maintain universal precautions.
High risk for alteration in fluid volume excess: related to positive water balance during mechanical ventilation.	• Maintain water balance and normal electrolyte values.	1. Monitor ventilator temperature and humidifier q2–4h.
		2. Monitor input and output.
		3. Weigh patient daily.
		4. Calculate lung compliance q2–4h.
		5. Monitor serum sodium.
		6. Monitor CXR for signs of water retention.
		7. Check skin tugor and edema.
		8. Auscultate lungs for rales and wheezes q2h.
High risk for anxiety: related to critical illness, fear of death or disfigurement, role changes within social setting or permanent disability.	• Patient will be able to express anxieties to appropriate resource person.	1. Provide environment that encourages open expression of emotional issues.
		2. Mobilize patient's support system and involve these resources as appropriate.
		3. Allow time for patient to express self.
		4. Identify possible hospital resources for patient/family support.
		5. Encourage open family-to-nurse communications regarding emotional issues.
		6. Validate patient and family knowledge base regarding the critical illness.
		7. Involve religious support systems as appropriate.
		8. Allow patient control over some care, when able.

TABLE 19–22
Troubleshooting the Ventilator

Problem	Possible Causes	Action
Volume or pressure alarm on	*Patient-Related*	
	Patient disconnected from ventilator	Reconnect stat.
	Loss of delivered V_T	Occlude endotracheal tube adaptor—if alarm goes off, there is a patient problem; if not, there is a ventilator problem
		Auscultate neck for possible leak around ET cuff
		Review chest film for endotracheal tube placement—may be too high
		Check for loss of V_T through chest tube
	Decrease in patient-initiated breaths	Evaluate patient for cause: check respiratory rate, ABGs, last sedation dosage
	Increased compliance	Good news! May be due to clearing of secretions or relief of bronchospasms
	Ventilator-Related	
	Leaks	Check all tubing for loss of connection, starting at patient and moving toward the ventilator
		Tighten cascade humidifier
		Determine whether ventilator settings have changed
		Check for interference with spirometer dipstick
		Calibrate spirometer or pressure alarm
		If all else fails, replace exhalation valve (*Note:* If problem is not corrected stat, bag-breathe patient until respirator problem is corrected)
	Decreased pressure to ventilator on pressure-driven ventilator (*eg,* Monaghan or Bird)	Have engineering department check pressure line; must deliver 50 psi
High-pressure or peak-pressure alarm	*Patient-Related*	
	Decreased compliance	
	Increased dynamic pressures	Suction patient
		Administer inhaled β-agonists
		If sudden, evaluate for pneumothorax
		Alleviate coughing with sedation or lidocaine
		Try to change patient's position
		Evaluate chest film for endotracheal tube placement in right main stem bronchus
		Sedate if patient is bucking the ventilator or biting the ET tube
	Increased static pressures	Evaluate ABGs for hypoxia, fluids for overload, chest film for atelectasis
		Auscultate breath sounds
	Ventilator-Related	
	Tubing kinked	Check tubing
	Tubing filled with water	Empty water into a receptacle; do not drain back into the humidifier (*Note:* Water in tubing will increase PEEP levels)
	Patient–ventilator asynchrony	Recheck sensitivity and peak flow settings
Abnormal ABGs	*Patient-Related*	
Hypoxia	Secretions	Suction
	Increase in disease pathology	Evaluate patient and chest film
	Positive fluid balance	Evaluate intake and output
Hypocapnia	Hypoxia	Evaluate ABGs and patient
	Increased lung compliance	Good news; evaluate for weaning potential
Hypercapnia	Sedation	Increase respiratory rate or V_T settings on ventilator
	Fatigue	
	Ventilator-Related	

(continued)

TABLE 19–22
Troubleshooting the Ventilator (Continued)

Problem	Possible Causes	Action
Hypoxia	F_IO_2 drift	Check ventilator with oxygen analyzer
		Possible blender piping failure
		Check oxygen source for failure
		Check oxygen reservoir for leaks
Hypocapnia	Settings not set correctly	Decrease respiratory rate, V_T, or MV settings. Consider dead space if assist–control is used
Hypercapnia	Settings not set correctly	Increase respiratory rate, V_T, or MV settings
Heater alarm	Addition of cool water to humidifier	Wait
	Altered setting	Reset
	Faulty temperature gauge	Replace gauge
	Thermostat failure	Replace heater

traffic and noise. See Nursing Care Plan 19–1: The Mechanically Ventilated Patient.

REFERENCES

Bronchial Hygiene

1. Gallon A: Evaluation of chest percussion in the treatment of patients with copious sputum production. Respir Med 85:45–51, 1991
2. Stiller K, Geake T et al: Acute lobar atelectasis: A comparison of two chest physiotherapy regimens. Chest 98:1336–1340, 1990
3. Kinlay S, Olson LG: Patterns of use of chest physiotherapy in a teaching hospital. Aust Clin Rev 11:154–158, 1991

Chest Tubes

4. Gift A, Bolgiano C et al: Sensations during chest tube removal. Heart Lung 20:131–137, 1991
5. Teplitz, L: Update: Are milking and stripping chest tubes necessary? Focus Crit Care 18: 506–511, 1991

Pharmacologic Agents

6. Gever M: Top 25 discharge drugs. Nursing 21(6):53–58, 1991
7. Mathewson H: Adrenergic bronchodilators: Trends in drug design. Respir Care 36(8):861–863, 1991
8. Jederlinic P, Irwin R: Status Asthmaticus. In Rippe J et al: Intensive Care Medicine, pp 545–568. Boston, Little, Brown & Co, 1991
9. Niederman M, Fein A: Acute infectious pneumonia. In Rippe J et al: Intensive Care Medicine, pp 713–728. Boston, Little, Brown & Co, 1991

Ventilatory Support

10. Sauret J, Guitart A: Intermittent short-term negative pressure ventilation and increased oxygenation in COPD patients with severe hypercapnic respiratory failure. Chest 100:455–59, 1991

11. Petty TL: A historical perspective of mechanical ventilation. Crit Care Clin 6:489–504, 1990
12. Petty TL: A historical perspective of mechanical ventilation. Crit Care Clin 6:489–504, 1990
13. Consensus Conference on Artificial Airways in Patients Receiving Mechanical Ventilation. 96:178–81, July 1989
14. Craven DE, Daschner FD: Nosocomial pneumonia in the intubated patient: Role of gastric colonization. Eur J Clin Microbiol Infect Dis :40–50, 1989
15. Meijer K, Hendrik KF van S et al: Infection control in patients undergoing mechanical ventilation: Traditional approach versus a new development-selective decontamination of the digestive tract. Heart Lung 19:11–20, 1990
16. Dellinger PR: Pathophysiology, monitoring, and management of the ventilator-dependent patient: Considerations for drug therapy, emphasis on stress ulcer prophylaxis. DICP 24: , 1990
17. Kappstein I, Schulgen G et al: Incidence of pneumonia in mechanically ventilated patients treated with Sucralfate or cimetidine as prophylaxis for stress bleeding: Bacterial colonization of the stomach. Am J Med 91:2A-125–131, 1991
18. Pingleton S: Enteral nutrition and infection in the intensive care unit. Semin Respir Infect 5:185–90, 1990
19. Hunt L: Eye risks for ventilated or unconscious patients. Am Soc Ophthal Reg Nurse 14:7, 1991

BIBLIOGRAPHY

Bronchial Hygiene

Fedorovich C, Littleton MT: Chest physiotherapy: Evaluating the effectiveness. Dimens Crit Care Nurs 9(2):68–74, 1990
Gursli S, Haanes OC: Lung physiology in cystic fibrosis. Tidsskr Nor Laegeforen 111:720–722, 1991
Mortensen J, Falk M et al: The effects of postural drainage and positive expiratory pressure physiotherapy on tracheobronchial clearance in cystic fibrosis. Chest 100:1350–1357, 1991
Pennza PT: Aspiration pneumonia, necrotizing pneumonia, and lung abscess. Northeast Ohio Universities, College of Medi-

cine, Rootstown. REVIEW ARTICLE: 58 REFS. Emerg Med Clin North Am 7:279–307, 1989

Shim C, Santos GH et al: Percutaneous drainage of lung abscess. Lung 168:201–207, 1990

Vandenplas Y, Diericx A et al: Esophageal pH monitoring data during chest physiotherapy. J Pediatr Gastroenterol Nutr 13:23–26, 1991

Villeneuve MJ, Hodnett ED: Cerebrovascular status and Trendelenburg position in severe head injury. Axon 11:64–67, 1990

Artificial Airways

Advanced Cardiac Life Support, 4th ed. American Heart Association, 1990

Consensus conference on artificial airways in patients receiving mechanical ventilation. Chest 96:178–180, 1989

Habib M: Physiologic implications of artificial airways. Chest 96: 180–186, 1989

Levine SA, Niederman MA: The impact of tracheal intubation on host defenses and risks for nosocomial pneumonia. Clin Chest Med 12:523–543, 1991

Miracle VA, Allnutt DR: How to perform basic airway management. Nursing 20(4):55–60, 1990

Somerson SJ, Sicilia MR: Emergency oxygen administration and airway management. [Continuing education credit.] Crit Care Nurse 12:(4)23–31, 1992

Stone K: Ventilator versus manual resuscitation bag as the method for delivering hyperoxygenation before endotracheal suctioning. AACN Clin Issues Crit Care Nurs 1:289–299, 1990

Stone K, Talaganis S et al: Effect of lung hyperinflation and endotracheal suctioning on heart rate and rhythm in patients after coronary artery bypass graft surgery. Respir Crit Care 20: 443–449, 1991

Chest Tubes

Pierce JD, Piazza D et al: Effects of two chest tube clearance protocols on drainage in patients after myocardial revascularization surgery. Heart Lung 20(2):125–130, 1991

Williams T: To clamp or not to clamp? Nurs Times 88(18):33, 1992

Pharmacologic Agents

Lindell K, Mazzocco M: Breaking bronchospasm's grip with metered dose inhalers. Am J Nurs 90(3):34–41, 1990

McFadden ER: When to use high-dose inhaled steroids. J Respir Dis 12(11):1005–1012, 1991

Olin B: Drug Facts and Comparisons. St. Louis, Facts and Comparisons, Wolters Kluwer Company, 1992

Ventilatory Support

Briones TL: Pressure support ventilation: New ventilatory technique. Crit Care Nurse 12(4):51–58, 1992

Carrieri-Kohlman V: Dyspnea in the weaning patient: Assessment and intervention. REVIEW ARTICLE: 69 REFS. AACN Clin Issues Crit Care Nurs 2(3):462–473, 1991

Dettenmeier PA, Johnson TM: The art and science of mechanical ventilator adjustments. Crit Care Nurs Clin North Am 3(4):575–583, 1991

Halloran T: Use of sedation and neuromuscular paralysis during mechanical ventilation. Crit Care Nurs Clin North Am 3(4):651–657, 1991

Henneman EA: The art and science of weaning from mechanical ventilation. REVIEW ARTICLE: 82 REFS. Focus Crit Care 18(6):490–501, 1991

Knebel AR: Weaning from mechanical ventilation: Current controversies. University of California, San Francisco. REVIEW ARTICLE: 61 REFS. Heart Lung 20(4):321–331, 1991

Smith C et al: Diarrhea Associated with Tube Feeding in Mechanically Ventilated Critically Ill patients. Nursing Research, 1990, 39 (3), 148–152.

Stewart KH, Kewman S, Adamczyk MA, Grondin L: Quality of care in weaning from mechanical ventilation. J Nurs Care Qual 6(4):44–50, 1992

Weilitz PB: Weaning from mechanical ventilation: Old and new strategies. Crit Care Nurs Clin North Am 3(4):585–590, 1991

STUDY QUESTIONS

Bronchial Hygiene

1. The objectives of deep-breathing and coughing exercises include
   a. promotion of lung expansion and relief of bronchial edema
   b. prevention of pneumonia and increase in general activity level
   c. mobilization of secretions and prevention of the side effects of retained secretions
   d. prevention of the side effects of retained secretions and increase in activity level

2. Which two conditions of the following are not contraindications for postural drainage?
   a. osteoporosis
   b. increased intracranial pressure
   c. immediately after a meal
   d. fractured rib
   e. acute heart disease

3. What are the two most common potential hazards associated with inhaled moisture treatments?

    a. bronchospasm in patients with hyperactive airways
    b. infection from contaminated equipment
    c. bronchodilatation
    d. pneumothorax

Artificial Airways

1. The purposes for an artificial airway are to

    a. establish a patent airway
    b. provide for continuous ventilatory assistance
    c. collect scientific data for further research
    d. both a & b

2. One of the complications of tracheal intubation is

    a. airway patency
    b. ineffective airway clearance
    c. displacement of the tube and aspiration
    d. enteral feedings

Chest Tubes

1. Indications for chest tube placement include

    a. hemothorax, pneumothorax, cancer
    b. pleural effusion, lung disease, cancer
    c. chylothorax, pleural effusion, hemothorax
    d. tension pneumothorax, hemothorax, asthma

2. The underwater seal in a chest tube drainage system functions to

    a. allow air to escape from the chest to the outside air
    b. allow drainage to escape from the chest
    c. provide a "seal" to re-establish intrapleural negative pressure
    d. all of the above

3. Chest tubes are clamped

    a. as a routine measure to equalize lung pressures
    b. to locate an air leak in the chest tube drainage system
    c. during patient transport
    d. chest tubes are never clamped

Pharmacologic Agents

1. The first line bronchodilator used in moderate to severe bronchospasm is

    a. atropine sulphate
    b. theophylline
    c. methylprednisolone
    d. gentamycin

2. In most clinical settings, the degree of hypoxemia that warrants supplemental oxygen is a PaO_2 less than

    a. 40mm Hg
    b. 50mm Hg
    c. 60mm Hg
    d. 70mm Hg

Ventilatory Support

1. Indications for mechanical ventilation include

   a. RR > 40/min with signs of fatigue
   b. pH < 7.25, $PaCO_2$ > 50 mm Hg, PaO_2 < 50 mm Hg on O_2
   c. diminished or no breath sounds
   d. all of the above

2. Assist–control mode is defined as

   a. a basic rate is set but the patient can trigger more breaths from the ventilator; each breath is at the set volume on the ventilator
   b. the ventilator controls the rate and volume of patient delivered breaths
   c. only the breaths triggered by the patient are delivered to the patient at the volume set on the ventilator
   d. the mode that allows the patient to breathe at his own rate and tidal volume in addition to the rate and volume set on the ventilator

3. The physiological impact of the ventilator on a patient who is hypovolemic includes the following:

   a. decreased blood return to the heart
   b. decreased cardiac output
   c. predisposing the patient to barotrauma
   d. all of the above

4. A patient is considered "ready to wean" when

   a. the doctor writes the order
   b. the patient says he or she is ready
   c. the cause of respiratory failure is corrected
   d. none of the above

5. Assessment criteria that can terminate weaning from mechanical ventilation include

   a. pulse increase or decrease of 20 beats/min
   b. change of 10 breaths/min
   c. dysrhythmias
   d. all of the above

CHAPTER 20

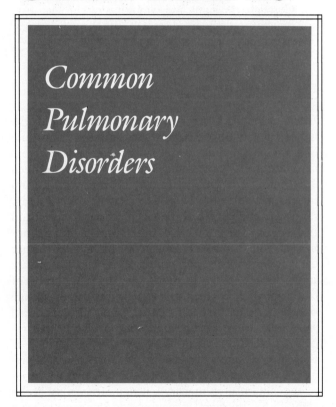

Common Pulmonary Disorders

(continued)

Hudak: Critical Care Nursing:
A Holistic Approach, 6th ed. © 1994
J. B. Lippincott Company.

BEHAVIORAL OBJECTIVES

Based on the content in this chapter, the reader should be able to:

1. Compare and contrast three causes of atelectasis.
2. Outline the signs and symptoms frequently seen with atelectasis.
3. Describe the pathophysiology and anticipated management of pneumonia, bronchospasm, pulmonary emboli, pneumothorax, pleural effusion, and flail chest.
4. Correlate the signs and symptoms of chronic obstructive pulmonary disease (COPD) to the anticipated medical management.

Description

Alarming statistics reveal that lung disease is not only the third leading cause of death but also the fastest rising cause of death in the United States. The number of deaths from chronic obstructive pulmonary disease (COPD) between 1968 and 1978 showed a 60% increase, with a 10% increase per year since 1978. The specialty of critical care nursing continually challenges its practitioners to expand their scope to meet the needs of the patient with pulmonary disease. Increased accountability for nursing practice demands continual development of the knowledge base from which the critical care nurse operates. The purpose of this chapter is to enable nurses to enhance their knowledge of normal pulmonary function and apply it to abnormal situations when assessing, applying, and evaluating therapeutic modalities. Patient observation and recognition of the signs of pulmonary insufficiency—tachypnea, tachycardia, diaphoresis, and anxiety—are the keys to recognizing abnormal pulmonary function. The ability of the clinician to anticipate, recognize, and intervene to treat pulmonary disorders can modify or prevent common lung disorders.

Atelectasis

Atelectasis can be defined as a diminution of volume or collapse of lung units. Several etiologic factors can precipitate atelectasis.

Reabsorption atelectasis occurs if communications between the alveoli and trachea are obstructed, for example, by plugging of a bronchus with mucus. The alveolar gas is rapidly absorbed into the circulation and because of the obstruction cannot be replenished; alveolar collapse ensues.

Passive atelectasis occurs if air or fluid in the pleural space prevents normal alveolar filling.

Compression atelectasis occurs in the presence of a space-occupying lesion such as a pulmonary mass. Atelectasis can also occur in patches, which can be caused by mucous plugging or altered compliance in the atelectatic area.

Atelectasis results in a pathological shunting of blood from the right side of the heart to the left, resulting in desaturation of blood entering the systemic circulation. The degree of shunt present depends on the severity of the atelectasis. In the normal lung, there is a small amount of unoxygenated blood entering the systemic circulation. Contributing to the normal shunt are those vessels whose venous outflow bypasses pulmonary capillaries. Shunting is increased by atelectasis because blood flow passes through the pulmonary capillaries that are in contact with nonventilated alveoli (Fig. 20–1).

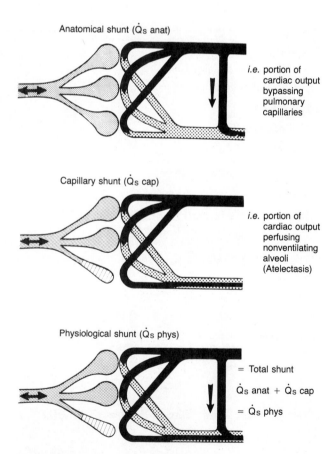

Anatomical shunt ($\dot{Q}_S$ anat)

i.e. portion of cardiac output bypassing pulmonary capillaries

Capillary shunt ($\dot{Q}_S$ cap)

i.e. portion of cardiac output perfusing nonventilating alveoli (Atelectasis)

Physiological shunt ($\dot{Q}_S$ phys)

= Total shunt

$\dot{Q}_S$ anat + $\dot{Q}_S$ cap

= $\dot{Q}_S$ phys

FIGURE 20–1
Subdivisions of the physiological shunt. (Bendixen HH et al: Respiratory Care. St. Louis, CV Mosby).

Clinical Manifestations

Signs and symptoms vary with the severity of atelectasis and degree of shunt present. With severe shunts (ie, large areas of atelectasis) cyanosis may become evident. Arterial blood gases (ABGs) reflect the degree of hypoxemia and the adequacy of alveolar ventilation. There is frequently roentgenographic evidence of atelectasis. In compression atelectasis, there is roentgenographic evidence of air or fluid collection in the pleural space. All the roentgen signs are based on diminished volume of the affected lobe or segment. Cyanosis may become evident as atelectasis increases. Large areas of atelectasis can cause a shift of the mediastinal structures toward the affected side, which can be demonstrated roentgenographically. Auscultatory examination reveals decreased breath sounds over the atelectatic lung. There may be diminished chest expansion of the affected side. The patient may complain of shortness of breath, dyspnea on exertion, and weakness. Tachypnea, tachycardia, fever, anxiety, restlessness, and confusion may be present.

Management

Treatment is based on the etiology of the atelectasis. Meticulous bronchial hygiene (see Chapter 19), mobilization of the patient if appropriate, and administration of oxygen in pharmacologic doses constitute the basic framework of therapy.

Pneumonia

Pneumonia is an inflammatory process in which alveolar gas is replaced by cellular material. The cause can be viral, bacterial, fungal, protozoan, or rickettsial, or hypersensitivity can result in the primary presenting illness. Pneumonia can also result from aspiration.

Clinical Manifestations

The signs and symptoms depend on the location and extent of involvement (ie, segmental or lobar) and the cause of the pneumonia.[1] Subjective findings include dyspnea, tachypnea, pleuritic chest pain, fever, chills, hemoptysis, and cough productive of rusty or purulent sputum. Objective findings include fever, splinting of involved hemithorax, hypoxemia, percussion dullness, coarse inspiratory rales, and diminished breath sounds over the involved area.

Management

The management of pneumonia depends on the cause. Observation of the patient for tachycardia, tachypnea, diaphoresis, restlessness, and confusion (signs of hypoxemia), increased sputum production, and increased splinting is essential in determination of progression or regression of the process. Careful attention must be directed toward improving ventilation through adequate pain medication followed by bronchial hygiene.

Complications of pneumonia include abscess formation, pleural effusion, empyema, bacteremia, and septicemia. Superinfection can occur as a complication of pharmacologic treatment.

Bronchospasm

Bronchospasm implies a narrowing of the airways resulting in increased airway resistance, and it can be caused by a variety of mechanisms: (1) inhalation of toxic or irritating substances, such as smoke, pollens, dust, and noxious gases; (2) bronchitis; (3) severe coughing episodes; (4) extreme cold; and (5) exercise. Although bronchospasm is usually associated with asthma, these mechanisms can precipitate bronchospasm in anyone.

Clinical Research

Roberts J, Barnes W, Pennock M, Browne G. Diagnostic accuracy of fever as a measure of postoperative pulmonary complications. Heart Lung 17(2):166–170, 1988

The diagnostic accuracy of fever as a measure of atelectasis in 270 postoperative elective abdominal surgery patients was studied. Fever was present in 40%. Fever was present in only 56% of patients with radiographic evidence of atelectasis. The researchers concluded that neither the presence nor absence of fever is a useful indicator of postoperative complications such as atelectasis.

Clinical Manifestations

Signs and symptoms vary with the degree of bronchospasm. The patient may complain of shortness of breath associated with wheezing respirations. Additional findings include tachycardia, tachypnea, retractions, restlessness, anxiety, inspiratory/expiratory wheezing, hypoxemia, hypercapnia, cyanosis, and coughing. One must be aware that a decrease in wheezing does not necessarily mean decreased bronchospasm, but rather progression of airway narrowing and markedly decreased ventilation.

Management

Treatment is directed at removing the cause of bronchospasm and initiating bronchodilator therapy (see Chapter 19, Table 19–12). The patient must be observed for increasing bronchospasm and deteriorating pulmonary function manifested by a rising PCO_2.

Pulmonary Embolism

Pulmonary emboli can occur as a complication of many medical conditions that predispose to venous thrombosis, including postoperative states, prolonged bed rest, and trauma. Deep venous thrombosis, particularly in the lower extremities, is the main predisposing factor for pulmonary emboli.[2]

Both pulmonary and hemodynamic changes occur as a result of occlusion of a pulmonary artery by an embolus. Alveoli are ventilated but not perfused, thereby producing areas of ineffective ventilation, that is, increased respiratory dead space (Fig. 20–2).

Pneumoconstriction resulting from a lack of carbon dioxide normally present in pulmonary arterial blood shifts ventilation from the underperfused alveoli. The decrease in pulmonary blood flow due to an embolus results in deficient nutrients for surfactant production, ultimately resulting in atelectasis. The severity of hemodynamic changes depends on the size of the embolus. Increased pulmonary vascular resistance occurs, which, if pulmonary blood flow remains constant, can result in right ventricular failure. Pulmonary emboli can resolve or infrequently can lead to death of tissue, that is, pulmonary infarction.

Clinical Manifestations

The symptom complex of a pulmonary embolus depends on its size. Dyspnea, one of the most frequent complaints, is often out of proportion to the physical findings. Ta-

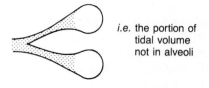

Anatomical dead space (V_D anat)

i.e. the portion of tidal volume not in alveoli

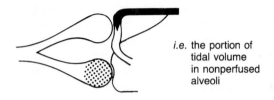

Alveolar dead space (V_D alv)

i.e. the portion of tidal volume in nonperfused alveoli

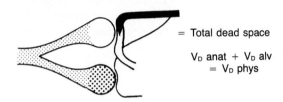

Physiological dead space (V_D phys)

= Total dead space

V_D anat + V_D alv
= V_D phys

FIGURE 20–2
Subdivisions of physiological dead space. Only that part of the volume of ventilation that enters perfused alveoli is effective in blood–gas exchange and is labeled *alveolar ventilation*. The remainder is wasted, or dead space, ventilation. Total ventilation may be subdivided accordingly.

Total ventilation (V)	−	Alveolar ventilation (V_A)	=	Dead space ventilation (V_D)

This division applies equally to minute ventilation and to the individual tidal volumes. Dividing by the respiratory frequency we get

Tidal volume (V_T)	−	Alveolar tidal volume	=	Physiological dead space ($V_{Dphys.}$)

(Bendixen HH et al: Respiratory Care, St. Louis, CV Mosby.)

chypnea and tachycardia may be present in varying degrees. Mild fever may exist, although leukocytosis is rare. Pleuritic chest pain and hemoptysis are associated with pulmonary infarction rather than with pulmonary embolus.

Massive pulmonary embolization results in a more dramatic clinical manifestation of acute illness. The patient develops pronounced tachypnea, usually with cyanosis, tachycardia, restlessness, confusion, and hypotension. The resulting shock state produces concomitant changes of decreased urinary output and cold, clammy skin.

Management

A suspected pulmonary embolus can be confirmed by radioactive lung scanning and pulmonary angiography. Management includes anticoagulation and correction of predisposing causes of venous thrombosis. Anticoagulant therapy is administered in various ways in different institutions. The nurse must be aware that multiple drug interactions can occur with use of anticoagulant therapy.

Hemothorax/Pneumothorax

A pneumothorax occurs if air enters the pleural space between the visceral and parietal pleurae. Blood in this location is called a *hemothorax*. There are two types of pneumothorax: spontaneous pneumothorax and tension pneumothorax.

A *spontaneous pneumothorax* can result from the rupture of a subpleural alveolar cyst or an emphysematous bleb. The signs and symptoms vary with the size of the pneumothorax and can range from mild shortness of breath to chest pain and signs of increasing respiratory distress. Physical examination reveals decreased breath sounds and decreased respiratory movement on the affected side.[3] The diagnosis is confirmed by roentgenography.

Chest trauma, intermittent positive pressure breathing (IPPB), positive end-expiratory pressure (PEEP), cardiopulmonary resuscitation, thoracic and high abdominal surgery, and thoracentesis can precipitate an iatrogenic pneumothorax or hemothorax. A pneumothorax, regardless of cause, becomes life-threatening as tension in the pleural space occurs.

If a *tension pneumothorax* develops, the tear in lung bronchus or chest wall acts as a one-way valve that allows air to enter the pleural space on inspiration, but not to escape on expiration.[4] If it is not immediately recognized and treated, massive atelectasis results. In addition, the mediastinal structures are displaced toward the unaffected side, and tracheal deviation can be especially prominent. This mediastinal shift results in a decreased venous return, decreased cardiac output, and ultimately death.

Clinical Manifestations

Clinically, the patient manifests severe respiratory distress. Agitation, cyanosis, and tachypnea are severe. Tachycardia and the initial increase in blood pressure are followed by hypotension as cardiac output decreases. The diagnosis is based on the clinical manifestations as well as the clinical setting. Any patient who is being ventilated and suddenly develops acute respiratory distress during ventilation evidenced by markedly increased inspiratory pressures is possibly experiencing a tension pneumothorax.

Management

Treatment must be immediate. A 16- to 18-gauge needle is inserted into the second, third, or fourth intercostal space at the midclavicular line on the affected side to relieve the pressure. After this has been accomplished, a chest tube should be inserted and underwater seal drainage instituted to prevent any further development of tension.

Pleural Effusion

The pleural space is a potential space between the visceral and parietal pleurae that line the lungs and interior chest wall. This space normally contains a small amount of fluid.[5] Excess fluid can accumulate in neoplastic, thromboembolic, cardiovascular, and infectious disease processes. This is caused by at least one of four basic mechanisms:

- increased pressure in subpleural capillaries or lymphatics;
- decreased colloid osmotic pressure of the blood;
- increased intrapleural negative pressure;
- inflammatory or neoplastic involvement of the pleura.

Clinical Manifestations

Subjective findings include shortness of breath and pleuritic chest pain, depending on the amount of fluid accumulation. Objective findings include tachypnea and hypoxemia if ventilation is impaired, dullness to percussion, and decreased breath sounds over the involved area.

Management

Removal of the pleural effusion by thoracentesis or chest tubes is palliative treatment. Major treatment is directed toward the underlying cause.

Empyema

Empyema is a collection of purulent material in the pleural space secondary to an inflammatory process of the mediastinum, lung, esophagus, or subdiaphragmatic space.

Clinical Manifestations

The symptom complex can include shortness of breath and pleuritic chest pain. A major objective finding is continued fever during antibiotic administration. Other findings include those of pleural effusion.

Management

Treatment consists of rigorous antibiotic therapy and chest tube drainage (see discussion of chest tubes in Chapter 19). A serious complication of empyema is irreversible fibrotic changes that compromise pulmonary ventilation, caused by trapping of the lung on the involved side.

Flail Chest

Flail chest, a consequence of trauma to the thorax, is caused by the disruption of the normally semirigid structure of the chest cage resulting from (1) fracture of three or more adjoining ribs in one or more places; (2) rib fracture(s) with costochondral separation; or (3) sternal fractures. Wherever fractures occur, that segment loses continuity with the remaining intact chest wall and subsequent paradoxical movement occurs.

Clinical Manifestations

During paradoxical ventilation, as the intact chest expands, the injured "flail" segment is depressed, thereby limiting the amount of negative intrathoracic pressure needed to move air into the lungs. During expiration the flail segment bulges outward, interfering with exhalation. The degree of ventilatory impairment that results from a flail chest is proportional to the extent of injury. The occurrence of concomitant hemothorax/pneumothorax further impairs ventilation.

During inspiration, the intrapleural pressures on the unaffected side are greater, thus displacing the mediastinum toward it. Conversely, during expiration the negative pressure on the unaffected side is less than on the affected side, and the mediastinum shifts toward the affected side. This phenomenon, known as *mediastinal flutter*, further impairs ventilation and cardiac output. Normally, venous return to the right heart is enhanced during inspiration. Reduced intrapleural negative pressure during inspiration impairs circulation dynamics, decreasing venous return to the heart, right atrial filling, and ultimately cardiac output.

Frequent patient assessment, including anterior and posterior visual inspection of chest movement, is essential to evaluation and intervention in the treatment of a patient with a flail chest.

Management

Treatment is directed toward improvement of ventilation and oxygenation and stabilization of the chest wall. The increased effort that is needed for adequate ventilation is difficult for the patient to maintain because of the pain caused by injury. A mechanically controlled volume ventilator, which enhances chest wall stability and improves alveolar ventilation, is the treatment of choice. Ventilatory support is needed for approximately 14 to 21 days or until the chest is adequately stabilized. A hemothorax or pneumothorax is treated by chest tubes, underwater seal drainage, and surgical intervention if repair of structural damage is necessary. Chest tubes with underwater seal drainage systems are usually maintained during the entire time the patient needs ventilatory assistance, to manage not only the initial hemothorax/pneumothorax but any that occur as a complication during positive pressure mechanical ventilation (see p. 435).

Acute Respiratory Failure

Acute respiratory failure (ARF) can be defined as respiratory dysfunction of such a degree that gas exchange is no longer adequate to maintain normal ABGs. Quantitatively, ARF can be defined as a PO_2 less than 50 mm Hg with or without a PCO_2 greater than 50 mm Hg (Fig. 20–3). See discussion of respiratory failure in Chapter 19 under Indications for Ventilatory Support.

ARF can result from a variety of insults including pneumonia, atelectasis, and pneumothorax. Neuromuscular disease, drugs, toxins, and trauma can also lead to ARF.

Management

The key to treatment of ARF is anticipation of its subsequent development in the face of a precipitating event. Management goals for the patient with ARF are twofold:

- establishment of adequate arterial oxygenation, thereby providing adequate tissue perfusion;
- amelioration of the underlying cause(s) of ARF.

Chronic Obstructive Pulmonary Disease

The common pulmonary disorders discussed previously are potentially reversible causes of respiratory insufficiency, but several disease entities result in COPD. These include chronic bronchitis, bronchiectasis, emphysema, and asthma.[6] Of major importance to the health care team is the fact that COPD is the most common cause of respiratory insufficiency.

Chronic Bronchitis

Chronic infection or irritation of the bronchi can result in bronchitis. The mucus-secreting glands of the tracheobronchial tree become thickened and encroach on the

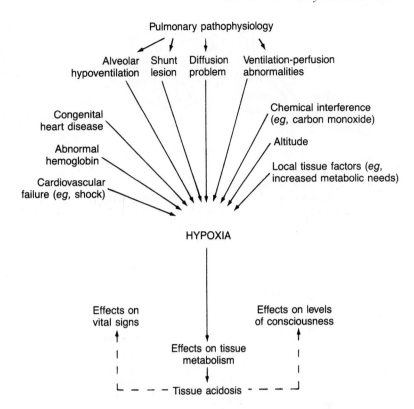

FIGURE 20–3
Hypoxia; mechanisms and effects. (Brannin P: "Oxygen therapy and measures of bronchial hygiene." Nurs Clin North Am.)

diameter of the airway lumen (Fig. 20–4). In addition, there is increased mucus production in peripheral airways. By far the most common cause is tobacco smoking.

The two most common bacterial organisms isolated from the secretions of the chronic bronchitic are *Haemophilus influenzae* and *Pneumococcus* spp. Exacerbation of chronic bronchitis with resultant respiratory insufficiency most often is caused by an acute bacterial inflammation of the bronchial tree. (See Display Box 20–1.) An essential prophylactic measure in preventing an acute inflammatory process is rigorous bronchial hygiene to promote clearance of secretions that provide an ideal medium for bacterial growth in the peripheral airways. In contrast to

emphysema, chronic bronchitis can have a reversible component if the source of chronic infection or irritation is treated.

Bronchiectasis

The term *bronchiectasis* means an irreversible dilatation of the bronchi that can be caused by repeated or prolonged episodes of pneumonitis, foreign body aspiration, or a mass (ie, neoplasm) encroaching on the bronchial lumen with resultant obstruction. The majority of cases are associated with severe chronic bronchitis. A hallmark of the

Clinical Research

DeVito A: Dyspnea during hospitalizations for acute phase of illness as recalled by patients with chronic obstructive pulmonary disease. Heart Lung 19(2):186–191, 1990

Using an interview, 96 adults with COPD were interviewed during a non-acute phase of their illness. Questions were asked regarding their feelings during an acute phase of dyspnea. Content analysis revealed several themes associated with the experience of dyspnea. The most universal response was fear. Helplessness commonly emerged as patients found they could not control their respiratory pattern. Other themes were the real threat to life, preoccupation with the dyspnea, and the desire to have the health care team consider their dyspnea legitimate.

Nurses can apply the findings of this study through acknowledgment of the patient's fear, role playing breathing patterns for the patient to imitate, reducing self-care activities, and handling the clinical situation with solemnity and competence.

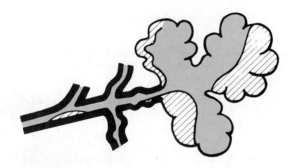

FIGURE 20–4
Bronchitis inflammation and thickening produce narrowing of airways. Lined areas indicate secretions.

disease is the production of copious amounts of mucopurulent, often foul-smelling, sputum that settles out into three layers: cloudy mucus on top, clear saliva in the middle, and a cloudy purulent residue on the bottom. The diagnosis is made largely from the history and is confirmed by bronchography. The primary treatment modality is *rigorous* bronchial hygiene several times daily. This therapy is essential because effective secretion clearance is altered in these patients as the result of abnormal widening of the airways.

Emphysema

Emphysema is an irreversible dilatation of the acinus accompanied by destructive changes of acinar walls, with resultant loss of elastic recoil of the lung. Experimental

---

studies have confirmed the key role of injury to the elastic fiber network in the structural changes of emphysema. Two possible sources of elastolytic activity are neutrophils and alveolar macrophages, both of which are increased in cigarette smokers. Cigarette smoking is a major factor in the development of emphysema. In addition, elastase can be released from neutrophils because of components of smoke. Therefore, this factor may play a role in an imbalance of an elastase/anti-elastase system.

Extensive reported research provides the potential for development and testing, initially in experimental animals and then in humans, of new hypotheses leading to new methods for prevention of emphysema, a major cause of lung disease, disability, and death. The destructive process resulting in airway obstruction develops insidiously. In contrast to the chronic bronchitic, patients with emphysema usually have mild chronic hypoxemia because destruction of acinar walls is accompanied by destruction of corresponding vasculature. The ratio of ventilated to perfused lung tissue remains stable (Fig. 20–5).

The majority of patients with COPD have a mixture of chronic bronchitis and emphysema rather than "pure" bronchitis or emphysema (Table 20–1).

Asthma

In comparison with emphysema and, to a lesser extent, chronic bronchitis, asthma is an acute reversible airway disease that occurs because of bronchospasm resulting from a variety of causes (eg, allergens, infections, exercise). Bronchospasm actually includes smooth muscle constriction, mucosal edema, and excessive mucus with plugging of the conducting airways in the advanced stages. Figure 20–6 illustrates a series of events that can become a vicious cycle resulting in life-threatening status asthmaticus unless bronchospasm is controlled.

Spontaneous remission of bronchospasm can occur; however, use of bronchodilating agents (see Table 19–12) in addition to rigorous bronchial hygiene is the usual mode of treatment. The potential severity of an asthma attack is frequently minimized by these means.

Status Asthmaticus

Status asthmaticus, a medical emergency, is an attack of acute asthma that is refractory—that is, it has not responded to rigorous therapy with β-adrenergic compounds or intravenous theophylline. The patient manifests a dramatic picture of acute anxiety, marked labored breathing, tachycardia, and diaphoresis. Deterioration of pulmonary function results in alveolar hypoventilation with subsequent hypoxemia, hypercapnia, and acidemia.[7] A rising PCO_2 in a patient with an acute asthmatic attack is often the first objective indication of status asthmaticus.

DISPLAY BOX 20–1
Manifestations of Severe Exacerbations of Chronic Bronchitis

Constitutional Signs

Temperature frequently subnormal
WBC varies—may be slightly ↑, normal, or ↓

CNS Disturbances

Headache
Confusion
Hallucinations
Depression
Drowsiness
Somnolence
Coma
Papilledema

Cardiovascular Signs

Diaphoresis
Tachycardia
Blood pressure varies: Normal, ↑, or ↓
Vasoconstriction initially followed by vasodilation

Neuromuscular Signs

Fine tremors
Asterixis
Flaccidity
Convulsions

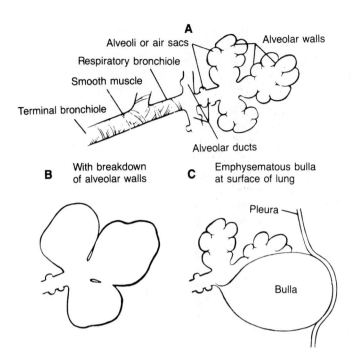

Multiple therapeutic modalities must be instituted. All patients in status asthmaticus demonstrate hypoxemia and require oxygen therapy. Dehydration usually exists and requires correction. Pharmacologic agents consist of methylxanthines, sympathomimetic amines, and corticosteroids. If pulmonary function cannot be improved and respiratory failure ensues, the patient may require intubation and assisted ventilation.

For the purpose of teaching and learning, distinct pathophysiological differences among emphysema, chronic bronchitis, and asthma have been presented. There are times when the health care provider is uncertain whether the problem is asthma or chronic bronchitis. The asthmatic is often a nonsmoker; gives a history of a nonproductive cough possibly associated with chest tightness; states that symptoms are frequently triggered by allergens, cold air, exercise, or irritants; and tends to hyperventilate (defined by $PaCO_2$) and blow off carbon dioxide in acute attacks. The chronic bronchitic usually gives a history of smoking; has experienced cough at least 2 months per year for 2 or more years with excessive sputum production; may have right heart failure secondary to hypoxemia; and tends to hypoventilate and retain carbon dioxide. There are certain signs and symptoms that can overlap. Some of these are chronic cough, shortness of breath, wheezing,

FIGURE 20–5
Emphysema. Airway showing normal primary lobule (**A**) and emphysematous lobule (**B** and **C**). (Introduction to Lung Diseases, 6th ed, New York, American Lung Association.)

TABLE 20–1
COPD: *Features that Distinguish Bronchitis and Emphysema*

Features	Bronchitis	Emphysema
Primary Location of Pathology	Airways	Air sacs
Clinical Examination		
Subjective Data	Frequent recurrent chest infections	Frequently only insidious dyspnea—initially with exercise only, then progressing
	Sputum production	
	Cough	
Objective Data		
Appearance	"Blue bloaters"	"Pink puffers"
Chest examination	Noisy chest, *slight* overdistention	Quiet chest, marked overdistention
Sputum	Frequently copious and purulent	Usually scant and mucoid
Chronic cor pulmonale	Common—may occur relatively early	Infrequent until terminal stages
Laboratory Tests		
ABGs		
Chronic hypoxemia	Often significant	Usually mild
Chronic hypercapnia	Common	Uncommon
Spirometry		
FEV_1/FVC	Decreased	Decreased
FEV_1	Decreased	Decreased
Therapeutic Modalities		
Bronchial hygiene (measures to enhance secretion clearance)	Very important	Less important unless patient has respiratory infection

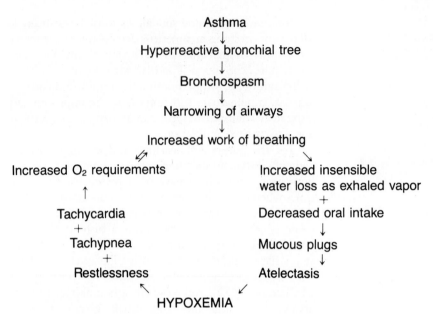

FIGURE 20–6
Sequence of events leading from asthma to hypoxemia.

airway obstruction, hyperinflation, and hypoxemia secondary to ventilation/perfusion ($\dot{V}/\dot{Q}$) mismatching and altered gas exchange.

The key to successful management of the asthmatic is *identification* and *prevention* of all possible factors that trigger bronchospasm. If a known cause of an asthma attack is exercise, the patient should be educated to take an inhaled bronchodilator treatment before starting. The adult patient should always have an inhaled bronchodilator (ie, metered dose) device such as a metaproterenol inhaler or a dose of bronchodilator in a hand-powered nebulizer that is stored in a purse or pocket.

Sleep Apnea Syndrome

A disorder that is prevalent in patients with COPD is sleep apnea syndrome (SAS). This condition is more common in men than in women, although the incidence increases in women after the menopause, suggesting that female hormones are in some way protective. The patient's bed partner, if questioned directly, or the nurse in attendance for hospitalized patients, usually describe intermittent loud snoring followed by silence (apnea) lasting 10 to 100 seconds or longer.

Three classifications of apnea are (1) *obstructive*—associated with absence of airflow despite ventilatory efforts; (2) *central*—associated with absence of both airflow and ventilatory efforts; and (3) *mixed*—during which there is an initial period of central apnea followed by obstructive apnea. The site of obstruction in obstructive apnea is the oropharynx, and it is apparently related to an abrupt loss of tone in the muscles surrounding the oropharynx just before the onset of inspiration. It is believed that a decreased ventilatory drive exists, for unknown reasons, in both central and obstructive apnea; ventilatory responsiveness to both hypoxemia and hypercarbia is depressed.

In the obstructive type of sleep apnea caused by laryngeal obstruction by the tongue or other neck structures, the patient often has struggling respirations but no airflow, followed by loud snoring.[8] However, in the central apneas, the reduced central nervous system drive to breathe is not associated with characteristic loud snoring. The obstructive apneas are more common.

Clinical Manifestations

Signs and symptoms of SAS include hypersomnolence, snoring, insomnia, abnormal motor activity during sleep,

---

DISPLAY BOX 20–2
Signs and Symptoms of Sleep Apnea

Daytime drowsiness
Headache on awakening
Intermittent loud snoring
Apnea spells of 10 to 100 sec or longer
Difficulty concentrating
Personality changes
Reduced libido
Restless sleep
Cardiac rhythm disturbances
Pulmonary hypertension
Hypoxemia
Right ventricular failure

morning headache, personality and intellectual changes, altered relationships (ie, social, family, or job), bizarre behavior, sexual impotence, systemic hypertension, pulmonary hypertension and cor pulmonale, secondary erythrocytosis, cardiac dysrhythmias, and sudden nocturnal death. (See Display Box 20–2.) Most cases of SAS occur in middle-aged men between 40 and 60 years of age. Suspicion of SAS is based on a middle-aged man who gives a history of sleep disturbance that may be accompanied by the previously mentioned signs and symptoms. A definitive diagnosis is based on the results of polysomnography.

Conditions that can be predisposing to secondary sleep apnea include obesity, myxedema, acromegaly, anatomical upper airway obstruction (ie, nasal deformity with resultant obstruction), brain stem lesions, cervical spine injury, encephalitis, and myotonic dystrophy.

Management

Treatment of SAS is based on the type of apnea and the severity of symptoms. For example, a tracheostomy for obstructive apnea may resolve all symptoms. Before this drastic measure is performed—unless the condition is life-threatening—a protriptyline trial is warranted. Protriptyline is a nonsedating tricyclic antidepressant that evidently improves pharyngeal muscle tone during inspiration. The usual dose is 10 to 30 mg taken at bedtime. If successful, this agent decreases somnolence, but patients continue to have abnormal sleep patterns associated with many apneas and arousals. Other forms of treatment include medroxyprogesterone acetate (very useful in obesity–hypoventilation syndrome), continuous positive airway pressure (CPAP), and surgical enlargement of the pharyngeal airway by resection of excessive mucosa. By far the simplest treatment is nocturnal oxygen administration, which often prevents the nocturnal desaturation and many of the other symptoms.

CASE STUDY

Tom Blair, a 58-year-old white male, was well known to the critical care nursing staff. His emphysema was brought on by a 32-year history of cigarette smoking. He was admitted four months ago for respiratory failure and received a tracheostomy during his three weeks of mechanical ventilation. Although discharged on home oxygen therapy, Tom continued to smoke one pack of cigarettes per day.

Six days ago, Mr. Blair presented in his physician's office with increasing shortness of breath, increased yellow tinged secretions, and a very poor activity tolerance. He was sent home on erythromycin syrup, O_2 4 liters per minute by nasal cannula, and home care by respiratory therapy. Tom managed his care adequately until last night. At 9:00 PM he developed shaking chills and severe shortness of breath. He increased his oxygen to 6 liters per minute. His daughter found him unresponsive at 10:35 PM and called the paramedics.

On presenting in the emergency department, he was orally intubated by the paramedics, had a liter of normal saline infusing via a left antecubital #18 gauge angiocath and was barely responsive to deep pain. His initial vital signs were: BP—98/52 mm Hg; heart rate—108, sinus tachycardia; respiratory rate—20 per Ambu bag at 100% FIO_2; temperature—102°F per rectum. Tom was once again admitted to the ICU on a mechanical ventilator with the diagnosis of COPD exacerbation and pneumonia.

After he was settled in the ICU, routine laboratory tests were done. This included serum chemistry tests, a complete blood count, an ABG, urinalysis, serum toxicology screen, and coagulation studies. A portable chest film was completed. After performing a thorough bedside physical assessment, the critical care nurse reviewed all the pertinent findings. Tom was barely arousable. His weight had dropped 15 pounds since his last admission. His breath sounds were very coarse, with rhonchi throughout all anterior and lateral lung fields. Thick yellow secretions were suctioned out of the endotracheal tube. His vital signs were similar to the findings in the emergency department.

The lab results were normal except for the following:

ABG on 100% FIO_2, tidal volume 650 cc, assist–control rate of 14:

pH	7.30
PCO_2	58
PO_2	81
O_2 Saturation	90%
HCO_3^-	35

Serum chemistry:

K	3.4
Glucose	154

CBC:

Hemoglobin	11.4
Hematocrit	32%

Toxicology Screen:

Negative for sedatives, barbiturates, alcohol and cocaine

The chest radiograph showed white fluffy infiltrates in all lung fields and confirmed adequate endotracheal tube placement. The chest film showed rib changes consistent with COPD and a mild enlargement of the cardiac shadow. A comparison of this film to previous studies was not available.

The nurse medicated Mr. Blair with a Tylenol suppository 650 mg and collected a sputum culture specimen. A Foley catheter and nasal gastric tube (to lower intermittent wall suction) were placed. The intravenous fluid was changed to 5% Dextrose/.45% Normal Saline with 40 mEq KCl at 125 cc/h. Bilateral soft wrist restraints were placed and secured to the bed frame. Continuous oxygen saturation was monitored with a finger pulse oximeter. A rectal probe was placed for verification of body temperature, and a second intravenous site was initiated, although capped with a dead end plug. These interventions took about one hour to perform, and after they were completed Tom was awake, alert, and cooperative with the care in progress.

The Gram stain of the sputum specimen showed gram-positive cocci, most likely *Haemophilus influenzae*. Augmentin

500 mg, IVPB q8h was begun. Respiratory therapy began to titrate down the FIO_2 as long as the SaO_2 was equal to or greater than 92%. By morning the FIO_2 was at 50%. His temperature responded to antipyretics and fell to 100°F per rectum.

By mid-morning, Tom was very comfortable on the ventilator. His secretions remained thick yellow but were decreasing in amount. He was cooperative with all of his care, communicating by writing notes. Whenever weaning from the ventilator was mentioned, Tom became very frightened, tachypneic, and tachycardic. He did not want the support discontinued. It took extra time for the respiratory therapists to perform routine ventilator checks because Tom was so fearful they were decreasing his support. Finally, the medical team choose not to increase his work of breathing by weaning the ventilator until he had rested thoroughly.

The next morning, all attempts to increase Tom's work of breathing failed. He would panic, rapidly increasing his respiratory and heart rates while decreasing his SaO_2. His chest radiograph showed some response to antibiotic therapy. His supportive care included sitting in the chair, physical therapy exercises, occupational therapy for mental stimulation, IV aminophylline, maintenance intravenous fluids, ice chips for oral comfort, and aerosol treatments every four hours. Tom was comfortable and wrote notes that he was not short of breath for the first time since his discharge from the ICU months ago.

Recognizing the chronicity of Tom's disease, it was decided to provide nutrition through a feeding tube. A low, acid ash formula was started at half strength at 30 cc/h. This was to be advanced by 10 cc every two hours until at 75 cc/h. The nurses checked for gastric residual every 4 hours or if Tom complained of feeling full. He tolerated the tube feedings well. It seemed like another long stay was in order for Tom.

Tom's hospital course was unremarkable for several days. He was very comfortable on the ventilator and little progress was made in weaning attempts. The discharge planning team decided to meet with him and discuss placement in a nursing home. Tom found this idea totally unacceptable, and he agreed to participate in ventilator weans immediately.

Weans began with decreasing the FIO_2 to 35%. Because the SaO_2 remained above 92%, the assist–control respiratory rate was slowly dropped to 8, and his total respiratory rate stayed in the low 20s. Tom was allowed to rest overnight, and weaning resumed in the morning. Again, the weaning process was tolerated well. By that evening, the sixth hospital day, Tom was performing all of his own work of breathing on a 35% T-piece adapter. Again he rested on the ventilator overnight.

Tom was extubated at 10:00 AM on the seventh day of his hospital stay. His antibiotic course was complete. His only request was to have some ice cream for lunch! His post-extubation ABG revealed:

pH	7.38
PCO_2	52
PO_2	78
O_2 Saturation	91%
HCO_3^-	36

The nurses were confused about his sudden cooperation with the ventilator weans and decided to confront him about the radical behavior change. Tom revealed that the only thing that frightened him more than being short of breath was to lose his independence. He saw nursing homes as a place to go to die. He admitted that the ventilator and ICU setting provided him with confidence and a feeling of ease. He did not realize that this "service" could not be provided indefinitely.

Nursing Care Plan

Nursing Care Plan 20–1 summarizes the important aspects of care for the patient with COPD.

Interstitial Lung Disease

The phrase *interstitial lung disease* (ILD) has become widely acceptable because many of the diseases in this extensive category are accompanied by an increase in connective tissue of the lung. These diseases include, but are not limited to, hypersensitivity pneumonitis, asbestosis, pneumoconiosis, sarcoidosis, pulmonary vasculitis, and connective tissue diseases such as rheumatoid arthritis, systemic lupus erythematosus, scleroderma, and ankylosing spondylitis.

Many use the term *pulmonary interstitium* in reference to alveolar walls. However, ILD is comprehensively defined as an inflammatory process involving each component of the alveolar wall. These components are the connective tissue of the blood vessels, the connective tissue of the pleura, the bronchi, and the respiratory airspace walls. The inflammatory process can heal completely or can result in subsequent development of excess connective tissue (diffuse scarring or fibrosis) accompanied by significant distortion of lung structure.

Numerous ILD disorders have been described; however, it is not within the scope of this discussion to address each one. Fundamental pathology, pathogenesis, pathophysiology, clinical features, diagnostic approaches, and management are presented in Table 20–2.

Nonpulmonary Respiratory Complications

Postoperative Pulmonary Compromise

Patients who have surgery, notably high abdominal thoracic and low abdominal resection, are especially susceptible to respiratory embarrassment.[9] The mechanism of pulmonary compromise is a restrictive entity in which there is a reduction of vital capacity (VC), resulting in a limited ventilatory reserve. The major restrictive insult occurs in the first 24 hours postoperatively. Patients without complications gradually resume their preoperative ventilatory status.

Postoperative pulmonary complications can be avoided

(*Text continues on page 498*)

NURSING CARE PLAN 20–1:
The Patient With COPD

NURSING DIAGNOSIS	OUTCOME CRITERIA/ PATIENT GOALS	NURSING INTERVENTIONS
Impaired gas exchange: related to CO_2 retention, increased secretions, increased work of breathing, disease process.	• Patient will maintain adequate gas exchange and oxygenation.	1. Assess ABGs and monitor oxygenation with oximetry. 2. Assess breath sounds q4h and after interventions such as suctioning or inhalation treatments. 3. Provide supplemental O_2 as ordered. 4. Assess mentation q4h and prn. 5. Carefully evaluate agitation/lethargy. Avoid sedation if possible. 6. Assess respiratory rate, pattern and depth. 7. Have patient describe his/her work of breathing. Establish baseline desciption. 8. Turn bedridden patient q2h. 9. Cough and deep breathe q2h. 10. Prepare for and assist with intubation prn.
Ineffective breathing pattern: related to COPD, chest wall distention, fatigue, work of breathing.	• Patient will demonstrate an effective breathing pattern.	1. Monitor rate, rhythm and depth of respiration. 2. Position patient to facilitate breathing, ie, ↑ HOB. 3. Avoid sedation or narcotic analgesics if possible. 4. Minimize gastric distention, if present. 5. Assess respirations during sleep. Note any sleep apnea or Cheyne-Stokes patterns. 6. Have patient describe his/her work of breathing. 7. Reassure patient and give support during times of dyspnea.
Ineffective airway clearance: related to COPD, increased secretions, decreased cough mechanism, fatigue.	• Patient will maintain a patent airway.	1. Assess breath sounds q4h. 2. Assistant patient with cough and deep breathing. 3. Suction airway prn. 4. Use humidified O_2 systems. 5. Avoid sedatives and narcotic analgesics.

(continued)

NURSING DIAGNOSIS	OUTCOME CRITERIA/ PATIENT GOALS	NURSING INTERVENTIONS
		6. Mobilize patient to chair ASAP or consider air filled, self-turning bed.
		7. Maintain adequate systemic hydration with IV fluids prn, as ordered.
		8. Avoid milk products because dairy products thicken sputum.
		9. Administer bronchodilators as ordered.
		10. Provide chest physical therapy as ordered.
		11. Prepare for and assist intubation if indicated.
Knowledge deficit: related to self-management of chronic disease.	• Patient will be able to state disease cause, course, treatment and symptoms to report to MD.	1. Evaluate patient readiness to learn.
		2. Present content with family members in attendance.
		3. Explain all procedures and treatments before performing them.
		4. Utilize available community and hospital teaching materials.
		5. Have patient demonstrate behaviors such as applying O_2, set-up to face, resting in high Fowler's position, etc.
		6. Document content presented and patient's level of understanding.
		7. Continue patient teaching after transfer from ICU.
Anxiety: related to critical illness, fear of death, role changes within social setting, or permanent disability.	• Patient will be able to express anxieties to appropriate resource person.	1. Provide environment that encourages open discussion of emotional issues.
		2. Mobilize patient's support system and involve these resources as appropriate.
		3. Allow time for patient to express self.
		4. Identify possible hospital resources for patient/family support.
		5. Validate patient and family knowledge base regarding the critical illness.
		6. Involve religious support systems as appropriate.

(continued)

NURSING DIAGNOSIS	OUTCOME CRITERIA/ PATIENT GOALS	NURSING INTERVENTIONS
High risk for fluid volume excess: related to cor pulmonale, IV infusions, pulmonary capillary permeability increase, bedrest.	• Patient will be uvolemic and not experience weight gain.	1. Assess intake and output. 2. Monitor hemodynamics if available: PAP, PCWP, CO, CI, CVP. 3. Assess breath sounds for crackles q4h. 4. Assess for edema. 5. Evaluate neck vein distention and S_3 heart sound. 6. Evaluate and report electrolytes, hematocrit, renal and liver function tests. 7. Weigh daily. 8. Maintain fluid restriction as ordered.
High risk for altered tissue perfusion: related to high hematocrit, pulmonary congestion, poor nutrition with low serum albumin, CO_2 retention, and hypoxemia.	• Patient will maintain function of all organs.	1. Assess breath sounds q4h. 2. Assess abdomen for distention, liver tenderness q8h. 3. Assess urine output and report <30 cc/h. 4. Assess mentation q4h and prn. 5. Assess peripheral pulses and edema q4h. 6. Record daily weights. 7. Monitor oxygenation with oximetry. 8. Monitor lab reports on hematocrit, electrolytes, BUN, creatinine, and liver function tests.
High risk for infection: related to retained secretions, ineffective cough, immobility.	• Patient will not acquire a nosocomial infection.	1. Monitor temperature q4h. 2. Use sterile technique with all IV lines, catheters, and suctioning. 3. Maintain universal precautions. 4. Monitor WBC and report abnormalities. 5. Inspect and record color, tenacity, and amount of secretions. 6. Maintain adequate nutrition. 7. Administer antibiotics as ordered.
High risk for altered nutrition, less than body requirements: related to chronic illness, high metabolic rates, dyspnea when eating, anxiety.	• Patient will have nutritional needs met.	1. Evaluate nutritional status. 2. Consult dietician for calorie count, educational resources. 3. Evaluate caloric intake.

(continued)

NURSING CARE PLAN 20–1: (Continued)
The Patient With COPD

NURSING DIAGNOSIS	OUTCOME CRITERIA/ PATIENT GOALS	NURSING INTERVENTIONS
		4. Provide high calorie, low acid ash supplements.
		5. Tube feed if unable to orally meet needs.
		6. Use hyperalimentation if unable to meet caloric needs via PO or tube-fed meals.
		7. Weigh patient daily.
		8. Evaluate electrolyte imbalances via lab work. Provide supplements prn, especially potassium.
High risk for fatigue: related to CO_2 retention, hypoxemia, emotional focus on breathing, sleep apnea, chronicity of illness.	• Patient will obtain the amount of rest needed to maintain wakeful energy levels.	1. Provide uninterrupted rest.
		2. Plan activities with rest breaks.
		3. Careful use of sedatives or hypnotics in presence of CO_2 retention problems.
		4. Gradually increase participation in ADLs.
		5. Maintain O_2 supplements when exercising.
		6. Allow the patient to control some aspects of care while working toward ADL independence.

or minimized by adequate preoperative cardiopulmonary evaluation by the critical care nurse. The nurse can thereby institute measures to monitor pulmonary status and provide modalities aimed at improving VC.

Pharmacotherapy Complications

Appropriate administration of narcotics and sedatives is a necessary adjunct to pulmonary care. The use of these drugs must be guided by the patient's clinical status. The aim of pharmacologic therapy is to minimize pain so the patient can tolerate respiratory therapy and other therapeutic modalities. However, overzealous use of these drugs can result in respiratory depression and ARF.

The patient with a sedative or narcotic overdose presents with respiratory insufficiency. The severity of the respiratory insufficiency depends on the specific type and amount of drug(s) ingested, time of ingestion, and rate of metabolism of the drug(s).

Factors that can alter drug effects include multiple

drug ingestion, hepatic or renal function abnormalities, and preexisting pulmonary disease such as COPD.

Care of patients with drug overdose is guided by this information and by the knowledge that patients with certain types of drug ingestion (eg, glutethimide) can show a fluctuation in level of consciousness. This presents a problem in the maintenance of an adequate airway. It must not be assumed that a patient who at one time appears alert and able to maintain the airway will continue to do so.

There are also drugs that in normal pharmacologic doses can cause neuromuscular blockage with resultant respiratory paralysis. These include kanamycin, gentamicin, streptomycin, neomycin, and polymyxin B.

Neuromuscular Involvement

Disease states or trauma involving the neuromuscular system can affect pulmonary function. The degree of dysfunction depends on the extent of respiratory muscle involvement.

In certain neurologic diseases, gag and cough reflexes

TABLE 20-2
Summary: Interstitial Lung Disease

I. *Pathology of ILD*
    A. Primary process—active inflammation (alveolitis)
    B. Secondary process—fibrosis

II. *Pathophysiology*
    A. Alveolitis involving lymphocytes—exposure to an antigen is the initiating event
    B. Alveolitis involving neutrophils—production of chemical mediators potentially toxic to components of alveolar walls

III. *Pathophysiology basic to majority of ILD*
    Inflammation and fibrosis of alveolar wall components:
    A. Decreased pulmonary compliance (increased stiffness) due to significant inflammatory and fibrotic process
    B. Generalized decrease in lung volume due to change in compliance (stiffness) of the lung
    C. Impaired diffusion of O_2 and CO_2 due to destruction of alveolar–capillary walls with resultant decrease of available surface area for gas exchange
    D. Disturbances in gas exchange (primarily ↓ PaO_2) secondary to disruption of normal matching of ventilation and perfusion

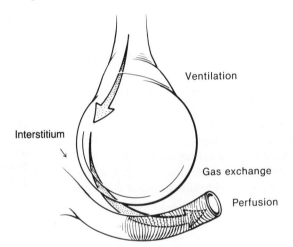

    E. Pulmonary hypertension—ultimate sequelae with severe ILD secondary to:
        (1) bronchoconstriction associated with hypoxemia and (2) destruction of small pulmonary vessels by the alveolar wall fibrotic process

IV. *Clinical features/assessment*
    A. Dyspnea on exertion progressing to dyspnea at rest
    B. Cough—usually nonproductive
    C. Velcro (dry) crackles—most prominent at base of lungs

V. *Diagnosis*
    A. Chest roentgenogram
    B. Bronchoscopy/biopsy/lavage—as indicated
    C. Open lung biopsy—as indicated/appropriate

VI. *Management*
    A. Corticosteroids—↓ inflammatory process
    B. Immunosuppressive agents—eg, Imuran

can be diminished, resulting in aspiration of food, fluid, or secretions. The aspirated contents can cause atelectasis and pneumonia, which, if not recognized, lead to progressive respiratory failure. As impairment of respiratory muscles progresses, there is a resultant decrease in VC.

Taking serial measurements of the VC is an important method of assessing adequacy of pulmonary function. This assessment can be done quite readily by the nurse. Cardinal signs of respiratory embarrassment, pulmonary function measurements, and ABG analysis must be correlated with the clinical status of the patient.

Long-term management of a patient with a neuromuscular disorder includes maintenance of a patent airway, rigorous clearance of secretions, treatment of infections, maximal mobilization of the patient, and ventilatory assistance if indicated.

Restrictive Disorders

Several entities restrict chest wall expansion, with resultant compromised pulmonary function. These include kyphoscoliosis, rheumatoid spondylitis, scleroderma, pectus excavatum, and use of orthopedic appliances such as spica casts. Patients with these conditions can, in a stable environment, have normal pulmonary function. A crisis such as trauma, or a major medical illness such as drug overdose, can precipitate severe respiratory impairment. In the management of these patients the nurse must use measures that maximize ventilation and minimize pulmonary complications.

Noncardiac Pulmonary Edema

This type of pulmonary congestion occurs without cardiac malfunction. As opposed to cardiac pulmonary edema, the findings of heart failure are absent. Neck veins are not distended, there is no left ventricular gallop, and the pulmonary artery pressure is normal (ie, <18 cm H_2O).

See Chapter 21 for a detailed discussion of possible pathophysiology, therapeutic modalities, and sequelae of noncardiac pulmonary edema, or adult respiratory distress syndrome.

Summary

Common pulmonary disorders and the less known and understood interstitial lung diseases provide the critical care nurse with unlimited academic and patient-oriented challenges. The nurse is encouraged to watch for new developments regarding expanded etiology, pathology, pathogenesis, and treatment of ILD; longitudinal analysis of the effects of cigarette smoking; risk factors of airway-obstructive disease; the contribution of occupational ex-

posure to chronic airway obstruction; predictors of spirometric changes and mortality in the latter; breathing during sleep and chronic airway obstruction; mechanism of arterial desaturation during sleep; respiratory muscles in COPD; diaphragm fatigue and the strategy of breathing in COPD; effect of daily intermittent rest on respiratory muscles in patients with COPD; nutrition and COPD; and the effects of ventilatory muscle training and pulmonary rehabilitation. These important issues can have a great effect during the patient's critical care hospitalization.

REFERENCES

1. Niederman M, Fein A: Acute infectious pneumonia. In Rippe J et al: Intensive Care Medicine, pp 713–729. Boston, Little, Brown & Co, 1991
2. Benotti J et al: Pulmonary embolism. In Rippe J et al: Intensive Care Medicine, pp 308–315. Boston, Little, Brown & Co, 1991
3. Young N, Gorzeman J: Managing pneumothorax and hemothorax. Nursing 21(4):56–57, 1991
4. Waxman K: Pleural disorders. In Shoemaker W et al: Textbook of Critical Care, pp 599–605. Philadelphia, WB Saunders, 1989
5. Waxman K: Pleural disorders. In Shoemaker W et al: Textbook of Critical Care, pp 599–605. Philadelphia, WB Saunders, 1989
6. Irwin R: Chronic obstructive pulmonary disease. In Rippe J: Intensive Care Medicine, pp 468–476. Boston, Little, Brown & Co, 1991
7. Murray R, Panettieri R: Management of asthma: The changing approach. In Fishman A: Update: Pulmonary Diseases and Disorders, pp 67–82. New York, McGraw-Hill, 1992
8. Hudgel D, Cherniack N: Sleep and breathing. In Fishman A: Update: Pulmonary Diseases and Disorders, pp 249–261. New York, McGraw-Hill, 1992
9. Litwack K et al: Postoperative pulmonary complications. Crit Care Clin North Am 3(1):77–81, 1991

BIBLIOGRAPHY

DeVito A: Dyspnea during hospitalizations for acute phase of illness as recalled by patients with chronic obstructive pulmonary disease. Heart Lung 19(2):186–191, 1990

Downs J, Douglas M: Physiologic effects of respiratory therapy. In Shoemaker W et al: Textbook of Critical Care Medicine, pp 599–605. Philadelphia, WB Saunders, 1989

Janson-Bjerklie S et al: Clinical markers of asthma severity and risk: Importance of subjective as well as objective factors. Heart Lung 21:265–272, 1992

Roberts J, Barnes W, Pennock M, Brown G: Diagnostic accuracy of fever as a measure of postoperative pulmonary complications. Heart Lung 17(2):166–170, 1988

Stevenson G: Operation Cleanup: Infection risks in respiratory therapy. Nursing Stand 6(18):32–3, 1992

Suddarth D: The Lippincott Manual of Nursing Practice, 5th ed. Philadelphia, JB Lippincott, 1991

STUDY QUESTIONS

1. Which of the following is *not* a symptom of atelectasis?

   a. tachycardia and tachypnea
   b. asymmetric chest expansion
   c. pain on deep inspiration
   d. shortness of breath or dyspnea on exertion

2. The best definition of pulmonary emboli is

   a. increased dead space from ventilation past a non-perfused alveolus
   b. an expansion of the normal ventilation/perfusion mismatch
   c. perfusion of a nonventilated alveolar area, causing an increased ventilation/perfusion mismatch
   d. a showering of multiple small emboli to the distal pulmonary capillary beds

3. All of the following statements are true except

   a. cor pulmonale occurs more often with bronchitis than with emphysema
   b. bronchial hygiene is crucial to the management of emphysema
   c. asthma management focuses on preventing the attack, and the cause of the attacks should be avoided
   d. sleep apnea occurs most often in men between 40 and 60 years of age and in women past menopause

4. Which of the following statements about sleep apnea syndrome is not true?

   a. it is more common in men than in women
   b. female hormones may be a protective factor in women
   c. the apnea can be obstructive, central or mixed
   d. it occurs most commonly in men 60 to 70 years of age

CHAPTER 21

Adult Respiratory Distress Syndrome (ARDS)

BEHAVIORAL OBJECTIVES

Based on the content in this chapter, the reader should be able to:

1. Relate the assessment findings in ARDS to the pathophysiological process.
2. List the major components of the anticipated medical management.
3. Describe four key nursing diagnoses applicable to the patient with ARDS and outline the nursing interventions for each diagnosis.

Hudak: Critical Care Nursing:
A Holistic Approach, 6th ed. © 1994
J. B. Lippincott Company.

Description

The adult respiratory distress syndrome (ARDS) is a pulmonary emergency that is a sudden and severe form of respiratory failure, usually occurring in previously healthy people who have been exposed to various pulmonary or nonpulmonary insults. Some precipitating factors include near drowning, fat emboli, sepsis, pancreatitis, pulmonary emboli, aspiration, hemorrhage, and trauma of any kind. The two groups who appear to be at greatest risk for the syndrome are those who have the sepsis syndrome and those who have aspirated large amounts of gastric fluid with a low pH. Most sepsis cases that result in ARDS and multiple organ failure are associated with infection by gram-negative aerobic bacilli. The precipitating event usually occurs 1 to 96 hours before the onset of ARDS. Display Box 21–1 provides an extensive list of disorders associated with ARDS.

Adult respiratory distress syndrome was first described as a clinical syndrome in 1967. It involves an increased pulmonary capillary permeability, resulting in noncardiac pulmonary edema. Adult respiratory distress syndrome is defined as diffuse acute pulmonary infiltrates associated with a large oxygenation problem despite supplemental oxygen and a pulmonary arterial wedge pressure (PAWP) of less than 18 mm Hg. The PAWP is necessary to rule out cardiac or hydrostatic pulmonary edema.

Adult respiratory distress syndrome frequently occurs in combination with multiple organ injury and is likely to become part of multiple organ failure. The prevalence of ARDS is estimated to be at least 150,000 cases per year. Until there is an effective reporting mechanism based on a consistent definition, however, the true incidence of ARDS will remain unknown. The mortality rate depends on the etiology and therefore is variable. Adult respiratory distress syndrome is a major cause of death among trauma and septic patients, with an overall mortality rate of approximately 50% to 70%.[1] This distinct clinical syndrome of diverse etiology appears to manifest a common pathogenesis regardless of causative factors.

DISPLAY BOX 21–1
Disorders Predisposing to ARDS

Systemic
  Shock, of any etiology
  Gram-negative sepsis
  Hypothermia
  Hyperthermia
  Drug overdose
    Narcotic
    Salicylate
    Tricyclic
    Paraquat
    Methadone
    Bleomycin
  Hematologic disorders
    Disseminated intravascular coagulation
    Massive transfusion
    Cardiopulmonary bypass
  Eclampsia
  Burns
Pulmonary
  Pneumonia
    Viral
    Bacterial
    Fungal
    Pneumocystic carinii
  Trauma
    Fat emboli
    Lung contusion
  Aspiration
    Gastric fluids
    Near-drowning
    Hydrocarbon fluids
  Pneumonitis
Nonpulmonary
  Head injury
  Increased intracranial pressure
  Postcardioversion
  Pancreatitis
  Uremia

Pathophysiological Principles

Despite a wide spectrum of precipitating events associated with ARDS, the common pathogenesis is diffuse damage to the alveolocapillary membrane, postulated to be due to one of two primary categories of mechanisms:

1. Aspiration of certain chemicals or inhalation of noxious gases into the airways is directly toxic to the alveolar epithelium, resulting in destruction and increased permeability of the alveolocapillary membrane.
2. Damage to the alveolocapillary membrane can be initiated in the pulmonary microvasculature.

Regardless of the mechanism of lung injury, the common denominator is increased permeability at the level of the alveolocapillary membrane with resultant leakage of fluid in a two-stage process.[2] First, a disruption of the capillary endothelium occurs; fluid leaks into the interstitial space. Second, a disruption of the alveolar epithelium occurs; fluid leaks into the alveoli. Fluid in the interstitium and alveoli interferes significantly with gas transport; therefore, hypoxemia occurs. Lung compliance is decreased, causing pulmonary vascular resistance to rise.

An increase in alveolocapillary membrane permeability leads to interstitial and alveolar edema and alveolar atelectasis. Thus, the amount of air remaining in the lungs at the end of a normal expiration, functional residual capacity (FRC), is decreased.

Mechanical properties of the lungs change. Lung distensibility (compliance) is decreased. The lung become stiff. Therefore, greater than normal ventilator pressures will be needed to maintain adequate minute ventilation.

The ultimate outcome in the pathogenesis of ARDS is profound hypoxemia, which exists in spite of high inspired oxygen fractions (FIO_2). This cardinal feature may be secondary to extensive interstitial and alveolar edema, surfactant abnormalities, massive atelectasis, shunting, or ventilation–perfusion ($\dot{V}/\dot{Q}$) imbalance (Fig. 21–1).

Recent studies show that surfactant, usually responsible for alveolar antiedema and alveolar surface tension lowering, is abnormal in function, levels, and composition in ARDS.[3] Further research on human subjects is needed in this area.

A febrile, acidemic, and catabolic state frequently is present in the patient with multiple organ failure. This is coupled with abnormalities of the coagulation and inflammatory responses. Investigations have addressed the latter systems, paying particular attention to the interactions of platelets, complement, and polymorphonuclear leukocytes. Perhaps the emphasis of future studies should be to look for major mediator cells such as phagocytic and vascular endothelial cells. This might explain, at least partially, the metabolic effects of multiple organ injury and thus suggest new possibilities for therapeutic intervention.

Assessment

Clinical Manifestations

The clinical presentation and manifestations of ARDS will be a function of the acute pulmonary or nonpulmonary event that caused the syndrome. Unfortunately, in contrast to the magnitude of this medical emergency, the physical examination usually is not very revealing. Hallmarks of assessment are respiratory distress, profound

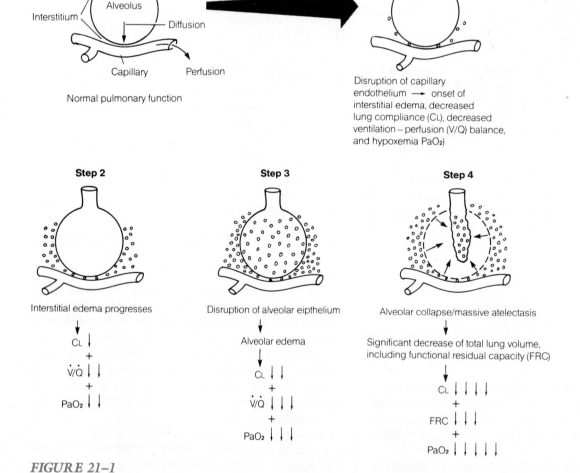

FIGURE 21–1
Pathogenesis of ARDS.

hypoxemia, and diffuse bilateral alveolar infiltrates on the chest film. The last is secondary to increased alveolocapillary permeability with associated flux of fluid and protein into interstitium and alveoli.

Cardinal signs of respiratory distress and profound hypoxemia are changes in level of mental acuity, restlessness, tachycardia, and tachypnea.[4] The respiratory rate frequently increases significantly with a high minute ventilation. Dyspnea with labored respirations and associated intercostal retractions is common. Cyanosis may or may not be present. It must be remembered that cyanosis is neither an early nor a reliable sign of hypoxemia.

Chest auscultation reveals few, if any, abnormalities. The bubbling crackles of cardiogenic pulmonary edema are not present. Rhonchi secondary to secretions in large airways do not occur. Cardiac auscultation usually reveals normal heart sounds without gallops or murmurs, unless myocardial disease is present or trauma has occurred.

Because the physical examination frequently is not revealing, one of the most powerful assessment tools is the constant awareness of the multiple causes of ARDS. The nurse must maintain a high level of suspicion, and strive to be an astute observer. Essential baseline data should be gathered; changes and trends that can be early clues of abnormal lung function—in vital signs, sensorium, and arterial blood gases (ABGs)—should be noted. A gradual increase in respiratory rate without apparent accompanying symptoms or signs may be the first clue. The clinical onset of ARDS may be insidious or sudden. The nurse should develop and learn to follow his or her index of suspicion. Prevention should be the major point of management.

Diagnostic Studies

Arterial blood gases document the severity of hypoxemia. The degree of hypoxemia becomes more severe (ie, $PaO_2 < 50$ mm) as the process continues—despite increasing concentrations of supplemental oxygen. In contrast to refractory hypoxemia, the $PaCO_2$ is low. The latter finding reflects the significant compensatory increase of minute ventilation ($\dot{V}_E$) in an attempt to maintain PaO_2, which exists until the patient becomes fatigued. Display Box 21–2 provides a summary of ARDS, from clinical presentation through the management process.

Management

Therapeutic modalities for ARDS have remained static for the past 20 years. At the time of this writing, treatment is supportive and consists of assisted ventilation and positive end-expiratory pressure (PEEP), in the hopes of buying time for the patient until contributing factors can be corrected and some healing of the lungs can occur.

The primary goal of treatment is to reverse the imme-

DISPLAY BOX 21–2
ARDS: Summary of Clinical Assessment Through Management Process

A. Precipitating pulmonary or nonpulmonary event
B. Clinical signs/assessment
 1. Tachypnea
 2. Tachycardia
 3. Labored respirations
 4. Use of accessory muscles
C. Laboratory findings
 1. ABG analysis: $\downarrow\downarrow$ PaO_2 (ie, < 50 mm with supplemental O_2) $\downarrow$ $PaCO_2$
 2. Chest radiograph: diffuse bilateral pulmonary infiltrates
 3. High $\dot{V}_E$ (ie, >20 L/min)
 4. Low left atrial pressure via pulmonary artery catheter
D. Management
 1. Establishment of definitive airway: endotracheal tube/tracheostomy
 2. Mechanical ventilation: volume ventilator with high pressure and flow capabilities
 3. PEEP
 4. Monitoring for adequate arterial oxygenation
 5. Fluids
 6. Pharmacological agents (ie, O_2 and diuretics; antibiotics for documented infection)
 7. Airway maintenance
 8. Prevention of infection
 9. Nutritional support
 10. Monitor *all* systems for response to therapy and potential complications
 11. Treatment of underlying condition
E. Prognosis: approximately 50% to 70% mortality
F. Sequelae on recovery: infrequent

---

diate life-threatening problem: inadequate delivery of oxygen to the tissues secondary to the inability of the lungs to oxygenate, which is caused by severe $\dot{V}/\dot{Q}$ abnormalities and shunting. Oxygen delivery is determined by the amount of oxygen in the blood and the cardiac output. A second goal of treatment is to minimize pulmonary vascular pressures to prevent or inhibit the leakage of fluid at the alveolar capillary membrane (see Nursing Care Plan 21–1).

Oxygen Therapy

Oxygen is a drug with essential therapeutic properties and potentially toxic side effects. Patients without underlying lung disease apparently tolerate 100% oxygen for 24 to 72 hours without physiological abnormalities of clinical importance. High FIO_2 (ie, >0.5) over a long period of time, however, may cause increased permeability of endothelium and epithelium. The amount of oxygen prescribed for ARDS should be the lowest FIO_2 that produces an adequate oxygen content (ie, oxyhemoglobin content >90%). Intubation almost always is indicated to maintain constant high FIO_2.

Mechanical Ventilation

An important aspect of treatment of true ARDS is mechanical ventilation. (For a detailed discussion of general and specific principles of ventilatory management, refer to the ventilatory section of Chapter 19.) A therapeutic goal of this treatment modality is to provide ventilatory support until the integrity of the alveolocapillary membrane is reestablished. Two additional goals are:

- Maintenance of adequate ventilation and oxygenation during the critical period of severe hypoxemia
- Reversal of the etiologic factors that initially caused the respiratory distress

To facilitate reversal or prevention of atelectasis, tidal volumes (V_T) of 10 to 15 ml/kg body weight are recommended.

Positive End-Expiratory Pressure

Adequate ventilation and oxygenation are provided by volume ventilator with high pressure and flow capabilities, to which PEEP may be added. Positive end-expiratory pressure is maintained in the alveoli throughout the entire respiratory cycle, thereby preventing or minimizing alveolar collapse at the end of expiration (Fig. 21–2). Positive end-expiratory pressure results in restored FRC with improved airway resistance and compliance. The goal of continuous PEEP is improved oxygenation with a subsequent decrease in the inspired oxygen concentration needed to correct life-threatening hypoxemia.

The major complications of PEEP are decreased cardiac output and barotrauma. Subcutaneous emphysema, pneumothorax, and pneumomediastinum occurring during mechanical ventilation are termed *barotrauma*. It occurs more frequently when patients are ventilated with V_T above 15 ml/kg or with high levels of PEEP. Patients with status asthmaticus and chronic obstructive pulmonary disease with associated high lung volumes are also at risk for development of barotrauma during mechanical ventilation. Emergency chest tube thoracostomy equipment should be readily available.

Decreased cardiac output secondary to PEEP results from decreased venous return or increased pulmonary vascular resistance. Careful monitoring of the patient's blood pressure, pulse, urine output, and sensorium is

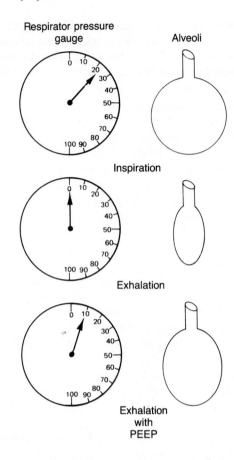

PEEP: Desired effect is: ↑ FRC (Functional residual capacity)
↓ FIO_2 (Fraction of inspired oxygen)

FIGURE 21–2
With PEEP, the alveoli have more gas remaining after exhalation for O_2/CO_2 exchange to take place.

necessary. Dopamine or nitroprusside have been used to return cardiac output to normal. Infusion of additional volume also would restore cardiac output but ultimately would increase lung water content.

The degree of PEEP for ARDS is highly controversial. The goal of PEEP is to correct life-threatening hypoxemia while using the safest therapeutic approach. Several pulmonologists use, for most patients, low levels of PEEP (ie, <15 cm H_2O). Owing to the potential cardiac effects of PEEP, additions and reductions in amount should be accomplished in 3- to 5-cm H_2O increments or decrements. Blood pressure should be noted before and after each change. Arterial blood gases will provide documentation for the effectiveness of PEEP (ie, improved oxygenation).

Hemoglobin Levels

Most of the volume of oxygen is transported to the tissues in combination with hemoglobin. If anemia is present, oxygen content in the blood is reduced. As a result, the effects of mechanical ventilation, PEEP, and supplemental oxygen would be minimized. Serial hemoglobin measurements are necessary for calculation of oxygen content, which will determine the need for transfusing red blood cells.

Fluid Titration

The pathogenetic mechanism of increased alveolocapillary permeability results in interstitial and alveolar edema. Excessive administration of fluid in normal people can produce pulmonary edema and respiratory failure. The choice of colloid versus crystalloid fluid for replacement therapy remains controversial. In spite of advanced technology, an accurate *daily weight* (note trend) frequently is the most important indicator of fluid balance. The primary goal of fluid therapy is to maintain normal physiologic parameters (see Chapter 12, section on Hemodynamic Pressure Monitoring).

Pharmacologic Therapy

The use of corticosteroids is controversial. Previously, antibiotic therapy was initiated for prophylaxis, but experience demonstrated that this did not prevent dangerous gram-negative sepsis. Routine prophylactic antibiotic therapy is no longer acceptable.

Surfactant replacement therapy may be available in the future. Current studies of animal, human, and synthetic surfactant substances are well underway.[3] The data are encouraging, but the therapy is unlikely to be widely available for some time.

Nutritional Management

The critically ill patient's demand for energy and protein increases while supply all too often decreases—a classic dilemma in the critical care setting. Malnutrition is a relatively common problem in critically ill patients who are receiving ventilatory support. Nutritional management of ARDS commonly is overlooked during the early, as well as late, stages. Optimal nutrition during this pulmonary emergency may be difficult to achieve, but the establishment and maintenance of an adequate nutritional support program will be imperative for the successful management of every patient with this syndrome.

One of the most outstanding effects of malnutrition on pulmonary function is to decrease the ability of patients to sustain appropriate levels of ventilation. This occurs secondary to the effects of nutritional deficit on both the central nervous system and the respiratory muscles. The diaphragm is the major muscle of respiration. There are two ways in which the diaphragm is weakened secondary to malnutrition: (1) actual muscle mass is reduced, and (2) marked reduction of the contractile strength of the remaining muscle fibers occurs.

A discussion of individual nutrients and minerals is beyond the scope of this chapter. It would be advantageous, however, to discuss briefly proteins and the mineral phosphorus because both are essential to adequate nutritional balance.

Protein is stored as a nitrogen reservoir. Each molecule of protein is either part of the contractile force in muscle, part of the cellular content or membrane, or an enzyme. Protein depletion results in loss of essential function. Skeletal muscle undergoes the largest part of protein loss in starvation, with a resultant poor energy supply of less than 1 calorie/g muscle.

The mineral element, phosphorus, probably has more functions than any other. It is necessary for building bones and teeth, nucleic acids of all cells, phospholipids that regulate absorption and transportation of fats, enzymes involved in energy metabolism, buffer salts in the regulation of acid–base balance, and compounds involved in the sequential phases of muscle contraction. In other words, this mineral is involved in many metabolic pathways. The normal serum phosphate level is 2 to 5 mg/dl. Hypophosphatemia is said to occur with a serum level less than 1 mg/dl.

Assessment of nutritional status is crucial. Body weight and body height are the most simple measurements. The nurse must be aware that a major change in weight may be secondary to fluid shifts or to changes in body fat. Assessment of protein reserves includes lymphocyte count (normal, 1,800/mm³), cumulative nitrogen balance, albumin (normal, 3 g/dl), total protein (normal, 6 g/dl), and maximum voluntary ventilation (100% of predicted) to test respiratory muscle strength. Variance from norms should be considered as protein depletion.

Total parenteral nutrition (intravenous hyperalimentation) or enthusiastic tube feeding can correct the malnutrition and allow patients to avoid respiratory failure due to poor nutrition of inspiratory muscles.[5] Certainly, malnourished patients with respiratory failure are difficult or impossible to wean from a ventilator until their malnutrition is corrected. In addition to calories and protein, phosphate must be supplied to allow the muscles to function properly (see Chapter 35).

Occasionally, a patient in respiratory failure who is receiving total parenteral nutrition has difficulty weaning from the ventilator because such a high percentage of total calories is being given as carbohydrates that the patient converts the excess carbohydrate to fat (lipogenesis), which produces a large amount of carbon dioxide.[6] Sometimes, this excessive carbon dioxide is more than the body can eliminate without the assistance of a ventilator.

Equipment that accurately can measure oxygen consumption and carbon dioxide production is available and useful in making sure that the patient is nourished correctly, especially when it is combined with nitrogen balance studies. Some new ventilators have a device for measuring carbon dioxide production that is sold as an accessory.

The nitrogen balance study is simple to do and is perhaps the best easy measure of adequate nutrition, particularly with regard to protein. The nitrogen in protein intake is calculated according to the formula in Figure 21–3. It is assumed that 4 g of protein is lost daily in the stool and skin. Positive nitrogen balance (more protein nitrogen in than out) means positive protein balance.

Airway Maintenance

A definitive airway—either an endotracheal or tracheostomy tube—is established not only as an airway but also as a means of protecting the airway (with the cuff intact), providing for continuous ventilatory support, and sustaining oxygen concentrations. Maintenance of the airway involves knowing *when* to suction; meticulous suctioning technique; adequate cuff pressures; prevention of pressure necrosis from endotracheal and oropharyngeal tubes; nasal and oral care to remove accumulated secretions, which, if aspirated into the lower respiratory tract, can cause secondary pulmonary infection; and constant monitoring of upper airway and tracheal secretions as well as the tracheostomy site for evidence of infections. This care is crucial. The new or inexperienced nurse should observe this process demonstrated and, in turn, demonstrate *both* assessment and technical skills before becoming responsible for this aspect of intensive therapy. It should be remembered that an artificial airway and ventilatory support buy time for the patient—*time* for the underlying conditions that precipitate ARDS to be treated, and, it is hoped, *time* for ARDS to resolve. Maintenance of the airway and associated prevention of infection are paramount for recovery.

Surveillance for and Prevention of Infection

The importance of attention to upper and lower respiratory tract secretions and prevention of infection through meticulous suctioning techniques has been addressed. Nosocomial infections are hospital-acquired infections. It is estimated that a staggering 2 million nosocomial infections occur annually in the United States. The tremendous impact of such infections on the economy (ie, extra hospital days) needs to be appreciated.

Most common sites of infection are the urinary tract, surgical wound infections, lower respiratory tract, and skin. The cause of infection may be exogenous (pathogen from any source other than the patient) or endogenous (patient's own microbial flora). Usually the localized primary sites of infection progress to an overwhelming generalized sepsis or bacteremia. Some of the important signs and symptoms of infection that the nurse should be alert to include pain, fever, redness, warmth, or swelling associated with joints or wounds, and change in drainage or secretions (ie, amount, consistency, color, or odor) and an elevated white blood count.

Monitoring Respiratory Function

Hemodynamic indices of the patient in respiratory failure usually are monitored on a routine basis. The type of monitoring that is too commonly minimized—or completely overlooked (because of hemodynamic monitoring devices)—is that which is most simple. Astute *observation* by qualified personnel of pulmonary function (and the total patient) over time is vitally important. Physical diagnosis and radiologic examination of the chest continue to

Protein intake		minus	Protein output	=	Balance
Grams of protein $\dfrac{\text{eaten}}{6.25}$	$+$ Grams of protein $\dfrac{\text{in TPN}}{6.25}$	$-$	Urinary N_2 + 4 g (stool and skin N_2)	=	Balance

Example of patient in negative nitrogen balance					
$\dfrac{60}{6.25}$		$-$	$8 + 4$	$=$	
9.6		$-$	12	$=$	-2.4

FIGURE 21–3
Nitrogen balance formula.

Clinical Research

Stone K, et al: *Effects of lung hyperinflation on mean arterial pressure and postsuctioning hypoxemia.* Heart Lung 18:377–385, 1989

Using 12 patients with normal lung function, the process of three hyperinflations before suctioning was examined. In the study, the volumes of each hyperinflation varied from 12 to 18 ml/kg. Affects of the hyperinflations on mean arterial pressure and postsuctioning hypoxemia were measured. The mean arterial pressure increased 15 mm hg. The PaO$_2$ had a significant increase after suctioning and returned to normal within 5 minutes. Although this study is limited by size, it did demonstrate that postsuctioning oxygenation was improved with any hyperinflation of 12–18 ml/kg.

be fundamental techniques that must be used. Technology should be considered a means of enhancing physical and radiographic findings rather than replacing them.

Physical examination of the intubated patient must include an attempt to elicit subjective information. If the patient is able to cooperate and write, paper and pen will provide a means for response to questions such as the following:

- How do you feel?
- How is your breathing?
- Are you getting enough air?
- Where are you?
- What are the date and time?
- Who is the president of the United States?

The deleterious effects of hypoxemia on central nervous system function must be kept in mind. Asking questions of the patient in an attempt to determine mental acuity is an important part of assessment.

Objective assessment is next. Pulse rate is a nonspecific cardiopulmonary variable that, when elevated, can suggest hypoxemia, blood volume or flow deficits, fever, anxiety, cardiac impairment, and so forth. An increased respiratory rate is one of the earliest responses to either a decreased PaO$_2$ or an increased PaCO$_2$. When the rate exceeds 20/minute with an upward trend, the nurse must be aware of the likelihood of severe respiratory distress.

General assessment of ventilatory effectiveness can be gleaned by observation of chest movement. The nurse should stand at the foot of the bed with the patient's chest exposed, and observe the thorax for symmetry. Asymmetry can occur with right main stem bronchus intubation, pneumothorax, and atelectasis. Chest auscultation may or may not reveal unequal ventilation, depending on degree.

Assessment of breath sounds allows detection of ventilatory fluid and secretions, need for or adequacy of suctioning, and adequacy of tracheostomy or endotracheal tube cuff inflation. Wheezes, crackles, and dullness to percussion usually are considered late signs of respiratory failure. Again, the nurse must remember the importance of the physical examination as an essential counterpart of roentgenography and physiological studies in following

the trend of ARDS, the underlying condition, and the course of treatment.

Chest roentgenography is an important way to document appropriate placement of an endotracheal tube and to determine the presence of pneumothorax after procedures such as thoracentesis and subclavian venous catheterization, after trauma, and secondary to PEEP. Chest radiography also is useful in following the course of ARDS and in detecting complications such as pneumonia and atelectasis. The nurse should develop a habit of reviewing and discussing chest films for the patient with the physician. Findings on the chest film may assist in selecting proper positioning for postural drainage.

Cardiac dysrhythmias usually are latent manifestations of pulmonary problems. It is important to monitor the patient with continuous cardiac monitoring. In addition to dysrhythmia detection, the direct visibility of a cardiac monitor will assist the nurse in the delivery of patient care. The nurse should glance at the monitor before, during, and after endotracheal suctioning. Evaluation of heart rate and rhythm should be ongoing and is a useful measure of the patient's response to treatments.

Other equally important guides for monitoring bedside parameters of respiratory function in a patient with ARDS include ABGs, V$_T$, and V$_E$. The nurse must learn to integrate each aspect of care with normal pulmonary anatomy and function, altered lung function (in this case, ARDS), and associated therapeutic modalities. A summary of bedside measurements of respiratory function has been developed as a guide for patient care and communication of patient information (ie, nursing report and patient record; see Display Box 21–3).

Complications

The significance of ARDS as an extreme pulmonary emergency with an average mortality of 50% to 70% could well indicate multiple sequelae on recovery, yet the long-term prognosis appears to be good. Mild to moderate physiological abnormalities that have been reported are restrictive–obstructive abnormalities (airflow limitation), moderate diffusion defects, and shift hypoxemia during exercise. The positive outcome for those who recover from ARDS

DISPLAY BOX 21–3
Bedside Measurements
of Respiratory Function

Physical Examination

Subjective information (what patient says/writes)
Objective information (what nurse observes)
    Daily weight
    Urine output/specific gravity
    Vital signs
    CNS: mental acuity, behavior
    Mouth: color of mucosa → ? central cyanosis
    Neck: ? prominent neck veins; ? supple
    Cardiopulmonary: heart sounds, breath sounds
    Abdomen: tenderness or distention?
    Extremities: ? cyanosis or clubbing

Pt/Ventilator

Tidal volume (V_T)
Minute ventilation ($\dot{V}_E$)
Inspiratory pressure
Compliance (C_L)

Laboratory

CXR
ECG
ABG
Hgb/Hct
Albumin/Total protein
WBC
Electrolytes

---

is most likely a threefold function of the abilities of the health care team to protect the lung from further insult during the life support period, prevention of oxygen toxicity, and meticulous attention to sepsis reduction.

CASE STUDY

Anita Weiss was a 43-year-old woman who was admitted to a medical floor 2 days ago. Her temperature was 103°F on admission, and she felt very "weak." Blood cultures done at the time of admission showed gram-negative rods. In spite of a normal chest radiograph, she manifested an increasing heart rate, increasing respiratory rate, and severe anxiety. She was transferred to the Critical Care Unit for further observation.

The critical care nurse's initial assessment included:

BP: 102/64 mm Hg

HR: 132/min

Rhythm: sinus tachycardia

RR: 28/min

Breath sounds: slightly decreased in right anterior fields

T: 100.4°F, orally

O_2: 35% Venturi mask

IV: D5 0.45 NS at 50 ml/hr

The nurse found Anita to be oriented to person, place, and time, but very restless. The nurse decided to find an O_2 saturation monitor to check Anita's progress and placed a call to her physician due to concern about her restlessness.

Placing the monitor on her finger, the nurse noticed that Anita's hand is cool, although not diaphoretic. The SaO_2 reads 74%. The nurse stayed with Anita and called for an ABG kit. The results were called to the unit at the same time the physician arrived:

    pH: 7.34

    PCO_2: 28

    PO_2: 48

    O_2 SAT: 76%

    HCO_3^-: 24

Throughout the nurse's shift, Anita's supplemental oxygen was titrated up, in the attempt to reach > 90% SaO_2. When the nurse left, Anita was on 100%, nonrebreather mask. She appeared exhausted. Her respirations were > 30/min and she was using accessory muscles. Her skin was cool and damp, although her heart rate and rhythm were unchanged. Her SaO_2 was 86%. The physician was talking to Anita's husband, obtaining permission for an elective intubation.

On the nurse's arrival the next morning, Anita was on a mechanical ventilator. Her face looked relaxed. Her respirations were still in the high 20s, and her rhythm was sinus tachycardia. During report, the nurse found that although the intubation went well, Anita's BP fell dramatically when placed on the ventilator. She received 1,500 ml of extra IV fluid to keep her systolic pressure above 95 mm Hg. She had very few secretions. Her chest film was essentially unchanged. Her ventilator was set: TV 800 cc, RR 16 IMV, FiO_2 80%, PEEP + 10 cm. Her postintubation and ventilation ABG was: pH 7.39, PCO_2 30, PO_2 72, O_2 SAT 85%, and HCO_3^- 25

She was on a theophylline infusion of 800 mg/hr, gentamycin 120 mg BID, ancef (cefazolin sodium) 1 g q6h, solumedrol 24 mg q6h. Albuterol inhalation treatments q4h. The nurse placed a call to Anita's physician.

When the physician returned the call, the nurse offered several suggestions. The sensitivity report on the blood cultures was available for the physician to select an antibiotic specific for Anita's infection. The nurse suggested that an increase in the PEEP may allow Anita's FiO_2 to be decreased, and suggested the placement of a central line with three lumens to facilitate intravenous medications and allow for hyperalimentaion. The nurse also secured an order for a mild sedative, to be given if Anita was not able to rest.

After 4 days of ventilation with PEEP, attempts were made to wean Anita from the ventilator. Her FiO_2 was decreased first, until it was 50%. Next, her PEEP was slowly decreased to +5 cm. Her work of breathing was increased as she was changed to 15-minute intervals of spontaneous breathing, supported with CPAP. In 8 days, Anita was able to leave the Critical Care Unit. She will have approximately 5 more hospital days, but she will be able to return to her home without permanent disability.

Nursing Care Plan

Nursing Care Plan 21–1 outlines the important features of care for the patient with ARDS.

(Text continues on page 514)

NURSING DIAGNOSIS	OUTCOME CRITERIA/ PATIENT GOALS	NURSING INTERVENTIONS
Impaired gas exchange: related to refractory hypoxemia and pulmonary interstitial/alveolar leaks found in alveolar capillary injury states.	• Adequate oxygenation.	1. Assess breath sounds q2–4h. 2. Assess for signs of respiratory distress: increased heart rate, agitation, diaphoresis, cyanosis. 3. Assess chest excursion/symmetry. 4. Monitor input and output, observing effects of diuresis and fluid administration. 5. Assess rhythm/dysrhythmias by ECG monitoring. 6. Check ABGs for ↓ PaO_2, ↑ $PaCO_2$. 7. Administer and monitor bronchodilator therapy (eg, theophylline and sympathomimetic agents), as ordered. 8. Maintain mechanical ventilation. 9. Follow serial chest radiograph reports.
Ineffective airway clearance: related to increased secretion production and decreased ciliary motion.	• Maintain patent airway. • Aspiration will not occur • Secretions will remain liquid and readily cleared.	1. Assess breath sounds q2–4h and prn. 2. Maintain proper position of tracheostomy or endotracheal tube. 3. Suction tracheostomy/endotracheal tube, oral and nasal cavities, using sterile technique. Note color, amount, and consistency of secretions. 4. Postural drainage and chest percussion when appropriate to augment secretion clearance. 5. Position to facilitate good gas exchange q2h. 6. Monitor for signs of respiratory distress. 7. Maintain adequate cuff pressures/minimal leak technique to avoid aspiration of secretions and tissue necrosis. 8. Elevate head of bed during tube feedings. 9. Provide supplemental humidification. 10. Prepare for bronchoscopy, as ordered.

(continued)

NURSING CARE PLAN 21–1: (Continued)
The Patient With Adult Respiratory Distress Syndrome

NURSING DIAGNOSIS	OUTCOME CRITERIA/ PATIENT GOALS	NURSING INTERVENTIONS
Fluid volume excess: related to noncardiac pulmonary edema, PEEP causing a decreased venous return/cardiac output, or diuretic therapy.	• Maintain hemodynamic stability.	1. Weigh patient daily. 2. Monitor total input and output hourly. 3. Assess signs and symptoms of decreased cardiac output: elevated pulse, decreased BP, decreased urine output, change in mentation, decreased PCO_2. 4. Assess signs of fluid overload: dependent edema, increased weight, pulmonary crackles, respiratory distress, increased CVP. 5. Monitor hemodynamic parameters: MAP, PCWP, and cardiac output. 6. Administer/monitor IV fluid and electrolyte therapy, as ordered.
	• Urine output will be adequate	7. Monitor total input and output hourly. 8. Report urine output <30 ml/hr to physician. 9. Administer diuretics as ordered. 10. Evaluate BUN and serum creatinine as ordered.
Altered tissue perfusion: related to decreased venous return and decreased cardiac output with PEEP therapy, edema from volume overload, hypotension from shock and ventilation/perfusion mismatch, resulting in hypoxemia.	• Patient will be awake and alert. • Patient will have warm skin and not be diaphoretic. • Patient will have normal bowel sounds and abdomen will not be tender. • Maintain adequate distal peripheral pulses.	1. Assess mental status. 2. Allow patient to make some care decisions. 3. Assess for decreased perfusion to skin. 4. Assess hemodynamic status (PAP, PCWP, CVP). 5. Assess ECG rhythm. 6. Assess GI system: bowel sounds, nausea, vomiting, tenderness. 7. Assess nutritional status. 8. Assess dorsalis pedis, posterior tibial, and radial artery pulses for quality q4h. 9. Evaluate capillary refill time.
Ineffective breathing pattern: related to inadequate gas exchange, increased secretions, decreased ability to oxygenate adequately, fear or exhaustion.	• Work of breathing will be minimized by maintaining bed rest or low level ADLs.	1. Monitor meticulously for onset/progress of signs of respiratory distress.

(continued)

NURSING CARE PLAN 21–1: *(Continued)*
The Patient With Adult Respiratory Distress Syndrome

NURSING DIAGNOSIS	OUTCOME CRITERIA/ PATIENT GOALS	NURSING INTERVENTIONS
		2. Position to facilitate breathing, usually with head of bed elevated.
		3. Reassure patient by confident and calming approach. Stay with patient.
		4. Review serial radiograph reports.
		5. Monitor serial ABGs.
		6. Administer oxygen as indicated.
		7. Use oximetric device to evaluate O_2 saturation during activity.
		8. Sedation, as ordered, prn.
		9. Evaluate all subjective complaints.
		10. Turn, cough, deep breathe q2h.
		11. Suction prn.
		12. Analgesics for pain prn, as ordered.
		13. If patient is ventilated, develop alternate communication system and use soft restraints as needed, if agitated.
High risk for anxiety: related to critical illness, fear of death or disfigurement, role changes within social setting, or permanent disability.	• Patient will be able to express anxieties to appropriate resource person.	1. Establish effective communication with ventilated patient (ie, writing notes).
		2. Provide environment that encourages open discussion of emotional issues.
		3. Mobilize patient's support system and involve these resources as appropriate.
		4. Allow time for patient to express self.
		5. Identify possible hospital resources for patient/family support.
		6. Encourage open family-to-nurse communications regarding emotional issues.
		7. Validate patient and family knowledge base regarding the critical illness.
		8. Involve religious support systems as appropriate.

REFERENCES

1. Rinaldo J: Adult respiratory distress syndrome. In Shoemaker W (ed): Textbook of Critical Care, pp 500–505. Philadelphia, WB Saunders, 1989
2. Albelda S: The alveolar–capillary barrier in adult respiratory distress syndrome. In Fishman A (ed): Update: Pulmonary Diseases and Disorders, pp 197–211. New York, McGraw-Hill, 1992
3. Pattishall E, Long W: Surfactant treatment of the adult respiratory distress syndrome. In Fishman A (ed): Update: Pulmonary Diseases and Disorders, pp 225–236. New York, McGraw-Hill, 1992
4. Rinaldo J: Adult respiratory distress syndrome. In Rippe J (ed): Intensive Care Medicine, pp 476–481. Boston, Little, Brown & Co., 1992
5. Perry A, Potter P: Clinical Nursing Skills and Techniques, pp 625–630. St. Louis, CV Mosby, 1990
6. Rothkopf M: Nutritional support in respiratory failure. Nutrition in Clinical Practice 4(5):166–172, 1989

BIBLIOGRAPHY

Litwack K, et al: Postoperative pulmonary complications. Critical Care Nursing Clinics of North America 3:77–82, 1991
Ranieri V, Elissa N, Corbeil C, Chasse M, et al: Effects of positive end-expiratory pressure on alveolar recruitment and gas exchange in patients with the adult respiratory distress syndrome. Am Rev Respir Dis 144:544–551, 1991
Stone K: Endotracheal suctioning. Annual Review of Nursing Research 7:27–49, 1989

STUDY QUESTIONS

1. The leaking of the alveolar/capillary membrane in ARDS leads to all of the following *except*

   a. pulmonary capillary wedge pressure greater than 18
   b. alveolar atelectasis
   c. decreased functional residual capacity
   d. decreased pulmonary compliance

2. Which assessment is likely to be within normal limits in ARDS?

   a. mental status
   b. heart rate
   c. lung auscultation
   d. respiratory rate and work of breathing

3. Mr. Smith is a 163-pound patient with ARDS. Which ventilator settings would be the most appropriate?

   a. TV: 400 cc; RR: 20; FiO_2: 65%; PEEP: +5 cm
   b. TV: 800 cc; RR: 20; FiO_2: 65%; PEEP: +10 cm
   c. TV: 800 cc; RR: 20; FiO_2: 35%; PEEP: 0
   d. TV: 800 cc; RR: 20; FiO_2: 50%; PEEP: +25 cm

4. Which of the following nursing interventions are *not* performed to maintain a patent airway?

   a. therapeutic positioning of the patient in bed
   b. hyperinflation and suctioning
   c. evaluation of daily chest radiograph
   d. adequate nutrition and hydration

UNIT III

Renal System

BEHAVIORAL OBJECTIVES

Based on the content in this chapter, the reader should be able to:

1. Identify the structures comprising the nephron: the glomerulus, proximal tubule, loop of Henle, distal and collecting tubules.
2. Describe the functions of the nephron, including glomerular filtration, passive and active transport, tubular secretion, and clearance.
3. Discuss normal fluid pressures in the nephron and how they affect glomerular filtration rate.
4. Explain the relationship of antidiuretic hormone, renin, and aldosterone to fluid regulation by the kidneys.
5. Describe the mechanisms by which the kidneys help maintain homeostasis.

CHAPTER 22

Anatomy and Physiology of the Renal System

Hudak: Critical Care Nursing:
A Holistic Approach, 6th ed. © 1994
J. B. Lippincott Company.

Normal Structure of the Kidney

The regulation and concentration of solutes in the extracellular fluid of the body are the primary functions of the kidney. The kidneys remove metabolic waste products and excess concentrations of constituents and conserve those substances present in normal or low quantities. Figure 22–1 is a schematic representation of the general macroscopic and microscopic structure of the kidney.

Urine, the end product of kidney function, is formed from the blood by the nephron. A nephron is composed of one glomerulus, proximal tubule, loop of Henle, and distal tubule. Several distal tubules drain into a collecting tubule. From the collecting tubules, urine flows to the pelvis of the kidney. From there, it leaves the kidney by way of the ureter and flows into the urinary bladder. Each human kidney consists of about 1 million nephrons, all of which function identically, and thus kidney function can be explained by describing the function of one nephron.

Figure 22–2 is a composite drawing of a functional nephron. Each nephron is made up of two major components: (1) the glomerulus and Bowman's capsule, in which water and solutes are filtered from the blood; and (2) the tubules, which reabsorb essential materials from the filtrate and permit waste substances and unneeded materials to remain in the filtrate and flow into the renal pelvis as urine.

The glomerulus consists of a tuft of capillaries fed by the afferent arteriole, drained by the efferent arteriole. The glomerulus is surrounded by Bowman's capsule. The efferent arteriole supplies blood to the peritubular capillaries. Fluid that is filtered from the capillaries into this capsule then flows into the tubular system, which is divided into four sections: (1) the proximal tubule, (2) the loop of Henle, (3) the distal tubule, and (4) the collecting tubule.

Most of the water and electrolytes are reabsorbed into the blood in the peritubular capillaries. The end products of metabolism pass into the urine.

The nephron is so arranged that the initial portion of the distal tubule lies at the juncture of the afferent and efferent arterioles, which is very near the glomerulus. Here, macula densa cells of the distal tubule lie in approximation to the juxtaglomerular cells of the wall of the afferent arteriole. Both these cell types plus some connective tissue cells constitute the juxtaglomerular apparatus.

Normal Renal Physiology

Glomerular Filtration

Like other body capillaries, the glomerular capillaries are relatively impermeable to large plasma proteins and are quite permeable to water and smaller solutes such as electrolytes, amino acids, glucose, and nitrogenous waste.

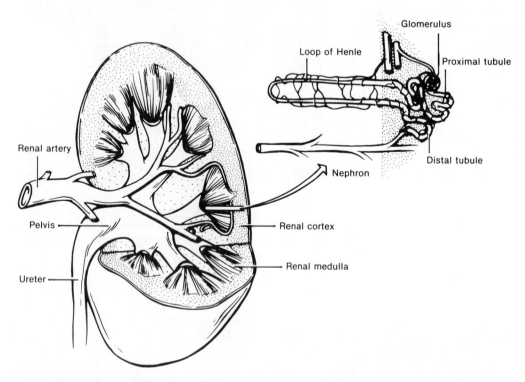

FIGURE 22–1
General characteristics of kidney structure. One nephron contains a glomerulus, located in the renal cortex, and a proximal, distal, and collecting tubule, located in the renal medulla.

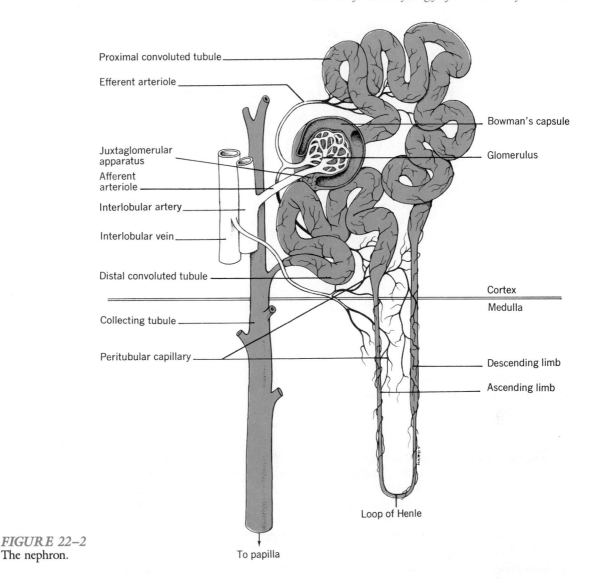

Proximal convoluted tubule

Efferent arteriole

Juxtaglomerular apparatus

Afferent arteriole

Interlobular artery

Interlobular vein

Distal convoluted tubule

Collecting tubule

Peritubular capillary

Bowman's capsule

Glomerulus

Cortex

Medulla

Descending limb

Ascending limb

Loop of Henle

To papilla

FIGURE 22–2
The nephron.

Unlike other capillaries in the body, the glomerular capillaries have an elevated blood pressure (90 mm Hg versus 10–30 mm Hg). This elevated pressure occurs because the afferent arteriole leading to the glomerular capillaries is larger in diameter and offers less resistance than other capillaries. In particular, the afferent arteriole is proportionately larger in diameter than the efferent arteriole. Blood literally is squeezed into a smaller and smaller space, forcing the water and small solute particles of the plasma to exude into Bowman's capsule. This pressure of blood against vessel walls is called *hydrostatic pressure* (HP). The movement of exudate into Bowman's capsule is termed *glomerular filtration*, and the material entering Bowman's capsule is called *filtrate*.

The HP of the glomerulus does not operate unopposed. Three other factors participate in filtration: the HP and the osmotic pressure (OP) of the filtrate in Bowman's capsule, and the plasma OP. Figure 22–3 illustrates the interaction of these factors. Osmotic pressure is the pressure exerted by water (or any solvent) on a semipermeable

membrane as it attempts to cross the membrane into an area containing more molecules that cannot cross the semipermeable membrane. The pores in the glomerular capillary make it a semipermeable membrane that permits smaller molecules and water to cross but prevents larger molecules (eg, plasma proteins) from crossing. Filtrate HP, about 15 mm Hg, results from the presence of filtrate in the capsule, and opposes blood HP. The filtrate also exerts an OP of 1 to 3 mm Hg, which opposes plasma OP. The difference between the OPs of the plasma and fluid in Bowman's capsule reflects a difference in protein concentrations. This difference occurs because the capillary pores prevent most plasma proteins from being filtered. Indeed, the filtrate in Bowman's capsule contains only 0.03% protein. Plasma HP (90 mm Hg) and Bowman's capsule filtrate OP (1–3 mm Hg) cooperate to promote the movement of water and small permeable molecules from the plasma into Bowman's capsule. Plasma OP (32 mm Hg) and the HP of the filtrate (15 mm Hg) within Bowman's capsule, together, prompt the movement of water and

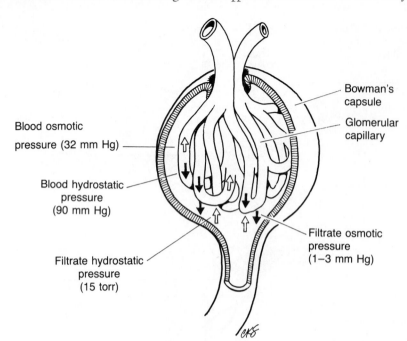

Blood osmotic pressure (32 mm Hg)

Blood hydrostatic pressure (90 mm Hg)

Filtrate hydrostatic pressure (15 torr)

Bowman's capsule

Glomerular capillary

Filtrate osmotic pressure (1–3 mm Hg)

FIGURE 22–3
Opposing pressures in glomerular capillaries and Bowman's capsule that result in renal filtration.

permeable molecules from Bowman's capsule back into the capillary. The sum of these pressures is the net gradient of 46 mm Hg ([90 + 3] − [32 + 15] = 46) that favors movement of filtrate from the bloodstream into Bowman's capsule.

The rate at which the filtrate is formed is termed the *glomerular filtration rate* (*GFR*). In the typical healthy person, this amounts to the formation of 125 ml of filtrate per minute. Major clinical factors that influence the GFR are the blood HP and filtrate OP. Hypoproteinemia, as in starvation, will lower filtrate OP and increase the GFR. The GFR decreases with severe hypotension, due to a drop in blood HP. Other factors that decrease the HP and thus the GFR are afferent arteriole constriction and renal artery stenosis.

Because of the influence of HP on the GFR, the kidneys long were thought to function in the normal homeostasis of systemic blood pressure. But we now know that the GFR is relatively stable over a wide range of arterial blood pressures. The reason for this stability is that the afferent arterioles adjust their diameter in response to the pressure of blood coming to them. If the blood pressure decreases, the smooth muscles of the afferent arterioles relax. This causes dilation of these arterioles, which, in turn, increases the perfusion of the glomeruli and maintains the GFR at its normal rate; conversely, with an increase in blood pressure, these vessels constrict. There is a limit, however, to this autoregulatory mechanism. Below a mean arterial pressure of 90 mm Hg and above a mean of 250 mm Hg, GFR is proportional to perfusion pressure. For example, if the system blood pressure falls greatly, such as in shock, the GFR will fall to near zero, thereby producing near anuria.

Tubular Reabsorption and Secretion

Roughly 23% of the cardiac output goes to the kidneys in a resting adult. From this, about 125 ml of filtrate is produced each minute. This totals 180 liters/day and is about 4.5 times the total amount of fluid in the body. Of course, not all this filtrate is excreted as urine. As this filtrate passes from Bowman's capsule through the remainder of the nephrons, all but about 1.5 L/day will be returned to the bloodstream. Similarly, at plasma glucose levels of less than 200 mg/dl, none of the filtered glucose is found in the urine when it enters the collecting tubules. The volume and content of the urine are the result of tubular reabsorption and tubular secretion. Reabsorption is accomplished by active transport, osmosis, and diffusion. It occurs in all parts of the nephron. Secretion involves active transport and is performed only by distal tubule cells.

Active transport involves the binding of a molecule of a substance to a carrier, which then moves the molecule from one side of the membrane to the other against the concentration gradient of that substance. Because it helps molecules to move in a direction opposite to the direction they would move by simple diffusion, the carrier acts somewhat like a pump. In tubular cells, the carrier is located in the cell membrane nearest the peritubular capillaries, and it transports material out of the tubular cell into the peritubular fluid. This lowers the intracellular concentration of the type of molecule being transported. The decreased concentration enables more of those molecules to diffuse from the urine (filtrate) into the tubule cell. These molecules, in turn, exit the cell and enter the peritubular fluid by active transport. The movement of molecules increases the peritubular fluid concentration of the molecule, and this increase in turn stimulates the diffusion of the molecule into the peritubular capillaries. Thus, in the nephrons, active transport removes molecules from the filtrate (urine) back to the bloodstream.

Because active transport involves carrier molecules and energy exchanges, there is an upper limit to the number of molecules of a substance that can be transported at one time. This maximum limit for reabsorption rates is called T_{max}. Glucose is an example of a molecule that will appear in the same concentrations that it appears in the blood. As serum glucose rises, filtrate glucose also rises. The renal tubules will reabsorb the filtered glucose at faster and faster rates, until this molecule's active transport mechanisms all are being used. At this T_{max}, more glucose is appearing in the filtrate than can be reabsorbed, and glucose will be excreted in the urine. This "spilling" of glucose into the urine indicates serum levels higher than T_{max}.

Urea is an example of a molecule that is reabsorbed by diffusion. Under the high pressures in the glomerular capillaries, urea is filtered. In the tubules, as water is reabsorbed into the bloodstream, urea follows by simple diffusion. No selective permeability prevents its return to the bloodstream, and no transport mechanism is required. The reabsorption rates of urea range from 40% to 60% of that which is filtered, and depend entirely on water reabsorption rates.

The active transport of sodium is responsible for the osmotic reabsorption of water from the filtrate both here in the proximal and later in the distal tubule. As sodium ions are actively transported out of the cell and into the peritubular fluid, they make the osmotic pressure of this peritubular fluid higher than that of the cell or tubule fluid. Water is thus osmotically "pulled out" of the tubular fluid. Both water and sodium then diffuse into peritubular capillaries and thus are returned to the bloodstream. This movement of positively charged sodium ions also creates an electrochemical gradient that draws negatively charged ions—especially chloride—out of the tubular fluid and back into the bloodstream.

Tubular secretion involves the active transport of molecules from the bloodstream through tubule cells into the filtrate. Many substances that are secreted do not occur naturally in the body (eg, penicillin). Naturally occurring bodily substances that are secreted include uric acid and potassium and hydrogen ions.

In the distal tubule, the active transport of sodium uses a carrier system that also is involved in the tubular secretion of hydrogen and potassium ions (Fig. 22–4). In this relationship, every time the carrier transports sodium out of the tubular fluid, it carries *either* a hydrogen *or* a potassium ion into the tubular fluid on its "return trip." Thus, for every sodium ion reabsorbed, a hydrogen *or* potassium must be secreted, and *vice versa*. The choice

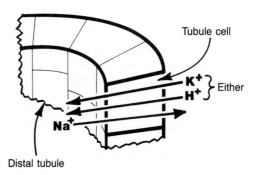

FIGURE 22–4
Cation exchange in the distal tubule.

of cation to be secreted depends on the extracellular fluid (ECF) concentration of these ions (hydrogen and potassium).

Knowledge of this cation exchange system in the distal tubule helps us understand some of the relationships that these electrolytes have with one another. For example, we can understand why an aldosterone blocker may cause hyperkalemia or why there can be an initial fall in plasma potassium as severe acidosis is corrected therapeutically.*

Overview of Nephron Function

Approximately 80% of the filtrate is returned to the bloodstream by reabsorption in the proximal tubule. In the normal healthy person, all the filtered glucose and amino acids plus much sodium, chloride, and other electrolytes as well as uric acid are reabsorbed here. The proximal tubule cells also secrete urea, creatinine, hydrogen, and ammonia into the urine (filtrate).

In the loop of Henle the filtrate (urine) becomes highly concentrated. This part of the nephron is composed of a thin-walled descending portion and a thick-walled ascending portion. Loops of Henle belonging to juxtamedullary nephrons dip into the medulla of the kidney, which contains a highly concentrated interstitial fluid. (The thin walls of the descending portion are quite permeable.) This permeability, together with the high concentration of the interstitial fluid at this point, causes water to osmose from the filtrate into the interstitial fluid. This makes the filtrate

---

* The aldosterone blocker reduces sodium reabsorption. Such reduced reabsorption of sodium also reduces the tubular secretion of either hydrogen or potassium. The hydrogen excess can be buffered, but the potassium simply rises to above-normal levels. In severe acidosis, the nephrons have been attempting to compensate by increasing their hydrogen ion secretion rates. As acidosis is therapeutically corrected (*e.g.*, by sodium bicarbonate administration), one change is secretion of potassium ions (another concerns a shift of potassium into cells). As hydrogen ions no longer need to be secreted, potassium ions become the sole exchange for sodium ions, leading, it is thought, to a reduction in plasma potassium.

quite concentrated by the time it reaches the ascending limb of the loop.

The thicker-walled ascending limb is relatively impermeable to water, but it contains ion carriers that actively transport chloride ions out of the filtrate. This creates an electrochemical gradient that "pulls" the positively charged sodium ions out of the filtrate as well. This exit of electrolytes without water now makes the filtrate more dilute than before.

In the distal tubule, sodium again is reabsorbed by active transport, and hydrogen, potassium, and uric acid can be added to the urine by tubular secretion.

The collecting ducts or collecting tubules receive the contents from many distal tubules. There is no further electrolyte reabsorption or secretion, and in the well hydrated person, no further water reabsorption as well. Water reabsorption without electrolyte reabsorption can occur in the collecting ducts under the stimulus of anti-diuretic hormone (ADH).

Hormonal Influences

Through the reabsorption of sodium, and the passive "following" of water and chloride, it is possible to make urine of the same osmolality as blood. Under conditions of dehydration, however, urine is very concentrated, whereas if a great deal of water is drunk, urine will be more dilute than blood. This final regulation of urine, and thus serum osmolality and volume, is regulated by three hormones.

Osmoreceptors in the hypothalamus are sensitive to serum osmolality (Fig. 22–5). During dehydration, when serum osmolality rises, osmoreceptors in the hypothalamus respond by stimulating the hypothalamus to secrete ADH, which increases the permeability of collecting tubule cells to water. This permits the reabsorption of water alone (without electrolytes), which in turn will decrease the concentration of the ECF. Negative feedback loops regulate ADH secretion. This means that as the concentration of the ECF returns to normal, the stimulus to ADH secretion disappears, and ADH secretion is stopped.

Another hormone that influences urine concentration is renin. When GFR falls owing to dehydration or blood loss, the juxtaglomerular apparatus will secrete renin. Subnormal sodium levels in the filtrate also stimulate renin secretion. Renin converts angiotensin, which is secreted by the liver, into angiotensin I. Pulmonary capillary cells, in turn, convert this into angiotensin II.

Angiotensin II constricts the smooth muscle sur-

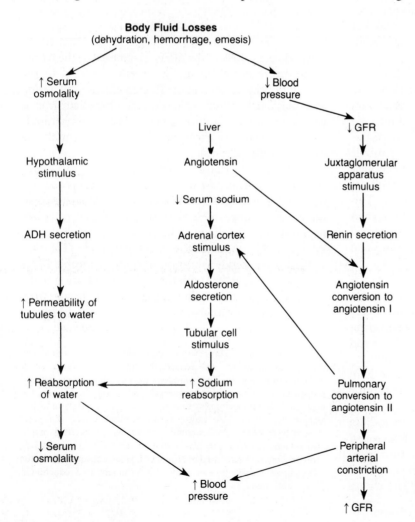

FIGURE 22–5
Relationship of ADH, renin, and aldosterone to fluid regulation by the kidneys.

rounding arterioles. This increases blood pressure, which in turn increases the GFR. Angiotensin II also triggers the secretion of aldosterone, the third hormone that influences urine osmolality. The adrenal cortex, when stimulated by angiotensin II, secretes aldosterone. By increasing sodium reabsorption in distal tubule cells, aldosterone causes an increase in renal water reabsorption. This increases blood pressure, and decreases serum osmolality. Aldosterone also is secreted in response to subnormal serum sodium levels.

Clearance

From the previous discussion, a very important concept in renal function emerges—that of *clearance*. As the filtrate moves along the nephron, a large proportion of metabolic end products remains in it, unreabsorbed. These products thus are removed (cleared) from the blood and exit the body in the urine. Indeed, of each 125 ml of glomerular filtrate formed per minute, about one half, or 60 ml, returns to the blood without urea, and about one half is excreted with urea. Stated another way, 60 ml of plasma is "cleared" of urea each minute in normally functioning kidneys. In the same way, 125 ml of plasma is cleared of creatinine, 12 ml of uric acid, 12 ml of potassium, 25 ml of sulfate, 25 ml of phosphate, and so forth each minute.

It is possible to calculate renal clearance by simultaneously sampling urine and plasma. By dividing the quantity of substance found in each milliliter of plasma into the quantity found in the urine, the milliliters cleared per minute can be calculated. This method is used as one means of testing kidney function.

Other methods of assessing renal function involve chemicals that are known to be either filtered only or both filtered and secreted. *Inulin*, for example, is filtered only, and neither absorbed nor secreted. Thus, the clearance of inulin provides a measure of glomerular filtration. *Mannitol* can be used similarly. Para-aminohippurate (PAH) or iodopyracet (Diodrast) are drugs that are secreted in addition to being filtered. As such, their clearance provides an index of plasma flow through the kidneys. They also can be used together with a filtered-only drug in assessing tubular secretion and thus the health of tubular cells.

The sodium concentration in the urine also can serve as an index of tubular health in certain situations. For example, in acute renal failure, an increased clearance of sodium can indicate acute tubular necrosis. Accordingly, supernormal blood levels of filtered substances (creatinine and other nitrogenous wastes) indicate a fall in glomerular filtration and thus in nephron health.

Renal Regulatory Functions

In addition to excreting nitrogenous wastes as urea and other by-products of metabolism, the kidneys can func-

tion in regulating the electrolyte concentration and the pH of the ECFs (blood and interstitial fluids) of the body.

Electrolyte Concentration

Decreased ECF sodium concentrations will stimulate aldosterone secretion directly from the adrenal cortex. Because decreased ECF sodium also can cause a decrease in tubular sodium, it may stimulate the juxtaglomerular secretion of renin, which will increase aldosterone levels indirectly. Aldosterone stimulates sodium reabsorption of the distal tubule cells. Thus, sodium homeostasis is restored. A rise in ECF sodium can cause the reverse.

The kidneys also function in the homeostasis of plasma potassium levels. If there are high levels of potassium in the face of normal sodium levels, the distal tubules and collecting ducts actively secrete (reverse of active reabsorption) potassium back into the urine. Specific reabsorption mechanisms exist for divalent ions such as calcium, magnesium, and phosphates, and regulate the plasma concentrations of these ions as well.

The regulation of the monovalent anions, chloride and bicarbonate, is secondary to sodium ion regulation. As the positively charged cation, sodium, is reabsorbed, a negatively charged ion is carried along electrochemically. This maintains electroneutrality. Whether the negative ion is bicarbonate or chloride depends on the pH of the ECF, which also is regulated by buffers and respiratory and renal mechanisms.

pH Regulation

If buffers and the respiratory mechanism for pH homeostasis are insufficient, the kidneys then take part, although much more slowly than the respiratory system. Although respiratory control of carbon dioxide, and therefore hydrogen ion levels, can take only seconds to achieve, 48 to 72 hours may pass before the renal system can change serum acid–base balance significantly.

Alkalosis occurs as a result of too few hydrogen ions or too many bicarbonate ions. To compensate, the body must conserve hydrogen ions. In renal compensation for alkalosis, tubular reabsorption of hydrogen ions is increased and secretion is decreased. This increases the hydrogen ion concentration of the ECF and thereby decreases the alkalosis.

Acidosis occurs as a result of too many hydrogen ions and too few bicarbonate ions. To compensate, the body must secrete hydrogen ions. Renal compensation for acidosis involves an increase in the hydrogen ion secretion of the tubule cells, especially in the distal tubule cells. Now, bicarbonate and sodium ions are being filtered from continually the glomerulus. Also, as has been stated, hydrogen ion secretion by distal tubule cells causes an increase in

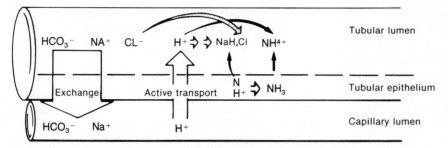

FIGURE 22–6
Renal compensation for acidosis. Hydrogen is moved from blood into filtrate by secretion, and exits the body as ammonium and sodium hydrochloride. In exchange, sodium and bicarbonate enter the blood.

sodium reabsorption. Such sodium reabsorption can increase bicarbonate reabsorption electrochemically. Thus, as hydrogen ions are being eliminated from the ECF, sodium and bicarbonate ions are being added to it. Both will decrease the acidosis (Fig. 22–6).

Urine can be acidified (by hydrogen ion secretion) only to a pH level of 4.0 to 4.5. If the tubular secretion of hydrogen ions was the only mechanism operating, only a few hydrogen ions could be secreted before the critical shut-off level of 4.0 was reached, because hydrogen would combine with urinary chloride to make hydrochloric acid (HCl). Not many of these strong HCl molecules are needed to make the urine pH 4.0. The formation of HCl would then stop tubular hydrogen ion secretion before sufficient compensation for acidosis could be obtained. This does not occur because tubule cells deaminate certain amino acids and secrete the nitrogenous component as ammonia (NH_3). This ammonia combines with hydrogen in the urine to form ammonium (NH_4^+). Because tubule membranes are not permeable to NH_4^+, much of it is secreted in this form. Some ammonia combines with chloride to form ammonium chloride (NH_4Cl).

Summary of Nephron Function

The total blood flow into the nephrons of both kidneys is estimated to be about 1,200 ml/minute. Of this total amount, about 650 ml is plasma. Approximately one fifth of the plasma filters through the glomerular membranes into the Bowman's capsules, forming 125 ml of glomerular filtrate per minute. This filtrate is essentially plasma minus proteins. The pH of glomerular filtrate is equal to that of plasma, or 7.4.

As the glomerular filtrate passes through the proximal tubules, nearly 80% of the water and electrolytes, all of the glucose and proteins, and most of the amino acids are reabsorbed. The glomerular filtrate passes on through remaining tubules, where water and electrolytes are reabsorbed, depending on the need of body fluids and the effectiveness of the regulatory mechanism responsible for maintaining their normal levels.

The pH of the forming urine may rise or fall, depending on the relative amount of acidic and basic ions that are reabsorbed by the tubule walls. The osmotic pressure of the tubular fluid depends on the amounts of electrolytes and water that are reabsorbed. Because of those factors, urine pH may vary from 4.5 to 8.2, and osmotic pressure may vary from one fourth that of plasma to approximately four times plasma pressure.

The amount of urine delivered to the renal pelvis usually is about 1/125 the amount of glomerular filtrate produced or about 1 ml/minute. This 1 ml of urine will contain nearly one half the urea contained in the original 125 ml of glomerular filtrate, all of the creatinine, and large proportions of uric acid, phosphate, potassium, sulfates, nitrates, and phenols.

Although all glucose and proteins, nearly all amino acids, and large amounts of water and sodium in the original glomerular filtrate are reabsorbed, a very large proportion of the waste products are never reabsorbed and are found in the urine in highly concentrated form.

In addition to waste excretion, the kidneys function in the regulation of the OP, volume, electrolyte concentrations, and pH of body fluids.

Other Renal Functions Not Associated With Urine Formation

Renal interstitial (not nephron) cells manufacture and secrete two hormones, calcitriol and erythropoietin, the actions of which are unrelated to urine formation. These hormones are discussed in Chapter 39.

BIBLIOGRAPHY

Ganong WF: Review of Medical Physiology, 15th ed. Norwalk, CT, Appleton & Lange Medical Publications, 1991

Guyton AC: Textbook of Medical Physiology, 8th ed. Philadelphia, WB Saunders, 1991

McCance KL, Huether SE: Pathophysiology: The Biologic Basis for Disease in Adults and Children. St. Louis, CV Mosby, 1990

Prezbindowski KS, Tortora GJ: Learning Guide to Accompany *Principles of Anatomy and Physiology*. New York, Harper and Row, 1990

Tortora GJ, Anagnostakos NP: Principles of Anatomy and Physiology. New York, Harper and Row, 1990

STUDY QUESTIONS

1. In the glomerulus, urine is formed by

   a. secretion
   b. filtration
   c. reabsorption
   d. b & c

2. Aldosterone stimulates increased sodium reabsorption by distal tubule cells. One consequence of elevated plasma aldosterone levels would be

   a. metabolic acidosis
   b. hyperkalemia
   c. metabolic alkalosis
   d. supernormal urine sodium levels

3. Hyperglycemia increases the osmotic pressure of the filtered urine in the nephron. This would cause

   a. increased sodium and water reabsorption, leading to oliguria
   b. decreased sodium and water reabsorption, leading to diuresis
   c. decreased glomerular filtration, leading to prerenal azotemia
   d. increased glomerular secretion of proteins into the filtrate

4. Severe hypotension would cause elevated blood urea nitrogen (BUN) levels (prerenal azotemia) by

   a. decreasing glomerular filtration
   b. increasing glomerular filtration
   c. increasing BUN and water reabsorption
   d. increased sodium and water reabsorption

CHAPTER 23

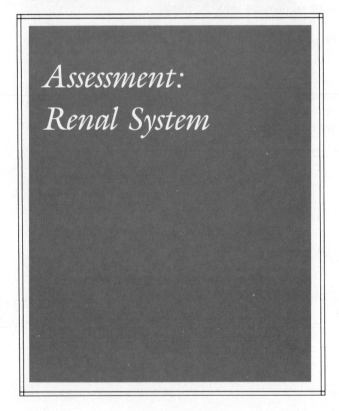

Assessment:
Renal System

BEHAVIORAL OBJECTIVES

Based on the content in this chapter, the reader should be able to:

1. Describe the pathophysiology of fluid and electrolyte disorders.

2. Identify manifestations of fluid and electrolyte imbalances.
3. Describe the diagnostic tests used in the evaluation of renal status.
4. Describe the nursing assessment and management of patients with fluid and electrolyte disorders.
5. Formulate a nursing care plan for the patient with hyponatremia.

Description

The nurse plays a vital role in the assessment and management of fluid and electrolyte disorders in the critically ill patient. Careful monitoring of the patient's symptoms and general appearance, weight, and vital signs, along with interpretation of laboratory results, may provide early clues to the diagnosis of disorders of water and volume imbalance as well as other complications of renal dysfunction. An understanding *both* of the factors involved in the body's regulation of water and volume homeostasis and of the processes that alter those homeostatic mechanisms is paramount in providing high-quality nursing care.

Pathophysiological Principles

Alterations in Urinary Output and Solute Load

The *normal kidney* can maintain solute balance when urine volume is reduced to between 5 and 600 ml/day because the kidneys can increase the urine concentration from 1,000 to 1,200 mOsm/kg. In the average person producing 600 mOsm of metabolic solute from dietary intake and metabolic conversion, approximately 500 ml of urine is required to excrete this if solute urine-concentrating ability is normal. If, however, solute load is increased as a result of increased intake (eg, from high protein diets, hyperalimentation, or hypercatabolism), a greater urine volume will be required to excrete the metabolic solute load.

Because the urinary concentrating ability normally decreases progressively after 40 years of age, older people will require a greater urine volume to maintain homeostasis in the face of "normal" intakes. Even if urine-concentrating ability is reduced to 600 mOsm/kg, however, only 1,000 ml of urine would be required to excrete an "average" 600 mOsm solute load generated per day. Older people probably eat considerably less and therefore a smaller urine volume is required to maintain homeostasis. The same sort of decreased urinary concentrating ability is noted in patients with chronic renal disease as their disease progresses. In addition to increased solute load from hyperalimenation, glycosuria associated both with poorly controlled diabetes and radiologic contrast agents can result in a solute diuresis, with a greater urine volume than normal.

In *chronic renal disease*, the kidneys have the ability to adapt significantly to maintain water and electrolyte levels that are equivalent to normal levels, until the glomerular filtration rate (GFR) drops below 15 to 20 ml/minute. This is accomplished through increased solute and water excretion per nephron and is modulated in part by changes in systemic and local intrarenal hormone production, possibly by the so-called natriuretic factor.

When either too much or too little sodium and water are taken in, the kidney's ability to compensate may be restricted in chronic renal failure. For example, when sodium intake decreases abruptly, the kidneys may take longer than the normal 2 to 3 days to adapt, and a relative state of "salt wasting" may occur. Some patients may actually have true sodium wasting and require greater than normal sodium intake to maintain sodium balance. This is rare, however, and most patients with chronic renal failure can adapt if sodium restriction takes place slowly. In addition, unless acidosis is present, as with hyporeninemic hypoaldosteronism or with more severe decreases in GFR, serum potassium levels and the ability to excrete potassium also are maintained. When the GFR decreases to below 10 ml/minute, patients with end-stage renal disease may require restriction of sodium, potassium, and water intake to maintain balance. This usually requires major adjustments in the diet.

Acute renal failure (ARF) is quite different from chronic renal disease. Because patients with classic ARF have oliguria or anuria (<500 ml/day or <100 ml/day, respectively), they demand much more attention to electrolyte and water balance than patients with comparable degrees of chronic renal failure. Sodium and water restriction, as well as protein and potassium restriction, become necessary because of the limited capacity of the kidney to excrete these substances. In addition, the hypercatabolic state, with generation of excess metabolic water and with shifts of solutes between intracellular and extracellular compartments as a result of acidosis, adds to the effects of uremia in most patients with ARF.

Those at risk for decreased output include patients with:

- Increased solute intake (eg, hyperalimentation)
- Decreased ability to concentrate urine (eg, elderly)
- Chronic renal failure
- Acute renal failure

Disorders of Water Balance

Primary disorders of water balance, *hyponatremia* and *hypernatremia*, occur when water is retained or lost from the body in excess of sodium.

Hyponatremia

In a number of disease states, the serum sodium concentration may be reduced (hyponatremia) because of an inability of the kidneys to excrete free water. This is due to either a persistent release of antidiuretic hormone (ADH) in response to a decrease in the total or effective intravascular volume, or to inappropriate stimulation of ADH release. States of actual or effective intravascular volume depletion also contribute to the hyponatremia by decreasing distal delivery of fluid in the nephron, thereby limiting the amount of water that can be excreted.

Hyponatremia may be associated with (1) an increased total body sodium and edema; (2) a decreased total body sodium and hypovolemia; or (3) a normal or slightly increased total body sodium and increased blood volume, depending on the clinical disorder that gives rise to the hyponatremia.

In patients with edema due to cirrhosis, congestive heart failure, or the nephrotic syndrome, hyponatremia occurs frequently and may be enhanced by the use of diuretics. In these conditions, although there is an overall increase in body sodium and water, ADH release is stimulated because the *effective* blood volume is decreased. As a result, the kidneys tend to reabsorb a greater percentage of filtered fluid in the proximal tubule. This causes further fluid retention and hyponatremia, especially if the patient has unlimited access to water, because the little fluid reaching the distal tubule is reabsorbed more completely owing to the high plasma ADH level.

Treatment with thiazide diuretics, furosemide, or ethacrynic acid can produce or seriously compound the hyponatremia because these drugs (1) may decrease further the effective blood volume, and (2) they decrease sodium transport in the ascending loop of Henle, which is necessary for the kidneys' ability to excrete free water and maximally dilute the urine.

Patients with volume depletion due to loss of sodium or blood also may have hyponatremia when the volume depletion is great enough to stimulate ADH release. In this situation, body sodium and blood volume are reduced, and edema is not present. Diuretic administration, renal salt wasting, adrenal insufficiency, and hemorrhage are examples of this type of condition. Antidiuretic hormone release occurs and stimulates water reabsorption in an attempt to restore intravascular volume, regardless of serum osmolality. If the patient ingests water without salt, or if hypotonic fluids are administered intravenously, hyponatremia will result.

In addition, the following situations can cause hyponatremia: increased thirst from central nervous system (CNS) disease, and decreased renal water excretion resulting from the use of drugs that stimulate vasopressin release (eg, cyclophosphamide and diazepam) or drugs that interfere with the action of vasopressin on the kidney (eg, chlorpropamide and nonsteroidal anti-inflammatory drugs).

Hypervolemia

Hypervolemia occurs when there is excess extracellular fluid. It may occur in the patient with heart failure, because decreased blood flow to the kidneys results in decreased excretion of urine. The patient with renal dysfunction also may have hypervolemia because of fluid and sodium retention. Liver disease may result in hypervolemia secondary to hypoproteinemia; the hypoproteinemia causes decreased production of albumin, which results in decreased serum colloid osmotic pressure. In turn, this causes leakage of interstitial fluid from capillaries.

Hyponatremia: Accompanying Factors and Causes

Increased total body sodium and edema:
    Congestive heart failure
    Decompensated cirrhosis
    Nephrotic syndrome
Decreased total body sodium and hypovolemia:
    Diuretics
    Renal salt wasting
    Adrenal insufficiency
    Hemorrhage
Normal total body sodium and hypervolemia:
    Syndrome of inappropriate ADH secretion, which may accompany CNS and pulmonary disease, tumors, porphyria, use of certain drugs, psychiatric disorders, myxedema

---

Hypernatremia

Hypernatremia occurs when the sodium level in the extracellular fluid is above normal. It almost always is associated with a loss of body fluids in excess of sodium. For example, it may occur as a result of inadequate fluid intake or profuse diarrhea. Aldosteronism, which causes increased sodium retention by the kidneys, is another cause of hypernatremia. Inhalation of salt water in a near drowning incident can result in hypernatremia because of absorption of salt water from the alveoli into the pulmonary capillaries. Finally, therapies such as hypertonic tube feedings, drugs such as steroids, lithium, and doxycycline, and overzealous infusion of intravenous saline solution all may result in hypernatremia. These circumstances all interfere with the kidney's ability to conserve water by responding appropriately to vasopressin.

Hypovolemia

Hypovolemia is caused by a deficit in extracellular fluid that usually is accompanied by a loss of electrolytes. Hypovolemia also may be referred to as dehydration. When it is accompanied by a loss of electrolytes (often combined water and sodium deficits), it usually is referred to as volume depletion. Patients with the following clinical conditions are at risk for becoming hypovolemic:

1. Decreased oral intake because of physical or mental debilitation or difficulty in swallowing
2. Increased output from renal losses (eg, diuretics) gastrointestinal losses (diarrhea, vomiting, or suctioning) or skin losses (diaphoresis or draining wounds)
3. Blood loss
4. Impaired renal function
   a. kidneys are unable to concentrate urine
   b. too much fluid is removed during dialysis
5. Diabetes insipidus (decreased secretion of ADH)
6. Collection of third space fluids (eg, effusions, decreased osmotic pressure that causes capillary leakage, ascites).

History

Assessing the renal system involves determining how well the kidneys perform their many functions. Assessment, therefore, involves gathering information about many systems. Kidney dysfunction may be the primary problem, or it may be secondary to a preexisting condition. Table 23–1

TABLE 23–1
Renal Assessment

1. History
   A. Chief complaint
      1. Description
      2. Signs and symptoms
      3. Treatments and response to treatments
   B. Systems review
   C. Medical history
   D. Family history
2. Physical examination
   A. Skin: turgor, temperature, dryness/moisture, scratches, lesions
   B. Mucous membranes
   C. Presence of edema, ascites
   D. Respiratory rate, lung sounds
   E. Blood pressure, heart rate, rhythm, sounds
   F. Behavioral changes, mental status
   G. Test for tetany: Chvostek's, Trousseau's signs
   H. Paresthesias, numbness, weakness, tremors of extremities
3. Additional findings
   A. Laboratory values
      1. Serum creatinine, urea nitrogen, osmolality
      2. Urine specific gravity, sodium, osmolality
      3. Serum electrolytes
   B. Radiographic studies
   C. Electrocardiogram tracing
   D. Intake and output records
   E. Weight records

outlines a format for renal assessment. The initial patient history is important in determining the cause, severity, and treatment of the dysfunction. Begin by asking the patient's perception of the chief complaint. The description should include onset, location, duration, and factors that lessen or aggravate the problem. Ask what treatments and medications the patient has used to alleviate symptoms. Conduct a systems review. Some specific questions to ask are:

1. Has the patient ever had any dysuria, nocturia, polyuria, or incontinence?
2. Has the patient ever experienced any flank pain? Hematuria?
3. Has the patient ever passed a renal stone?
4. Has there been a change in the amount or pattern of voiding?
5. Has there been a change in weight?

After obtaining the history of the present problem, inquire about past medical history and family history. This information may offer clues to the underlying cause of the problem. A history of polycystic kidney disease, renal calculi, or hereditary nephritis is common in patients with kidney disease. Certain systemic diseases also may contribute to the development of renal failure, such as:

- Diabetes mellitus
- Systemic lupus erythematosus
- Hypertension
- Sickle cell anemia
- Wegener's granulomatosis
- Goodpasture's syndrome

Another common cause of kidney disease is exposure to nephrotoxic agents, such as aminoglycosides, furosemide, radiographic dyes, and other drugs and chemical agents. There also are some unrelated medical conditions that can result in renal failure. One is low cardiac output (eg, cardiac arrest, congestive heart failure, or shock), in which there is a lack of kidney perfusion that may result in kidney damage. Another is rhabdomyolysis. Severe trauma resulting in skeletal muscle destruction alters cell integrity, allowing intracellular content to escape into the plasma. Cellular contents that may be nephrotoxic at high levels include myoglobin, potassium, organic acids, and phosphorus. The myoglobin is responsible for acute renal failure in patients with rhabdomyolysis (see discussion of rhabdomyolysis and myoglobinuria in Chapter 31).

Physical Examination

Objective data are obtained in the physical examination and are used to substantiate and clarify the history. The history also guides the physical examination and helps determine areas of the examination that may require more depth. Table 23–1 lists the parameters often used for assessing the renal system.

When evaluating the patient's volume status, observe the mucous membranes, examine skin turgor, and note whether edema is present. Take the blood pressure, pulse, respirations, and temperature; examine jugular venous pressure and listen to lung sounds. Observe mental status and behavioral changes. If the patient is experiencing symptoms of hypocalcemia, hypomagnesemia, or both, look for positive Chvostek's or Trousseau's signs. Neuromuscular abnormalities such as paresthesia and weakness also may indicate electrolyte imbalances. Other signs for specific electrolyte imbalances are listed in Tables 23–5 through 23–9.

Diagnostic Tests

Tests That Assess Renal Function

The patient whose condition is serious enough to warrant observation in the critical care unit frequently will manifest abnormalities of renal function. These abnormalities include:

1. Impaired ability to excrete nitrogenous waste products, toxins, and drugs
2. Inability to handle water and electrolyte loads efficiently
3. Inability to regulate acid–base balance
4. Inadequate production of erythropoietin

Therefore, certain aspects of renal function will be monitored on an intermittent or continuing basis to detect complications early and institute appropriate therapy.

Laboratory Tests

The first group of tests includes:

- Creatinine
- Blood urea nitrogen (BUN)
- Specific gravity
- Osmolality (blood and urine)
- Urinary sodium concentration
- Fractional excretion of sodium

Creatinine and Creatinine Clearance

The most commonly used tests of renal function are the serum creatinine and the BUN, but the most accurate test readily available is the creatinine clearance. Creatinine is formed as a by-product of normal muscle metabolism and is excreted in the urine primarily as the result of glomerular filtration, with a small percentage secreted into the urine by the kidney tubules. It therefore is a useful indicator of the GFR. The amount of creatinine excreted in the urine of any given person is related to muscle mass and will remain quite constant unless muscle wasting occurs.

The actual creatinine clearance is calculated by the following formula:

$$\text{creatinine clearance} = \frac{UV}{PC}$$

where U is the urine creatinine concentration, V the urine volume, and P the plasma creatinine concentration. The most important technical aspect of this test is the *accuracy of the urine collection*; it is important to know the exact time it took to form the sample and the exact amount of creatinine present.

The expression UV tells how much creatinine appears in the urine during the period of collection, and this can be converted readily to milligrams per minute, which is the standard reference point. Dividing this value by the plasma creatinine concentration (which must be converted from mg/100 ml to mg/ml) tells the minimum number of milliliters of plasma that must have been filtered by the glomeruli to produce the measured amount of creatinine in the urine. The final result is expressed in milliliters per minute, and the normal range varies between 80 and 120, depending on the person's size and age. The results should be corrected to a standard body size of 1.73 m^2 (body surface area [BSA]), which can be derived from standard tables if the patient's height and weight are known, and averages 120 to 125 ml/minute/1.73 m^2 BSA.

Interpretation of Creatinine. If the kidneys are damaged by some disease process, the creatinine clearance will decrease, and the serum creatinine concentration will rise. The urine creatinine excretion will decrease initially until the blood level rises to a point at which the amount of creatinine appearing in the urine is again equal to the amount being produced by the body. For example, a normal person with a serum creatinine concentration of 1 mg/dl and a creatinine excretion of 1 mg/minute has a creatinine clearance of 100 ml/minute. If renal disease develops, with 50% loss of renal function, serum creatinine will rise to 2 mg/dl, and the patient will continue to excrete 1 mg of creatinine in the urine per minute when balance is restored. In many situations in which the patient has rapidly changing renal function and oliguria (eg, ARF), the creatinine clearance becomes less reliable until the situation becomes more stable. It therefore is useful to follow the serum creatinine concentration as an indicator of the rate and direction of change until stability occurs. In patients with rhabdomyolysis, the serum creatinine will be elevated out of proportion to the reduction of GFR as the result of chemical conversion of muscle creatine to creatinine, and is less reliable as an indicator of renal function.

Blood Urea Nitrogen

The BUN also has been used for many years as an indicator of kidney function, but, unlike the serum creatinine, its level tends to be influenced by a great many factors.

Urea has a clearance rate less than that of creatinine, largely because some urea diffuses out of the tubule back into the bloodstream. This is particularly true at low urine flow rates, at which more sodium and water, and, consequently, more urea are being reabsorbed. Therefore, in states of relative or absolute volume depletion, the BUN will tend to rise out of proportion to any change in renal function. In addition, the amount of urea produced per day, unlike the quantity of creatinine, is quite variable, especially in seriously ill patients.

Interpretation of BUN. Increased urea production can result from increased protein intake (tube feedings and some forms of hyperalimentation) or increased tissue breakdown, as with crush injuries, febrile illnesses, steroid or tetracycline administration, and reabsorption of blood from the intestine in a patient with intestinal hemorrhage. The BUN also may be elevated in the dehydrated patient because the lack of fluid volume causes a concentrated value. The patient in shock and the patient with congestive heart failure may have an elevated BUN secondary to decreased renal perfusion. All these factors may cause an increase in urea production and an increase in BUN, even though renal function might be normal; and they also would contribute to the rate of rise in BUN in a person with renal failure.

BUN will rise with:

- Increased protein intake
- Increased tissue breakdown
- Dehydration
- Shock
- Congestive heart failure

The opposite is true for patients with decreased protein intake or liver disease (both of which reduce urea production) and for patients with large urine volumes secondary to excessive fluid intake.

The BUN therefore is less useful as a guide to changes in renal function than is the serum creatinine in most circumstances. The BUN still is of significant value, however, especially when looked at in comparison to the serum creatinine concentration. Normally, these are present in a ratio of 10:1 (urea:creatinine). Discrepancies in this ratio might suggest a potentially correctable situation, as noted in Table 23–2.

Specific Gravity

The specific gravity of the urine is the time-honored test of the kidneys' ability to concentrate and dilute the urine. The specific gravity measures the buoyancy of a solution compared to water, and depends on the number of particles in solution as well as their size and weight.

Two methods have been used to obtain this measurement in clinical practice, the *hydrometer* and the *refractometer* (or TS meter, as it frequently is called). The hydrometer has been in clinical use for many years and is the less

TABLE 23–2
Facts Affecting Serum Urea:
Creatinine Ratio

A. Decreased urea: creatinine (<10:1)
　1. Liver disease
　2. Protein restriction
　3. Excessive fluid intake
B. Increased urea: creatinine (>10:1)
　1. Volume depletion
　2. Decreased "effective" blood volume
　3. Catabolic states
　4. Excessive protein intake

---

preferred of the two methods because it requires a much larger volume of urine, its results are less reproducible, and it requires a greater amount of time.

The refractometer gives highly reproducible results and requires only a drop of urine for the measurement. In addition, this instrument can be used to measure the total solids in plasma (hence the name, "TS" meter), which is a good indicator of the plasma protein concentration and a useful indicator of the state of a patient's fluid balance, especially when serial determinations are made. The refractometer, because of its advantages, should replace the hydrometer for specific gravity determinations and should be used in the critical care unit.

Interpretation of Specific Gravity. The normal kidney has the capacity to dilute the urine to a specific gravity of 1.001 and to concentrate the urine to at least 1.022 (higher values are not unusual). Normally, a person's water balance will determine whether the urine is concentrated or dilute, with a dilute urine being an indicator of water excess, and a concentrated urine an indicator of water deficit. In many renal diseases, the ability of the kidneys to form a concentrated urine is lost, and the specific gravity becomes "fixed" at 1.010, a finding that might be seen in acute tubular necrosis, acute nephritis, or chronic renal disease.

Like many simple laboratory tests, the specific gravity determination has limited accuracy. The specific gravity is not always the most accurate indicator of the ability of the kidneys to concentrate the urine because this ability is a reflection of the concentration of particles in the urine. In addition to the concentration of particles, the size and weight of the particles in solution reflect, in part, the specific gravity. Therefore, a falsely high specific gravity determination will be found when high-molecular-weight substances such as protein, glucose, mannitol, and radiographic contrast material are present in the urine. A greater degree of accuracy can be obtained with urine osmolality determinations.

Osmolality

The *osmolality* of a solution is an expression of the total number (concentration) of particles in solution and is independent of the size, molecular weight, and electrical charge of the molecules. All substances in solution contribute to the osmolality to a certain degree. For example, a mol (gram molecular weight) of sodium chloride dissociates incompletely into Na^+ and Cl^- ions and produces 1.86 osmols when dissolved in a kilogram of solvent (such as plasma). A mole of nonionic solute (eg, glucose or urea) produces only 1 osmol when dissolved in a kilogram of solvent. The total concentration of particles in a solution is the osmolality, and is reported in units of osmols per kilogram of solvent. In clinical situations, because we are dealing with much smaller concentrations, the osmolality is reported in milliosmols (thousandth of an osmol, abbreviated mOsm) per kilogram of solvent (plasma or serum).

The normal *serum osmolality* consists primarily of sodium and its accompanying anions, with urea and glucose contributing about 5 mOsm each. Therefore, given known serum sodium, urea, and glucose concentrations, the osmolality of plasma can be calculated by the formula:

$$\text{osmolality} = 2\,Na + \frac{BUN}{2.6} + \frac{glucose}{18}$$

The calculated osmolality normally will be within 10 mOsm of the measured osmolality, which normally averages 290 ± 5 mOsm/kg. The plasma osmolality in normal people is quite constant from day to day.

Because water permeates freely between the blood, interstitial fluid, and tissues, change in the osmolality of one body compartment will produce a shift in body fluids. Therefore, the osmolality of the plasma is always the same as that of the other body compartments, except in the most rapidly changing conditions, where a slight lag may occur.

The *significance* of the plasma osmolality is that it is the main regulator of the release of ADH. When sufficient water is not being taken in, the osmolality will rise, stimulating the release of ADH, which signals the kidneys to conserve water and produce a more concentrated urine. When excessive amounts of water are ingested, the osmolality decreases, ADH release is inhibited, and the urine becomes more dilute. Under maximum ADH stimulation, the kidneys can concentrate the urine to approximately 1,200 mOsm/kg, and with maximum ADH suppression (water load), the kidneys can dilute the urine to approximately 50 mOsm/kg.

Thus, there is no single normal urine osmolality, but a range in which predicted values might be expected, depending on the clinical setting. Also, when compared to the plasma osmolality, the urine osmolality depends less on the urine sodium concentration, and other substances such as urea play a more important role. In renal disease, one of the first renal functions to be lost is the ability to concentrate urine. As a reflection of this, the urine osmolality becomes fixed within +50 mOsm of the simultaneously determined serum osmolality. Therefore, the osmolality is a useful parameter of renal function.

A decrease in the serum osmolality can occur only when the serum sodium is decreased. An increase in the serum osmolality can occur whenever the serum sodium, urea, or glucose is elevated or when there are abnormal compounds present in the blood, including drugs, poisons, or metabolic waste products that usually are not measured, such as lactic acid. Symptoms due to increased osmolality usually occur when the osmolality is greater than 350 mOsm, and coma occurs when the osmolality is in approximately 400 mOsm or greater (see section on serum sodium balance).

The usual close correlation between the measured and calculated osmolality has been mentioned. In certain circumstances, the measured serum osmolality might be significantly higher than the calculated osmolality when substances of an unusual nature are present in the blood. Many drugs and toxins such as aspirin and alcohol raise the serum osmolality. In a comatose patient, a discrepancy between the measured and calculated serum osmolalities might lead to the appropriate drug screen to provide the correct diagnosis. In patients with heart failure, hepatic disease, or shock, a discrepancy of 40 or more mOsm between the measured and calculated osmolalities, due to unknown metabolites, has been correlated with a mortality rate of 95% or greater.

Urinary Sodium Concentration

In the differentiation of the oliguria of ARF from that due to prerenal causes, the urinary sodium excretion is used frequently as one indicator of intact renal function. States of underperfusion of the kidney are associated with a decrease in urinary sodium concentration (usually <10 mEq/L), whereas in ARF, because of damage to the tubular transport mechanisms, urine sodium concentration generally is above 30 to 40 mEq/L despite oliguria. When the urine pH is alkaline, however, urine sodium concentration will not reflect sodium balance accurately, and the chloride concentration becomes a better indicator of volume depletion.

Fractional Excretion of Sodium Test

Another test of renal function, used for the same purpose as the urine sodium concentration, is the fractional excretion of sodium (FE_{Na}). This test gives a more precise estimation of the amount of filtered sodium that remains in the urine and is more accurate in predicting tubular injury than the urinary sodium concentration. It is calculated by the formula:

$$(U/P)\,Na/(U/P)\,Cr \times 100$$

in which U and P are the urinary and plasma concentrations of sodium and creatinine, respectively. (Although volume measurements are necessary to derive the absolute urinary excretion of both sodium and creatinine, these cancel out in deriving this formula.)

The test therefore requires the determination of both serum and urinary sodium and creatinine concentrations on simultaneously obtained samples. Values less than 1% indicate prerenal azotemia, or underperfusion. Values greater than 1% (and frequently greater than 3%) are indicative of ARF.

This test appears to be a little more discriminating in detecting cases of ARF than is measurement of urinary sodium concentration alone, especially in those patients who have borderline urinary sodium concentration values.

Radiologic Studies

Radiologic studies of the kidneys that may be useful in evaluating renal abnormalities include roentgenography, ultrasonography, and radionuclide studies. These studies and their purposes are summarized in Table 23–3.

Surgical Studies

Renal Biopsy

Renal biopsy is the ultimate diagnostic tool in renal evaluation. It may provide an accurate histologic classification of the cause of renal dysfunction, but, except in certain

circumstances, cannot provide an etiologic diagnosis, although it may be suggestive or confirmatory. Renal biopsy is performed to define the histologic counterpart of the clinical picture, provide for etiologic clues or diagnosis, assess prognosis, guide therapy, and provide assessment for insurability, employment, or disability.

The indications for renal biopsy depend on the clinical problem, and opinions about the procedure vary among physicians. Even when there is relative agreement among nephrologists as to when to perform a renal biopsy, there generally are few controlled studies to document how much a renal biopsy aids in therapy or prognosis above and beyond the other clinical parameters in a given clinical setting. The general indications for renal biopsy are given in Table 23–4. In each category, the timing of a renal biopsy will depend on the other clinical characteristics in each case. For instance, in the nephrotic syndrome in the pediatric age group, renal biopsy generally is not done unless the patient is steroid resistant or has some other findings that suggest a primary renal disease or systemic disease other than lipoid nephrosis, the most common etiology of nephrotic syndrome in this age group. In

TABLE 23–3
Radiologic Study of Kidneys

Diagnostic Test	Purpose
1. Roentgenography	
a. Radiograph of kidney–ureter–bladder (KUB)	a. To detect abnormal calcifications, renal size
b. Tomography	b. To determine renal outlines and abnormalities
c. Intravenous pyelography (IVP)	c. To detect anatomic abnormalities of the kidneys and ureters
d. Retrograde pyelography	d. To assess renal size, to evaluate ureteral obstruction, to localize and diagnose tumors, obstructions
e. Antegrade pyelography	e. To distinguish cysts from hydronephrosis
f. Renal arteriography and venography	f. To evaluate possible renal arterial stenosis, renal mass lesions, renal vein thrombosis, and venous extension of renal cell carcinoma
g. Digital subtraction angiography	g. To visualize major arterial vessels
2. Ultrasonography	
	a. To delineate renal outlines
	b. To measure longitudinal and transverse dimensions of the kidneys
	c. To evaluate mass lesions
	d. To examine perinephric area
	e. To detect and grade hydronephrosis
3. Radionuclide scintillation imaging (renal scan)	
a. Static imaging	a. To evaluate location, size, and contour of functional renal tissue; may reveal areas of inhomogeneity or filling defects
b. Dynamic imaging	b. To monitor the passage of a radiopharmaceutical agent through the vascular, renal parenchymal, and urinary tract compartments
4. Magnetic resonance imaging	
	a. To determine anatomic abnormalities

TABLE 23–4
Indications for Renal Biopsy

Clinical Condition	Biopsy Indicated	Expected Gain
Orthostatic proteinuria	No	—
Isolated hematuria and/or-proteinuria	No*	—
Hematuria and/or proteinuria with ↓ GFR	Yes	D,P,T
Nephrotic syndrome	Yes	D,P,T
Systemic disease with renal abnormalities	Yes†	D,P,T
Classic ARF	No	—
ARF with 1. azotemia >3 wk	Yes	D,P
2. moderate proteinuria	Yes	D,T
3. anuria	Yes	D,T
4. eosinophilia or eosinophiluria	Yes	D,T
Post-transplant ↓ in GFR	Yes	D,P,T

GFR, glomerular filtration rate; D, diagnosis; P, prognosis; T, therapy; ARF, acute renal failure.
* Biopsy may be indicated for insurance, administrative reasons, and so forth.
† Biopsy may or may not be indicated, depending on clinical picture.

adults with the nephrotic syndrome, renal biopsy usually is performed before therapy is started (although this is a subject of considerable debate). In certain patients (eg, an adult diabetic with the nephrotic syndrome and a benign urine sediment), however, renal biopsy is not performed universally. If clinical characteristics of other than diabetic nephropathy are present (eg, RBC casts), a biopsy may be indicated. Similar caveats may be used in the other listed categories, depending on the circumstances. Thus, there are no general absolute indications for renal biopsy.

Contraindications for renal biopsy are relative. A serious bleeding disorder is the single generally accepted contraindication. Relative contraindications include excessive obesity, severe hypertension until blood pressure is controlled, uncooperativeness, renal malignancies, and inability to tolerate the procedure because of other serious medical conditions.

Procedure. Although renal biopsies generally performed are percutaneously with a biopsy needle, open renal biopsy under general anesthesia still is performed when percutaneous biopsy is impractical. Percutaneous renal biopsy usually is performed under either fluoroscopic or ultrasonographic control in the radiology department. The procedure generally requires about 30 minutes in the average patient when a regular routine is established.

Preparation for a renal biopsy should include the usual informed consent, prebiopsy clotting studies, some form of sedation (diazepam, 5–10 mg, is sufficient in most patients), establishment of an intravenous access for treat-

ment or prevention of complications, and preoperative blood typing in case replacement is necessary.

After biopsy, the patient's vital signs should be checked regularly every 15 minutes for the first 2 hours, hourly for 4 hours, and then every 4 hours for the first 24 hours. The postoperative urine should be examined for blood. The major complication is bleeding, occurring either retroperitoneally or into the urinary tract. Although bleeding rarely is sufficient to require transfusion, it can be massive, and, if occurring into the urinary tract, can result in clot formation and ureteral colic or obstruction. Intravenous fluids for maintenance of urinary flow can decrease the incidence of the latter two complications. Other complications include biopsy of other abdominal viscera (bowel, pancreas, liver, spleen, and vessels) and tears in the diaphragm or pleura.

Death occurs in fewer than 0.5% of cases. A late complication is infection in a perinephric hematoma, which can result in death if not diagnosed and treated adequately.

Tests That Assess Electrolyte Balance

The role of the kidney is central in maintaining fluid volume and ionic composition of body fluids. When the kidneys properly regulate the excretion of water and ions, homeostasis is achieved. When they fail to adapt adequately, imbalances occur. Electrolyte values and signs and symptoms of imbalance are listed in Tables 23-5 through 23-9. The following tests will be described:

> Acid–base balance
> Anion gap
> Sodium balance
> Potassium balance
> Calcium and phosphate balance
> Magnesium balance

Acid–Base Balance

The acidity or alkalinity of the body fluid is expressed as pH, with 7.35 to 7.45 being the normal range. The body maintains acid–base balance by the buffer system, the respiratory system, and the renal system. The buffer and respiratory systems react quickly to changes in body pH. The kidneys take more time to adjust to changes in body pH.

There are five major processes associated with regulation of acid–base balance by the renal system: (1) hydrogen ion excretion; (2) sodium ion reabsorption; (3) bicarbonate ion generation and reabsorption; (4) phosphate salt and titratable acid excretion; and (5) ammonia synthesis and ammonium excretion. Acid–base imbalances may result when the kidneys are unable to perform those processes adequately (Table 23–5).

TABLE 23–5
Electrolyte Abnormalities: Acid–Base Balance

Electrolyte	Abnormality	Assessment Findings	Causes
Acid–base balance	Metabolic acidosis pH below 7.35 HCO_3 below 22 $PaCO_2$ normal	Tachypnea (Kussmaul's respiration), headache, confusion, drowsiness, cold, clammy skin; vasodilation, which leads to low cardiac output and hypotension	• Renal failure • DKA • Starvation • Poisoning • Diarrhea • Lactic acidosis • Intestinal fistulas
	Metabolic alkalosis pH above 7.45 HCO_3 above 26 $PaCO_2$ normal	Increased neuromuscular irritability, paresthesias; tetany, seizures; dysrhythmias; hypoventilation	• Vomiting • Gastrointestinal suctioning • Diuretic therapy • Cushing's syndrome • Excessive antacid ingestion

DKA, diabetic ketoacidosis.

The Anion Gap

To maintain chemical neutrality, the total concentration of cations and anions in the blood (as well as other body fluids) must be equivalent in terms of milliequivalents per liter. Because there are a number of anions and cations present in blood that are not routinely measured, however, a "gap" exists between the total concentration of cations and anions and the concentration normally measured in plasma:

$$Na + K \text{ vs } Cl + HCO_3$$

This gap is composed primarily of an excess of unmeasured anions, including plasma proteins, inorganic phosphates and sulfates, and organic acids. The unmeasured cations that exist in smaller concentration are primarily calcium and magnesium.

The anion gap generally is calculated by the following formula:

$$Na - (Cl + HCO_3)$$

and has a normal mean of approximately 12 mEq/L (range, 8–16 mEq/L). Potassium is generally, but not always, omitted from the formula because of its relatively low concentration and narrow range of fluctuation. Departures from this "normal" anion gap may have important diagnostic significance in acid–base disorders, especially metabolic acidoses, and also may assist in the diagnosis of other disorders.

The most common abnormality of the anion gap is an increase that is due most frequently to increased concentrations of lactate, ketone bodies, or inorganic phosphate and sulfate that are found in lactic acidosis, ketoacidosis, and uremia, respectively. Other forms of acidosis associated with ingestion of toxins such as ethylene glycol, methanol, paraldehyde, and salicylates also may produce significant increases in the anion gap. Increases in anion gap due to a decrease in unmeasured cations are rare but can be observed.

Decreases in the anion gap are less common but equally important, and can occur because of increases in unmeasured cations or because of decreases in unmeasured anions, such as hypoalbuminemia. Causes are listed in Display Box 23–1.

Alterations of the anion gap also may be caused by laboratory error in measuring the electrolytes; measurements always must be verified to avoid confusion and diagnostic error. Simultaneous occurrences of two disorders having opposite effects on the anion gap also could obscure any potential diagnostic change.

Sodium Balance

The serum sodium concentration generally is maintained in a narrow range (135–145 mEq/L). It is regulated by the kidneys and depends on the sodium concentration in the extracellular fluid. When the concentration rises, the kidneys retain water in response to ADH. When the concentration falls, aldosterone promotes sodium retention by the kidneys (see Figure 22-5). When the kidneys malfunction, this balance is not maintained. Generally, sodium is relatively constant in a normal person who is not exposed to physiological stress. A low serum sodium usually indicates water intake in excess of sodium and is characterized by an increase in body weight. A high serum sodium usually indicates water loss in excess of sodium and is reflected in weight loss. Sodium is essential for maintaining the osmolality of extracellular fluids, neuromuscular function, acid–base balance, and various other cellular chemical reactions. In addition to foods and preservatives, sodium also may be found in both prescription and nonprescription drugs (Table 23–6).

```
┌─────────────────────────────────────────┐
│ ═══════════════════════════════════════ │
│  DISPLAY BOX 23–1                         │
│  Causes of an Altered Anion Gap           │
│ ═══════════════════════════════════════ │
│                                           │
│  Increased Anion Gap                      │
│    I. Laboratory error                    │
│   II. Increased unmeasured anions         │
│       A. Endogenous metabolic acidosis    │
│          1. Lactic acidosis               │
│          2. Ketoacidosis                  │
│          3. Uremic acidosis               │
│       B. Exogenous anion ingestion        │
│          1. Ethylene glycol               │
│          2. Methanol                      │
│          3. Paraldehyde                   │
│       C. Therapeutic agents               │
│          1. Paraldehyde                   │
│          2. Penicillin                    │
│          3. Carbenicillin                 │
│       D. Increased plasma proteins        │
│          1. Hyperalbuminemia              │
│  III. Decreased unmeasured cations        │
│       A. Hypokalemia                      │
│       B. Hypocalcemia                     │
│       C. Hypomagnesemia                   │
│                                           │
│  Decreased Anion Gap                      │
│    I. Laboratory error                    │
│   II. Increased unmeasured cations        │
│       A. Normal cations                   │
│          1. Hypercalcemia                 │
│          2. Hyperkalemia                  │
│          3. Hypermagnesemia               │
│       B. Abnormal cations                 │
│          1. Increased globulins           │
│             (myeloma, etc.)               │
│          2. TRIS buffer                   │
│          3. Lithium                       │
│  III. Decreased unmeasured anions         │
│       A. Hypoalbuminemia                  │
│                                           │
└─────────────────────────────────────────┘
```

Potassium Balance

Potassium affects numerous body functions, including intracellular osmolality and acid–base balance. It is very important in regulating nerve impulse conduction and muscle contraction.

Normal serum potassium concentration is 3.5 to 5.0 mEq/L. Under normal conditions, potassium balance depends on dietary intake and renal excretion. Ninety-eight percent of potassium is located in the skeletal muscle; therefore, the balance of this electrolyte also is strongly tied to the exchanges between the intracellular and extracellular compartments in the body.

Hypokalemia can result from inadequate potassium intake, excessive potassium loss through the kidneys, gastrointestinal loss, and extracellular-to-intracellular potassium shifts. Diuretic therapy usually contributes to potassium excretion. Diuretics, having a locus of action before the late distal tubule, cause a concomitant potassium loss through the urine.

Hyperkalemia may be caused by a decrease in the renal excretion of potassium or transcellular shifts of potassium. This is seen most often in acidosis, cell injury or destruction, and hyperglycemia (Table 23–7).

Calcium and Phosphate Balance

Calcium and phosphate are regulated reciprocally in the body by vitamin D, parathyroid, and calcitonin. The calcium and phosphate salts are deposited in the bone, and when calcium levels are high, phosphate levels are low. In renal failure, the kidneys are unable to eliminate phosphate, so renal failure patients often have high phosphate and low calcium levels.

Calcium's primary function is maintenance of bone and teeth strength. It also influences myocardial and skeletal contractility. In addition, calcium maintains cellular permeability and assists in blood coagulation.

Normal serum concentration of calcium is 8.5 to 10.5 mg/dl. Serum calcium consists of ultrafilterable calcium as well as the calcium that is bound to protein, primarily albumin. Ultrafilterable calcium includes ionized calcium and the calcium complexed to bicarbonate, citrate, and phosphate. The physiological processes involved in serum calcium level maintenance are (1) absorption of calcium from the gastrointestinal tract, (2) changes in calcium excretion from the kidneys, and (3) mobilization of calcium from the bone. Calcium reabsorption in the kidneys occurs throughout the nephron, and, proximal to the loop of Henle, is parallel to the reabsorption of sodium. Distal to this point, sodium and calcium reabsorption are influenced independently.

Disturbances in calcium metabolism that result in hypocalcemia occur in renal failure, and are thought to involve impaired absorption of dietary calcium and resistance to the action of vitamin D.

Phosphate's primary function is in the formation of adenosine triphosphate. Phosphate also assists in the maintenance of cell membrane structure, oxygen delivery, and cellular immunity. The normal phosphate level is 3.0 to 4.5 mg/dl. Absorption of phosphorus takes place in the gastrointestinal tract, and excretion occurs via the kidneys (Table 23–8).

Magnesium Balance

The magnesium ion, which is the second major intracellular ion, has a normal serum concentration of 1.8 to 2.1 mEq/L. Magnesium balance is necessary for the functional integrity of the neuromuscular system. The parathyroid glands regulate both magnesium and calcium, and the presence of the sodium ion is necessary for magnesium reabsorption. Magnesium, sodium, potassium, and calcium all are required in the proper ratio for the regulation of most body cells.

TABLE 23–6
Electrolyte Abnormalities: Sodium

Electrolyte	Abnormality	Assessment Findings	Causes
Sodium	Hypernatremia Na > 145 mEq/L	Sticky or dry oral mucous membranes; thirst; hypotension; firm body tissues; tachycardia, oliguria or anuria, anxiety	• Increased sodium intake or decreased water intake (ie, aldosteronism) • Inhalation of salt water in near drowning • Hypertonic tube feedings • High-dose steroids • Excessive infusion of saline solutions
	Hyponatremia Na < 135 mEq/L 135–125 mEq/L	Generally none	• Increased water intake with decreased sodium intake (ie, diuretics, excess IV D5W, gastric suction [especially with tap water irrigation or ice chip ingestion]) • Vomiting • Diarrhea
	125–110 mEq/L	Headache, apathy, lethargy, weakness, disorientation	• Repeated tap water enemas • Water replacement without salt replacement in a hot environment that causes diaphoresis
	110–100 mEq/L	Confusion, hostility; lethargy or violence; nausea and vomiting; areflexia	• Addison's disease • SIADH that occurs in patient's with CNS disturbances, patients on ventilators, and those with oat cell cancer
	100–95 mEq/L	Delirium, convulsions, coma, hypothermia; Cheyne–Stokes respiration; death	• Excessive beer intake • Inhalation of fresh water in near drowning

D5W, Dextrose 5% in water; SIADH, syndrome of inappropriate antidiuretic hormone secretion; CNS, central nervous system.

TABLE 23–7
Electrolyte Abnormalities: Potassium

Electrolyte	Abnormality	Assessment Findings	Causes
Potassium	Hyperkalemia K > 5.0 mEq/L	Irritability and restlessness; anxiety; nausea, vomiting, and diarrhea; muscle cramps, weakness; paresthesias; ECG changes with cardiac irregularities; peaked T waves, ventricular fibrillation, cardiac arrest	• Renal failure • Excessive K^+ replacement • Initial reaction to massive tissue damage (ie, burns, trauma, metabolic acidosis) • Hypoaldosteronism • Potassium-sparing diuretics
	Hypokalemia K < 3.5 mEq/L	Fatigue that progresses to paralysis; paresthesias; nausea, vomiting, anorexia, dizziness; confusion; ventricular ectopy, cardiac arrest; increased sensitivity to digitalis	• Inadequate intake • Vomiting, diarrhea, suctioning, wound drainage • Excessive diaphoresis • Metabolic alkalosis • Hyperaldosteronism • Diuretic phase of renal failure • Insulin drip for DKA

ECG, electrocardiograph; DKA, diabetic ketoacidosis.

TABLE 23–8
Electrolyte Abnormalities: Calcium and Phosphate

Electrolyte	Abnormality	Assessment Findings	Causes
Calcium	Hypercalcemia Ca > 10.5 mg/dl	Muscle weakness/atrophy; lethargy, coma; personality or behavioral changes; pathologic fractures; bone pain; polyuria; excessive thirst; anorexia, nausea, vomiting, constipation; hypertension; ECG changes (ie, shortened QT, AV block)	• Increased intestinal absorption • Excessive vitamin D • Increased bone resorption • Immobility • Thiazide diuretics • Hyperparathyroidism • Multiple fractures • Decreased phosphorus
	Hypocalcemia Ca < 8.5 mg/dl	Paresthesias, tetany, seizures, abdominal spasms, cramps; skeletal muscle cramps; laryngeal spasm; positive Chvostek's and Trousseau's signs, impaired memory, irritability; decreased cardiac output; bleeding	• Renal failure • Protein malnutrition or malabsorption • Decreased intake • Burns or infection • Hypoparathyroidism • Diarrhea • Excessive antacid use • Multiple blood transfusions • Acute pancreatitis • Liver disease • Vitamin D intoxication • Elevated phosphate
Phosphate	Hyperphosphatemia > 4.5 mg/dl	Tachycardia; nausea, diarrhea, abdominal cramps; muscle weakness, paralysis, increased reflexes; decreased calcium	• Renal failure • Hypoparathyroidism • Lactic acidosis • Chemotherapy, certain malignancies • Hypocalcemia, vitamin D intoxication
	Hypophosphatemia < 3 mg/dl	Ataxia, paresthesias, confusion, coma, seizures; muscle weakness, joint stiffness, bone pain; anorexia, dysphagia; anemia, platelet dysfunction, impaired immunity	• Decreased intake or malabsorption • DKA • Excessive antacid use • Lack of vitamin D • Alkalosis, hyperparathyroidism, renal tubule defects • Insulin therapy in DKA, alcoholism

AV, atrioventricular; DKA, diabetic ketoacidosis.

The patient with renal insufficiency often has high magnesium levels because of the kidneys' inability to excrete it. Magnesium accumulates in the serum, bone, and muscle in renal failure and may be involved, along with calcium and phosphorus, in the bone problems accompanying chronic renal failure (Table 23–9).

Nonspecific Tests

The following laboratory values are nondiagnostic by themselves; however, they are important in determining severity of renal impairment and treatment.

Hematocrit and Hemoglobin

The normal hemoglobin in men is between 13.5 to 17.5 g/dl, and is 12 to 16 g/dl in women. The normal hematocrit is between 40% to 52% for adult men and 37% to 48% for adult women. An elevated hematocrit may be seen in the dehydrated patient because of the concentration of body fluids. A low hematocrit may be a dilutional value because of hypervolemia. The kidney is the primary site for the production of erythropoietin, which acts on the bone marrow to stimulate production and release of red blood cells. People with renal failure produce insufficient amounts of erythropoietin, resulting in chronic anemia. Some pa-

TABLE 23–9
Electrolyte Abnormalities: Magnesium

Electrolyte	Abnormality	Assessment Findings	Causes
Magnesium	Hypermag-nesemia > 2.1 mEq/L	CNS depression, respiratory paralysis; lethargy, coma; bradycardia, hypotension	• Renal insufficiency • Excessive intake from antacids and laxatives, severe dehydration with oliguria
	Hypomag-nesemia < 1.4 mEq/L	Tremors, tetany, seizures; positive Chvostek's or Trousseau's signs; tachycardia, hypertension, ventricular arrhythmias; personality changes	• Malnutrition • Alcoholism • Diuretics • Diarrhea • Dehydration

CNS, central nervous system.

tients with renal failure also have a bleeding tendency because of impaired platelet function. In addition, immunologic abnormalities decrease the renal patient's efficiency in responding to infection. Thus, clotting studies and complete blood count differentials also should be monitored.

Uric Acid

Uric acid is excreted by the kidneys, and uric acid therefore may be elevated in renal failure. The normal uric acid serum level is between 2 and 8.5 mg/dl.

Assessment and Management

The nurse's role in the assessment and management of problems of fluid balance includes accurate measurement of intake and output, weight, and vital signs. The most sensitive indices of changes in body water content are serial weights and intake and output patterns. Although vital signs provide supporting data, they may not be abnormal until significant volume or water deficits occur. Assessment of fluid imbalance is based on observation and recognition of pertinent symptoms, and nursing intervention involves replacement or restriction of fluids. Knowing how the patient's health status and medications may affect fluid balance is important in predicting which patients are at risk and require closer supervision.

Intake and Output

An accurate intake and output record provides valuable data for evaluating and treating fluid and electrolyte imbalances. It is important that the nurse instruct the patient and visitors in this activity. The severity of the circumstances will dictate how exact the record should be and what data will be included. For example, in a postsurgical patient who has no complications, fluid replacement may be projected on estimated and actual losses for a 24-hour period. All measurable intake and output is recorded and totaled at the end of every shift.

In the presence of excessive losses or deterioration of cardiac, hepatic, renal, or respiratory function, more detailed recording of every source of fluid intake and output is necessary, and calculations may be required every 1 to 4 hours.

Intake includes not only pure liquids such as water and juices but also those foods that are high in water content (eg, oranges, grapefruit, gelatin, and ice cream). Patients and their families must be reminded frequently that ice and water are the same and that ice therefore must be included in the measurements. It is useful to keep a list of equivalents for fruits, ice cubes, and other sources of water and electrolytes. Output should include intestinal and renal as well as respiratory and cutaneous losses if the patient's temperature or the ambient temperature is high. If enteric, thoracic, abdominal, or ileostomy drainage is present, it also should be recorded.

In severe electrolyte and fluid imbalances, the time and type of fluid intake as well as the time and amount of each voiding should be recorded. In the event that renal function decreases because of prerenal azotemia or ARF, this information may aid immeasurably in the diagnosis and possible prevention of ARF.

Sources of Excessive Loss

Fever. A patient with a fever of 104°F (40°C) and a respiratory rate of 40 breaths/minute can lose as much as 2,500 ml of fluid in a 24-hour period from the respiratory tract and from the skin.

Environment. Hot, dry climates can increase evaporative sweat losses to 1,500 ml/hour to maintain body evaporative heat loss. This can increase to between 2 and 2.5 L/hour for short times in acclimatized people exercising in hot climates.

Hyperventilation. Hyperventilation can increase respiratory water losses as the result of either disease or use of nonhumidified respirators.

Gastrointestinal tract. Vomiting, nasogastric suction, diarrhea, and enterocutaneous drainage or fistulas can increase gastrointestinal losses.

Third-spacing. Formation of pleural or peritoneal effusions and edema from liver, renal, or hepatic disease or from the diffuse capillary leak syndrome can result in a loss of effective intravascular volume. Drainage of peritoneal or pleural fluid, when formation of these third spaces still is occurring, can result in further effective intravascular losses because of continued fluid shifts from the vascular compartment to the third space.

Burns. Fluid loss into burned tissues can result in a significant decrease in effective intravascular volume. Because both evaporative and transudative losses through the burned skin can result in absolute losses of 1,000 to 2,000 ml/day, the burned patient requires special attention to maintain fluid and electrolyte balance.

Renal losses. Inappropriate solute and fluid loss from the kidneys can occur because of renal salt wasting, as seen in the diuretic phase of acute tubular necrosis, in some rare patients with true renal salt wasting, and as the result of excessive diuretic administration. It also may occur as the result of solute diuresis from high-protein or high-saline enteral and parenteral alimentation and from administration of osmotic agents, such as mannitol and radiocontrast agents. Finally, there can be fluid loss during the generation phase of metabolic alkalosis, in which compensatory urinary bicarbonate excretion obligates renal sodium excretion, frequently in the face of volume depletion.

Weight

Rapid daily gains and losses in weight usually are related to changes in fluid volume. Because of the difficulties in obtaining accurate figures for intake and output records, serial weights often are more reliable. In addition, *weight changes usually will pick up imbalances before symptoms are apparent*.

As with intake and output records, the weighing procedure should be consistent. The patient should be weighed on the same scale with the same attire, preferably in the morning before breakfast and after voiding. Variations in the procedure should be noted and made known to the physician.

A kilogram scale provides for greater accuracy because drug, fluid, and diet measurement are calculated with the metric system, and conversion from pounds to kilograms may lead to discrepancies.

Normally, a patient with a balanced nutritional intake will maintain weight. A patient whose protein intake is limited or who is catabolic will lose about 2.2 lb/day (1 kg/day). A weight gain of more than 2.2 kg/day (1 lb/day)

suggests fluid retention. *A generally accepted guide is that 473 ml (1 pt) of fluid is reflected in 0.5 kg (1.1 lb) of weight gained.*

Nursing Assessment of Hypovolemia and Hypervolemia

The nurse must be continually on the alert to detect early changes in the patient's volume status. Seldom is the diagnosis made on the basis of one diagnostic parameter. The first clue may be the patient's general appearance; after observing this, the nurse should seek and note more specific parameters.

Symptoms vary with the degree of imbalance; some are seen early in imbalance states and others are not evident until severe imbalances have occurred. Table 23–10 lists the signs and symptoms of hypovolemia and hypervolemia.

In volume depletion, the patient may complain of orthostatic light-headedness when assuming the sitting or standing position (this also can occur from inactivity and autonomic dysfunction). Development of tachycardia on assuming the upright position and a decrease in blood pressure (orthostatic hypotension), as opposed to the normal rise, are frequent early findings. Later, the pulse may become rapid, weak, and thready. There may be early dryness of the skin, with loss of elasticity, sunken eyes, loss of axillary sweating, and dry, coated tongue. The patient in renal failure often has rough, dry skin with deposits of urate crystals present. This is referred to as "uremic frost." When severe volume depletion occurs, thirst, decreased urine volume, and weight loss may be noted; however, weight loss and orthostatic blood pressure and pulse changes may be the only findings present.

Laboratory studies such as a high urine osmolality and low urinary sodium may facilitate the diagnosis. Other guidelines such as a raised hematocrit, decreased central venous pressure, and decreased pulmonary wedge pressure may corroborate the diagnosis.

In fluid overload, the patient, if alert, may complain of puffiness or stiffness in the hands and feet or state that rings or shoes feel tight. Later, periorbital edema or puffiness, followed by pitting edema of the dependent parts (feet and ankles if upright; sacral area and posterior thighs if supine) will occur, followed by dyspnea or ascites, depending on etiology (ie, cardiac decompensation and systemic fluid overload versus hepatic disease). Urine volume and urine sodium may be normal, increased, or decreased, depending on the etiology. In most diseases with fluid retention, except for the syndrome of inappropriate ADH secretion, urine sodium will be reduced. The hematocrit will be decreased, reflecting hemodilution.

The pulse may be rapid and auscultation of the heart may reveal the presence of S_3, S_4, or a murmur secondary to volume overload. Respirations may be increased because of pulmonary congestion, and auscultation of the chest may reveal rales. A chest film may reveal pulmonary

TABLE 23-10
Signs and Symptoms of Hypovolemia and Hypervolemia

Parameters	Hypovolemia	Hypervolemia
Skin and subcutaneous tissues	Dry; less elastic	Warm, moist, pitting edema over bony prominences; wrinkled skin from pressure of clothing
Face	Sunken eyes (late symptom)	Periorbital edema
Tongue	Dry, coated (early symptom); fissured (late symptom)	Moist
Saliva	Thick, scanty	Excessive, frothy
Thirst	Present	May not be significant
Temperature	May be elevated	May not be significant
Pulse	Rapid, weak, thready	Rapid
Respirations	Rapid, shallow	Rapid dyspnea, moist rales, cough
Blood pressure	Low, orthostatic hypotension; small pulse pressure	Normal to high
Weight	Loss	Gain

vascular congestion, increased alveolar lung markings, cardiac dilatation, frank pulmonary congestion, and pleural effusions.

All data should be evaluated in the light of other evidence. Trends usually are more significant than isolated values. For example, when a decrease in urine output is noted, a systematic assessment should be done to determine why this is happening and what nursing interventions are most appropriate. Factors affecting water balance are listed in Table 23-11.

Nursing Management of Hypovolemia and Hypervolemia

After reviewing the intake and output records for both the current and the previous day and evaluating the symptoms and parameters just discussed, the nurse can make a decision about whether to increase or decrease fluid intake. In the absence of symptoms of fluid retention, when intravenous fluids are behind schedule and intake is inadequate for the patient's condition, missed fluids should be given. The nurse should watch the patient's fluid status closely for the next few hours, especially urine output, to evaluate whether or not the increase in fluid intake corrected the patient's fluid balance. If, however, urine output is zero or diminished in the presence of adequate fluid intake, no more fluids are given, and the physician is notified immediately. If a patient presents any of the symptoms of fluid overload discussed earlier, all fluid intake is restricted, and the physician is notified immediately.

Fluid replacement can be calculated for any given period of time, depending on the severity of the situation. For example, a 24-hour calculation of intake for a patient who is oliguric with normal insensible losses could be as follows:

Previous 24-hour urine output:	100 ml
Insensible loss replacement:	500 ml
Total 24-hour fluid allowance:	600 ml

Although the physician will specify the total amount of fluid replacement, the details of distribution often are decided by the nurse. Priority is given to fluid needed for administration of drugs, both intravenous and oral. Distribution of the remaining fluid is then made according to patient preference. The nurse guides the selection to help the patient avoid using up the entire day's allowance early in the day. Because sodium and potassium may be restricted in the patient with renal failure, fluids such as ginger ale, 7-Up, and Kool Aid, which are low in sodium and potassium, are given.

Assessment and Management of Hyponatremia

Hyponatremia is important because it can produce a wide range of neurologic symptoms, including death. The severity of symptoms depends on the degree of hyponatremia and on the rate at which it has developed. Generally, symptoms do not occur until the serum sodium is below 120 mEq/L. Table 23-6 depicts the symptoms to be expected in several ranges of hyponatremia. It is important to remember that for each level of sodium concentration, the severity of symptoms encountered will depend on how rapidly the sodium concentration was lowered.

Treatment of hyponatremia depends on the level of serum sodium, the patient's symptoms, and the cause.

TABLE 23–11
Factors Affecting Water Balance

		Water Excess	Water Deficiency
Intake			
	Thirst	Decreased thirst threshold	Increased thirst threshold
		Increased osmolality	Decreased osmolality
		Potassium depletion	Lack of access
		Hypercalcemia	Psychiatric disorders
		Fever	
		Dry mucous membranes	
		Poor oral hygiene	
		Unmisted O_2 administration	
		Hypotension	
		Psychiatric disorders	
	Parenteral fluids	Excessive D5W	Deficient replacement
			Osmotic loads
			Hyperalimentation
			Hyperglycemia
			Mannitol
			Radiographic contrast agents
Output			
	Sweating		High ambient temperature
			High altitude
			Fever
	Renal excretion	Inappropriate ADH release	Excess excretion
		Appropriate ADH release	Central
		Congestive failure	Nephrogenic
		Decompensated cirrhosis	Potassium depletion
		Volume depletion	Hypercalcemia
		Adrenal insufficiency	Lithium administration
		Renal salt-wasting	Declomicin
		Hemorrhage	Penthrane
		Diuretics	
		Burns	
		Hypothyroidism	
		Renal disease	
		ARF	
		Chronic renal failure	
		Nephrotic syndrome	
		Acute glomerulonephritis	
		Nonsteroidal anti-inflammatory agents	

D5W, Dextrose 5% in water; ADH, antidiuretic hormone; ARF, acute renal failure.

In most cases of mild hyponatremia associated with congestive heart failure, fluid restriction to approximately 1,000 ml/day usually is the only treatment recommended. In cases associated with true volume depletion, however, normal saline usually will correct the volume deficit and restore the sodium concentration to normal. For the most severe degrees of hyponatremia, with potentially life-threatening symptoms, hypertonic (3%) sodium chloride given intravenously may be necessary.

If fluid overload also is a problem, water restriction and intravenous furosemide or ethacrynic acid, both of which cause water loss in excess of sodium, may be the therapy of choice, sometimes with concomitant replacement with hypertonic saline. This type of therapy requires hourly urine collections and accurate measurements of electrolyte losses so that serious electrolyte disturbances are prevented.

Assessment and Management of Hypernatremia

Symptoms of hypernatremia generally are the same as those of hyperosmolality and result from CNS dehydration.

Mental confusion, stupor, seizures, coma, and death may occur, in addition to other signs of dehydration such as fatigue, muscle weakness and cramps, and anorexia. The serum osmolality generally is above 350 mOsm/L before significant symptoms are noted. This corresponds to a serum sodium of 165 to 170 mEq/L.

Treatment consists of administering free water (without salt) by mouth (or, if necessary, 5% dextrose in water intravenously). The correction should be made slowly to prevent hypertonicity and CNS dysfunction. Vasopressin (Pitressin; Parke-Davis, Morris Plains, NJ) also is given in those cases due to pituitary diabetes insipidus along with eliminating conditions known to produce nephrogenic diabetes insipidus (hypercalcemia, hypokalemia, demeclocycline, and lithium administration).

Summary

The nurse plays a critical role in the assessment and management of patients with fluid and electrolyte disorders. Careful monitoring of patients' symptoms, general appearance, and changes in weight, blood pressure, and pulse may provide early clues to changes in volume status and to disorders of water balance. Knowledgeable application and interpretation of laboratory studies will facilitate the diagnosis and treatment of fluid and electrolyte disorders as well as other complications of renal dysfunction in the seriously ill patient.

CASE STUDY

Mr. Ellis, a 46-year-old man, was admitted with a 48-hour history of jaundice and increasing mental confusion. Mr. Ellis indicated he has a history of alcoholism and had been drinking heavily during the past few weeks. For 2 weeks he had noted increasing edema and increasing abdominal girth. During physical examination, he was moderately obtunded but arousable. Blood pressure was 98/68 mm Hg, pulse was 92/min, and temperature was 97°F. Mr. Ellis had marked scleral icterus, tense abdominal ascites, and diffuse pitting edema below the waist. Initial laboratory studies revealed the following:

Serum:

Na: 115 mEq/L
Cl: 75 mEq/L
K: 2.8 mEq/L
CO_2: 30 mEq/L
BUN: 10 mg/dl
Creatinine: 0.8 mg/dl
Albumin: 2.4 g/dl

Urine:

Specific gravity: 1.028; pH 6.8
U_{osm}: 890 mOsm/L
U_{Na}: 8 mEq/L
U_K: 33 mEq/L
U_{Cl}: 2 mEq/L

The serum bilirubin, aspartate aminotransferase, alkaline phosphatase, and lactate dehydrogenase levels all were elevated, but the blood ammonium level was normal

Discussion

Mr. Ellis had severe hyponatremia in the face of an increase in total body sodium and water, as reflected by the pronounced edema. Sodium retention is due to the combined effects of decreased renal perfusion secondary to (1) hypovolemia from hypoalbuminemia and ascites formation, (2) alcoholic peripheral vasodilation, and (3) secondary hypoaldosteronism. The hyponatremia is due to the combined effects of volume-mediated vasopressin release, as reflected in the high urine specific gravity and osmolality, and to decreased distal nephron sodium and water delivery due to renal underperfusion.

Mr. Ellis had acute alcoholic hepatitis and was treated with enteral hyperalimentation via a nasogastric tube. Initial treatment of his hyponatremia consisted of water restriction and a combination of a thiazide diuretic and aldactone, resulting in slow correction of his serum sodium.

In addition to his hyponatremia, Mr. Ellis also had a hypokalemic metabolic alkalosis, probably resulting from the combined effects of volume and potassium depletion. His urinary sodium of 8 mEq/L was considerably higher than his urine chloride concentration, probably due to spilling of bicarbonate in the urine. Bicarbonaturia obligates urinary sodium excretion, even in the face of volume depletion. In this situation, the urinary chloride concentration is a better indication of volume depletion than is the urinary sodium concentration, as was noted in this patient.

NURSING CARE PLAN 23–1:
The Patient with Hyponatremia

NURSING DIAGNOSIS	OUTCOME CRITERIA/ PATIENT GOALS	NURSING INTERVENTIONS
Altered tissue perfusion, Renal: related to sodium retention, acid–base imbalance, and excessive alcoholic intake.	• Maintain perfusion to kidney for adequate fluid and electrolyte balance.	1. Carry out physician's orders for hyperalimentation. 2. Restrict water intake, as ordered. 3. Administer diuretic therapy, as ordered. 4. Monitor for signs and symptoms of hyponatremia: cold, clammy, poor skin turgor, edema of sternum, sunken eyes, tachycardia, thready pulse, weight loss, anorexia, vomiting, nausea, abdominal cramps, diarrhea, oliguria to anuria, headache, seizures, shock, lethargy, fatigue, irritable, weak, twitchy and hyporeflexive muscle tone, anxiety, confusion, apathy. 5. Assess intake and output balance. 6. Initiate nursing care precautions for potential seizures, including safety precautions. 7. Keep bed at lowest height level. 8. Pad and elevate bed side rails. 9. Assist patient with ambulation and repositioning. 10. Keep call light within patient's easy reach. 11. Monitor for signs and symptoms of hypokalemia: cyanotic skin, weak, faint, and irregular pulse, shallow respirations, hypertension, ECG changes (elevated P wave, flattened T or inverted, prolonged QT interval), weak voice, flabby to flaccid paralysis, absent reflexes, apathy, depression, lethargy, intermittent tetany, Chvostek's sign. 12. Monitor for signs and symptoms of metabolic alkalosis: cyanotic skin, slow, shallow respirations, ECG changes (flattened T wave, elevated P wave), hypertonic tetany, personality changes, weakness.

(continued)

NURSING CARE PLAN 23–1: *(Continued)*
The Patient with Hyponatremia

NURSING DIAGNOSIS	OUTCOME CRITERIA/ PATIENT GOALS	NURSING INTERVENTIONS
High risk for injury: related to alcohol withdrawal.	• Patient will recover from alcohol withdrawal with as few adverse effects as possible.	1. Monitor for signs and symptoms of alcohol withdrawal: restlessness, agitation, irrational behavior, increased blood pressure and pulse, fever, insomnia, anorexia, weight loss, dehydration, electrolyte imbalance, decreased analgesic effect from pain medication, hand tremors, gastric discomfort, abdominal cramps, hallucinations, delirium tremens. 2. Maintain safe environment. 3. Evaluate the need for chemical or physical restraint. 4. Provide emotional support. 5. Check BP, pulse and respirations q4h. 6. Medicate with tranquilizers as ordered.

BIBLIOGRAPHY

Brenner BM, Rector FC: The Kidney, 4th ed, vols I and II. Philadelphia, WB Saunders, 1991

Burrell LO: Adult Nursing in Hospital and Community Settings. Norwalk, CT, Appleton & Lange, 1992

Corbett JV: Laboratory Tests and Diagnostic Procedures With Nursing Diagnosis. Norwalk, CT, Appleton & Lange, 1992

Innerarity SA: Electrolyte emergencies in the critically ill renal patient. Critical Care Nursing Clinics of North America 2(1):89–99, 1990

Innerarity SA: Hyperkalemic emergencies. Critical Care Nursing Clinics of North America 14(4):32–39, 1992

Jones A, Moseley M, Halfmann S, Health A, Henkelman W, Ciaccia J, Belcar B: Fluid volume dynamics. Critical Care Nurse 11(4):74–76, 1991

Terry J: The other electrolytes: Magnesium, calcium and phosphorus. Journal of Intravenous Nursing 14(3):167–176, 1991

Ulrich BT: Nephrology Nursing: Concepts and Strategies. Norwalk, CT, Appleton & Lange, 1989

Yarnell RP, Craig M: Detecting hypomagnesemia: The most overlooked electrolyte imbalance. Nursing 21(7):55–57, 1991

STUDY QUESTIONS

1. Which laboratory value is most useful in assessing renal function?

   a. potassium
   b. BUN
   c. creatinine
   d. uric acid

2. The following laboratory values will be elevated in renal failure

   a. potassium, phosphate, and magnesium
   b. calcium, potassium, and phosphate

    c. calcium and magnesium
    d. bicarbonate and chloride

3. Signs and symptoms of hypernatremia include

    a. edema, dry skin, bradycardia
    b. thirst, high specific gravity, hypotension
    c. increased blood pressure and central venous pressure
    d. ECG changes, flaccid paralysis

4. Treatment of mild hyponatremia includes

    a. water restriction
    b. IV fluid administration of D5W
    c. IV fluid administration of 0.45 NS
    d. bed rest and NPO

CHAPTER 24

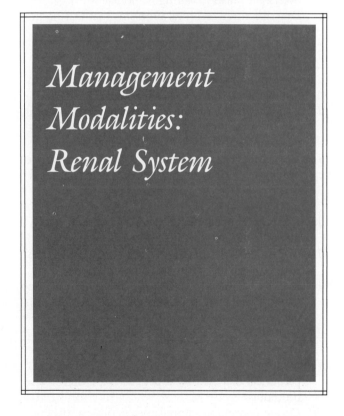

Management Modalities: Renal System

BEHAVIORAL OBJECTIVES

Based on the content in this chapter, the reader should be able to:

1. List four functions of the artificial kidney system.
2. Describe how the artificial kidney interacts with

(*continued*)

Hudak: Critical Care Nursing:
A Holistic Approach, 6th ed. © 1994
J. B. Lippincott Company.

BEHAVIORAL OBJECTIVES (*Continued*)

a dialyzing solution to achieve desired changes in blood components.

3. Describe three variables that should be included in the predialysis assessment.
4. Define ultrafiltration and the circumstances in which this process is used to correct fluid imbalances.
5. Identify one situation in which a patient could benefit from a continuous renal replacement therapy to achieve fluid balance.
6. List three reasons why a patient might experience hypotension during hemodialysis.
7. Identify one electrolyte whose level usually is corrected during hemodialysis and one electrolyte that usually is restored.
8. Describe the role of oral calcium compounds in correcting hyperphosphatemia.
9. Identify two methods the nurse can use to avoid overheparinization during hemodialysis.
10. Describe three technical problems that can occur during hemodialysis.
11. Explain the difference between the arteriovenous fistula and polytetrafluoroethylene graft.
12. Identify two common sites for insertion of central vein catheters for hemodialysis use.
13. Explain why hemodialysis nurses sometimes are involved in performance of therapies such as hemoperfusion and therapeutic plasma exchange.
14. Describe the psychological needs of the patient receiving hemodialysis therapy for acute renal failure versus those of the person who is on chronic hemodialysis.
15. Define peritoneal dialysis and two ways in which it differs from hemodialysis.
16. List four essential features of nursing care for the patient receiving peritoneal dialysis.
17. Identify two reasons why peritoneal fluid retention may occur during peritoneal dialysis and two nursing measures to alleviate this problem.
18. State three common signs or symptoms of peritonitis.
19. Identify two reasons why the patient receiving peritoneal dialysis may experience pain during the procedure.
20. Define continuous ambulatory peritoneal dialysis and continuous cyclic peritoneal dialysis.

Hemodialysis

Description

Dialysis refers to the diffusion of dissolved particles from one fluid compartment to another across a semipermeable membrane. In *hemodialysis*, the blood is one fluid compartment and the dialysate is the other.

The semipermeable membrane is a thin, porous sheet made of a cellulose or synthetic material. The pore size of the membrane permits diffusion of low–molecular-weight substances such as urea, creatinine, and uric acid. Water molecules also are very small and move freely through the membrane, but most plasma proteins, bacteria, and blood cells are too large to pass through the pores of the membrane. The difference in the concentration of the substances in the two compartments is called the *concentration gradient*.

The blood, which contains waste products such as urea and creatinine, flows into the blood compartment of the dialyzer, or artificial kidney, where it comes into contact with the dialysate, which contains no urea or creatinine. A maximum gradient is established so that these substances move from the blood to the dialysate. Repeated passages of the blood through the dialyzer at a rate ranging from 200 to 400 ml/minute over 2 to 4 hours reduces the level of these waste products to a more normal state. Hemodialysis is indicated in acute renal failure (ARF) and chronic renal failure, drug and chemical intoxications, severe fluid and electrolyte imbalances, and hepatorenal syndrome.

The artificial kidney system:

- Removes the by-products of protein metabolism such as urea, creatinine, and uric acid
- Removes excess water by effecting a pressure differential between the blood and fluid compartments, usually consisting of positive pressure in the blood path and negative (suction) pressure in the dialysate compartment (process of ultrafiltration)
- Maintains or restores the body buffer system
- Maintains or restores the level of electrolytes in the body

Equipment Features

The Dialyzer or Artificial Kidney

This component encases the dialyzing membrane separating the blood and dialysate compartments. Dialyzers vary in size, physical structure, and type of membrane used to construct the blood compartment. All these factors determine the potential efficiency of the dialyzer, which refers to its ability to remove water (ultrafiltration) and waste products (clearance).

The two types of dialyzer designs currently available are the parallel plate and hollow fiber. These designs differ in structure of the dialyzing pathway and come in different sizes, varying according to the needs of the patient. Both designs meet the desired characteristics of an artificial kidney—a low blood volume, maximum solute clearance, and predictable ultrafiltration. Because biocompatibility of the membrane with the patient also is gaining favor, such materials have been developed and are being used increasingly to satisfy this need.

There are relative advantages and disadvantages to each dialyzer that must be considered when a selection is being made. Parallel plates may be used when:

- Usual amounts of heparinization are contraindicated for patients with active or potential bleeding problems
- Compliance of the blood compartment is desirable, as with a single vascular access for both blood inflow to, and blood outflow from, the dialyzer

The parallel-plate configuration is not used as commonly as the hollow-fiber dialyzer. More efficient hollow-fiber dialyzers generally are used when:

- A highly efficient, shorter dialysis is preferred, as in patients who require rapid removal of excess fluid, electrolytes, or waste products
- Extracorporeal blood volume is the major concern (because this dialyzer design has the lowest priming volume)
- Chronic dialysis requires the most blood clearance in the shortest amount of time (to save time for both patients and staff)

Another consideration is dialyzer size. Smaller, low-blood-volume dialyzers are preferable for children and some geriatric patients. Dialyzers with more surface area (and therefore more solute clearance) are used for large patients, for those who can benefit from high-efficiency, short dialysis, and for those who require increased amounts of ultrafiltration. Traditionally, dialyzers have been made of Cuprophane and other cellulose membranes. Due to studies reporting some short- and long-term incompatibility to cellulose,[1] however, membranes now are available that are made of any one of several synthetic materials.

The size and type of dialyzers depend on the aforementioned factors as well as the experience and philosophy of personnel in charge of the hemodialysis unit.

Dialysate or Dialyzing Solution

The dialysate, or "bath," is a solution composed of water and the major electrolytes of normal serum. It is made in a clean system with filtered tap water and chemicals. It is not a sterile system, because bacteria are too large to pass through the membrane and the potential for infection of the patient is minimal. Because bacteria by-products, however, can cause pyrogenic reactions, especially in highly permeable membranes, water used to make dialysate must be bacteriologically safe. Dialysate concentrates usually are provided by commercial manufacturers. A "standard" bath generally is used in chronic units, but variations may be made to meet specific patient needs.

Dialysate Delivery System

A single delivery unit provides dialysate for one patient; the multiple delivery system may supply as many as 20 patient units. In either system, an automatic proportioning device and metering and monitoring devices ensure precise control of the water–concentrate ratio.

The single delivery unit usually is used in acute dialyses. It is a mobile unit, and dialysate requirements are tailored easily to meet individual patient needs.

Accessory Equipment

Hardware used in most dialysis systems includes a blood pump, infusion pumps for heparin delivery, and monitoring devices for detection of unsafe temperatures, dialysate concentration, pressure changes, air, and blood leaks. All dialysis delivery systems currently consist of a single compact unit that includes both the dialysate delivery equipment as well as blood monitoring components (Fig. 24–1). Disposable items used in addition to the artificial kidney include dialysis tubing for transport of blood between the dialyzer and patient, pressure transducers for protection of

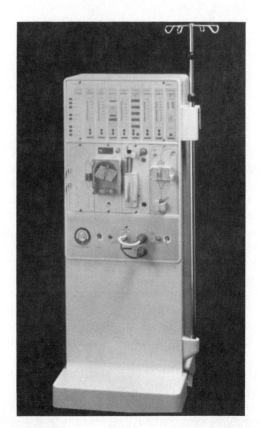

FIGURE 24–1
Hemodialysis delivery unit. Includes automatic blood pressure cuff, heparin infusion pump, and blood pump. Displays continuous readout of ultrafiltration goal, rate, and total fluid removed. Monitors dialysate temperature and conductivity; can vary dialysate sodium concentration (Fresenius 2008E, Fresenius VSA, Inc., Concord, CA).

monitoring devices from blood exposure, and a normal saline bag and tubing for priming the system before use.

The Human Component

Expertise in the use of highly technical equipment is gained through theoretical and practical training in the clinical setting. The operation and monitoring of various kinds of dialysis equipment will differ, however. Reference to the manufacturer's instruction manuals will give the nurse guidelines for the safe operation of equipment. Although the technical aspects of hemodialysis may at first seem overwhelming, they can be learned fairly rapidly. A more critical aspect, one that takes long to achieve, consists of the understanding and knowledge that the nurse will use in caring for patients during dialysis.

Assessment and Management

Because hemodialysis is a dynamic procedure, alterations in blood chemistries and fluid balance occur quickly. Therefore, the nursing process is in continued use throughout the treatment, with the nurse changing the plan of care according to changes in objective and subjective data. The nurse's observation skills, assessment of symptoms, and appropriate actions can make the difference between a smooth dialysis with minimal problems and one fraught with a series of crises for the patient and the nurse.

Predialysis Assessment

The degree and complexity of problems arising during hemodialysis will vary among patients and will depend on many factors. Important variables are the patient's diagnosis, stage of illness, age, other medical problems, fluid and electrolyte balance, and emotional state. Because more people older than age 60 are receiving dialysis, it also is important to consider the normal decreases in cardiac function as well as other system changes due to the aging process.

The essential first step in the hemodialysis procedure consists of a review of the patient's history, clinical records, response to previous dialysis treatment, consultation with other caregivers, laboratory reports, and, finally, the nurse's observations of the patient.

After reviewing the data and while consulting with the physician, the dialysis nurse will *establish objectives* for the dialysis treatment. The objectives will vary from one dialysis to the next in the ARF patient, whose condition may change rapidly. For example, fluid removal may take precedence over correction of an electrolyte imbalance or *vice versa*. Bleeding problems—actual or potential—will determine the type and degree of anticoagulation.

The patient's emotional state should be included in this initial evaluation. Anxiety and apprehension, especially during the first dialysis, may contribute to change in

blood pressure, restlessness, and gastrointestinal upsets. The security provided by the presence of a nurse during the first dialysis probably is more desirable than administration of a drug that might precipitate changes in vital signs.

A basic explanation of the procedure and its place in the total care plan for the patient also may allay some of the anxiety experienced by the patient and family. It is important that they understand that dialysis is being used to support normal body function rather than "cure" the kidney problem.

Predialysis

Assessment

Diagnosis
Stage of illness
Other health problems
Fluid and electrolyte balance
Laboratory values
Other clinical findings
Response to previous dialysis treatment
Emotional state
Observations

Plan

Prepare patient and family
Determine objectives for treatment
Safety check of equipment

Procedure

After the predialysis assessment, development of objectives, and a safety check of equipment, the nurse is ready to begin hemodialysis. Access to the circulatory system is gained by one of several options: the arteriovenous (AV) fistula or graft, or a dual-lumen hemodialysis catheter. Two large-gauge (15- or 16-gauge) needles are needed to cannulate a graft or fistula. The dual-lumen catheters, placed either in the subclavian, internal jugular, or femoral veins, will need to be opened under aseptic conditions according to institutional policy.

Once vascular access is established, blood begins to flow, assisted by the blood pump. The part of the disposable circuit before the dialyzer is designated the "arterial" line, both to distinguish the blood in it as blood that has not yet reached the dialyzer, and in reference to needle placement: the "arterial" needle is placed closest to the AV anastomosis in a graft or fistula to maximize blood flow. A clamped saline bag always is attached to the circuit just before the blood pump. In episodes of hypotension, blood flow from the patient can be clamped while the saline is opened and allowed to infuse rapidly to correct blood pressure. Blood transfusions and plasma expanders also can be attached to the circuit at this point and allowed to drip in, assisted by the blood pump. Heparin infusions may be located either before or after the blood pump, depending on the equipment in use.

The dialyzer is the next important component of the circuit. Blood flows into the blood compartment of the dialyzer, where exchange of fluid and waste products takes place. Blood leaving the dialyzer passes through an air and foam detector that will clamp off and shut down the blood pump should any air be detected. At this point in the pathway, any medications that can be given on dialysis are infused via a medication port. It is important to remember, however, that most medications are held until after dialysis unless otherwise ordered (Fig. 24–2).

Blood that has passed through the dialyzer returns to the patient through the "venous," or postdialyzer line. After the prescribed treatment time, dialysis is terminated

by clamping off blood from the patient, opening the saline line, and rinsing the circuit to return the patient's blood. The lines and dialyzer are disposable in the acute setting, although chronic dialysis programs often purchase equipment to clean and reuse dialyzers.

Universal precautions should be followed scrupulously throughout the dialysis treatment because of the exposure to blood. A protective face shield and gloves are mandatory for the nurse performing hemodialysis.

Interpretation of Results

The results of a dialysis treatment should be interpreted by assessing the amount of fluid removed and correction of electrolyte and acid–base disorders. Blood drawn immediately postdialysis may show falsely low levels of electro-

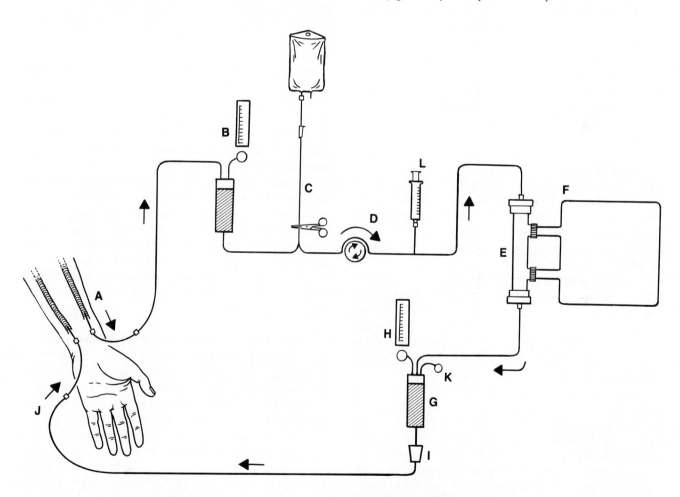

A. Arterial needle
B. Arterial pressure monitor
C. Saline line
D. Blood pump
E. Dialyzer
F. Dialysate delivery system

G. Venous drip chamber
H. Venous pressure monitor
I. Air and foam detector and clamp
J. Venous needle
K. Medication administration port
L. Heparin infusion

FIGURE 24–2
Hemodialysis circuit.

lytes, blood urea nitrogen, and creatinine. The process of equilibration is thought to continue for some time after dialysis, as these substances move from inside the cell to the plasma.

Complications

Fluid Imbalances

It is necessary to evaluate fluid balance before dialysis so that corrective measures may be initiated at the beginning of the procedure. Parameters such as blood pressure, pulse, weight, intake and output, tissue turgor, and other symptoms will assist the nurse in estimating fluid overload or depletion. Monitoring tools such as pulmonary artery pressure also are indispensable in determining the cardiovascular fluid load.

The term *dry* or *ideal* weight is used to express the weight at which fluid volume is in a normal range for the patient who is free of the symptoms of fluid imbalance. The figure is not an absolute one, but it provides a guideline for fluid removal or replacement. It requires frequent review and revision, especially in the newly dialyzed patient, in whom frequent changes in weight are occurring due to fluid removal or accumulation and to tissue gains or losses.

Hypervolemia

The following findings may suggest fluid overload: blood pressure elevation, increased pulse and respiratory rate, increased central venous pressure, dyspnea, moist rales, cough, edema, excessive weight gain since last dialysis, and a history or record of excessive fluid intake in the absence of adequate losses.

A chest roentgenogram to assess heart size or pulmonary congestion may confirm the diagnosis of fluid overload but may not be essential in the presence of overt symptoms. Increase in abdominal girth will suggest accumulation of fluid in the abdominal cavity. If ascites is present, measurement of the abdominal girth will help determine how to correct the problem.

Analyzing the causes of the fluid overload can help prevent recurrences. Only after the causes are determined can a nursing diagnosis of "fluid volume excess related to . . ." be made accurately. Nursing interventions then can be planned appropriately. The intake and output record may provide a clue. For example, the patient may have been given excessive intravenous fluids in a "keep open" line, or fluids used as a vehicle for intravenous medications may not have been calculated in the intake. The patient may not have adhered to the fluid restriction or may have had a decrease in fluid losses—for example, gastric suction may have been discontinued. Often, after the institution of chronic dialysis, urinary output decreases. If the patient continues normal fluid intake, fluid overload will occur. In the chronic hemodialysis patient, fluid overload may be related to the intake of high-sodium foods. Moderate restriction is necessary for all patients so that extracellular fluid overload is prevented. Change in weight provides an indication of water load; an acceptable weight gain is 0.5 kg for each 24 hours between dialyses.

Treatment of fluid overload during dialysis is directed toward the removal of the excess water. Because this removal depends on shifting of fluid to the vascular space from other body compartments, care must taken during dialysis to avoid removing fluid so rapidly that it leads to volume depletion. Excessive fluid removal may lead to hypotension, and little is gained if intravenous fluids are given to correct the problem. Thus, it is better to reduce the volume overload over a period of two or three dialyses, unless pulmonary congestion is life-threatening.

Ultrafiltration

Excessive water is removed from the vascular compartment by the process of ultrafiltration. This is accomplished by application of negative pressure to the effluent dialysate. This creates a "siphoning" effect on the dialysate, with water molecules being pulled across the membrane into the dialysate. As much as 4 to 5 kg (approximately 10 lb) of water may be removed in a 2- to 6-hour period. The amount of negative pressure that is applied is based on the ultrafiltration capability of the dialyzer, the amount of fluid that needs to be removed, and the individual patient's tolerance.

In some newer dialysis systems using highly permeable membranes, ultrafiltration can be excessive and must be aggressively managed. These systems are equipped with *volumetric control monitors*, which limit ultrafiltration by controlling the size of ultrafiltration chambers and constantly monitoring cumulative fluid removal.

Symptoms of excessive ultrafiltration are similar to those of shock: hypotension, nausea, vomiting, diaphoresis, dizziness, and fainting.

Sequential Ultrafiltration (Diafiltration)

Aggressive ultrafiltration for the purpose of relieving or preventing hypertension, congestive heart failure, pulmonary edema, and other complications associated with fluid overload often is limited by the patient's tolerance of manipulations of intravascular volume.

Observation by several investigators suggests that there is a significant increase in patient tolerance to large, rapid fluid volume removal when the ultrafiltration process occurs in the absence of diffuse mass transfer. This has resulted in a mode of therapy designated *sequential ultrafiltration*, or *diafiltration*, in which the removal of body fluid is separated from the total dialysis procedure. This is accomplished by (1) initiation of dialysis without a dialysate flow, (2) maintenance of negative pressure in the dialysate compartment, and (3) return to the usual dialysis procedure after a predetermined amount of ultrafiltration time. It is thought that this technique is effective because plasma osmolality is kept constant without solute removal during ultrafiltration, thus enhancing fluid shifts from extravascular spaces.

Hypovolemia

Assessment of hypovolemia also is based on the evaluation of trends in vital signs and symptoms. Clues to hypovolemia include falling blood pressure, increasing pulse and respiration rates, loss of skin turgor, dry mouth, a falling central venous pressure, and a decreasing urine output. A history of excessive fluid loss through profuse perspiration, vomiting, diarrhea, and gastric suctioning with resulting weight loss will further substantiate the nursing diagnosis of fluid deficit.

Intervention is directed toward the replacement of previous losses and the prevention of further losses during dialysis. In some cases, constant monitoring of the patient's weight during dialysis is available to assist in determining need for fluid removal or replacement. This is possible using special bed or chair weighing systems that provide constant readouts of the patient's weight, with or without bed or chair.

It is usual practice to phlebotomize the patient at the onset of dialysis. The patient's blood is pumped through the dialyzer, displacing the priming normal saline solution. In the hypovolemic patient, the nurse can connect the venous return blood line immediately and infuse the normal saline into the patient. The 200 ml of solution might be sufficient to restore balance or at least prevent further hypotension. Ultrafiltration will be avoided in the hypovolemic patient, and additional fluids may even be required.

Normal saline is the solution used most frequently to replace depleted fluids during dialysis because small volumes usually produce the desired effect. Replacement in 100- to 200-ml increments is suggested, with frequent monitoring of blood pressure.

Blood volume expanders such as albumin sometimes are used in patients with a low serum protein. The treatment is expensive when the underlying cause of the hypoproteinemia is not corrected and repeated infusions become necessary.

Hypotension

Hypotension during dialysis may be caused by preexisting hypovolemia, excessive ultrafiltration, loss of blood into the dialyzer, dialyzer membrane incompatibility, and antihypertensive drug therapy. Hypotension at the beginning of dialysis may occur in patients with a small blood volume, such as children and small adults. Use of a small-volume dialyzer or administration of normal saline on initiation of dialysis may prevent or minimize problems. In some cases, a Doppler stethoscope or automatic blood pressure monitor may be needed to assess low blood pressure accurately. These nursing interventions should be included in the patient's care plan, if effective, and linked with the appropriate nursing diagnosis, such as "potential for decreased cardiac output related to blood removal during initiation of dialysis."

Hypotension later in dialysis usually is due to excessive or too rapid ultrafiltration. This may be confirmed by weighing the patient and estimating fluid loss. Keeping the patient in a horizontal position and reducing the ultrafiltration rate may return the blood pressure to normal. If hypotension persists, saline or other plasma expanders may be administered. Intravenous fluids should be kept to a minimum and discontinued as soon as the patient is normotensive. If hypotension persists despite adequate fluid replacement, other medical causes for hypotension should be considered. In some computerized dialysis systems, ultrafiltration is stopped automatically when targeted fluid removal is reached. This avoids hypovolemia and hypotension.

Clinicians have found that elevation of the sodium level of the dialysis bath also can help prevent hypotensive episodes and muscle cramps during and after the treatment. Dialysate sodium levels often are kept between 138 and 145 mEq/L, depending on the patient's serum sodium. Personnel in some units also are experimenting with varying the dialysate sodium levels during the treatment, so as not to leave the patient with a high serum sodium at the end of dialysis (this can lead to increased thirst and excessive weight gains).

It also is well documented that dialysis systems using acetate in the bath as the base buffer may cause vasodilation with subsequent symptomatic hypotension.[2] Most dialysis units have found that a switch to bicarbonate dialysis has improved the cardiovascular stability of their patients.

Nurse researchers also are beginning to identify those types of patients at high risk for hypotensive episodes during dialysis, such as patients with impaired cardiovascular function. Interventions such as careful monitoring of vital signs and observation of specific symptoms can help limit the occurrence and severity of hypotensive episodes in these patients.

Blood loss due to technical problems such as membrane leaks and line separations also may lead to hypotension. The use of blood leak detectors and other monitoring devices has reduced the risk of excessive blood loss due to these causes, but it can occur. If separation of blood lines occurs, clamping the arterial blood line and stopping the blood pump immediately will minimize further blood loss.

The incidence of membrane leaks has decreased owing to improvements in dialyzer technology and the use of negative-pressure dialyzers. In these systems, excessive pressure is not exerted in the blood compartment, so leaks are unusual unless the membrane already is damaged. If gross leaks do occur, dialysate may cross the membrane into the blood compartment. In this situation, the blood may be returned to the patient, who should be observed for pyrogenic reactions. If the patient's hematocrit is low, the risk of blood loss may be greater than the possibility of dialysate contamination. Some units have standing policies to cover this contingency; however, decisions may be made according to individual circumstances. In isolated instances, patients may exhibit symptoms of immunologic reaction to standard cellulose dialysis membranes. These symptoms include hypotension, chest pain, shortness of breath, and muscle cramping, and often occur at dialysis initiation when the patient's blood comes in contact with the dialyzer. Switching to a more biocompatible synthetic membrane dialyzer will help determine if this is the cause of otherwise unexplainable hypotension when dialysis begins.

The use of *antihypertensive drugs* in the dialysis patient may precipitate hypotension during dialysis. To avoid this, many units make it standard practice to omit antihypertensive drugs 4 to 6 hours before dialysis. Fluids and sodium restrictions are more desirable controls for hypertension. *Sedatives* and *tranquilizers* also may cause hypotension and should be avoided if possible.

Hypertension

The most frequent causes of hypertension during dialysis are fluid overload, disequilibrium syndrome, renin response to ultrafiltration, and anxiety.

Hypertension during dialysis usually is caused by sodium and water excesses. This can be confirmed by comparing the patient's present weight to ideal, or dry, weight. If fluid overload is the cause of hypertension, ultrafiltration usually will bring about a reduction in the blood pressure.

Some patients who may be normotensive before dialysis become hypertensive during dialysis. The rise may occur either gradually or abruptly. Although the cause is not well understood, it may be the result of renin production in response to ultrafiltration and an increase in renal ischemia. Careful monitoring of these patients is important because the vasoconstriction caused by the renin response is limited. Once a decrease in blood volume surpasses the ability to maintain blood pressure through vasoconstriction, hypotension can occur precipitously.

Hypertension is a common finding in dialysis disequilibrium syndrome (see following discussion) and usually will respond to correction of that condition. If the diastolic blood pressure is over 120 mm Hg or the patient has symptoms, small doses of hydralazine (Apresoline; Ciba Pharmaceutical Co., Summit, NJ) may be given intravenously. An initial dose of 10 mg may bring about a favorable response. Hydralazine is preferred to methyldopa (Aldomet; Merck Sharp & Dohme, West Point, PA) because its effect is more rapid. Blood pressure is monitored at frequent intervals after the administration of antihypertensive drugs.

Anxiety, fear, and apprehension, especially during the first dialysis, may cause transient and erratic hypertension. Sedatives may be necessary, but confidence in the staff and a smooth, problem-free dialysis will help reduce anxiety during subsequent treatments.

Dialysis Disequilibrium Syndrome

Dialysis disequilibrium syndrome is manifested by a group of symptoms suggestive of cerebral dysfunction. Symptoms range in severity from mild nausea, vomiting, headache, and hypertension to agitation, twitching, mental confusion, and convulsions. It is thought that rapid, efficient dialysis results in shifts in water, pH, and osmolality between cerebrospinal fluid and blood, which cause the symptoms.[3]

Slow dialysis for short periods daily for two or three treatments may prevent disequilibrium syndrome in the acutely uremic patient. Phenytoin (Dilantin; Parke-Davis, Morris Plains, NJ) sometimes is used before and during dialysis in the new patient to reduce the risk of central nervous system symptoms.

Restlessness, confusion, twitching, nausea, and vomiting may suggest early disequilibrium. Reduction of the blood flow rate and administration of sedatives may prevent more severe symptoms, but it may be necessary to discontinue dialysis if symptoms persist or worsen.

Electrolyte Imbalances

With the trend toward early and adequate dialysis, the severe extremes of electrolyte imbalances are not seen with the same frequency as before the widespread use of hemodialysis.

Maintenance and restoration of electrolyte balance in the dialysis patient are accomplished primarily with dialysis and to a lesser degree with dietary controls. Most of the dialysate electrolyte concentrations are standard for all patients, but the potassium concentration is determined according to the patient's individual serum level. Changes often are made in the calcium and sodium levels as well, depending on the variety of dialysate concentrates available and sophistication of the machinery used.

Laboratory tests for evaluation of electrolyte status are performed before and sometimes after each dialysis in ARF. If laboratory studies are desired postdialysis, they should be performed at least 1 hour after dialysis is completed to allow for equilibration of the vascular, tissue, and cell compartments. Otherwise, false values, derived from the blood compartment only, will be obtained. The nurse's role includes:

- knowing normal values
- recognizing symptoms of imbalance
- evaluating probable causes

In many institutions, nursing intervention also includes taking the necessary corrective measures as defined by the policies of the critical care unit. For example, a patient complains of extreme muscle weakness. The nurse notes excessive amounts of gastric drainage during the previous 24-hour period. The situation suggests hypokalemia, and the nurse orders a stat serum K^+ level. If the result is low, the nurse increases the potassium level in the dialysate from the standard 2 mEq/L to 3.5 mEq/L.

The nurse also monitors the patient for possible cardiac dysrhythmias during the procedure.

The electrolytes of main concern in dialysis, which normally are corrected during the procedure, are sodium, potassium, bicarbonate, calcium, phosphorus, and magnesium.

Serum Sodium

Although serum sodium extremes usually are not seen in the adequately dialyzed patient, thirst may indicate sodium excess. The patient who is thirsty because of excessive sodium intake will drink excessive amounts of water, which can lead to hypertension and fluid overload. Evaluation of sodium intake should be made in the patient who retains excessive amounts of fluid between dialyses. Again, the recommended weight gain is approximately 2.2 lb (1 kg) for each day between dialysis. Shifts in sodium and water during hemodialysis may lead to muscle cramping. This can be alleviated by reducing the flow rate and ultrafiltration, or supplementing the serum osmolality with an intravenous medication. Preparations frequently used to relieve muscle cramping include hypertonic saline, sodium bicarbonate, and 50% dextrose.

Potassium

Rapid correction of serum potassium in either direction should be avoided. Rapid lowering of the potassium level during dialysis can lead to hypokalemia, to increased effects of digitalis, and possibly to serious and sometimes fatal dysrhythmias. The potassium level in the bath is kept at 2 to 3.5 mEq/L, whichever is more appropriate for the individual patient. Patients with overt or potential problems should be monitored for cardiac function during dialysis.

Bicarbonate

Bicarbonate protects the body from excessive acid loads. Normal concentration varies between 25 and 30 mEq/L.

In uremia, the bicarbonate is depleted because it has been used to buffer the acidosis resulting from the inability of the kidneys to excrete acids. Acidosis in the uremic patient who has not been started on dialysis is corrected by administration of sodium bicarbonate.

During dialysis, acidosis is corrected by addition of either acetate or bicarbonate to the dialysate. Acetate diffuses into the blood, where it is metabolized to form bicarbonate. This used to be the most common form of base buffer used in dialysis concentrates, but it has been shown that some patients are either intolerant of the acetate itself or unable to use it effectively as a buffer. Acetate intolerance is exhibited by impairment of the cardiac contractile force, which leads to a drop in blood pressure as well as nausea, vomiting, headache, and other neurologic symptoms.

Because dialysis of the critically ill patient can be complicated further by these symptoms, bicarbonate dialysis usually is used. Depending on the type of dialysis machinery used, the production of bicarbonate bath usually requires special equipment, concentrates, and procedures.

Calcium

The dialysate calcium is kept at 3 to 3.5 mEq/L to prevent the loss of calcium from the blood to the dialysate. Dialysis, however, does not seem to correct the bone problems that occur in the chronic patient as a result of calcium–phosphorus imbalances (see Chapter 26). These must be controlled by a combination of dietary intervention and medications.

Phosphorus

In chronic renal failure, antacids or calcium compounds are used to bind phosphorus in the intestinal tract and prevent its absorption. The lowered serum phosphorus reduces the risk of calcium–phosphorus imbalances and resulting bone problems.

Aluminum-based hydroxide antacids such as Basaljel (Wyeth Laboratories, Philadelphia, PA) traditionally had been used to bind phosphorus. Evidence has shown, however, that constant exposure of the dialysis patient to aluminum in water used for dialysis or phosphate binders exacerbates bone disease and produces faulty mineralization. Subsequently, calcium compounds such as calcium carbonate and calcium acetate have been shown not only to supplement serum calcium levels but also to bind phosphorus.[4] These compounds now are the preferred method of phosphate control for chronic renal failure.

Phosphate binders usually are given during or after meals. A high serum phosphorus indicates to the nurse that the patient is not taking the phosphate binder or is taking it at the wrong times. Occasionally, patients with gastric distress will take too much of the binder because these also are used as antacids, in which case a very low phosphate level will be seen.

In either case, nursing interventions should include additional teaching and consultation with the physician, if needed.

Magnesium

Magnesium generally is maintained at an acceptable level with regular dialysis, but its intake should be limited so that symptoms of hypermagnesemia are avoided. Because it is difficult to reduce magnesium intake in the diet and provide palatable and nutritious meals, dietary limitations are problematic.

The regular use of magnesium-containing drugs should be avoided. Dialysis patients should be taught to avoid antacids or laxatives with a magnesium base such as Gelusil (Parke-Davis), milk of magnesia, or Maalox (Rorer Consumer Pharmaceuticals, Fort Washington, PA).

Infection

The uremic patient has a lowered resistance to infection, which is thought to be due to a decreased immunologic response. Therefore, all possible foci of infection should be eliminated. Indwelling urinary catheters and intracatheters should be removed as soon as possible, or their use should be avoided altogether. Strict aseptic technique is essential in catheterizations, venipunctures, catheter and wound dressings, and tracheal suctioning. Usual physiological responses to infection also may be altered in uremia. This effect is exhibited by a basal temperature that is lower than normal and by the absence of a usual temperature rise when infection is present.

Pulmonary infections are a leading cause of death in the acute uremic patient. Contributing factors include depression of the cough reflex and respiratory effort due to central nervous system disturbances, increased viscosity of pulmonary secretions due to dehydration and mouth breathing (especially in the unresponsive patient), and pulmonary congestion due to fluid overload. Fluid in the lungs not only acts as a medium for growing bacteria but also impedes respiratory excursion.

Nursing techniques that prevent or minimize pulmonary complications cannot be overlooked during the hemodialysis procedure. They include frequent turning, deep breathing and coughing, early ambulation, adequate humidification, hydration, tracheal aspiration, use of intermittent positive pressure machines, and oxygen therapy.

Oral hygiene is important because bleeding from the oral mucous membrane and the accumulation of dry secretions promote growth of bacteria in the mouth, which can lead to pneumonia.

Bleeding and Heparinization

Bleeding during dialysis may be due to an underlying medical condition such as an ulcer or gastritis or may be the result of excessive anticoagulation. Blood in the extracorporeal system, such as the dialyzer and blood lines, clots rapidly unless some method of anticoagulation is used. *Heparin* is the drug of choice because it is simple to administer, increases clotting time rapidly, is monitored easily, and may be reversed with protamine.

Specific heparinization procedures vary, but the primary goal in any method is to prevent clotting in the dialyzer with the least amount of heparin. Two methods commonly are used, intermittent and constant infusion. In both cases, an initial priming dose of heparin usually is given, followed by smaller doses either at intervals or at a constant rate by an infusion pump; the resulting effect is *systemic heparinization*, in which the clotting times of the patient and the dialyzer essentially are the same.

Absolute guidelines are difficult to provide because methods and dialyzer requirements vary. The normal clotting time of 6 to 10 minutes may be increased to the range of 30 to 60 minutes. The effect of heparin usually is monitored at the bedside by the activated clotting time or whole blood partial thromboplastin time. These tests have replaced the use of the Lee White method because they

can provide results in seconds, which gives the dialysis nurse the opportunity to make rapid adjustments in heparin administration.

Predialysis assessment of the patient's need for heparinization should be performed routinely to help determine an appropriate beginning heparin dose, especially in the critically ill patient who may be actively bleeding or have an increased potential for bleeding. The patient's platelet count, serum calcium level, and results of any coagulation studies are valuable in assessing current function of the clotting process. Often, little to no heparin can be used for the patient who already has serious derangements of one or more factors needed for effective clotting.

Systemic heparinization usually presents no risk unless the patient has overt bleeding (eg, gastrointestinal bleeding, epistaxis, or hemoptysis), is 3 to 7 days postsurgery, or has uremic pericarditis. In these situations, other methods to prevent clotting of the extracorporeal system can be used. With *regional heparinization*, the patient's clotting time is kept normal while that of the dialyzer is increased. This is accomplished by infusing heparin at a constant rate into the dialyzer and simultaneously neutralizing its effects with protamine sulfate before the blood returns to the patient.

Like systemic heparinization, regional heparinization has no associated standard heparin–protamine ratio. Frequent monitoring of the clotting times is the best way to achieve effective regional heparinization. Because of the rebound phenomenon that has been reported after regional heparinization and the use of activated coagulation time methods, many dialysis units have switched to low-dose heparinization, even in the presence of overt bleeding. With this method, minimal heparin doses are used throughout dialysis. Although some clotting may take place in the dialyzer, the small blood loss is preferable to the risk of profound bleeding.

Bleeding problems occasionally occur because of accidental heparin overdose. This may be caused by infusion pump malfunction or carelessness in setting the delivery rate. Because of the hazards, the importance of careful, frequent monitoring of heparin delivery cannot be overemphasized.

Recently, nurses have been instrumental in devising and perfecting other ways to prevent dialyzer clotting and reduce the risk of bleeding due to heparin use. Infusion of a very small initial heparin dose (eg, 250 U) and frequent normal saline flushes of the extracorporeal system can prevent clotting successfully for some patients.

Other dialysis centers are performing regional citrate anticoagulation in which citrate is infused into the system before the dialyzer binds calcium, obstructing the normal clotting pathway. The citrate–calcium complex is then cleared from the blood by the dialyzer, and the anticoagulant effect is reversed by infusion of calcium chloride before the blood returns to the patient. Although some problems are inherent in this type of anticoagulation, more experience may perfect its application and use by the dialysis community.

Troubleshooting

Equipment Problems

One of the major objectives of a dialysis unit is the prevention of complications resulting from the treatment itself. Hemodialysis involves the use of highly technical equipment. The efficiency of the dialysis, as well as the patient's comfort and safety, is compromised if both the patient and the equipment are not adequately monitored. Mechanical monitors provide a margin of safety but should not replace the observations and actions of the nurse.

Monitoring devices are designed to monitor many parameters, the most important of which are flow, concentration, and temperature of the dialysate, flow and leakage of blood, and air in the dialysis circuit. The design and operation of dialysis equipment and monitoring devices vary greatly; however, they have a common purpose.

Dialysate Flow

Inadequate dialysate flow will not harm the patient, but it will compromise dialysis efficiency. Flow is maintained at the rate recommended for the type of dialyzer, rate of blood flow, or method of dialysis being used. Traditionally dialysis flow is usually maintained at 500 ml/minute, although more rapid flows may be used in high-efficiency, short dialysis where blood flow rates also are high.

The nurse usually checks the flow at least every hour and makes adjustments as necessary.

Dialysate Concentrate

Sudden or rapid changes in dialysate concentration may result in red blood cell damage and cerebral disturbances. Mild symptoms include nausea, vomiting, and headache. In severe cases, convulsions, coma, and death may ensue. If a central delivery system is used to supply dialysis bath to several patients at the same time, the patients will manifest similar symptoms simultaneously. If this occurs, dialysate concentrate imbalance should be thought of immediately. If a patient is accidentally dialyzed against water or a hypotonic solution, hemolysis will occur, and the first symptom may be sudden severe pain in the returning vein. Because of hemolysis, blood will immediately appear a clear cherry red in the dialysis return lines. When this occurs, dialysis is discontinued at once.

In a single-delivery, proportioning system, monitoring devices are built into the system, and the concentrate is monitored continuously. If the concentrate exceeds the predetermined limits, dialysate automatically bypasses the dialyzer until the problem is corrected. The problem may have been caused by an interruption in the water or concentrate delivery. Inflow lines should be checked for kinking, and the concentrate container should be inspected for quantity.

In a central delivery system, the electrolyte concentration also is checked continuously by a meter that measures the electrical conductivity of the solution. If the solution exceeds the limits, the transfer valve is closed automatically so that no solution in unsafe concentrations is delivered to the bedside. The solution is bypassed, and a system of visual and audible alarms alerts dialysis personnel to problems. This alarm condition should not be reset to function unless the problem has been corrected.

Temperature

Most dialysate delivery systems use a heating element to maintain dialysate temperature at optimal levels (98°F to 101°F, or 36.7°C to 38.3°C). All modern systems include visual or audible alarms when preset temperature limits are violated.

Excessively cool temperatures may cause chilling and vessel spasm. Sometimes, chilling in the patient is the first indication of a drop in dialysate temperature. In some cases, lowering of the dialysis temperature to 36°C decreases the incidence of hypotension and other symptoms that can occur during rapid fluid removal. If this is successful, it must be balanced against the effects of chilling the patient.

High temperatures (over 101°F, or 38.3°C) may produce fever and discomfort in the patient, whereas extremely high temperatures (110°F, or 43.3°C) will cause hemolysis. Corrections should be made as soon as the temperature reaches 101°F (38.3°C).

Blood Flow

Monitoring adequate blood flow rate throughout dialysis is essential to dialysis efficiency. Hemodialysis usually requires a blood flow rate of 200 to 300 ml/minute in adult patients; a somewhat lower rate usually is prescribed for children or very frail geriatric patients. If high-efficiency, short dialysis is being used, blood flow rates are raised to 300 to 400 ml/minute to take advantage of high dialyzer clearance rates. Factors that influence blood flow rate are blood pressure, fistula and catheter function, and the extracorporeal circuit. A manometer connected to the drip chamber is used to measure the pressure in the blood lines. Changes in blood line pressures are transmitted to the drip chamber and register on the manometer as high- or low-pressure alarms.

A high-pressure alarm indicates a problem in the venous blood line, a clot in the venous needle or catheter, or a clotted vein. If clotting is suspected in any portion of the venous line or blood access, immediate flushing with normal saline solution may help to determine where the clot is and whether the clot can be removed, thereby reducing the pressure.

A low-pressure alarm reflects an obstruction to blood flow from the patient. Arterial spasm, clotting, displacement of a fistula needle, and a drop in blood pressure are possible causes. Correction again is directed to the cause.

Blood Leaks

A blood leak detector is invaluable when outflow dialysate is not visible, as in a single-pass delivery system. One type of blood leak detector is a color-sensitive photocell that picks up color variations in the outflow dialysate. Any foreign material, such as blood, will be detected, and an alarm will be set off. Because false alarms sometimes are set off by air bubbles, the nurse will check the dialysate visually for a gross leak and with a hemastix (Miles Inc., Diagnostic Division, Elkhart, IN) for smaller leaks.

Dialysis usually is discontinued immediately with a gross leak. Whether or not the blood is returned to the patient is either a matter of unit policy or a determination based on individual circumstances. If the patient is severely anemic, the risk of losing the blood in the dialyzer may outweigh the risk of a reaction to dialysate-contaminated blood. Sometimes minor leaks, in which there is no visible blood in the dialysate and only a small hemastix reaction, seal over, and dialysis is continued.

Air Embolism

The risk of air embolism is one of the most serious patient safety problems in the hemodialysis unit. Air can enter the patient's circulation through defective blood tubing, faulty blood line connections, vented intravenous fluid containers, or accidental displacement of the arterial needle.

The use of air and foam detectors and nonvented plastic fluid containers has minimized air embolus risks, but the prevention of potential problems by strict attention to technical details and visual monitoring cannot be overemphasized.

Access to Circulation

Successful repeated hemodialysis depends on access to the patient's circulation. Methods commonly used are the internal AV fistula, autografts or synthetic grafts, and central vein catheters.

Arteriovenous Fistula

The AV fistula technique was developed in 1966 by Cimino and Brescia in an effort to provide long-term use of an access for hemodialysis. Although the AV shunt had been used since 1960, complications such as clotting and infection limited its long-term availability for some patients.

To create the AV fistula, the surgeon anastomoses an artery and a vein, creating a fistula or artificial opening between them. Arterial blood flowing into the venous system results in marked dilation of the veins, which are then punctured easily with dialysis fistula needles, usually 15- or 16-gauge in size. Two venipunctures are made at the time of dialysis, one for a blood source and one for a return.

The arterial needle is inserted toward the fistula to obtain the best blood flow, but the tip should not be placed closer than 2.5 to 4 cm from the fistula. A traumatic puncture might lead to damage and closure of the fistula. The venous needle is directed away from the fistula in the direction of normal venous flow. It may be placed in the vessel, in another vein in the same arm, or even in another extremity.

If both needles are inserted into the same vessel, the tips should be at least 8 to 10 cm apart to avoid mixing of the blood, which would result in inadequate dialysis. If it is necessary to place the needles close to each other, a tourniquet applied between the two needles may help prevent mixing.

Fistulated veins that have not matured well present a challenge to dialysis nurses, whose goals are successful venipuncture and adequate blood flow rate. Inadequate arterial flow from AV fistula due to vessel immaturity is a common problem for these patients. Appropriate interventions include increased exercise of the fistulated arm, application of warm soaks to the arm during dialysis, and investigation of fistula revision if other measures fail.

Once the suture lines from the operative procedure have healed, care of the AV fistula is relatively uncomplicated. Normal showering or bathing with soap provides adequate skin cleansing. Traumatic venipunctures or repetition in the same site should be avoided because these lead to excessive bleeding, hematoma, and scar formation. Excessive manipulation and adjustment of the needles also should be avoided for the same reasons. Postdialysis care includes adequate pressure on the puncture sites after the needles are removed.

Most AV fistulas are developed and ready to use in 1 to 3 months after surgery. Patients are taught to exercise the arm after initial healing has occurred to assist in vessel maturation. They also are encouraged to become familiar with the quality of the "thrill" felt at the site of anastomosis so that they can report any deviation in its presence or strength.

Blood pressures and venipunctures should *not* be done on the arm with the fistula. A loud, swishing sound termed the *bruit* indicates a functioning fistula.

Although AV fistulas usually have a long life, complications can occur. These include thrombosis, aneurysm or pseudoaneurysm, or arterial insufficiency causing a "steal syndrome." This syndrome occurs when shunting of blood from the artery to the vein produces ischemia of the hand, causing pain or coldness in the hand. Surgical intervention can remedy all of these problems and restore adequate fistula flow.

Autografts

When suitable veins are not available for creation of an AV fistula, one alternative is use of a portion of the patient's own saphenous vein for fistula construction. A portion of this vein can be transplanted to another extremity and interposed between an available artery and vein. If the patient's arms already have been used for previous access surgeries, the thigh may be used with the saphenous vein attached to one or both femoral vessels. This is a technique used sometimes when smaller vessels cannot provide adequate blood flow to maintain access patency.

Autografts are not used frequently because of the availability of synthetic grafts. Although use of the patient's vein avoids problems encountered with foreign graft material, some centers have found that the saphenous vein cannot withstand the abuse of hemodialysis.

Synthetic Grafts

As an alternative to autograft use, synthetic grafts were developed in response to a need for blood access in those patients with inadequate blood vessels of their own. The synthetic material currently used is polytetrafluoroethylene (PTFE), a prosthetic material manufactured from an expanded, highly porous form of Teflon. The graft is anastomosed between an artery and a vein. After a suitable healing period, the vessel is used in the same manner as an AV fistula.

PTFE grafts have been shown to be extremely valuable for many patients whose own vessels are not adequate for fistula formation. PTFE segments also are used to patch areas of AV grafts or fistulas that have stenosed or developed areas of aneurysm. It is preferable to avoid venipuncture in new PTFE grafts while growth of the patient's tissue into the graft is occurring, which usually lasts 2 to 4 weeks. If tissue growth is allowed to progress satisfactorily, the graft has an endothelium and wall composition similar to the patient's own vessels.

The procedures for prevention of complications in grafts are the same as those used for AV fistulas; however, certain complications are seen more frequently with grafts than with fistulas, including thrombosis, infection, aneurysm formation, and stenosis at the site of anastomosis.

Dual-Lumen Central Vein Catheters

Catheters inserted into large veins are used for hemodialysis when no other means of access to the circulation are available. Veins commonly used are the subclavian, femoral, or internal jugular vein. The site chosen depends on the patient's anatomy and vein accessibility, as well as the physician's experience and site preference. Dual-lumen central vein catheters also are used temporarily for acute dialysis patients who are critically ill or chronic patients who are waiting for a more permanent access to mature. The advantages of large-vein catheters are that they can be inserted at the bedside and do not produce permanent vessel alteration. Although usually thought of as a temporary means, subclavian or internal jugular vein catheters

are being used by some centers as a permanent means of access in patients in whom there is absolutely no other available vascular route of access and in whom peritoneal dialysis is contraindicated. These catheters frequently include an implantable Dacron cuff that adheres to subcutaneous tissue to provide a barrier to infection.

Subclavian vein catheters (SVC) have gained wide acceptance as a temporary means of access because the location is more accessible, and there are fewer complications than with femoral vein catheters. It even is possible to send patients home with a SVC in place, once careful instruction is given. Subclavian catheters are available with either a single lumen for use with a single-needle device or a double lumen, which provides avenues for both blood supply and blood return (Fig. 24–3). Insertion of the SVC is similar to that for any central line and must be performed by an experienced physician so that complications such as pneumothorax and pulmonary embolization are avoided. Proper placement of the SVC always should be verified by chest film before dialysis is initiated.

Although the SVCs have numerous advantages, evidence is mounting to show that they cause stenosis in the subclavian vein, which can thwart future efforts to create fistulas or grafts in the affected side. For this reason, use of the internal jugular vein for temporary access is growing in favor.[5]

The internal jugular vein is used routinely in some centers, especially for insertion of permanent catheters such as the Hemocath or Hickman catheter (Bard Access Division, Salt Lake City, UT). Although the right internal jugular vein is preferred, the left internal jugular vein or right external jugular vein also can be used. A softer catheter can be used for insertion into the jugular vein in contrast to the subclavian vein, allowing for longer use and avoiding problems such as pneumothorax. Central vein thromboses also are less common, as are catheter kinking and poor flow, which can occur frequently with more rigid SVCs.

Whenever central vein catheters are used, care must be taken to avoid accidental slippage and dislodgement during hemodialysis. Femoral catheters usually are secured to the leg with tape; SVCs and jugular catheters are sutured to the skin. The length of time for which catheters are left in place depends on catheter function and policy of the physician or institution or both. Subclavian vein catheters generally can be used for up to 3 to 4 weeks, but femoral

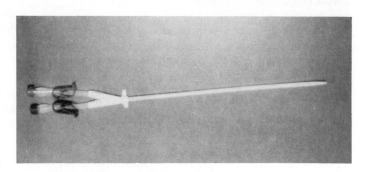

FIGURE 24–3
Dual-lumen subclavian catheter.

catheters usually are removed within 24 to 48 hours after insertion to avoid infection. More permanent internal jugular vein catheters often function for up to 9 months before problems force their removal. Catheters left in place between dialysis treatments usually are filled with a concentrated heparin–saline solution after dialysis and plugged to prevent clotting. Cleansing and dressing of the insertion site are the same as with other central lines. These catheters should *never* be used for any purpose other than hemodialysis without first checking with dialysis unit personnel.

If the catheters are removed at the end of dialysis, pressure is applied to the puncture sites until complete clotting occurs. The site is checked for several hours thereafter so that any recurrent bleeding can be detected.

Removal of the more permanent internal jugular Hemocath or Hickman catheter requires use of local anesthetic at the exit site and careful dissection around the Dacron cuff to free it from the attached subcutaneous tissue. Table 24–1 lists the care of the hemodialysis access.

Use of Streptokinase/Urokinase

One of the more exciting advances made in preserving vascular access is the use of streptokinase or urokinase to dissolve clots in either internal vascular accesses or external catheters. These enzymes, derived from streptococcal bacteria, are capable of activating the fibrinolytic system and dissolving intravascular thrombi. Experience with these enzymes has shown that their use can limit the need for surgery or catheter reinsertion.

Despite these advantages, there are risks and side

TABLE 24–1
Care of the Hemodialysis Access

AV Fistula or Graft
1. No blood pressures or blood drawing from the access limb.
2. Listen for bruit and palpate for thrill each shift.
3. No tight clothing or restraints on the access limb.
4. In the event of postdialysis bleeding from the needle site, apply just enough pressure to stop the flow of blood and hold till bleeding stops. NEVER occlude the vessel.
5. Hypotension can predispose to clotting; therefore, check more frequently for patency.

Dual-Lumen Access Catheter
1. Subclavian and internal jugular vein catheters must have placement verified radiographically before use.
2. A central line dressing is used to cover the insertion site and is cared for according to institutional policy.
3. Both limbs of the catheter usually are filled with concentrated heparin; therefore, *never* inject any other medication into the catheter.
4. *Never unclamp the catheter*—this can cause blood to back up into the lumen and clot.

effects inherent in the use of streptokinase and urokinase. These include local pain, bleeding, and an allergic response (eg, fever, chills). In addition, there is a substantial expense incurred with the use of these drugs. Continued experience and refinement of these enzymes may increase their usefulness on a more routine basis when thrombosis occurs.

Continuous Renal Replacement Therapies

Hemodialysis often is difficult to perform on the hemodynamically unstable patient, or on the patient who needs more than the usual 3- to 4-hour treatment to correct the metabolic imbalances of ARF. Continuous renal replacement therapies offer an alternative to hemodialysis in the critical care setting.

Continuous renal replacement therapy describes circulation of the blood outside the body through a highly porous filter. Much as in hemodialysis, water, electrolytes, and small- to middle-sized molecules are removed by ultrafiltration. This process occurs over an extended period of time, with the patient's arterial pressure usually serving as the driving force for blood passage through the extracorporeal circuit, although in some cases a blood pump is used to expedite the process (Fig. 24–4).[6]

Continuous renal replacement therapies ideally are used for patients with a high risk for hemodynamic instability who would not tolerate the rapid fluid shifts occurring with hemodialysis, and for those who require large amounts of hourly intravenous fluids or parenteral nutrition. The various continuous renal replacement therapy options can be performed by critical care nurses who are not trained in hemodialysis.

Continuous arteriovenous hemofiltration (CAVH) and continuous arteriovenous hemodialysis (CAVHD) both require arterial and venous access sites. Arterial pressure propels blood through the extracorporeal circuit, which includes tubing and the hemofilter. The tubing is short to minimize extracorporeal volume and should come equipped with a heparin infusion line and lines for replacement fluid both before and after the filter. For the process to be successful, the patient's mean arterial pressure should be greater than 70 mm Hg and hematocrit less than 40%.[6,7] Blood will flow through the filter at a rate of 40 to 90 ml/minute, yielding about 500 ml/hour of fluid. A hemodynamically compromised patient normally cannot tolerate this amount of fluid shift, so fluid replacement generally is ordered based on a net fluid loss goal. Replacement fluid is likely to be customized for the patient and may be infused either before or after the filter, depending on institutional practice.

Peritoneal dialysate can be added to the CAVH filter, where it remains separated from blood in the filter by the semipermeable membrane. Similar to hemodialysis, this process, now called CAVHD, yields removal of small molecules, depending on their concentration gradient. Con-

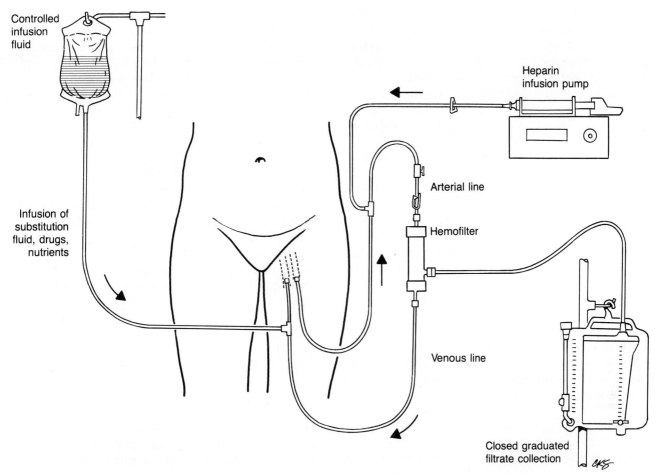

Controlled infusion fluid

Infusion of substitution fluid, drugs, nutrients

Heparin infusion pump

Arterial line

Hemofilter

Venous line

Closed graduated filtrate collection

FIGURE 24–4
Continuous arteriovenous hemofiltration.

tinuous arteriovenous hemodialysis is used when aggressive management of uremia is necessary, as with the highly catabolic patient. Nursing management is similar to that in CAVH; however, the nurse must keep track of the exact amount of dialysate that flows through the hemofilter and subtract this number from the fluid in the collection device to determine the total quantity of fluid removed from the patient.

Both CAVH and CAVHD depend on adequate arterial blood flow and blood pressure. Clearances of substances from the blood as well as fluid removal will increase or decrease in proportion to blood flow. Slow blood flow also greatly increases the risk of clotting the filter, which will be obvious when the rate of ultrafiltration diminishes while blood flow remains constant. To solve some of these problems, continuous venovenous hemofiltration (CVVH) and continuous venovenous hemodialysis (CVVHD) have been developed and are in widespread use in Europe.[8]

In CVVH, a dual-lumen access catheter is placed in one of the subclavian, internal jugular, or femoral veins to provide blood flow. A blood pump is added to the circuit to assist blood flow and maintain it at a rate of 100 to 150 ml/minute. This system is reported to manage uremia and remove fluid without the problems of clotted filters and the risks of arterial cannulation. The addition of dialysate to the circuit (CVVHD) increases the ability to remove uremic wastes. Disadvantages include an added piece of equipment which incorporates the blood pump, a venous pressure monitor, and an air leak detector. Critical care nurses will need some education to operate the equipment, but once learned, CVVH or CVVHD is said to be managed easily by the nursing staff.[9]

Hemodialysis Use With Other Therapies

The technical equipment and knowledge needed to perform hemodialysis often are applied to other therapies that involve an extracorporeal blood process, such as hemoperfusion and therapeutic apheresis. Although they are not used for the treatment of renal failure, nephrologic personnel often are recruited to perform these techniques, because the principles of altering blood components outside of the body are similar to those used in hemodialysis.

Hemoperfusion is used primarily for the treatment of drug overdose. Blood is pumped from the body and perfused through a column of charcoal or other absorbent materials. These bind the drug, leading to a rapid reduction in serum levels and avoiding potential tissue damage caused by an abnormally high drug level. This therapy is particularly useful for drugs that are fat bound or whose molecular structure is too large to be removed by hemodialysis. A hemodialysis blood pump and air detector often are used with hemoperfusion cartridges and tubing to perform the procedure.

Therapeutic plasma exchange, or apheresis, is another therapy that can be performed using standard hemodialysis equipment and supplies in conjunction with a plasma separator cell and replacement fluids. Apheresis is used to treat diseases caused or complicated by circulating immune complexes or other abnormal proteins. During the procedure, whole blood is separated into its major components, with subsequent removal of one or more of the offending components.

Hemodialysis also has been performed during cardiopulmonary bypass, allowing for expeditious surgery without waiting for preoperative dialytic stabilization. Although not yet common, this combination of extracorporeal therapies is one example of performing hemodialysis while blood already is being treated outside of the body for another patient need.

Psychological Aspects

The psychological impact of ARF is quite different from that of chronic renal failure. Even though the patient depends on a machine in both situations, the expectation in ARF is that the patient may recover renal function. Thus, concerns usually focus on the discomfort associated with insertion of the temporary vascular access and the dialysis treatment itself. Once these situations are dealt with, the patient and family then must cope with the uncertainty of how long renal failure will last and how long dialysis will be necessary.

Patients with chronic renal failure must deal with the fact that renal replacement therapy will be necessary for the rest of their lives. It is not uncommon for patients to deny a great deal of what is happening to them at first. This may continue over time and prevent some patients from accepting necessary aspects of their medical regimen. Other patients who feel considerably better after starting dialysis may enter a "honeymoon phase" and appear quite euphoric for a while. It is hoped that the normal grieving stages of depression will be followed by acceptance, with patients using their own coping mechanisms to deal with the chronicity of their treatment.

Issues of dependence versus independence also exist because the patient relies on equipment and personnel to maintain life. Education about their disease and involvement in the planning and implementation of care help most patients combat feelings of dependence and become motivated to keep themselves as well as possible. These aspects are outlined in Nursing Care Plan 24–1.

Peritoneal Dialysis

Description

Peritoneal dialysis and hemodialysis accomplish the same function and operate on the same principle of diffusion. In peritoneal dialysis, however, the peritoneum is the semipermeable membrane, and osmosis is used to effect fluid removal, rather than the pressure differentials used in hemodialysis.

Intermittent peritoneal dialysis is an effective alternative method of treating ARF when hemodialysis is not available or when access to the bloodstream is not possible. It sometimes is used as an initial treatment for renal failure while the patient is being evaluated for a hemodialysis program (Table 24–2).

Clinical Research

Rydholm L, Pauling J: Contrasting feelings of helplessness in peritoneal and hemodialysis patients: A pilot study. ANNA J 18:183–187, 1991

The purpose of this study was to compare levels of helplessness perceived by continuous ambulatory peritoneal dialysis (CAPD) versus hemodialysis patients. A newly developed tool, the Learned Helplessness Scale, was used to measure perceptions of the nursing diagnosis "helplessness." Working with only a small sample of patients, the authors administered the tool and found that hemodialysis patients experience a significantly higher degree of helplessness than do their CAPD counterparts. Although not implicating hemodialysis as the cause of helplessness, the results imply that patients receiving chronic hemodialysis may be in greater need of nursing interventions that foster a perceived sense of control. Descriptions of behaviors supporting the nursing diagnosis of "helplessness" also are included. Suggestions are offered for nursing interventions that might foster perceived control in the care of the hemodialysis patient.

NURSING DIAGNOSIS	OUTCOME CRITERIA/ PATIENT GOALS	NURSING INTERVENTIONS
Fluid volume deficit: related to effect of ultrafiltration during dialysis.	• Patient will remain hemodynamically stable during and after hemodialysis.	1. Assess vital signs, central venous pressure (CVP) readings (if available), breath sounds, heart sounds, weight, and intake and output predialysis.
		2. Assess degree of fluid accumulation in tissues predialysis.
		3. Determine appropriate degree and rate of ultrafiltration for the treatment.
		4. Monitor response to ultrafiltration (BP every $1/2$ hr or more often, apical rate and CVP readings as indicated).
		5. Adjust degree and rate of ultrafiltration according to patient response.
		6. Administer replacement fluids, as ordered and indicated.
		7. Consult with physician to adjust or institute vasoactive drug if indicated.
		8. Consult with physician to consider use of plasma expanders if hypotension persists and edema is present.
		9. Check levels of K^+, Na^+, Ca^{++}, and CO_2 predialysis.
		10. Consult with physician if serum levels indicate need for change in dialysate bath components.
		11. Observe patient for signs of hypokalemia (ECG changes, muscle weakness).
		12. Observe for intolerance to fluid removal if bath sodium level lower than serum level (cramps, hypotension).
		13. Observe for signs of acetate intolerance if bicarbonate bath is not used or unavailable (hypotension, nausea, backache).
		14. Allow time for equilibrium between blood and tissue spaces if postdialysis serum levels are ordered.
		15. Record predialysis and postdialysis weights.

(continued)

NURSING CARE PLAN 24–1: (Continued)
The Patient Undergoing Hemodialysis

NURSING DIAGNOSIS	OUTCOME CRITERIA/ PATIENT GOALS	NURSING INTERVENTIONS
Knowledge deficit: related to illness and need for dialysis.	• Patient and family will state realistic expectation for recovery of renal function.	1. Assess patient's or family's level of knowledge regarding kidney function, disease, reasons for dialysis, and prospect for recovery. 2. Assess ability and readiness to learn. 3. Identify barriers to learning. 4. Provide information appropriate to readiness and ability to learn, including major functions of kidney; reasons for patient's loss of function; signs and symptoms related to renal function loss; objectives of current treatment plan, including dialysis; realistic prospects for recovery of renal function. 5. Encourage verbalization of questions, fears, anxiety.
Powerlessness: related to feelings of lack of control, dependency on dialysis, chronicity of disease.	• Patient will describe realistic expectations regarding return of kidney function and need for dialysis.	1. Spend time discussing patient's feelings; reassure that such feelings are normal. 2. Support patient and family through grieving process. 3. Explore with patient and family successful coping mechanisms used in past; assist with use of these in current situation. 4. Offer and obtain assistance from other health professionals as necessary. 5. Teach and reinforce information about disease process and need for dialysis. 6. Assist patient in remaining oriented to reality; remain optimistic that renal function will return if appropriate. 7. Encourage patient to be involved in learning and following dialysis-related care if this will enhance feelings of control. 8. Plan for the same nurses to care for the patient.

(continued)

NURSING CARE PLAN 24–1: *(Continued)*
The Patient Undergoing Hemodialysis

NURSING DIAGNOSIS	OUTCOME CRITERIA/ PATIENT GOALS	NURSING INTERVENTIONS
High risk for injury: related to vascular access and complications secondary to insertion and maintenance of vascular access.	• Patient will be free from complications after catheter insertion.	1. Maintain sterile environment during catheter insertion.
		2. Obtain chest radiograph after subclavian vein catheter insertion. Observe for signs of pneumothorax, cardiac irregularities, excessive bleeding. Check for bilateral breath sounds.
		3. Change catheter dressings routinely per unit policy.
		4. Maintain sterile technique in handling vascular access.
		5. Observe catheter exit site routinely for signs of inflammation, purulent drainage, catheter kinking.
		6. Assess catheter for patency at least q2d.
		7. Heparinize catheter between dialysis treatments per unit policy.
		8. Notify physician of observed complications.
		9. Do not use hemodialysis access catheters for intravenous fluids/medications.
High risk for fluid volume deficit: related to blood loss or inappropriate heparinization during dialysis.	• Excessive bleeding of catheter site, wounds, or mucous membranes will not occur.	1. Assess integrity of patient's coagulation system predialysis (eg, platelet count, prothrombin time, partial thromboplastin time, history of recent bleeding).
		2. Use low-dose regional heparinization if there is evidence of actual or potential bleeding.
		3. Obtain bedside clotting time values predialysis and frequently during dialysis to assess degree of heparinization needed.
		4. Visually assess patency of extracorporeal system frequently during dialysis.
		5. Adjust heparin, as ordered.

(continued)

NURSING CARE PLAN 24–1: (Continued)
The Patient Undergoing Hemodialysis

NURSING DIAGNOSIS	OUTCOME CRITERIA/ PATIENT GOALS	NURSING INTERVENTIONS
High risk for fluid volume deficit: related to technical problems during dialysis resulting in blood loss.	• Blood loss due to technical problems with the extracorporeal circuit will be absent or minimal.	1. Ensure that dialyzer and line connections are secure before initiating dialysis. 2. Educate patient about role in keeping connection between vascular access and dialysis lines intact. 3. Provide constant visual and audible monitoring of patient and dialysis system. 4. Use techniques to minimize blood loss if integrity of dialysis system is broken.
High risk for injury: related to air embolism.	• Symptoms of air embolism will be absent during dialysis: shortness of breath, cyanosis, loss of consciousness.	1. Ensure adequate clamping of all potential air entry ports during dialysis. 2. Use proper techniques when initiating or terminating dialysis and when administering solutions or medications during the procedure. 3. Ensure that air detector is armed and functioning properly during dialysis. 4. Use appropriate emergency interventions if air embolism is suspected: stop infusion of air and clamp blood lines; position patient on left side with head lower than chest; administer oxygen; notify physician.
High risk for injury: related to inappropriate dialysate concentration or temperature.	• Patient will receive dialysis using correct solutions at proper temperatures.	1. Use safety measures designed to reduce the risk of and prevent dialysate error: check conductivity and temperature settings; verify that correct dialysate concentrate is being used; verify that machine alarms are functioning properly; set temperature parameters within appropriate limits. 2. Monitor vital signs and patient's general status throughout treatment. 3. Use appropriate emergency measures if symptoms due to dialysate error occur.

TABLE 24–2
Comparison of Hemodialysis and Peritoneal Dialysis as Treatment for Acute Renal Failure

	Peritoneal	Hemodialysis
Access	Peritoneal catheter	AV Arteriovenous fistula or graft, Dual-lumen venous catheter
Heparin requirements	Not required	Systemic
Length of treatment	Continuous or intermittent exchanges	3–4 hours, three to five times per week, depending on patient acuity
Complications	Peritonitis, dialysate leaks, exit site or tunnel infections, inability to infuse or drain, hernias	Hypotension, muscle cramps, bleeding, cardiac instability during treatment, clotted accesses, machine malfunction
Advantages	Continuous removal of wastes and fluid, better hemodynamic stability, fewer dietary restrictions	Quick, efficient removal of metabolic wastes and excess fluid; useful for overdoses and poisonings
Disadvantages	Contraindicated after abdominal surgery or in presence of many scars; removal of waste products may be too slow in a very catabolic patient	May require frequent vascular access procedures, places strain on a compromised cardiovascular system, potential blood loss from bleeding or clotted lines

Peritoneal dialysis has some advantages over hemodialysis. First, the required technical equipment and supplies are less complicated and more available. Second, there is less need for highly skilled personnel. Third, the adverse effects associated with the more efficient hemodialysis are minimized, which may be important in patients who cannot tolerate rapid hemodynamic changes, such as those with severe cardiac disease.

There also are a few disadvantages associated with peritoneal dialysis. It requires more time to remove metabolic wastes adequately and to restore electrolyte and fluid balance than does hemodialysis. In addition, repeated treatments may lead to peritonitis, and long periods of immobility may result in such complications as pulmonary congestion and venous stasis. Because fluid is introduced into the peritoneal cavity, peritoneal dialysis is contraindicated in patients who have existing peritonitis, in those who have undergone recent or extensive abdominal surgery, and in those who have abdominal adhesions. In the event of a cardiac arrest, the patient's abdomen should be drained immediately to maximize the efficiency of chest compressions.

Equipment Features

Solutions. As in hemodialysis, peritoneal dialysis solutions contain "ideal" concentrations of electrolytes but lack urea, creatinine, and other substances that are to be removed. Unlike dialysate used in hemodialysis, solutions must be sterile.

Dextrose concentrations of the solutions vary; a 1.5%, 2.5%, or 4.25% dextrose solution can be used. Use of 2.5% or 4.25% solutions usually is reserved for more fluid removal and occasionally for better solute clearance. Peritoneal dialysate usually contains no potassium, so potassium chloride may have to be added to the dialysate to prevent hypokalemia. The patient's serum potassium must be monitored closely to regulate the amount of potassium to be added.

Peritoneal dialysis administration set.

Peritoneal dialysis catheter set, which includes the catheter, a connecting tube for connecting the catheter to the administration set, and a metal stylet.

Trocar set of the physician's choice.

Ancillary drugs:
Local anesthetic solution—2% lidocaine
Aqueous heparin—1,000 units/ml
Potassium chloride
Broad-spectrum antibiotics

Procedure

Preliminary Steps

1. Prepare the patient for catheter insertion and the dialysis procedure by giving a thorough explanation of the procedure. A consent form may be signed according to hospital policy.

2. The bladder should be emptied just before the procedure to avoid accidental puncture with the trocar.
3. The patient may receive a preoperative medication to enhance relaxation during the procedure.
4. The dialyzing fluid is warmed to body temperature or slightly warmer, using a device manufactured solely for this purpose. It is not recommended that peritoneal dialysate be warmed in microwave ovens due to uneven heating of the fluid and inconsistency from one microwave to another.
5. Baseline vital signs, such as temperature, pulse, respirations, and weight, are recorded. An in-bed scale is ideal for frequent monitoring of the patient's weight, and so should be used if possible. Moving a lethargic or disoriented patient to a scale may create problems such as catheter displacement.
6. A physical assessment of the abdomen is performed, and a history of abdominal surgery or trauma is obtained before the catheter is inserted.
7. Specific orders regarding fluid removal, replacement, and drug administration should be written by the physician before the procedure.

Technique

Under sterile conditions, a small midline incision is made just below the umbilicus. A trocar is inserted through the incision into the peritoneal cavity. The obturator is removed and the catheter secured.

The dialysis solution flows into the abdominal cavity by gravity as rapidly as possible (5–10 minutes). If it flows in too slowly, the catheter may need repositioning. When the solution is infused, the tubing is clamped, and the solution remains in the abdominal cavity for 30 to 45 minutes. Next, the solution bottles or bags are placed below the abdominal cavity, and the fluid is drained out of the peritoneal cavity by gravity. If the system is patent and the catheter well placed, the fluid will drain in a steady, forceful stream. Drainage should take no more than 20 minutes.

This cycle is repeated continuously for the prescribed number of hours, which varies from 12 to 36, depending on the purpose of the treatment, the patient's condition, and the proper functioning of the system (Fig. 24–5).

Dialysis effluent is considered a contaminated fluid and gloves should be worn while handling it.

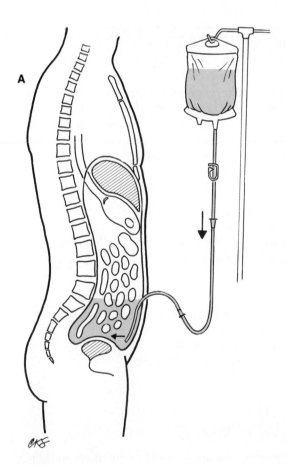
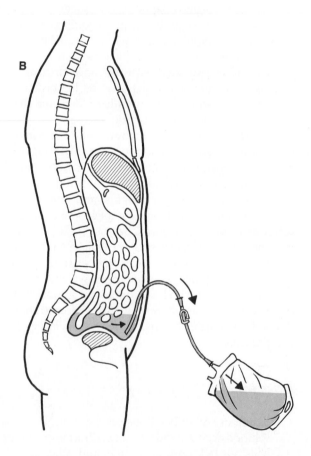

FIGURE 24–5
Periotoneal dialysis. (**A**) Dialysate flowing in. (**B**) Dialysate draining.

Automated Peritoneal Dialysis Systems

Automated peritoneal dialysis systems have built-in monitors and a system of automatic timing devices that cycle the infusion and removal of peritoneal fluid.

Automated peritoneal delivery systems are more appropriately used for chronic peritoneal dialysis in which a permanent, indwelling peritoneal catheter is used. Less sophisticated devices that minimize the necessity for manual bottle exchanges are more appropriate for the unit in which only an occasional peritoneal dialysis is performed.

Assessment and Management

Essential Features of Nursing Care

- *Maintaining accurate intake and output records as well as accurate records of weights* obtained from the same scale for assessment of volume depletion or overload.
- *Frequent monitoring of blood pressure and pulse.* Orthostatic blood pressure changes and increased pulse rate are valuable clues that help the nurse evaluate the patient's volume status.
- *Detecting signs and symptoms of peritonitis early.* Low-grade fever, abdominal pain, and cloudy peritoneal fluid all are possible signs of infection.
- *Maintaining the sterility of the peritoneal system.* Masks and sterile gloves must be worn while the abdominal dressing is being changed. Solution bags or bottles should be changed in as controlled a physical environment as possible to avoid contamination (eg, avoiding areas of high traffic and high air flow).
- *Detecting and correcting technical difficulties early* before they result in physiological problems. Slow outflow of the peritoneal fluid may indicate early problems with the patency of the peritoneal catheter.
- *Preventing the complications of bed rest* and providing an environment that will assist the patient in *accepting bed rest* for prolonged periods of time.
- *Preventing constipation.* Difficult or infrequent defecation will decrease the clearance of waste products and cause the patient more discomfort and distention.

Complications

Technical Complications

Incomplete Recovery of Fluid

The fluid that is removed should equal or exceed the amount inserted. Commercially prepared dialysate contains approximately 1,000 to 2,000 ml of fluid. If after several exchanges the volume drained is less (by 500 ml or more) than the amount inserted, an evaluation must be made.

Signs of fluid retention include abdominal distention or complaint of fullness. The most accurate indication of the amount of unrecovered fluid is weight.

If the fluid drains slowly, the catheter tip may be buried in the omentum or be clogged with fibrin. Turning the patient from side to side, elevating the head of the bed, and gently massaging the abdomen may facilitate drainage.

If fibrin or blood exists in the outflow drainage, heparin will need to be added to the dialysate. The specific dose, which is ordered by the physician, will be in the range of 5,000 to 1,000 U/L.

Leakage Around the Catheter

Superficial leakage after surgery may be controlled with extra sutures and a decrease in the amount of dialysate instilled into the peritoneum. Nursing studies have shown that increases in intra-abdominal pressure also may cause dialysate leaks. Therefore, continued vomiting, coughing, and jarring movements should be avoided during the initial postoperative period.

A catheter that is suspected of leaking should be corrected because it acts as a pathway for bacteria to enter the peritoneum. "High risk for infection . . . " is an appropriate nursing diagnosis in this situation. The abdominal dressing must be checked frequently so that any leakage can be detected. Dialysate leakage can be distinguished from other clear fluids by checking with a dextrose test strip. Because of the dextrose content in dialysate, this action will yield a positive result.

Blood-Tinged Peritoneal Fluid

This is expected in the initial outflow but should clear after a few passes. Gross bleeding at any time is an indication of a more serious problem and should be investigated immediately.

Physiological Complications

Peritonitis

This is a serious but manageable complication of peritoneal dialysis. Because peritonitis is a potential problem for any patient with a peritoneal catheter, it should be included on the patient's care plan. Early detection and initiation of treatment will lessen the patient's discomfort and prevent more serious complications.

Signs of peritonitis include low-grade fever, abdominal pain when fluid is being inserted, and cloudy peritoneal drainage fluid.

Treatment should begin as soon as a sample of peritoneal fluid is obtained. The specimen should be sent to the laboratory for culture and sensitivity. The patient then should be started on a broad-spectrum antibiotic, which usually is added to the dialysate solution, although it also can be given intravenously. Depending on the severity of the infection, the patient's condition should improve dramatically within 8 hours of initiation of antibiotic therapy.

Catheter Infection

During the daily dressing change, the exit site should be examined closely for signs of infection, such as tenderness, redness, and drainage around the catheter. In the absence of peritonitis, a catheter infection generally is treated with an oral, broad-spectrum antibiotic.

Hypotension

This complication may occur if excessive fluid is removed. Vital signs are monitored frequently, especially if a hypertonic solution is used. Lying and sitting blood pressure readings are especially useful in evaluation of fluid status. A progressive drop in blood pressure and weight should alert the nurse to the potential problem of fluid deficit.

Hypertension and Fluid Overload

These problems may occur if all the fluid is not removed in each cycle. An increase in weight requires an assessment of the catheter and dialysate solutions. The exact amount in the bottles should be noted. Some manufacturers add 50 ml to a 1,000-ml bottle. Over a period of hours, this can make a considerable difference.

The nurse should observe the patient for signs of respiratory distress, which may indicate pulmonary congestion. In the absence of other symptoms of fluid overload, hypertension may be the result of anxiety and apprehension. Reassurance of the patient and prompt correction of problems are preferable to the administration of sedatives and tranquilizers.

Blood Urea Nitrogen and Creatinine

Close monitoring of the serum blood urea nitrogen and creatinine will assist in the evaluation of the effectiveness of the dialysis. Inadequate clearance of waste products needs prompt attention.

Hypokalemia

This is a common complication of peritoneal dialysis. Close monitoring of the serum potassium will indicate the need to add potassium chloride to the dialysate as well as the amount to be added.

Glucose

Blood glucose levels should be monitored closely in patients with diabetes mellitus and hepatic disease, in addition to observing for signs of hypoglycemia or hyperglycemia. If needed, supplemental insulin can be added to the dialysate to control hyperglycemia.

Pain

Mild abdominal discomfort may be experienced by the patient at any time during the procedure and probably is related to the constant distention or chemical irritation of the peritoneum. If a mild analgesic does not provide relief, insertion of 5 ml of 2% lidocaine directly into the catheter may help.

The patient may be less uncomfortable if nourishment is given in small amounts, when the fluid is draining out rather than when the abdominal cavity is distended.

Severe pain may indicate more serious problems of infection or paralytic ileus. Infection is not likely in the first 24 hours. Aseptic technique and the use of prophylactic antibiotics minimize the risk of infection. Periodic cultures of the outflowing fluid will assist in the early detection of pathogenic organisms.

Immobility

Immobility may lead to hypostatic pneumonia, especially in the debilitated or elderly patient. Deep breathing, turning, and coughing should be encouraged during the procedure. Leg exercises and the use of elastic stockings may prevent the development of venous thrombi and emboli.

Discomfort

Because peritoneal dialysis results in slower clearance of waste products than does hemodialysis, it rarely is associated with the disequilibrium seen with hemodialysis. Because the treatment is longer, however, boredom is a frequent problem.

Nursing measures are directed toward making the patient as comfortable as possible. Diversions such as having visitors, reading, and watching television should be encouraged. Educating the patient about peritoneal dialysis and involving the patient in the care may reduce some of the anxiety and discomfort (see Nursing Care Plan 24–2).

Chronic Forms of Peritoneal Dialysis

Peritoneal dialysis has gained popularity as a chronic form of dialysis therapy, especially since *continuous ambulatory peritoneal dialysis* (CAPD) has become available. *Intermittent peritoneal dialysis* (IPD) has been used for chronic therapy for quite a few years, but it requires the patient to remain stationary for 10 to 14 hours three times per week. Because of this inconvenience to the patient and the increased staff time needed if this therapy is performed in-center, it seldom is used and is not available in many dialysis centers.

Continuous ambulatory peritoneal dialysis is taught easily to patients and does not limit ambulation between dialysate fluid exchanges. It uses the dialysis fluid that is continuously present in the peritoneal cavity, 24 hours a day, 7 days a week. Dialysis fluid is drained by the patient and replaced with fresh solution three to five times per day. The number of solution exchanges needed per day depends on the patient's individual needs. Although the patient is required to perform dialysis techniques every

NURSING CARE PLAN 24–2:
The Patient Undergoing Peritoneal Dialysis

NURSING DIAGNOSIS	OUTCOME CRITERIA/ PATIENT GOALS	NURSING INTERVENTIONS
Fluid volume excess: related to poor drainage, inaccurate fluid calculations, inappropriate use of hypotonic dialysate.	• Minimal positive fluid balance in dialysate exchanges will occur.	1. Calculate fluid balance accurately with each exchange. 2. Correct any possible drainage problems if positive fluid balance occurs. 3. Correlate all sources of fluid intake with output. 4. Assess vital signs frequently. 5. Assess respiratory status and evidence of peripheral edema. 6. If significant positive fluid balance occurs: limit fluid intake; decrease dwell times; consider the use of more hypertonic dialysate; weigh frequently; reassess frequently. 7. If respiratory status is impaired, dialyze in more upright position and decrease volume of dialysate.
Pain: related to air entry during catheter insertion, misplaced catheter, abdominal distention.	• Patient will not have abdominal discomfort.	1. After catheter insertion, observe for signs of bowel or bladder perforation if abdominal pain occurs. Signs and symptoms of bowel perforation include flatus or feces in effluent; diarrhea; abrupt onset of peritonitis. Signs and symptoms of bladder perforation are abrupt onset of polyuria; incomplete dialysate drainage; glycosuria (due to dextrose in dialysate mixed with urine). 2. If perforation is suspected, notify physician at once. Prepare for catheter removal and other appropriate therapy. 3. Pinpoint location of pain and level of severity during exchange process to help determine if catheter tip is misplaced (toward liver or on bladder or bowel). If so, pain will intensify during dialysate infusion.

(continued)

NURSING CARE PLAN 24–2: (Continued)
The Patient Undergoing Peritoneal Dialysis

NURSING DIAGNOSIS	OUTCOME CRITERIA/ PATIENT GOALS	NURSING INTERVENTIONS
		4. To avoid entrance of air into peritoneal cavity, keep all tubings primed and connections tight. Keep small reservoir of dialysate in peritoneal cavity until therapy is discontinued.
		5. If air is suspected, keep patient in upright position. Confirm air on radiograph if necessary. Assist patient to expel air by coughing or performing Valsalva maneuver while lying down, with dialysate inflow clamp closed and outflow clamp open.
High risk for infection: related to poor aseptic technique, break in dialysis system, catheter or tunnel infection, peritonitis.	• Patient will not acquire a nosocomial infection.	1. Maintain aseptic technique throughout dialysis procedure.
		2. Use sealed plastic dialysate bags instead of vented glass bottles.
		3. Change dialysis tubing regularly per protocol.
		4. Swab or soak tubing connections and injection ports with bactericidal solution before adding medications or breaking closed system.
		5. Assess patient continuously for signs and symptoms of peritonitis (pain, cloudy effluent, fever).
		6. Change exit site dressing daily using aseptic technique until healing occurs. Assess daily for increase in inflammation or drainage.
		7. If infection is suspected, obtain appropriate culture and begin antibiotic according to protocol or physician's order.
		8. Administer prophylactic antibiotics, as ordered.

day, CAPD is attractive to many end-stage renal disease patients because they can accomplish it easily and independently. It also may be the preferred therapy for patients who benefit from a slow, continuous removal of sodium and water, as in those with refractory congestive heart failure.

Another variation of chronic peritoneal dialysis therapy is *continuous cyclic peritoneal dialysis (CCPD)*. Patients who choose this form of therapy perform IPD at night during sleep using a cycling machine and in the morning instill dialysis fluid, which remains in the abdomen during the whole day. This is most convenient for those who require the help of working family members to perform their exchanges.

As with acute peritoneal dialysis, peritonitis is the greatest potential problem with chronic forms of dialysis. The peritoneal catheters that are used are permanent and inserted in the operating room. They have one or two Teflon cuffs that the surgeon sutures to the abdominal wall or subcutaneous tissue or both to anchor the catheter and provide a permanent seal against invading bacteria. Patients are taught how to recognize any potential problem associated with the catheter or treatment and to seek help from the CAPD team when needed.

Patients who perform IPD, CAPD, or CCPD at home generally visit the dialysis unit every 4 to 8 weeks. At this time, a nursing assessment is done, techniques are reviewed, and required blood studies are drawn. All health team members, including the physician, nurse, dietitian, and social worker, work together with the patient and family to ensure successful adaptation to the chosen mode of treatment.

REFERENCES

1. Schulman G, Hakim R: Recent advances in the biocompatibility of haemodialysis membranes. Nephrol Dial Transplant 6:14–17, 1991
2. Palmer BF: The effect of dialysate composition on systemic hemodynamics. Seminars in Dialysis 5:54–60, 1992
3. Keen M, Lancaster L, Binkley LS: Concepts and principles of hemodialysis. In Lancaster L (ed): Core Curriculum for Nephrology Nursing, 2nd ed., pp. 199–254. Pitman, NJ, AJ Jannetti, 1990
4. Schaefer K, Scheer J, Asmus G, Umlauf E, Hagemann J, von Herrath D: The treatment of uremic hyperphosphatemia with calcium acetate and calcium carbonate: A comparative study. Nephrol Dial Transplant 6:176–179, 1991
5. Schillinger F, Schillinger D, Montagnac R, Milicent T: Post catheterization vein stenosis in hemodialysis: Comparative angiographic study of 50 subclavian and 50 internal jugular accesses. Nephrol Dial Transplant 6:722–724, 1991
6. Price C: Continuous renal replacement therapy: The treatment of choice for acute renal failure. ANNA J 18:239–244, 1991
7. Brundage D: Surgical and therapeutic procedures. In Brundage D (ed): Renal Disorders, pp. 134–177. St. Louis, Mosby Year Book, 1992
8. Canaud B, Laurie JG, Christol JP, Aubas S, Beraud JJ, Mion C: Pump assisted continuous venovenous hemofiltration for treating acute uremia. Kidney Int 33(Suppl 24):s154–s156, 1988
9. Wedon F, Smithles M, Sheppard K, Bullen J, Tinkes J, Bihari D: Continuous high volume venous-venous haemofiltration in acute renal failure. Intensive Care Med 15:358–363, 1989

BIBLIOGRAPHY

Covalesky R: Myths and facts . . . about peritoneal dialysis. Nursing 20(4):91, 1990
Gallagher NM: Peritoneal dialysis: Monitoring and evaluating therapy, review of clinical indicators and use of data collection tools. ANNA J 18:284–287, 1991
Lancaster L (ed): Core Curriculum for Nephrology Nursing, 2nd ed. Pitman, NJ, AJ Jannetti, 1990
Levine D (ed): Care of the Renal Patient, 2nd ed. Philadelphia, WB Saunders, 1991
Maher J (ed): Replacement of Renal Function by Dialysis, 3rd ed. Boston, Kluwer Academic Publishers, 1989
Nissenson A, et al (eds): Clinical Dialysis. Norwalk, CT, Appleton and Lange, 1990
Stark JL: Dialysis options in the critical ill patient: Hemodialysis, peritoneal dialysis, continuous renal replacement therapy. Critical Care Nursing Quarterly 14(4):40–44, 1992

STUDY QUESTIONS

1. Which statement about hemodialysis is *not* true?

   a. it is indicated in acute renal failure
   b. it cannot restore the level of electrolytes in the body
   c. it removes excess body water by effecting a pressure differential between the blood and fluid compartments
   d. it can restore the body buffer system

2. Which components of the predialysis assessment must the nurse consider when establishing treatment objectives?

   1. review of patient history
   2. most recent laboratory reports
   3. response to previous dialysis treatment
   4. nurse's observations of the patient

      a. 1 and 2
      b. 1, 2, and 4

  c. all of the above
  d. none of the above

3. Which statements about hemodialysis technique are true?

   1. access to the bloodstream is necessary to initiate treatment
   2. at the end of treatment, all blood is discarded
   3. there is no way to prevent air from entering the bloodstream—the nurse therefore must be very vigilant
   4. the portion of the dialysis circuit before the dialyzer is called the arterial side

      a. all of the above
      b. none of the above
      c. 1 and 4
      d. 1, 2, and 4

4. The term *dry* or *ideal* weight refers to

   a. an absolute measure of the patient's weight
   b. the patient's weight without clothes on
   c. the patient's weight with clothes on
   d. the weight at which fluid volume is in normal range for a patient who is free of symptoms of fluid imbalance

5. Continuous renal replacement therapies are used when

   a. hemodialysis presents high risk for hemodynamic instability
   b. rapid removal of fluid is desired
   c. the patient's blood pressure is lower than normal
   d. high blood flows are desired

6. Which electrolyte would be increased in the dialysate if the patient has had excessive gastric drainage over the past 24 hours and complains of muscle weakness?

   a. bicarbonate
   b. calcium
   c. sodium
   d. potassium

7. Which statement about heparinization during hemodialysis is *not* true?

   a. the primary goal of any heparinization method is to prevent clotting in the dialyzer
   b. any amount of heparin may be used as long as the nurse monitors activated clotting times
   c. protamine may be used to reverse the effects of heparin
   d. little or no heparin can be used for the patient who has underlying derangements of clotting factors

8. Which statement about AV fistulas and grafts is *not* true?

   a. blood pressures may be taken in the arm with the graft or fistula
   b. steal syndrome from the shunting of blood from an artery to a vein produces ischemia in the limb distal to the fistula
   c. a 2- to 4-week waiting period is recommended before performing venipuncture on a graft
   d. presence of a bruit and thrill indicates that the fistula or graft is functioning

9. Peritoneal dialysis would be an appropriate choice if

    a. the patient is dangerously hyperkalemic
    b. pulmonary edema is present
    c. severe cardiac disease is present
    d. the patient has had multiple abdominal surgeries

10. An appropriate intervention for cloudy peritoneal drainage would be

    a. infuse another bag of dialysate, wait 4 hours, and carefully observe the next drainage
    b. send a specimen of the fluid to the laboratory for culturing and sensitivity tests
    c. begin oral antibiotics
    d. do nothing—cloudiness is normal

CHAPTER 25

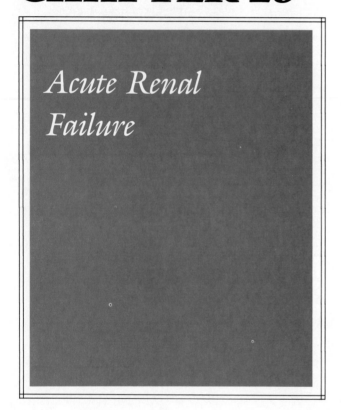

Acute Renal Failure

Hudak: Critical Care Nursing:
A Holistic Approach, 6th ed. © 1994
J. B. Lippincott Company.

BEHAVIORAL OBJECTIVES

BEHAVIORAL OBJECTIVES

Based on the content in this chapter, the reader should be able to:

1. Demonstrate knowledge of the causes of acute renal failure (ARF).
2. Describe urine production during the nonoliguric, oliguric, and diuretic stages of ARF.
3. Identify the clinical manifestations of hypoperfusion that can lead to ARF: decreased cardiac output, altered peripheral vascular resistance, and hypovolemia and hemorrhage.
4. Identify the clinical manifestations of ARF according to their categories: prerenal, intrarenal, and postrenal.
5. Discuss nursing assessment parameters used to identify the alteration in ARF.
6. Develop a nursing care plan for managing the shock and postshock states of ARF.

Description

Acute renal failure (ARF) refers to the sudden (hours to a few days) loss of renal function characterized by an increase in blood urea nitrogen (BUN) and serum creatinine. Although no exact criteria for BUN and creatinine can be set, an increase in BUN from 15 to 30 mg/dl and a rise in creatinine from 1 to 2 mg/dl suggest ARF in patients with preexisting normal renal function. In patients with preexisting renal disease, larger variations may be required to suggest the diagnosis because small changes in renal function, not related to ARF, may be magnified when nephron loss already is present. Early awareness of the diagnosis, however, is critical because of the persistent high mortality rate (60%–65%) associated with ARF despite the general availability of hemodialysis.

Categories of Renal Failure

Acute renal failure is classified into three general categories, according to the precipitating factors and the symptoms manifested by the disease. These categories are prerenal, intrarenal, and postrenal. The ability to distinguish among these categories is essential to the nurse.

Prerenal

Prerenal causes of ARF include physiological events that result in decreased circulation (ischemia) to the kidneys. Most commonly, these include hypovolemia and cardiovascular failure; however, any other event that leads to an acute decrease in the oxygenation of the kidneys can fall into this category, which sometimes is described as prerenal azotemia (Table 25–1).

TABLE 25–1
General Categories of Acute Renal Failure

Prerenal Failure	Intrarenal Failure	Postrenal Failure
Dehydration	Acute glomerulonephritis	Kidney stones
Sepsis/shock	Severe renal ischemia	Clots
Hypovolemic shock	Chemicals (radiographics dyes, commercial chemicals, etc)	Structure malformation
Vena cava obstruction		Tumors
Trauma with bleeding	Certain drugs (ie, anti-inflammatory drugs, antibiotics)	Prostatitism
Sequestration (burns, peritonitis)	Neoplasms	Rupture of the bladder
Hypovolemia (ie, diuretics)	Malignant hypertension	Ureteral obstruction
Cardiovascular failure (ie, myocardial failure, tamponade, vascular pooling, congestive heart failure, dysrhythmia)	Systemic lupus erythematosus	Retroperitoneal fibrosis
	Diabetes mellitus	Bilateral renal venous occlusion
	Complications of pregnancy (ie, eclampsia)	Neurogenic bladder
Hemorrhage	Streptococcal infections	
Gastrointestinal losses (diarrhea, vomiting)	Vasopressors	
Extreme acidosis	Microangiopathy	
Anaphylaxis/shock	Hyperviscosity states	
Renal artery stenosis or thrombosis	Hypercalcemia	
	Postrenal transplant	
	Myeloma	
	Interstitial nephritis	
	Transfusion reactions	
	HIV nephropathy	
	Heroin nephropathy	

Intrarenal

The intrarenal category of ARF includes physiological events directly affecting kidney tissue structure and function. These often include events causing damage to the interstitium and the nephron tissue. The kidneys lose their ability to excrete nitrogen waste produced by protein metabolism. Tubule damage leads to an inability to concentrate the urine. Also, when conditions causing prerenal failure create kidney tissue destruction, the disease progresses to the intrarenal stage (see Table 25–1). Acute tubular necrosis (ATN) is a common example of this category of ARF.

Postrenal

The postrenal category includes any obstruction in urine flow from the collection ducts in the kidney to the external urethral orifice, or venous blood flow from the kidney.

The obstructions may be from anatomic or functional causes. Anatomic causes usually are events such as strictures, tumors, or stones. Functional causes can include drugs, such as ganglionic blocking agents that interrupt autonomic supply to the urinary system. Bilateral renal venous obstruction is rare; however, it also is categorized as a postrenal cause of ARF. It is seen most often secondary to intra-abdominal neoplasms and iatrogenic causes (see Table 25–1).

Summary

The ability to distinguish the fine differences among patient conditions associated specifically with these ARF categories will enable the nurse to provide more individualized care (see Nursing Care Plans 25–1, 25–2, and 25–3).

Pathophysiological Principles

Prerenal Azotemia

The adverse effect of reduced renal perfusion on renal function is distinct. Because of the large amount of renal blood flow required to maintain normal renal function, changes in urinary composition occur early when renal perfusion is decreased.

When renal blood flow is severely compromised as a result of either reduction in effective blood volume, fall in cardiac output, or decrease in blood pressure below 80 mm Hg, characteristic changes occur in renal function. The capacity for complete autoregulation is exceeded. The glomerular filtration rate (GFR) falls. The amount of tubular fluid is reduced, and the fluid travels through the tubule more slowly. This results in increased sodium and

water reabsorption. Because of the reduced renal circulation, the solutes reabsorbed from the tubular fluid are removed more slowly than normal from the interstitium of the renal medulla. This results in increased medullary tonicity, which in turn further augments water reabsorption from the distal tubular fluid. Therefore, the urinary changes are typical in the underperfused state. The urinary volume is reduced to less than 400 ml/day (17 ml/hour), urinary specific gravity is increased, and urinary sodium concentration is low (usually less than 5 mEq/L; Fig. 25–1).

In addition, substances such as creatinine and urea, which normally are filtered but poorly reabsorbed from the renal tubule, are present in high concentration in the urine as a result of the increased water reabsorption. Because of the characteristic changes associated with renal underperfusion, measurement of urinary volume and specific gravity is a simple method of determining the effect of management on renal perfusion.

An increase in systemic blood pressure does not necessarily imply improvement in renal perfusion. This may be especially evident when drugs such as norepinephrine (Levophed; Winthrop Pharmaceuticals, New York, NY) are used to correct the hypotension associated with states of volume depletion. These drugs may be associated with further reduction in renal blood flow as a consequence of constriction of renal arteries. This is manifested by a further fall in urinary volume and rise in specific gravity.

In turn, if the hypoperfusion state is more appro-

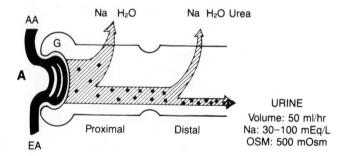

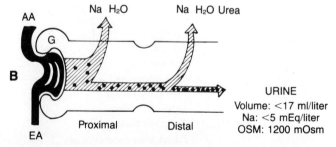

FIGURE 25–1

(**A**) Normal perfusion of the kidney compared with (**B**) underperfusion. Underperfusion of the kidney results in decreased renal blood flow and glomerular filtration; increase in the fraction of filtrate reabsorbed in the proximal tubule; and low urine flow with low sodium content and increased concentration. **B** characterizes the prerenal category of ARF.

priately and specifically treated by replacement of volume, improvement of cardiac output, correction of dysrhythmias, or administration of low-dose dopamine (Intropin; American Critical Care, McGraw Park, IL) at 0.5 mg/kg, the improved renal perfusion will be manifested as an increased urinary volume and a fall in specific gravity of the urine.

Intrarenal Acute Renal Failure

When renal underperfusion persists for a sufficient period of time (the exact duration of which is unpredictable and varies with the clinical circumstances), the kidneys may become damaged so that restoration of renal perfusion no longer effects an improvement in glomerular filtration. In this situation, intrinsic renal failure (intrarenal category, such as ATN, vasomotor nephropathy, and lower nephron nephrosis) occurs. This effect may be exaggerated by concomitant administration of nephrotoxic drugs or antibiotics such as the aminoglycosides. Alternatively, these agents and an increasing number of nephrotoxic substances may produce ARF, even in the absence of systemic hypotension and renal ischemia, as a direct result of their toxic effects on the kidney. In both situations, the kidney may or may not reveal significant morphologic changes associated with the inciting insult. For example, in postischemic ARF, the kidney may appear edematous and swollen but show only minor histologic changes on microscopic examination. In nephrotoxic ARF, however, histologic changes, most commonly in the late proximal convoluted tubule and pars recta, may be seen more frequently in association with distal tubular dilation and accumulation of cellular debris and intraluminal casts. Despite severe reduction in renal function, pathologic changes may be minimal and may not reflect the nature of the underlying process unless detailed evaluation of the fine renal architecture is made by electron microscopy. Regardless of the extent of histologic damage, most patients recover complete renal function. Recovery time varies from a period of days to weeks, depending on the severity and etiology of the process.

The exact mechanism that reduces glomerular filtration in any given patient with ARF may be difficult to ascertain owing to the complexity of clinical circumstances. The mechanisms that will be discussed subsequently represent those proposed for relatively pure circumstances of hypoperfusion-induced (prerenal) and nephrotoxin-induced (intrarenal) renal failure, as defined by both human and laboratory animal studies. Even so, despite years of investigation, there is no overwhelming evidence that supports one potential mechanism over another, and it is likely that several operate together in any given clinical or experimental setting.

Renal blood flow has been found to be reduced to approximately one third of normal in ATN, whereas the GFR is almost completely suppressed. This is in contrast to other states in which a similar reduction in renal blood flow is accompanied by much better maintenance of glomerular filtration and renal function.

Numerous animal studies have suggested that intratubular obstruction from casts and cellular debris may be involved in the suppression of glomerular filtration. If this obstruction is relieved, renal function returns. Other studies have suggested that there is disruption of the tubule epithelium with excessive back flow of the filtrate out of the tubule lumen, thus explaining the lack of urine formation in the face of continuing, although reduced, renal blood flow (Fig. 25–2).

The mechanism responsible for the decreased superficial cortical blood flow in the kidney with ATN has not been defined. Earlier, discovery of converting enzyme in the kidney suggested that renin–angiotensin may play a role in this phenomenon. Subsequent studies, however, clearly have ruled out the renin–angiotensin system as the sole mediator of renal vasoconstriction and the decrease in GFR. Rather, the abnormalities are mediated by excesses or deficiencies of numerous vasoactive substances, both vasoconstrictors and vasodilators, and by lack of intrinsic myogenic tone in the renal vasculature. It is likely that no single factor, but rather an imbalance of vasoconstrictors and vasodilators acting in unison on the glomerular vasculature, is at fault in the observed renal ischemia (Fig. 25–3). In certain cases, increases of angiotensin II or vasopressin or decreases in prostaglandins or bradykinin may be the overriding phenomenon that disrupts the maintenance of renal blood flow and GFR. Prostaglandin inhibitors, for example, may decrease renal blood flow and GFR in states of stress, such as volume depletion, and further induce ARF. Prostaglandin inhibitors also may enhance renal failure caused by gentamicin and myoglobin, at least in the experimental setting. More studies are needed to define these etiologic associations.

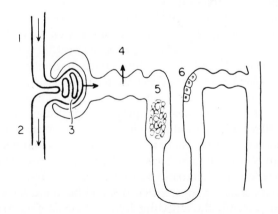

FIGURE 25–2
Potential mechanisms causing ARF include decreased filtration pressure because of constriction in the renal arterioles (*1* and *2*); decreased glomerular capillary permeability (*3*); increased permeability of the proximal tubules with back-leak of filtrate (*4*); obstruction of urine flow by necrotic tubular cells (*5*); increased sodium delivery to the macula densa (*6*); which causes an increase in renin–angiotensin production and vasoconstriction at the glomerular level.

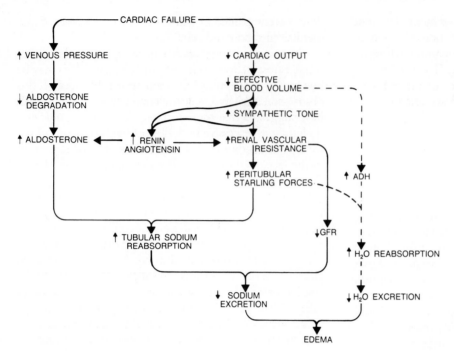

FIGURE 25–3
Factors affecting sodium reabsorption with decreased cardiac output.

Regardless of the mechanism, there are measurable physiological changes that predictably occur. First, urine volume generally is reduced in most cases produced by ischemic and nephrotoxic etiologies. Exceptions do occur, however, especially with nephrotoxic ARF caused by aminoglycosides, in which azotemia can occur without the urine flow rate ever being interrupted. The decreased GFR is accompanied by a rising serum creatinine and BUN and by characteristic urinary findings that differ from those seen in prerenal azotemia. First, urinary concentration (osmolality or specific gravity) falls to levels similar to plasma concentration, and the urine concentrations of urea and especially of creatinine are decreased, in contrast to findings made in the prerenal state of azotemia. Both reflect failure of distal tubules to concentrate the urine appropriately. The mechanism may be direct distal tubular toxicity or ischemia, or it may be disruption of the normal medullary solute concentration gradient necessary to produce a concentrated urine. Also, urinary sodium concentration no longer reflects systemic volume status and becomes disproportionately high (usually > 30 mEq/L), indicating an inability to modulate sodium concentration appropriate for the clinical circumstance. This is assessed more accurately by the fractional sodium excretion (or, alternatively, by the renal failure index), which usually is greater than 1% and often greater than 3%, probably also reflecting decreased tubular function in residual filtering nephrons.

Main Causes of Intrarenal Acute Renal Failure

The causes of ARF are numerous but can be divided into two main groups: *ischemic* (prerenal) and *nephrotoxic* (intrarenal) (Table 25–2).

Ischemic Acute Renal Failure

As indicated in Table 25–2, anything that reduces renal blood flow as a result of intravascular volume depletion can result in ARF. In traumatic shock, both the duration and severity of hypotension play major roles in the development of ARF. The incidence and average duration of shock have been reduced because of prompt and effective therapy with blood products and volume expanders. Acute renal failure is more likely to occur *after* hospitalization as a result of septic complications or nephrotoxic antibiotic administration than as a result of the shock itself.

Nephrotoxic Acute Renal Failure

A large number of diverse chemicals and drugs have been implicated in the production of ARF (see Table 25–2). In the hospitalized patient, the most common offending nephrotoxic agents are the antibiotics, especially the aminoglycosides. Examples of these agents are as follows, listed in decreasing order of the severity with which they produce dose-dependent damage to the proximal tubule: neomycin > tobramycin > kanamycin > gentamicin > amikacin > secomicin > netilmicin > streptomycin. Aminoglycoside nephrotoxicity accounts for up to 16% of all cases of ARF, usually is nonoliguric, and frequently improves after cessation of the antibiotic therapy. Because these agents accumulate preferentially in the renal cortex and are excreted slowly, however, they sometimes do not produce measurable toxicity until up to 1 week after cessation of administration. Routine monitoring of BUN and creatinine therefore are necessary when these agents are administered. Also, because these agents are eliminated from the body primarily by the kidneys, dosage must be adjusted in patients with preexisting renal function impairment. Peak and trough blood levels must be measured

TABLE 25–2
Common Causes of Acute Renal Failure

Ischemic (prerenal)	Nephrotoxic (intrarenal)
Hemorrhagic hypotension	Antibiotics: aminoglycosides, penicillins, tetracycline, amphotericin
Severe volume depletion	
Surgical aortic cross-clamping	Heavy metals: mercury, lead, *cis*-platinum, uranium, cadmium, bismuth, arsenic
Cardiac and biliary surgery	
Defective cardiac output, including open heart surgery	Hemoglobinuria (from hemolysis)
	Myoglobinuria (rhabdomyolysis)
Septic shock	Radiologic contrast agents
Pregnancy	Drugs: phenytoin, phenylbutazone, cimetidine, cyclosporine
Pancreatitis	Organic solvents: carbon tetrachloride
	Fungicides and pesticides
	Uric acid
	Ethylene glycol
	Anesthetics (methoxyflurane)
	Disseminated intravascular coagulation
	Plant and animal substances (mushrooms, snake venom)

frequently so that drug dosage can be adjusted to the correct therapeutic range.

Nephrotoxicity associated with radiocontrast media administration also must be considered in the critical care setting. Patients at the greatest risk for development of renal failure after a load of contrast dye are those with diabetes, and especially diabetics with underlying renal failure.[1] This type of renal failure usually is mild, nonoliguric, and reversible. Serum creatinine rises within 48 hours after contrast administration, peaks in 3 to 5 days, and returns to baseline in 7 to 10 days. If the oliguric episode is more severe, it may take 5 to 10 days for the creatinine to reach peak levels, and baseline renal function may not be reached for 2 to 4 weeks. The need to provide temporary or permanent dialysis is rare except in patients with advanced underlying renal insufficiency.

The risk of contrast media-associated nephrotoxicity may be lowered by reducing the total dose of contrast media, by volume expansion before the injection, by mannitol infusion in conjunction with the dye, or by administration of loop diuretics and calcium channel blockers. Some authors now advocate the use of low-osmolality contrast media because of the reduced incidence of adverse effects.[2]

In addition to diabetics with underlying renal failure, other risk factors are recognized for the development of radiocontrast-associated nephrotoxicity. These are dehydration, large contrast loads, prior episodes of contrast associated nephrotoxicity, congestive heart failure, repeated contrast exposure, and multiple myeloma.

The nonsteroidal anti-inflammatory agents also may induce ARF in patients with diabetes, particularly in the presence of congestive heart failure due to coronary artery disease. Baseline renal function should be restored when the drug is discontinued.

Postrenal Acute Renal Failure

Any condition that blocks the flow of urine from the kidneys to the exterior can result in postrenal azotemia. Obstruction can occur at any point in the urinary tract. When urine cannot get around the obstruction, resulting congestion will cause retrograde pressure through the collecting system and nephrons. This slows the rate of tubular fluid flow and lowers the GFR. As a result, the reabsorption of sodium, water, and urea is increased, leading to lowered urine sodium, and an increase in urine osmolality and BUN. Serum creatinine also will rise. With prolonged pressure from urinary obstruction, the entire collecting system will dilate, compressing and damaging nephrons. This unfortunate circumstance can be avoided by prompt removal of the obstruction.[3]

Assessment

Clinical Course

Nonoliguric Acute Renal Failure

Classically, patients have oliguria in association with ATN; however, this is not always so. A group of patients presents with acute nonoliguric (partially reversible) renal failure. This state is especially common in patients receiving nephrotoxic antibiotics. If antibiotics are discontinued before renal function is reduced markedly, the patient frequently sustains moderate functional impairment for 7 to 10 days with gradual return to normal. In general, patients with nonoliguric ARF have few symptoms, and the disease is much less serious than the oliguric form of ATN.

Oliguric Acute Renal Failure

The more classic or oliguric form of ATN begins with an acute precipitating event immediately followed by oliguria (urine volume less than 400 ml/day). The mean duration of oliguria is approximately 12 days, although it may last only 2 to 3 days or as long as 30 days. This is accompanied by a usual rise in BUN of 25 to 30 mg/100 ml/day and an increase in creatinine of 1.5 to 2 mg/100 ml/day. The most common complication in this period is overhydration with resulting cardiac failure, pulmonary edema, and death. In addition, the patient may have acidosis, hyperkalemia, and symptoms of uremia.

Diuretic Stage

The oliguric phase is followed by gradual return of renal function as manifested by a stepwise increase in urine volume (the diuretic stage). The degree of diuresis is determined primarily by the state of hydration at the time the patient enters the diuretic stage. If the patient is markedly overloaded, urinary volume eventually may exceed 4 to 5 L/day. This could result in marked sodium wasting, with death resulting from electrolyte depletion in a few patients.

Because of the slow return of renal function during the diuretic phase, the degree of azotemia may increase during the early part of the diuretic period, and the patient will have complications that are similar to those noted in the oliguric phase. A period of several months is required for full recovery of renal function after the end of the diuretic period.

Diagnostic Findings

Intrarenal ARF must be differentiated from prerenal azotemia, or decreased perfusion, and from obstruction. The latter can be distinguished by history and the appropriate use of ultrasonography and abdominal computed tomography scanning. In current practice, very rarely will retrograde catheterization of the urinary tract be necessary to exclude this diagnosis.

Differentiation of intrarenal ARF from prerenal azotemia may be clinically difficult in many patients because both conditions frequently are accompanied by oliguria. A carefully collected urine sample, however, may provide significant clues in making the distinction. By itself, the routine urine analysis may be of little diagnostic aid because mild proteinuria may be present in both conditions, in association with a few cellular elements and granular casts on microscopic examination. The latter are much more numerous in ARF than in prerenal azotemia and also tend to be pigmented; these are highly characteristic but not diagnostic.

Procurement of a urine specimen for diagnostic chemistries and indices as indicated in Table 25–3 is invaluable in establishing the diagnosis of ARF. This urine sample should be obtained *before* a diagnostic challenge of diuretics because these agents may alter the urine chemical composition. Urinary chemistry determinations distinguish between underperfusion of the kidney, in which most solutes except for sodium tend to be concentrated, and intrarenal ARF, in which there tends to be a reduced solute concentration resulting from an inability of the injured tubules to alter the urine composition. Thus, in

TABLE 25–3
Use of Laboratory Values in Differentiating Acute Tubular Necrosis from Decreased Renal Perfusion

Test	Acute Tubular Necrosis	Reduced Renal Blood Flow
Urine		
Volume	<400 ml/24 hr	<400 ml/24 hr
Sodium	40–10 mEq/L	<5 mEq/L
Specific gravity	1.010	Usually >1.020
Osmolality	250–350 mOsm/L	Usually >400 mOsm/L
Urea	200–300 mg/100 ml	Usually >600 mg/100 ml
Creatinine	<60 mg/100 ml	Usually >150 mg/100 ml
Fe_{Na}	>3.0%	<1.0%
Blood		
BUN:Cr	10:1	Usually >20:1
Responses to Mannitol	None	None or flow increases to >40 ml/hr
Furosemide	None	Flow increases to >40 ml/hr

FE_{Na}, fractional excretion of sodium; BUN:Cr, blood urea nitrogen–creatinine ratio.

Differential Diagnosis of Acute Renal Failure

1. Prerenal azotemia
   a. Hypovolemia
   b. Cardiovascular failure
      1. Myocardial failure
      2. Vascular pooling
   c. Hepatorenal syndrome
2. Vascular obstruction
   a. Arterial obstruction
      1. Embolization
      2. Thrombosis
      3. Dissection
   b. Venous obstruction
3. Intrinsic renal disease
   a. Glomerulonephritis
   b. Vasculitis
   c. Microangiopathic disease
      1. Hemolytic uremic syndrome
      2. Thrombotic thrombocytopenic purpura
   d. Malignant nephrosclerosis
4. Postrenal azotemia
   a. Obstructive uropathy
   b. Bladder rupture

TABLE 25–4
Diagnostic Clues in Acute Renal Failure

Urine

- *Urate crystals:* Tumor lysis, especially lymphoma (urate nephropathy)
- *Oxalate crystals:* Ethylene glycol nephrotoxicity, methoxyflurane nephrotoxicity
- *Eosinophils:* Allergic interstitial nephritis, especially methicillin
- *Positive benzidene without RBCs:* Hemoglobinuria or myoglobinuria
- *Pigmented casts:* Hemoglobinuria or myoglobinuria
- *Massive proteinuria:* Acute interstitial nephritis, thiazide diuretics, hemorrhagic fevers (Korean, Scandinavian, etc.)
- *Anuria:* Renal cortical necrosis, bilateral obstruction, hemolytic uremic syndrome, rapidly progressive glomerulonephritis

Plasma

- *Marked hyperkalemia:* Rhabdomyolysis, tissue necrosis, hemolysis
- *Marked hypocalcemia:* Rhabdomyolysis
- *Hypercalcemia:* Hypercalcemic nephropathy
- *Hyperuricemia:* Tumor lysis, rhabdomyolysis, toxin ingestion
- *Marked acidosis:* Ethylene glycol, methyl alcohol
- *Eosinophilia:* Allergic interstitial nephritis

RBCs, red blood cells.

prerenal azotemia the urinary sodium is low, as are the renal failure index and fractional excretion of sodium (Fe_{Na}), whereas the urine osmolality and concentration of nonreabsorbable solutes are high. In intrarenal ARF, urine sodium is greater than 30 mEq/L, the renal failure index and Fe_{Na} are greater than 1%, and the urine osmolality is close to that of plasma, reflecting the inability of the damaged kidney to reabsorb sodium and concentrate the urine.

Acute tubular necrosis also must be distinguished from all other intrinsic renal diseases that can rapidly reduce renal function. Many of these can be differentiated by their clinical picture and urine analyses. In some circumstances, the diagnosis may be difficult, such as with rapidly progressive glomerulonephritis without significant urine sediment abnormalities. In this situation, urine chemistries look more like those seen in prerenal azotemia than those observed in ATN, and should serve as a clue to the diagnosis. There frequently are subtle clues that will aid in the diagnosis of ARF, and these should be sought carefully (Table 25–4).

Management

Primary management of renal function impairment is directed at the adequate and specific management of the hypoperfused state. The three most common causes for reduced renal perfusion are decreased cardiac output, altered peripheral vascular resistance, and hypovolemia.

Managing Decreased Cardiac Output

Factors such as cardiac dysrhythmias, acute myocardial infarction, and acute pericardial tamponade, all of which decrease cardiac output, may be associated with a reduction in renal blood flow. The reversibility of the renal failure thus depends on the ability to improve cardiac function.

In these conditions, cardiac output usually is acutely and severely compromised. When cardiac output is impaired to a lesser extent over a longer period of time, however, features of congestive heart failure occur. Again, there is reduced renal perfusion, although to a lesser extent. The major feature of this state, from the renal aspect, is avid sodium reabsorption, which results in increased extracellular fluid volume, elevation of central venous pressure, and edema.

Several mechanisms are responsible for the increased tubular reabsorption of sodium (see Figure 25–3). First, there is a greater reduction in renal blood flow than in glomerular filtration, bringing into play the mechanisms discussed earlier. Second, it has been suggested that blood flow to the superficial cortex is reduced, whereas blood flow to the inner cortical area is increased. In addition, it is thought that the nephrons in the inner cortical region reabsorb a greater percentage of the filtered sodium than the nephrons in the outer cortex of the kidney.

Other factors include increased proximal and distal tubule sodium reabsorption. The mechanisms responsible for the increased proximal tubule sodium reabsorption are dependent largely on increased postglomerular oncotic pressure; however, aldosterone mostly is responsible for the increased distal tubule sodium reabsorption. It can be seen that numerous mechanisms are responsible for the increased tubular reabsorption of sodium in congestive heart failure.

Therapy is directed largely at increasing urinary sodium excretion. At times, this can be accomplished by improvement of cardiac output, which in turn increases renal perfusion. This is not always possible, however.

Diuretics are used frequently to increase sodium excretion. These agents directly inhibit sodium reabsorption in the renal tubule. The potency of a diuretic is determined primarily by the site in the renal tubule where sodium reabsorption is blocked.

The two most potent diuretics currently available are furosemide (Lasix; Hoechst-Roussel Pharmaceuticals, Somerville, NJ) and ethacrynic acid (Edecrin; Merck Sharp & Dohme, West Point, PA). These agents block sodium reabsorption in the ascending limb of the loop of Henle and in the distal tubule. It still is unclear whether they have an effect in the proximal tubule as well. The thiazide diuretics have their major site of action in the distal tubule and are therefore somewhat less potent than the above agents.

Another commonly used diuretic is spironolactone (Aldactone; Searle Laboratories, Chicago, IL), which increases urinary sodium by blocking the renal tubular effect of aldosterone.

Spironolactone should be used with caution in patients with severe decreases in cardiac output and renal underperfusion because it decreases potassium excretion and can produce life-threatening hyperkalemia in such patients. The same is true of triamterene, another potassium-sparing diuretic.

Managing Altered Peripheral Vascular Resistance

Renal perfusion is compromised in these states as a result of increased size of the intravascular compartment and redistribution of blood volume. This may be a consequence of gram-negative septicemia, certain drug overdoses, anaphylactic reactions, and electrolyte disturbances such as acidosis.

Management is directed primarily at treating the basic disturbance with appropriate specific therapy plus fluid,

electrolyte, and colloid replacement. The controversy over the use of steroids and various pressor agents in gram-negative sepsis is beyond the scope of this discussion.

Managing Hypovolemia and Hemorrhage

Restoration of extracellular fluid and blood volume is of major importance in the management of any hypoperfused state. Evidence for extracellular volume depletion usually is obtained from the history and physical examination.

Historically, the patient may give evidence of external sodium and water loss as a result of vomiting, diarrhea, excessive sweating, or surgical procedures. Blood volume also may be compromised as a result of fluid redistribution, as seen both with burns and with inflammatory processes in the abdomen, such as pancreatitis or peritonitis. The physical findings associated with extracellular volume depletion are sunken eyes, dry mouth, loss of skin turgor, and tachycardia. Postural hypotension also may be noted.

Therapy is directed at sodium and water replacement or blood when hemorrhage is the cause. Response to treatment can be judged by changes in urinary volume, specific gravity, central venous pressure, and the aforementioned physical findings.

Maintaining Urinary Flow

At times, despite adequate treatment, urinary volume remains low. This may be a result of either continuing functional impairment in the post-hypoperfusion period or parenchymal renal damage resulting from the hypoperfusion. It is necessary to differentiate these two states from each other because prolonged oliguria, if allowed to persist, eventually may lead to ATN. Mannitol and furosemide have been used in this situation for both diagnosis and maintenance of urinary function.

Mannitol is the reduced form of the six-carbon sugar, mannose. It is distributed in the extracellular fluid and essentially is not metabolized. It is freely filtered at the glomerulus and not reabsorbed by the tubule. Because of its small molecular size, it exerts a significant osmotic effect and, in turn, increases urinary flow.

Mannitol usually is infused rather rapidly. The more rapid the infusion, the higher the blood level and, in turn, the filtered load. Urinary flow depends on the amount of mannitol filtered, and if the infusion is too slow, changes in urinary flow rate will be delayed and less apparent.

The usual test is 0.2 g/kg given intravenously as a 25% solution over 3 to 5 minutes. If urine flow increases to greater than 40 ml/hour, the patient is thought to have reversible renal failure, and urine volume is then maintained at 100 ml/hour with additional mannitol and fluid replacement as indicated.

More recently, *furosemide* and *ethacrynic acid* largely have replaced mannitol in the diagnosis of reversible renal failure. A number of patients who fail to have diuresis after infusion of mannitol will have an acceptable increase in urinary volume after administration of furosemide or ethacrynic acid.

After correction of volume depletion, furosemide in dosages of 200 to 1,000 mg is given intravenously. The peak diuresis usually occurs within 2 hours of its administration. If furosemide is effective in increasing urinary volume, it is repeated at 4- to 6-hour intervals to maintain the urinary flow rate as long as fluids are administered to maintain urine.

In patients failing to respond to furosemide, a diagnosis of ATN must be considered. In patients who respond to furosemide and mannitol, it is important to replace sodium and water losses to avoid depletion. Usually, urine volume is replaced by half-strength normal saline. In addition, potassium replacement frequently is required.

Complications

Preventing Acute Tubular Necrosis

Because ATN continues to be associated with a high mortality, the major objective is preventing this complication. Acute tubular necrosis can be prevented in patients with major traumatic injuries by rapid replacement of blood loss and correction of fluid and electrolyte disturbances.

Similarly, patients receiving potentially nephrotoxic agents should undergo serial determinations to evaluate renal function during the course of the administration of these agents. This is accomplished most easily by measuring serum creatinine levels on an every-other-day schedule. If the serum creatinine begins to rise, the drug should be discontinued. In most patients, functional deterioration stabilizes, and the patient recovers without the development of severe impairment of renal function.

There still is considerable debate with regard to the effectiveness of mannitol and furosemide in the prevention of ARF. In fact, some evidence has been accumulated that suggests that furosemide actually may increase the toxicity of certain nephrotoxic agents. Most authors, however, agree that a trial of furosemide up to 500 mg intravenously should be used. Often, this may correct oliguric to nonoliguric ARF, which is easier to manage clinically.

Managing Acute Tubular Necrosis

Volume Replacement

After development of ATN, the primary consideration is maintenance of fluid and electrolyte balance. During the oliguric phase, urinary volume usually is less than 300 ml/day. Insensible losses average 800 to 1,000 ml/day and are virtually free of electrolytes.

In general, fluid replacement should be approximately 500 ml/day. Additional water will be obtained from the water present in foods plus the water of oxidation from metabolism. Because of the use of body proteins and fats, the patient ideally should lose approximately 2.2 lb (1 kg) a day to maintain water balance. The *danger of fluid overload* with resulting congestive heart failure and pulmonary edema exists throughout the oliguric period. In contrast, during the diuretic phase of ATN, extensive *sodium wasting* may occur in association with the increased urinary volumes. It thus is necessary to keep accurate intake and output records as well as daily weights during both phases. This is especially important when there are other avenues of fluid and electrolyte losses such as vomiting, diarrhea, nasogastric suction, and drainages from fistulas. In general, losses occurring as a result of these problems should be replaced in full.

Nutritional Therapy

Besides replacing fluids and electrolytes, intake is directed at supplying the patient with calories in the form of carbohydrates and fats to decrease the rate of breakdown of body protein. Because 1 g of urea is formed from every 6 g of protein metabolized, protein intake usually is restricted to prevent the BUN from rising at too fast a rate.

With the development of nutritional teams, there has been a growing tendency to provide more calories and protein in the form of parenteral or enteral hyperalimentation in attempts to improve the overall condition of the patient and to hasten recovery of renal function. Diets containing 2,000 to 3,000 calories/day with 40 to 60 g of protein or essential amino acids have been used with increased frequency. These diets contain more than the 500 ml of fluid recommended earlier. Therefore, hyperalimentation requires more frequent dialysis, especially in the oliguric period, often in combination with hemofiltration.

Control of Acidosis

Metabolic acidosis of moderate severity usually is present in patients with renal failure. This results from the inability of the kidneys to excrete fixed acids (eg, H_2PO_4) produced from normal metabolic processes.

The acidosis usually can be controlled easily by giving the patient 30 to 60 mEq of sodium bicarbonate daily but does not require treatment unless the HCO_3^- falls below 12 to 15 mEq/L.

Control of Hyperkalemia

Hyperkalemia commonly occurs in patients with ATN. This is a consequence of both the reduced ability of the kidneys to excrete potassium and the release of intracellular potassium because of acidosis and tissue breakdown.

The acidosis results in movement of the hydrogen ion into the cell, thus displacing potassium into the extracellular fluid. This maintains electrical neutrality but increases the hyperkalemic state.

An additional mechanism for producing hyperkalemia, often overlooked in acutely ill patients, is caloric restriction, especially glucose restriction. Transport of glucose and amino acids into cells is accompanied by potassium. In acutely ill, catabolic patients, when dietary intake is restricted or intravenous fluid therapy inadvertently disrupted, failure of transport of potassium intracellularly may contribute to hyperkalemia. Because this process requires insulin, insulin deficiency may have the same consequences, and diabetics may therefore be more prone to acute disturbances in potassium balance when renal failure occurs.

By interfering with catecholamine-induced translocation of potassium into cells, β-blockers also can enhance hyperkalemia and should be avoided in patients with ARF.

Hyperkalemia is manifested clinically by cardiac and neuromuscular changes. Both cardiac conduction disturbances and acute flaccid quadriplegia are life-threatening complications. These hyperkalemic changes are reversed rapidly by administration of intravenous calcium gluconate, which has a direct antagonist effect on the action of potassium. Serum potassium can be reduced by intravenous administration of sodium bicarbonate for treatment of acidosis. In addition, administration of glucose and insulin frequently is used as an additional method of shifting extracellular potassium to intracellular pools.

Sodium polystyrene sulfonate resin (Kayexalate; Winthrop Pharmaceuticals) given orally (25 g four times a day in 10 ml of 10% sorbitol) may reduce the body potassium burden more slowly and should be instituted when hyperkalemia begins to develop. In addition, when life-threatening hyperkalemia develops and these treatments fail or do not restore serum potassium to normal, emergency intervention, either hemodialysis or peritoneal dialysis, should be instituted. Although hemodialysis will reduce body burden of potassium to a greater degree than peritoneal dialysis, peritoneal dialysis generally can be instituted much more quickly. Because plasma potassium equilibrates rapidly with peritoneal fluid, serum potassium can be reduced promptly.

Hyperkalemia usually can be prevented by avoidance of potassium supplements, institution of chronic therapy for acidosis, and use of sodium polystyrene sulfonate resin when serum potassium is even slightly elevated.

Sodium and Water Diuresis

During the oliguric phase of ATN, sodium retention may occur. With the onset of the diuretic period, however, urinary volume and sodium excretion may increase markedly.

Urinary volume largely is determined by the state of hydration at the onset of the diuretic period. Because urinary sodium concentration is relatively fixed, sodium losses are determined mostly by urinary volume. Therefore, if the patient is markedly overhydrated at the onset of the diuretic phase, sodium losses may be severe. Clinically, sodium depletion is characterized by either extracellular volume depletion, as manifested by tachycardia and postural hypotension, or water intoxication when sodium losses exceed water losses. This latter syndrome is characterized by markedly reduced serum sodium concentrations in association with personality changes, convulsions, coma, and death if allowed to progress untreated.

With acute water intoxication, treatment is directed at elevating the serum sodium concentration by administering hypertonic (3%–5%) sodium chloride intravenously.

Uremic Syndrome

In addition to electrolyte disturbances, the patient may have symptoms of uremia. Early findings are nausea, anorexia, and vomiting. Later, stupor, convulsions, and coma develop. In addition, bleeding abnormalities, uremic pneumonitis, pericarditis, and pleuritis, may occur.

Dialysis is indicated before the development of clinical symptoms of uremia. With the availability of hemodialysis or peritoneal dialysis, the clinical features of uremia do not usually occur in patients with ATN. Most patients having oliguria for more than 4 to 5 days will require dialysis sometime during the course of ATN. Dialysis has improved survival in patients with ATN. Continuous hemofiltration also has been used to treat ATN.

Prognosis is determined largely by the primary event that led to the development of ATN. Among patients with ATN due to medical causes (eg, transfusion reactions, myoglobinuria, nephrotoxic agents, and simple volume depletion), the mortality rate is approximately 25%, whereas cases resulting from trauma and severe surgical complications are associated with a 60% to 70% mortality rate. Death usually results as a complication of poor wound healing and sepsis or the underlying disease.

Drug Precautions

Certain drugs should be avoided or dosage reduced in any patient with markedly impaired renal function. Because of the possibility of magnesium intoxication, *antacids* containing magnesium should be avoided. Because of the reduced renal function, *digitalis* excretion may be reduced. Dosage should be altered to avoid excessively high blood levels. In addition, certain *antibiotics* should be given in much smaller dosages than usual, as indicated in Table 25–5. Table 25–5 lists most commonly used antibiotics and gives general guidelines as to how dosage should be modified based on the GFR level. Modifications may be made based on the dosage interval (I) or on alterations of the percentage of the normal dose (D) given at standard dosage intervals. In many cases, the modifications listed are only rough approximations and, when possible, serum levels also should be measured so that dosage can be

TABLE 25–5
Recommended Antibiotic Dosage in Renal Failure

Antibiotic Group	Method	Adjustment for Renal Failure GFR (ml/min) >50	10–50	<10	Dialysis Supplement
Aminoglycosides	I*	12–18	12	24	Yes
Amikacin					
Gentamicin					
Kanamicin					
Netilmicin					
Streptomycin					
Tobramicin					
Cephalosporins					Yes
All except Cefoperozone require reduction, but adjustments vary significantly between drugs.					
Cefaclor	D†	100	50–100	33	Yes
Cefadroxil	I	8	12–24	24–48	Yes
Cefamandole	I	6	6–8	8	Yes
Cefazolin	I	8	12	24–48	Yes
Cefoperazone	I	—	None‡	—	Yes
Ceforanide	I	12	24–48	48–72	Yes
Cefotaximine	I	6–8	8–12	12–24	Yes
Cefoxitin	I	8	8–12	24–48	Yes
Cefroxadine	D	65–100	15–65	10–15	?
Cefuroxime	I	8–12	24–48	48–72	Yes
Cefsulodin	D	50–100	15–50	10–15	Yes
Ceftizoxime	D	45–100	10–45	5–10	?
Cephalothin	I	6	6	8–12	Yes
Cephalexin	I	6	6–8	12	Yes
Cephapirin	I	6	6–8	12	Yes
Cephradine	D	100	50	25	Yes
Moxalactam	I	8	12	12–24	Yes
Clindamycin	D	—	None	—	Yes
Erythromycin	D	—	None	—	Yes
Lincomycin	I	6	12	24	Yes
Methenanime mandelate	D	100	Avoid§	Avoid	—
Nalidixic acid	D	100	Avoid	Avoid	—
Nitrofurantoin	D	100	Avoid	Avoid	—
Penicillins					
Amoxicillin	I	6	6–12	12–16	Yes
Ampicillin	I	6	6–12	12–16	Yes
Azlocillin	I	4–6	6–8	8	Yes
Carbenicillin	I	8–12	12–24	24–48	Yes
Cloxacillin	D	—	None	—	No‖
Cyclacillin	I	6	6–12	12–24	Yes
Dicloxacillin	I	—	None	—	No
Methicillin	I	4	4–8	8–12	No
Mezlocillin	I	4–6	6–8	8	Yes
Nafcillin	D	—	None	—	No
Oxacillin	D	—	None	—	No
Penicillin G	I	6–8	8–12	12–16	Yes
Piperacillin	I	4–6	6–8	8	Yes
Ticarcillin	I	8–12	12–24	24–48	Yes
Sulfonamides and trimethoprim					
Sulfamethoxazole	I	12	18	24	Yes
Sulfisoxazole	I	6	8–12	12–24	Yes
Trimethoprim	I	12	18	24	Yes

(continued)

TABLE 25–5
Recommended Antibiotic Dosage in Renal Failure (Continued)

		Adjustment for Renal Failure			
		GFR (ml/min)			Dialysis Supplement
Antibiotic Group	*Method*	>50	10–50	<10	
Tetracyclines					
Doxycycline	I	12	12–18	18–24	No
Minocycline	D	—	None	—	No
Vancomycin	I	24–72	72–240	240	No

*I refers to alteration in dosage interval in hours.
†D refers to percentage of alteration of usual dose.
‡None means no dosage adjustment is necessary.
§Avoid means drugs toxic in renal failure.
‖No means that hemodialysis does not significantly alter kinetics of the drug.
Modified from Bennett WM, et al: Drug prescribing in renal failure: Dosing guidelines for adults. Am J Kidney Dis 3:155–193, 1983.

determined more accurately. Table 25–6 lists antibiotics that may require supplemental doses because of their removal by hemodialysis.

Before administering a drug to a patient with renal failure, the following questions should be reviewed:

- Does the drug depend on the kidney for excretion?
- Does an excess blood level affect the kidney?
- Does the drug add chemically to the pool of urea nitrogen?
- Does the effect of the drug alter electrolyte balance?
- Is the patient more susceptible to the drug because of kidney disease?

As new drugs are introduced into the clinical setting, it is imperative that nurses working with renal patients review the need to modify drug dosages or frequencies to avoid toxicity or to provide necessary supplementation.

Because GFRs can change rapidly with certain physiological dysfunctions and multisystem involvement, the nurse should monitor laboratory data, assessment parameters, and patient response closely to anticipate needed adjustments in drug therapy. Likewise, in patients receiving dialysis, the same precaution should be taken to ensure that serum levels remain therapeutic.

Summary

A knowledge of the causes and manifestations of ARF will enable the nurse to assess a patient's problems throughout the stages of illness, develop a comprehensive care plan to manage the patient's changing needs, and evaluate the patient's response to the nursing and medical regimen. The nurse's ability to manage care innovatively and appropriately during rapidly changing stages in health status is critical to patient recovery.

TABLE 25–6
*Supplemental Antibiotic Dosages for Patients on Hemodialysis**

Drug	Dosage Modification
Antifungal Drugs	
Amphotericin B	None
Fluconazole	100 mg
Miconazole	None
Antitubercular Drugs	
Ethambutol	15 mg/kg
Isoniazid	5 mg/kg
Rifampin	None
Antiviral Drugs	
Acyclovir	5 mg/kg
Amantadine	None
Ganciclovir	2.5 mg/kg
Zidovudine	200 mg
Carbapenem	
Imipenem	0.5 g
Quinolones	
Ciprofloxacin	None
Norfloxacin	Avoid
Ofloxacin	100 mg
Miscellaneous	
Aztreonam	125 mg
Chloramphenicol	None
Clindamycin	None
Erythromycin	None
Metronidazole	250 mg

* Give all supplements *after* dialysis.
Modified from Cutler R, Forland S: Removal of drugs by hemodialysis and continuous ambulatory peritoneal dialysis: Suggested dosing modifications. Dialysis and Transplantation 20(12):759–761, 1991.

NURSING CARE PLAN 25–1:
The Patient With Acute Renal Failure: Prerenal Azotemia

NURSING DIAGNOSIS	OUTCOME CRITERIA/ PATIENT GOALS	NURSING INTERVENTIONS
Altered tissue perfusion: related to hypovolemia secondary to ARF.	• Patient will be hemodynamically stable.	1. Monitor BP, pulse, respirations, PAP, PCWP, CVP, CO, CI, every hour until stable, then q2h.
		2. Monitor laboratory reports (Na, K, Hgb, Hct, WBC coagulation studies).
		3. Monitor for dry mucous membranes.
		4. Maintain intake and output record.
		5. Daily weights.
		6. Administer fluid and blood per physician's order.
		7. Monitor for fluid overload and/ or transfusion reaction.
		8. Weigh patient daily.
		9. Instruct to increase fluid intake to 2,000 ml/day.
		10. Monitor for signs and symptoms of hyponatremia.
		11. Monitor urine output for adequate volume q1h until output is >30 ml/hr, then take q2h and then q4h.
		12. Test urine for specific gravity every shift. Report abnormalities.
		13. Initiate measures to improve circulation (position changes, maintain warmth).
		14. Monitor temperature and skin color q1h until stable, then q2h.
		15. Monitor for mentation changes (lethargy, stupor).
		16. Reorient to reality frequently. Call by name, tell patient your name, orient to surroundings.

CASE STUDY

Mrs. Landry, an 85-year-old woman with calcific aortic stenosis, was admitted with mild congestive heart failure. She complained of weakness, fatigue, and loss of appetite. She stated that she lived alone and had great difficulty caring for herself. Admission examination revealed that the elderly woman, who appeared chronically ill, was mildly dyspneic but not edematous. Her mucous membranes were very dry, her tongue was coated, and her skin was dry and flaky. She reported two-pillow orthopnea and had been spending most of her time in bed over the last 2 weeks. Her weight was 53.3 kg, blood pressure was 120/60, pulse was 98 beats/min, temperature 97.8°F, and respirations were 24/min. BUN was 13.4 mg/dl, and serum creatinine was

NURSING CARE PLAN 25–2:
The Patient With Acute Renal Failure: Intrarenal

NURSING DIAGNOSIS	OUTCOME CRITERIA/ PATIENT GOALS	NURSING INTERVENTIONS
Altered tissue perfusion: related to renal ischemia secondary to acute glomerulonephritis.	• Patient will maintain fluid and electrolyte balance.	1. Maintain intake and output record. 2. Regulate hydration and avoid dehydration. 3. Observe for signs and symptoms of fluid retention (ie, swelling of ankles). 4. Monitor P, BP, RR. 5. Observe for signs of hyperkalemia; monitor ECG reports. 6. Monitor laboratory values: Na, K, Cl, acid–base balance; administer necessary replacements. 7. Administer Kayexalate as ordered.
High risk for infection: related to ARF.	• Patient will not acquire a nosocomial infection.	1. Observe for signs and symptoms of infection; elevated temperature and WBC. 2. Monitor RR, breath sounds. 3. Observe IV insertion sites for signs of inflammation. 4. Turn, cough, deep-breathe q2h.
High risk for injury: related to anemia secondary to renal failure.	• Patient will not have anemia.	1. Monitor HBF, HCT. 2. Observe for signs of bleeding; hematest urine and stool. 3. Observe for symptoms of anemia; increased fatigue, pallor, dyspnea, altered consciousness. 4. Provide adequate nutrition and rest.
Fluid volume excess: related to ARF, poor filtration, and IV intake.	• Patient will maintain fluid balance. • Patient's status will be maintained.	1. Monitor urine output. 2. Record and assess intake and output. 3. Assess urine for hematuria, specific gravity. 4. Provide for safety if BUN and creatinine levels are elevated. 5. Monitor for signs and symptoms of toxic drug accumulation. 6. Assess lung sounds for crackles and periphery for edema.

NURSING CARE PLAN 25-3:
The Patient With Acute Renal Failure: Postrenal

NURSING DIAGNOSIS	OUTCOME CRITERIA/ PATIENT GOALS	NURSING INTERVENTIONS
Altered urinary elimination: related to obstruction secondary to cancer of prostate, urethral obstruction.	• Patient will be able to maintain urinary elimination.	1. Observe voiding pattern. 2. Maintain patency of urinary catheters. 3. Palpate bladder for retention, catheterize if necessary per physician's order. 4. Take measures to prevent calculi (ie, change position q2h, administer urine-acidifying juices). 5. Inspect urine for hematuria and stones. 6. Provide for privacy during procedures.
	• Patient will maintain fluid and electrolyte balance.	1. Maintain accurate intake and output record. 2. Replace sodium, potassium, and chloride losses. 3. Weigh patient daily. 4. Encourage fluids per physician's order.
High risk for altered comfort: related to ineffective urinary elimination, full bladder.	• Patient will be able to maintain comfort during urinary elimination.	1. Monitor for favorable or adverse responses to treatment regimen. 2. Administer pain medication per physician's order. 3. Instruct in nonpharmacologic means of pain relief (ie, relaxation techniques). 4. Allow patient time and privacy during urination.

0.4 mg/dl. Mrs. Landry was maintained on her normal dose of digoxin (0.125 mg/day) and placed on a 1,200-calorie, 2-g sodium diet and given hydrochlorothiazide, 50 mg two times a day.

Mrs. Landry's cardiovascular symptoms gradually improved, but 1 week later she was slightly confused and complained of dizziness on sitting up. Her blood pressure was 150/60, pulse was 108 beats/min, and weight was 47.7 kg. She did not recall voiding in the past 24 hours. A Foley catheter was inserted and 15 ml of dark yellow urine was obtained. The following laboratory values were obtained:

Serum
  Na: 149 mEq/L
  Cl: 112 mEq/L
  CO$_2$: 29 mEq/L
  K: 3.5 mEq/L
  BUN: 144 mg/dl

  Creatinine: 2.1 mg/dl
  Osmolality: 303 mOsm/L

Urine
  Na: 11 mEq/dl
  K: 33 mEq/dl
  Osmolality: 482 mOsm/L
  Creatinine: 89 mg/dl

Case Study Discussion
The hypernatremia suggested mild dehydration. BUN was alarmingly high, and the serum creatinine of 2.1 mg/dl, although seemingly low in relation to the BUN, was four times greater than the value recorded on admission, suggesting a loss of 75% of initial renal function. A diagnosis of ARF secondary to volume depletion was considered. When urine chemistries returned, however, the low urinary sodium, the urinary osmolality (which

NURSING CARE PLAN 25–4:
The Patient With Congestive Heart Failure and Prerenal Azotemia

NURSING DIAGNOSIS	OUTCOME CRITERIA/ PATIENT GOALS	NURSING INTERVENTIONS
Self-care deficit: feeding, bathing, hygiene and ambulation related to weakness and fatigue secondary to congestive heart failure.	• Patient will show increased independence in carrying out hygiene activities. • Patient will have increased endurance in completing self-care activities.	1. Observe functional level every shift and report any changes. 2. Encourage patient to verbalize concerns about self-care deficits. 3. Monitor completion of bathing and hygiene activities daily. 4. Provide assistance with ambulation as needed. 5. Instruct on bathing techniques that conserve energy. 6. Assist with feeding. 7. Apply lotion to dry, flaky skin areas.
Altered tissue perfusion: related to volume depletion secondary to prerenal azotemia.	• Maintain fluid and electrolyte balance. • Maintain serum sodium within normal limits.	1. Observe voiding pattern. 2. Hydrate per physician's order. 3. Monitor BP, pulse, respirations, and temperature q2h and then q4h. 4. Maintain intake and output record. 5. Observe character of urine. 6. Monitor laboratory reports. 7. Instruct regarding sodium-restricted diet. 8. Assist with ambulation when ordered. 9. Weigh patient daily. 10. Check skin turgor q4h.
Altered nutrition: less than body requirements: related to loss of appetite and fatigue secondary to congestive heart failure and prerenal azotemia.	• Adequate dietary intake will be promoted. • Patient will adhere to 1,200-calorie, 2-g sodium diet. • Patient will demonstrate knowledge about need for adequate food and fluid intake. • Patient's energy levels will be maintained.	1. Weigh patient daily. 2. Assist with all meals and snacks. 3. Arrange in a comfortable sitting position. 4. Remove all noxious stimuli. 5. Arrange for family member to be present at meal times. 6. Instruct on rationale for six-meal-a-day diet plan and adequate fluid intake. 7. Arrange for dietitian also to instruct on prescribed diet. 8. Provide for frequent rest before each meal period. 9. Perform range of motion exercises q2h.

was 1.6 × that of plasma), and the U/P creatinine ratio of 42/1 suggested intact renal function. The fractional excretion of sodium (U:P Na/U:P creatinine × 100) was calculated as follows: $Fe_{Na} = 11:149/89:2.1 \times 100 = 0.17\%$

This also was consistent with volume depletion and prerenal azotemia.

Mrs. Landry could have had either (1) ARF resulting from excessive volume depletion or from emboli due to cardiac disease, or (2) prerenal azotemia resulting from volume depletion.

A challenge with 500 ml normal saline (N/S) IV over 1 hour produced a urine flow of 40 ml in the next hour. A slow infusion of N/S, 2 L/day, was given over the next 4 days and followed by increasing urine volumes. Mrs. Landry's weight increased to 51.1 kg, and the BUN and creatinine dropped to 22.4 and 0.9 mg/dl, respectively, without increased signs of cardiac decompensation. This dramatic response confirmed the laboratory-supported diagnosis of prerenal azotemia.

A nursing care plan for Mrs. Landry was developed (see Nursing Care Plan 25–4).

REFERENCES

1. Glassock R, Adler S: Diabetic nephropathy. In Levine D (ed): Care of the Renal Patient, 2nd ed. Philadelphia, WB Saunders, 1991
2. Berns J, Rudnick M: Radiocontrast media associated nephropathy. The Kidney 24(4):1–5, 1992
3. Lancaster L: Manifestations of renal failure. In Lancaster L (ed): Core Curriculum for Nephrology Nursing, 2nd ed., pp. 79–107. Pitman, NJ, AJ Jannetti, 1990

BIBLIOGRAPHY

Baer CL: Acute renal failure: Recognizing and reversing its deadly course. Nursing 20(6):34–40, 1990
Baer CL, Lancaster L: Acute renal failure. Critical Care Nursing Quarterly 14(4):1–21, 1992
Brundage D: Renal Disorders. St. Louis, Mosby Year Book, 1992
Cutler R, Forland C: Removal of drugs by hemodialysis and continuous ambulatory peritoneal dialysis: Suggested dosing modifications. Dial Transplant 20 (12):759–761, 1991
Dolleris PM: Diuretic and vasopressor usage in acute renal failure: A synopsis. Critical Care Nursing Quarterly 14(4): 28–31, 1992
Handerhan B: Understanding acute tubular necrosis. Nursing 21(1):20–21, 23, 1991
Lancaster LE: Renal response to shock. Critical Care Nursing Clinics of North America 2:221–233, 1990
Levine D: Care of the Renal Patient, 2nd ed. Philadelphia, WB Saunders, 1991
Murphy T, Bennett E: Low tech, high touch perfusion assessment. Am J Nurs 92(5):36–46, 1992
Toto KH: Acute renal failure: A question of location. Am J Nurs 92(11):44–53, 1992

STUDY QUESTIONS

1. In prerenal azotemia, the events that lead to a decline in function occur
   a. between the bladder and the ureters
   b. in the renal cortex
   c. at the level of the glomeruli
   d. before circulation reaches the kidney

2. Events that cause kidney tissue damage along with renal failure are categorized as
   a. severe renal ischemia
   b. hyperviscosity states
   c. intrarenal acute renal failure
   d. post renal acute renal failure

3. The primary focus of treating prerenal azotemia is to
   a. restore renal circulation
   b. control serum sodium and potassium
   c. remove the enlarged prostate
   d. inspect urine for hematuria and stones

4. Your patient is an elderly woman with diabetes and a serum creatinine of 2.0 mg/dl. She is to have an angiogram to rule out coronary artery disease. What should your care plan include up to the first 3 days post?
   1. meticulous monitoring of intake and output before and after the procedure
   2. request an order for preprocedure hydration

   3. daily weights
   4. measure BUN and creatinine daily

      a. 1 and 2
      b. 2 and 3
      c. 2, 3, and 4
      d. all of the above

5. What is the most common complication of oliguric renal failure?

   a. respiratory acidosis
   b. overhydration
   c. metabolic acidosis
   d. hyperglycemia

6. The most important aspect of nursing care during the diuretic phase of acute renal failure is

   a. relieving symptoms of uremia
   b. measuring serial potassium levels
   c. monitoring oxygen saturation
   d. maintaining fluid balance

7. The primary danger of not correcting prerenal acute renal failure is

   a. cardiovascular collapse
   b. progression to intrarenal acute renal failure
   c. pulmonary edema
   d. cerebral hemorrhage

CHAPTER 26

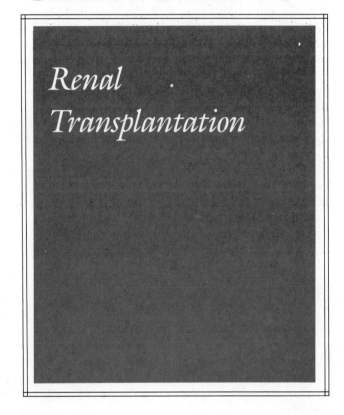

Renal Transplantation

BEHAVIORAL OBJECTIVES

Based on the content in this chapter, the reader should be able to:

1. Define end-stage renal disease (ESRD).
2. Describe the altered body functions created by ESRD.
3. Compare and contrast the degrees to which dialysis and transplant manage various alterations created by ESRD.
4. List the criteria for selecting a kidney donor.

(continued)

5. Recognize the signs and symptoms of postoperative transplantation complications, including acute and chronic rejection, infection, and altered urinary output.
6. Describe the immunosuppression drug therapy regimens.
7. Develop care plans for the pretransplant, postoperative, and long-term phases of the transplantation process.

Description

Transplantation research began in the early 1900s, although it was not until the early 1950s that transplantation became a realistic and therapeutic approach for chronic renal failure in humans.

Originally, kidneys were grafted into the thigh, with the femoral vessels used for vascularization. Experience with this procedure was limited to a very few patients. Because this site obviously was not practical for long-term graft survival, surgeons began grafting kidneys into the iliac fossa in the mid-1950s, the site still used today.

Since that time, renal transplantation has been performed as definitive therapy for end-stage renal disease (ESRD). As more centers evolved, so too have a multitude of approaches and philosophies, with the major differences revolving around immunosuppressive therapy and immunoalteration.

This chapter does not encompass all possible management approaches, but will, however, cover the major aspects of transplantation and care common to all centers and well documented in the literature. It will provide the critical care nurse with sufficient information to provide competent care for the transplant recipient.

End-Stage Renal Disease

Pathophysiological Principles

Renal failure is rarely an "all-or-none" phenomenon but instead is a gradual loss of function involving either some or all of the nephrons, depending on the basic disease process.

When a patient has minimal renal damage, the body may compensate for certain lost functions, and symptoms will not be manifest. If the process is acute and reversible, the effects of long-term failure (eg, anemia, osteodystrophy) will not be seen. For many patients, however, the process is long and exhausting, and affects all body systems.

It is not until irreversible damage occurs to most of the nephrons (which total approximately 2 million) and the glomerular filtration rate (GFR) decreases to 10 ml/minute that a patient is considered to have ESRD.

Once a patient reaches ESRD, three options are available: no treatment and death, chronic dialysis (either peritoneal dialysis or hemodialysis), or transplantation (Fig. 26–1). The option of no treatment and certain death is considered and occasionally chosen; however, most people choose to receive treatment. Although dialysis and transplant are separate treatment options, each of these therapies is an integral part of the other. Dialysis support must be available for pretransplant and possible post-transplant application. If the transplant fails, these recipients have a chance to continue life support with the aid of dialysis.

Both ESRD and replacement therapy change the patient's previous state of being. Therefore, the alterations created by the disease and their therapies must be considered because some alterations may persist post-transplant. Table 26–1 outlines the altered body functions created by ESRD and the effects on them when managed by dialysis or a well functioning transplant.

Alterations Created by End-Stage Renal Disease

Body Fluids

In ESRD, the GFR and urinary output are grossly diminished, creating an excess of body fluids. Consequently, renal filtration occurs only during dialysis. With a well-functioning renal graft, however, renal filtration is constant.

Nutrition

All people receiving dialysis have dietary restrictions, although individual requirements vary widely. The restrictions for patients receiving hemodialysis, which include protein, sodium, potassium, and fluid, are necessary because the equivalent of renal filtration occurs for only a limited number of hours per week. Patients undergoing peritoneal dialysis have less extensive dietary restrictions. To follow the diet, a lifetime of eating habits must be changed, placing severe limits on the patient's social activities. Gross nonadherance to the diet can result in malignant hypertension, congestive heart failure, pulmonary edema, hyperkalemia, and, potentially, cardiac arrest.

Sodium restriction may be necessary after successful transplantation because steroids and cyclosporine can cause

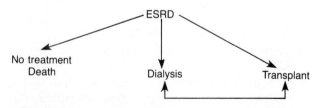

FIGURE 26–1
Options facing a person with end-stage renal disease (ESRD).

TABLE 26–1
Alterations Created by End-Stage Renal Disease
Managed by Dialysis and Well Functioning Transplant

Function	Dialysis	Well-Functioning Transplant
Body fluids	Excess body fluids	Alteration in fluids resolved
	Renal filtration occurs only during dialysis	Acid–base balance maintained
	Metabolic acidosis	
Nutrition	Na, K, protein and fluid restrictions	Possible Na and K restriction for up to 1 yr after transplant
		Possible alterations in diet for hyperglycemia
Hematologic system	Anemia, fatigue	Normal RBC and Hct
	Shortened RBC survival	
	Prolonged clotting time	Normal clotting time
Physical mobility Bone disease	Renal osteodystrophy:	No further bone resorption
	Osteomalacia	Steroid-induced osteoporosis
	Osteoporosis	Possible tertiary hyperparathyroidism
	Osteitis fibrosa cystica	Avascular/aseptic necrosis
	Possible secondary hyperparathyroidism	
Decreased muscle strength	Decreased muscle mass due to dietary limits	Myopathy that improves when steroid dosage decreases and patient's activity increases
	Decreased exercise tolerance	
Nervous system control	Peripheral, gastrointestinal, and genitourinary neuropathy	Neuropathy will not progress and may improve
	Autonomic nervous system neuropathy	
Hepatic function	Increased risk of hepatitis from extracorporeal circulation in hemodialysis patient	Risk of hepatitis due to azathioprine or cyclosporine therapy
	Increased risk of hepatitis B or non-A, non-B hepatitis from transfusions	Risk of hepatitis B or C from transfusions
		Increased susceptibility to viral hepatitis
Cardiovascular system	Risk of vascular access infection, clotting, exsanguination, and frequent site changes	No need for vascular access
	Accelerated atherosclerosis	Effect on atherosclerotic process uncertain
	Hypertriglyceridemia	Increased cholesterol levels
	Ventricular hypertrophy, heart failure	Ventricular size sometimes returns to normal
	Uremic pericarditis	
	Cardiac tamponade	
Gastrointestinal function	Increased gastric acid production	Increased risk of ulceration
	Increased incidence of diverticulosis	Diverticulosis predisposes to perforation
	Constipation	
Immune response	Increased susceptibility to infection from uremia	Increased susceptibility to infection from immunosuppressive drugs
		Increased incidence of malignancy (especially skin, lymph, and cervix)
Gas exchange	Risk of pulmonary edema, congestive heart failure	Risk of pulmonary infections secondary to immunosuppressive therapy
Self-concept and body image	Dependent on machine and solutions to support life	Dependent on medications to support renal function
	Gradual, subtle physical changes (eg, change in skin color, muscle loss)	Rapid, abrupt early physical changes (eg, cushingoid appearance, hirsutism, gingival hyperplasia, acne)
Sexual function	Impotence	Persistent impotence often secondary to other medicines, (eg, antihypertensives)
	Decreased libido	Libido usually improves
	Amenorrhea	Ovulation and menses usually return (age appropriate)

RBC, red blood cell; Hct, hematocrit.

sodium retention; the use of cyclosporine also may necessitate a potassium restriction.

Rather than having fluids restricted, patients with normal urine output may drink 2 liters of fluid a day. Protein is not restricted when renal function is normal. If the recipient has diabetes mellitus (or has iatrogenic diabetes from steroids or cyclosporine), a diabetic diet will be incorporated into the existing diet plan.

Hematologic System

Anemia is common to all patients with ESRD. Because the kidney no longer is able to produce adequate amounts of erythropoietic stimulating factor, red blood cell production is low. This, along with shorter red blood cell survival in the uremic patient, causes hematocrits one half of normal. This anemia is thought to cause the fatigue that can be one of the most frustrating problems for the ESRD patient.

The use of iron and androgen therapy historically benefited many patients, but the current use of human recombinant erythropoietin (epoetin alfa or EPO) therapy has been far more successful, and with fewer side effects. It is necessary to monitor the hematocrits of ESRD patients to titrate the proper dosage of EPO, but patients now have hematocrits of 30% to 36% without the need for transfusions. Some patients, however, fail to achieve or maintain a target hematocrit. This may result from infections or other inflammatory conditions, malignant processes, pericarditis, hematologic diseases, hemolysis, or osteitis fibrosa cystica.[1] Transfusions for this group of patients still may be necessary. Patients who respond favorably to EPO may deplete iron stores quickly in the manufacture of hemoglobin, and therefore should receive iron replacement.

The dramatic decrease in the use of blood transfusions to treat anemia has reduced the degree to which transplant recipients become sensitized to tissue antigens. Some clinicians still believe that transfusions are beneficial before transplantation for the purposes of immunoalteration, although this process is becoming much less common.

Several months after the transplant, anemia is seldom a problem, and the patient will have a near normal, if not normal, hematocrit. Although the kidney was denervated when transplanted, this does not affect the erythropoiesis of the graft. Although blood loss from laboratory tests is appreciable immediately after the transplant, it is markedly reduced after hospital discharge. The patient should have a normal protein intake, an increased ability to absorb iron, and normal red blood cell survival time, all increasing the ability to maintain the hematocrit at a higher level.

Physical Mobility

Bone Disease

The kidneys play a major role in maintaining calcium–phosphorus balance in the body. They accomplish this function by excreting these elements and also by converting vitamin D to its active form, cholecalciferol. Loss of nephron (kidney) function, therefore, is accompanied by gross disturbances in calcium metabolism and the development of a complex set of comorbidity problems that are referred to commonly as *renal osteodystrophy*. Renal osteodystrophy refers to three bone disease processes that are caused by the malfunctioning kidneys, as opposed to other etiologies: osteomalacia, osteoporosis, and osteofibrosa cystitis.

The ESRD patient may exhibit one or all three processes concurrently. The first process, *osteomalacia*, is defined as a softening of the bones. This process can cause bones to become so brittle that spontaneous fractures may occur. The second process is *osteoporosis*, which is defined as increased porosity of the bone and which occurs as bones continue to lose calcium.

Both osteomalacia and osteoporosis are caused by the lack of activated vitamin D to assist in maintaining calcium hemostasis. Activated vitamin D or D_3 acts by increasing renal calcium reabsorption and intestinal transport of calcium into the bloodstream as well as by assisting in calcium mobilization from the bone in conjunction with parathyroid hormone (PTH). Vitamin D is acquired from sunlight or dietary sources, but requires a functioning renal mass for complete activation.

In renal failure, dietary calcium is restricted, lessening the availability of this element to maintain serum calcium values. In addition, the continued serum phosphorus elevation is thought to shut off vitamin D conversion and to increase skeletal resistance to the effect of PTH. The long-term effect of this skeletal resistance is that the parathyroid gland enlarges to secrete enough PTH to increase serum calcium.

The enlargement of the parathyroid causes hyperplasia, or secondary hyperparathyroidism, and *osteitis fibrosa cystica*, the third bone disease process. Symptoms may include itching, metastatic soft tissue calcifications around joints and tendons, vascular calcifications of the large and small blood vessels, and diffuse or local skeletal pain. Continued gland enlargement can lead to tertiary or autonomic hyperparathyroidism diagnosed by hypercalcemia.

Medical management of these problems should be provided early in the course of renal failure. Foods containing calcium and phosphorus should be restricted, although it is difficult adequately to limit their intake because they are present in so many foods. The use of aluminum-containing phosphorus binders should be avoided owing to the potential accumulation of aluminum to toxic levels. The administration of the synthetic form of active vitamin D in combination with calcium supplements helps to maintain the serum calcium and phosphorus at more normal levels. Caution should be used to avoid hypercalcemia, which may lead to the formation of calcium phosphate deposits.

Once the patient is on dialysis, the active form of vitamin D may be given either orally or intravenously, to allow the patient to absorb calcium more normally. Calcium carbonate may be given to provide calcium without phosphorus (because the elements usually are found in the same foods) so that the calcium can be absorbed while keeping the phosphorus down. Even with adequate therapy, bone disease may continue, and a subtotal parathyroidectomy may be required to halt the progression of bone changes.

A successful renal transplant stops many of the osteodystrophic changes produced by ESRD because the kidney can again take an active role in calcium metabolism. Occasionally, the parathyroid glands continue to enlarge, causing tertiary hyperparathyroidism. In addition, the catabolic nature of the steroid medication contributes to the development of osteoporosis and aseptic necrosis of major joints.

Decreased Muscular Strength

A loss of muscle mass is common with ESRD. Limited dietary intake and inability to exert oneself due to the fatigue associated with anemia probably are the major contributing factors. When EPO is used and a normal or near normal hematocrit is maintained, the loss may be minimized.

The transplant recipient frequently will experience myopathies due to steroid therapy. This loss in muscle mass can be recovered with exercise, particularly when the dose of steroids is reduced. In an attempt to avoid severe myopathies, the transplant recipient is encouraged to walk, climb stairs, and exercise as much as possible.

Nervous System Control

Although the mechanism is poorly understood, neuropathies may develop in the presence of severe or chronic uremia. This is especially prevalent among those with long-standing diabetes mellitus. The neuropathies cause muscle weakness, which sometimes requires the use of braces, walkers, or crutches for ambulation. Functions of the autonomic nervous system may be impaired to the extent that the gastrointestinal tract may be affected and blood pressure control is poor. Patients actually may have chronic hypotension from autonomic nervous system neuropathy.

Neuropathy should not increase in severity after transplantation; and depending on its severity, partial or total reversal may occur after successful transplantation.

Sexual Dysfunction

Impotence is prevalent among dialysis patients. Although women may be physically capable of engaging in sexual intercourse, libido often is decreased markedly, lowering their desire for sexual activity.

Most male patients are impotent, perhaps because of their disease or because of antihypertensive medications. The etiology of this complication probably is physiological as well as psychological. Research data suggest that certain trace elements (eg, zinc) may be implicated in sexual dysfunction. Marriages and other comparable relationships can be adversely affected, and the long-term effects can be devastating.

Some patients remain impotent after transplantation, although this is associated most frequently with antihypertensive medication and steroid therapy. The libido, which is decreased while the patient is on dialysis, seems to return to normal after transplantation.

Women usually stop having menstrual periods while on dialysis, but after transplantation once again will ovulate and menstruate. Therefore, some means of contraception should be used for 2 years post-transplantation, when renal function is stable and immunosuppression is at a minimum dosage. There is additional risk for the mother and fetus if pregnancy occurs during periods of unstable renal function and higher doses of immunosuppressive medications.

Hepatic Function

Problems associated with the dialysis treatments alone are considerable. Hepatitis is an ever-present threat due to the frequent extracorporeal circulation in the hemodialysis patient. If the transplant recipient receives blood transfusions before transplantation, the patient has the added risk of acquiring hepatitis from the transfusions. This risk includes hepatitis B virus, hepatitis C virus, and the human immunodeficiency virus (HIV). Although blood donors are screened for hepatitis B and HIV, screening for hepatitis C remains ill defined, causing it to be a threat to the integrity of hepatic function.

After the initial postoperative period, transplant recipients rarely receive transfusions. Both azathioprine and cyclosporine are potentially hepatotoxic, however, as reflected by an elevation in the results of liver function studies. When azathioprine is responsible for the alteration of function, the drug is withdrawn while steroids and cyclosporine are continued. On rare occasions, cyclophosphamide may be substituted for azathioprine. In either case, withdrawal of the drug allows for reversal of liver abnormalities. If it is necessary to decrease or stop cyclosporine, steroid therapy may be initiated or increased.

Cardiovascular Function

Perhaps the most dramatic complication of ESRD is the rate of accelerated atherosclerosis. The etiology is not understood, but the greatest cause of mortality in long-term dialysis patients is cardiovascular accidents.

Some of the most advanced atherosclerosis seen at postmortem examination has been in long-term dialysis patients. Many ESRD patients have type IV hyperlipidemia, with elevated levels of triglycerides. Diet, weight reduction, and exercise are the preferred ways to reduce the levels of very-low-density lipoproteins and increase the levels of high-density lipoproteins. Saturated fats such as whole milk, cream, cream cheese, and animal fats are discouraged; monounsaturated and polyunsaturated fats are allowed. Foods such as oat bran and drugs such as lovastatin have been shown to reduce serum cholesterol levels as much as 30% to 40%. Attaining ideal body weight also may help control hyperlipidemia. Even light exercise (eg, exercising to 50% of the target pulse rate) can be effective in reducing cholesterol and limiting cardiovascular disease. Patients can perform light exercise and can experience emotional as well as cardiovascular benefits from a structured exercise program.

The effect of transplantation on atherosclerosis is uncertain but is under investigation. It is thought, however, that cholesterol levels increase after transplantation. The return to a normal diet can decrease the dietary contributions to atherosclerotic changes.

Depending on the underlying pathologic cause of renal failure and the degree of residual renal function, dialysis patients may have little or no urine output. Consequently, any fluid consumed between dialysis treatments is retained, other than insensible losses. The degree to which the patients follow their fluid restriction will influence the fluid volume status directly. Excessive intake of fluids can tax the cardiopulmonary system as hypervolemia develops. Congestive heart failure or pulmonary edema may develop, and must be treated by rapid removal of fluid by dialysis. This expansion and rapid contraction of fluids in the vasculature adds to the stress under which the cardiovascular system is functioning, and may contribute significantly to hypertension, followed by hypotension.

Hypervolemia can develop in the transplant recipient when decreased urinary output occurs as the result of rejection episodes or acute tubular necrosis (ATN). It is managed with diuretic therapy or dialysis support.

Uremic pericarditis is another complication that occurs in ESRD patients. The specific mechanism that causes this is unclear. Depending on the severity and chronicity of pericarditis, a pericardial window or a pericardectomy sometimes is necessary to control this problem. A pericardial rub may not be heard when hypervolemia is secondary to fluid contained in the pericardial sac. What seems to be an appropriate therapy—dialyzing to remove excess fluid—actually can increase the patient's pain because the fluid is removed, and the friction is increased. At this point, a rub is very prominent.

Gastrointestinal Function

Gastric acid production is increased in many ESRD patients. High levels of PTH and decreased degradation of gastrin by the diseased kidneys both contribute to this.

Although these dysfunctions can be reversed by replacement of normal renal function, the risk of ulceration is increased post-transplantation. This risk is greatest during a period of compromised renal function (ie, during a rejection episode), when the patient also is receiving higher doses of immunosuppressants. It has not been observed during periods of normal renal function and lower-dosage drug therapy.

The presence of diverticulosis before transplant predisposes the patient to bowel perforation after transplant. To reduce the risk of this serious problem, a colon resection is done before transplantation. Limited fluid intake and the use of phosphorus binders not only contribute to constipation, but also can lead to the development of an antacid bezoar, causing impaction, possible perforation, and possible death. Elevated serum amylase levels are common in those receiving dialysis and are not necessarily indicative of acute pancreatitis.

Immune System

Both dialysis and transplant patients are more susceptible to infections, the former from uremia and the latter from medications that alter the immune response.

There also is an increased incidence of malignancy among transplant patients, especially of the skin, lymphatic system, and cervix. The data for dialysis patients are obscure, controversial, and difficult to correlate with the disease or the treatment.

All organ donors are screened for the presence of HIV to ensure that it is not transmitted to the recipient by the transplanted kidney. Recipients also usually are screened for HIV. There is disagreement, however, about whether a positive HIV without clinical manifestation of acquired immune deficiency syndrome (AIDS) should negate the prospect of transplantation.

Gas Exchange

Hypervolemia as the result of ESRD can cause congestive heart failure, pulmonary congestion, and pulmonary edema. After transplantation, the risk of congestive heart failure and pulmonary edema diminishes because fluid balance can be maintained by the functioning kidney graft. Hypervolemia, however, may occur due to acute renal failure, cyclosporine toxicity, or rejection. Treatment of hypervolemia with diuretics or dialysis is essential before a patient receives Orthoclone OKT3 (Ortho Pharmaceutical Corp., Raritan, NJ) to treat rejection. Dyspnea, wheezing, chest pain, and pulmonary edema will occur if the patient is not normovolemic when OKT3 is administered, particularly with the first dose. The risk of pulmonary infection is increased after transplantation as a result of immunosuppressive therapy.

Self-Concept and Body Image

Patients with ESRD need dialysis to live and therefore are physiologically dependent on a machine or solutions. This can alter the concept of one's self as an independent person. The average time spent on hemodialysis can vary from 6 to 12 hours per week. A patient on peritoneal dialysis may spend several hours a day executing the exchanges, or perhaps overnight (or the equivalent) if a cycling machine is used to perform the dialysis.

Because of the life-sustaining value of dialysis as well as the time devoted to the procedure, patients have varying degrees of emotional dependence on the treatment.

For some, dependence is kept in perspective by treating the time spent on dialysis as a part-time job, continuing with other facets of life in as normal a manner as circumstances permit. Others, however, may allow their lives to be consumed by their need for life-support treatment. Their emotional energy may be centered on the dialysis treatment and the personnel providing it. They also may develop a sense of community and social contacts within the treatment setting. They may become so attached to this setting that the option of transplantation and freedom from life-support therapy is unattractive and undesirable. Those who assume this sick role and become comfortable with it actually may do poorly after transplantation, when independence is encouraged and the emphasis has shifted from sickness to wellness. When such patients receive transplants, compliance with immunosuppressive therapy may be jeopardized by the desire to return to the sick role, thus threatening the potential for maintaining a viable, successful, kidney transplant.

Conversely, the transplant recipient is no longer dependent on a machine, but on medication to support the function of the graft. Although dependence on medications generally is more acceptable than dependence on mechanical support, it still may be unacceptable to some. Failure of kidney transplants from medication noncompliance probably is much greater than existing data suggest. This noncompliance may result from rejecting the sick role because of feeling healthy and normal—and therefore having no further need for medication. This clearly represents a view opposite from that of the sick role group, but nonetheless is as dangerous with regard to potential for long-term survival with a functioning kidney.

Changes in body image are more abrupt after transplantation because of the immunosuppressive drugs. The changes seen with chronic dialysis (eg, skin color changes associated with anemia and uremia as well as muscle wasting) are more gradual and subtle.

Summary

End-stage renal disease is chronic and complex and presents a multitude of problems for the patient, family, and the health care team, regardless of whether the decision is for continued dialysis or transplantation. Those who elect to pursue transplantation must then consider the evaluation and preparation required.

Renal Transplantation

Indications and Evaluation

The following general criteria guide the selection for kidney transplantation.

- Age is evaluated individually, although recipients usually are younger than age 60. Those older than age 50 may be at increased risk for complications. Children younger than age 5 are considered in pediatric centers.
- Gastrointestinal disease, liver disease, and acute or chronic infection including AIDS are absent or have been treated.
- Patient must be motivated for transplantation.
- Patient has normal function of lower urinary tract; exceptions include neurogenic bladder secondary to diabetes mellitus. Other exceptions exist and require evaluation.

Medical problems that prohibit safe transplantation include advanced or uncorrectable cardiac disease, advanced pulmonary disease (eg, chronic obstructive pulmonary disease), chronic or recurrent infection or inflammatory disease that could become disseminated when immunosuppressants are given, and malignancy, unless 2 years or more have passed without recurrence. Routine evaluation and preparation include the following:

- ABO typing
- Tissue typing
- Transfusion history
- Tuberculosis skin test
- Hepatitis screening
- HIV screening
- Liver function studies
- Leukocyte and platelet count $\times$ 3
- Administration of Pneumovax (Merck Sharp & Dohme, West Point, PA) vaccine if patient has never received it
- Chest x-ray
- Dental evaluation to rule out infections
- Gynecologic examination
- Social history, review of patient motivation, and ability to follow postoperative regime, possible psychological evaluation

Possible additional studies include radiologic studies of the gastrointestinal tract and bladder and studies of the gallbladder.

Once a person has been selected for transplantation, the search begins for a suitable donor.

Donor Selection

Determining Compatibility

There are several requirements for the selection of donor–recipient pairs for kidney transplantation. Red blood cell compatibility between donor and recipient is essential to avoid reactions that could cause organ loss. Histocompatibility testing (tissue typing) also is performed to determine further the compatibility between the donor and recipient and improve the chances of acceptance of an organ. Antigens that comprise a person's tissue type are coded for by the major histocompatibility complex (MHC) genes. These genes contain the genetic information for cell surface antigens that differentiate self from nonself. These antigens are referred to as human leukocyte antigens (HLA), and are found on the surface of lymphocytes. Lymphocytes isolated from peripheral blood, lymph nodes, or spleen are a source of tissue-typing material for these antigens. The MHC encodes for several major allelic systems including A, B, and DR (D-related) that have been found to be of importance in transplantation. Each person has two A-locus, B-locus, and DR-locus antigens. These are inherited as a haplotype from each parent that contains one A-locus, B-locus, and DR-locus antigen. Many possible antigens may occur at each locus, resulting in a very large number of possible combinations of expressed HLAs. Therefore, it is rare that unrelated people will have identical antigens. With histocompatibility typing, however, better-matched donor and recipient pairs may be chosen for transplantation.

Crossmatch testing between potential donors and recipients also must be performed before transplantation. This test screens recipient serum for preformed antibodies to donor antigens that are present on donor lymphocytes. The recipient may have produced antibodies from prior exposure to antigens in pregnancy, transfusion, or previous transplantation. A crossmatch will take 6 to 8 hours to complete. A positive crossmatch is a contraindication to transplantation because the potential recipient has an antibody that will attack the donor graft. A negative crossmatch is needed for recipient selection.

A test used to identify compatibility at another locus, the D locus, of the MHC is the mixed lymphocyte culture, or mixed lymphocyte response. A mixed lymphocyte culture is a complex test that measures the reaction between donor and recipient when their lymphocytes are grown together in a culture. This test is not suitable for selection of cadaver kidney recipients because the test requires 5 to 7 days for cellular stimulation and division to occur.

There has been a trend to administer blood transfusions to potential recipients before transplantation. Although the mechanism of action of the transfusions on the immune system still is under study, many centers have observed improvement in graft survival. As immunosuppression is improved, however, the beneficial effect of transfusions may be superseded.

Laboratory testing and treatment protocols are attempts to improve the results of organ transplantation. The complexity of the immune system and its role in graft acceptance, however, continue to be areas of investigation in transplantation.

Living Donors

As the term indicates, a living person can donate a kidney. Historically, most living donors were relatives (ie, a sibling, parent, or child). More recently, however, kidneys from "emotionally related" donors (eg, a spouse or significant other) are being transplanted. This is the result of the shortage of cadaveric organ donors and of the improved results with current immunosuppression.

The greatest potential for a successful transplant exists when the donor and recipient have inherited identical antigens from their parents. The inheritance of identical antigens, a two-haplotype match, occurs only in siblings. Other possible matches include a one-haplotype match, in which half of the antigens in the donor and recipient are identical; a no-antigen match, in which there are no shared haplotypes or antigens; or a range of matches between one and six.

Once a potential living donor is identified, a thorough medical evaluation is performed to determine that the donor is free of underlying disease, has two kidneys, and that donation could in no obvious way jeopardize the donor's well-being. Once this evaluation is completed successfully, a living donor transplant may be performed.

Donor-specific transfusion (DST) is a technique of altering the immune responsiveness in living donor situations. The technique involves transfusing blood from a potential living donor to the recipient one to three times before transplanting the kidney. Depending on the transplant program's protocol, 50 to 100 ml of donor blood is administered to the recipient once or at 2-week intervals, two or three times. Donor-specific transfusion is thought to improve graft survival by (1) identifying recipients who would have reacted strongly to the antigens of the donor before actual transplantation; and (2) inducing acceptance of the donor tissue, probably by stimulating the development of suppressor T cells. The risk in performing DST before transplantation is that the recipient will become sensitized (ie, antibodies will develop) against the potential donor, thus eliminating that person as a donor. If sensitization does not occur and the transplant is performed, 1-year graft survival in a one-haplotype-matched living related donor and recipient exceeds 90%. Donor-specific transfusion has been used less frequently since cyclosporine has become widely used. The drug achieves about the same results without the risk of recipient sensitization that occurs with DST.

Ethical questions continue to be raised about the use of living donors. Long-term studies of living donors have demonstrated no adverse effects of donation and, in fact, some have found beneficial psychological effects from donation. Opponents of the use of living donors believe the improved results of cadaveric donation make the risks for living donors unjustifiable.

Cadaveric Donors

Despite the increasing frequency of living donor transplants, the supply of organs does not meet the demand. In 1991, the national waiting list for organ transplants reached 25,000. In the same year, there were 4,534 cadaveric organ donors in the United States.[2] Estimates based on age, cause of death, and other criteria indicate that 14,000 of the 2.2 million Americans who die each year could be organ donors.[3] Clearly, there is a large discrepancy between the number of potential versus actual organ donors. The reasons for this discrepancy are varied, and include lack of information on the part of the public. Polls, however, show that 84% of those surveyed approve of organ donation; almost 75% would want their own organs donated after death.[4]

Another reason for the lack of donors is that health care professionals often do not inform families of potential donors about the option of donation. Lack of knowledge about donation and how to discuss donation with the family often are cited as reasons for not addressing this with families. As a result, routine inquiry (or required request) legislation has been implemented. This legislation requires that families of appropriate potential organ donors be given the opportunity to donate organs. In an effort to decrease the reluctance to discuss donation with families, some laws also require training for those who are in the position to speak with families about the option of donation.

The United Network for Organ Sharing (UNOS) is the federally funded organization that coordinates organ sharing. UNOS maintains a computer network for matching donors and recipients. Current national policy mandates that all kidneys that are perfectly matched to a recipient be offered to that recipient. UNOS also facilitates the sharing between organ procurement organizations so that the number of transplanted kidneys (and other organs) is maximized.

Identification of Potential Cadaveric Organ Donors

Any health care professional can identify a patient as a potential cadaveric organ donor. Criteria for organ donation vary widely, depending on the particular transplant center and the organ(s) to be donated. Therefore, it is recommended that any patient for whom the possibility of donation is considered be referred to the local Organ Procurement Organization.

Potential donors often are victims of trauma or cerebral aneurysm as well as a variety of other circumstances. Most organ donors are between the ages of newborn and 65 years. There are a variety of factors that preclude organ donation. When these exist, organ donation is not discussed with the family. These factors include:

1. Current malignancy (except primary brain or skin tumors).
2. Transmissible infectious diseases (hepatitis, HIV-positive, or positive risk factors for HIV infection).
3. Sepsis.

Determination of Death

With current technology, death can be determined in two ways, based on the absence of cardiopulmonary function or based on the absence of brain function. The absence of cardiopulmonary function is the better known method; however, the absence of brain function (brain death) also is a common method of determining death (see Chapter 28 for neurologic criteria for determining death). Most patients who are organ donors are pronounced dead based on the absence of brain function. The critical care nurse should be familiar with the laws in his or her state related to "brain death," and also with the institutional policies for the determination of death. Most policies require two physical examinations documenting the absence of brain function. Some require a confirmatory test (eg, an electroencephalogram or a radionuclide blood flow study). To avoid conflict-of-interest issues, the physicians caring for the potential donor and pronouncing death cannot be involved in the removal or transportation of organs.

The Nurse's Role

Critical care nurses are an integral part of the organ donation team. Almost all organ donors die in critical care units; thus, the critical care nurse is a key person in identifying potential donors. Moreover, the nurse plays an important role as advocate by making certain that all efforts are made to determine and act on the patient's wishes regarding donation. Nurses also play a vital role in supporting the family psychologically, particularly when they are trying to accept the donor's death. When a decision is made for organ donation, the nurse also plays an important role in supporting the donor physiologically.

When caring for a potential donor, it is essential to maintain hemodynamic stability so that vital organs are perfused adequately. To do this, hypotension is first treated by administering fluids and plasma volume expanders. Next, if vasopressors are necessary, dopamine is administered in doses less than 10 μg/kg to maintain systolic blood pressure above 100 mm Hg. When vasopressors are required to maintain blood pressure for more than 24 hours, cardiac donation may be precluded.

It also is essential to assess urine output hourly to detect diabetes insipidus. This is common in organ donors and is due to failure of the posterior pituitary to produce or release antidiuretic hormones. Aqueous vasopressin or desmopressin acetate may be ordered to reduce urine output and help maintain fluid balance.

The Transplant Coordinator's Role

The role of the transplant coordinator has evolved as a result of the need to make more organs available for transplantation. Although kidneys are the most commonly transplanted organs, the coordinator is involved in the coordination and procurement of all transplantable organs. A person may donate kidneys, heart, lungs, liver, pancreas, corneas, skin, bone, and perhaps other organs or tissue. The role of the transplant coordinator usually includes ensuring that the family has the information necessary to give informed consent and providing them with bereavement support. They also serve as a resource for the health care team and as a liaison between the transplant program and the critical care area. Cooperation between the critical care staff and the transplant program will help ensure that the option of donation is offered to families of all potential donors.

Assessment and Management

The transplant recipient usually is cared for in a specially designated area throughout both acute and convalescent phases of recovery. This eliminates patient transfer, decreases fragmentation of care, and reduces exposure to infection for this immunosuppressed patient. The transplant recipient usually is not critically ill and therefore many times does not fit the criteria for admission to a critical care area. Nevertheless, at times transplant patients will be cared for in a critical care area, especially if complications occur during the acute postoperative phases.

Preoperative Phase of Care

Preparation for kidney transplantation begins long before the phase immediately preceding surgery. It includes assessment and intervention with regard to the patient's level of anxiety, knowledge about the transplant procedure, and physiological status. In the immediate preoperative phase, preparation includes comprehensive blood work, an electrocardiogram, a chest x-ray, and dialysis within 24 hours of surgery. This dialysis is to return blood chemistries to as near normal levels as possible, reverse alteration in platelet aggregation created by uremia, and eliminate excess fluid. Immunosuppression may be initiated before surgery as well. The amount of time available to complete this preparation is dictated largely by the donor source. When there is a living related donor, preparation can occur over the course of the day before transplantation, whereas with a cadaveric donor all preparation must be completed in a matter of hours.

The Surgical Procedure

The kidney is placed retroperitoneal, in the iliac fossa. The vascular anastomoses are accomplished most commonly using the hypogastric or internal artery and the external iliac vein. When it is mechanically difficult to access these vessels, as with children, it may be necessary to anastomose the renal vessels to the inferior vena cava and aorta.

There are two types of ureteral anastomoses that can be performed. In the first, the donor ureter is implanted into the recipient's bladder by a vertical cystotomy and a submucosal antireflux tunnel, because the ureter will lack innervation and normal peristalsis.[5] In the second, much less frequently used type, the donor kidney is anastomosed at the ureteropelvic junction to the recipient ureter. A Foley catheter is used for both types of anastomoses, and occasionally a ureteral stent may be used. In either case, hematuria will be present for several days. In the more common procedure, clots may be seen in the urine, because of the vascular nature of the bladder. In the latter procedure, the urine will change to pink within the first postoperative day because there are no sutures in the bladder.

Postoperative Phase of Care

Immediately after surgery, the transplant recipient is cared for in a closely monitored area until stable. As the patient arrives in this postanesthesia care unit or intensive care area, make the following assessments:

1. Blood pressure, apical pulse, respirations, temperature, and central venous pressure (CVP). Blood pressure should be taken on the extremity that does not have a functioning vascular access site because even momentary interference with arterial blood flow may lead to access malfunction.
2. The patient's level of consciousness and degree of pain.
3. The number of intravenous lines present, noting the site, type of solution, and flow rate.
4. The abdominal dressing for drainage, noting whether a Hemovac or drain is present.
5. The presence of Foley and possible placement of ureteral catheters, and observe the patency and urinary drainage of each.
6. Locate the vascular access and determine its patency by placing either fingers or a stethoscope directly over the access site and feeling or listening for a characteristically loud, pulsating noise called a *bruit*.
7. If the patient has been maintained on peritoneal dialysis and the catheter is in place, make certain the catheter system remains sterile and is capped.
8. If a nasogastric tube is present, attach it to an appropriate drainage system.
9. Obtain a baseline weight within 24 hours of surgery.
10. Measure abdominal girth at the iliac crest. This is baseline information used at a later time for assessment of complications (eg, ureteral leak, lymphocele, or bleeding).

11. Monitor a child more frequently than an adult because of the dynamic nature of a child's fluid and cardiovascular status (ie, blood pressures, weights, and CVPs).

Answers to the following questions will provide additional baseline information:

- Are the patient's own kidneys present in addition to the graft, and, if so, how much urine do they produce daily? This information will help determine how much of the urine produced is from the transplanted kidney. If the chart does not provide answers, the patient and family can. In addition, flank scars usually indicate that nephrectomies have been done.
- When was the last dialysis treatment? The nurse should pay particular attention to the metabolic status if the patient has not been dialyzed within 24 hours of surgery.
- What are the preoperative results of laboratory tests (serum electrolytes, urea nitrogen, creatinine, liver function, calcium, phosphorus, complete blood count with differential and platelet counts, urine electrolytes, specific gravity, creatinine clearance)?
- How much and what kind of intravenous fluid has the patient received?
- Did the patient receive a loading dose of immunosuppressive drugs preoperatively?
- Is the patient to receive steroids, cyclosporine, azathioprine, antilymphocyte globulin (ALG), murine monoclonal antibody (muromonab) CD3 (Orthoclone OKT3), or other immunosuppressive therapy? This drug information helps not only to clarify the regimen but also to estimate the degree of immunosuppression.
- Were any of these agents administered in the operating room and, if so, what is the dosage schedule?
- What preoperative teaching has been done? Patients who are well informed tend to be less anxious and more cooperative because they know what to expect.
- Which physician is to be called—how, where and when—for ongoing medical care? Clarifying and recording this information may enhance communication and efficiency, especially in case of emergency. See Figures 26–2 and 26–3.

Many nursing responsibilities revolve around

- Observing the function of the transplanted kidney
- Monitoring fluid and electrolyte balance
- Helping the patient avoid sources of infection
- Detecting early signs of complications
- Supporting the patient and family through the recovery phase

Nursing care of the patient undergoing kidney transplantation is described in Nursing Care Plan 26–1.

Monitoring Renal Graft Function

The transplanted kidney may function immediately after revascularization and produce large amounts of urine (200–1,000 ml/hour), small amounts of urine (<20 ml/hour), or no urine at all, based on the following factors.

The Effect of Ischemic Time. The amount of urine produced is related to the length of time the donor kidney was ischemic. Because the ischemic time tends to be shorter in living related transplantation than in cadaver transplantation, the living related donor kidney has less damage and tends to produce more urine in the initial recovery phase.

The hourly production of large amounts of urine, however, is called post-transplantation diuresis and is thought to be the result of a proximal tubular defect. The proximal tubule is responsible for 80% reabsorption of water, electrolytes, and glucose, and interference with its function allows more filtrate than normal to be excreted. This is a reversible state in which tubular reabsorptive functions are temporarily lost or greatly diminished because of an ischemic time period that begins with clamping the renal artery in the donor and concludes with the end of the venous revascularization of the recipient.

Preservation Time. Ischemic time is prolonged in the cadaver donor situation because after the donor nephrectomies have been completed, tissue typing and crossmatching for the most suitable recipient takes several hours. During this time, the kidneys are placed on an organ preservation machine or in a preservation solution until recipients are identified. The kidneys are then transported to the appropriate transplant centers.

Desirable preservation time is fewer than 50 hours, although as much as 72 hours may be acceptable. This preservation time added to hypotensive periods in some cadaver donors explains the possibility of tissue damage and low urine output in the early transplant periods. In this situation, the graft may produce little or no urine for up to 4 weeks after the transplant operation. This is ATN and usually is reversible.

Renal Function Tests. The quantity of urine does not have to correlate with the quality of graft function. Renal function is assessed by periodic serum urea nitrogen and creatinine levels and in some centers by a β_2-microglobulin test. This low-molecular-weight globulin is filtered readily by the glomerular basement membrane and is reabsorbed and metabolized almost completely by the proximal renal tubules.

A renal scan is a radionuclide test used to determine renal perfusion, filtration, and excretion. It is done frequently in the first 24 hours for baseline data and periodically thereafter when laboratory values or clinical changes suggest an alteration in renal function. A renal biopsy also may be done to determine the cause of the graft dysfunction.

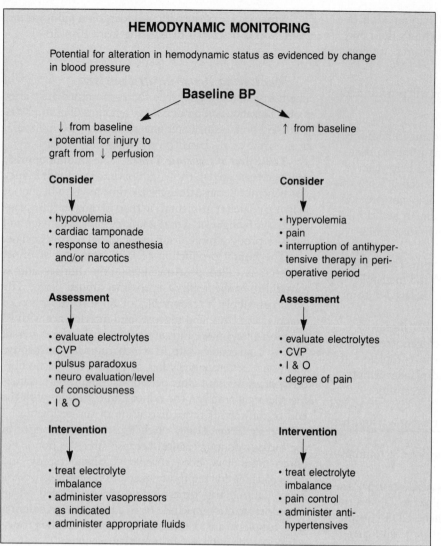

HEMODYNAMIC MONITORING

Potential for alteration in hemodynamic status as evidenced by change in blood pressure

Baseline BP

↓ from baseline
• potential for injury to graft from ↓ perfusion

↑ from baseline

Consider

• hypovolemia
• cardiac tamponade
• response to anesthesia and/or narcotics

Consider

• hypervolemia
• pain
• interruption of antihypertensive therapy in perioperative period

Assessment

• evaluate electrolytes
• CVP
• pulsus paradoxus
• neuro evaluation/level of consciousness
• I & O

Assessment

• evaluate electrolytes
• CVP
• I & O
• degree of pain

Intervention

• treat electrolyte imbalance
• administer vasopressors as indicated
• administer appropriate fluids

Intervention

• treat electrolyte imbalance
• pain control
• administer antihypertensives

FIGURE 26–2
Renal transplantation, postoperative hemodynamic monitoring.

Urinary Drainage Problems. When a change in urinary output occurs, such as a large volume one hour to a diminished amount the next, mechanical factors that interfere with urinary drainage should be suspected. Clotted, kinked, or compressed tubing in the urinary drainage system may be the cause of the decreased output. When the catheter is occluded by a clot, the patient may complain of pain, feel an urgency to void, or have bloody leakage around the catheter. Milking is the preferred way to dislodge clots because irrigation, even under aseptic conditions, increases the risk of infection. Gentle irrigation with strict aseptic technique may be necessary, however. Small amounts of irrigant (no more than 30 ml) are recommended because recipients commonly have small bladders. Vigorous irrigation also could cause extravasation at the ureteral anastomotic site.

Urinary Leakage. Urinary leakage on the abdominal dressing and severe abdominal discomfort or distention may indicate retroperitoneal leakage from the ureteral anastomosis site.

Decreased urinary output or severe abdominal pain in the presence of good renal function and adequate pain medication should be reported because technical and surgical complications can result in loss of graft function.

Maintaining Fluid and Electrolyte Balance
Maintaining fluid and electrolyte balance follows the same principles outlined in Chapter 23. Intake is provided intravenously until the patient is able to take fluids by mouth.

Flow Rate. A standard maintenance solution of 600 to 1,200 ml/24 hour for an adult is based on insensible water losses, whereas replacement solution is calculated for each patient according to urine output, gastric and wound drainage, and CVP readings. When urinary output is high, as in post-transplantation diuresis, replacement will be large. Replacement fluid volumes will be smaller when oliguric or anuric states exist. The solutions used most often include 0.9% normal saline, 5% dextrose in water, 0.45% saline, and 2.5% dextrose in water. Centers use a variety of total parenteral nutrition solutions,

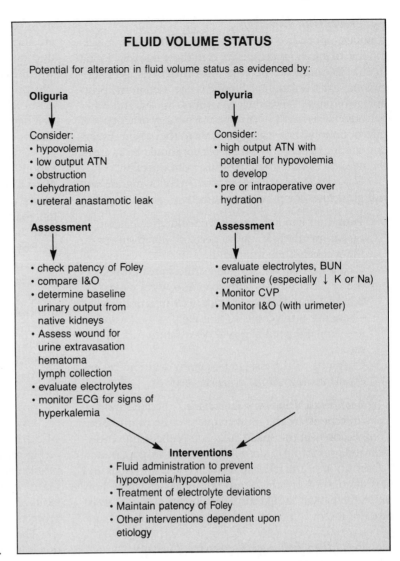

FLUID VOLUME STATUS

Potential for alteration in fluid volume status as evidenced by:

Oliguria

Consider:
• hypovolemia
• low output ATN
• obstruction
• dehydration
• ureteral anastamotic leak

Assessment

• check patency of Foley
• compare I&O
• determine baseline
  urinary output from
  native kidneys
• Assess wound for
  urine extravasation
  hematoma
  lymph collection
• evaluate electrolytes
• monitor ECG for signs of
  hyperkalemia

Polyuria

Consider:
• high output ATN with
  potential for hypovolemia
  to develop
• pre or intraoperative over
  hydration

Assessment

• evaluate electrolytes, BUN
  creatinine (especially ↓ K or Na)
• Monitor CVP
• Monitor I&O (with urimeter)

Interventions
• Fluid administration to prevent
  hypovolemia/hypovolemia
• Treatment of electrolyte deviations
• Maintain patency of Foley
• Other interventions dependent upon
  etiology

FIGURE 26–3
Renal transplantation, postoperative monitoring.

occasionally referred to as "renal failure fluid." Short-chain amino acid solutions (eg, Nephramine; American McGaw, Santa Ana, CA) promote osmotic diuresis from the higher dextrose content, control potassium, with the dextrose acting as the transport mechanism for keeping the serum potassium within acceptable limits, and minimize urea nitrogen production by using simple amino acids, generating minimum waste.

Infusion Site. The maintenance intravenous solution, or renal failure fluid, may be infused through a CVP line. When peripheral sites are necessary, they should *not* be in the extremity having a vascular access site. All efforts should be made to preserve an existing, patent vascular access, in the event that further hemodialysis is necessary.

Electrolyte Values. Serum electrolytes are measured shortly after the patient arrives in the unit. The frequency of these tests usually depends on graft function. If the patient has a large volume of output, laboratory tests may be done every 4 to 6 hours for the first 24 to 36 hours. If the patient is anuric but otherwise stable, tests for

electrolytes are done daily except for potassium, which may be ordered more frequently.

Blood drawing should be kept to a minimum because the recipient is anemic in the initial recovery phase secondary to ESRD.

The most frequent electrolyte disturbance in the acute postoperative phase is hyperkalemia. Most transplant recipients are dialyzed within 24 hours before surgery and therefore have a normal serum potassium in the operating room. If the graft functions and excretes a high volume of urine, it generally also is able to excrete the excessive serum potassium created by surgical tissue damage. If the patient is oliguric or anuric after surgery, the serum potassium may increase to unacceptable levels. Interventions include administration of glucose and insulin to transport potassium into the cell and administration of polystyrene sulfonate (Kayexalate; Winthrop Pharmaceuticals, New York, NY) either orally or as an enema. Polystyrene sulfonate is no longer the preferred treatment because of its potential for causing gastrointestinal complications.

Preventing Infection

Immunosuppressive therapy renders patients more susceptible to infectious organisms, even those normally found in the environment. Because most infections are endogenous, strict isolation technique is not used in the postoperative phase. Nevertheless, visitors, nurses, and other personnel who have upper respiratory or any other type of infection should not visit or give care to the patient. Everyone coming in contact with the patient should be aware of the need to protect these patients from infection.

General Preventive Measures. Following are several guidelines for preventing infection:

- Thorough handwashing before and after patient care is an effective way to decrease organisms in the recipient's environment.
- Cleansing the catheter and perineal area around the urethral meatus with soap and water every 8 hours may decrease urinary tract infections.
- Changing intravenous tubing daily as well as when it is contaminated also will decrease the risk of sepsis.
- Changing wet dressings frequently will remove an excellent medium for organism growth.

Avoiding Pulmonary Infections. Because pulmonary infections are the most frequent cause of infectious complications in transplant recipients, enhancing ventilation and promoting drainage of secretions are paramount. Observation of the rate and character of respirations and auscultation of breath sounds will help determine how often the patient should turn, deep breathe, cough, walk, use the incentive spirometer, or need postural drainage.

Providing Immunosuppressive Therapy

The transplanted kidney is a foreign antigen implanted in a recipient. Eventually, the recipient's body will recognize the kidney as a foreign antigen and mobilize its defense system to try to rid itself of this foreign substance. Therefore, immunosuppressive therapy is necessary to suppress the immune response to permit acceptance of transplanted organs, most often with a type of tissue at least partially different from that of the recipient. The difficulty of this therapy is in providing enough suppression to prevent rejection without rendering the recipient grossly susceptible to opportunistic infections.

Drugs. The drugs given to control the immune response are methylprednisolone (Solu-Medrol; Upjohn, Kalamazoo, MI), prednisone, azathioprine (Imuran; Burroughs Wellcome Co., Research Triangle Park, NC), cyclosporine (Sandimmune; Sandoz Pharmaceuticals, East Hanover, NJ), muromonab-CD3 (Orthoclone OKT3), ALG or antithymocyte globulin (ATG), and cyclophosphamide (Cytoxan; Bristol-Meyers, Evansville, IN). Major points about these drugs are summarized in Table 26–2.

Methylprednisolone is the parenteral steroid used in the initial postoperative period, and prednisone is the most commonly used oral steroid. These corticosteroids are anti-inflammatory agents, but also decrease the production of activated T-helper cells and cytotoxic cells, which help decrease the antigenic activity of the graft. Prednisone may be given in a variety of schedules and doses, and the philosophy varies from center to center, just as it does with the use of methylprednisolone in the treatment of rejection episodes.

Treatment of rejection episodes may include intravenous injections of methylprednisolone in boluses from 40 to 1,000 mg. It is recommended that a bolus be administered over 20 to 30 minutes. This is particularly important because several cardiac arrests have been reported after the administration of 1 g methylprednisolone delivered by intravenous push.

Azathioprine, one of the first drugs developed for immunosuppression, is an antimetabolite. It interrupts DNA synthesis and inhibits cellular division of immunocompetent cells. In doing so, the growth of activated B lymphocytes and cytotoxic T cells is inhibited. The patient's ability to tolerate 2 to 3 mg/kg consistently is important for long-term graft survival. Azathioprine cannot be increased to treat rejection because of its bone marrow suppression effects and its cumulative effects in the presence of little or no renal function.

Cyclosporine, a fungal metabolite, is much more specific than steroids or azathioprine. It prevents rejection by acting on T-helper cells, preventing them from secreting interleukin-2 (IL-2) and IL-1 from macrophages. By acting in such a specific manner, it appears to spare other facets of a person's immune system, thus allowing for some protection from infectious organisms.

The usefulness of cyclosporine in renal transplantation is limited by its adverse effects, most notably nephrotoxicity. Other major known side effects include hepatotoxicity, marked hirsutism, tremors, hyperglycemia, and gum hypertrophy. Cyclosporine is available as a capsule or liquid. The liquid must be measured precisely and mixed in a glass container with juice or milk.

Both the nephrotoxicity and the cost of this drug have led to the development of protocols called triple and quadruple therapy, which use several drugs in combination with cyclosporine.

FK 506 is the newest immunosuppressant drug. It decreases the production of IL-2 and other lymphokines that help T cells proliferate. Although the best method of using FK 506 has yet to be determined, it usually is used in combination with at least one other immunosuppressant, often steroids. The method of action for FK 506 is similar to cyclosporine's, so the two are not often used in combination.[7] FK 506 is available in intravenous or oral form. Side effects include nephrotoxicity, neurotoxicity, increased risk of infection, hypertension, lymphoproliferative disorders, and diabetogenesis.

Muromonab-CD3, or OKT3, is a monoclonal antibody specifically directed against the T lymphocyte. As a monoclonal antibody, it has a number of advantages: ho-

TABLE 26–2
Immunosuppressive Drugs Used in Renal Transplantation

Drug	Adverse Reactions	Dosage	Comments
Methylprednisolone (Solu-Medrol) (IV) Prednisone (PO)	Increased susceptibility to infection	Initial: 0.5 to 3 mg/kg of body weight, tapered to an adequate oral maintenance dose	Methylprednisolone is given up to 1 wk
	Masks symptoms of infection Peptic ulcer, GI bleeding		An antacid is given while patient is on steroids to reduce the risk of gastric irritation and ulceration; cimetidine may also be used to decrease ulcerogenic tendencies
	Increased appetite, weight gain		
		During rejection, methylprednisolone may be given in IV boluses up to 1 g/dose	Cardiac arrest can occur if IV bolus of 1 g is given rapidly
	Increased sodium and water retention, which exaggerate hypertension Delayed healing Negative nitrogen balance Adrenal gland suppression Behavior and personality changes Diabetogenic effect Muscle weakness Osteoporosis with long-term therapy Skin atrophy, striae Easy bruising Glaucoma, cataracts Hirsutism Acne Avascular/aseptic necrosis		Sodium restriction may be necessary when steroid dosage is high or when fluid retention increases
Azathioprine (Imuran) (IV or PO)	Bone marrow suppression: leukopenia, thrombocytopenia, anemia, pancytopenia Rash Alopecia Liver damage, jaundice Increased susceptibility to infection	Regulated to keep WBC 5,000 to 10,000. Drug usually stopped when WBC is 3,000 or less Initial 2–5 mg/kg of body weight Maintenance: 2–3 mg/kg of body weight During rejection: maximum of 3 mg/kg of body weight, dose not usually increased with rejection	Lower doses are given when 1. Renal function is poor 2. WBC is low 3. Given concurrently with allopurinol, which delays metabolism of azathioprine (allopurinol and azathioprine are synergistic)
Cyclosporine (Sandimmune) (IV or PO)	Nephrotoxicity Hepatotoxicity	Initial: 4 mg/kg/day (IV) Maintenance: 5–15 mg/kg/day PO may be used as part of triple therapy regime (prednisone, azathioprine, cyclosporine), or quadruple therapy regime (same as triple therapy plus ALG or OKT3)	Initially, nephrotoxicity and hepatotoxicity seem to be dose-related and respond to dose reduction Long-term nephrotoxicity is a major concern Nephrotoxicity sometimes difficult to differentiate from rejection or ATN

(continued)

TABLE 26–2
Immunosuppressive Drugs Used in Renal Transplantation (Continued)

Drug	Adverse Reactions	Dosage	Comments
			Metabolized by cytochrome P-450 enzymes. Drugs that are inducers or inhibitors for P-450 enzymes may increase or decrease cyclosporine concentrations.[6]
		Dosage is altered by monitoring drug levels at least during initial period	Trough levels done to monitor and filtrate dosage
	Hypertension Hirsutism Gum hyperplasia Malignancy		Administration: liquid form; must be mixed with juice or milk
			Administer in glass container only, must be precisely measured
	Nausea, vomiting, diarrhea Tremors/seizures Diabetogenic effects Anaphylactic reactions have been seen with IV administration		Risk of anaphylaxis is reduced if slow continuous infusion is given
Monoclonal antibody muromonab-CD3 (Orthoclone OKT3)	Febrile reactions; fever, chills, tremor Respiratory: dyspnea, chest pain, wheezing, pulmonary edema GI: nausea, vomiting, diarrhea	2.5–5 mg/day IV bolus over 30–60 sec, for 10–14 days	Reactions greatest with first dose Reactions occur within 30–60 min To minimize first dose reaction, pretreat with methylprednisolone, acetaminophen, and diphenhydramine hydrochloride Monitor vital signs q15m for 2 hr, then q30m first two doses Have emergency equipment and cooling blanket available
Antilymphocyte globulin (ALG)	Anaphylactic shock due to hypersensitivity to animal serum	Skin test for hypersensitivity to animal serum performed before initial dose	
Antithymocyte globulin (ATG) Antilymphocyte serum (ALS)	Fever (up to 105°F or 40.6°C) and chills Increased susceptibility to infections due to decreased lymphocytes	Dosage may vary	Lymphocytes or platelets decrease sharply with drug admnistration; therefore, blood work for lymphocyte and platelet counts should be drawn before infusion is started
Antithymocyte serum (ATS) (usually IV, IM, or deep SC)	IM or deep SC injection site may be swollen, red, and painful, with abscess formation Difficulty walking if IM or SC injection given in thigh		Usually given only for short period of time to either prevent or treat rejection; not a long-term immunosuppressant
Cyclophosphamide (Cytoxan)	Leukopenia, thrombocytopenia Increased susceptibility to infections	1 to 2 mg/kg (or ½ to ⅔ of Imuran dosage)	Given in place of azathioprine when it causes hepatotoxicity

(continued)

TABLE 26–2
Immunosuppressive Drugs Used in Renal Transplantation (*Continued*)

Drug	Adverse Reactions	Dosage	Comments
	Metabolites are direct irritants to bladder mucosa and may cause hemorrhagic cystitis		Administer upon awakening to avoid accumulation of metabolites in bladder while sleeping
			Observe for hematuria
			Fluid intake should be encouraged to dilute metabolites
F-K 506	Alopecia Infection Nephrotoxicity Neurotoxicity Hypertension Diabetogenesis	Dosage varies 0.10 mg/kg/day IV 0.30 mg/kg/day PO (given in divided doses)	May be able to discontinue steroids Monitor renal and liver function P-450 enzyme system affected

IV, intravenous; PO, oral; WBC, white blood count; ATN, acute tubular necrosis; IM, intramuscular; SC, subcutaneous.

mogenicity, specificity, consistent potency, and predictable adverse reactions and efficacy. OKT3 is administered as an intravenous bolus drug as a prophylaxis for rejection. It also is used in the treatment of acute rejection episodes as "rescue" therapy when rejection has failed to respond to other efforts.

OKT3 removes most T lymphocytes from circulation. Those remaining are rendered unresponsive to the antigenic stimulation of the graft. OKT3 is used for a 10- to 14-day course of therapy. Because it is made in mice, sensitivity to OKT3 may occur.

Antilymphocyte globulin, ATG, antilymphocyte serum, and antithymocyte serum are used in a number of centers in an effort to prevent rejection by providing the patient with antibodies against lymphocytes or thymocytes, which are the cells responsible for rejection. These polyclonal antibodies are produced by injection of human lymph or thymus cells into an animal (horse, rabbit, or goat), which then produces antibodies against these cells. These antibodies against human T cells are administered for 14 to 21 days, either via intramuscular or intravenous route. Sensitivity against the agent usually develops after one course, and the drug cannot be reintroduced unless the animal source used to produce the drug is different.

Cyclophosphamide decreases serum immunoglobulins and destroys proliferative lymphoid cells. Rarely used since the addition of cyclosporine to immunosuppressive regimens, cyclophosphamide may replace azathioprine when hepatotoxicity develops. Cyclophosphamide is inferior to azathioprine in prolonging graft survival and can cause such serious side effects as hemorrhagic cystitis and bladder fibrosis. Hemorrhagic cystitis increases the risk for development of bladder cancer and necessitates discontinuation of therapy.

Triple therapy is a combination of low-dose prednisone, azathioprine, and cyclosporine or FK 506. These drugs are used in lower dosages so patients experience fewer side effects than from any one agent. For example, the risk of aseptic necrosis, diabetes mellitus, cataracts, and gastrointestinal complications attributed to chronic steroid therapy is greatly reduced. Because the dosage of azathioprine is low, the potential for hepatotoxicity and leukopenia is less. Problems associated with higher doses of cyclosporine, including lymphoma, hirsutism, hepatotoxicity, gingival hyperplasia, seizures, or gastrointestinal disturbances, rarely are seen.

Another advantage includes greater flexibility in altering dosage if problems occur with any one medication. For example, the specific drug causing a problem can be reduced in dosage, and the others slightly increased to maintain optimal immunosuppression. A final advantage is that cyclosporine, which is very costly, is used with two other agents, allowing it to be given in smaller, less expensive doses.

Quadruple or sequential therapy uses the same three agents as in triple therapy, plus antithymocyte antibody preparations or monoclonal antibody, OKT3. Cyclosporine may not be added to the regimen until renal function is present. All four drugs are given for several days, after which the polyclonal or monoclonal antibody preparation is discontinued. A triple-drug regime is used for maintenance therapy. The primary advantage of quadruple therapy is that cyclosporine can be withheld in the absence of renal function. Because of cyclosporine's nephrotoxicity and its cumulative effect in the absence of renal function, both broad and specific immunosuppression can be accomplished without it. The disadvantage of quadruple therapy is the potential inability to use the polyclonal or monoclonal antibody preparation for treatment of rejection or rescue therapy. These regimes demonstrate the increasing options available to individualize immunosuppression based on each patient's needs.

Radiation. Radiation therapy given locally to the graft sometimes is used as an adjunct to conventional immunosuppressive therapy during a rejection episode. This therapy has been used since the 1960s, and reports of its efficacy have ranged from beneficial to ineffective. It continues to be used in some centers.

Thoracic Duct Drainage. Thoracic duct drainage (TDD) has been used since the 1960s by a diminishing number of centers. Thoracic duct drainage involves cannulation of the left thoracic duct to remove lymph fluid. The purpose of lymph removal is to reduce the number of lymphocytes available that could become involved in the rejection process. The procedure usually is carried out for several weeks to 1 month before transplantation, depending on the amount of lymph fluid removed.

Thoracic duct drainage requires hospitalization for the duration of drainage because the patient's physiological status must be monitored carefully. Replacement of fluids and protein is required, and thus close monitoring of the fluid and electrolyte balance is necessary; some patients may drain as much as 1 L/hour.

Inclusion of TDD as part of the immunosuppressive protocol has been disappointing in that improved graft survival has not been demonstrated consistently. In addition, it is unrealistic to to attempt it when using a cadaver donor because its efficacy is greatest when the transplant is performed very shortly after completing TDD. Furthermore, it is costly, increases risk to the patient, and prolongs the patient's hospitalization.

Total Lymphoid Irradiation. Sublethal levels of total lymphoid irradiation have been used by a very few centers to improve the results of renal transplantation. This technique remains investigational and now is used rarely. Alternate, safer, and more effective means of immunosuppression and immunoalteration are available, making this technique less attractive.

For the Future. Many new drugs for immunosuppression are in the developmental stages. These drugs include rapamycin, deoxyspergualin, RS 61443, mizoribine, brequinar sodium, and new monoclonal antibodies. It remains to be seen which of these drugs will have clinical usefulness and what the side effects will be in humans. The potential advantage to these new immunosuppressants is that the treatment options will expand and possibly lead to improved results in organ transplantation.

Complications

Rejection of the Transplanted Kidney

The most frequently occurring noninfectious complication is graft rejection. This process can be confusing because, like renal failure, graft rejection is rarely an "all-or-none" phenomenon.

Rejection can vary in degree from mild to severe reversible rejection (ie, rejection episode) to complete or irreversible rejection. Rejection episodes are reversible when treated with a variety of antirejection therapies.

Categories of Rejection

The four basic categories of rejection are

- Hyperacute
- Accelerated
- Acute
- Chronic

Hyperacute Rejection. This type of rejection can occur within minutes to hours after transplantation. This may occur either because of a major blood group incompatibility or, more commonly, because preformed antibodies ("humoral immunity") existed in titers too low to be detected in the tissue-typing tests. There is no treatment for hyperacute rejection, and it always results in loss of the graft, which must be removed. With improved tissue-typing methods, hyperacute rejection is very uncommon.

Accelerated Rejection. This type of rejection occurs within a few days to approximately 1 week after transplantation. It is due either to preformed antibodies against the donor antigens in the recipient's blood or to lymphocytes in the recipient, which already are sensitized to some of the donor antigens. Accelerated rejection, like hyperacute rejection, is seen infrequently because of improved techniques of tissue typing and crossmatching. If it occurs, accelerated rejection must be treated aggressively with immunosuppressive medications. Even then, it may not respond to therapy and usually results in loss of the transplanted kidney.

Acute Rejection. This occurs after the first postoperative week. It is the most frequently seen form of rejection and fortunately the type that responds best to therapy. The nurse must *assess* for the following signs and symptoms because the patient may experience any, all, or none of the following during an acute rejection episode:

- decrease in urine output
- weight gain
- edema
- a temperature of 100°F (37.8°C) or greater
- tenderness over the graft site, with possible swelling of the kidney itself
- general malaise
- increased blood pressure

Other findings indicating an acute rejection episode include:

- increased serum creatinine
- decreased urine creatinine and creatinine clearance
- possible decrease in urine sodium
- increased BUN
- increased serum β-2 microglobulin
- increased urine β-2 microglobulin
- decreased blood flow as demonstrated on renal scan

Changes in laboratory values usually are the earliest and most reliable indicators that graft function is deteriorating. Clinical manifestations of rejection often are more subtle, require keen observation, and may not be seen initially.

Chronic Rejection. This is a gradual deterioration of kidney function and is the result of repeated insults from acute rejection episodes. The symptoms are similar to those of acute rejection except that fever and graft enlargement may not occur.

Chronic rejection results in scarring of renal tissue and infarction of renal vessels from the vasculitis accompanying acute rejection. Therefore, in chronic rejection the inflammatory signs are absent.

Laboratory findings are similar in both acute and chronic rejection, but chronic rejection also includes those changes consistent with chronic renal failure, including declining hematocrit, calcium–phosphorus imbalance, and so forth. The rate of deterioration in chronic rejection can vary, and the patient may have adequate renal function from a few months to years before replacement therapy is indicated.

There is no known effective therapy to treat this type of rejection. Unlike other forms of rejection, chronic rejection does not always require a transplant nephrectomy because the kidney does not always become necrotic and cause a life-threatening situation.

Infection

One of the greatest threats to recipient survival is sepsis. Its origin may be the blood (septicemia); a single organ, such as the liver, lungs, or pancreas; or the entire body (ie, a disseminated infection).

The pathogens vary from the more commonly seen bacterial organisms to fungal, viral, or even protozoan organisms. The last three groups of organisms are referred to as opportunistic pathogens. Infections occurring in the first month after transplantation usually are bacterial and may originate from such sites as intravenous lines, Foley catheters, wounds, or from postoperative pneumonia. Those seen beyond a month are more likely from opportunistic pathogens such as the cytomegalovirus and herpes simplex. These organisms, normally found in humans and in the environment, generally are considered harmless. The patient with a compromised immune system, however, is susceptible to infections from these organisms. The microorganisms "take advantage" of the decreased host defenses—thus the term "opportunistic." Specific examples of these opportunistic infections include herpes simplex, herpes zoster, *Candida albicans*, *Aspergillus*, *Cryptococcus*, *Nocardia*, *Pneumocystis carinii*, and cytomegalovirus. The presence of any of these infections should be monitored closely because they can pose life-threatening crises.

Immunosuppressive drugs are discontinued in the presence of a severe infection so that the patient can mobilize the immune response. Consequently, the graft may be sacrificed to save the patient. The immunosuppressive drugs decrease the patient's defense system as they work to prolong graft survival.

Recent advances in antimicrobial therapy include an-

tiviral agents, such as acyclovir (Zovirax; Burroughs Wellcome, Research Triangle Park, NC) and gancyclovir (Cytovene, Syntex Laboratories, Palo Alto, CA), so that viral illnesses that previously were not amenable to therapy now can be treated successfully. These drugs also can be used prophylactically. Additionally, antifungal agents, such as fluconazole (Diflucan; Roerig, New York, NY), can treat fungal infections with fewer side effects than with previously available therapy.

The nephrotoxicity associated with the use of many antibiotics and antifungal agents causes difficult management problems that require close monitoring of renal function. An example is amphotericin B therapy, used for the treatment of systemic fungal infections. The decreased renal perfusion associated with the use of this drug can pose a risk to renal transplant recipients. The use of mannitol with amphotericin B can counteract or minimize this problem by increasing renal perfusion.

Serious infections often can be prevented by careful surveillance for and treatment of localized infection. For example, oral candidial infections are common. Precautions should be taken, however, to prevent the progression to candidial esophagitis, a serious infectious complication. Precautions include daily observation of the mouth and prophylactic treatment of oral candidiasis with an appropriate locally acting antifungal agent, such as nystatin or clotrimazole.

Hematologic Complications

A variety of hematologic complications can occur, including alterations in hemoglobin and hematocrit and white blood count. The white blood count is monitored daily, primarily to detect any sudden or gradual decline in the white blood count. Leukopenia can occur as a result of bone marrow depression secondary to immunosuppression, a side effect of other medications, or as a result of viral infection. Changes in medications or a viral work-up may be initiated in response to leukopenia.

As in any postoperative patient, a decrease in the hemoglobin or hematocrit can indicate bleeding or changes in the fluid status of the patient. Because renal transplant recipients often have a hemoglobin or hematocrit that is below normal, careful attention must be paid to the recipient's preoperative baseline values. Lack of information about baseline laboratory results can lead to the mistaken conclusion that the patient is bleeding or has other problems with fluid status.

Cardiovascular Complications

Since the early 1970s, high-risk patients, such as those with diabetes, vasculitis, systemic lupus erythematosus, and those ages 50 to 70, have received transplants. These diseases are associated with a high rate of cardiovascular pathologic conditions. In fact, patients with cardiac disease treated by coronary bypass surgery have later received renal transplants. Perhaps these higher risks have contributed to an increase in death from vascular complications. Because there is an increasing patient population 15 years or more post-transplantation, there is more opportunity to study the long-term cardiovascular complications.

Hypertension

Hypertension is a common but often transitory complication after renal transplantation. Many patients requiring chronic antihypertensive therapy are hypertensive before the transplant, and their hypertension is made worse by post-transplantation steroid and cyclosporine therapy. Various factors responsible for post-transplantation hypertension are described in the following sections.

Steroid-Induced Hypertension

Transplant recipients are placed on steroids, usually prednisone or methylprednisolone. Although these are glucocorticoids, they are converted into mineralocorticoids and cause sodium and water retention. Even for patients on a sodium-restricted diet, drug therapy often is necessary. Spironolactone, an aldosterone-blocking agent, often is useful in treating steroid-induced hypertension, along with the diuretics, hydrochlorothiazide and furosemide. Nurses must monitor for potential electrolyte imbalances (specifically, hyponatremia and hypokalemia) and instruct the patient and the family about the signs and symptoms of these imbalances and what to do if they occur.

The effect of these drugs does not occur immediately, and therefore electrolyte imbalances usually are not seen until several days after the medications are started. At this time, a brisk diuresis may follow, increasing the potential for both hypovolemia and electrolyte imbalances. Because rapid fluid loss will result in weight loss, the patient's weight should be recorded carefully.

Renin-Dependent Hypertension

Steroid treatment is only one mechanism that causes post-transplantation hypertension. A second mechanism, excessive renin production, is seen rather frequently. It may result from ischemia, rejection, and renal artery stenosis.

Immediately after the transplant procedure, the recipient may have markedly elevated blood pressure. The ischemic injury that occurs to the organ between time of removal and time of implantation may cause excessive amounts of renin to be released. Once adequate circulation has been established within the organ, this mechanism should "turn off," resulting in a return of the blood pressure to the preoperative level within a few days after the transplant.

Hypertension may be one of the first clinical manifestations of rejection. The basis of this hypertension also is excessive renin production. Because rejection is an inflammatory response, vasculitis within the kidney impedes normal circulation and results in elevated renin

levels. Renin levels are elevated in virtually all patients who have hypertension during an acute rejection episode. This phenomenon occurs in chronic rejection as well. Therefore, the nurse should pose the question of ensuing rejection when first detecting an elevated blood pressure.

Renal artery stenosis also can result in renin-dependent hypertension. The stenosis may cause a decrease in renal perfusion, leading to increased renin production. When this occurs, an abdominal bruit may be auscultated lateral to the midline and medial to the kidney. The sudden appearance of a bruit or an increase in an abdominal bruit previously present is strongly suggestive of a renal artery stenosis.

Diagnosis of renal artery stenosis is made with angiography or Doppler ultrasound. Computer enhancement (digital subtraction angiography) allows a smaller amount of contrast material to be used. This is beneficial because the contrast material potentially is nephrotoxic. Once a transplant artery has been found to be stenotic, generally either surgical repair or balloon angioplasty is indicated to correct the problem. There is a risk of loss of some renal function or even of loss of the graft itself with either technique. The long-term adverse effects of uncontrolled hypertension resulting from an unrepaired renal artery stenosis, however, generally are thought to be more serious threats to the patient than the risks of repairing the lesion. In fact, deterioration of renal function is more likely to occur if the stenosis is not corrected.

Drug Therapy

β-Blocking agents, such as metoprolol tartrate (Lopressor; Geigy Pharmaceuticals, Ardsley, NJ) and propranolol (Inderal; Ayerst Laboratories, New York, NY) often are used to treat renin-dependent hypertension because they act as renin inhibitors. Because these drugs are cardiac depressants, congestive heart failure may result from prolonged use. The use of a diuretic may help prevent this complication. The use of catecholamine-depleting agents such as reserpine, however, is unwise because the patient is unable to respond to a sympathetic drive, owing to the adrenergic blocking effects.

Minoxidil has been effective in treating renin-dependent hypertension that does not respond to therapy with a sympathetic blocker alone. A potent vasodilator, it usually is given with a diuretic such as furosemide because of the sodium and fluid retention it causes. A sympathetic blocker also is advisable to offset the tachycardia minoxidil creates. Hirsutism, the major obvious side effect of minoxidil, can be very distressing to the patient and may actually affect compliance with this therapeutic regimen.

Angiotensin-converting enzyme inhibitors (eg, captopril) are useful in the treatment of renin-dependent hypertension. A rapid drop in blood pressure can occur with even small doses of these medications. Patients must be monitored closely when drug therapy is initiated. The most serious side effect of such medications is bone marrow suppression. White blood counts and platelet counts must be watched carefully.

Volume-Dependent Hypertension

Volume-dependent hypertension is another problem for the transplant recipient. During rejection episodes or periods of ATN, the patient may become fluid-overloaded because of inadequate fluid output from the kidney.

If the patient does not respond to diuretic therapy, the use of dialysis may be indicated for further control of the hypervolemic and hypertensive state until renal function recovers. The development of malignant hypertension precipitating hypertensive crisis is managed as with any other patient.

Drug Precautions

Many other antihypertensive medications are appropriate and useful; those mentioned earlier are some examples. Problems associated with antihypertensive therapy, however, are not unique to the transplant patient. Lethargy, impotence, and orthostatic hypotension are just some of the untoward effects of such therapy. In addition, many antihypertensive medications require multiple doses throughout the day. It is not surprising that noncompliance sometimes is a problem. Once renal function has stabilized, the steroid and cyclosporine doses have been reduced, and urine output is satisfactory, however, the need for antihypertensive medications is reduced markedly.

Gastrointestinal Complications

Gastrointestinal complications may pose serious and even life-threatening situations for the recipient. Chronic steroid therapy increases the risk of peptic ulceration and erosive gastritis because it increases the secretion of hydrochloric acid and pepsinogen. Massive gastrointestinal bleeding may occur not only from steroid therapy, but also from stress and decreased tissue viability due to long-term protein restriction.

For these reasons, patients usually are given antacids. The degree of renal function dictates which antacid is selected. Liquid preparations are considered more effective. Histamine antagonists such as cimetidine or ranitidine also may be prescribed to prevent ulceration.

Other serious gastrointestinal complications include acute pancreatitis, obstruction from bowel adhesions, and ulcerative colitis. If the patient has an intestinal perforation, infection becomes an added risk. Ischemic bowel disease has been observed in the early post-transplantation period and is a result of dehydration. During the dialysis immediately before surgery, ultrafiltration is used to remove fluid and achieve a "dry weight." A low circulating blood volume combined with anesthesia and blood loss may result in hypovolemia and hypotension and, in turn, possible ischemia to the bowel.

Transplant recipients may have more than one complication occurring simultaneously. In addition, signs and symptoms of gastrointestinal bleeding or perforation may be obscured by the anti-inflammatory effects of steroids. Therefore, complaints or changes in the patient's progress must be assessed thoroughly and promptly.

A Patient's View

How do patients who have experienced many complications view their decision to have a renal transplant? One patient received a cadaver transplant that was chronically rejected after 3½ years, underwent bilateral total hip replacements for aseptic necrosis, and had impaired vision resulting from cataracts. When asked if it had been worth it to him to be off dialysis and whether he would like to

(*Text continues on page 621*)

Clinical Research

Hauser ML, Williams J, Strong M, Ganza M, Hathaway D: Predicted and actual quality of life changes following renal transplantation. ANNA Journal 18:295–304, 1991

The purpose of this study was to determine the changes in quality of life in patients after renal transplantation, and to determine who anticipated the changes more accurately, staff members or the patients. An exploratory/descriptive survey design was used. This study was a follow-up study of renal transplant recipients, 16–26 months after transplantation; patients who rejected the transplant were excluded from the study. The sample size was 39 patients; they were asked open-ended questions via telephone interview. Also for each patient in the study, three staff nurses were asked to predict how they would expect the patient's quality of life to change. Specific areas studied included quality of life, post-transplantation quality of life expectations, fulfilled expectations, and unfulfilled expectations. Results showed that patients underestimated the number of positive and negative changes ($P < 0.001$) and staff anticipated more positive changes than actually occured ($P = 0.001$). The staff predictions were closer to what actually occured than were the patient predictions.

NURSING CARE PLAN 26–1:
The Patient Undergoing Renal Transplantation

NURSING DIAGNOSIS	OUTCOME CRITERIA/ PATIENT GOALS	NURSING INTERVENTIONS
Anxiety: related to securing a suitable kidney donor.	• Patient will develop realistic expectations for transplantation.	1. Determine patient's previous coping styles, support systems, and level of anxiety. 2. Determine understanding of histocompatibility testing and donor selection. 3. Provide clear, simple explanations of histocompatibility testing and donor selection. 4. Allow patient to ask questions about pretransplant screening. 5. Assist patient to discuss donation with eligible family members. 6. Allow verbalization of fears about lack of a suitable donor. 7. Offer a realistic appraisal and acknowledge the uncertainty about the amount of time to wait for a suitable cadaver donor.
Knowledge deficit: related to surgical procedure of kidney transplantation.	• Patient can state the process of renal transplantation.	1. Describe preoperative preparation to the patient including NPO status, enemas, IVs, dialysis, and preoperative medications. 2. Explain the surgical procedure including where the kidney will be located in the abdomen, how the kidney will function, and the duration of surgery. 3. State that dialysis might be necessary temporarily after a successful transplant. 4. Describe the presence of post operative IVs, drains, and catheters. 5. Discuss incisional pain. Assure patient that methods will be available to reduce pain including medications and splinting of the incision. 6. Practice coughing, deep breathing, turning, and using the incentive spirometer. 7. Allow patient to express anxiety about the surgery, verbalize any uncertainties, and ask questions.

(continued)

NURSING CARE PLAN 26–1: (Continued)
The Patient Undergoing Renal Transplantation

NURSING DIAGNOSIS	OUTCOME CRITERIA/ PATIENT GOALS	NURSING INTERVENTIONS
		8. Use simple statements; repeat and rephrase content as necessary.
		9. Encourage involvement with a group of patients who have already had transplants.
		10. Offer the opportunity for the patient to confer with those who have had successful and unsuccessful renal transplants.
High risk for infection: related to immunosuppression.	• Patient will have normal tissue healing.	1. Perform thorough handwashing before, during, and after care.
		2. Use scrupulous aseptic technique in the care of all catheters, central lines, endotracheal tubes, and peripheral lines.
		3. Cleanse bladder catheter and urethral meatus with soap and water q8h.
		4. Remove catheters as soon as possible, as ordered.
		5. Maintain a clean environment.
		6. Encourage coughing and deep breathing using incentive spirometer q1–2h.
		7. Discouage visitors and caretakers with active upper respiratory infections from coming in contact with the patient.
		8. Maintain skin integrity.
		9. Change wet dressings promptly to limit the media for organisms.
		10. Provide adequate nutrition.
		11. Check temperature q4h.
		12. Monitor laboratory values, especially WBC and differential.
		13. Inspect the oral and anal mucosa daily for evidence of monilial infections.
		14. Examine surgical incisions and insertion sites of all IVs for signs of inflammation; pain, redness, swelling, heat, drainage.
		15. Auscultate lungs at least q4h.

(*continued*)

NURSING CARE PLAN 26–1: (Continued)
The Patient Undergoing Renal Transplantation

NURSING DIAGNOSIS	OUTCOME CRITERIA/ PATIENT GOALS	NURSING INTERVENTIONS
		16. Notify physician of any indications of infection.
		17. Adminsister antimicrobials, as ordered.
		18. Closely monitor renal function when nephrotoxic antimicrobials must be used.
		19. Maintain universal precautions or protective isolation, per unit protocol.
High risk for injury: related to graft rejection, immunosuppression, or need for further hemodialysis.	• Patient will maintain kidney function.	1. Monitor for signs of acute rejection.
		2. Monitor urine output q1h then q4h as indicated.
		3. Weigh patient daily.
		4. Check BP q1–4h, note any increase in BP of 10–20 mm Hg.
		5. Check temperature q4h.
		6. Examine sacrum and extremities for edema.
		7. Palpate gently to determine tenderness or swelling over graft site every shift.
		8. Ask patient about feelings of weakness, tiredness, or general malaise.
		9. Assess serum creatinine.
		10. Assess urine creatinine and creatinine clearance.
		11. Assess urine sodium.
		12. Assess BUN.
		13. Administer methylprednisone, as ordered.
		14. Monitor patient closely for signs of infection, fluid retention, and GI bleeding.
		15. Administer antacids and antihistamines, as ordered to prevent gastric irritation.
		16. If Orthoclone OKT3 is used:
		• Assess patient's hydration status, weight, and chest x-ray. If weight 3% > dry weight or signs of volume overload, alert physician, prepare to administer diuretics or treatment as ordered.

(continued)

NURSING CARE PLAN 26–1: *(Continued)*
The Patient Undergoing Renal Transplantation

NURSING DIAGNOSIS	OUTCOME CRITERIA/ PATIENT GOALS	NURSING INTERVENTIONS

		• Advise patient that flulike reaction with fever, chills, and GI symptoms will occur on first and second days of therapy.
		• Premedicate patient with IV steroids, Benadryl, and Tylenol as ordered.
		17. If cyclosporine is used monitor cyclosporine trough levels. If nephrotoxicity or hepatotoxicity occur, notify physician so dosage may be adjusted.
		18. If azathioprine is used, monitor CBC and renal function closely.
		19. Assess patency of dialysis access.
		  • Listen for bruit and feel for thrill.
		  • Avoid constrictive clothing, tourniquets, or BP cuffs above vascular access.
		  • Maintain sterility and patency of access if appropriate.

Altered urinary elimination: related to transplantation, rejection, nephrotoxic drugs, renal failure.	• Patient will maintain an adequate urinary output.	1. Observe for and maintain patency and urinary drainage of each catheter. 2. Check urine output q1h initially. 3. Note color of urine and presence of clots. 4. Maintain high volume IV fluids to flush kidneys, as ordered. 5. Notify physician of urinary leakage on abdominal dressing, severe abdominal pain, or distention. 6. If patient has progressive oliguria, examine renal function studies and cyclosporine trough levels, assess hydration status, and notify physician.
Fluid volume excess: related to decreased urinary output, renal failure, transplant rejection, high volume IV fluids.	• Patient will have adequate urine output and not retain fluid.	1. Measure urine output q1h. 2. Monitor BP and pulse q1h. 3. Auscultate lungs each shift and as indicated. 4. Maintain accurate input and output records. 5. Weigh patient daily.

(continued)

NURSING CARE PLAN 26–1: (Continued)
The Patient Undergoing Renal Transplantation

NURSING DIAGNOSIS	OUTCOME CRITERIA/ PATIENT GOALS	NURSING INTERVENTIONS
		6. Encourage fluids, as prescribed.
		7. Administer diuretics, as ordered.
		8. Maintain sodium intake, as indicated.
		9. Report all abnormal findings.
Knowledge deficit: related to administration of immunosuppressive agents, lack of retention of pretransplantation teaching.	• Patient will understand safe, accurate administration of medication.	1. Encourage the patient to avoid infection.
		2. Teach the patient to observe for and report signs of infection.
		3. Emphasize that although doses and drugs may be varied to manage side and adverse effects, immunosuppressives must always be taken.
		4. Teach the patient taking prednisone to: • Take medication with food or an antacid. • Avoid adding salt to foods. • Walk or exercise daily to limit muscle wasting. • Report hip or knee pain on weight-bearing because it may indicate septic necrosis of the hip. • Report any visual disturbance and schedule yearly eye examination to detect cataract formation.
		5. Teach the patient taking azathioprine to: • Report for scheduled CBCs and liver function tests. • Report any abnormal bleeding, bruising, or mucosal ulceration.
		6. Teach the patient taking cyclophosphamide to: • Take the medication on arising in the morning. • Report hematuria immediately as hemorrhagic cystitis may occur. • Maintain a fluid intake of at least 2,000 ml/day.

(continued)

NURSING CARE PLAN 26–1: (Continued)
The Patient Undergoing Renal Transplantation

NURSING DIAGNOSIS	OUTCOME CRITERIA/ PATIENT GOALS	NURSING INTERVENTIONS
		7. Teach the patient taking liquid cyclosporine to: • Measure the dose with a graduated syringe, place it in a glass container, and add a consistent volume and type of diluent immediately before taking it. • Try a change of diluent if nausea and vomiting are a consistent problem. • Take the medication 1 hr before or 2 hr after eating. • Report for scheduled cyclosporine trough levels as well as renal and liver function tests. • Report any reduction in urine output, increase in weight and BP. • Practice excellent oral hygiene to limit gingival hyperplasia.
Knowledge deficit: related to signs of rejection, lack of recall of pretransplantation teaching.	• Patient will know when to obtain medical assistance.	1. Teach patient to recognize signs of rejection including: weight gain, decreased urine output, temperature more than 100°F, tenderness or swelling over the graft site, and feelings of general malaise. 2. Daily weights are recorded by patient. 3. encourage patient to take BP weekly. 4. Discuss follow-up schedule for evaluation visits at regular intervals. 5. Give patient access to resource information around the clock (physician office number, clinic number, etc.).

receive a new kidney graft, he responded without question or hesitation with an emphatic "Absolutely!"

People who have had successful renal transplantation, even in the face of complications, state unequivocally that they would not alter their decision to have received a renal graft. Both the success of such patients and their appreciation of new lives make transplantation a challenging and richly rewarding field.

REFERENCES

1. Prowant BF: Nephrology nursing care plan and patient education for the patient receiving Epogen. ANNA J 18: 188–194, 1991
2. UNOS, May 1992, vol. 8, Issue 5, pp. 1–2. United Network for Organ Sharing, Richmond, VA
3. United States Department of Health and Human Services:

The Surgeon General's Workshop on Increasing Organ Donation. Rockville, MD, United States Department of Health
and Human Services, 233, 1991

4. The Partnership for Organ Donation: Solving the Organ
Donor Shortage. Boston, The Partnership for Organ Donation, 1991

5. Perryman J, Stillerman P: Kidney transplantation. In Smith
SL (ed): Kidney Transplantation, pp 192–193. St. Louis,
CV Mosby, 1990

6. Yee G: Pharmacokinetic interactions between cyclosporine
and other drugs. Transplant Proc 22:1203–1207, 1990

7. Johansson A, Moller E: Evidence that immunosuppressive
effects of KF 506 and cyclosporine are identical. Transplantation 50:1001–1007, 1990

BIBLIOGRAPHY

Almond PS, Gillingham K, Sibley R, Manivel C, Najarian JS,
Matas AJ: Impact of cyclosporine and cyclosporine nephro-
toxicity on long-term renal allograft function. Dialysis and
Transplantation 21:682–685, 1992

Bass M: Infection in renal transplantation: The first six months.
Critical Care Nursing Clinics of North America 2:133–188,
1990

Berg J: Assessing for pericarditis in the end-stage renal disease
patient. Dimensions of Critical Care Nursing 9:266–271,
1990

Campton CM: Oral care for the renal transplant patient. ANNA
J 18:39–41, 1991

Cunningham N, Boteler S, Windham S: Renal transplantation.
Critical Care Nursing Clinics of North America 4:79–88
1992

Cunningham N, Smith SL: Postoperative care of the renal transplant patient. Critical Care Nurse 10(9):74–81, 1990

Duffy MA, Nestor A: Nursing guidelines for muromonab—
CD3 (OKT3). ANNA J 19:493–495, 1992

Emmett M, et al: Calcium acetate control of serum phosphorus

in hemodialysis patients. Am J Kidney Dis 17:544–550,
1991

Gallagher-Lepak S: Functional capacity and activity level before
and after renal transplantation. ANNA J 18:378–382, 406,
1991

Gharbieh PA: Renal transplant surgical and psychologic hazards.
Critical Care Nurse 8(6):58–71, 1988

Jones KR: Risk of hospitalization for chronic hemodialysis patients. Image 24(2):88–94, 1992

Kiberd MC, et al: Nursing attitudes toward organ donation,
procurement, and transplantation. Heart Lung 21:106–111,
1992

Kirlin L: Case management of the anemic patient: Epoetin alfa:
Focus on hematocrit. ANNA J 19:66–67, 1992

Lange S: Psychosocial, legal, ethical, and cultural aspects of
organ donation and transplantation. Critical Care Nursing
Clinics of North America 4:25–42, 1992

Nuttal A: ESRD and cardiovascular instability. ANNA J 17:
192–193, 1990

Pezze JL, Whiteman K: Transplantation's newest weapon, FK506.
Am J Nurs 91(10):40–42, 1991

Sigardson-Poor KM, Haggety LM (eds): Nursing Care: The
Transplant Recipient. Philadelphia, WB Saunders, 1990

Special Report: The end-stage renal disease program: A report
from the Institute of Medicine. N Engl J Med 324:1143–
1148, 1991

Staschak-Chico SM, Zamerlan K, Thomson AW: An overview
of FK 506 in transplantation and autoimmune disease.
Dialysis and Transplantation 21(8):500–504, 531, 1992

Swanson MA, Palmeri D, Vossler ED, Bartus SA, Hull D,
Schweizer RT: Non-compliance in organ transplant recipients. Pharmacotherapy 11(6):174S, 1991

Trusler LA: Management of the patient receiving simultaneous
kidney-pancreas transplantation. Critical Care Nursing Clinics of North America 4:89–96, 1992

Willis R, Skelly L: Serving the needs of donor families: The role
of the critical care nurse. Critical Care Nursing Clinics of
North America 4:63–78, 1992

STUDY QUESTIONS

Case Study

Gary Smith is a 21-year-old black man with end-stage renal disease secondary to glomerulonephritis. Gary began hemodialysis treatments 10 months ago. Family members were
evaluated as potential living donors; however, due to medical problems and blood type
incompatibility, no family member could donate a kidney. Gary received a cadaveric renal
transplant 3 weeks ago. The kidney was a three-antigen match. After a brief period of
ATN, the kidney began to function well. He now has normal renal function and is ready
to be discharged from the hospital.

1. Which of the following factors are not considered in donor recipient matching?

   a. ABO compatibility
   b. negative crossmatch
   c. number of antigens matched for
   d. Rh compatibility

2. When Gary came to the hospital for his renal transplant, which of the following assessments would have been the most appropriate?

    a. assessment of laboratory studies
    b. last dialysis treatment
    c. psychosocial readiness for transplant
    d. all of the above

3. In the PACU, the nurse notes a decrease in urine output from 150 ml/hour to 30 ml/hour. What is the most appropriate initial assessment and/or consideration?

    a. check patency of Foley catheter
    b. assess lung sounds
    c. measure CVP
    d. notify physician

4. As part of education before discharge, Gary learned about rejection of the kidney transplant. What type of rejection is Gary most likely to experience?

    a. chronic
    b. accelerated
    c. acute
    d. hyperacute

5. Gary had postoperative ATN of the transplant. Which symptoms might you expect to find?

    a. low urine output
    b. increasing BUN and creatinine associated with fever
    c. tenderness over the kidney
    d. leukopenia

6. Which drug is the most likely cause of leukopenia?

    a. steroids
    b. epoetin alfa
    c. azathioprine
    d. fluconazole

UNIT IV

Nervous System

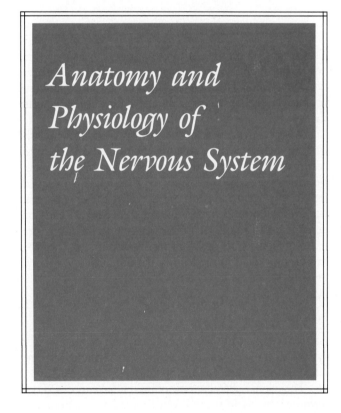

CHAPTER 27

Anatomy and Physiology of the Nervous System

BEHAVIORAL OBJECTIVES

Based on the content in this chapter, the reader should be able to:

1. List the cellular units of the nervous system.
2. Briefly explain the physiology of a nerve impulse.
3. List two functions of cerebrospinal fluid.
4. Explain the functions of the thalamus.
5. Define the reticular activating system.
6. Briefly define the sensory system and the motor system.
7. List and explain three cord reflexes.
8. Explain the physiology of pain and the gate theory of pain regulation.

Hudak: Critical Care Nursing:
A Holistic Approach, 6th ed. © 1994
J. B. Lippincott Company.

Description

The nervous system traditionally is discussed in both anatomic and functional divisions. Anatomic components are the central nervous system (CNS; brain and spinal cord) and the peripheral nervous system (spinal and cranial nerves). Functional divisions are the sensory, interpretive, and motor (somatic and autonomic) divisions.

Content will be ordered according to both divisions. First, however, cell anatomy and physiology and the meninges will be discussed.

Anatomy and Physiology of Cells of the Nervous System

The cellular units are the *neuron*—the basic functional unit—and its attendant cells, the *neuroglias* and *Schwann cells*. It may, perhaps, be easier to treat the attendant cells first and then proceed to neuronal functioning.

Neuroglial Cells

The neuroglial cells constitute the supportive tissue that lies within the CNS around the neurons. There are three types of glial cells: microglia, astrocytes, and oligodendroglia. These last cells are thought to produce the myelin that covers nerve fibers within the CNS.

Whereas neurons lose their ability to undergo mitosis early in the life of the individual, neuroglial cells seem to retain mitotic abilities throughout a person's life span. Because of this, nonmetastatic CNS lesions involve glial cells rather than neurons. As the glial tumor enlarges, however, it does adversely affect adjacent neurons early by exerting pressure and later by promoting an inflammatory reaction along with the pressure. The counterpart of the myelin-producing oligodendroglial cell in the peripheral nervous system is the cell of Schwann.

Neurons

As stated earlier, the basic functional unit of the nervous system is the *neuron*, and all information and activity, whether sensory, motor, or integrative, is processed by it.

The precise characteristic of individual neurons is determined by their specific function. Some neurons are extremely large and may give rise to extremely long nerve fibers. Transmission velocities in the long fibers may be as high as 100 m/second, whereas smaller neurons with very small fibers demonstrate velocities of 1 m/second. Some neurons connect to many different neurons in a "network," and still others have few connections to other cells of the nervous system.

It has been estimated that there are 12 billion neurons in the CNS. Three-fourths of these neurons are located in the cerebral cortex, where information transmitted

through the nervous system is processed. This processing, as already indicated, includes not only the determination of appropriate and effective responses but also the storage of memory and the development of associative motor and thought patterns.

Neuron Structure and Function

The neuron is also termed a *nerve cell*. It consists of a nerve cell body that contains nuclear and cytoplasmic material and processes arising from this. These processes are functionally differentiated into axons and dendrites (Fig. 27–1). *Axons* normally carry nervous impulses away from the cell body, whereas *dendrites* conduct the impulse toward the cell body. Axons and dendrites may be merely microscopic knobs or areas on the cell body surface, or they may be cylindrical processes that can, in certain cases, extend to over 1 m (4 ft) in length.

Neurons do not connect to one another. There are spaces between the axon (or axons) of one neuron and the dendrite (or dendrites) of another. This space is termed the *synapse*. Axons and dendrites may branch, enabling the axon of one neuron to synapse with dendrites of more than one other neuron. Similarly, axons from several neurons may synapse with a single neuron. The former is an example of divergence; the latter exemplifies convergence.

Nerves and Ganglia

Axons and dendrites are referred to collectively as *nerve fibers*. A bundle of nerve fibers together with their coverings is termed a *nerve*. A *ganglion* is a group of cell bodies.

Nerve Fiber Coverings

Within the CNS, some fibers are covered with a lipid–protein sheath termed the *myelin sheath*. This appears to be formed by the action of oligodendrocytes. Other fibers remain unmyelinated. Peripheral nerve fibers all are covered by a *neurilemma*. This is a sheath formed by the cells of Schwann, which wrap themselves around the fiber. The Schwann cells around some fibers also secrete myelin; others do not (see Figure 27–1). The neurilemma of myelinated fibers comes in contact with the fiber at periodic intervals. These periodic constrictions of the neurilemmal sheath are termed the *nodes of Ranvier*. Such nodes produce a faster impulse conduction.

Fiber Regeneration

If a nerve fiber is severed, the portion distal to the cell body will die. That part still attached to the cell body will regenerate. In peripheral neurons, the neurilemma itself provides a channel that can be followed by a regenerating fiber so that it may become reattached to its original anatomic connection (Fig. 27–2). Regeneration also occurs in the absence of a neurilemma, as in the case of CNS neurons. Because there is no channel to ensure correct anatomic reconnection, most such regeneration does not

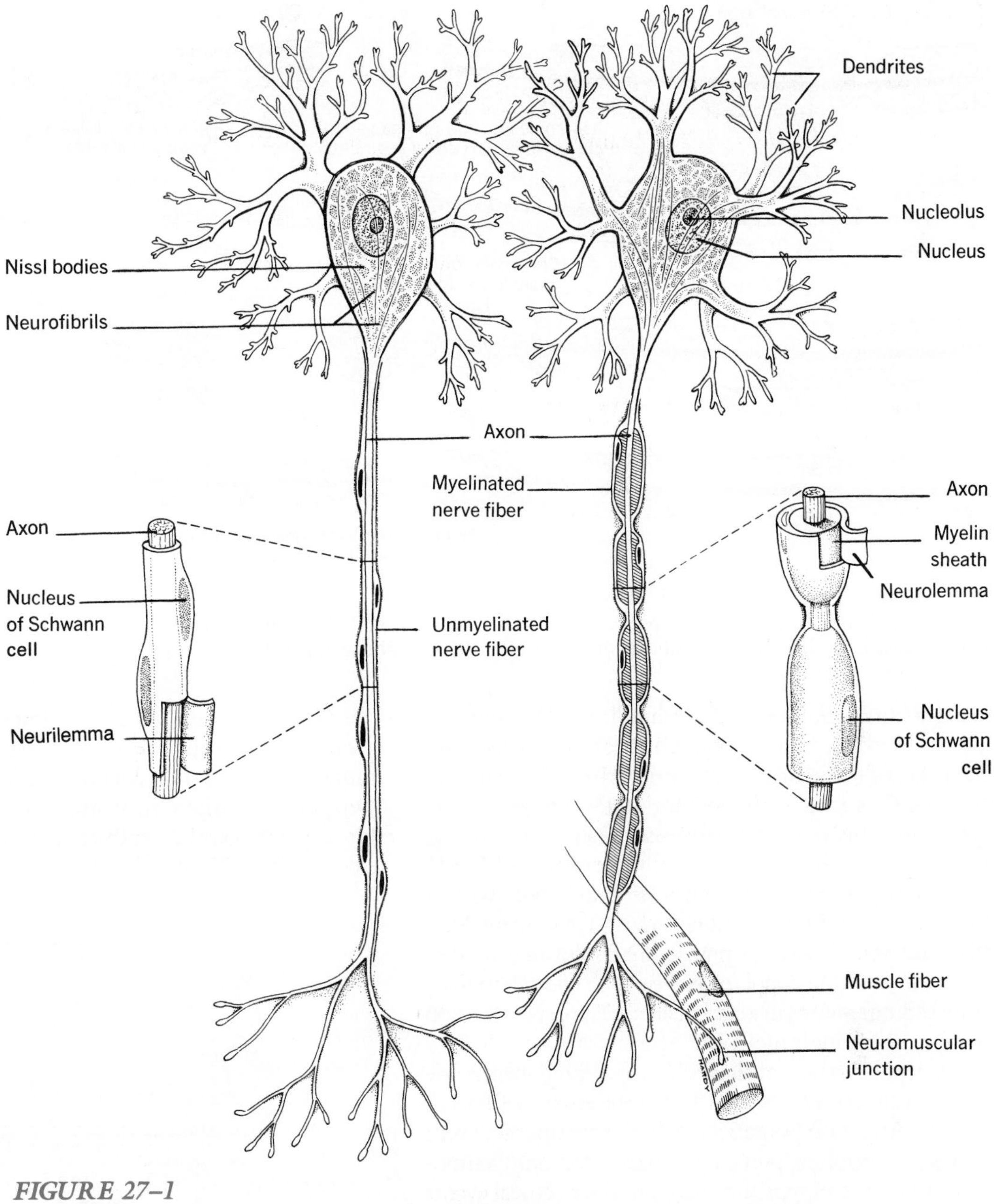

FIGURE 27–1

Typical efferent neurons. *Left*, unmyelinated fiber; *right*, myelinated fiber (Chaffee EE, Lytle IM: Basic Physiology and Anatomy, 4th ed. Philadelphia: JB Lippincott).

produce recovered function. The regrowing stump may wind aimlessly among other structures or curl into a useless tangle. A bigger hindrance to functional regeneration within the CNS has been discovered, however—an overgrowth of neurologic cells that occurs in response to injury. This produces a glial thicket that acts as a barrier to the reconnection of severed neuronal networks.

Nerve Impulse

The essence of the nerve impulse is the action potential and its self-propagated conduction, as described in Chapter 11. The neuronal membrane contains sodium–

potassium pumps that keep the inside of the neuron more negatively charged than the outside interstitial fluid. As in cardiac tissue, the cytoplasm of the neuron contains anions (negatively charged particles) that are too large to leave the cell. These electrochemically attract, in part, positively charged potassium ions and positively charged sodium ions as well. If this were all that happened, the influx of positively charged ions would counterbalance the negatively charged ones, electroneutrality would be established within the neuron, and nothing further could occur. The active transport enzyme system within the neuronal membrane, however, pumps sodium out of the cell almost as

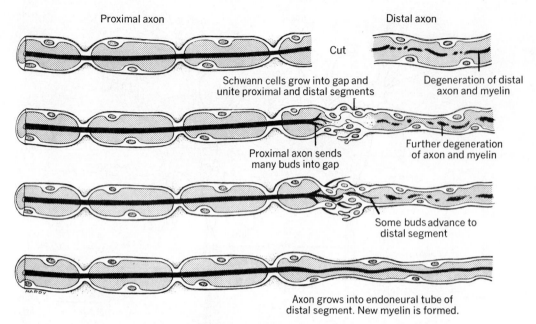

Proximal axon

Distal axon

Cut

Schwann cells grow into gap and unite proximal and distal segments

Degeneration of distal axon and myelin

Proximal axon sends many buds into gap

Further degeneration of axon and myelin

Some buds advance to distal segment

Axon grows into endoneural tube of distal segment. New myelin is formed.

FIGURE 27–2
Diagram of changes that occur in a nerve fiber that has been cut and then regenerates (Chaffee EE, Lytle IM: Basic Physiology and Anatomy, 4th ed. Philadelphia, JB Lippincott).

fast as it enters. Although potassium is pumped into the cell, this is insufficient to counterbalance the anions. Thus the inside of the neuron remains negative with respect to the outside as long as the sodium–potassium pumps are operating. This internal relative negativity is the *resting polarity* of the neuron and typically measures -85 mV.

A stimulus acts locally to turn off sodium pumps. This causes a local influx of sodium and a consequent local *depolarization*. If enough pumps are inactivated temporarily, the resulting depolarization is large enough to inactivate sodium pumps in adjacent areas. The depolarization can spread through the entire neuron.

A depolarization of such self-propagating magnitude is termed an *action potential*, which is the essence of a nerve impulse. An action potential is a discrete temporary event because the sodium pumps are inactivated only temporarily. Once the pumps turn back on, the electrical events reverse, and the resting potential is restored (Fig. 27–3).

The electrical activity embodied in the action potential can be monitored in certain clinical situations. For example, the electroencephalogram depicts multiple action potentials from surface neurons of the brain.

Synaptic Transmission

A synapse is made up of a presynaptic element, a postsynaptic element, and a small (150–1,000 A) space between elements called a synaptic cleft. A presynaptic element is any terminal portion of a neuron; a postsynaptic element is any part of another neuron in close proximity to the presynaptic element. One neuron stimulates or inhibits another by chemical transmission across the synapse. This involves the synthesis of the transmitter by the first neuron. Transmitter packets are then stored in the

presynaptic element. As a nerve impulse passes down the axon, it triggers the release of a certain number of transmitter packets. These chemicals then diffuse across the synaptic cleft, where they attach temporarily to receptor binding sites on the dendrite surface of the postsynaptic element (Fig. 27–4).

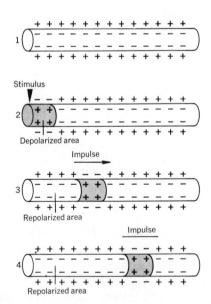

FIGURE 27–3
Propagation of impulses. (1) Resting membrane. (2) Action potential, first stage: stimulation of fiber results in depolarization. (3) Action potential, second stage: repolarization occurs as the resting potential is restored. (4) Propagation of impulses continues in direction of arrow (Chaffee EE, Lytle IM: Basic Physiology and Anatomy, 4th ed. Philadelphia, JB Lippincott).

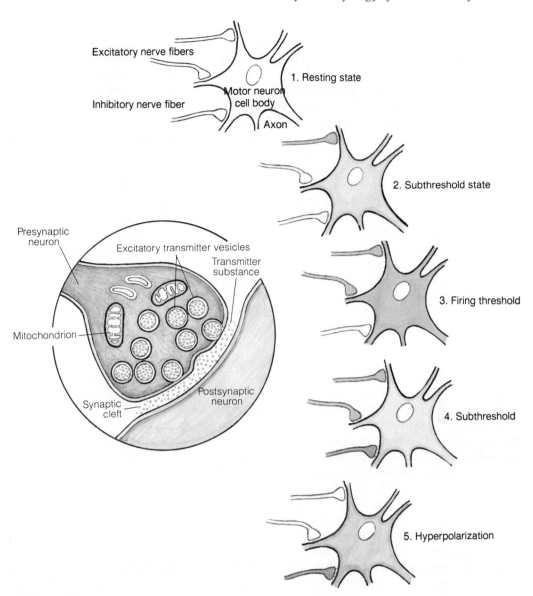

FIGURE 27–4

Conduction at synapses. *Left,* enlarged view of liberation of chemical transmitter substance at a synapse; *right,* diagrams illustrating how a neuron may be excited or inhibited by transmitter substances liberated by presynaptic nerve fiber endings. Two excitatory and one inhibitory fiber are shown: (1) resting state; (2) subthreshold state; impulses from only one excitatory fiber cannot cause the postsynaptic neuron to fire; (3) firing threshold is reached by the addition of impulses from a second excitatory fiber; (4) subthreshold state is restored by impulses from an inhibitory fiber; (5) when the inhibitory fiber alone is carrying impulses, the postsynaptic neuron is in a state of hyperpolarization and is unable to fire (Chaffee EE, Lytle IM: Basic Physiology and Anatomy, 4th ed. Philadelphia, JB Lippincott).

While the transmitter is bound to the receptor site, the dendrite area is either stimulated (depolarized or hypopolarized) or inhibited (hyperpolarized). Most chemical transmitters are stimulators. Only one, γ-aminobutyric acid (GABA), is known to hyperpolarize a neuron.

Within an extremely short interval (millionths of a second), the transmitter detaches from the receptor site. It may then reattach or be inactivated. Inactivation occurs in two basic ways, depending on the chemical. The transmitter norepinephrine diffuses back into the axon to be re-

used. The transmitter acetylcholine is destroyed by an enzyme present in the synaptic cleft. In either case, the availability of a transmitter that can attach to the receptor sites is restricted temporarily. This enables rapid, repetitive, discrete stimulation (or inhibition) of neurons, a necessary factor in the functioning of the nervous system. From this picture, it can be see that synaptic transmission is a one-way street—from the axon across the synaptic cleft to the dendrite of the next neuron. It cannot proceed in the opposite direction. It also can be seen that decreased destruction of transmitter can increase the effect of this transmitter on the postsynaptic membrane. Similarly, increased destruction of transmitter reduces its postsynaptic effects.

The best known synaptic transmitters are acetylcholine and norepinephrine. Other transmitters include dopamine, serotonin, histamine, endogenous opiates, and GABA. Most of these act to excite, or hypopolarize, the postsynaptic neuronal membrane; GABA and possibly some endogenous opiates act to inhibit, or hyperpolarize, the postsynaptic neuronal membrane.

It was not until the 1970s that it was known that peptides could act as neurotransmitters. Examples of these neuropeptides are the endorphins, enkephalins, and substance P, which appear to be involved in pain sensation. The endorphins and enkephalins, often described as the body's own morphine, contribute to a decrease in pain sensation. Substance P excites spinal neurons that respond to painful stimuli, so it is thought to be involved in transmission of pain information from the periphery to the CNS.

Neuronal Thresholds

In the CNS (and sympathetic ganglia), the axons of several neurons may synapse with the dendrites or cell body of a single neuron. Some may release excitatory synaptic transmitters, whereas others may release an inhibitory transmitter. The excitatory transmitter released from a single axon often is insufficient to trigger an action potential in the postsynaptic neuron (ie, to excite the postsynaptic cell fully). Rather, it may be sufficient to depolarize, or excite, the postsynaptic membrane only partially. As such it is termed a *subthreshold stimulus*. The partial depolarization, or hypopolarization, it produces renders the postsynaptic neuron more easily excitable by subsequent excitatory transmitter stimuli from other axons, provided such transmitters arrive while the postsynaptic membrane is hypopolarized. Thus, this initial subthreshold excitatory stimulus is said to "lower the threshold" of the postsynaptic neuron for stimulation by another presynaptic neuron. Full excitation of a postsynaptic membrane is prerequisite to establishment of an action potential and thus the firing of a nerve impulse along the postsynaptic neuron. It may require the near-simultaneous depolarization produced by excitatory transmitters from two or more presynaptic neurons.

If the synaptic transmitter is an inhibitory one (eg, GABA), it will hyperpolarize, or "raise the threshold" of the postsynaptic neuron. This renders it more difficult to excite fully by excitatory transmitters. Figure 27–4 illustrates the action of three convergent presynaptic neurons on the threshold of a single postsynaptic neuron.

These principles underlie much of the normal functioning of cord neurons and spinal reflexes. For example, certain descending fibers from the brain stem deliver a low-level subthreshold stimulation to certain cord neu-rons. Although this stimulation is insufficient to activate cord neurons, it is enough of a background stimulus to make it easier for other input to excite these neurons fully. Such subthreshold stimuli would be said to be *facilitatory*. When the cord is severed, the distal portion also is separated from receipt of such facilitatory brain stem influences. As a result, it takes greater stimuli to cause action potentials in the neurons in this part of the cord than before. Indeed, when initially separated from the brain, these cord neurons do not function noticeably at all for a few weeks. Such a condition is termed *cord shock*. In it, no reflexes are possible.

Neuronal thresholds can also be influenced by hormones. *Thyroxine* lowers thresholds of certain neurons, and one sign of hyperthyroidism is the presence of exaggerated cord reflexes, such as the knee jerk and ankle jerk.

Meninges

The CNS is covered by three layers of tissue called, collectively, the *meninges*, and consisting of the pia mater, the arachnoid layer, and the dura mater. The *pia mater* is the layer that lies next to the CNS. Next is the *arachnoid layer*, which contains a substantial vascular supply. Last is the *dura mater*, the thickest layer of all, lying next to the bones surrounding the CNS.

Cerebrospinal Fluid

Cerebrospinal fluid (CSF) functions as a fluid shock absorber, keeping the delicate CNS tissues from impacting against surrounding bony structures and being mechanically injured. It also functions in the exchange of nutrients between the plasma and cellular compartments. Cerebrospinal fluid is a plasma filtrate that is exuded by the capillaries in the roofs of each of the four ventricles of the brain. As such, it is similar to plasma minus the large plasma proteins, which stay behind in the bloodstream. Most of this fluid is made in the lateral ventricles, which are located in each cerebral hemisphere. It moves from there through ducts into the third ventricle of the diencephalon. From here it travels through the aqueduct of Sylvius of the midbrain and enters the fourth ventricle of the medulla. Then most of it passes through holes (foramina) in the roof of this ventricle and enters the subarachnoid space. (A small amount diffuses down into the spinal canal.) In the subarachnoid space, the CSF is reabsorbed back into the bloodstream at certain points called the *subarachnoid plexus*.

The formation and reabsorption of CSF are governed by the same hydrostatic and colloid osmotic forces that regulate the movements of fluid and small particles between the plasma and interstitial fluid compartments of the body. Briefly reviewed, the action of these forces is as follows. Two opposing teams of push–pull forces influence the movement of water and small particles through the semipermeable capillary membranes. One team is composed of plasma osmotic pressure and CSF hydrostatic pressure. It favors movement of water from the CSF compartment into the plasma. The movement of water in the opposite direction is influenced by the team of plasma hydrostatic pressure and CSF osmotic pressure. Team influences are exerted simultaneously and continually. In the ventricles, the flow of CSF reduces CSF hydrostatic pressure. This tips the collective team influence in favor of the movement of water and small particles from plasma to ventricles. The low plasma hydrostatic pressure of blood in the venous sinuses next to the arachnoid villi tips the scales in favor of the movement of water and solute from the CSF compartment back into the bloodstream. Death of cells lining the CSF compartment will spill proteins into the CSF. This elevates CSF osmotic pressure and retards reabsorption (while also hastening formation if the damage is in ventricle walls). Increased CSF proteins from this or other causes can provoke or exacerbate a condition of excess CSF called *hydrocephalus*.

Central Nervous System

The purpose of this section is to consider major functions briefly so that their abnormalities can be associated with specific brain damage discussed in other chapters. The reader is referred to the Bibliography for sources of indepth discussions.

The CNS comprises the brain and spinal cord. It receives sensory input by way of sensory fibers (dendrites) within spinal and cranial nerves and sends out motor impulses by way of axons in these same nerves. The CNS also contains large numbers of neurons that are entirely contained within it. These neurons are termed *internuncial neurons*, or *interneurons*, and may exist within brain and cord or connect one with the other. Each of the seven major parts of the brain and then the spinal cord will be examined briefly.

Brain

Basic anatomy of the brain is illustrated in Figure 27–5. The parts of the brain, in descending order, are the cerebral hemispheres, diencephalon, midbrain, pons, medulla, and cerebellum. The general appearance of the brain can be viewed as a stem extending upward from the spinal cord with an inferior small flowering overgrowth (cerebellum) covering the lower part of the stem and a large superior flowering overgrowth (cerebrum) covering most of the upper portion of the stem. The medulla, pons, and midbrain compose the brain stem. Some authors include the diencephalon.

Cerebrum

Each of the two cerebral hemispheres (left and right) has a layer of cortex covering the surface. This cortical layer is made of several different types of unmyelinated neurons and glial cells arranged in six distinctive layers according to cell type and function. Underneath the cortex is white

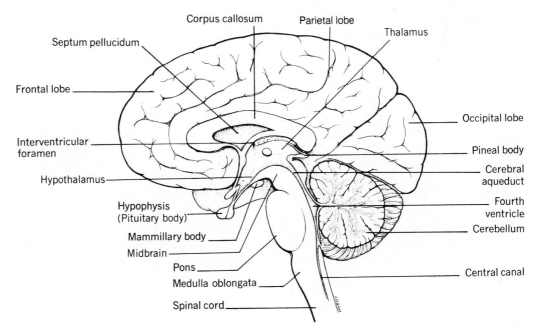

FIGURE 27–5
Midsagittal section of the brain.

matter (myelinated nerve fibers). Deep within each hemisphere are several collections of nerve cell bodies, termed the *basal ganglia*, and a lateral ventricle containing CSF. The left and right hemispheres are connected and communicate with each other by a transverse band of nerve fibers termed the *corpus callosum*. Each hemisphere has four lobes named for and generally underlying each of the following skull bones: frontal, parietal, temporal, and occipital. For the most part, each hemisphere serves the contralateral side of the body (fibers cross over in the CNS).

One notable exception is Broca's speech area. This area of cortex subserves all motor speech functions and is located in a posterolateral area of the left frontal lobe for all right-handed and many left-handed persons. Damage to this area in an adult produces motor dysphasia.

Cortex

The cortex is thought to operate in all higher mental functions such as judgment, language, memory, creativity, and abstract thinking. It also functions in the perception, localization, and interpretation of all sensations and governs all voluntary and especially discrete motor activities (Fig. 27–6). Various areas of the cortex have been identified as having different motor and sensory functions, but some of these areas are being implicated in other functions as well (eg, the occipital area is now known to function in some learning processes of blind people). Many areas of the cerebrum operate together to produce coordinated human function; the process of communication provides a good example of this.

Verbal communication depends on the ability to interpret speech and to translate thought into speech. Ideas usually are communicated between people by either spoken or written word. With the spoken word, the sensory input of information occurs through the primary auditory cortex. In auditory association areas, the sounds are interpreted as words and the words as sentences. These sentences are then interpreted by a common integrative area of the cerebral cortex as thoughts.

The common integrative area also develops thoughts to be communicated. Letters seen by the eyes are associated as words, thoughts, and sentences in the visual association area and integrated into thought in this area as well. Operating in conjunction with facial regions of the somesthetic sensory area, the common integrative area initiates a series of impulses, each representing a syllable or word, and transmits them to the secondary motor area controlling the larynx and mouth.

The speech center, in addition to controlling motor activity of the larynx and mouth, sends impulses to the respiratory center of the secondary motor cortex to provide appropriate breath patterns for the speech process.

Basal Ganglia

The basal ganglia function in cooperation with other lower brain parts in providing circuitry for basic and subconscious bodily movements. They provide (1) the necessary background muscle tone for discrete voluntary movements, (2) smoothness and coordination in functions of muscle antagonists, and (3) the basic automatic subconscious rhythmic movements involved in walking and equilibrium maintenance. Lesions of these basal ganglia will produce various clinical abnormalities such as chorea, hemiballismus, and Parkinson's disease.

Diencephalon

Below the cerebrum lies the next brain area, the diencephalon. This area contains the third ventricle and the thalamus. Below is the hypothalamus and above is the epithalamus or pineal gland (see Figure 27–5). The diencephalon is the most superior portion of what most authors call the *brain stem* (diencephalon, midbrain, pons, and medulla).

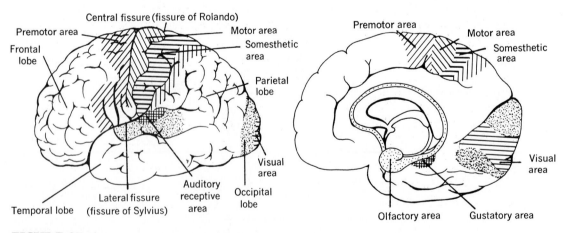

FIGURE 27–6
Diagram of the localization of function in the cerebral hemisphere. Various functional areas are shown in relation to the lobes and fissures: *Left*, lateral view; *right*, medial view.

The *thalamus* functions as a sensory and motor relay center. It relays sensory impulses, including those of sight and sound, up to the cortex. It also functions in the gross awareness of certain sensations, most notably pain. Discrete localization and the finer perceptual details are cortical functions, but the remaining awareness occurs at the thalamic and even midbrain areas.

The thalamus also has other cells, the axons of which travel to association areas of the cortex. The function of these cells and the cortical areas to which they attach are unknown.

Last, the thalamus possesses some of the fiber tracts of the reticular activating systems (RAS) that function in promoting wakefulness and consciousness, and possibly some aspects of attention.

The *hypothalamus* is the seat of neuroendocrine interaction. It is here that various neurosecretory substances are produced—hormones that previously were attributed to the posterior pituitary (antidiuretic hormone and oxytocin) and that stimulate or inhibit the secretion of anterior pituitary hormones.

This area of the brain also contains centers for (1) coordinated parasympathetic and sympathetic stimulation; (2) temperature regulation; (3) appetite regulation; (4) regulation of water balance by antidiuretic hormone; and (5) regulation of certain rhythmic psychobiologic activities (eg, sleep).

Limbic System

The hypothalamus, cingulate, gyrus of the cortex, the amygdala and hippocampus within the temporal lobes, and the septum and interconnecting fiber tracts among these areas compose a functional unit of the brain called the *limbic system*. This system provides a neural substrate for emotions (terror, intense pleasure, eroticism, and so forth).

This region of the brain is involved in emotional experience and in the control of emotion-related behavior. Also, it is here that neural pathways provide a connection between higher brain functioning and endocrinologic–autonomic activities.

Midbrain

The midbrain lies between the diencephalon and the pons of the brain stem. It contains the aqueduct of Sylvius, many ascending and descending nerve fiber tracts, and centers for auditory and visually stimulated nerve impulses. It is here that the *Edinger–Westphal nucleus* is located. This nucleus contains the autonomic reflex centers for pupillary accommodations to light. It receives fibers from the retina by way of cranial nerve II and emits motor impulses by way of sympathetic and parasympathetic (cranial nerve III) fibers to the smooth muscles of the iris. Impaired pupillary accommodation signifies that at least one of these inputs or outputs is damaged or that the midbrain itself is suffering insult (often from tentorial herniation or stroke).

Pons

The *pons varolli* lies between the midbrain and the medulla oblongata of the brain stem and has cell bodies of fibers contained in cranial nerves V, VI, VII, and VIII. It contains pneumotaxic and apneustic respiratory centers and fiber tracts connecting higher and lower centers, including the cerebellum.

Medulla

The *medulla* lies between the pons and the cord. It contains autonomic centers that regulate such vital functions as breathing, cardiac rate, and vasomotor tone as well as centers for vomiting, gagging, coughing, and sneezing reflex behaviors. It also contains the fourth ventricle. Cranial nerves IX to XII have their cell bodies in this area. Impairment of any of these vital functions or reflexes suggests medullary damage.

Cerebellum

The cerebellum is located just superior and posterior to the medulla. It receives "samples" of all ascending somesthetic sensory input as well as of all descending motor impulses. Use of these connections enables the cerebellum to match intended motor stimuli (before they reach the muscles) with actual sensory data. This ensures optimal match for voluntary motor "intention" with actual motor action, with time to alter the motor message in case of error. It sends its own messages up to the basal ganglia and cortex, as well as to parts of the brain stem, to perform three basic subconscious functions.

The cerebellum functions to (1) produce smooth, steady, harmonious, and coordinated skeletal muscle actions; (2) maintain equilibrium; and (3) control posture without any jerky or uncompensated movements or swaying.

Cerebellum disease can produce certain symptoms, the most prominent of which are disturbances of gait, equilibrium ataxia (overstability or understability of the walk), and tremors.

Functionally Integrated Systems

There are three networks within the brain stem that bear mention here. They are the integrated systems responsible for consciousness, sleep, and posture–equilibrium.

Bulboreticular Formation

This is a network of neurons in the brain stem that functions in maintaining bodily support against gravity and equilibrium. Figure 27–7 illustrates the anatomic location

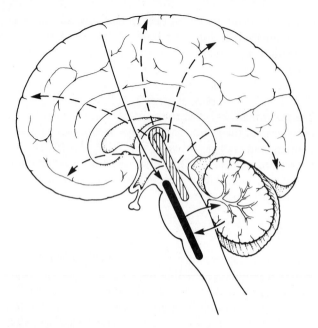

FIGURE 27–7
Bulboreticular and reticular activating systems. *Black area*, bulboreticular system; *striped area*, reticular activating system.

of the bulboreticular formation. This area receives information from a variety of sources that include all areas of the peripheral sensory receptors via the spinal cord, the cerebellum, the inner ear equilibrium apparatus, the motor cortex, and the basal ganglia. The bulboreticular formation, then, is an integrative area for sensory information, motor information from the cerebral cortex, equilibrium information from the vestibular apparatus, and proprioceptive information from the cerebellum. Output from the bulboreticular formation travels down descending fibers to internuncial neurons in the cord. This output alters the tonus of muscles maintaining equilibrium and the positions of major body parts (trunk, appendages) necessary for the performance of discrete actions (eg, writing at a table, walking).

Reticular Activating System

The RAS is an ascending fiber system originating in the midbrain and thalamus (see Figure 27–7). Branches extend up to the cortex. In this way, the RAS can stimulate the cortex. The RAS itself is stimulated by the arrival of a variety of sensory impulses and chemical stimuli from various sources. These include input from the optic and acoustic cranial nerves, somesthetic impulses from the dorsal column and spinothalamic pathways, and fibers from the cerebral cortex. In addition, it is stimulated by norepinephrine and epinephrine.

The stimulation of the cortex by the RAS seems to be the major physiological basis for consciousness, alertness, and attention to various environmental stimuli. Some of the aforementioned stimuli (eg, pain, noise), however, also can increase one's level of consciousness, at least

temporarily. Decreased activity of the RAS produces decreased alertness or levels of consciousness, including stupor and coma. Inactivation of the RAS can result from anything that interrupts the entry of a critical amount of sensory input or by any damage that prevents the RAS fibers from sending impulses to the cortex. Normal inactivation of the cortex occurs during sleep.

Sleep Centers

The release of stored serotonin from the diencephalon, medulla, thalamus, and a small forebrain area (DMTF) results in inactivation of the RAS and activation of the DMTF. DMTF activity results in the first four stages of sleep, stages I, II, III, and IV. It is during stages III and IV that parasympathetic activity (with decreased heart rate, respiratory rate, and so forth) predominates and that sleepwalking and talking and nocturnal enuresis occur.

Rhythmic discharges (about four to eight times/night, from 10–20 minutes/episode) from the pontine nuclei during sleep result in rapid eye movement sleep, during which about 80% of all dreaming occurs and sympathetic nervous system activity predominates.

Based on circadian rhythmicity and decreasing cerebral serotonin levels, the RAS is reactivated in the morning, after 6 to 8 hours of sleep.

Spinal Cord

The spinal cord lies within the neural canal of the vertebral column, extending down and filling the neural canal to the level of the second lumbar vertebra. A pair of spinal nerves exists between adjacent vertebrae the entire length of the vertebral column. Below the point at which the cord terminates, the neural canal is filled with spinal nerves, extending to their point of exit (Fig. 27–8). Because neurons occupy less space in the canal at lower lumbar levels, it is here that spinal taps may be performed most safely. This anatomic fact also explains why injuries to lumbar and lower thoracic vertebrae can produce impairment at disproportionately lower body levels.

Within the cord lie interneurons, ascending sensory fibers, descending motor fibers, and the nerve cell bodies and dendrites of the second-order somatic (voluntary) and first-order autonomic motor neurons. The central area of the cord, the gray matter, contains nerve cell bodies and internuncial neurons (ie, nerve cells contained entirely within the cord). The gray matter has left and right dorsal and ventral projections, giving it an H-shaped appearance. Nerve cell bodies of motor neurons supplying skeletal muscles lie in the ventral horns. Left and right lateral projections or horns of gray matter exist in the thoracic, lumbar, and sacral cord. Within those lie the nerve cell bodies of autonomic neurons. Surrounding the gray matter is the white matter of the cord. It contains ascending and descending fiber tracts as well as fibers entering or leaving the cord. Its white color comes from the myelin that covers these fibers.

Spinal nerves contain both sensory and motor fibers. Each spinal nerve attaches to the cord by a dorsal and ventral root. The dorsal root houses the nerve cell bodies and fibers of sensory neurons. Motor fibers (whose nerve cell bodies lie within the gray matter) traverse the ventral root. Thus, damage to one root may impair sensory function without impairing motor function, or vice versa. A spinal nerve injury could damage both sensory function and motor functioning.

Sensory Division

The sensory division of the nervous system is composed of sensory receptors, sensory neurons, sensory tracts, and perceptive areas of the brain.

Sensations and Receptors

A wide variety of structures respond to diverse stimuli. They range in structure and function from light-sensitive retinal cells to stretch-sensitive structures in muscles and tendons. Stimulation of a sensory receptor initiates an electrical charge (generator potential), which in turn stimulates the sensory neuron synapsing with the receptor. A series of nerve impulses travels along the sensory neuron to the CNS, where they in turn stimulate neurons in either brain or cord tracts to carry impulses to the appropriate centers in the brain (thalamus and cortex), where the sensation finally may be perceived consciously.

Sensations often are divided into those of the major senses (eg, vision, hearing, and smell) and those termed somesthetic sensations (eg, pain, touch, and stretch). Somesthetic sensations provide information on such things as body position and conditions of the immediate external environment, as well as conditions of the internal environment. These are called proprioceptive, exteroceptive, and visceral sensations, respectively. In this chapter, only somesthetic sensations will be discussed.

Proprioceptive sensations describe the physical position state of the body, such as tension in muscle, flexion or extension of joints, tendon tension, and deep pressure in dependent parts like the feet while one is standing or the buttocks while one is seated. *Exteroceptive sensations* monitor the conditions on the body surface. These include temperature and pain. *Visceral sensations* are like exteroceptive sensations except that they originate from within and monitor pain, pressure, and fullness from internal organs.

The sensory receptors for somesthetic sensations include both free nerve endings and specialized end-organs. Free nerve endings are nothing more than small, filamentous branches of the dendritic fibers. They detect crude sensations of touch, pain, heat, and cold. The precision is crude because there are many interconnections between

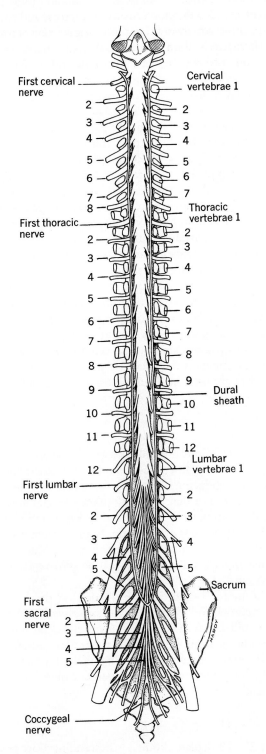

FIGURE 27–8
Spinal cord lying within the vertebral canal. Spinous processes and laminae have been removed; dura and arachnoid have been opened. Spinal nerves are numbered on the left side; vertebrae are numbered on the right side. Note the site of origin of each spinal nerve in the cord and its point of exit from the vertebral column.

the free endings of different neurons. They are the most profusely distributed and perform the general discriminatory functions, however, whereas the more specialized receptors discriminate between very slight differences in degrees of touch, heat, and cold.

Structurally, the special exteroceptive end-organs for detection of cold, warmth, and light touch differ from one another and are quite specific in their function. The physiological basis for this specific function has not been determined but is presumed to be based on some specific physical effect on the organ itself.

There are three proprioceptive receptors. Joint kinesthetic receptors are found in the joint capsules and provide data on the angulation of a joint and the rate at which it is changing. Information from muscles concerning the degree of stretch is transmitted to the nervous system from the muscle spindle apparatus, whereas the Golgi tendon determines the overall tension applied to the tendons.

When a sensory receptor is stimulated, it responds with an increased frequency of firing (generator potential). At first there is a burst of impulses; if the stimulus persists, the frequency of impulses transmitted begins to decrease. All sensory receptors show this phenomenon of *adaptation* to varying degrees and at different rates. Adaptations to light touch and pressure occur in a few seconds, whereas pain and proprioceptive sensation adapt very little, if at all, and at a very slow rate. The determination of the intensity of sensation is made on a relative rather than an absolute basis and follows a logarithmic response. Therefore, the intensity of a sensation increases logarithmically, whereas the frequency of response in the nerve ending increases linearly.

Although there are structurally different receptors for detecting each type of sensation, it is the area of the brain to which the information is transmitted that determines the *modality*, or type of sensation a person feels. The thalamus and somesthetic areas of the cortex operate together to attribute various sensory qualities and intensities to the nerve impulse information they receive.

Sensory Neurons

Stimulation of sensory receptors creates nerve impulses (action potentials) in sensory neurons. These neurons conduct such impulses to the CNS.

Sensory Pathways

Depending on the type of somesthetic receptor involved, fibers of sensory neurons may, on entering the cord, do one of three things. They may travel the white matter of the cord on the same side of the body as the sensory receptor. There they will synapse with a second set of neurons that then cross over to the opposite side of the brain and travel to the thalamus. This pathway is termed the *dorsal column* or *posterior column pathway* (Fig. 27–9) and is used for the conduction of impulses originating from stimulation of (1) muscle, tendon, and joint proprioceptors; (2) vibration-sensitive receptors; and (3) receptors in the skin involved in precise localization of touch.

Alternatively, the sensory neuron may synapse immediately on entering the cord with a second neuron that then immediately crosses over to the opposite side of the cord. Fibers from this second neuron then travel up the white matter of the cord to the thalamus. This is called the *spinothalamic pathway* (see Figure 27–9). It conducts impulses concerned with pain, temperature, poorly localized touch, and sex organ sensations. In the thalamus, neurons of both the spinothalamic pathway and the dorsal column pathway synapse with other neurons that transmit impulses to the appropriate area of the somesthetic cortex. Because of this, impulses from either pathway give rise to consciously perceived sensations.

Last, certain sensory neurons may synapse with a neuron belonging to the *spinocerebellar* pathway. Spinocerebellar neurons do not cross over, and they carry impulses only as far as the cerebellum (and possibly lower brain stem). This pathway carries impulses originating from stimulation of muscle, tendon, and joint proprioceptors. Because this pathway ends at the cerebellum, it transmits sensory information that never is perceived consciously. These data are used in reflex postural adjustments.

Motor System

The motor system technically comprises the areas of the brain, descending fiber tracts, and the motor neurons involved in producing or altering movement or adjusting tonus of skeletal cardiac and smooth muscles and in regulating the secretions of the various exocrine and certain endocrine gland cells of the body. In practical terms, the heart usually is excluded from this system. Muscle and glandular tissues are referred to as the *effective organs* of this system.

The motor system can be divided on the basis of motor neurons and effector organs into *somatic* and *autonomic* subdivisions. The former involve skeletal muscles and motor neurons innervating them. The autonomic subdivision is composed of smooth muscle and gland cells plus the sympathetic and parasympathetic fibers innervating them.

Somatic Motor Division

Figure 27–10 depicts the major descending fiber tracts from motor areas of the cerebral cortex. Some of these fibers cross over to the opposite side of the body in the brain. Many cross in the medulla. A few cross over in the cord centers. Descending fibers from motor areas of the cortex ultimately stimulate somatic motor neurons, the nerve cell bodies of which lie in the anterior (ventral)

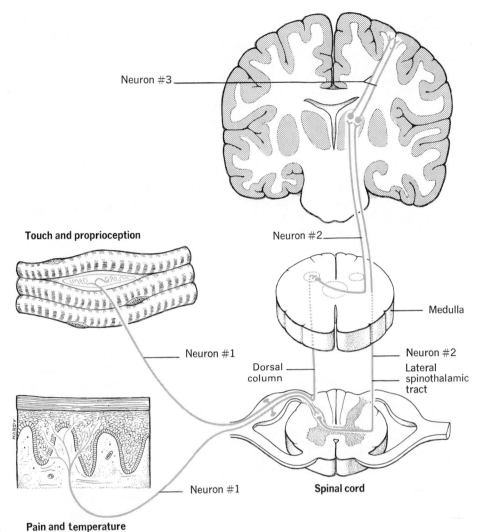

Touch and proprioception

Neuron #3

Neuron #2

Neuron #1

Neuron #1

Medulla

Dorsal column

Neuron #2
Lateral spinothalamic tract

Spinal cord

Pain and temperature

FIGURE 27–9
Diagrammatic representation of the decussation (crossing) of ascending tracts. First-order neurons for touch and proprioception ascend in the dorsal columns to the medulla; here they synapse with second-order neurons that cross to the opposite side before ascending to the thalamus. First-order neurons for pain and temperature enter the dorsal gray matter of the cord; here they synapse with second-order neurons that cross to the opposite side and ascend in the lateral spinothalamic tract to the thalamus. Third-order neurons connect the thalamus with the cerebral cortex.

horn of the gray matter in the cord. The axons of these motor neurons travel within spinal nerves and terminate adjacent to the membranes of skeletal muscle cells. The space between the somatic motor neuron axon and the muscle cell is termed the *myoneural junction*. When stimulated, somatic motor neurons conduct impulses to the ends of their axons. As the impulse arrives there, it triggers the release of a certain number of acetylcholine molecules that are stored in the terminal bouton. The acetylcholine diffuses across the myoneural junction and binds with receptor sites on a skeletal muscle cell. This triggers a chain of events leading to contraction. Thus, willed intentional motor movements are enacted.

Not shown in Figure 27–10 are descending fiber tracts that stimulate motor neurons responsible for the movement of skeletal muscles of the head (eg, tongue, face, jaw). The general pattern and myoneural transmitter are the same, except the somatic motor neuron nerve cell bodies lie within certain areas of the brain.

Also not shown in Figure 27–10 are several extrapyramidal tracts that arise from brain stem centers (eg,

bulboreticular formation, midbrain). Some of these cross over, whereas others do not. Fibers in these tracts descend the cord and ultimately stimulate either somatic motor neurons, which stimulate skeletal muscle cells, or other motor neurons (gamma efferent) that alter the tension of stretch receptor organelles (spindles) within the skeletal muscles. Alteration of spindle tension provokes a spinal reflex arc that efficiently and indirectly alters skeletal muscle tonus. These extrapyramidal pathways conduct impulses that produce the automatic coordinated alterations in skeletal muscle tonus and movement that are necessary for gross motor movements (eg, walking) and for appropriate posture for conduction of finer movements (eg, sitting at a desk with arm flexed in preparation for writing; standing).

Autonomic Motor Division

The autonomic division comprises both *sympathetic* and *parasympathetic motor fibers*. They are responsible for contraction and relaxation of smooth muscle, rate of contrac-

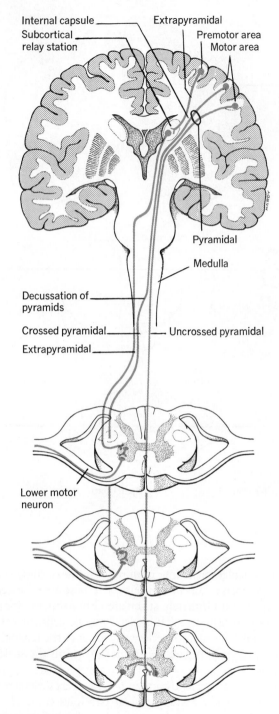

FIGURE 27–10
Diagram of motor pathways between the cerebral cortex, one of the subcortical relay centers, and lower motor neurons in the spinal cord. Decussation (crossing) of fibers means that each side of the brain controls skeletal muscles on the opposite side of the body.

tion of cardiac tissue, secretion of exocrine glands, and secretion of the adrenal medulla and islets of Langerhans in the pancreas.

The sympathetic and parasympathetic sections differ on the basis of (1) the anatomic distribution of nerve fibers, (2) the secretion of two different neural transmitters by the postganglionic fibers of the two divisions, and (3) the antagonistic effects of the two divisions on some of the organs they innervate. Figure 27–11 shows the anatomy of the sympathetic and parasympathetic nervous systems. It is important to understand that 80% of parasympathetic activity occurs by way of cranial nerve X, the vagus nerve, and about 20% occurs by way of the pelvic nerve. Unopposed vagus activity accounts for the bradycardia (and so on) seen in the early weeks of spinal cord injuries, when cord activity below the level of injury temporarily ceases.

Both the sympathetic and parasympathetic motor pathways essentially are composed of a chain of two neurons carrying nerve impulses from the CNS to the effector organ. The first neuron in the chain is termed the *preganglionic neuron* and the second one is called the *postganglionic neuron*. Nerve cell bodies of preganglionic sympathetic neurons lie in the lateral horns of the gray matter of the thoracic and lumbar segments of the cord; those of preganglionic parasympathetic neurons lie either in certain areas of the brain or in the lateral horns of gray matter in the sacral cord.

Axons of preganglionic sympathetic neurons exit the cord and enter the ventral roots of spinal nerves. They then leave the spinal nerve to enter a nearby sympathetic ganglion (by way of a connecting pathway termed a *ramus*). Within a ganglion, the preganglionic neuron synapses with a postganglionic one. The postganglionic sympathetic neuron then may reenter the spinal nerve or exit the ganglion by a special sympathetic nerve and travel to the effector organ.

Parasympathetic preganglionic axons leave the CNS by certain cranial or spinal nerves and travel to the effector organ. At or near the effector organ, they synapse with the postganglionic neuron, which in turn innervates the effector organ.

Acetylcholine is the neurotransmitter at *all* synapses between preganglionic and postganglionic autonomic neurons—both parasympathetic and sympathetic. It also is the transmitter secreted by the axons of postsynaptic parasympathetic neurons. For this reason, these axons are called *cholinergic fibers.* Sympathetic postganglionic fibers are called *adrenergic fibers* because they secrete noradrenalin (norepinephrine). The actions of these two arms of the autonomic division and their chemical transmitters are summarized in Table 27–1.

The neurotransmitters balance each other. When there is a disruption in the production or destruction of one, clinical manifestations may become apparent. For example, in Parkinson's disease there is a neurochemical imbalance. A dopaminergic pathway, the nigrostriatal pathway, connects the substantia nigra to the striatum. This pathway is thought to be inhibitory to the striatal neurons that communicate with the motor cortex. The striatum also contains cholinergic interneurons that functionally oppose

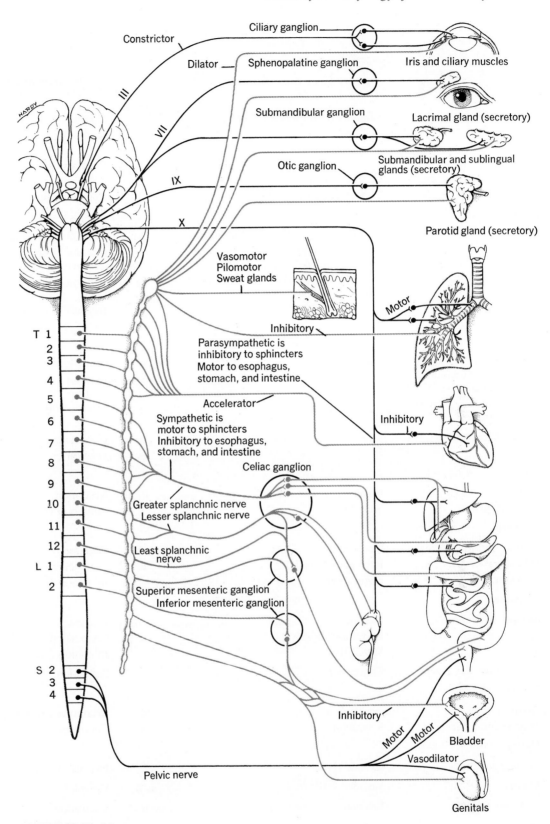

FIGURE 27–11

Diagram of the autonomic nervous system. Parasympathetic, or craniosacral, fibers are shown in black, and the sympathetic, or thoracolumbar, fibers are shaded. Note that most organs have a double nerve supply.

TABLE 27–1
Responses of Effector Organs to Autonomic Nerve Impulses and Circulating Catecholamines

Effector Organs	Cholinergic Impulses Response	Noradrenergic Impulses	
		Receptor Type	Response
Eye			
Radial muscle of iris	—	α	Contraction (mydriasis)
Sphincter muscle of iris	Contraction (miosis)		
Ciliary muscle	Contraction for near vision	β	Relaxation for far vision
Heart			
SA node	Decrease in heart rate; vagal arrest	β_1	Increase in heart rate
Atria	Decrease in contractility and (usually) increase in conduction velocity	β_1	Increase in contractility and conduction velocity
AV node and conduction system	Decrease in conduction velocity; AV block	β_1	Increase in conduction velocity
Ventricles	—	β_1	Increase in contractility and conduction velocity
Arterioles			
Coronary, skeletal muscle, pulmonary, abdominal viscera, renal	Dilation	α β_2	Constriction Dilation
Skin and mucosa, cerebral, salivary glands	—	α	Constriction
Systemic Veins	—	α β_2	Constriction Dilation
Lung			
Bronchial muscle	Contraction	β_2	Relaxation
Bronchial glands	Stimulation	?	Inhibition (?)
Stomach			
Motility and tone	Increase	α, β_2	Decrease (usually)
Sphincters	Relaxation (usually)	α	Contraction (usually)
Secretion	Stimulation		Inhibition (?)
Intestine			
Motility and tone	Increase	α, β_2	Decrease
Sphincters	Relaxation (usually)	α	Contraction (usually)
Secretion	Stimulation		Inhibition (?)
Gallbladder and Ducts	Contraction		Relaxation
Urinary Bladder			
Detrusor	Contraction	β	Relaxation (usually)
Trigone and sphincter	Relaxation	α	Contraction
Ureter			
Motility and tone	Increase (?)	α	Increase (usually)
Uterus	Variable*	α, β_2	Variable*
Male Sex Organs	Erection	α	Ejaculation
Skin			
Pilomotor muscles	—	α	Contraction
Sweat glands	Generalized secretion	α	Slight, localized secretion†
Spleen Capsule	—	α β_2	Contraction Relaxation

(continued)

TABLE 27–1
Responses of Effector Organs to Autonomic Nerve Impulses and Circulating Catecholamines
(*Continued*)

Effector Organs	Cholinergic Impulses Response	Noradrenergic Impulses	
		Receptor Type	*Response*
Adrenal Medulla	Secretion of epinephrine and nor-epinephrine		—
Liver	—	α, β$_2$	Glycogenolysis
Pancreas			
Acini	Secretion	α	Decreased secretion
Islets	Insulin and glucagon secretion	α	Inhibition of insulin and glucagon secretion
		β$_2$	Insulin and glucagon secretion
Salivary Glands	Profuse, watery secretion	α	Thick, viscous secretion
		β$_2$	Amylase secretion
Lacrimal Glands	Secretion		—
Nasopharyngeal Glands	Secretion		—
Adipose Tissue	—	β$_1$	Lipolysis
Juxtaglomerular Cells	—	β(β$_1$?)	Renin secretion
Pineal Gland	—	β	Melatonin synthesis and secretion

AV, atrioventricular.
*Depends on stage of menstrual cycle, amount of circulating estrogen and progesterone, pregnancy, and other factors.
†On palms of hands and in some other locations ("adrenergic sweating").
(From Ganong WF: Review of Medical Physiology, 11th ed. Los Altos, Lange Medical Publications, 1983)

the dopaminergic input. Parkinsonism involves a defect in the nigrostriatal pathway. As a result, the dopamine that normally is secreted in the striatum no longer is present. The neurons that secrete acetylcholine remain functional, and in the absence of dopamine, become overactive, contributing to the motor symptoms of parkinsonism.

In addition to the two subdivisions of the autonomic motor division, there are three different actions of adrenergically (sympathetically) stimulated effector organs. These actions are determined by the type of receptor site in the effector organ. Receptor sites may be α, β$_1$, or β$_2$.

Patterns of autonomic function can be regulated or triggered by centers in the hypothalamus, medulla, and bulboreticular formations. Autonomic functioning, however, does not seem limited to the stem. Stimulation of certain cortical nerves can trigger both discrete and widespread autonomic changes. Exact mechanisms for these interactions await research. These centers in the CNS send impulses along descending fibers to the appropriate preganglionic autonomic neuron. In the cord, such fibers would travel by special descending tracts in the white matter until they reached the appropriate level of the cord. Thus, any interruption of these descending fibers (eg, transection of cervical tracts) would impede or prevent stimulation of

preganglionic autonomic neurons in the thoracic, lumbar, and sacral regions of the cord.

Reflexes

Basically, a reflex is an instantaneous and automatic motor response to a sensory input. It arises from a special anatomic relationship among sensory receptors, sensory neurons, interneurons, somatic or autonomic motor neurons, and effector organs. The effector is the end-organ that receives the motor impulse, such as skeletal, smooth, or cardiac muscles, or an exocrine or endocrine gland.

Somesthetic sensory neurons involved in a reflex arc usually have branching axons: one branch participates in the arc, whereas the other travels up to the cerebrum by way of the dorsal column or spinothalamic tracts. This enables the person to perceive the sensation involved; however, such perception is not part of, nor requisite for, the operation of a reflex arc. Because it takes slightly longer for sensory data to reach the cortex than to reach an interneuron, a person often becomes aware of the sensation only during or after the occurrence of the reflex arc. Also, a cord reflex can occur even if the cord is transected

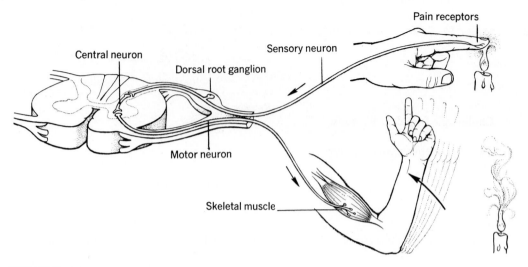

FIGURE 27–12
Diagram of withdrawal reflex.

above the level required for the reflex so that no sensory information can get to the brain. Reflexes may involve the cord or the brain; the former will be considered first.

Cord Reflexes

One type of common cord reflex is the *withdrawal reflex* (Fig. 27–12). Pain is the sensation that triggers this reflex. It stimulates sensory neurons, which in turn stimulate "central" interneurons, which stimulate motor fibers that innervate skeletal muscles. When contracted, the skeletal muscles will produce withdrawal of the body part (here, a hand) from the painful stimulus. Its occurrence depends on the appropriate anatomic connections, or "wiring," along sensory and motor neurons within the cord. If these become nonfunctional (eg, cord shock or physical trauma), the reflex will not be possible.

Reflex withdrawal of one foot is associated with another reflex, the *crossed extensor reflex* (Fig. 27–13). This reflex involves stimulation of various extensor muscles in the opposite leg so that the person's weight is fully supported while one lower extremity is withdrawn from a painful stimulus. Such a reflex is very complex and involves many levels of the cord. Any imbalance, however slight, during the operation of this reflex in a normal person will trigger the occurrence of additional reflexes involving the bulboreticular formation, cerebellum, and various muscles of arms and trunk so as to maintain balance and posture.

Another cord reflex is the *stretch reflex*, most commonly illustrated by the clinical test of the knee jerk reflex (Fig. 27–14). Because of anatomic connections within the cord, the stimulation of stretch receptors in a muscle or a tendon automatically triggers an immediate contraction of the muscle. In the knee jerk reflex, the hammer blow stretches the tendon of the quadriceps. This reflexively causes contraction of the quadriceps, which causes the lower leg to "kick forward." Other stretch reflexes of clinical importance are the ankle jerk and the biceps and triceps reflexes. All involve stretching the muscle by a hammer tap of its tendon.

An important feature of all cord reflexes involving skeletal muscles is *reciprocal inhibition*, which occurs in the antagonist muscle of the one stimulated. For example, when a flexor reflex stimulates the biceps, it also inhibits its antagonist, the triceps, and provides for more efficient performance of motor activities in the upper arm.

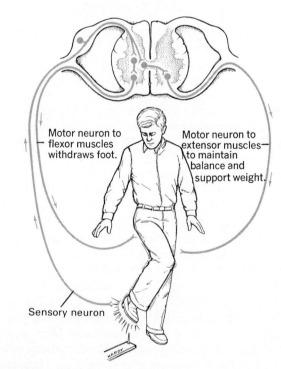

FIGURE 27–13
Diagram of flexor and crossed extensor reflexes.

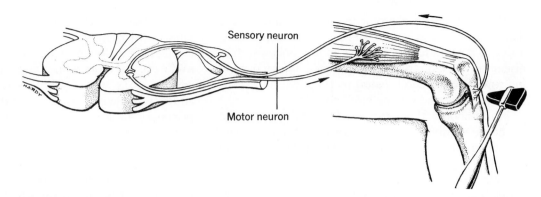

FIGURE 27–14
Diagram of a stretch reflex.

Spinal cord activities also include reflex circuits, which aid in the *control of visceral functions* of the body. Sensory input arises from visceral sensory receptors and is transmitted to the spinal cord, where reflex patterns appropriate to the sensory input are determined. The signals are then transmitted to autonomic motor neurons in the gray matter of the spinal cord, which send impulses to the sympathetic nerves innervating visceral motor end-organs. A most important autonomic reflex is the *peritoneal reflex*. Tissue damage in any portion of the peritoneum results in the response of this reflex, which slows or stops all motor activity in the nearby viscera. Other autonomic cord reflexes are capable of *modifying local blood flow* in response to cold, pain, and heat. This vascular control by autonomic reflexes in the spinal cord can operate as a backup mechanism for the usual brain stem control patterns in patients with transectional injuries at the brain stem.

Also included in the autonomic reflexes of the spinal cord are those causing the *emptying of the urinary bladder and the rectum*. When the bowel or bladder becomes distended, sensory signals from stretch receptors in the bowel or bladder wall are transmitted by sensory neurons to the internuncial neurons of the upper sacral and lower lumbar segments of the cord. These neurons in turn stimulate parasympathetic motor neurons innervating the wall of the bowel or bladder and its internal sphincter. Somatic motor neurons innervating the extrinsic sphincter muscles also are reflexively stimulated by the internuncials. The net result of such motor neuron stimulation is a reflex contraction of bowel or bladder and an opening of the sphincters, thereby permitting defecation or micturition.

Descending fibers from the cerebral cortex also synapse with the internuncials. These fibers act to inhibit the reflex emptying of bowel or bladder at times or places deemed inappropriate by the person. Toilet training of infants must await the functional maturation of these descending fibers. Cord transections or other damage above the level of the cord housing the neurons for the bowel or bladder evacuation reflexes will interrupt some or all of these descending fibers. This produces a condition wherein the patient cannot consciously control (ie, prevent) the emptying of the bowel or bladder or both. Damage to or interrupted function of that level of the cord housing the anatomic neuronal connections for these reflexes (eg, spina bifida, cord shock, severe injuries to the sacral lower or lumbar cord) will prevent reflex evacuation of bowel or bladder or both. Such a patient may exhibit retention with overflow but will not possess any effective mechanism for emptying the bowel or bladder or both.

Brain Reflexes

Brain reflexes operate in the same way as do cord reflexes, except that the brain houses the connection, not the cord. Brain reflexes include those involving the *cardioreaulatory and vasomotor centers* of the medulla, plus the pupillary adjustment center, which involves the midbrain. Because the sensory and motor arms of the heart rate and vasopressure reflexes are commonly known, only the *pupillary reflex* will be discussed

Light in the retina causes stimulation of the optic nerve. Fibers in this nerve travel to the Edinger–Westphal nucleus in the midbrain. Here the sensory fibers synapse with interneurons. The result is outgoing autonomic motor impulses to the smooth muscles of the iris. Increases in parasympathetic impulses (by way of cranial nerve III) or decreases in sympathetic impulses cause pupillary constriction in response to the light. As the light stimulus of the retina decreases, this reflex causes pupillary dilation. Lack of this reflex signifies damage to the midbrain–optic fiber connection or to the oculomotor nerve (cranial nerve III).

Pain

The sensation of pain warrants special consideration because it plays such an important protective role for the body. Whenever there is tissue damage, nerve endings are stimulated and the sensation of pain is felt. This sensation usually is felt during the time that tissue is undergoing damage and ceases when the damage ends. This condition is due to the release of chemicals and metabolites such as histamine and kinin from damaged cells. Typical damaging stimuli are physical trauma (cutting, crushing, tearing), ischemia, and intense heat and cold.

In addition to these stimuli, acidity of the tissue fluid at the nerve fiber ending is known to stimulate pain sensations, which can be eliminated by making this fluid alkaline.

Variation in pain thresholds both among different people and within the same person at different times has been long known. (This is in addition to the wide variation in people's reactions to pain.) It was thought formerly that the sensation of pain depended in large part on the number of "pain receptor endings" that were simultaneously and continuously stimulated as well as on variations in cortical or brain stem thresholds.

Although the exact mechanism for the transmission and perception of pain is not clear, neurophysiological, psychological, and sociologic research has contributed to formulation of pain theories.

Gate Theory

More recent evidence, however, points to the existence of gating mechanisms in the substantia gelatinosa at all levels of the spinal cord, which are capable of regulating the amount of pain impulses that can enter the spinothalamic tract and travel to the brain. This cord level of pain regulation opens new avenues to the treatment of pain.

Briefly, two types of fibers are involved. One is a small-diameter (S) fiber that carries impulses responsible for the sensation of pain (pain impulses). The other is a large-diameter (L) fiber that carries impulses responsible for cutaneous tactile sensations. The S and L fibers each synapse with two other cells—a gate cell and a T cell of the spinothalamic tract. The gate cell also synapses with the T cell and acts to *inhibit* (by hyperpolarization) the T cell. L-fiber impulses stimulate the gate cell, thereby hyperpolarizing the T cell to a certain degree. S-fiber impulses inhibit the gate cell and stimulate the T cell. When the gate cell is inhibited, the T cell is stimulated. Thus, by itself, the S-fiber impulse readily gains access to the spinothalamic tract.

In theory, if tactile skin receptors *in the same dermatome* are stimulated simultaneously with S fibers, the action of the L fibers will (by way of the gate cell) hyperpolarize the T cell and thereby make it more difficult for S-fiber impulses to stimulate the T cell (gain access to the spinothalamic tract). Thus the relative S- to L-fiber activity can determine the degree of pain impulses that can enter the CNS at the level of the cord (Fig. 27–15).

Rubbing or other tactile sensation such as provided by transcutaneous nerve (skin) stimulation applied to a painful area may reduce the sensation of pain perceived by the patient.

Although much more remains to be learned, it is known that primitive sensations of pain occur once the ascending impulses from the spinothalamic tract reach the midbrain, and more refined and somewhat localized perception occurs at the level of the thalamus. Most refined and localized sensations, as well as their significance to the person, occur at the level of the cortex.

Other Pain Theories

The *specificity* theory was proposed in the early 1800s and was accepted for approximately 100 years as the most appropriate theory for explaining the pain phenomenon. This theory regards pain as a separate sensory modality evoked by the activity of specific receptors that transmit information to pain centers in the forebrain, where pain is experienced. This theory does not account for the multidimensionality of the pain experience.

Another group of theories is called collectively the *pattern theory*. In this theory, two primary pain fibers are identified: a rapidly conducting fiber and a slowly conducting one. Both fibers synapse in the spinal cord and send information to the brain. As small fibers converge at the level of the spinal cord, the summation of these impulses is relayed to the brain. The amount, intensity, and type of sensory input to the brain allow for interpretation of the character and quantity of the pain input. This theory, like the specificity theory, fails to account for the factors that change the perception of pain, such as anxiety and depression. The theories also do not explain why pain may continue after surgical transection of the pain pathways and spinal cord.

Referred Pain

This type of pain is perceived as arising from a site that is different from its true point of origin. Well known examples include the referring of pain from severe cardiac ischemia to the left arm or the referring of diaphragmatic pain to the neck and shoulder. The "true point of origin" for this type of pain usually is some visceral organ or deep somatic structure and the "point of reference" is some area of the body surface. A knowledge of the embryologic development of various parts of the body provides an understanding of the physiological basis of referred pain. The true point of origin and its common referred-to areas were, at one time, embryologically close together and are innervated by sensory neurons that enter the same segment of the spinal cord. Although the two areas move farther apart in the normal growth and development of a person, their innervation persists. Thus, sensory impulses originating from painful stimuli in either the "true" or "referred" body areas will enter the same level of the cord and synapse with the same neurons of the spinothalamic pathway at this level. There is no way for the cerebral cortex to "know" whether a given spinothalamic neuron was stimulated originally by pain from the true point of

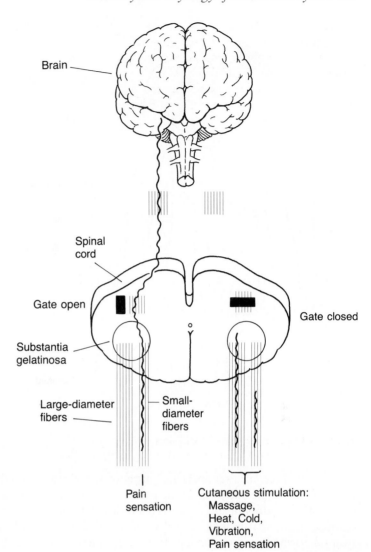

Brain

Spinal cord

Gate open

Gate closed

Substantia gelatinosa

Large-diameter fibers

Small-diameter fibers

Pain sensation

Cutaneous stimulation:
Massage,
Heat, Cold,
Vibration,
Pain sensation

FIGURE 27–15
Gate control theory of pain.

origin or the referred-to area. In localizing the source of the pain stimulus, the cortex relies on prior experience regarding the person's geographic knowledge of his or her own body. Because surface areas are more familiar to a person than the locations of the visceral or deep somatic structures, the referred-to locale is used preferentially over the more unfamiliar but true point of origin (Fig. 27–16).

Endogenous Opiates

These are substances that in terms of molecular structure and action resemble opiate drugs. Two types are known: enkephalins and endorphins. Enkephalins are pentapeptides synthesized by certain CNS neurons. They appear to function as inhibitory neurotransmitters in pathways conducting impulses concerning pain (nociception). Stimulation of "enkephalinergic neurons" produces analgesia similar to that produced by opiate drugs. Enkephalins bind to opiate receptors on the postsynaptic membrane. In most cases, this inhibits (hyperpolarizes) the postsynaptic neuron by decreasing its sodium influx.

Opiate receptors and enkephalins have been discov-ered in various locations with the CNS. These locations function in the conduction of "pain impulses" up the cord and brain stem to the cortex, in areas associated with emotional effects produced by opiates, or in "analgesic centers" within the brain stem. One location is that part of the dorsal horn of gray matter housing the "spinal gate." Here, enkephalinergic neurons, which receive impulses from descending fibers of the nucleus raphe magnus in the medulla, in turn act on sensory neurons to inhibit the stimulation of T cells by small fibers. This inhibits the entry of "pain impulses" into the spinothalamic tract. Enkephalins and opiate receptors exist in the medullary respiratory center. The latter perhaps explains the potent action of opiate drugs on respiration. They also are found in certain limbic system structures (eg, amygdala). This may explain the emotional effects produced by natural and synthetic opiate drugs. It also suggests that endogenous opiates may function in naturally evoked feelings of pleasure or well-being. The role of enkephalins and opiate receptors found in other brain centers, such as the basal ganglia and neocortex, is unclear at this time.

Enkephalins and opiate receptors also are richly dis-

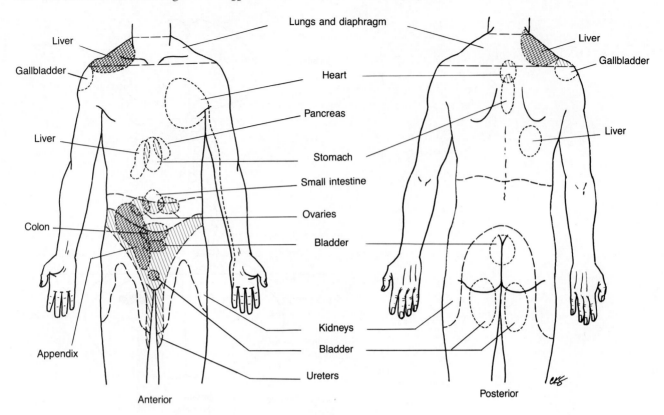

FIGURE 27–16
Anterior and posterior referred pain sites.

tributed in three "central analgesic" areas of the brain stem: (1) the raphe magnus, (2) the periaqueductal gray matter of the midbrain, and (3) areas bordering the third ventricle in the thalamus. Electrical stimulation of these areas is known to produce varying but strong, widespread analgesic effects. Electrical stimulation of the first two areas produces a systemic analgesia that lasts for hours after the stimulation is stopped. It is one current modality for the treatment of intractable pain, but its effects are limited because (1) patients develop tolerance to therapy as they do to narcotics; and (2) there is cross-tolerance between such "electrical stimulation-produced analgesia" and narcotic drugs. The exact manner by which these areas produce analgesia is not known, but enkephalins clearly are involved as mediators because opiate-blocking drugs such as naloxone will inhibit such electrical stimulation-produced analgesia.

The raphe magnus (in the medulla) functions in regulating the spinal gates. Descending fibers from the raphe synapse at all levels of the cord with enkephalinergic internuncial neurons that regulate the ability of "pain-stimulated" sensory neurons to stimulate spinothalamic neurons. Thus, the raphe magnus controls the entry of pain impulses into the pain conduction system in the first place. What cannot enter cannot be perceived. It is not clear whether this raphe is, in turn, regulated by either of the two higher analgesic centers.

Opiate drugs exert their effects by binding with the opiate receptors in many or all of these areas—depending on dosage. Acupuncture and various "placebo analgesics" seem to act by causing a release of endogenous opiates because, in double-blind studies, their analgesic effects are blocked by naloxone. The parts of the CNS involved in such analgesia are unknown. Differing levels of enkephalinergic neuron activity (especially in central analgesic areas) may provide a physiological basis for individual differences in pain reports and tolerances.

Endorphins are part of the pro-opiomelanocortin (POMC) molecule that is secreted by the corticotrophic cells of the anterior pituitary (see Chapter 39). They consist of any segment of this POMC that also contains the five-amino-acid enkephalin sequence (represented by amino acids numbers 61 to 65). They bind to various opiate receptors in the brain, especially the basal ganglia and the limbic system, and seem to function in endogenously produced analgesia. Their exact role or roles are unknown.

BIBLIOGRAPHY

Guyton A: Textbook of Medical Physiology, 8th ed. Philadelphia, WB Saunders, 1991

Hole J Jr: Human Anatomy and Physiology. Dubuque, IA, William C. Brown Publishers, 1992

Noback C, Strominger N, Demarest R (eds): The Human Nervous System: Introduction and Review, 4th ed. Malvern, PA, Lea & Febiger, 1991

Porth C: Pathophysiology: Concepts of Altered Health States. Philadelphia, JB Lippincott, 1990

STUDY QUESTIONS

1. Which statement is true regarding the structure of neurons?

   a. axons carry impulses toward the cell body
   b. dendrites carry impulses toward the cell body
   c. neurons connect one to the other
   d. the synapse is the space between two axons

2. Which brain structure connects the two cerebral hemispheres, allowing communication between the two?

   a. cortex
   b. pons
   c. reticular activating system
   d. corpus callosum

3. Which is *not* a function of the autonomic nervous system?

   a. to regulate rate of cardiac contraction
   b. to regulate secretion of the adrenal medulla and islets of Langerhans
   c. to receive sensory input from dendrites and send out motor impulses via axons
   d. to regulate contraction and relaxation of smooth muscle

4. Which is an example of a cord reflex?

   a. withdrawal reflex
   b. pupillary reflex
   c. corneal reflex
   d. action potential depolarization

5. Cholinergic responses would include

   a. an increase in heart rate
   b. pupillary dilation
   c. increased stomach motility
   d. arteriole contraction

6. A major function of the brain stem is to

   a. provide a neural pathway for emotions
   b. control posture and balance
   c. stimulate sensory neurons, which in turn stimulate interneurons, which stimulate motor fibers that innervate skeletal muscles
   d. control respirations, cardiac rate, and blood vessel diameter

CHAPTER 28

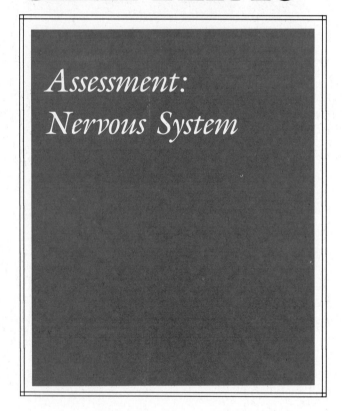

*Assessment:
Nervous System*

BEHAVIORAL OBJECTIVES

Based on the content in this chapter, the reader should be able to:

1. Discuss the value of gathering neurologic data in an orderly and objective manner.
2. Correlate such data over time.
3. Recognize those patterns of assessment findings that imply a significant change in pathologic condition for the patient.
4. Relate the procedure of selected neurodiagnostic tests to nursing implications for patient care.

5. Evaluate the effect of neurologic dysfunction on the patient's living patterns.
6. Define brain death.

Description

For many critical care nurses, assessment and care of a patient with a neurologic problem constitute one of the biggest challenges—and one of the biggest headaches! In basic nursing education and in many critical care courses, an assessment of nervous system functioning frequently is covered last and not to the depth or complexity of other body systems. It is not uncommon, then, for even the experienced caregiver to feel confused when gathering data about the nervous system.

There are three major goals in the nursing assessment of a patient with a real or potential neurologic problem. The first goal is to gather data about nervous system functioning in an objective and orderly manner. Data can be considered objective if several examiners, seeing the same phenomenon or behavior, would give similar descriptions. A standard neurologic check sheet should be used by all the nursing staff, with clearly defined grading scales or terms to be used (eg, "stuporous" to one person may mean "lethargic" to another).

The second objective of neurologic assessment is to correlate the data over time. For such a correlation to be of value, the results of history, physical assessment, and diagnostic tests must be interrelated. Consideration of the information in a patterned format will help in the establishment of both medical and nursing diagnoses and guide the nurse in choosing and evaluating therapy.

The third objective of the neurologic nursing assessment is to determine the effect of dysfunction on the patient's daily living and ability to care for self. To this point, the goals of both physicians and nurses in the care of a patient with a neurologic problem are similar. Each discipline uses many of the same questions and techniques to determine normal and abnormal nervous system functioning. But in contrast to medicine, the focus of nursing is to assist patients in coping with real or potential changes in daily living and self-care.

History

Neurologic assessment begins at the first encounter. Conversation with the patient and family is a vital source of data needed to evaluate overall functioning. The focus of such an interview is twofold: analysis of the current problem bringing the patient to the health care facility, and a general survey of other systems to determine if other problem areas exist in addition to those identified by the patient. In gathering this information, the nurse also should ask questions geared to the detection of neurologic prob-

lems and their effect on the patient. It is helpful to have a family member or friend present who can confirm and clarify the patient's responses.

What to Ask About

- Recent trauma that could affect the nervous system, (eg, a fall or an automobile accident)
- Recent infections, including sinusitis and ear or tooth infections
- Recent headaches and problems with concentration and memory
- Feelings of dizziness, loss of balance, "black-out" spells, tinnitus, and hearing problems
- Clumsiness or weakness of the extremities and difficulty walking
- Sensory distortions (eg, numbness, tingling, hypersensitivity, pain) or sensory loss in face, trunk, or extremities
- Impotence or difficulty in urination
- Recent difficulties in performing everyday activities
- Effects of problem on usual pattern of living, job performance, social interactions
- Tobacco, alcohol, and drug use
- Medication use, both prescription and over-the-counter forms, including dose, schedule, and therapeutic and adverse effects.

Physical Examination

Level of Consciousness

The quality of a patient's consciousness is the most basic and most critical parameter requiring assessment. The level of a patient's awareness of, and response to, the environment is the most sensitive indicator of nervous system dysfunction.

Several systems are used for grading alterations in arousal and awareness. Terms such as *lethargic*, *stuporous*, and *semicomatose* are in common use in many areas (Table 28–1).

In an acute care setting where time for gathering data is limited, the Glasgow Coma Scale can provide a useful shortcut. Such a scale allows the examiner to grade objectively the patient's three major responses to the environment: eye opening, verbalization, and movement. In each category, the best response is scored. Maximum total score for a fully awake and alert person is 15. A minimum score of 3 is indicative of a completely unresponsive patient. An overall score of 8 or below is associated with coma; if maintained over time it may be one predictor of a poor functional recovery. This scoring system was designed as a guide to rapid evaluation of the acutely ill or severely injured patient whose status may change quickly. It is not

TABLE 28–1
A Method of Grading Responsiveness

Alert: normal

Awake: may sleep more than usual or be somewhat confused on first awakening, but fully oriented when aroused

Lethargic: drowsy but follows simple commands when stimulated

Stuporous: very hard to arouse; inconsistently may follow simple commands or speak single words or short phrases

Semicomatose: movements are purposeful when stimulated; does not follow commands or speak coherently

Comatose: may respond with reflexive posturing when stimulated or may have no response to any stimulus.

useful as a guide for evaluation of patients in long-standing comas or during prolonged recovery from severe brain injury (Table 28–2).

An alternative to grading scales is to describe what stimulus is used and what the patient's response was. A suggested order of stimuli is:

1. Call the patient by name.
2. Call name louder.
3. Combine calling name with light touch.
4. Combine calling name with vigorous touch ("shake and shout").
5. Create pain.

TABLE 28–2
The Glasgow Coma Scale

Best Eye-Opening Response	Score
Spontaneously	4
To speech	3
To pain	2
No response	1

Best Verbal Response	Score
Oriented	5
Confused conversation	4
Inappropriate words	3
Garbled sounds	2
No response	1

Best Motor Response	Score
Obeys commands	6
Localizes stimuli	5
Withdrawal from stimulus	4
Abnormal flexion (decorticate)	3
Abnormal extension (decerebrate)	2
No response	1

When noxious stimuli are needed to evoke a response, the nurse should pay careful attention to where the painful stimulus is applied. It is not unknown for a misplaced examiner's hand to cause serious skin or tissue injury. Areas to avoid include the skin of the nipples and genital area. Instead, one should apply pain to the big toenail, the knuckles or nails of the fingers, the sternum, or the supraorbital ridge. When stimulating the last area, one should take care to not damage the eye itself (Table 28–3).

More information about nervous system functioning may be obtained by gathering data about the patient's ability to integrate attention, memory, and thought processes. Such a mental status examination also may uncover clues about the presence of additional problems affecting the patient's lifestyle (Table 28–4).

In gathering such a wealth of data, assessment of the patient's ability to communicate becomes paramount. Language use requires comprehension of verbal and nonverbal symbols, as well as the ability to use those symbols to communicate with others. Evaluation of the patient's understanding normally is accomplished through the spoken word. Speech dysfunctions may make such evaluations exceedingly difficult (Table 28–5).

Movement, Strength, and Coordination

Muscle weakness is a cardinal sign of dysfunction in many neurologic disorders. The nurse can test strength of extremities by offering resistance to various muscle groups, by using the nurse's own muscles or by using gravity. As a quick test to detect weakness of the upper extremities, the nurse can have the patient hold the arms straight out with palms upward, with eyes closed. Observe for any drift downward or pronation of the forearms. A similar test for the lower extremities includes having the patient raise the legs straight off the bed against the examiner's resistance. Weakness noted in any of these tests may indicate damage to the motor neuron pathways of the pyramidal system, which transmits commands for voluntary movement (Table 28–6).

Hemiparesis (weakness) and hemiplegia (paralysis) is unilateral dysfunction that results from a lesion contralateral to the corticospinal tract. Paraplegia may result from bilateral spinal cord or peripheral nerve dysfunctions. Quadriplegia is associated with bilateral spinal cord lesions, brain stem dysfunction, and with large bilateral lesions in the cerebrum.

Assessment of size, muscle tone, and smoothness of passive movement also should be made for each extremity. Dysfunctions noted here may indicate problems in the basal ganglia (also called the extrapyramidal system). These pathways normally suppress involuntary movements through controlled inhibition. Assessment findings may include the "clasp-knife" phenomenon, in which initially strong resistance to passive movement suddenly decreases.

TABLE 28–3
A Stimulus-Reaction Level Scale

Level	Description
1	Alert; no delay in response.
2	Drowsy but responsive to gentle stimulation. Confused about either name, place, or time.
3	Very drowsy; responds to strong stimulation with orienting eye movements, obeying commands or localizing, and actively attempting to remove stimulus.
4	Unconscious. Localizes but not successful in removing stimulus.
5	Unconscious. Withdrawal movements to any stimulation.
6	Unconscious. Stereotypical flexion movements to pain.
7	Unconscious. Stereotypical extension movements to pain.
8	Unconscious. No response to pain stimulation.

Alternatively, "lead-pipe" rigidity may be present, which is steady, continuous resistance to passive movement and is characteristic of diffuse hemispheric damage.

The nurse also should be alert for the presence of involuntary movements, from mild fasciculation to the violent, flailing movement of an extremity (Table 28–7).

The cerebellum is responsible for smooth synchronization, balance, and ordering of movements. It does *not* initiate any movements, so a patient with cerebellar dysfunction is not paralyzed. Instead, ataxia, dysmetria, and lack of synchronization of movement are common manifestations.

Some of the more common tests for cerebellar synchronization of movement with balance include the following:

- *Romberg test*—performed by having the patient stand with feet together, first with eyes open, then with eyes closed. Observe for sway or direction of falling and be prepared to catch the patient if necessary.
- *Finger to nose test*—performed by having the patient touch one finger to the examiner's finger, then touch own nose. Overshooting or past-pointing the mark is called *dysmetria*. Both sides are tested individually.
- *Rapidly alternating movement (RAM)*—checked on each side by having the patient oppose each finger and thumb in rapid succession or by performing rapid pronation and supination of the hand on the leg. Inability to perform RAM is termed *adiadokokinesia*.

Assessment of movement and strength in a patient who cannot follow commands or is unresponsive can be difficult. For such a patient it is important to note what, if any, stimuli initiate a response and to describe or grade the type of response obtained.

Motor response in the comatose person may be appropriate, inappropriate, or absent (Fig. 28–1). Appropriate responses, such as localization or withdrawal, mean that the sensory pathways and corticospinal pathways are functioning (see Figure 28–1A, B). There may be monoplegia or hemiplegia, indicating that the corticospinal pathways are interrupted on one side.

Inappropriate responses include decorticate rigidity and decerebrate rigidity. *Decorticate* rigidity results from lesions of the internal capsule, basal ganglia, thalamus, or cerebral hemisphere that interrupt corticospinal pathways. It is characterized by flexion of the arms, wrists, and fingers, by adduction of the upper extremities, and by extension, internal rotation, and plantar flexion of the lower extremities (see Figure 28–1C).

Decerebrate rigidity consists of extension, adduction,

TABLE 28–4
Format for Mental Status Examination

Attention
Digit span forward and backward

Remembering
Short-term: recall of three items after 5 min
Long-term: recall of mother's maiden name, recall of breakfast menu, events of previous day, etc.

Feeling (affective)
Observe for facial, body expression of mood
Verbal description of affect
Congruence of verbal, body indicators of mood

Language
Content and quantity of spontaneous speech
Naming common objects, parts of objects
Repetition of phrases
Ability to read and explain short passage in newspaper, magazine
Ability to write to dictation, spontaneously

Thinking
Fund of information (example: current president, preceding three)
Knowledge of current events
Orientation to person, place, time (tested as part of arousal, see consciousness)
Calculation: add two numbers, subtract 7 from 100
Problem-solving: What would you do if you found a stamped envelope on the street? What would you do if you smelled smoke in a theater?

Spatial Perception
Copy drawings: square, cross, three-dimensional cube
Draw clock face, map of room
Point out right and left side of self
Demonstrate: putting on a coat, blowing out match, using a toothbrush

(Mitchell PH, Cammermeyer M, et al: Neurological Assessment for Nursing Practice, p 35. Reston, VA, Reston Publishing Co., 1984)

TABLE 28–5
Patterns of Speech Deficits

Type	Deficit Location	Speech Patterns
Fluent dysphasia	Left parietal–temporal lobes (Wernicke's area)	• Fluent speech that lacks coherent content • Impaired understanding of spoken word in spite of normal hearing • May have normal-sounding speech rhythm but no intelligible words • May use invented meaningless words (neologism) or word substitution (paraphasia), or repetition of words (perseveration, echolalia)
Nonfluent dysphasia	Left frontal area (Broca's area)	• Slow speech with poor articulation • Inability to initiate sounds • Comprehension usually intact • Usually associated with impaired writing skills
Global dysphasia	Diffuse involvement of frontal, partietal, and occipital areas	• Nonfluent speech • Inability to understand spoken or written words
Dysarthria	Corticobulbar tracts; cerebellum	• Loss of articulation, phonation • Loss of control of muscles of lips, tongue, palate • Slurred, jerky, or irregular speech but with appropriate content

and hyperpronation of the upper extremities and extension of the lower extremities, with plantar flexion of the feet (see Figure 28–1D). Many times, the person also is opisthotonic, with clenched teeth. Injury to the midbrain and pons results in decerebration. At times, the inappropriate responses of decortication and decerebration may switch back and forth. If there is no response to noxious stimuli or very weak flexor responses, the person probably has extensive brain stem dysfunction (see Figure 28–1E).

Reflexes

A reflex occurs when a sensory stimulus evokes a motor response. Cerebral control and consciousness are not re-

TABLE 28–6
A Grading Scale for Muscle Strength

0 = No muscle contraction
1 = Flicker or trace of contraction
2 = Moves but cannot overcome gravity
3 = Moves against gravity but cannot overcome resistance of examiner's muscles
4 = Moves with some weakness against resistance of examiner's muscles
5 = Normal power and strength

TABLE 28–7
Types of Involuntary Movements

Tremor	Purposeless movement
Resting	Lesion in basal ganglia
Intention	Lesion in cerebellum
Asterixis	Metabolic derangement
Physiologic	Due to fatigue or stress
Fasciculation	Twitching of resting muscles; due to peripheral nerve or spinal cord lesion or to metabolic influences such as cold or anesthetic agents.
Clonus	Repetitive movement; elicited with stretch reflex and implies lesion of the corticospinal tracts.
Myoclonus	Nonrhythmic movement; single jerk-like movements, symmetrical, unknown etiology
Hemiballismus	Flailing movement of extremity; violent movement; not present during sleep; lesion in subthalamic nuclei of basal ganglia
Chorea	Irregular movements; involves limbs and facial muscles; asymmetric movements at rest; involuntary movements may increase when purposeful movement attempted
Athetosis	Slow, writhing movements

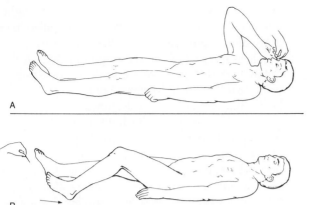

(A) Localizing pain. An appropriate response is to reach up above shoulder level toward the stimulus. Remember, a focal motor deficit such as hemiplegia may prevent a bilateral response.

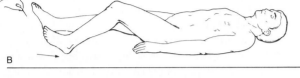

(B) Withdrawal. An appropriate response is to pull the extremity or body away from the stimulus. As brain stem involvement increases, your patient may respond by assuming one of the following postures. Each one shows more advanced deterioration.

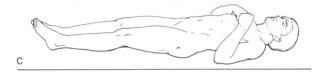

(C) Decorticate posturing. One or both arms in full flexion on the chest. Legs may be stiffly extended.

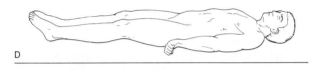

(D) Decerebrate posturing. One or both arms stiffly extended. Possible extension of the legs.

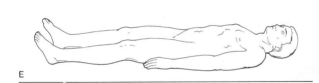

(E) Flaccid. No motor response in any extremity. An extremely ominous sign.

FIGURE 28–1
Motor responses to pain. When a painful stimulus is applied to an unconscious patient's supraorbital notch, the response will be in one of these ways.

quired for a reflex to occur. Superficial and deep reflexes are tested on symmetrical sides of the body and compared by reference to the strength of contraction elicited.

Muscle stretch reflexes, also called deep tendon reflexes, are elicited by a brisk tap with a reflex hammer. The target for this sensory stimulus is a stretched tendon of a muscle group. The desired motor response is contraction of the muscle group that was stimulated. Deep tendon reflexes commonly are graded on a scale of 0 to 4, where grade 2 is indicative of normal response (Table 28–8).

Cutaneous or superficial reflexes occur when certain areas of skin are lightly stroked or tapped, causing contraction of the muscle groups beneath. Such reflexes are graded simply as normal, abnormal (pathologic), or absent. An example is the plantar reflex. The sensory stimulus is applied by briskly stroking the outer edge of the sole and across the ball of the foot with a dull object such as a tongue blade or key. The normal motor response is down-

ward or plantar flexion of the toes. An abnormal response (Babinski's sign) is upward or dorsiflexion of the big toe, with or without fanning of the other toes.

A "shorthand" method of documentation of reflex responses is to draw a stick figure with grades or direction of responses indicated (Fig. 28–2).

TABLE 28–8
Deep or Muscle Stretch Reflex Grades

4+—Very brisk response; evidence of disease and/or electrolyte imbalance; associated with clonus
3+—A brisk response, possibly indicative of disease
2+—A normal, average response
1+—A response in low-normal range
0 —No response; possibly evidence of disease or electrolyte imbalance

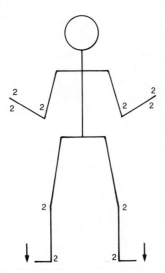

FIGURE 28–2
Documentation of selected deep and cutaneous reflexes. Reflexes shown here at major muscle stretch reflex sites are normal and symmetrical.

Pupillary Changes

Pupils should be examined for their size (best specified in millimeters) and shape. Have the patient focus on a distant point in the room. The examiner should place the edge of one hand along the patient's nose. Direct a bright light into one eye and note the briskness of pupillary constriction (direct response). Note that the other pupil also should constrict (consensual response). Repeat the procedure with the other eye. *Aniscoria* (unequal pupils) may be normal in a small percentage of the population or may be an indication of neural dysfunction.

To test accommodation, hold an object 8 to 12 inches in front of the patient's face. Have the patient focus on the object as the examiner moves it in toward the patient's nose. The pupils should constrict as the object gets closer and the eyes turn inward to maintain a clear image. The normal response to testing may be documented as PERRLA, or pupils equal, round, reactive to light, and accommodation.

Some important pupillary abnormalities are shown in Figure 28–3. Causes of small reactive pupils include metabolic abnormalities and bilateral dysfunction in the diencephalon. Large, fixed pupils (5–6 mm) that may show slight rhythmic constriction and dilation when stimulated may indicate midbrain damage. Midposition-fixed pupils (4–5 mm) also may indicate midbrain dysfunction, with both sympathetic and parasympathetic pathways interrupted. Pinpoint, nonreactive pupils are seen after damage to the pons area of the brain stem, with selected eye medications, and with opiate administration. A unilaterally dilated, nonreactive ("blown") pupil will be seen with

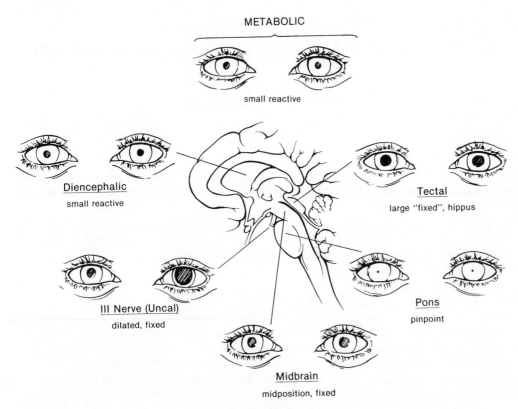

FIGURE 28–3
Abnormal pupils (Adapted from Plum F, Posner, J: The Diagnosis of Stupor and Coma, 3rd ed. Philadelphia, FA Davis).

TABLE 28–9
Quick Guide to Causes of Pupil Size Changes

Pinpoint pupils
  Drugs: opiates
  Drops: medications for glaucoma
  "Nearly dead": damage in the pons area of the brain stem

Dilated pupils
  Fear: panic attack, extreme anxiety
  "Fits": seizures
  "Fast living": cocaine, crack, phencyclidine (PCP) use

third cranial (oculomotor) nerve damage when the uncal portion of the temporal lobe herniates through the small opening in the tentorium. When structures are compressed around the opening in the tentorium or fold of dura that separates the cerebrum from the cerebellum and brain stem, loss of functioning of the parasympathetic nerves to the pupil on that side results in an ipsilaterally dilated pupil (Table 28–9).

Vital Signs

Classic signs of *increased intracranial pressure* include an elevated systolic pressure in conjunction with a widening pulse pressure, slow bounding pulse, and respiratory irregularities.

After any emergency treatment that may be indicated (eg, maintenance of the airway for adequate ventilation), vital signs should be taken immediately and followed frequently. Any indication of shock should alert the nurse to search for signs of thoracic and intra-abdominal injuries. It must be remembered that vital signs are only signs, and are not infallible in determining the patient's neurologic status (Fig. 28–4).

Hypoventilation after cerebral trauma can lead to respiratory acidosis. As the blood carbon dioxide increases and blood oxygen decreases, cerebral hypoxia and edema can result in secondary brain trauma. *Hyperventilation* after cerebral trauma produces respiratory alkalosis with increased blood oxygen and decreased blood carbon dioxide levels. This causes vasoconstriction of cerebral vessels and decreases oxygen consumption, resulting in cerebral hypoxia.

Because temperature elevation increases cellular metabolism, measures should be implemented to maintain temperature in the normal range, or hypothermia may be induced if indicated.

Cranial Nerves

I. Olfactory. The first cranial nerve contains sensory fibers for the sense of smell. This test usually is deferred unless the patient complains of an inability to smell. One tests the nerve, with the patient's eyes closed, by placing

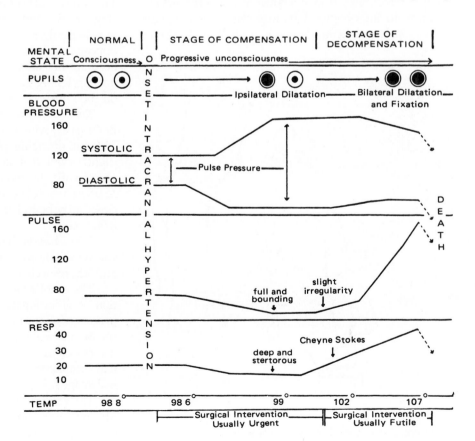

FIGURE 28–4
Vital sign changes during IICP. Chart showing changes in mental state, pupils, blood pressure, pulse rate, respiratory rate, and temperature before and after the onset of fatal IICP.

aromatic substances near the nose for identification. Fragrances that have a distinct smell (eg, soap, coffee, or cinnamon) should be used. Ammonia should not be used because the patient will respond to irritation of the nasal mucosa rather than the odor. Each nostril is checked separately. Loss of smell may be caused by a fracture of the cribriform plate or a fracture in the ethmoid area.

The patient also may have anosomia (loss of sense of smell) from a shearing injury to the olfactory bulb after a basilar skull fracture or from cerebrospinal fluid (CSF) rhinorrhea.

II. Optic. Gross visual acuity is checked by having the patient read ordinary newsprint. The patient's preinjury need for glasses should be noted. Visual field can be tested by having the patient look straight ahead with one eye covered. The examiner will move a finger from the periphery of each quadrant of vision toward the patient's center of vision. The patient should indicate when the examiner's finger is seen. This is done for both eyes, and the results are compared to the examiner's visual fields, which are assumed to be normal (Fig. 28–5). Damage to the retina will produce a blind spot. An optic nerve lesion will produce partial or complete blindness on the same side. Damage to the optic chiasm results in bitemporal hemianopsia, blindness in both lateral visual fields. Pressure on the optic tract can cause homonymous hemianopsia, half blindness on the opposite side of the lesion in both eyes. A lesion in the parietal or temporal lobe may produce contralateral blindness in the upper or lower quadrant of vision, respectively, in both eyes (this is known as *quadrant deficit*). Damage in the occipital lobe may cause homonymous hemianopsia with central vision sparing (Fig. 28–6).

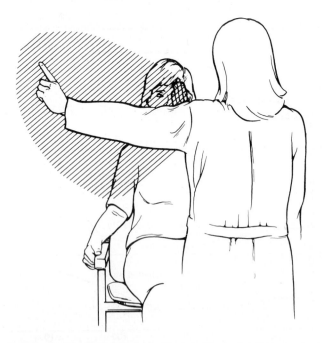

FIGURE 28–5
Confrontational method of testing visual fields.

III. Oculomotor; IV. Trochlear; VI. Abducens. These cranial nerves are checked together because they all innervate extraocular muscles. The parasympathetic fibers of the oculomotor nerve are responsible for lens accommodation and pupil size through control of the ciliary muscles. The motor fibers of the oculomotor nerve innervate the muscles that elevate the eyelid as well as those that move the eyes up, down, and medially. These include the superior rectus, inferior oblique, inferior rectus, and medial rectus muscles. The trochlear nerve innervates the superior oblique muscle to move the eyes down and in. The lateral rectus muscle moves the eyes laterally and is innervated by the abducens nerve. Diplopia, nystagmus, conjugate deviation, and ptosis may indicate dysfunction of these cranial nerves. These nerves are tested by having the patient follow the examiner's finger as it is moved in all directions of gaze (Fig. 28–7).

V. Trigeminal. The trigeminal nerve has three divisions: ophthalmic, maxillary, and mandibular. The sensory portion of this nerve controls sensation to the face and cornea. The motor portion controls the muscles of mastication. This nerve is partially tested by checking the corneal reflex; if it is intact, the patient will blink when the cornea is stroked with a wisp of cotton. Facial sensation can be tested by comparing light touch and pinprick on symmetrical sides of the face. The ability to chew or clench the jaw also should be observed.

VII. Facial. The sensory portion of this nerve is concerned with taste on the anterior two thirds of the tongue. The motor portion controls muscles of facial expression (Fig. 28–8). With a central (supranuclear) lesion, there is muscle paralysis of the lower half of the face on the side opposite the lesion. The muscles about the eyes and forehead are not affected. In a peripheral (nuclear or infranuclear) lesion, there is complete paralysis of facial muscles on the same side as the lesion.

The most common type of peripheral facial paralysis is Bell's palsy, which consists of ipsilateral facial paralysis. There is drooping of the upper lid with the lower lid slightly everted. Facial lines on the same side are obliterated with the mouth drawn toward the normal side. Artificial tears or ophthalmic ointment and taping the eye closed may be indicated to prevent corneal abrasion and irritation.

VIII. Acoustic. This nerve is divided into the cochlear and vestibular branches, which control hearing and equilibrium, respectively.

The cochlear nerve is tested by air and bone conduction. A vibrating tuning fork is placed on the mastoid process; after the patient can no longer hear the fork, he or she should be able to hear it for a few seconds longer when it is placed in front of the ear (Rinne's test). The patient may complain of tinnitus or decreased hearing if this nerve is damaged.

The vestibular nerve may not be evaluated routinely. The nurse should be alert, however, to complaints of dizziness or vertigo from the patient.

VISUAL FIELD DEFICITS AND NEUROANATOMIC CORRELATES

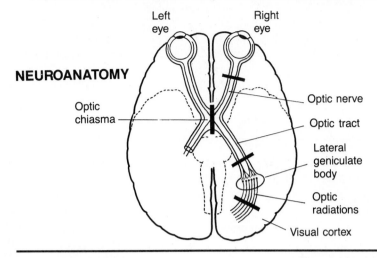

NEUROANATOMY

Left eye

Right eye

Optic nerve

Optic chiasma

Optic tract

Lateral geniculate body

Optic radiations

Visual cortex

FIELD DEFECTS

DESCRIPTION

Anopsia: blindness in one eye; due to complete lesion of the right optic nerve, as in trauma.

Bitemporal hemianopsia: also called central vision; due to lesions around the optic chiasm such as pituitary tumors or aneurysms of the anterior communicating artery.

Left homonymous hemianopsia: half-vision involving both eyes with loss of visual field on the same side of each eye; due to lesion of right temporal or occipital lobes with damage to the right optic tract or optic radiations.

Left eye

Right eye

FIGURE 28–6
Visual field defects associated with lesions of the visual system.

IX. Glossopharyngeal; X. Vagus. These cranial nerves usually are tested together. The glossopharyngeal nerve supplies sensory fibers to the posterior third of the tongue as well as the uvula and soft palate. The vagus innervates the larynx, pharynx, and soft palate and conveys autonomic responses to the heart, stomach, lungs, and small intestines. Autonomic vagal functions usually are not tested because they are checked during the general physical examination. These nerves can be tested by eliciting a gag reflex, observing the uvula for symmetrical movement when the patient says "ah," or observing midline elevation of the uvula when both sides are stroked. Inability to

cough forcefully, difficulty with swallowing, and hoarseness may be signs of dysfunction.

XI. Spinal Accessory. This nerve controls the trapezius and sternocleidomastoid muscles. The examiner tests this nerve by having the patient shrug the shoulders or turn the head from side to side against resistance.

XII. Hypoglossal. This nerve controls tongue movement. It can be checked by having the patient protrude the tongue. Check for deviation from midline, tremor, and atrophy. If deviation is noted secondary to damage of the nerve, it will be to the side of the lesion.

Testing cranial nerve function completely is time-

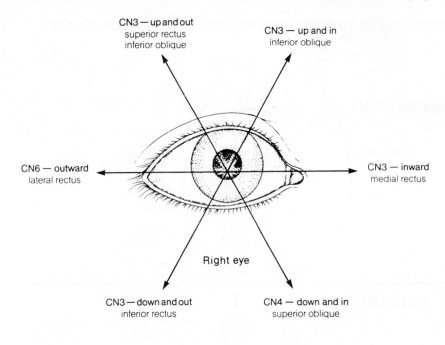

CN3 — up and out
superior rectus
inferior oblique

CN3 — up and in
inferior oblique

CN6 — outward
lateral rectus

CN3 — inward
medial rectus

Right eye

CN3 — down and out
inferior rectus

CN4 — down and in
superior oblique

FIGURE 28-7
Muscles used in conjugate eye movements in the six cardinal directions of gaze (Adapted from Bates B: A Guide to Physical Examination, 3rd ed, p 59. Philadelphia, JB Lippincott, 1983).

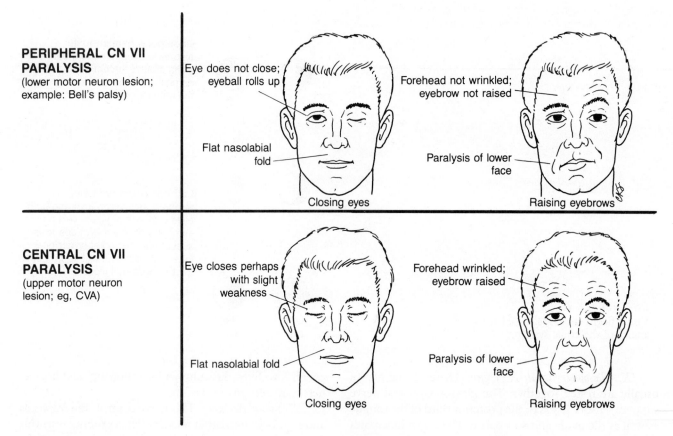

PERIPHERAL CN VII PARALYSIS
(lower motor neuron lesion; example: Bell's palsy)

Eye does not close; eyeball rolls up

Forehead not wrinkled; eyebrow not raised

Flat nasolabial fold

Paralysis of lower face

Closing eyes

Raising eyebrows

CENTRAL CN VII PARALYSIS
(upper motor neuron lesion; eg, CVA)

Eye closes perhaps with slight weakness

Forehead wrinkled; eyebrow raised

Flat nasolabial fold

Paralysis of lower face

Closing eyes

Raising eyebrows

FIGURE 28-8
Facial movements with upper and lower motor neuron facial paralysis (Adapted from Bates B: A Guide to Physical Examination, 5th ed, pp 550–551. Philadelphia, JB Lippincott, 1991).

TABLE 28–10
A Quick Screening Test for Cranial Nerve Function

	Nerve	Reflex	Procedure
II III	Optic Oculomotor	Pupil constriction (protection of the retina)	Shine a light into each eye and note if the pupil on that side constricts (direct response). Next, shine a light into each eye and note if the opposite pupil constricts (consensual response).
V VII	Trigeminal Facial	Corneal reflex (protection of the cornea)	Approaching the eye from the side and avoiding the eyelashes, touch the cornea with a wisp of cotton. Alternatively, a drop of sterile water or normal saline may be used. A blink response should be present.
IX X	Glossopharyngeal Vagus	Airway protection	Touch the back of the throat with a tongue depressor. A gag or cough response should be present.

consuming and exacting. A partial and quicker screening assessment may be performed, focusing on those nerves where dysfunction may indicate serious problems or interfere with activities of daily living. The cranial nerves of primary importance in a screening examination are the optic (CN II) and oculomotor (CN III), trigeminal (CN V) and facial (CN VII), and glossopharyngeal (CN IX) and vagus (CN X) (Table 28–10).

Ocular Signs in the Unconscious Patient

Ocular position and movement are among the most useful guides to the site of brain dysfunction in the comatose person. When observing the eyes at rest, it is not uncommon to note a slight divergence of gaze. If both eyes are conjugately deviated to one side, there is possible dysfunction either in the frontal lobe on that side or in the contralateral pontine area of the brain stem. Downward deviation suggests a dysfunction in the midbrain.

"Doll's Eyes" and Caloric Reflex

Although the unconscious patient cannot participate in the examination by moving the eyes through fields of gaze voluntarily, the examiner still can test the range of ocular movement using the oculocephalic ("doll's eyes") and oculovestibular (caloric) reflexes.

The oculocephalic reflex can be assessed by quickly rotating the patient's head to one side and observing the position of the eyes (Fig. 28–9). This maneuver must *never* be performed in a person with possible cervical spine injury. A normal response consists of initial conjugate deviation of the eyes in the opposite direction, then, within a few seconds, smooth and simultaneous movement of both eyes back to midline position.

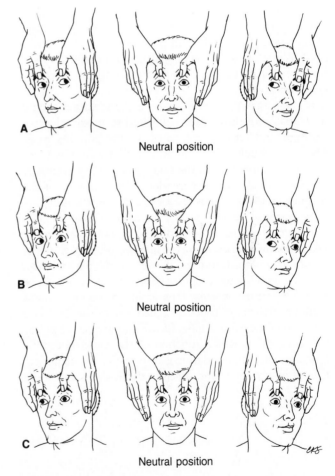

A Neutral position

B Neutral position

C Neutral position

FIGURE 28–9
Test for oculocephalic reflex response (doll's eyes phenomenon). (**A**) Normal response—when the head is rotated, the eyes turn together to the side opposite to the head movement. (**B**) Abnormal response—when the head is rotated, the eyes do not turn in a conjugate manner. (**C**) Absent response—as head position is changed, eyes do not move in the sockets.

An abnormal reflex response occurs when one eye does not follow the normal response pattern. Absence of any ocular movement when the head is rotated briskly to either side or up and down indicates an absent reflex and portends severe brain stem dysfunction.

The examiner tests oculovestibular reflex (caloric test) by elevating the patient's head 30° and irrigating each ear separately with 30 to 50 ml of iced water (Fig. 28–10). This test never should be performed in a patient who does not have an intact eardrum or who has blood or fluid collected behind it. In an unconscious patient with an intact brain stem, the eyes will exhibit horizontal nystagmus with slow, conjugate movement toward the irrigated ear followed by rapid movement away from the stimulus. When the reflex is absent, both eyes remain fixed in midline position, indicating midbrain and pons dysfunction.

Sensation

The primary forms of sensation are tested first. These include perception of touch (cotton wisp), pain (pin prick), temperature (hot, cold), and proprioception (limb position). With the patient's eyes closed, multiple and symmetrical areas of the body are tested, including the trunk and extremities.

The patient's ability to perceive the sensation should be noted, with distal areas compared to proximal areas, and right and left sides compared at corresponding areas. The nurse should determine whether sensory change involves one entire side of the body. Abnormal results may indicate damage somewhere along the pathways of the receptors in the skin, muscles, joints and tendons, spinothalamic tracts, or sensory area of the cortex (Table 28–11).

Cortical forms of sensation also should be tested. Disturbances of these forms, when the primary forms of sensation are intact, indicate damage to the parietal lobe.

The inability to recognize objects by sight, touch, or sound is termed *agnosia*. The ability to recognize and identify objects by touch is called *stereognosis* and is a function of the parietal lobe. Identification of an object by the sense of sight is a function of the parieto-occipital junction. The temporal lobe is responsible for identification of objects by sound. Each of these senses should be tested separately. For example, a patient may not be able to identify a whistle by its sound but may recognize it immediately if he or she holds it or looks at it.

Other cortical forms of sensation include the following:

- *Graphesthesia*—the ability to recognize numbers or letters traced lightly on the skin. Bilateral sides are compared.
- *Point localization*—the ability to locate the precise spot on the body touched by the examiner. One version of dysfunction in this area is called *extinction phenomenon*, the inability to recognize bilateral sensations when the examiner simultaneously touches two symmetrical areas on opposite sides of the body.
- *Two-point discrimination*—tested by using two sharp objects and determining the smallest area in which two points can be perceived.
- *Texture discrimination*—the ability to recognize materials such as cotton, burlap, and wool by feeling them.

Other Observations

- *Battle's sign*—bruising over the mastoid areas, suggests basal skull fracture.
- *Raccoon's eye*—periorbital edema and bruising, suggests frontobasilar fracture.
- *Rhinorrhea*—drainage of CSF from the nose suggests fracture of the cribriform plate with herniation of a fragment of the dura and arachnoid through the fracture.
- *Otorrhea*—drainage of CSF from the ear usually is associated with fracture of the petrous portion of the temporal bone.
- *Meningeal irritation*—can be detected by the presence of nuchal rigidity in conjunction with fever, headache, and photophobia. A positive Kernig's sign, pain in the neck when the thigh is flexed on the abdomen and the leg extended at the knee, also may be present. Brudzinski's sign, involuntary flexion of the hips when the neck is flexed toward the chest, is another indication of meningeal inflammation (Fig. 28–11).

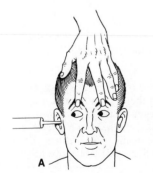
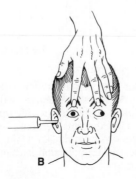
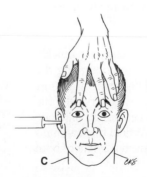

FIGURE 28–10
Test for oculovestibular reflex response (caloric ice-water test). (**A**) Normal response—ice water infusion in the ear produces conjugate eye movements. (**B**) Abnormal response—infusion produces dysconjugate or asymmetric eye movements. (**C**) Absent response—infusion produces no eye movements.

TABLE 28-11
Testing Superficial and Deep Sensations

Sensation	Stimuli	Dysfunction
Spinothalamic tracts carry impulses for		
Pain	Alternate sharp and dull ends of a pin, asking patient to discriminate between the two (superficial pain). Squeeze nail beds, apply pressure on the orbital rim, rub sternum (deep pain).	• Ipsilateral sensory loss implies a peripheral nerve lesion. • Contralateral sensory loss is seen with lesions of the spinothalamic tract or in the thalamus.
Light touch	Use a wisp of cotton on skin and ask patient to identify when it touches.	• Bilateral sensory loss may indicate a spinal cord lesion. • Paresthesia is an abnormal sensation such as itching or tingling.
Temperature	Use test tubes filled with hot and cold water or use small metal plates of varying temperatures. (Test only if pain and light touch sensations are abnormal.)	• Causalgia is a burning sensation that can be caused by peripheral nerve irritation.
Posterior columns carry impulses for		
Vibration	Apply a vibrating tuning fork on bony prominences and note patient's ability to sense and locate vibrations bilaterally.	• Ipsilateral sensory loss may be due to spinal cord injury or to peripheral neuropathy.
Proprioception	Move the patient's finger or toe up and down and ask patient to identify final resting position.	• Contralateral loss may occur from lesions of the thalamus or of the parietal lobes.

Evaluation of Dysfunction in Patient's Living Patterns

Neurologic nursing assessment would be incomplete if the process consisted solely of gathering data and identifying abnormal functions. Nursing expertise should expand the scope to include an evaluation of the impact of dysfunction on the patient's living patterns and ability to care for self. For example, diplopia (double vision) is an abnormal finding and may be an indicator of problems with the ocular muscles or with the nervous system. But it also may be a clue suggesting difficulty in carrying out daily activities.

Neurodiagnostic Tests and Normal Values

A considerable number of diagnostic tests are now available to assist in the diagnosis of neurologic and neurosurgical problems. Such neurodiagnostic testing is performed in conjunction with a thorough neurologic examination. The ease of availability and the diagnostic accuracy of current technology benefits the patient in an acute setting by shortening the time required to arrive at a diagnosis and institute therapy. The choice of which investigative test to perform should be based on the examiner's ability to integrate the findings with neurologic assessment and locate the cause of the abnormality.

The nurse's role in neurodiagnostic testing involves patient and family preparation and monitoring the critical patient during and after the procedure for potential complications. Although there has been a definite increase in the number of tests that can be performed at the bedside, there still are many that require the patient to be transported to the imaging department or even out of the institution, further expanding the role of the critical care nurse. Table 28-12 summarizes some of the diagnostic tests and outlines nursing implications.

Neuroradiologic Techniques

Plain x-rays of the skull and spine are used frequently to identify fractures, dislocations, and other bony anomalies, especially in the setting of acute trauma. In addition, plain

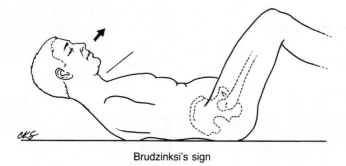

Brudzinksi's sign

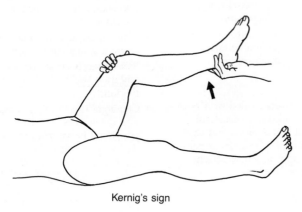

Kernig's sign

FIGURE 28-11
Two signs of meningeal irritation.

x-rays may be diagnostic when displacement of the calcified pineal gland is visible, which is an immediate clue to the presence of a space-occupying lesion. The presence of air inside the skull also allows diagnosis of an open skull fracture, such as a frontal or basilar skull fracture, that may not be readily apparent externally. Plain x-rays of the skull also may demonstrate infection or neoplasm manifested by changes in the bone density or other intracranial calcification.

The procedure for plain films of the skull and spine requires careful patient positioning and is relatively painless. The nurse's role involves monitoring the patient and attendant equipment during the procedure and being alert for complications related to patient position and the length of the procedure.

Computed Axial Tomography

Computed tomographic (CT) scanning has been in use in the United States since 1973. It permits more refined measurement of the density of tissues, blood, and bone within the body. The value of this technique is illustrated best in the trauma setting, where the ability rapidly and accurately to image the intracranial contents and position of vertebrae and spinal cord has dramatically changed the treatment of neurologic patients. Computed tomographic scanning can detect reliably such conditions as skull frac-

tures, tissue swelling, hematomas, and tumors and abscesses. The use of radiographic contrast material allows better visualization of vascular areas and enhances lesions previously seen on noncontrast films. Sometimes, two technologies are used in combination, such as myelography with CT scanning, to provide a more refined image of anatomic structures of the spinal cord and vertebral column. With current technology, a routine scan now takes less than 5 minutes to survey the patient, analyze the data, and display a finished image.

Magnetic Resonance Imaging

Magnetic resonance imaging (MRI), known in the past as nuclear magnetic resonance (NMR) imaging, has become widely available in medium and large medical centers. This modality uses nonionizing forms of radiation to produce computerized cross-sectional images in much the same fashion as a CT scan. It provides much more finely detailed images, however, that look remarkably like anatomic slices of the body. The MRI is superior to CT in the early diagnosis of cerebral infarction and in the detection of demyelinating disorders such as multiple sclerosis. Traditional CT scanning is superior at scanning for bony abnormalities, which visualize poorly on MRI.

Magnetic resonance imaging, although superior in many ways to CT scanning, has its limitations. The powerful magnetic fields interfere with the functioning of devices such as cardiac pacemakers. Patients with surgical clips and prosthetic implants made of ferrous metal cannot be scanned. It also is difficult to study patients on life-support equipment because most ventilators and monitors are constructed in part of ferrous metal. If emergency therapy is needed, the patient must be removed from both the scanning chamber and the imaging suite before resuscitation can begin.

Positron Emission Tomography and Single-Photon Emission Computed Tomography

Positron emission tomography is a process by which molecules labeled with radioactive isotopes are located within the brain and recorded by radiation-sensitive detectors outside the head. It has the capacity to measure cerebral blood flow and cerebral metabolism, as the isotope-labeled glucose or oxygen is used within the body. It is superior to previous technologies that could image structure only, and not function. But the complexity of the testing, the cost of nearly $5,000 per scan, as well as the need to have a cyclotron nearby to produce the short-lived radioactive isotopes, makes this modality impractical and unwieldy in the clinical setting.

(*Text continues on page 668*)

TABLE 28–12
Neurodiagnostic Tests

Diagnostic Test	What It Is	What It Tells You	Nursing Implications
A. Computed axial tomography, or CT scan (invasive and noninvasive)	A larger scanner takes a series of radiographic images all around the same axial plane. A computer than creates a composite picture of various tissue densities visualized. The images may be enhanced with the use of IV contrast dye.	CT scans give detailed outlines of bone, tissue, and fluid structures of the body. They can indicate shift of structures due to tumors, hematomas, or hydrocephalus. A CT scan is limited in that it gives information only about structure of tissues, not about functional status.	Instruct the patient to lie flat on a table with the machine surrounding, but not touching, the area to be scanned. Patient also must remain as immobile as possible; sedation may be required. The scan may not be of the best quality if the patient moves during the test or if the x-ray beams were deflected by any metal object in or around the patient (ie, traction tongs, ICP monitoring devices).
B. Magnetic resonance imaging (MRI)	A selected area of the patient's body is placed inside a powerful magnetic field. The hydrogen atoms inside the patient are temporarily "excited" and caused to oscillate by a sequence of radiofrequency pulsations. The sensitive scanner measures these minute oscillations, and a computer-enhanced image is created.	An MRI scan creates a graphic image of bone, fluid, and soft tissue structures. It gives a more defined image of anatomic details and may help one diagnose small tumors or early infarction syndromes.	Risk factors for this new technique are not well identified. This test is contraindicated in patients with previous surgeries where hemostatic or aneurysm clips were implanted. The powerful magnetic field can cause such clips to move out of position, placing the patient at risk for bleeding or hemorrhage. Inform patient the procedure is very noisy. Use caution if patient is claustrophobic. Other contraindications include patients with: cardiac pacemakers, valve prosthesis, bullet fragments, orthopedic pins. The patient (and any caregivers in the room) must remove all metal objects with magnetic characteristics (eg, scissors, stethoscope).
C. Positron Emission Tomography (PET); Single-Photon Emission Computer Tomography (SPECT)	The patient either inhales or receives by injection radioactively tagged substances such as oxygen or glucose. A gamma scanner measures the radioactive uptake of these substances, and a computer produces a composite image, indicating where the radioactive material is located, corresponding to areas of cellular metabolism.	These diagnostic tests are the only ones to measure physiological and biochemical processes in the nervous system. Specific areas can be identified as to functioning and nonfunctioning. Cerebral metabolism and cerebral blood flow can be measured regionally. PET and SPECT scans help diagnose abnormalities (tumors, vascular disease), and also behavioral disturbances such as dementia and schizophrenia that may have a physiological basis.	The patient receives only minimal radiation exposure because the half-life of the radionuclides used is from a few minutes to 2 hr. Testing may take a few hours. The patient must remain very still and immobile. Procedure is very expensive.

(continued)

TABLE 28–12
Neurodiagnostic Tests (*Continued*)

Diagnostic Test	What It Is	What It Tells You	Nursing Implications
D. Cerebral angiography (invasive)	This is a radiographic contrast study in which radiopaque dye is injected by a catheter into the patient's cerebral arterial circulation. The contrast medium is directed into each common carotid artery and each vertebral artery and serial radiographs are then taken.	The contrast dye illuminates the structure of the cerebral circulation. The vessel pathways are examined for patency, narrowing, and occlusion as well as structural abnormalities (aneurysms), vessel displacement (tumors, edema), and alterations in blood flow (tumors, AV malformations)	In preparation for this test, inform the patient as to the location of the catheter insertion (femoral artery is a common site) and that a local anesthetic will be used. Also warn that a warm, flushed feeling will occur when the dye is injected. After this procedure, assess the puncture site for swelling, redness, and bleeding. Also check the skin color, temperature, and peripheral pulses of the extremity distal to the site for signs of arterial insufficiency due to vasospasm or clotting. A large amount of contrast medium may be needed during this test, with resulting increased osmotic diuresis and risk of dehydration and renal tubular occlusion. Other complications include: temporary or permanent neurologic deficit, anaphylaxis, bleeding or hematoma at insertion site, and impaired circulation to the extremity used for injection.
E. Digital subtraction angiography (invasive)	In this test, a plain radiograph is taken of the patient's cranium. Then, radioopaque dye is injected into a large vein and serial radiographs are taken. A computer converts the images into digital form and "subtracts" the plain radiograph from the ones with the dye. The result is an enhanced radiographic image of contrast medium in the arterial vessels.	Extracranial circulation (arterial, capillary, and venous) can be examined. Vessel size, patency, narrowing, and degree of stenosis or displacement can be determined.	There is less risk to the patient for bleeding or vascular insufficiency because the injection of dye is intravenous rather than intraarterial. The patient must remain absolutely motionless during the examination (even swallowing will interfere with the results).
F. Myelography (invasive)	A myelogram is a radiographic study in which a contrast substance (either air or dye) is injected into the lumbar subarachnoid space. Fluoroscopy, conventional radiographs, or CT scans are used to visualize selected areas.	The spinal subarachnoid space is examined for partial or complete obstructions due to bone displacements, spinal cord compression, or herniated intervertebral discs.	Instruct the patient as for a lumbar puncture. In addition, advise that a special table will tilt up or down during the procedure. Postprocedure care is determined by the type of contrast material used.

(*continued*)

TABLE 28–12
Neurodiagnostic Tests (*Continued*)

Diagnostic Test	What It Is	What It Tells You	Nursing Implications
			Oil-based contrast dye: • flat in bed for 24 hr • force fluids • observe for headache, fever, back spasms, nausea and vomiting Water-based contrast dye: • head of bed elevated for 8 hr • keep patient quiet for first few hours • do not administer phenothiazines • observe for headache, fever, back spasms, nausea and vomiting, seizures
G. Electroencephalogram, or EEG (noninvasive)	An EEG is a recording of electrical impulses generated by the brain cortex that are sensed by electrodes on the surface of the scalp.	Analysis of the resulting tracings helps detect and localize abnormal electrical activity occurring in the cerebral cortex. It aids in seizure focus detection, localization of a source of irritation such as a tumor or abscess, and in the diagnosis of metabolic disturbances and sleep disorders.	Reassure the patient that he or she will not feel an electrical shock or pain during this test. The nurse also may need to clarify for the patient that the machine cannot "read minds" or indicate the presence of mental illness. The patient's scalp and hair should be free of oil, dirt, creams, and sprays because they can cause electrical interference and thus an inaccurate recording. Inform the EEG technician of electrical devices around the patient that may act as a source of interference during the procedure (eg, cardiac monitor, ventilator).
H. Cortical evoked potentials (noninvasive)	In this test, a specialized device senses central or cortical cerebral electrical activity by skin electrodes in response to peripheral stimulation of specific sensory receptors. The sensory receptors stimulated can be those for vision, hearing, or tactile sensation. The signals are graphically displayed by a computer, and characteristic peaks, and the intervals between them, are measured.	Cortical evoked potentials provide a detailed assessment of neuron transmission along particular pathways. It has value in determining the integrity of visual auditory and tactile pathways in patients with multiple sclerosis and spinal cord injury. This test also may be used in the assessment of a sensory pathway before, during, and after surgery.	This test may be used in conscious as well as unconscious patients and can be performed at the bedside. The patient must be as motionless as possible during some phases of this test to minimize musculoskeletal interference. Depending on the sensory pathway being tested, the patient may be instructed to watch a series of geometric designs or listen to a series of clicking noises.

(*continued*)

TABLE 28–12
Neurodiagnostic Tests (*Continued*)

Diagnostic Test	What It Is	What It Tells You	Nursing Implications
I. Transcranial Doppler sonography (TCD)	This is a test in which high-frequency ultrasonic waves are directed from a probe toward specific cerebral vessels. The ultrasonic energy is aimed through cranial "windows," areas in the skull where the bony table is thin (temporal zygoma) or where there are small gaps in the bone (orbit or foramen magnum). The reflected sound waves are analyzed for shifts in frequency, indicating flow velocity.	The speed or velocity at which blood travels through cerebral vessels is an indicator of the size of the vascular channel and the resistance to blood flow. An approximation of cerebral blood flow may be determined. Cerebral autoregulation can be monitored by observing the response of intracranial vessels to changes in arterial carbon dioxide and to the partial occlusion of the proximal vessels, as may occur in vasospasm.	The test is noninvasive and may be performed at the bedside by the physician or ultrasound technician in 30–60 min. There are no known adverse effects and the procedure may be repeated as often as necessary. The testing is accomplished with the patient initially supine, and later on his or her side, with the head flexed forward.
J. Lumbar puncture (invasive)	A hollow needle is positioned in the subarachnoid space at L3–4 or L4–5 level, and CSF is sampled. The pressure of the CSF also is measured. Normal pressure varies with age from 45 mm water in full-term newborns to 120 mm water in adults.	The CSF is examined for blood and for alterations in appearance, cell count, protein, and glucose. The opening pressure is roughly equivalent to the ICP for most patients, if done recumbent and no block is present.	This test is contraindicated in patients with suspected increased ICP because a sudden reduction in pressure from below may cause brain structures to herniate, leading to death. In preparation for this test, position the patient on side with knees and head flexed. Explain to the patient that some pressure may be felt as the needle is inserted and not to move suddenly or cough. After this procedure, keep the patient flat for 8 to 10 hours to prevent headache. Encourage liberal fluid intake.

ICP, intracranial pressure; IV intravenous; AV, atrioventricular.

The development of single-photon emission computed tomography (SPECT) combines the imaging ability of conventional nuclear medicine scanners with the technology of transaxial CT scanning to overcome some of those limitations. Using more stable radioisotopes, SPECT scanning has been able to detect diminished perfusion in an area of stroke before conventional CT evidence of infarction, as well as alterations in regional blood flow in patients with Alzheimer's disease.

Angiography and Digital Subtraction Angiography

Cerebral angiography remains the study of choice for evaluating cerebrovascular problems. It is the only test that can demonstrate large and small aneurysms and arteriovenous malformations and their relationship to adjacent structures and vessels. It involves the passage of a radiographic catheter via a large artery (usually femoral) to each of the arterial vessels bringing blood to the brain and spinal cord. Radiopaque contrast dye is then injected into each vessel in turn and a rapid sequence of films is taken, following the passage of the dye through small arterial branches, capillaries, and into the venous circulation.

Digital subtraction angiography makes use of radiographic contrast to illuminate the cerebral circulation, but in considerably smaller quantities than required for conventional angiography. The dye may be injected into either the arterial or the venous systems. Films are taken both before and after the dye injection and converted into digital information in the accompanying computer. The images are "subtracted" from each other, removing all images in common. The resultant image displays only the enhanced circulatory system, free of other anatomic distortion.

Myelography

Myelography is a contrast study of the spinal cord and surrounding structures. It involves the introduction of water-soluble material (metrizamide) into the CSF by way of a lumbar or cisternal puncture, performed under fluoroscopy. Because metrizamide is lighter than CSF, it allows for better visualization of nerve roots and surrounding structures. But because of its rapid dispersal into the subarachnoid space, the patient's position cannot be adjusted. At times, a heavier, oil-based preparation is used (Pantopaque; Alcon Surgical, Fort Worth, TX) that must be removed at the end of the procedure. Because metrizamide does not require removal, the patient should be kept well hydrated to facilitate dye excretion. It also is potentially toxic to cerebral tissue, as evidenced by grand mal seizures, so the patient must be maintained with the head up at least 30° to 45°, and phenothiazine medications, which increase the toxic symptoms, must be avoided.

Electrophysiological Studies

Electroencephalogram

Using electroencephalographs (EEG), a record is made of the brain's electrical activity. Small plate electrodes are placed in specific locations over the patient's scalp and 16 to 21 channels transcribe the electrical potentials generated by the brain. Waveforms are classified in terms of voltage and amplitude. It is most valuable in the diagnosis and treatment of patients with seizures. In addition, it may help in the localization of structural abnormalities such as tumors and abscesses, and aid in the differentiation of structural from metabolic abnormalities. It also may provide confirmatory criteria in the diagnosis of brain death. In recent years, a modified form of EEG is being used more at the bedside in critical care to monitor the effects of pharmacologic agents that reduce cerebral blood flow, and hence reduce electrical activity.

A computerized technique that dramatically compresses standard EEG data and converts them into a more easily interpreted and colorized form is called "compressed spectral array." This technique also is seen at the bedside in neurologic critical care units to monitor patients with severe head injuries.

Evoked Potentials

An evoked potential is an electrical manifestation of the brain's response to an external stimulus, be it auditory, visual, somatic, or a combination of these.[1] The measurement of the response evoked by a certain sensory stimulus provides an assessment of the function of neuropathways from the periphery through the spinal cord, brain stem, and finally to cortical structures (Fig. 28–12). This technique has been most helpful in the diagnosis of multiple sclerosis, Guillain–Barré syndrome, and in the prognosis of the reversibility of coma in the brain stem-injured patient.[2] It also may be used during surgery to monitor potential injury during manipulations of spinal nerves and structures.

Transcranial Doppler Sonography

Transcranial Doppler ultrasound studies provide a noninvasive means for monitoring intracranial hemodynamics at the bedside.[3] The examination is performed through cranial "windows," areas in the skull where the bone is relatively thin, such as the temporal area, or where there are small spaces between bones, such as the orbit (Fig. 28–13). The ultrasonic probe transmits sound waves at certain frequencies to a specified depth. The resultant reflected signal from blood traveling through cerebral vessels is interpreted for speed or velocity. As resistance or vascular size changes, it is reflected as a change in blood flow velocities. The data may be used to monitor therapy, aid in determining prognosis, and provide early recognition of cerebral vasospasm in patients after subarachnoid hemorrhage or severe head injury.

Lumbar Puncture/Cerebrospinal Fluid Examination

A lumbar puncture for CSF analysis may be performed to aid in the diagnosis of autoimmune disorders or infections. Occasionally, it is performed to verify subarachnoid hemorrhage, although the CT scan is the procedure of choice and is safer for such a patient. Cerebrospinal fluid is obtained by the insertion of a long, 18- to 22-gauge needle between the vertebrae at the L3–4 or L4–5 levels. The fluid is sent for content analysis as well as culture, sensitivity, and other serologic tests (Table 28–13).

Persistent Vegetative State

Vegetative state is a term used to describe a chronic condition that sometimes is the consequence of severe brain injury. It is characterized by a period of sleeplike coma followed by a return to the awake state but with a total lack of apparent cognition.[4] In persistent vegetative state, the higher cortical functions of the cerebral hemispheres have been damaged permanently, but the lower functions of the brain stem remain intact. The patient's eyes may open spontaneously, seemingly in response to verbal stimuli. Sleep–wake cycles exist. The patient maintains normal blood pressure and respiratory control. Also seen are involuntary lip-smacking, chewing, and roving eye movements.

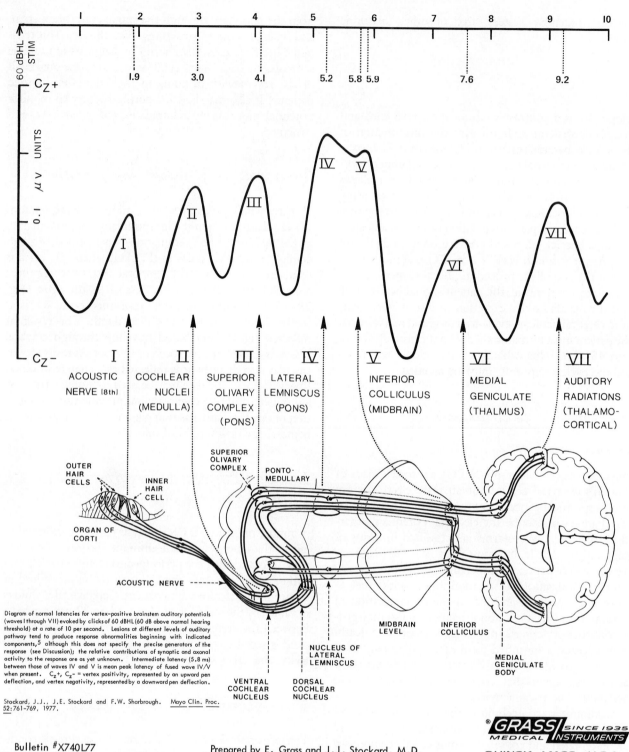

FIGURE 28–12
The waveform of a normal brain-stem auditory evoked response (Courtesy of Grass Instrument Company, Quincy, MA).

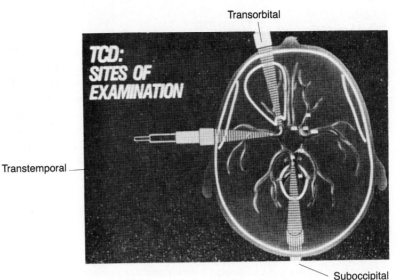

FIGURE 28–13
Transcranial Doppler: sites of examination via transcranial windows (Adapted from March K: Transcranial Doppler sonography: Non-invasive monitoring of intracranial vasculature. Journal of Neuroscience Nursing 22:113, 1990).

The issue of "chronic comatose-like" states first came to national attention in the early 1970s with the case of Karen Ann Quinlan, whose parents finally won a protracted legal battle to remove ventilatory support from their daughter. Even after the removal, Ms. Quinlan survived for several more years in a persistent vegetative state. More recently, the case of Nancy Cruzan was the first "right-to-die" case to be decided by the United States Supreme Court. In that landmark decision, the Court ruled that Ms. Cruzan's legal guardian, her father, had the right to request withdrawal of nutrition and hydration from his permanently brain-injured daughter, in accordance with "clear and convincing evidence" of her wishes.[5]

Caring for the patient in a persistent vegetative state

TABLE 28–13
Normal and Abnormal Values for Cerebrospinal Fluid

Characteristic	Normal	Abnormal
Color	Clear, colorless	Cloudy often due to presence of WBC or bacteria
		Xanthochromic due to presence of RBC
WBC	0–5/mm³, all mononuclear	Elevated count accompanies many conditions (tumor, meningitis, subarachnoid hemorrhage, infarct, abscess)
RBC	None	Presence may be due to traumatic tap or subarachnoid hemorrhage (SAH)
Chloride	120–130 mEq/L	Low concentration associated with meningeal infection and tuberculous meningitis
		Elevated level not neurologically significant
Glucose	50–75 mg/100 ml	Decreased level associated with presence of bacteria in CSF
		Elevated level not neurologically significant
Pressure	70–180 mm H₂O	Low pressure associated with inaccurate placement of needle, dehydration, or block along subarachnoid space or at foramen magnum
		Elevated pressure associated with benign intracranial hypertension; cerebral edema; CNS tumor, abscess or cyst; hydrocephalus; muscle tension or abdominal compression; subdural hematoma (SDH)
Protein	14–45 mg/100 ml	Decreased level not neurologically significant
		Increased level associated with demyelinating or degenerative disease, Guillain–Barré syndrome, hemorrhage, infection, spinal block, tumor

WBC, white blood cells; RBC, red blood cells; CSF, cerebrospinal fluid; CNS, central nervous system.
(From Cammermeyer M, Appeldorn C (eds): Core Curriculum for Neuroscience Nursing, 3rd ed, p. Vc7. Chicago, American Association of Neuroscience Nurses, 1990)

TABLE 28–14
Possible Clinical Criteria for Determining Brain Death

Nature of the Comatose State Must Be Determined

- Drugs must be excluded as a possible cause of the coma.
- The patient may not be hypothermic (ie, body temperature must exceed 33°C, or 91.4°F).
- There must be an appropriate period of observation of patient in comatose state for adequate assessment.

Absence of all Cortical/Brain Stem Function Must Be Established

- Absence of all cerebral responses to light, noise, motion, and pain.
- Absence of all reflexes or muscle activity unless the reflex activity is determined to be of spinal cord origin.
- Absence of spontaneous respirations with respirator disconnected for at least 3 min, with a PCO_2 of at least 55 mm Hg to stimulate respiratory response. Some institutions do not advocate arterial blood gases and do not recommend complete apnea for 3 min for fear of causing more neuronal death if viable brain function remains. In such institutions, high levels of oxygen are administered passively through endotracheal or tracheostomy tubes for rather prolonged periods without respiration for confirmation of apnea.
- Absence of cranial nerve reflexes: fixed pupils that do not react to light and absence of oculovestibular reflex (caloric ice test response).

In addition, other tests may be required, for example:

- Isoelectric electroencephalogram (EEG). Some institutions require only one isoelectric EEG; others require two, 12 hr apart.
- Absence of intracranial blood flow, as demonstrated by angiography, radioisotope techniques, echo pulsation, or computed tomography scan after administration of contrast medium.

(From Rudy ER: Brain death. Dimensions of Critical Care Nursing 1:183)

can be a physical and emotional challenge. Dealing with alternating cycles of hope and grief on the part of family and friends can be emotionally battering. The critical care nurse should use all available resources of pastoral care, social service, and various assistance programs to work through thoughts and feelings. Everyone involved in the care of such patients should have a realistic understanding of the prognosis of persistent vegetative state.

Brain Death

The patient's condition may be so severe that brain death is the final outcome (Table 28–14). The critical care nurse provides essential nursing care to such a patient as treatment is continued or as life-support measures are withdrawn. The nurse is involved in determining whether the patient has suffered brain death.

Many years ago, the common acceptable understanding of death was "total stoppage of the circulation of the blood and a cessation of vital functions such as respiration, pulsation, etc." In the 1960s, the advent of cardiopulmonary resuscitation measures made this criterion of death obsolete. In 1968, a landmark report was published by the Ad Hoc Committee of the Harvard Medical School to Examine the Definition of Death. This established the first widely accepted criteria to determine brain death. Finally, in 1979, the American Medical Association House of Delegates passed a model bill on the following definition of death:

An individual who has sustained either (a) irreversible cessation of circulatory and respiratory functions, or (b) irreversible cessation of all functions of the entire brain, should be considered dead. A determination of death shall be made in accordance with accepted medical standards.[6]

The first legal statute recognizing the concept of brain death was enacted in Kansas in the early 1970s. Since then, all states have passed similar statutes. The adoption of clinical criteria to determine brain death has been facilitated by larger medical centers and by institutions actively involved in organ transplant surgery.[7]

The role of the nurse who is caring for a potentially brain-dead patient is threefold:

- Question the possibility of brain death
- Assist in gathering data necessary to determine brain death
- Provide support, understanding, and empathy for the patient's family

These tasks become even more difficult for the critical care nurse. It often is very hard to "switch gears" from fighting for a person's life one day to accepting death the next day.

REFERENCES

1. Marshall SB, Marshall LF, et al: Neuroscience Critical Care. Philadelphia, WB Saunders, 1990
2. Barelli A, Valenti MR, et al: Serial multimodality evoked potentials in severely head injured patients: Diagnostic and prognostic implications. Crit Care Med 19:1374–1381, 1991
3. March K: Transcranial Doppler sonography: Non-invasive monitoring of intracranial vasculature. Journal of Neuroscience Nursing 22:113–116, 1990
4. Council on Scientific Affairs and Council on Ethical and Judicial Affairs: Persistent vegetative state and the decision to withdraw or withhold life support. JAMA 263:426, 1990
5. Lo B, Rouse F, Dornbrand L: Family decision making. N Engl J Med 322:1228–1232, 1990
6. American Medical Association: Model Bill. Chicago: American Medical Association, 1979
7. Younger SJ, Landenfeld S, Coulton CJ, et al: "Brain death" and organ retrieval. JAMA 262:2205, 1989

BIBLIOGRAPHY

Bates B: A Guide to Physical Examination and History Taking, 5th ed. Philadelphia, JB Lippincott, 1990
Cammermeyer M, Appledorn C (eds): Core Curriculum for Neuroscience Nursing, 3rd ed. Chicago, American Association of Neuroscience Nurses, 1990
Dimitrijevic MR, Hsu CY, McKay WB: Neurophysiological assessment of spinal cord and head injury. Journal of Neurotrauma 9(Suppl 1):S293–S300, 1992
Ditunno JF Jr: Functional assessment measures in CNS trauma. Journal of Neurotrauma 9(Suppl 1):S301–S305, 1992
Hilton G: Review of neurobehavioral assessment tools. Heart Lung 20(5 Pt 1):436–442, 1991
Weiner WJ: Emergent and Urgent Neurology. Philadelphia, JB Lippincott, 1992

STUDY QUESTIONS

1. The goals of nursing assessment of a patient with a neurologic problem include all of the following except

   a. to gather data about nervous system functioning in an orderly and objective fashion
   b. to correlate data over time
   c. to determine the effects of dysfunction on the patient's ability to care for self
   d. to develop one's own grading scale and terminology so there is individual nurse consistency

2. A patient whose movements are purposeful when stimulated but does not follow commands would be described as

   a. semicomatose
   b. stuporous
   c. comatose
   d. lethargic

3. All of the following may cause dilated pupils except

   a. fear
   b. seizure
   c. morphine
   d. cocaine

4. Approaching the eye from the side and touching the cornea to elicit a blink reflex tests which of the cranial nerves?

   a. optic
   b. facial
   c. oculomotor
   d. trigeminal

5. The most common cause for bitemporal hemianopsia is

   a. pyramidal tract damage
   b. pituitary tumor pressing on the optic chiasm
   c. lesion in the medulla
   d. bilateral dysfunction in the diencephalon

6. Tremor and deviation of the tongue indicate damage to cranial nerve

   a. X
   b. XI
   c. XII
   d. IX

CHAPTER 29

Management Modalities: Nervous System

(continued)

Hudak: Critical Care Nursing:
A Holistic Approach, 6th ed. © 1994
J. B. Lippincott Company.

BEHAVIORAL OBJECTIVES

Based on the content in this section, the reader should be able to:

1. Identify four indications for intracranial pressure (ICP) monitoring.
2. List four techniques for obtaining ICP measurements.
3. Define cerebral perfusion pressure.
4. Describe three interventions used to promote adequate cerebral blood flow in the presence of increased intracranial pressure (IICP).
5. List three possible nursing diagnoses for the patient with IICP and describe the nursing interventions for each diagnosis.

Description

Intracranial pressure (ICP) is the pressure exerted by the combined volume of the three intracranial components: brain tissue, cerebrospinal fluid (CSF), and blood. A normal ICP measurement varies between 0 and 15 mm Hg. Increased intracranial pressure (IICP, intracranial hypertension) is a serious complication that may result in herniation with respiratory and cardiac arrest and death. An ICP measurement greater than 15 mm Hg is considered IICP. Cerebral perfusion pressure (CPP) is an estimate of the adequacy of the cerebral circulation to deliver oxygen to brain tissue. A normal CPP is at least 60 mm Hg, with a range of 60 to 130 mm Hg. Intracranial pressure monitoring provides information that facilitates interventions to prevent cerebral ischemia and brain stem distortion.

Intracranial pressure monitoring used in conjunction with other invasive and noninvasive assessment techniques, such as magnetic resonance imaging, computed tomog-

raphy (CT) scanning, positron emission tomography, single-photon emission computed tomography, evoked potentials, and cerebral oximetry (Fig. 29–1) has aided significantly in the diagnosis, treatment, and prognosis of patients with a potential for development of intracranial hypertension.

Intracranial pressure measurement usually provides an indication of changes in ICP dynamics before such changes are clinically evident, facilitating the initiation of measures to reduce IICP.

The classic syndrome of IICP, which includes increased pulse pressure, decreased pulse, and decreased respirations with pupillary changes, usually occurs only in association with posterior fossa lesions and seldom with the more commonly observed supratentorial mass lesions, such as subdural hematoma. When these classic Kocker–Cushing signs do accompany a supratentorial lesion, they are associated with a sudden pressure increase and usually herald a state of decompensation. Brain damage usually is irreversible at this point, and death is imminent.

Between the onset of IICP and herniation is a stage in which a wide variety of treatments are available to reduce ICP. Therapies used to normalize ICP and maintain adequate cerebral perfusion include the use of hyperventilation to reduce intracerebral blood volume; CSF drainage to reduce intracerebral CSF volume; various pharmacologic agents to induce diuresis, sedation, or paralysis; and surgery.

Physiological Principles

Intracranial Dynamics

The Monro–Kellie hypothesis states that the volume of the intracranium is equal to the volume of the brain (80%–85% of intracranial contents) plus the volume of the cerebral blood (3%–10%) plus the volume of the CSF (8%–12%). Any alterations in the volume of any of these

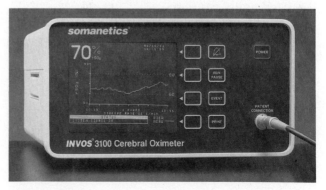

FIGURE 29–1
Cerebral oximeter for continuous noninvasive monitoring of cerebral oxygen (Courtesy of Somanetics Corporation, Troy, MI).

components of the cranial vault, as well as the addition of a lesion, may lead to an increase in ICP.

The normal brain has the ability to autoregulate cerebral blood flow (CBF), one of the three components affecting ICP. Normally, autoregulation ensures a constant blood flow through the cerebral vessels over a range of perfusion pressures by changing the diameter of vessels in response to changes in CPP. Factors that alter the ability of the cerebral vessels to constrict or dilate, such as ischemia, hypoxia, hypercapnia, and brain trauma, interfere with autoregulation. Carbon dioxide is the most potent vasodilator of cerebral vessels, causing increased CBF that can result in an increased volume within the cranium, leading to IICP. For autoregulation to be functional, carbon dioxide levels must be in an acceptable range and pressures within the following ranges: (1) CPP over 60 mm Hg, (2) a mean arterial pressure under 160 mm Hg and systolic pressure between 60 to 160 mm Hg, and (3) ICP under 30 mm Hg. Brain injury also may impair autoregulation. When autoregulation is impaired, the CBF fluctuates in correlation with the systemic blood pressure. In patients with impaired autoregulation, any activity that causes an increase in blood pressure, such as coughing, suctioning, and anxiety, can cause an increase in CBF that could increase ICP.

The brain can accommodate or compensate for minimal changes in volume by partial collapse of the cisterns, ventricles, and vascular systems, as well as decreasing production and increasing reabsorption of CSF (Display Box 29–1). During this compensatory period, the ICP remains fairly constant. When these compensatory mechanisms have been used fully, pressure increases rapidly until herniation occurs, and the blood supply to the medulla is cut off (Fig. 29–2). The ability of the intracranial contents to compensate depends on the location of the lesion, the rate of expansion, and the compliance or volume-buffering capacity of the system.

Volume–Pressure Curve

The intracranial volume–pressure curve, also referred to as a pressure–volume index, demonstrates the relationship between changes in volume and changes in intracranial

---

DISPLAY BOX 29–1
ICP Compensatory Mechanisms

• Shunting of CSF into the spinal subarachnoid space
• Increased CSF absorption
• Decreased CSF production
• Shunting of venous blood out of the skull

---

pressure. It may indicate the compressibility of the cerebrovascular system, providing an indication of the stiffness of vessel walls and intravascular pressure. The initial portion of the curve illustrates compliance, as the compensatory mechanisms maintain ICP in the normal range during increases in intracranial volume. Little change occurs in the ICP during the initial increase in volume, because the increase in volume added to the cranium is compensated for by volume displacement (Fig. 29–3A). As the compensatory mechanisms become exhausted, the volume added becomes greater than the volume displaced and there is a larger increase in ICP with a smaller volume increase. This is illustrated by the steeper portion of the curve (see Figure 29–3B). This disproportionate rise in pressure represents elastance, the opposite of compliance. In other words, high elastance is the same as low compliance and indicates that small changes in intracranial volume will cause large changes in ICP. The cranial contents become stiffer, and free communication of CSF between the lateral ventricles and infratentorium is lost. Drastic increases in ICP may result from hypercarbia, hypoxia, rapid eye movement sleep, pyrexia, or the administration of certain anesthetics. A major reason for controlling and decreasing ICP is the maintenance of cerebral oxygenation by adequate CBF, which is estimated clinically by the measurement of CPP.

Cerebral Perfusion Pressure

Normal CBF is provided by a CPP greater than 60 mm Hg. Below this level, blood supply to the brain is inadequate and neuronal hypoxia and cell death may occur. When perfusion pressure decreases, the cardiovascular response is a rise in systemic pressure. The autoregulation system for maintenance of constant blood flow does not function at pressures less than 40 mm Hg. A severe reduction in CPP is accompanied by an absence of brain stem auditory evoked potentials, indicating changes in brain stem function. Increased ICP leads to ischemia, brain shifts, and possible herniation (Fig. 29–4).

When brain damage is severe, as with widespread brain edema or when blood flow has been arrested in the brain, CBF may be reduced at relatively normal levels of CPP. This is due to impedance to the flow of blood across the cerebrovascular bed. Cerebral blood flow may not increase despite increases in CPP if autoregulation is impaired. This condition is referred to as *pressure–flow dissociation* or *vasomotor paralysis*.

CPP is determined by subtracting the mean ICP from the mean systemic arterial pressure (MAP):

$$CPP = MAP - ICP.$$

When the CPP is zero, there is no CBF. In other words, when ICP equals MAP, CPP equals zero and CBF is zero. Cerebral blood flow may cease totally at pressures somewhat above zero.

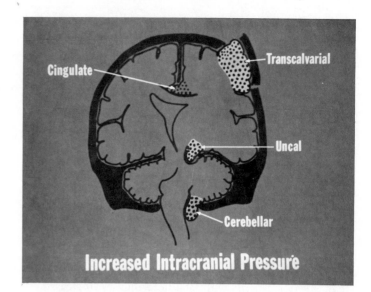

Increased Intracranial Pressure

FIGURE 29–2
The major types of cerebral herniation are (1) herniation of the cingulate gyrus under the falx; (2) herniation of the uncus of the temporal lobe beneath the free edge of the tentorium; (3) downward displacement of the midbrain through the tentorial notch; and (4) sometimes, with an open head injury, transcalvarial herniation.

Equipment Features

The proven value of ICP monitoring and the need for an accurate, reliable, and simple method of measurement has resulted in the development of numerous methods of monitoring ICP and a variety of devices to facilitate each method or technique. Intracranial pressure monitoring equipment may be categorized as internal or external measurement systems. The initial ICP monitoring systems consisted of an external pressure transducer (the same type used for systemic arterial blood pressure measurement) attached by a fluid-filled system of tubing and stopcocks to an intraventricular catheter, subarachnoid bolt, or epidural catheter device, with ICP waveforms and pressure displayed on a standard bedside monitor. These fluid-coupled external systems continue to be used widely. A variety of disposable ICP kits are available for placement of various ICP monitoring devices.

Internal measurement systems now are available that measure ICP directly from the site. Fiberoptic transducer-tipped catheters are inserted directly into the brain tissue, ventricles, or subdural–subarachnoid spaces, with the ICP waveforms and pressures displayed on a dedicated amplifier system. They eliminate the need for a fluid-filled system between the patient and the transducer. Both external and internal measurements systems are discussed in more detail in the discussion of ICP procedures that follows.

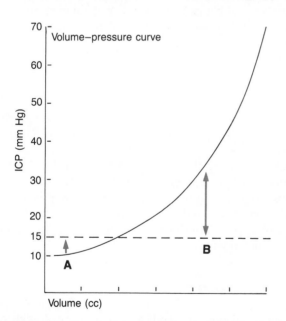

FIGURE 29–3
Volume–pressure curve. Volume–pressure response (VPR), also referred to as the pressure–volume index (PVI), provides a method of estimating the compensatory capacity of the intracranial cavity. Note that the ICP remains within the normal limit of 0–15 mm Hg as long as compliance is normal and fluid can be displaced by the additional volume (*a*). Once the compensatory system is exhausted, a small additional volume causes a greater increase in pressure (*b*). Acute changes can cause serious and sometimes fatal neurological deterioration.

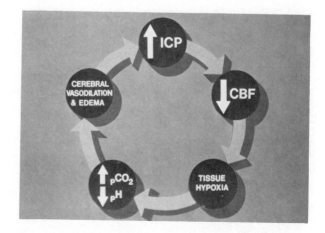

FIGURE 29–4
Cycle for malignant progressive brain swelling. As the ICP increases, CBF decreases, leading to tissue hypoxia, a decrease in pH, an increase in PCO_2, cerebral vasodilation, and edema, thus leading to further pressure increases. This malignant cycle continues until herniation occurs.

Indications for Intracranial Pressure Monitoring

Conditions that may be indications for ICP measurement include head injury, subarachnoid hemorrhage, brain tumors, cardiac arrest, strokes, surgery, and others (Display Box 29–2).

Head Injury

Intracranial hypertension develops almost universally in patients in whom intracranial mass lesions develop after head injury. Uncontrollable elevation of ICP is the cause of death in approximately half the fatally injured patients. Ischemic brain damage has been documented in more than 90% of patients with fatal head injuries. Increased morbidity is associated with patients exhibiting moderate elevations of ICP. Brain electrical dysfunction and disturbances of CBF frequently are associated with intracranial pressures greater than 40 mm Hg. Intracranial pressure monitoring has proven valuable in the detection of cerebral edema and hematoma formations. Various diagnostic studies, such as CT scans and cerebral angiography, differentiate between the two. Intracranial pressure monitoring also facilitates differentiation of brain stem dysfunction secondary to increases in ICP from primary brain stem injury, which is associated with a normal ICP.

DISPLAY BOX 29–2
Indications for ICP Monitoring

Increased Volume of Brain

Cerebral edema
Trauma
Surgery
Stroke
Tumor

Increased Volume of Blood

Hematomas
AV malformations
Aneurysm
Stroke
Increase in PCO_2

Increased Volume of CSF

Decreased CSF reabsorption
Congenital hydrocephalus

Lesions

Tumors
Abscesses

In addition, it has been recommended that continued monitoring be carried out for all patients with burr holes, patients who fail to regain consciousness within 48 hours after injury, and patients whose level of consciousness deteriorates, unless the patient has meningitis or a brain abscess.

Intracranial pressure monitoring may be indicated when head injury is associated with:

- inability to obey commands or utter recognizable words despite cardiopulmonary stabilization
- abnormal CT scan
- abnormal multimodality evoked potentials
- a Glasgow Coma Scale score of 9 or less

Patients with intracranial mass lesions after head injury often have early, severe intracranial hypertension; patients with acute subdural hematomas seem to be most prone to IICP; and patients who maintain ICPs of 45 to 60 mm Hg the first 48 hours after injury, despite all therapeutic intervention, have a mortality rate approaching 100%.

In patients with diffuse brain injury, any elevation above 10 mm Hg on admission results in a progressively worsening prognosis. The initial level of ICP is to some degree an indication of the extent of diffuse brain damage. Recurrent or persistent intracranial hypertension is more frequently a problem with intracerebral lesions, contusion, hematoma, and brain swelling than with discrete extracerebral hematomas, whether epidural or subdural. Recurrent or persistent intracranial hypertension is associated with a poorer outcome.

Subarachnoid Hemorrhage

The level of ICP correlates well with the clinical grade of the hemorrhage. The ICP is of value in determining the best time for surgery, predicting and detecting rebleeding, and determining the etiology of neurologic deterioration. Intracranial pressure monitoring facilitates the use of various drugs and other management techniques such as hyperventilation and continuous ventricular fluid drainage or a permanent shunt to compensate for CSF absorption impairment.

Brain Tumors

Intracranial pressure tends to remain normal, with episodic increases seen particularly at night. Elevations in ICP tend to occur when the mass has enlarged to the point at which the patient is demonstrating neurologic deterioration with papilledema, headache, and vomiting. Metastatic tumors can cause massive edema. Patients may be monitored before surgery to determine their response to the preoperative therapeutic regimen and to assist in determining the optimal time for surgery. After surgery, they may be monitored to assist with the diagnosis and treatment of diffuse generalized cerebral edema secondary to extensive manipulation of the brain during surgery.

Cardiac Arrest

Of long-term cardiac arrest survivors, 10% to 20% suffer permanent severe brain damage ranging from intellectual changes to vegetative states after global ischemic–anoxic insults. Intracranial pressure measurement has been of value in the development of new, specific neuron-saving therapies for "postresuscitation disease" to assist in the restoration of mentation.

Stroke

Increases in ICP are common with spontaneous intra-cerebral hemorrhage and routinely occur in comatose patients. In ischemic stroke, high ICP is likely after cerebral infarction has progressed to coma with midline brain shift. Intracranial pressure monitoring has been effective in the initiation and maintenance of therapeutic intervention. It also has provided valuable information for research on the mechanisms and amelioration of focal brain ischemia.

Surgery

During surgery, ICP monitoring provides assistance in determining the optimal position for the patient and the responses to various anesthetic agents and ventilatory support.

Contraindications

Systemic infection or a localized infection at the site of insertion of the ICP monitoring device may be considered contraindications to ICP monitoring.

Procedure

There are four basic techniques for measuring ICP: (1) intraventricular; (2) subarachnoid (subdural); (3) intra-parenchymal; and (4) epidural (extradural) (Fig. 29–5). All four methods require strict aseptic technique during insertion and maintenance.

The usual duration for ICP monitoring is 3 to 5 days. The diagnostic and therapeutic benefits of ICP monitoring far outweigh the minimal risk.

Intraventricular Technique

The intraventricular technique of ICP measurement was reported first in 1951 and remains the most frequently used method. It consists of placement of a catheter into the lateral ventricle. A twist drill hole or small burr hole is placed lateral to the midline at the level of the coronal suture, usually on the nondominant side. A ventriculostomy catheter is placed through the cerebrum into the anterior horn of the lateral ventricle. On occasion, the occipital horn is used. Connected to the ventricular catheter by a stopcock or pressure tubing is a pressure transducer. Sterile saline or Ringer's lactate solution is used to

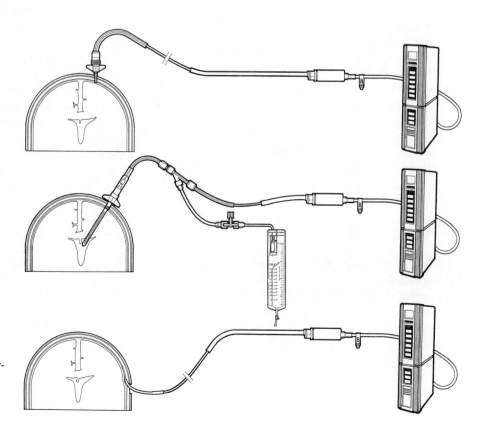

FIGURE 29–5
ICP monitoring systems. (1) Parenchymal; (2) ventricular ICP monitoring with ventriculostomy drainage; (3) subdural (Courtesy of Camino Laboratories, San Diego, CA).

provide the fluid column between the CSF and diaphragm of the transducer. A continuous-flush device is not used for ICP measurement.

The miniature transducer may be positioned directly on the patient's head. A standard-size transducer is mounted at the bedside, with the venting port positioned at the level of the foramen of Monro. External landmarks for this position are the edge of the brow or the tragus of the ear. For every 1 inch of discrepancy between the level of the transducer and the pressure source, there is an error of approximately 2 mm Hg.

A disposable fiberoptic transducer-tipped catheter may be used instead of an external transducer. This eliminates the need for the fluid-filled system required with external transducers. A Y-connector at the proximal end of the catheter facilitates attachment to the monitor and a CSF drainage system (see Figure 29–5).

The advantages and disadvantages of the intraventricular technique of ICP measurement are as follows.

Advantages

- Direct measurement of pressure from the CSF
- Access for CSF drainage or sampling
- Access for determining volume–pressure responses (VPRs)
- Access for instillation of drugs

Disadvantages

- Need to puncture the brain
- Difficulty in locating the lateral ventricle after midline shifting of the ventricle or collapse of the ventricle as a normal compensatory mechanism for increases in pressure
- Blockage of the catheter by fluid components or the ventricle wall
- Risks of intracranial hemorrhage and infection. During opening of the dura and puncturing of the ventricle there is a slight risk (less than 2%) of an intracranial hemorrhage. The risk of infection, related to the duration of monitoring and frequency of opening the system to the atmosphere, is reported between less than 1% up to 6%. An increased infection rate is associated with catheters in place for more than 5 days.

Subarachnoid Technique

The measurement of ICP by means of a subarachnoid screw or bolt was reported first in 1973. The screw device is inserted through a twist drill hole and extends into the subdural or subarachnoid space. Although the cerebrum is not penetrated, pressures, as with the intraventricular technique, are measured directly from the CSF. A transducer filled with saline or Ringer's lactate solution may be fastened directly to a stopcock on the screw or connected by pressure tubing. As with any technique for monitoring ICP, a continuous-flush device is contraindicated.

An alternate technique for monitoring subarachnoid pressure is the fiberoptic subarachnoid (subdural) catheter. The disposable fiberoptic transducer is introduced through a small subarachnoid–subdural bolt, with the catheter extending just beyond the tip of the bolt. Volume–pressure responses have been determined with these techniques. Subarachnoid pressures usually correlate well with intraventricular pressures.

The advantages and disadvantages of the subarachnoid technique are as follows.

Advantages

- Direct pressure measurement from CSF
- No need to penetrate cerebrum to locate ventricle
- Access for determining VPRs
- Access for CSF drainage and sampling
- Ease of insertion

Disadvantages

- Risk of complications comparable to those associated with intraventricular technique
- Need for closed skull
- Greater difficulty in VPR studies and with CSF drainage than with ventricular catheters
- Possible blockage of the measuring devices from high ICP
- Possible underestimation of ICP when it is elevated

Intraparenchymal Technique

The recent development of disposable fiberoptic transducer-tipped catheters and the improvement of catheter-tipped microtransducers has made intracerebral (intraparenchymal) pressure monitoring possible (see Figure 29–5).

The intraparenchymal technique provides a means of obtaining ICP recordings in patients with compressed and dislocated ventricles.

The catheter is inserted through a small subarachnoid bolt, and after puncture of the dura and coagulation of the arachnoid membranes, advanced several centimeters into the white matter of the brain. Brain tissue pressures correlate well with ventricular pressures.

The sensitivity and linearity of the fiberoptic transducer-tipped catheter are precalibrated. It is not necessary to balance the transducer after insertion. The mean ICP is displayed continuously on a portable monitor that interfaces with a standard monitoring system for oscilloscopic display and printout of ICP waveforms and values.

The advantages and disadvantages of the intraparenchymal technique are as follows.

Advantages

- Accurate—correlates well with ventricular pressures
- Ease of insertion
- No fluid- or air-filled system
- Eliminates effect of hydrostatic pressure on readings
- Minimizes artifact, leaks, drift, and infection

- No need to balance after insertion
- No calibration required
- No problem with transducer position

Disadvantages

- Catheter breakage with bending, tension, or rough manipulation
- No route for CSF drainage and sampling
- Inability to zero or calibrate after insertion
- Requires dedicated equipment

Epidural Technique

This technique involves placement of an epidural device such as a balloon with radionuclides, a radio transmitter, or a fiberoptic or pneumatic transducer between the skull and the dura. Some researchers believe that dural compression and surface tension, as well as thickening of the dura during prolonged monitoring, tend to cause inaccuracies in the pressure readings. Although subarachnoid and intraventricular pressures correlate well with each other, there have been inconsistent correlations between direct CSF pressure and pressure measurement using various epidural techniques.

The advantages and disadvantages of the epidural technique include:

Advantages

- Less invasive
- Usefulness of selected transducers for anterior fontanelle monitoring

Disadvantages

- Questionable reflection of CSF pressure; with high ICPs, epidural pressures may overread ventricular pressures considerably
- Slow response time; many systems are unable to pick up transient peaks caused by Valsalva maneuvers and respiratory changes
- No route for CSF drainage and sampling
- Infeasible VPRs
- Inability to zero and calibrate some systems after measurement is initiated
- Transducer placement. Transducer must touch but not indent the dura and must be parallel to, or coplanar with, the dura. If the dura is stretched, the pressure recording will be affected by dural compliance.

Telemetry Technique

Telemetry systems have been reported with both epidural and intraventricular devices. The two major uses of telemetry are reduction of the risk of infection and long-term monitoring. The latter is helpful in follow-up evaluation in long-term patients, such as those with hydrocephalus, some with metabolic encephalopathies, and those with brain tumors who are undergoing chemotherapy.

Interpretation of Results

Range

Intracranial pressure normally ranges between 0 and 10 mm Hg, with an upper limit of 15 mm Hg. During coughing or straining, a normal ICP may increase to 100 mm Hg. In acute situations, patients often become symptomatic at pressures ranging from 20 to 25 mm Hg.

The patient's tolerance of a change in ICP varies with the acuteness of its onset. Patients with a slower build-up of ICP, as occurs with certain brain tumors, are more tolerant of elevations in the ICP than patients in whom pressure changes rapidly, as seen in those with acute subdural hematoma. Uncontrolled ICP between 20 and 25 mm Hg is considered the "kiss of death" for the head-injured patient. Sustained intracranial hypertension greater than 60 mm Hg usually is fatal.

Intracranial pressure may rise to the level of the MAP. The greater the variations in the mean ICP, the more nearly exhausted are the compensatory mechanisms for intracranial volume increases.

Although protocols vary, measures to reduce ICP usually are initiated if the patient shows neurologic deterioration, such as a score of 7 or less on the Glasgow Coma Scale or an ICP of 15 mm Hg or greater.

Although ICP is monitored routinely as a mean pressure, systolic and diastolic pressures should be noted. Because there is a linear relationship between pulse pressure and ICP, pulse pressure may be used to estimate intracranial elastance, particularly in the patient with cerebral vasoparalysis.

For patients with head injury, the mortality rate is between 22% and 57%. Remaining comatose with an elevation of ICP within 72 hours of injury combined with a Glasgow Coma Scale score of less than 9, and older age, appear to be major factors associated with a poor outcome. In one study on elderly head-injured patients, there was an overall 6-month mortality rate of 75%. Patients with ICPs greater than 20 mm Hg had a mortality rate of 90%.[1]

Waveforms

Intracranial pressure waveforms provide an index of ICP dynamics. The appearance of ICP waveforms varies according to the technique of measurement being used and the patient's pathologic status. Hemodynamic and respiratory oscillations can be observed in ICP traces. Sometimes, the waveforms closely resemble arterial pressure waveforms; at other times, they resemble central venous pressure waveforms. To varying degrees, oscillations corresponding to the arterial pulsations are seen.

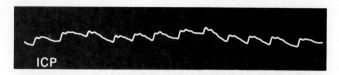

FIGURE 29–6
ICP waveform demonstrating hemodynamic and respiratory oscillations. Note the vascular pressure-type notches in the waveforms and the baseline variations that reflect respirations.

At times, a small "a" wave is superimposed on diastole, reflecting right atrial pressure.

Alterations in arterial driving force, disturbance of venous outflow, and cerebral vasodilation have been correlated with changes in waveform appearances.

In patients with ICP less than 20 mm Hg, a slower waveform, synchronous with respiration and caused by changes in intrathoracic pressure, can be seen (Fig. 29–6).

Some patients exhibit waveform variation, most commonly A, B, and C waves. *A waves*, also known as *plateau waves*, are spontaneous, rapid increases of pressure between 50 and 200 mm Hg, occurring at variable intervals (Fig. 29–7). They tend to occur in patients with moderate elevations of ICP, last 5 to 20 minutes, and fall spontaneously. The plateau waves usually are accompanied by a temporary increase in neurologic deficit. Although the mechanism of A waves has not been established firmly, it is thought that they indicate decreased intracranial compliance, and measures should be used to prevent their occurrence. They may result from an increase in blood volume with a simultaneous decrease in blood flow. The sudden reversal of high pressure may be caused by increased CSF absorption with reduction of CSF pressure. Falls in CPP with intact autoregulation and low intracranial compliance have been correlated with the initiating plateau waves. Plateau waves may be set off by a stimulus to vasodilation or by nonspecific stimuli such as hypoventilation or hyperventilation, pain, and aroused mental activities.

B waves are small, sharp rhythmic waves with pressures up to 50 mm Hg, occurring at a frequency of 0.5 to 2.0/minute. They correspond to changes in respiration, providing clues to periodic respiration related to poor cerebral compliance or pulmonary dysfunction. B waves often are seen with Cheyne–Stokes respirations. They may precede A waves and increase as compliance decreases. At times, they occur in patients with normal ICP and no papilledema. They may be secondary to oscillations of cerebral blood volume.

C waves are small, rhythmic waves with pressures up to 20 mm Hg, occurring at a rate of approximately 6/minute. They are related to the blood pressure. Like A waves, they indicate severe intracranial compression, with limited remaining volume residual within the intracranial space.

Management of Increased Intracranial Pressure

Most management techniques for IICP are oriented toward control of cerebral blood volume and CSF circulation, the two major mechanisms responsible for the regulation of intracranial pressure. Although protocols vary, measures to reduce ICP usually are initiated when the patient's ICP increases to approximately 15 mm Hg.

Hyperventilation, CSF drainage, osmotic diuretics, sedation, paralysis, steroids, and surgical decompression are among the measures used to treat intracranial hypertension. Although no one therapeutic regimen has been accepted universally, the goals in treatment of the patient with IICP remain

- to reduce ICP
- to improve CPP
- to reduce brain shift and distortion and the systemic effects that they induce.

The following discussion covers measures currently used in the management of IICP.

Surgical Decompression

Intracranial mass lesions are evacuated as early as possible, usually with replacement of the bone flap.

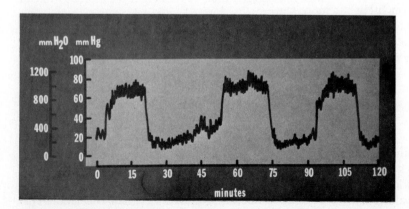

FIGURE 29–7
"A," or plateau, waves. Associated with decreased intracranial compliance, they may be secondary to an increase in blood volume with a simultaneous decrease in blood flow.

Ventilation

Maintaining adequate oxygenation and hypocapnea are essential in the patient with IICP. Neuronal damage or death may occur within 5 minutes of the onset of hypoxemia.[2] Uncorrected hypercapnia causes vasodilation of cerebral blood vessels with increased cerebral blood flow and increased ICP, leading to cerebral ischemia. With closed head injuries, it is recommended that the patient be manually hyperventilated with 100% O_2 before endotracheal tube suctioning and that the suctioning time be no more than 15 seconds, with 1 to 2 minutes of undisturbed rest between suction catheter passes.[2]

Endotracheal intubation usually is used with a tracheostomy performed by the third day if ventilation still is required. Intermittent positive pressure ventilation is indicated in head-injured patients in coma, patients with ICPs greater than 30 mm Hg after postcranial surgery, patients with chest injuries, and patients with decerebrate spasms or uncontrolled seizures secondary to brain damage. Reducing the arterial PCO_2 causes cerebral vasoconstriction, which reduces cerebral blood volume.

Ventilation usually is done at a slow rate (approximately 10–12 cycles/minute) with a high tidal volume (15 ml/kg body weight) to moderate hypocapnia (30–35 mm Hg). If necessary, small doses of chlorpromazine or morphine sulfate are used to phase the patient with the ventilator. For selected patients, paralyzing agents such as pancuronium bromide are used. When paralyzing or tranquilizing drugs are used, ICP monitoring is mandatory. With normally reacting blood vessels there is a 2- to 3-mm Hg decrease in ICP and a 1-mm Hg decrease in $PaCO_2$. Reduction of PCO_2 below 20 mm Hg causes no further vasoconstriction. Lowering PCO_2 below 25 mm Hg may increase lactic acid and dysrhythmias. Arterial PO_2 is maintained at over 70 mm Hg.

Positive end-expiratory pressure (PEEP) is used at levels up to 20 cm of water to improve oxygenation in patients with pulmonary dysfunction and requires ICP monitoring. The use of PEEP can increase ICP or reduce arterial blood pressure, thereby reducing CPP and decreasing CBF. This may be because PEEP causes a rise in intrathoracic pressure, which reduces cardiac filling pressure (preload), leading to a decrease in cardiac output. The circulatory compensation is incomplete and the blood pressure falls, causing a reduction in CPP. Intracranial pressure may be increased by impedance to cerebral venous outflow. In one study, significant increases in ICP occurred in approximately 50% of patients given PEEP. Patients with baseline ICPs greater than 25 mm Hg showed the most significant increases in ICP.

For optimal titration of PEEP in the patient who is at risk for development of intracranial hypertension, it is recommended that ICP and blood pressure be monitored continuously and measurements be made of neurologic status and intracranial and pulmonary compliance. Volume pressure responses and arterial blood gases therefore are indicated.

Position

The head is elevated 15° to 30° unless contraindicated by limb fractures or hepatorenal failure. In a study on patients with grade 4 hepatic coma, head elevation of less than 20° was associated with lowering ICP, whereas a greater than 20° elevation was associated with an increase in ICP and a decrease in CPP.[3] Decerebrate or decorticate posturing may increase ICP.

Flexion of the knees is contraindicated. A recent study documented that patients at risk for a pathologic increase in ICP should not be positioned with the neck in flexion or the head turned to either side.[4] These positions restrict venous drainage from the head through the internal jugular system and the vertebral venous plexus, increasing the total intracranial content. Rotation of the head to the right caused the greatest increase in ICP.

Hypothermia

Although hypothermia decreases the cerebral metabolic rate of oxygen consumption, used alone it may cause a reduction of CBF (Fig. 29–8). Except in patients in induced barbiturate coma, normothermia usually is used. Temperature elevations are treated promptly.

Hypothermia has been used successfully in conjunction with induced barbiturate coma. The combination may offer synergistic protection, acting through different mechanisms to control IICP.

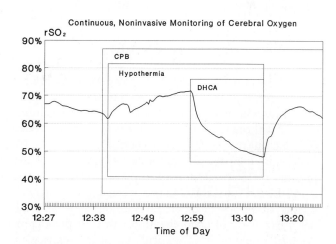

FIGURE 29–8
Intraoperative recording of cerebral O_2 saturation during posterior fossa aneurysm repair. Note that hypothermia reduced O_2 demand as reflected by the increase in rSO_2 between approximately 12:40 and 12:59 (Courtesy of Somanetics Corporation, Troy, MI).

Blood Pressure Control

Blood Pressure Reduction

When autoregulation is intact, a reduction in blood pressure causes an increase in ICP due to vasodilation and a subsequent increase in cerebral blood volume and brain stiffness. When autoregulation is defective, lowering blood pressure will decrease cerebral blood flow, which may cause cerebral ischemia (Fig. 29–9). Increased intracranial pressure and neurologic dysfunction can be aggravated by systemic vasodilator drugs such as sodium nitroprusside (Nipride; Roche Laboratories, Nutley, NJ). With a normal PCO_2, Nipride causes a significant increase in ICP with only a slight decrease in blood pressure. The use of hyperventilation attenuates but does not obliterate the ICP effect.

When induced hypotension is needed in the patient with IICP, Nipride administration should be titrated carefully. Ideally, the drug should be used in surgery only after the skull is opened.

Although high arterial blood pressure may be detrimental in patients with IICP, in patients with a very high ICP, a reduction in blood pressure may further reduce CBF. A study on patients with severe head injury indicates that even when blood pressure is high, a decline in blood pressure should be avoided.[5]

Reduction of arterial blood pressure is contraindicated in patients with brain edema when CBF already is reduced.

Blood Pressure Elevation

Postoperative intracranial aneurysm patients with cerebral ischemia secondary to severe intracranial vascular spasm have demonstrated marked clinical improvement after short periods of induced arterial hypertension.

Cerebrospinal Fluid Drainage

In situations involving impaired absorption of CSF, such as after a subarachnoid hemorrhage, impaired circulation of CSF, as with hydrocephalus and certain brain tumors, or IICP without total collapse of the ventricles, controlled CSF drainage may facilitate a reduction in ICP (Fig. 29–10). Ventricular drainage always should be against a positive pressure of 15 to 20 mm Hg to prevent ventricular collapse. Best results are obtained when there is bilateral dilation of the ventricles. Decompression should be gradual, particularly in children. Although CSF drainage is done routinely by intraventricular catheter (ventriculostomy), in selected patients CSF can be drained by a subarachnoid screw or bolt (Fig. 29–11). It is recommended that external ventricular drainage (ventriculostomy) systems be changed every 3 to 5 days, when three-quarters

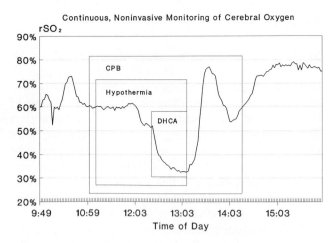

Continuous, Noninvasive Monitoring of Cerebral Oxygen

FIGURE 29–9
Intraoperative recording of cerebral O_2 saturation during middle cerebral artery aneurysm repair. Note the steep drop in rSO_2 between 12:03 and 13:03, when the patient's blood pressure was decreased to 31 mm Hg to control bleeding and the patient was in deep hypothermic circulatory arrest. (Courtesy of Somanetics Corporation, Troy, MI.) (CPB, cardiopulmonary bypass; DHCA, deep hypothermic circulatory arrest.)

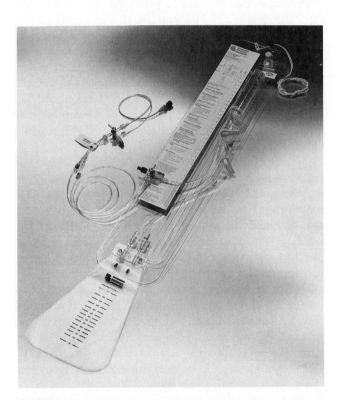

FIGURE 29–10
External ventricular drainage system (Becker External Drainage and Monitoring System II, Courtesy of Pudenz–Schulte Medical Corporation, Goleta, CA).

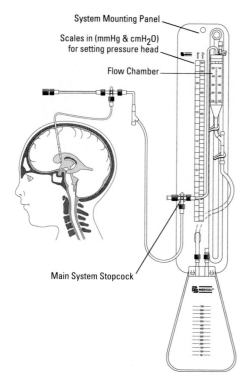

System Mounting Panel

Scales in (mmHg & cmH₂0)
for setting pressure head

Flow Chamber

Main System Stopcock

FIGURE 29–11
Becker EDMS for ICP monitoring and intermittent CSF drainage. A pressure transducer is attached to the intraventricular catheter or main system stopcock. Physician orders should specify the desired level of ICP and/or the volume of CSF to be drained (Courtesy of Pudenz–Schulte Medical Corporation, Goleta, CA).

filled or if the drainage becomes excessively bloody.[6] Strict sterile technique is required during catheter insertion, dressing changes, and drainage bag changes to reduce the risk of infection. It is important to minimize disruption of the drainage system.

Document the amount and appearance of CSF drainage and the condition of the catheter site after surgery.

Steroids

Glucocorticoids such as dexamethasone, betamethasone, and methylprednisolone have proved effective in reducing brain edema and ICP and in improving neurologic status, particularly in brain tumor patients with peritumoral edema. Clinical improvement usually is seen within 24 hours. An elevated resting ICP usually is not reduced until the second or third day of treatment. Steroid therapy has proved most effective in patients with focal chronic lesions. Standard doses of steroids have not been effective in reducing IICP associated with acute head injury, but higher doses of dexamethasone may be of value. In head-injured patients, steroids may be given for 3 days and, if improvement is seen, extended to 7 to 10 days.

Osmotherapy

Osmotic agents such as mannitol, urea and glycerol, and isosorbide may be used to assist in the management of IICP. They may decrease ICP by decreasing CSF volume and increasing CPP, and seem most effective in managing ICP elevations that have occurred within the previous hour. At times, loop diuretics such as furosemide (Lasix; Hoechst-Roussel Pharmaceuticals, Somerville, NJ) are used in conjunction with osmotherapy, requiring even more careful consideration of fluid and electrolyte balance. Although the osmotics have long been considered to introduce the risk of rebound, with ICP returning to or becoming higher than the pressure initially being treated, this phenomenon is now being questioned. Some investigators believe that rebound is unlikely when the drugs are managed properly. With diffuse head injury, an increase in CBF secondary to increased CPP may increase ICP. The effect of mannitol varies with the type of injury. Regardless of which agent is used, the optimal dose is the lowest dose that reduces ICP. Because the absolute effect of any drug cannot be determined in advance, continual monitoring of ICP is required to determine the correct dosage for a given patient. By titrating drug administration by means of ICP monitoring, the problem of increased osmolarity resulting from too high or too frequent dosages can be avoided.

The hyperosmotic agent most commonly used is 20% mannitol. Intravenous urea seldom is used because of the problem with severe local reaction if leakage occurs at the injection site. Mannitol therapy often is initiated if the patient's ICP has exceeded 15 to 20 mm Hg for at least 10 minutes. A dose of 0.25 to 1.00 g/kg of body weight is administered intravenously over a 10- to 15-minute period. Both bolus and continuous infusion techniques are used. The use of barbiturates reduces the mannitol requirement. Results should be evident within 15 minutes of completion of administration. Osmotherapy may increase CBF even when ICP is not reduced. In extremely ill patients, the administration of mannitol may cause parallel increases in blood pressure and ICP, with clinical deterioration.

Low normovolemia is maintained, usually two thirds of daily fluid requirements. Serum osmolarities often are maintained between 290 to 310 mOsm/ml. With IICP, colloid fluids such as albumin make maintenance of an adequate circulating volume possible. Solutions such as normal saline may promote brain edema secondary to a reduction in colloid osmotic pressure.

Calcium Antagonists (Blockers)

The effects of various calcium channel blockers such as nimodipine, nifedipine, verapamil, and diltiazem on the prevention and management of cerebral ischemia secondary to cerebral vasospasm are being investigated. It is hypothesized that these drugs inhibit large cerebral arteries from contracting by blocking the influx of extracellular calcium, resulting in the prevention of neurologic deficits secondary to cerebral arterial spasm. Because systemic arteries remain capable of contracting, calcium antagonists do not produce significant systemic hypotension.

Alkalizing Agents

The effects of alkalizing agents such as THAM (tromethamine; Abbott Laboratories, North Chicago, IL) and sodium bicarbonate in ICP reduction via suppression of brain swelling are being investigated. These agents may improve tissue acidosis, recover vascular tone, or act as hyperosmolar agents, preserving CBF in the ischemic lesion.

Induced Barbiturate Coma

Although somewhat controversial, induced barbiturate coma has been documented as increasing survival and decreasing morbidity, particularly in patients with head injuries and Reye's syndrome. Barbiturates suppress seizure activity and reduce cerebral metabolic activity and cerebral oxygen demand.

Mechanism

The mechanism by which ICP is reduced in barbiturate coma has not been established firmly. The barbiturate appears to have a direct, restrictive effect on cerebral vasculature, diverting small amounts of the blood from well perfused areas to ischemic areas, thereby improving cerebral pressure and collateral circulation. Vascular spasms are reduced, improving CBF. It lowers the systemic blood pressure, thereby decreasing blood–brain barrier disruption. Effects of noxious stimuli such as critical care unit noise are blunted, and patients are more tolerant of positioning and suctioning. The total muscle relaxation and immobilization reduce cerebral venous pressure. Both blood pressure and ICP become less labile.

Indications

Criteria vary extensively. Barbiturate coma may be initiated on head-injured patients with a Glasgow Coma Scale score of 7 or less and in whom the ICP reaches 25 mm Hg for longer than 10 minutes with the patient at rest while being treated with hyperventilation, steroids, mannitol, and CSF drainage.

Procedure

Before administration of the barbiturate (usually pentobarbital [Nembutal; Abbott Laboratories]) or thiopental (Pentothal; Abbott Laboratories), ICP, blood pressure, pulmonary artery pressure, and ECG monitoring with assisted ventilation are initiated. Baseline electroencephalogram (EEG) and brain stem auditory evoked responses (BAER) recordings are taken. An EEG is taken before initiation of barbiturate coma so that spontaneous electrocortical activity can be documented, and BAERs are recorded so that brain stem integrity can be assessed. The loading dose of pentobarbital is 5 to 10 mg/kg followed by 100 mg every hour until EEG burst suppression is documented. The EEG is used to titrate the barbiturates. Although high serum barbiturate levels will suppress electrocortical activity totally, BAER will remain as long as there is brain stem function. Because barbiturates are metabolized in the liver and excreted by the kidneys, impaired liver or kidney function will affect serum barbiturate levels.

Nursing Management

The patient in barbiturate coma becomes dependent. Clinical neurologic evaluation is almost impossible, making extensive, accurate monitoring of physiological responses to therapy mandatory. Artificial ventilation is required, and all vital functions must be maintained by the critical care team. Hypotension secondary to vasodilation and a reduction in cardiac output may occur. Serum blood levels of pentobarbital are maintained at 2.5 to 4.0 mg. The patient is at risk for deep venous thrombosis, pulmonary embolism, and hypostatic pneumonia. Treatment of IICP with high-dose barbiturates and mild hypothermia make it difficult to assess the patient for the complication of sepsis. Septic shock may be the first sign of sepsis recognized in the patient in barbiturate coma, adding the complication of hypotension to the morbidity associated with this intervention.

Indications for Discontinuing Barbiturate Coma

Barbiturate coma should be discontinued if any of the following exist: an ICP less than 15 mm Hg for 24 to 72 hours; a normal VPR (< 3 mm Hg/ml); a systolic blood pressure less than 90 mm Hg despite the use of vasopressors such as dopamine; lack of ICP response; progressive neurologic impairment such as deterioration of BAER; abolition of the need for vasodilator therapy to reduce systolic blood pressure below 160 mm Hg; and cardiac arrest.

The barbiturates are tapered gradually over a period lasting from 24 hours to several days. Arousal is gradual and prolonged, even after blood levels have been zero for several days. Patients must be weaned slowly and carefully from the respirator because of muscle weakness resulting from the therapy. The average length of treatment with pentobarbital coma is 72 hours.

Patients have vacuous facial expressions for several

DISPLAY BOX 29–3
Extracranial Causes of IICP

- Position of neck, head, and hips
- Cardiovascular instability
- Increased intrathoracic pressure
- Increased abdominal distention
- Decerebrate posturing and agitation
- Metabolic abnormalities
- Nontherapeutic touch and painful procedures
- Extraneous sounds
- Suctioning
- Hygienic measures
- Emotionally charged conversations

---

days despite normal blood barbiturate levels. Occasionally, during the first 24 hours, they have slow, abnormal movements that appear athetotic in nature. Dysarthria is common. Anticonvulsants are used for control of withdrawal seizures. Status epilepticus has been reported.

Nursing Care Considerations

Nursing care activity can compound the primary and secondary intracranial insults, contributing to rapid deterioration in the unstable patient who has lost intracranial compliance, autoregulation, and vasomotor tone. It is important to assess the patient for extracranial causes (Display Box 29–3) and potential causes of IICP and provide

---

DISPLAY BOX 29–4
ICP Monitoring Risk Factors: Infection

- Duration of ICP monitoring—the most significant risk factor; 85% of infections occur in patients monitored 5 days or longer.
- Maintenance of closed system: intermittent irrigations and tubing–stopcock changes may increase the risk.
- Aseptic technique during insertion and maintenance.
- ICP monitoring technique: intraventricular devices have a higher infection rate.
- Age and diagnosis: older patients and patients with open head trauma or intracerebral–intraventricular hemorrhage.
- Compliance with ICP monitoring protocols.

Modified from Hickman KM, Mayer BL, et al: Intracranial pressure monitoring: Review of risk factors associated with infection. Heart Lung 19:84–91, 1990

---

appropriate interventions to prevent elevations in ICP or to decrease ICP. For example, an interesting study on the effects of conversation on ICP in comatose patients demonstrated that in patients with Glasgow Coma Scale scores greater than 6, emotionally related conversation tended to

---

DISPLAY BOX 29–5
Intracranial–Extracranial Complications of Severe Head Injury

Intracranial Complications

- Intracranial hemorrhage secondary to interventions such as surgery or diagnostic procedures.
- Recurrent subdural–epidural hematomas.
- Cerebrospinal fluid leak resulting from interventions.
- Incorrect ICP measurements–catheter occlusion.
- Postsurgical ventriculitis–meningitis.
- Abscess at site of surgical or diagnostic intervention.
- Wound infection at intervention site.

Extracranial Complications

- Pulmonary: includes acute respiratory distress syndrome, atelectasis, pleural effusion, pulmonary embolus, respiratory failure, lung abscess, and empyema.
- Cardiovascular: includes cardiac arrhythmias, congestive heart failure, myocardial ischemia, systolic hypotension–hypertension.
- Peripheral vascular: deep venous thrombosis.
- Gastrointestinal: hemorrhage.
- Renal: acute renal failure.
- Hepatic: liver failure, hepatitis, cholangitis, and hepatic renal syndrome.
- Electrolyte abnormalities.
- Coagulopathy: determined by platelet count, prothrombin time, and partial thromboplastin time.
- Syndrome of inappropriate secretion of antidiuretic hormone.
- Diabetes insipidus: urine output over 200 ml/hr for 24 hours that does not respond to fluid restriction. Urine specific gravity <1.005, urine osmolality less than half that of plasma.
- Nonsurgical ventriculitis–meningitis: positive CSF culture or abnormal CSF cell count or CSF glucose.
- Pneumonia: diagnosed by chest x-ray and sputum cultures.
- Septicemia: positive blood culture and clinical findings of sepsis, including hyperthermia, hypotension.

Modified from Piek J, Chesnut RM, et al: Extracranial complications of severe head injury. J Neurosurg 77:901–907, 1992

increase ICP, probably due to increasing anxiety and stress. Conversations unrelated to the patient however, tended to decrease ICP.[7]

Complications

The monitoring and management of ICP are not without risks. Infection is the most common complication associated with ICP monitoring (Display Box 29–4). Infections may increase patient discomfort, prolong hospitalization, and increase the cost of care. A central nervous system infection, such as meningitis, brain abscess, or ventriculitis, may cause permanent disability or death. The incidence of reported ICP monitoring-related infection rates ranges from 0% to 26%.[8] The intraventricular catheter is associated with a higher rate of infection than alternate ICP monitoring devices. Factors that affect infection rates include the type of device used, differences in patient population, definitions of infection, methods of data analysis, and duration of monitoring. Patients monitored for 5 days or less have a negligible incidence of infection. With the use of external ventricular drainage, an infection rate from 4.5% to 27% has been reported.[6]

A multicenter study on the effect of intracranial and extracranial complications on recovery of patients with severe head injury indicated that intracranial complications did not alter outcome significantly, whereas extracranial complications were associated with an unfavorable outcome (Display Box 29–5).[9] The findings of this study indicated that prevention or reversal of pneumonia, hypotension, coagulopathy, and sepsis could improve outcome significantly in patients with severe head injury. Pulmonary, cardiovascular, coagulation, and electrolyte disorders occurred most frequently within 2 to 4 days, with infections peaking at 5 to 11 days. Although 59% of the patients in the four clinical centers in this study had electrolyte abnormalities, this complication did not affect outcome. Pulmonary infections were documented in 41% of the study patients, shock in 29%, coagulopathy in 19%, and septicemia in 10%. Rapid diagnosis and early treatment of pneumonia and sepsis were difficult in ICP-monitored patients being treated with barbiturate coma.

Troubleshooting Intracranial Pressure Lines

When the monitor indicates a change in ICP, the nurse must determine first whether the reading is accurate. If the reading is accurate, an attempt is then made to determine the reason for the pressure change. Table 29–1 provides a guide to troubleshooting ICP lines.

Nursing Care Plan

Nursing Care Plan 29–1 provides details of care for the patient with IICP.

Summary

From the foregoing discussion, it is apparent that numerous medical and nursing interventions are available for reducing the mortality and morbidity associated with IICP. Clinical assessment alone does not provide adequate information for giving optimal care to the critically ill patient with IICP. Correlating ICP, CPP, blood pressure, and pulmonary artery pressure measurements with other clinical assessments such as arterial blood gas levels often reduces the time required to obtain an accurate diagnosis, increases the time available for treatment, and provides continual feedback on the patient's response to selected treatments.

Nursing care activity can compound the primary and secondary intracranial insults, contributing to rapid deterioration in the unstable patient who has lost intracranial compliance, autoregulation, and vasomotor tone. It is important to assess the patient for extracranial causes and potential causes of IICP and provide appropriate interventions to prevent elevations in ICP or to decrease ICP.

(*Text continues on page 695*)

TABLE 29–1
Troubleshooting ICP Lines

Problem	Cause	Action
No ICP waveform	Air between the transducer diaphragm and pressure source	Eliminate air bubbles with sterile saline.
	Occlusion of intracranial measurement device with blood or debris	Flush intracranial catheter or screw as directed by physician: 0.25 ml sterile saline is often used.
	Transducer connected incorrectly	Check connection and be sure the appropriate connector for amplifier is in use.
	Fiberoptic catheter bent, broken	Replace fiberoptic catheter
	Incorrect gain setting for pressure or patient having plateau waves	Adjust gain setting for higher pressure range.
	Trace turned off	Turn power on to trace.

(*continued*)

TABLE 29–1
Troubleshooting ICP Lines (*Continued*)

Problem	Cause	Action
False high-pressure reading	Transducer too low	Place the venting port of the transducer at the level of the foramen of Monro. For every 2.54 cm (1 in) the transducer is below the pressure source, there is an error of approximately 2 mm Hg.
	Transducer incorrectly balanced	With transducer correctly positioned, rebalance.
		Transducer should be balanced every 2 to 4 hr and before the initiation of treatment based on a pressure change.
	Monitoring system incorrectly calibrated	Repeat calibration procedures.
	Air in system: air may attenuate or amplify pressure signal	Remove air from monitoring line.
High-pressure reading	Airway not patent: an increase in intrathoracic pressure may increase PCO_2	Suction patient.
		Position. Initiate chest physiotherapy.
	Ventilator setting incorrect	Check ventilator settings.
	PEEP	Draw arterial blood gases, because hypoxia and hypercarbia cause increases in ICP.
	Posture	Head should be elevated 15° to 30° unless contra-indicated by other problems such as fractures.
	Head and neck	The head should be positioned to facilitate venous drainage.
	Legs	Limit knee flexion.
	Decerebrate	Muscle relaxants or paralyzing agents sometimes are indicated.
	Excessive muscle activity during decerebrate posturing in patients with upper brain stem injury may increase ICP	
	Hyperthermia	Initiate measures to control muscle movement, infection, and pyrexia.
	Excessive muscle activity	
	Increased susceptibility to infection	
	Fluid and electrolyte imbalance secondary to fluid restrictions and diuretics	Draw blood for serum electrolytes, serum osmolality.
		Note pulmonary artery pressure.
		Evaluate input and output with specific gravity.
	Blood pressure: vasopressor responses occur in some patients with IICP	Use measures to maintain adequate CPP.
	Low BP associated with hypovolemia, shock, and barbiturate coma may increase cerebral ischemia	
False low-pressure reading	Air bubbles between transducer and CSF	Eliminate air bubbles with sterile saline
	Transducer level too high	Place the venting port of the transducer at the level of the foramen of Monro. For every 2.54 cm (1 in) the transducer is above the level of the pressure source, there will be an error of approximately 2 mm Hg.
	Zero or calibration incorrect	Rezero and calibrate monitoring system.
	Collapse of ventricles around catheter	If ventriculostomy is being used there may be inadequate positive pressure. Check to make sure a positive pressure of 15 to 20 mm Hg exists.
		Drain CSF slowly.
	Otorrhea or rhinorrhea	These conditions cause a false low-pressure reading secondary to decompression. Document the correlation between drainage and pressure changes.
	Leakage of fluid from connections	Eliminate all fluid leakage.
	Dislodgement of catheter from ventricle into brain	Contact physician regarding appropriate diagnostic studies and intervention. Use soft catheter designed for intraventricular measurement.
	Occlusion of the end of a subarachnoid screw by the necrotic brain	In most cases, remove screw.

ICP, intracranial pressure; PEEP, positive end-expiratory pressure; IICP, increased intracranial pressure; CPP, cerebral perfusion pressure; BP, blood pressure; CSF, cerebrospinal fluid.

NURSING CARE PLAN 29–1:
The Patient with Increased Intracranial Pressure

NURSING DIAGNOSIS	OUTCOME CRITERIA/ PATIENT GOALS	NURSING INTERVENTIONS
Altered tissue perfusion: related to decreased space for cerebral perfusion, cerebral tissue edema, decreased perfusion systemically, or absent cerebral perfusion due to embolus or cerebral vascular flow interruption.	• The patient's level of consciousness will be improved or maintained.	1. Accurately measure ICP and follow measurements continuously.
		2. Document ICP measurement q1h and as changes occur.
		3. Evaluate pattern of ICP monitoring to verify accuracy of the readings.
		4. Elevate head of bed 15°–30° at all times.
		5. Avoid flexion of the neck and head turning.
		6. Promote venous drainage of skull with alignment of the head.
		7. Use a consistent neurologic assessment system, such as the Glasgow Coma Scale. There must be consistency between nurses for an accurate trend of assessment data.
		8. Evaluate the following q1h and prn: Level of consciousness Pupil size Pupil reaction to light (briskness and size) Equality of pupils Movement of extremities Least stimulus to get reaction from the patient Appropriateness of patient's response to environment or stimuli Presence or absence of reflexes All involuntary motion such as seizures, twitching or asymmetry of motor function Blood pressure Heart rate and rhythm Respiratory rate and rhythm Hemodynamic parameters (PAP, PAd, PCWP, CVP, CO, CI) as available by invasive lines
		9. Calculate the CPP q1h and prn (CPP = MAP – ICP)

(continued)

NURSING CARE PLAN 29–1: *(Continued)*
The Patient with Increased Intracranial Pressure

NURSING DIAGNOSIS	OUTCOME CRITERIA/ PATIENT GOALS	NURSING INTERVENTIONS
		10. Report changes in assessment or CPP <70 or >90 mm Hg to physician.
		11. Avoid increases in intrathoracic pressure: avoid the use of PEEP on mechanical ventilators; avoid hip flexion; avoid coughing, vomiting, or Valsalva maneuvers.
		12. If ventilation is controlled with mechanical ventilator, keep PCO_2 low (18–25) to prevent cerebral vasodilatation.
		13. Control environment to decrease stimulation, limit contact with patient to necessary procedures.
		14. Administer corticosteroids, as ordered.
		15. Administer diuretics that decrease tissue volume (such as mannitol), as ordered.
		16. Maintain an accurate input and output, q8h.
		17. Limit fluid intake as much as possible.
		18. Anticipate dehydration, monitor urine and serum Na, osmolality.
		19. Maintain normal temperature, prevent shivering.
		20. Provide sedation or sedation and paralysis, as ordered, with barbiturates or Pavulon.
		21. Provide hyperventilation before removal from mechanical ventilator for suctioning.
Fluid volume deficit: related to diabetes insipidus (DI), potential diuretic therapy, high metabolic needs, diaphoresis, renal failure.	• Minimal intake and adequate output will be maintained.	1. Monitor the trends in serum and urine Na, osmolality, and creatinine levels.
		2. Keep accurate input and output q8h.
		3. Do not move patient to weigh (increased stimuli) unless absolutely necessary.
		4. Give medications (IVPB antibiotics) in minimal volumes.

(continued)

NURSING CARE PLAN 29–1: (Continued)
The Patient with Increased Intracranial Pressure

NURSING DIAGNOSIS	OUTCOME CRITERIA/ PATIENT GOALS	NURSING INTERVENTIONS
		5. Assess for DI: high urine output with low specific gravity.
		6. Replace electrolytes with supplemental therapy, as ordered.
		7. If DI present give Pitressin and DDAVP, as ordered.
		8. Monitor CVP and hemodynamic data, as available.
Ineffective breathing pattern: related to subdued level of consciousness, brain tissue injury near medulla or pons, inability to maintain adequate airway, lack of control over respiratory muscles, severe hypoventilation, or pulmonary complications.	• Patent airway will be maintained.	1. Assess ability to maintain patent airway.
		2. Assess reflexes necessary for adequate breathing: cough, gag, and swallow.
		3. Assess respirations for rate, depth, regularity, and chest expansion.
		4. Assess breath sounds for the movement of air to all lung fields.
		5. Maintain an elevated head of bed.
		6. Assess ABGs for evidence of adequate gas exchange, qd and prn.
		7. If mechanical ventilation is needed, maintain hyperventilation.
		8. Be aware of impact of depressant or sedative drugs on the respiratory drive.
		9. Suction, as needed, providing hyperventilation before the procedure.
		10. Monitor heart rate and rhythm.
		11. Follow results of daily chest x-ray reports.
		12. Monitor oxygenation with pulse oximetry.
High risk for altered body temperature: related to brain tissue injury or infection.	• Body temperature will stay within normal limits.	1. Check core temperature frequently.
		2. Prevent shivering by lowering an elevated temperature slowly.
		3. Use cooling blanket, as ordered.
		4. Administer antipyretics, such as Tylenol, as ordered.

(continued)

NURSING CARE PLAN 29–1: (*Continued*)
The Patient with Increased Intracranial Pressure

NURSING DIAGNOSIS	OUTCOME CRITERIA/ PATIENT GOALS	NURSING INTERVENTIONS
		5. Administer antibiotics, as ordered.
		6. Control the environmental temperature.
		7. Maintain aseptic technique with all procedures.
High risk for infection: related to invasive lines, decreased level of consciousness and immobility.	• Nosocomial infection will not occur.	1. Use strict sterile technique during insertion of ICP monitoring device, and maintenance of external ventricular drainage system.
		2. Perform sterile dressing changes at ICP monitoring device site, qd.
		3. Assess for symptoms of CNS infection: changes in LOC; increased WBC; elevated temperature; nuchal rigidity; photophobia; positive Kernig's sign.
		4. Obtain CSF cultures, as ordered.
		5. Administer antibiotics, as ordered.
		6. Monitor and record the presence of leaking CSF from nose, ears, or ICP monitoring device site.
High risk for injury: related to decreased level of consciousness, agitation, restlessness, or involuntary motion such as seizure activity.	• Patient will be free from injury.	1. Evaluate the patient's potential risk for injury, q8h and prn.
		2. If restless, pad side rails, keep both side rails up, keep bed in low position and restrain patient with soft wrist restraints or vest/jacket restraint, as needed.
		3. If subdued level of consciousness, turn q2h, position in anatomically functional positions, use soft wrist restraints, use device to decrease the stiffness of the mattress; keep side rails up and the bed in low position.
		4. Perform passive ROM exercises, if not contraindicated by increased ICP.
		5. Maintain bronchial hygiene.

(*continued*)

NURSING DIAGNOSIS	OUTCOME CRITERIA/ PATIENT GOALS	NURSING INTERVENTIONS
		6. Position to prevent aspirations.
		7. Use antiembolism stockings.
		8. Use high-top tennis shoes to prevent footdrop.
		9. Assess integrity of skin q8h.
		10. Keep skin clean, dry, free of harsh soaps or chemicals.
		11. Promote mobililty and place patient in the chair, as soon as medically cleared for increased activities.
High risk for altered nutrition: related to decreased level of consciousness, mechanical ventilation, or increased metabolic needs.	• Adequate nutrition will be maintained.	1. Maintain NPO status until full assessment is complete.
		2. Evaluate cough, gag, and swallow reflexes.
		3. Auscultate abdomen for bowel sounds q8h.
		4. If patient able to chew and swallow, feed patient a balanced diet including foods of the patient's choice.
		5. If unable to masticate and swallow, place thin, soft-walled feeding tube, as ordered.
		6. Verify feeding tube placement with radiography initially, and q8h with auscultation for injected air, aspiration of contents with syringe, or injection of water.
		7. Initiate tube feedings with small amounts and lower concentration. Increase amount and strength, as tolerated and as ordered.
		8. Stop any tube feeding if residual in stomach is large or regurgitation occurs.
		9. Maintain an elevated head of the bed during all tube feedings.
		10. Limit diarrhea with antidiarrheal agents.
		11. Give calories and free water, either by mouth or feeding tube.
		12. Weigh qd, when ICP has stabilized.
		13. Monitor fluid and electrolyte balance, qd and prn.

Hypothermia

BEHAVIORAL OBJECTIVES

Based on the content in this section, the reader should be able to:

1. Explain the rationale for using induced hypothermia in a clinical situation.
2. List and explain two methods for inducing hypothermia in the clinical setting.
3. Identify three causes of unintentional (accidental) hypothermia.
4. Describe three nursing diagnoses and their appropriate nursing interventions for the hypothermic patient.

Description

Hypothermia (lowered body temperature) occurs when the core temperature is less than 35°C (95°F) and may be classified as either induced or unintentional (accidental).

Moderate hypothermia may be classified as between 28°C to 33.5°C (82°–92.3°F). Heat loss may be secondary to conduction, convection, radiation, respiration, and evaporation. Although the decrease in metabolic rate associated with hypothermia affords a degree of cellular protection from ischemic injury, prolonged hypothermia with a core temperature below 30°C (86°F) has been associated with increased myocardial irritability, decreased cardiac output, increased clotting time, disseminated intravascular coagulation, hypokalemia, and severe metabolic acidosis.

Accidental hypothermia (an unintentional reduction in core temperature below 35°C [95°F]) is associated with conditions that decrease heat production, increase heat loss, or impair thermoregulation. Unintentional hypothermia may be caused by exposure to low ambient temperatures, water accidents, drug overdoses, and certain diseases, such as myxedema and hypopituitarism. Surgical patients may have hypothermia secondary to general anesthesia and the infusion of large volumes of cold crystalloids and blood products. The elderly patient appears to have a physiological predisposition to hypothermia. Aging is associated with autonomic dysfunction, with decreased resting peripheral blood flow, decreased heat production by shivering, diminished muscle mass and fat stores, impaired thermoperception, and decreased metabolism.

Other causes of hypothermia include open body wounds or cavities, pharmaceutical agents (vasodilators, barbiturates, phenothiazines, general anesthetics) decreased muscle activity, inhalation of cold gases, and sepsis.

The presence of fever (hyperthermia) in any patient produces greater cellular oxygen requirements because of the increased rate of metabolism. Each 1°C (33.8°F) elevation in temperature increases the metabolic rate 10% to 13%, causing an increase in oxygen consumption and carbon dioxide production.[10] This fact becomes especially significant in the patient whose vital centers already may be compromised because of cerebral edema that is surgically induced or the result of another form of insult such as hypoxia from cardiac arrest. It is to provide some margin of safety in these situations until injured tissue can recover that the body temperature is lowered or maintained at normothermic levels. Current emphasis is on prevention of marked elevations in body temperature as opposed to marked reduction of the temperature. Physiological responses to cold remain the same, and there are occasions when actual hypothermia is desirable.

Some studies indicate that in selected patients fever may have therapeutic effects, including the killing of some bacteria at temperatures of 40°C (104°F).[10] Uncontrolled fever is contraindicated in patients with or with the potential for intracranial hypertension.

Physiological Principles

Hypothermia causes physiological changes in all organ systems, with progressive depression of metabolic processes and nerve conduction, which may lead to death. In health, the hypothalamus controls body temperature within a narrow range, adjusting for both environmental and physiological temperature changes. Imbalances between heat dissipation and heat production can lead to hypothermia. Trauma patients are particularly at risk for development of accidental hypothermia. This may be due to shock-related decreases in heat production, decreases in oxygen transport to tissues secondary to hypovolemia, diaphoresis with heat loss through the skin, and respiratory heat loss associated with tachypnea. Shivering, the body's most effective method of heat production, may be inhibited in severely injured patients. With hypovolemic shock this may be related to decreased baroreceptor input to the brain or central nonadrenergic inhibition, or both. Alterations in thermoregulation also may be associated with the use of medications, including barbiturates, many narcotics, muscle relaxants, and sedatives. For example, skin heat loss secondary to vasodilation is associated with morphine sulfate. Burns and open wounds increase heat loss via convection and evaporation. Skin preparation, lavage, and irrigation, as well as vigorous blood and fluid replacement are instrumental in lowering core temperature. With traumatic brain injury, hypothalamic thermoregulatory structures may be damaged.

Neurologic effects of hypothermia include a 6% to 7% decrease in cerebral blood flow for every 1°C decrease in core temperature. At 30°C (86°F), a patient who is not shivering has a 54% reduction in brain metabolism, a 30% decrease in cerebral blood flow, and a 20% decrease in brain volume. The sensorium fades at 34° to 33°C (93°–91.4°F).

Hematologic effects of hypothermia include coagulopathy with prolongation of prothrombin time and partial thromboplastin time tests. There are decreased platelets and white blood cells, an increase in hemoglobin and hematocrit, and a left shift of the oxyhemoglobin curve, making the oxygen shift from red blood cells to tissue more difficult.

Because the critical care nurse usually is responsible for monitoring the hypothermic patient, it is important for the clinician to be aware of the physiological manifestations of the various phases of body cooling.

The body's initial reaction to cold exposure is an attempt to conserve body heat and to increase heat production. *Skin pallor* that occurs is due to a vasoconstrictor response that limits superficial blood flow and thus loss of body heat. Intense activity in the form of *shivering* occurs to maintain body heat. The effects of these compensatory responses will be reflected in the vital signs, and it is important that the nurse understand these transient variations and consider them in evaluating the patient.

During the first 15 to 20 minutes of hypothermia induction, all *vital signs* increase. Pulse and blood pressure rise in response to the increased venous return produced by vasoconstriction. Respiratory rate increases to meet the added oxygen requirements of increased metabolic activity produced by shivering and to eliminate the additional carbon dioxide produced. If the patient hyperventilates with shivering, respiratory alkalosis can develop. The initial rise in temperature is a reflection of this increased cellular activity.

Because the patient requiring hypothermia usually has an existing cellular oxygenation problem, the increased oxygen consumption induced by shivering is undesirable. For this reason, chlorpromazine (Thorazine; SmithKline Beckman, Philadelphia, PA) may be given at the beginning of induction to reduce hypothalamic response. *Hypoglycemia* is a potential occurrence during vigorous shivering because increased glucose is required for the increased metabolic activity.

After approximately 15 minutes, the vasoconstrictor effect is broken by means of a negative feedback loop, and warm blood flow to the body surface is reestablished. This accounts for the reddened skin color after initial skin pallor. (This same phenomenon can be seen by holding an ice cube in the hand for a short period of time.)

As superficial warm blood flow is reestablished, body heat is lost, and body temperature begins to drop. Because blood cooled at the body surface continues to circulate through the body core, downward drift of the temperature usually continues for approximately −17.2°C (1°F) after the cooling blanket is turned off.

When the desired level of induced hypothermia is achieved, usually around 32°C (89.6°F), other physiological changes become apparent. The vital signs at this stage all are diminished. The development of respiratory acidosis is a real possibility because, at deeper levels of hypothermia, ventilation falls off more rapidly than does reduced carbon dioxide production. Also, with increasing hypothermia the oxygen dissociation curve shifts to the left, and at lower tensions oxygen is not released readily by hemoglobin to the tissues. Because of the developing

---

Physiological Reactions During the First 15 to 20 Minutes of Hypothermia Induction

Skin: Pallor
Motor activity: Shivering
Pulse: Increased
Blood pressure: Increased
Respiratory rate: Increased
Temperature: May increase initially due to increased cellular activity

circulatory insufficiency and increased metabolic activity due to shivering, metabolic acidosis also is a possibility.

Secretion of antidiuretic hormone is inhibited, and an increase in urine output may be noted with a drop in the specific gravity. During hypothermia, water shifts from the intravascular spaces to the interstitial and intracellular spaces. This results from movement of sodium into the cell in exchange for potassium and movement of water with it. This fluid shift produces hemoconcentration.

Because all cellular activity diminishes with hypothermia, cerebral activity decreases and hearing fades at approximately 34° to 33°C (93°–91.4°F) due to reduced cochlear response. At 18° to 30°C (82°–86°F), there is no corneal or gag reflex, and pulse irregularities may be noted as the result of myocardial irritability, which probably occurs because of the movement of potassium into the cell.

Equipment Features

Warming and Cooling Systems

A variety of microprocessor-controlled systems are available for cooling and heating patients. In addition to the hyperthermia–hypothermia blanket systems, convective air-warming systems with an inflated warming tube and alarm system are available. Most commonly used with postoperative hypothermia, they provide a continuous flow of heated air to peripheral areas of the body. Convective warming therapy reduces the incidence of shivering.

Temperature Devices

For the measurement of temperature, a variety of peripheral and core techniques are available. Electronic thermometers are recommended for peripheral skin, oral, and rectal temperatures. In critical care, core temperatures are obtained most commonly via pulmonary artery thermistor catheters, urinary bladder thermistor catheters (temperature-sensing Foley catheters), and aural (ear, tympanic membrane) thermometers. Pulmonary artery and urinary bladder catheters provide continuous monitoring of core temperatures. An ear thermometer provides an intermittent core reading in 1 to 3 seconds (Fig. 29–12).

Indications

The use of induced hypothermia in clinical situations ranges from treatment of gastric hemorrhage to attempts to prevent irreversible cerebral damage. Decreased body temperature reduces cellular activity and consequently the oxygen requirement of tissues. Hypothermia therefore is induced in situations involving interrupted or reduced blood flow to vital areas to minimize tissue damage due to diminished oxygen delivery. This is the rationale for using hypothermia during open heart and neurosurgical procedures.

Procedure

Inducing Hypothermia

Although the method of inducing hypothermia will depend on the situation and the equipment available, essentially there are two ways to proceed—surface cooling and the more direct method of bloodstream cooling.

Surface cooling, which involves the use of blankets that circulate a refrigerant, is the method usually used in critical care units. The cooling blanket, with a disposable cover, may be placed directly against the patient. The important point here is to avoid placing any degree of

---

Physiological Effects of the Hypothermic State

	Response	Possible Complications
Skin	Decreased circulation leading to crystal formation in cells	Fat necrosis
Vital signs	Diminished	Respiratory acidosis Metabolic acidosis
Urinary output	Increased	
Fluid volume	Hemoconcentration	Embolization
Sensorium	Fades at 34°–33°C	Increased difficulty in determining mental status
Hearing	Fades at 34°–33°C	
Cardiac rhythm	Myocardial irritability below 28°C	Dysrhythmias

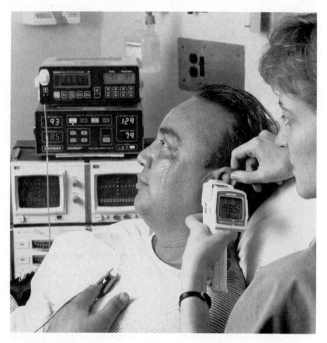

FIGURE 29–12
Use of infrared aural (ear, tympanic) thermometer for intermittent measurement of core, oral, rectal, or skin temperatures from the auditory canal. The ear thermometer offers a safe, fast, noninvasive method of measuring infrared emissions from the tympanic membrane, providing reflected core temperature readings within 3 seconds. (Diatek 9000 InstaTemp Infrared Aural Thermometer, courtesy of Diatek, Inc., a wholly owned subsidiary of Diatek Corporation, San Diego, CA.)

thickness between the patient and the blanket, because this will serve as an insulator and impede the cooling process.

When cooling is initiated, one blanket may be placed under the patient and another placed on top to hasten the cooling process. If a top blanket is used, exercise care in observing the patient's respiratory status because the weight of the cooling blanket may limit chest excursion. Keeping the blanket in contact with areas of superficial blood flow such as the axilla and groin also will expedite cooling. In the event that a cooling device is not available, apply ice bags to initiate the cooling process, using these same principles.

Bloodstream (core) *cooling* is the method used during open heart surgical procedures when the blood passes through the cooling coils in the cardiopulmonary bypass machine.

Rewarming

Once it is determined that the patient no longer requires the hypothermic state, rewarming can be accomplished by a number of methods, including surface rewarming (convective air warming), bloodstream rewarming, and natural rewarming. The last is the preferred method. The

cooling device is removed. A blanket may be used to cover the patient, but no artificial heat is used, and the patient is allowed to warm at his or her own rate. As the patient approaches normothermic levels, it is to be anticipated that vital signs will return to precooling levels due to reversal of the physiological events.

For profound, accidental hypothermia (core temperature below 30°C [86°F]), rewarming methods include active core (internal) warming such as extracorporeal bypass, active external rewarming such as convective warming, and passive or spontaneous rewarming such as blankets or a warm ambient room temperature.

Assessment and Management

The treatment and outcome of hypothermia are affected by length or type of exposure, nutritional status, infection, injury, age, state of health, and medication or intoxicant ingestion.

Cooling Phase

For the conscious patient, reduction of body temperature is at best an unpleasant experience. Adequate explanation and support for the patient and family are integral parts of nursing care.

In the obese patient, a greater degree of downward drift may be experienced after removal of a cooling blanket. For this reason, the cooling device should be turned off before the desired hypothermic level actually is attained. Temperature must be monitored closely to determine whether the trend remains downward or whether an increase in temperature occurs, requiring use of the blanket again.

Continuous temperature monitoring may be done with pulmonary artery thermistor catheters, urinary bladder thermistor catheters, and rectal probes.

Intermittent monitoring may be done with skin, esophageal, tympanic, or rectal probes, used in conjunction with various electronic thermometers.

For infection control, patient comfort, and convenience, disposable, moisture barrier, hyperthermia–hypothermia blankets, and disposable ear (tympanic), oral, skin rectal, and esophageal probes are available.

The measurement technique will affect the temperature reading. Because core temperatures are less influenced by external factors and more accurately reflect the mean temperature of vital organs, they are recommended for monitoring hypothermia patients (Display Box 29–6).

Because bladder temperatures are affected by urinary output, it is recommended that output be recorded when bladder thermistor catheters are used for core temperature monitoring. Because pulmonary artery temperatures are affected by inspired gas, notation of inspired gases is recommended.

DISPLAY BOX 29–6
Normal Temperature Ranges

Oral	97.6°–99.6°F
	36.5°–37.5°C
Core	98.2°–100.2°F
	36.8°–37.9°C
Rectal	98.6°–100.6°F
	37.0°–38.1°C

Skin care becomes particularly crucial due to the presence of cold and its circulatory effects. The clinician can change the patient's position to eliminate pressure points, taking care to move the blanket with the patient so that body contact is maintained with the cooling device.

To prevent embolization secondary to hemoconcentration, nursing measures such as passive range-of-motion exercises and frequent change of position are initiated.

For the neurologic patient who already has a depressed sensorium, other measures for evaluation of changes in the patient's level of response must be relied on, such as assessment of purposeful or nonpurposeful movements in response to painful stimuli and the degree of painful stimulus necessary to elicit a response.

Hypothermic Phase

When the patient has reached the desired hypothermic level, vital signs also will level out at reduced values. Changes in vital signs therefore must be evaluated in light of the patient's hypothermic state. For example, if the nurse is caring for a neurosurgical patient cooled to 32°C (89.6°F), and if the vital signs have decreased as would be expected normally, an increase in pulse, respirations, or blood pressure to "normal levels" must be interpreted in view of the hypothermic state. Is an infectious process present? Are changes occurring in the patient's neurologic status? Is ICP increasing?

If the patient is to be maintained at the hypothermic level for a prolonged period of time, this can be accomplished in a number of ways. The patient (after the temperature has risen several degrees) may need to be placed on the cooling blanket periodically and returned to the desired hypothermic level.

These nursing measures should be performed gently, with a minimal degree of activity on the patient's part to prevent an increase in body heat, such as when providing passive range-of-motion exercises. The nurse should bathe the patient with tepid or cool water to avoid increasing temperature in this manner.

Prevention of pulmonary problems in the hypothermic patient is dependent almost entirely on nursing care. Change of position allowing for postural drainage, measures to promote adequate ventilation, and suctioning to remove accumulated secretions all are extremely important in this patient.

Rewarming Phase

During the rewarming phase, the patient must be monitored closely for indications necessitating recooling. With the patient's normothermic status used as a baseline, these indications would include a fading sensorium, greater increase in pulse and respirations than normally would be expected with the warming process, and a drop in the blood pressure. Another important facet to be monitored is the cumulative effect of drugs given previously.

The necessity for interpretation of clinical changes in the patient on the basis of the physiological changes brought about through cooling and then rewarming cannot be overemphasized. The nurse must anticipate changes and findings based on the patient's pathologic condition and other variables present that would alter those findings.

Complications

Dysrhythmias

Ventricular fibrillation is a common occurrence at 28° to 30°C (82°–86°F), and consequently the patient usually is maintained at a hypothermic level around 32°C (89.6°F) so that cardiac problems are avoided. Defibrillation of patients with temperatures below 28° to 30°C (82.4°F–86°F) usually is unsuccessful. Many dysrhythmic, hypothermic patients will convert automatically to a sinus rhythm at a core temperature above 30°C (86°F).

Cumulative Drug Effects

Drugs tend to have a cumulative effect in the hypothermic patient. Decreased perfusion at the injection site and decreased enzyme activity result in slower chemical reactions. Therefore the intravenous route is preferred, and intramuscular or subcutaneous injections should be avoided. If a drug must be given hypodermically, it should be given deeply intramuscularly, and vigilance must be maintained during the rewarming phase for cumulative effects.

Fat Necrosis

Another potential occurrence during hypothermia is that of *fat necrosis*. This results from prolonged exposure to cold and decreased circulation, which allows crystals to form in the fluid elements of the cells, leading to necrosis and

NURSING CARE PLAN 29–2:
The Patient with Hypothermia

NURSING DIAGNOSIS	OUTCOME CRITERIA/ PATIENT GOALS	NURSING INTERVENTIONS
Hypothermia: related to prolonged exposure, decreased level of consciousness, rapid infusion of hypothermic intravenous solutions, or intentional cooling.	• Therapeutic temperature will be maintained.	1. Monitor temperature and ECG continuously. 2. Maintain prescribed warming or cooling method. 3. Check respirations if top blanket is used. 4. Assess vital signs. 5. Assess for cumulative effect of drugs. 6. Minimize patient activity. 7. Bathe patient with cool or tepid water. 8. Administer passive ROM exercises. 9. Change patient's position frequently. 10. Medicate to prevent shivering, as ordered.
Decreased cardiac output: related to decreased heart rate, peripheral vasoconstriction, or accelerated metabolic needs.	• Adequate systemic perfusion will be maintained.	1. Maintain hypothermic level around 32°C. 2. Monitor hemodynamics: cardiac output/index, especially during rewarming. 3. Monitor cardiac rate and rhythm.
Altered comfort: related to reduction in body temperature.	• Discomfort will be minimized.	1. Explain environment, all procedures, expectations, and equipment. 2. Allow patient to express self freely. 3. Include family in patient's care. 4. Alter temperature slowly. 5. Give sedatives, as ordered.
High risk for impaired skin integrity: related to ischemic skin areas, pressure points, or decreased cardiac output.	• Skin integrity will be maintained.	1. Check skin color, temperature q2h and prn. 2. Change patient's position to eliminate pressure points. 3. Consider therapeutic air bed for relief of pressure points on ischemic limbs.

(continued)

NURSING CARE PLAN 29–2: (Continued)
The Patient with Hypothermia

NURSING DIAGNOSIS	OUTCOME CRITERIA/ PATIENT GOALS	NURSING INTERVENTIONS
High risk for impaired gas exchange: related to increased metabolic needs, sedation, or discomfort/impaired chest wall motion.	• Adequate ventilation will be maintained.	1. Position to promote postural drainage. 2. Suction to remove accumulated secretions. 3. Assess breath sounds q2–4h. 4. Assess ABGs prn, for acid–base imbalances. 5. Evaluate chest radiography results/reports. 6. Provide supplemental O_2, as indicated. 7. Verify O_2 saturation with oximetry.
High risk for altered nutrition, less than body requirements: related to catabolism, nitrogen loss, and increased metabolic rate.	• Adequate nutrition will be maintained.	1. Assess nutrition and hydration, q4h and prn. 2. Maintain IV access and fluids. 3. Provide nutrition via hyperalimentation or tube feedings, as ordered. 4. Evaluate electrolytes and serum albumin levels. 5. Evaluate liver function tests and renal status (BUN/creatinine). 6. Assess all medications for hepatotoxicity or nephrotoxicity. 7. Monitor bowel elimination.

cellular death. Nursing measures that can minimize fat necrosis include turning the patient frequently, massaging the skin to increase circulation, and avoiding prolonged application of cold to any one area.

Rewarming Phase Problems

One of the hazards of artificially induced rewarming is that the skin and muscles may be warmed before the heart. The heart remains in a cooled state and is unable to maintain a sufficient cardiac output to meet the oxygen demands of the superficial areas. Further warming increases the dilation of peripheral vessels and blood pools, resulting in decreased circulating volume, decreased venous return, and therefore decreased cardiac output. This complication is referred to as "afterdrop," a form of rewarming shock. Core temperature may continue to drop up to 20 minutes after removal of the cold stimuli. Afterdrop is more prevalent in elderly and young patients, obese patients, and victims of cold water immersion. This sequence of events can be avoided if the heart is warmed first, as in the bloodstream method, or if the body is allowed to rewarm naturally.

Other complications that may occur during the rewarming process are hyperpyrexia, shock (for reasons just cited), and acidosis. The acidosis occurs as a result of the increase in metabolic activity in those areas already warmed and an insufficient circulation to meet the metabolic requirements of this increased activity. Oliguria also may result, probably because of antidiuretic hormone secretion.

Troubleshooting

Temperature Inaccuracies

For accurate temperature measurements, the thermometer probe specified by the instrument manufacturer should be used. This is particularly important for instruments that use temperature as a control input, such as warming and cooling blanket units.

When using an ear thermometer, it is important to remember that within the ear canal, the temperature between the opening of the ear canal and the area of the tympanic membrane can vary by as much as $-15°C$ (5°F). For accurate core temperature readings, it is important to measure the temperature near the tympanic membrane, which shares a common blood supply with the hypothalamus. Use of the manufacturer's guidelines for obtaining accurate ear temperatures is recommended.

Urinary bladder temperatures reflect the temperature of arterial and venous blood in the periureteral tissues. Because the temperature of the urine is partially a function of urine flow, urine output should be measured when urinary bladder temperatures are used to monitor core temperature. Urinary bladder temperatures usually are slightly higher than pulmonary artery temperatures.

Pulmonary artery temperatures reflect the temperature of mixed venous blood and are considered true core temperatures. They are affected by inspired gases and are higher when the patient is shivering. Because shivering does not affect the temperature of urine, there is an increase in the temperature gradient between the pulmonary artery temperature and urinary temperature during shivering.[11]

Nursing Care Plan

Nursing Care Plan 29–2 outlines the important aspects of care for the patient undergoing hypothermia.

REFERENCES

Intracranial Pressure Monitoring

1. Ross AM, Pitts LH, et al: Prognosticators of outcome after major head Injury in the elderly. Journal of Neuroscience Nursing 24(2):88–93, 1992
2. Crosby LJ, Parsons LC: Cerebrovascular response of closed head-injured patients to a standardized endotracheal tube suctioning and manual hyperventilation procedure. Journal of Neuroscience Nursing 24(1):40–49, 1992
3. Davenport A, Will EJ, et al: Effect of posture on intracranial pressure and cerebral perfusion pressure in patients with fulminant hepatic and renal failure after acetaminophen self-poisoning. Crit Care Med 18:286–289, 1990
4. Williams A, Coyne SM: Effects of neck position on intra-cranial pressure. American Journal of Critical Care 2(1): 68–71, 1993
5. Bouma GJ, Muizelaar JP, et al: Blood pressure and intra-cranial pressure-volume dynamics in severe head injury: Relationship with cerebral blood flow. J Neurosurg 77: 15–19, 1992
6. Cummings R: Understanding external ventricular drainage. Journal of Neuroscience Nursing 24(2):84–87, 1992
7. Johnson SM, Omery A, et al: Effects of conversation on intracranial pressure in comatose patients. Heart Lung 18: 56–63, 1989
8. Hickman KM, Mayer BL, et al: Intracranial pressure monitoring: Review of risk factors associated with infection. Heart Lung 19:84–91, 1990
9. Piek J, Chesnut RM, et al: Extracranial complications of severe head injury. J Neurosurg 77:901–907, 1992

Hypothermia

10. Segatore M: Fever after traumatic brain injury. Journal of Neuroscience Nursing 24(2):104–109, 1992
11. Earp JK, Finlayson DC: Urinary bladder/pulmonary artery temperature ratio of less than 1 and shivering in cardiac surgical patients. American Journal of Critical Care 1(2): 43–52, 1992

BIBLIOGRAPHY

Intracranial Pressure Monitoring

Bowton DL, Bertels NH, et al: Cerebral blood flow is reduced in patients with sepsis syndrome. Crit Care Med 17:399–403, 1989

Brucia JJ, Owen DC, et al: The effects of lidocaine on intracranial hypertension. Journal of Neuroscience Nursing 24(4): 205–214, 1992

Chan KH, Miller JD, et al: The effect of changes in cerebral perfusion pressure upon middle cerebral artery blood flow velocity and jugular bulb venous oxygen saturation after severe brain injury. J Nerurosurg 77:55–61, 1992

Davis M, Lucatorto M: The false localizing signs of increased intracranial pressure. Journal of Neuroscience Nursing 24(5):245–250, 1992

Mason PB: Neurodiagnostic testing in critically injured adults. Critical Care Nurse 12(6):64–75, 1992

McCormick PW, Stewart M, et al: Noninvasive cerebral optical spectroscopy for monitoring cerebral oxygen delivery and hemodynamics. Crit Care Med 19:89–97, 1991

Nierman DM: Core temperature measurement in the intensive care unit. Crit Care Med 19:818–823, 1991

Rosenwasser RH, Kleiner LI: Intracranial pressure monitoring in the posterior fossa: A preliminary report. J Neurosurg 71:503–505, 1989

Hypothermia

Clemmer TP, Fisher CJ, et al: Hypothermia in the sepsis syndrome and clinical outcome. Crit Care Med 20:1395–1401, 1992

Lawson LL: Hypothermia and trauma injury: Temperature monitoring and rewarming strategies. Critical Care Nursing Quarterly 15(1):21–32, 1992

Lennon RL, Hosking MP, et al: Evaluation of a forced-air system for warming hypothermic postoperative patients. Anesth Analg 70:424–427, 1990

Nicholson RW, Iserson KV: Core temperature measurement in hypovolemic resuscitation. Ann Emerg Med 20:62–65, 1991

Nierman DM: Core temperature measurement in the intensive care unit. Crit Care Med 19:818–823, 1991

Piek J, Chesnut R, et al: Extracranial complications of severe head injury. J Neurosurg 77:901–907, 1992

Rohrer MJ, Natale AM: Effect of hypothermia on the coagulation cascade. Crit Care Med 20:1402–1405, 1992

STUDY QUESTIONS

Intracranial Pressure Monitoring

1. Cerebral perfusion pressure (CPP)

   a. often increases with suctioning
   b. provides a clinical estimate of cerebral blood flow
   c. has a normal range of 11 to 15 mm Hg
   d. is the difference between the systolic and diastolic ICP

2. Initial treatment for increased intracranial pressure usually includes which of the following?

   a. craniectomy
   b. induced barbiturate coma
   c. pancuronium or curare
   d. diuretics, hyperventilation, and CSF drainage

3. Normal intracranial pressure is

   a. 50 to 60 mm Hg
   b. 0 to 15 mm Hg
   c. 20 to 40 cm of water
   d. approximately the same as mean systemic arterial blood pressure

4. Induced barbiturate coma

   a. should be preceded by ICP, blood pressure, pulmonary artery pressure, ECG monitoring, baseline recordings, and assisted ventilation
   b. produces the same clinical results as the use of pancuronium
   c. usually is initiated shortly after the patient's ICP exceeds 15 mm Hg
   d. contraindicates the use of hypothermia

5. Nursing measures that may prevent or reduce IICP include which of the following?

   a. frequent suctioning with aggressive hyperventilation
   b. flushing ICP line q1h and prn
   c. elimination of extracranial causes of IICP
   d. frequent turning and repositioning

6. Continuous-flush devices are not used for ICP monitoring because

   a. a small increase in the volume of fluid in the cranial vault of a decompensated patient may initiate herniation
   b. the infused flush solution is under too much pressure
   c. ICP may be greater than 300 mm Hg
   d. of high infection risk

7. Advantages of the intraventricular techniques include

   a. intact dura
   b. cerebrum not invaded
   c. the ability to drain CSF and do volume pressure responses
   d. the suitability for use in all neurosurgical patients

8. Plateau waves, also known as "A" waves

   a. may indicate decreased intracranial compliance
   b. are a preterminal sign
   c. usually have a duration of less than 5 minutes
   d. have no clinical significance

Hypothermia

1. Hypothermia may

   1. be induced or unintentional (accidental)
   2. provide cellular protection from ischemic injury
   3. cause hemoconcentration with an increased risk of embolization
   4. cause respiratory acidosis

      a. 1 and 2
      b. 2 and 3
      c. 3 and 4
      d. all of the above

2. Shivering

   1. is a compensatory response to maintain body heat
   2. increases oxygen consumption
   3. increases carbon dioxide production
   4. can result in hypoglycemia

      a. 1 and 2
      b. 2 only
      c. 2, 3, and 4
      d. all of the above

3. Rewarming shock

   1. can occur when hypothermia is terminated
   2. is associated with rapid rewarming
   3. involves a decrease in venous return and cardiac output caused by massive dilation of peripheral vessels
   4. usually can be avoided

      a. 1 and 2
      b. 2 and 3
      c. 3 and 4
      d. all of the above

CHAPTER 30

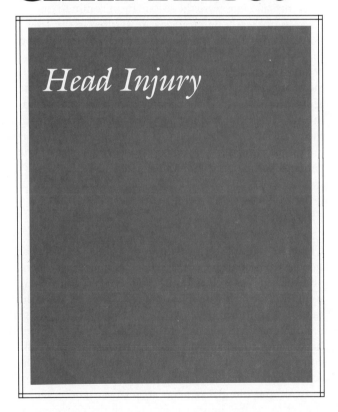

Head Injury

Hudak: Critical Care Nursing:
A Holistic Approach, 6th ed. © 1994
J. B. Lippincott Company.

BEHAVIORAL OBJECTIVES

Based on the content in this chapter, the reader should be able to:

1. Identify possible mechanisms of head injury associated with trauma.
2. Describe various types of head injuries and their associated symptomatology.
3. Explain the pathophysiologic process of potential patient problems resulting from head injuries.
4. Discuss the rationale for medical and nursing management in the therapy of the head-injured patient.

Description

Head injuries are among the most devastating and lethal catastrophes in humans. Of all cases of head injury in the United States in 1985, 49% were caused by motor vehicle accidents, and falls were the second most common cause.[1] Head injury was found to occur most often in the 15- to 24-year-old age group and to occur twice as often in men than in women.[2] The critical care nurse is in a central position to understand the psychological and physiological changes that head-injured patients undergo in the acute care setting. The nursing process uniquely helps the nurse identify nursing diagnoses and collaborate with the physician and other health care team members to focus on specific therapies based on the consequences of the patient's pathologic condition.

Descriptive Terms

There are multiple terms used to describe or classify patients with head injures. In earlier years, the terms "open" and "closed," as well as "coup" and "contra coup" were used. But the terms are misleading if used to describe the degree of injury severity. An "open" head injury could be a scalp laceration or a bullet through the brain. A "closed" head injury could apply equally to a patient with a mild concussion as to one with diffuse cerebral edema. The terms "coup" and "contra coup" describe the location of most of the internal damage in relation to the site of impact. A "coup" injury causes most of the damage relatively close to the impact site, whereas in a "contra coup" injury the damage is opposite to the site of impacting forces (Fig. 30–1). The Traumatic Coma Data Bank is a multinational effort begun in 1979 to gather data about the frequency of head injuries, their classification, and the role of therapy on outcome. The severity of head injury now is defined by the Traumatic Coma Data Bank on the basis of the Glasgow Coma Scale score (Table 30–1). The terms minor, moderate, and severe head injury are useful in relating assessment parameters to therapy and outcome

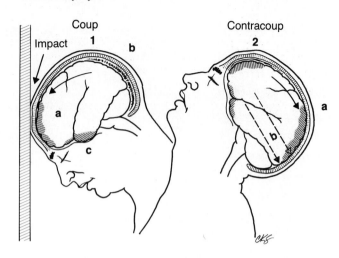

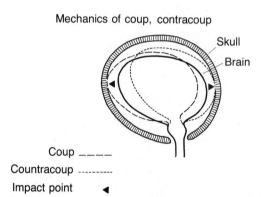

FIGURE 30–1
Coup and contrecoup head injury after blunt trauma. *1*, Coup injury: impact against object. *a*, Site of impact and direct trauma to brain; *b*, Shearing of subdural veins; *c*, Trauma to base of brain. *2*, Contrecoup injury: impact within skull. *a*, Site of impact from brain hitting opposite side of skull; *b*, Shearing forces throughout brain. These injuries occur in one continuous motion—the head strikes the wall (coup), then rebounds (contrecoup).

along a continuum of care. But the reader should not be misled into thinking a minor head injury will result in minor to absent problems for the patient. Such a patient may experience post-traumatic amnesia as well as memory problems that may significantly alter the patient's post-injury lifestyle.

Mechanisms of Injury

The mechanisms of injury play a large part in determining the pathophysiological consequences of head trauma. An acceleration injury occurs when a moving object strikes the stationary head, such as in a missile injury or one from a blunt object. A deceleration injury is one where the head strikes a relatively immobile object, such as an automobile frame or the ground. Both of these forces may occur together when there is sudden head movement without

TABLE 30–1
Categories Defining Head Injury Severity Based on Glascow Coma Scale (GCS) Score

Severity	Description	Frequency
Minor	GCS 13–15	55%
	May have loss of consciousness or amnesia but for less than 30 minutes.	
	No skull fracture, cerebral contusion, hematoma.	
Moderate	GCS 9–12	24%
	Loss of consciousness and/or amnesia occured for more than 30 minutes but less than 24 hours.	
	May have a skull fracture.	
Severe	GCS 3–8	21%
	Loss of consciousness and/or amnesia occured for more than 24 hours.	
	Also includes those with a cerebral contusion, laceration, or intracranial hematoma.	

direct contact, such as that produced when torso position is altered violently and rapidly. These forces may be combined with rotational displacement of the head, causing stretching and shearing injury to the white matter and the brain stem.

A primary injury, occurring at the time of impact, may be due to bruising on the brain surface, laceration of brain matter, or shearing injuries or hemorrhage. As a result, secondary injury may occur as cerebral autoregulatory ability is diminished or absent in the injured areas. The consequences include hyperemia (increased blood volume) in areas of increased capillary permeability, as well as arterial vasodilation, all leading to increased intracranial content and eventually increased intracranial pressure (ICP). Some conditions that may cause secondary brain injury include hypoxia, hypercarbia, and hypotension.[3]

Gennarelli and colleagues introduced "focal" and "diffuse" injuries as categories of severe head injuries in an attempt to trace outcome more specifically.[4] Focal injuries result from localized damage, including cerebral contusions and intracerebral hematomas, as well as secondary brain damage caused by expanding mass lesions, brain shifts, and herniation. Diffuse brain injuries are associated with more widespread damage and occur in four forms: diffuse axonal injury, hypoxic brain damage, diffuse brain swelling, and multiple small hemorrhages throughout the brain. These types of injury cause coma not by compression of the brain stem but by diffuse injury to the cerebral hemispheres, the brain stem, or both, a situation that occurs in almost 50% of patients who have sustained a severe nonmissile head injury.[5]

Specific Head–Brain Injuries

Skull Fracture

The arrangement of the layers of the skull along with the scalp help to dissipate energy from a head impact so that less force is transmitted to the brain surface. Nevertheless, skull fractures are common in severely head-injured patients, although the incidence varies from 12% to 80%, depending on the study reported. In general, children seem less susceptible than adults. Skull fractures occur in various patterns. *Linear fractures* are the most common and are caused by the application of forces over a relatively wide area of the skull.[6]

Basilar skull fractures may be limited to the floor of the skull or occur in association with fractures of the cranial vault, such as parts of the frontal or temporal bones. Fractures of the base of the skull are serious in that they may lead to contact between the cerebrospinal fluid (CSF) in the subarachnoid space and the air-containing sinuses of the face or skull. This communication may allow CSF to leak out through the sinus passages to the nose or ears and also allow bacteria contained within the sinus drainage to contaminate the spinal fluid.

Depressed skull fractures are caused by forces driving bone fragments downward toward the brain deeper than the thickness of the skull itself. These fractures are associated with laceration of the dura or brain in 60% of cases and with scalp lacerations in 90% of cases.

Cerebral Concussion

A concussion is a syndrome involving a mild form of diffuse brain injury. It is a temporary and reversible neurologic dysfunction with or without loss of consciousness. If there is loss of consciousness, it may be for a few seconds or minutes. Thereafter the patient may be disoriented and confused for a short period of time. Other symptoms include headache, inability to concentrate, memory problems, dizziness, and irritability. Some suffer a period of post-traumatic amnesia. Most patients recover completely and quickly, but a few develop postconcussion syndrome and may have continued symptoms for several months.

Cerebral Contusion

Cerebral contusion describes an area of the brain that is "bruised" without being punctured or lacerated. The bruise generally is on the surface and composed of an area of small hemorrhage that is diffused throughout the brain substance in that area, rather than being in one discrete location. Cerebral contusion is the most frequently seen lesion after head injury. The signs and symptoms of contusions vary, depending on the location and degree. There may be small, localized contusions resulting in focal neurologic deficits or there may be larger areas involved. These larger areas may expand over 2 to 3 days after the injury and create widespread dysfunctions as a result of increasing cerebral edema. It is this larger contused area that produces a mass effect seen on computed tomography scanning and may cause profound changes in ICP, raising the mortality rate to as high as 45%.

Epidural Hematoma

Epidural hematoma is an accumulation of blood in the space between the inner table of the skull and the outermost layer of meninges, the dura (Fig. 30–2). Such hematomas occur because of tearing of small branches of the middle meningeal artery or the frontal meningeal artery. Approximately 85% are associated with a linear skull fracture, usually of the temporal bone just in front and above the ear, which disturbs the artery imbedded in shallow depressions of the inner skull table. The incidence varies from 2% to 3% up to 9% in severely injured patients.[6] Patients with epidural hematoma compose a large group of those in the "talk and die" category. The "classic" signs and symptoms include a brief loss of consciousness at the time of impact followed by a relatively lucid period of minutes to hours. This "talk" period is then followed by rapid neurologic deterioration from confusion to coma, from purposeful movement to decorticate or decerebrate posturing, and from equal pupils to anisocoria. These all are signs of rapid herniation and must be treated quickly to prevent the patient's death.[7]

Subdural Hematoma

A subdural hematoma is an accumulation of blood below the dural meningeal layer and above the arachnoid covering of the brain (Fig. 30–3). The cause usually is tearing of surface veins or dislodgment of pools of venous blood (called "sinuses") that are found in this area. It often is associated with an underlying cerebral contusion from acceleration–deceleration and rotational forces of impact. Two adult patient groups in which this injury is seen more frequently are the elderly and alcoholics. Both groups have frequent falls in common as well as some degree of cortical atrophy that puts the bridging vein structure leading from the brain surface under more tension. Although blood in the subdural space is common to all types, subdural hematomas are classified as acute, subacute, and chronic based on the time from injury to symptom onset.

Patients with acute subdural hematoma manifest symptoms within 24 to 48 hours after injury. The manifestations

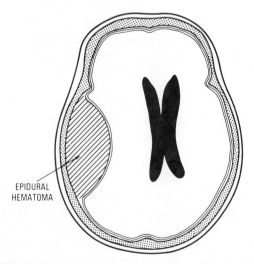

EPIDURAL
HEMATOMA

FIGURE 30–2
A large epidural hematoma showing the typical lenticular (lens) shape (Marshall SB, Marshall LF, et al: Neuroscience Critical Care, p 174. Philadelphia, WB Saunders, 1990).

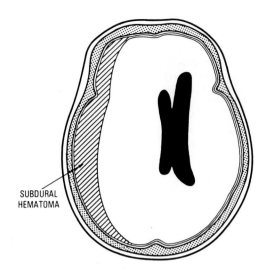

FIGURE 30–3
A large acute subdural hematoma covering the entire hemisphere and compressing the ipsilateral ventricle (Marshall SB, Marshall LF, et al: Neuroscience Critical Care, p 175. Philadelphia, WB Saunders, 1990).

are those of an expanding mass lesion and rapidly increasing ICP (IICP) and require emergent intervention. Patients with subacute subdural hematomas have clinical symptoms from 2 days to 2 weeks after injury. The onset of symptoms is slower and often more innocuous than in acute hematoma. The patients usually do not deteriorate to the point of herniation or brain stem compression.

Chronic subdural hematomas occur from 2 weeks to 3 to 4 months after the initial injury. The initial hemorrhage may be quite small. Within 1 week or so after the hemorrhage, the clot develops a fibrous membrane that encapsulates it. Further expansion of the mass occurs with slow capillary leaking, causing symptoms once it becomes large enough to put pressure on surrounding structures. Common symptoms include headache, lethargy, confusion, seizures, and occasionally dysphasia. If surgical intervention is required in the case of hematoma expansion and worsening symptoms, a craniotomy usually is required to remove both the fibrous capsule and the "jam-like" hematoma within. Drains may be placed in the bed of the hematoma and after surgery the head of the patient's bed may be ordered to be *flat* for the first 24 hours. This facilitates re-expansion of the brain, which may have been compressed for several weeks.

Intracerebral Hematoma

An intracerebral hematoma is a collection of blood 25 ml or more within the brain parenchyma. It is difficult to distinguish radiologically from a brain contusion with bleeding deep within the brain substance itself.[8] Traumatic causes include depressed skull fractures, penetrating missile injuries, and sudden acceleration–deceleration

movements. Treatment of patients with intracerebral hematomas is controversial as to whether surgery is indicated or medical management is the best course. In general, surgical intervention is used only if the lesion is continuing to expand and cause further neurologic deterioration.

Pathophysiological Principles

Breathing Patterns

Because the neurophysiology of respiration is so complex, a neurologic insult could produce problems at any number of levels. Numerous locations in both cerebral hemispheres regulate voluntary control over the muscles used in breathing, with the cerebellum synchronizing and coordinating the muscular effort. The cerebrum also has some control over the rate and rhythm of respiration. Nuclei in the pons and midbrain areas of the brain stem regulate the automaticity of respiration. Cells in these areas are responsive to small changes in pH and oxygen content of surrounding blood and tissues.

These centers can be injured by IICP and hypoxia as well as by direct trauma or interruption of blood supply. Cerebral trauma that alters the level of consciousness usually results in alveolar hypoventilation due to shallow respirations. These factors ultimately can lead to respiratory failure, which accounts for a high mortality rate among head-injured patients. Different respiratory patterns can be identified when there is an intracranial dysfunction (Fig. 30–4).

Cheyne–Stokes breathing is periodic breathing in which the depth of each breath increases to a peak and then decreases to a state of apnea. The hyperpneic phase usually lasts longer than the apneic phase. Cheyne–Stokes breathing patterns may be a normal result of aging when they occur in an older person during sleep. The pattern also may be seen with bilateral lesions located deep in the cerebral hemispheres. With traumatic brain injury, the onset of Cheyne–Stokes breathing might be due to herniation of the cerebral hemispheres through the tentorium, indicating a deteriorating neurologic condition. This herniation also can cause compression of the midbrain, and *central neurogenic hyperventilation* will be observed. This hyperventilation is sustained, regular, rapid, and fairly deep. It usually is caused by a lesion above the midbrain.

Apneustic breathing is characterized by respiration with a long pause at full inspiration or full expiration. The etiology of this pattern is loss of all cerebral and cerebellar control of breathing, with respiratory function at a brain stem level only.

Cluster breathing may be seen when the lesion is high in the medulla or low in the pons. This pattern of respiration is seen as gasping breaths with irregular pauses.

The critical centers of inspiration and expiration are located in the medulla oblongata. Any rapidly expanding

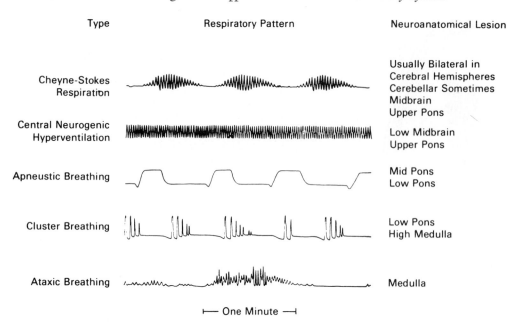

Type	Respiratory Pattern	Neuroanatomical Lesion
Cheyne-Stokes Respiration		Usually Bilateral in Cerebral Hemispheres Cerebellar Sometimes Midbrain Upper Pons
Central Neurogenic Hyperventilation		Low Midbrain Upper Pons
Apneustic Breathing		Mid Pons Low Pons
Cluster Breathing		Low Pons High Medulla
Ataxic Breathing		Medulla

├── One Minute ──┤

FIGURE 30–4
Respiratory patterns in neurologic dysfunctions (Gifford RRM, Plaut MR: Abnormal respiratory patterns in the comatose patient caused by intracranial dysfunction. J Neurosurg Nurs 7:58, 1975).

intracranial lesion, such as cerebellar hemorrhage, can compress the medulla, and *ataxic breathing* will result. This is totally irregular breathing consisting of both deep and shallow breaths associated with irregular pauses. When this pattern of respiration occurs, a ventilator should be available because neither respiratory rhythm nor continuation of respiration can be predicted.

Interference with some cranial nerves also can influence respiration. The brain stem centers receive information from chemoreceptors in the carotid artery and aorta and from stretch receptors in the lungs by way of the glossopharyngeal (IX) and the vagus (X) nerves. Outgoing information from the brain stem then travels by way of the phrenic nerve, which leaves the spinal cord with the third cervical nerve and activates the diaphragm. The intercostal muscles that expand the chest wall are activated by the intracostal nerves of the thoracic spinal cord.

Impaired Physical Mobility

A major result of severe brain injury can be its effect on body movement. Hemiparesis or hemiplegia may occur as a result of damage to the motor areas of the brain. In addition, the patient may have voluntary control over movements yet encounter difficulties in self-care and daily living related to abnormal posturing, spasticity, or contractures. Nursing interventions should be based on an assessment of the patient's motor functioning and impact on living patterns.

Voluntary movement occurs as a result of the synaps-

ing of two large groups of neurons. Nerve cells in the first group originate in the posterior portion of each frontal lobe, called the precentral gyrus, or "motor strip." Axons from these "upper" motor neurons terminate either in the brain stem or in the anterior gray horns at various levels in the spinal cord. Here they synapse with "lower" motor neurons, which travel from the brain stem or spinal cord to specific muscles. Each of these neuron groups transmits particular information on movement. Thus, the patient will exhibit specific symptoms if either of these two neuron pathways is injured (Table 30–2).

With bilateral hemispheric dysfunction or with dysfunction at the brain stem level, there is loss of cerebral inhibition of involuntary movements. There are disorders of muscle tone and the appearance of abnormal postures, which, in time, can create complications such as increased spasticity and contractures.

Hydration Balance

Nearly all severely head-injured patients will have a problem with maintenance of a balanced hydration state. For some, it will be a self-limiting response to the stress of trauma. In a physiological stress state, more antidiuretic hormone (ADH) and more aldosterone are produced, resulting in fluid and sodium retention. The process usually reverses itself within a day or two, when diuresis occurs.

In some patients with neurologic trauma—especially those with skull fractures, damage to the pituitary or

TABLE 30–2
A Comparison of Upper and Lower Motor Neuron Function

Neuron	Pathway/Names	Functions	Signs of Dysfunction

Neuron group no. 1, or "upper" motor neurons	From motor area of cerebral cortex to brain stem (corticobulbar tracts) or to spinal cord (corticospinal tracts)	Carries commands for voluntary movement of specific body parts
		Carries inhibition commands to control the response of the next neuron pathway
			Loss of voluntary muscle control
			Loss of inhibition of lower motor neurons, resulting in:
			  Preservation of reflex arcs
			  Pathologic reflex responses
			  Spastic muscles
			  Increased muscle tone
			  Little or no muscle atrophy

Neuron group no. 2, or "lower" motor neurons	From brain stem or spinal cord to specific muscle groups; names end in the word "nerve" (eg, femoral nerve, radial nerve)	Relays commands from the upper motor neurons to effect voluntary muscle movement
		Forms the effector response branch of the reflex arc
			Loss of voluntary muscle movement
			No reflex arc activity, resulting in:
			  Flaccid muscles
			  No pathologic reflex responses
			  Decreased muscle tone
			  Significant muscle atrophy

hypothalamus, or IICP—the clinical picture may be complicated by *diabetes insipidus*. In this condition, there is a dysfunction in the production and storage of ADH, with a subsequent decrease in the amount of ADH present in the blood. Without ADH, the kidneys excrete too much water, leading to dehydration. The same cerebral pathologic condition sometimes leads to an opposite problem of ADH being produced in excess of the body's needs. This *syndrome of inappropriate ADH (SIADH)* is characterized by fluid retention and consequent hemodilution (Table 30–3). See Chapter 41 for a discussion of SIADH and diabetes insipidus.

The Swallowing Act

Adequate nutrition plays a primary role in recovery from illness and often is neglected. A state of catabolism and negative nitrogen balance is a common finding in head-injured patients. Standard intravenous solutions generally are inadequate to prevent this problem. In addition, the body's demand for energy and substrates for repair and growth can cause breakdown of body proteins at an accelerated rate.

The acts of chewing and swallowing are integrated at the brain stem level through a complex feedback system involving multiple motor and sensory branches of several cranial nerves. For the most part, this is a reflex response to the presence of something in the mouth and pharynx.

Higher centers in the cerebral cortex, cerebellum, and basal ganglia participate in the speed and coordination of this reflex.

Swallowing is a three-stage process that begins with placement of food in the mouth. Solids are masticated and mixed with saliva to a softer consistency. In the oral stage, the tongue controls a bolus of food or liquid by pressing it against the soft palate and forming a seal around it (Fig. 30–5A). There is a respiratory pause on inspiration as the larynx moves up and forward to close and protect the airway. The seal around the bolus is broken as the soft palate elevates and closes the nasopharynx to prevent nasal regurgitation.

In the pharyngeal stage, with the soft palate elevated and the airway occluded, the tongue propels the bolus back against the posterior pharyngeal wall (see Figure 30–5B). The muscles of the pharynx contract sequentially to move the bolus downward, forcing the epiglottis closed over the tracheal opening (see Figure 30–5C). The cricopharyngeal sphincter relaxes and opens in the esophageal stage as the bolus of food enters the esophagus (see Figure 30–5D). Waves of peristalsis carry the bolus downward toward the stomach.

Disorders of the motor and sensory areas of the cerebral hemispheres impair the ability to detect the presence of food in the affected side of the mouth and to manipulate it by cheek and tongue movements. In addition, the brain stem reflexes of swallowing may be either hyperactive or diminished to absent. The functional result is choking,

TABLE 30–3
A Comparison of Diabetes Insipidus and the Syndrome of Inappropriate ADH Secretion

	Diabetes Insipidus (DI)	Syndrome of Inappropriate ADH (SIADH)
Clinical manifestations	Increased thirst drive in the awake patient Polyuria, usually more than 5 L/day Urine specific gravity 1.001 to 1.005 Volume depletion, as evidenced by slightly elevated hematocrit and serum sodium levels	Lethargy and confusion, leading to coma and seizures Decreased urine output, usually less than 500 ml/day Urine specific gravity usually greater than 1.025 Hemodilution, as evidence by decreased hematocrit and hyponatremia
Medical therapy	Appropriate fluid replacement PO or IV or both Supplemental ADH therapy using injectable pitressin or nasal spray solutions of desmopressin (DDAVP)	Fluid restriction Furosemide diuretics Drug therapy with demeclocycline hydrochloride (Declomycin), which blocks the effect of ADH on the kidney

ADH, antidiuretic hormone.

ineffective or absent coughing, and aspiration of food or fluid.

Communication Ability

The patient with cerebral trauma who presents with a breakdown in communication abilities is not alone. This dysfunction is the most frequently occurring handicap in head-injured persons. Such an impairment results from the combined effects of disorganized and confused language processing and specific aphasic disorders, if present.

Patients who have sustained injury to certain areas of the dominant cerebral hemisphere may evidence dysphasia, the loss of the ability to use language in some or all of its forms (Fig. 30–6). Language is the entire system of symbols that we learn as children to communicate efficiently with one another. This language system consists of

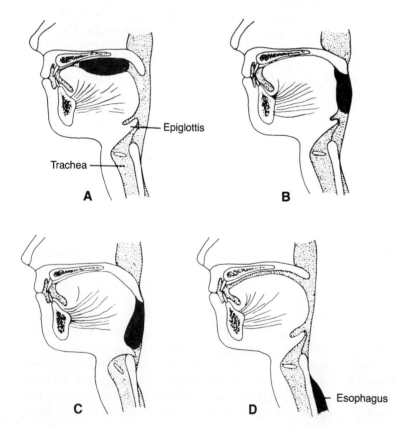

FIGURE 30–5
Stages of normal swallowing or deglutition (Mitchell PH, Cammermeyer M et al: Neurological Assessment for Nursing Practice. Reston, VA, Reston Publishing, 1984).

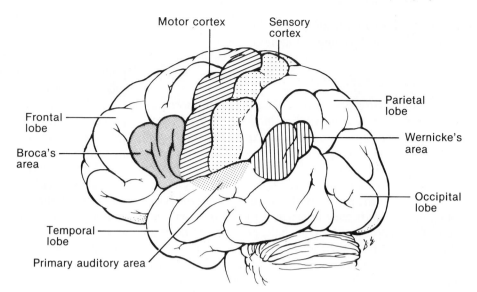

FIGURE 30–6
Cerebrocortical areas involved in communication. The frontal lobe contains the motor cortex, which controls voluntary movement, and Broca's area, which controls the output of language. The primary auditory cortex and Wernicke's area, which control comprehension of spoken and written language, are located in the temporal lobe. The occipital lobe contains the primary visual area, which serves to interpret written language and visual input.

our ability to interpret what sounds we hear as words, of the letters and numbers we learn to read and write to communicate without drawing detailed pictures of our environment, and of our ability to produce certain sounds to convey thoughts to other people. Speech is merely the sounds we make with our mouths to convey language.

Assessment and Management

Respiratory Problems

The patient should be positioned on the side or in the coma position (Fig. 30–7). Care must be taken to avoid extreme neck flexion because both the airway and ICP may be compromised. An oral airway may be used to prevent obstruction of the upper airway by the tongue. Frequent position changes or use of a rotokinetic bed will help prevent pooled secretions in dependent lung fields.

The nurse should assess the patient's respiratory rate and effort, as well as skin color, breath sounds, and chest expansion. If an abnormality is encountered, arterial blood gases (ABGs) should be measured to evaluate the effectiveness of ventilation. When suctioning is required, the patient should be hyperoxygenated before, during, and after the procedure so that secondary brain injury due to

hypoxia and IICP is minimized.[9] In addition, suctioning through the nasopharynx should be avoided in a patient with suspected basilar skull fracture.

The very critically ill head-injured patient may be managed initially on a ventilator. In such cases it frequently is not possible to determine a particular respiratory pattern or a definite rhythm or rate of respiration of the patient's own. One item of new technology that is increasingly useful in monitoring such patients is capnography. Capnography is the measurement and graphic display of the carbon dioxide level appearing at the airway entrance. A portable technology using infrared spectroscopy compares the amount of infrared light absorbed by a sample of patient gas to the amount of light absorbed in a chamber containing no carbon dioxide. This technology allows an approximation of the alveolar CO_2 and can be useful as an early warning device that ABGs need to be monitored so as to maintain arterial CO_2 levels within the desired range.

Mobility Problems

It is easier to "mold" a patient's posture and muscle tone early postinjury. Proper positioning helps inhibit abnormal tone and allows for easier handling by the physical and

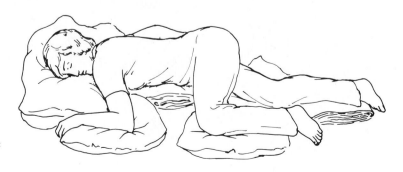

FIGURE 30–7
Positioning to reduce risk of aspiration. Shoulders are turned almost prone for better drainage of the oral and nasal passages.

occupational therapists and nurses who are helping the patient maintain full range of motion.

Abnormal Posturing

Most common in the brain-injured patient is opisthotonic posturing. This is a forward arching of the back and hyperextension of the head with all extremities rigid and straight or hyperextended. This posturing is exaggerated when the patient is supine. Trunk rotation and flexion of the lower extremities will help break up this posturing (Fig. 30–8). If the patient is left flat on the back with legs out straight, an increase in extensor muscle tone will be seen. Turning the hips to a side-lying position and flexing the knees will relax the tone.

Head positioning is important because of an asymmetrical tonic neck reflex. This reflex is demonstrated when the extremities on the same side to which the head is turned extend and the opposite extremities flex. Therefore, the nurse who is attempting to do range-of-motion exercises on a tightly drawn-up arm should try turning the head to that side and see whether the muscle tone decreases.

Each brain-injured patient will have different reflexive positioning, and the nurse must evaluate what positions can be accomplished. The goal of effective positioning is to break up reflexive patterns and decrease abnormal muscle tone.

Contractures

Passive range of motion is used to stretch muscles and to maintain joint mobility. With the immobile patient, the nurse should move each joint through its normal range of motion on a regular basis. The activity is accomplished easily during a bath. When limited joint mobility occurs due to increased muscle tone, "splinting" the joint in a functional position may help the patient regain lost range of motion.

Splints may be made of a variety of materials (plaster, acrylic) and padded to prevent skin irritation. Use of pillows or large foam pads is an easy and effective way to splint larger joints such as the knee or elbow. Extend the patient's extremity as far as possible and place two or more pillows or foam pads longitudinally across the affected joint. Secure in place tightly with an elastic bandage. The pillow splints may be left in place for up to an hour at a time if adequate circulation is not compromised. With proper use of splinting, range of motion in joints of the extremities can be increased and functional positioning maintained.

With a tight hand grip, either voluntary or involuntary, a cone can be used to decrease the development of hand contractures. Pressure on the insertion of a muscle inhibits muscle contraction; thus, use of a hand cone instead of a soft washcloth actually can cause relaxation of the hand and maintain normal functioning.

Skin Breakdown

With loss of motor function, the brain-injured patient is vulnerable to skin breakdown. The unconscious patient, and anyone who is immobilized, is prone to skin problems because of pressure, moisture, shearing forces, and diminished sensation.

One major rule must be followed to maintain skin integrity: prevent pressure. With current technology, numerous tools can help achieve this goal. Beds are available that distribute the patient's body weight evenly over the skin while giving support on a cushion of air. Beds are designed to change pressure areas constantly by keeping the patient in continual motion from side to side. Other beds facilitate turning while maintaining body alignment. There also are numerous items to be placed on a bed to make pressure less of a problem, such as alternating pressure air mattresses, water mattresses, gel pads, and sheepskins. The fact remains, however, that pressure sores can develop over time in an immobile patient who is not turned regularly, no matter what mattress is used. Each patient must be evaluated individually as to skin tolerance (how fast the skin turns red without the patient being turned). The average skin-pressure tolerance time for an acutely ill patient is less than 2 hours.

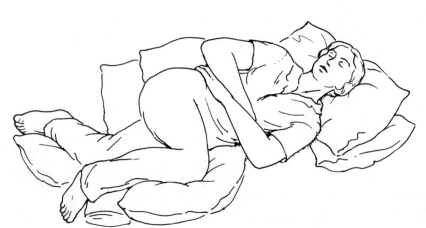

FIGURE 30–8
Positioning to relax extensor muscle tone in brain-injured patients. This position uses trunk rotation and lower extremity flexion to relax abnormal muscle tone.

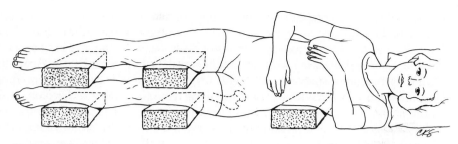

FIGURE 30–9
Positioning the patient in bed: side-lying position. Pads are used above and below the trochanter and lateral malleolus to relieve pressure.

Another technique that can help prevent pressure problems is the use of padding above and below prominent bony processes. For example, when the patient is on the side, the nurse can place a rectangular foam pad or small pillow above and below the hip trochanter and above the lateral malleolus of the ankle. Padding also should be placed between bony pressure points such as the knees (Fig. 30–9). The nurse should place a hand under the bony processes to confirm that pressure has been relieved. When the patient is on his or her back, the nurse should place a pad above and below the sacrum and above the heels (Fig. 30–10). Circular pads called "doughnuts" actually may impair circulation by causing circular pressure around the protected area. Use of rectangular pads allows for collateral circulation while relieving pressure. The pads should be made of firm, open-cell foam rather than rolled towels or blankets. They should be soft enough to redistribute the patient's weight evenly over a large area. Rolled towels or blankets apply pressure to only a narrow section of skin.

Skin massage with lotion is helpful in stimulating circulation to a pressure area, but the skin should be dried carefully because moisture can lead to irritation.

Another prime cause of a breakdown in skin integrity is the shearing effect of linen against skin. A lift sheet (folded draw-sheet or bath blanket) should be used to maneuver the patient in the bed. To shield the patient's elbows and heels, soft foam or sheepskin protectors should be used.

Hydration State Problems

Accurate measurement of intake and output and evaluations of changes in weight from day to day are essential to the assessment of fluid balance. The nurse also should assess the patient's skin and mucous membranes for drying and cracking, which predispose to further injury. Close observation of the patient's cardiovascular status is required with evaluation of the trends in vital signs, central venous pressure, pulmonary artery pressure, and cardiac output. In view of the alterations in fluid balance from trauma and the added effect of diuretic therapy, the critical care nurse must be vigilant for problems that could lead to a secondary neurologic injury.

Swallowing Problems

Factors to Consider Before Initiation of Oral Intake

Nursing literature supports the fact that inadequate nutrition is one of the head-injured patient's most significant outcomes. A 12% loss in body weight is common.[10]

Swallowing Ability
Swallowing ability should be evaluated and determined to be adequate without danger of aspiration. The most effective evaluation technique is fluoroscopy of a barium swal-

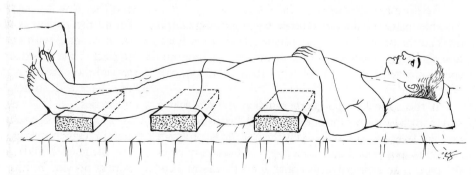

FIGURE 30–10
Positioning the patient in bed: supine position. Pads are used above and below the sacrum and above the heels to relieve pressure. A pad above the knees prevents hyperextension of the knees and relieves pressure on the popliteal space.

low recorded on videotape (videofluoroscopy) or movie film (cinefluoroscopy), with the patient in an upright position. Anteroposterior and lateral views of the passage of barium in the swallowing sequence readily reveal swallowing dysfunctions, such as poor tongue control, difficulty in initiation of the swallow, nasopharyngeal regurgitation, pharyngeal retention, inadequate relaxation of the cricopharyngeal area, or aspiration into the larynx. If cinefluoroscopy or videofluoroscopy demonstrates significant aspiration, an oral intake program is contraindicated.

Swallowing function may be evaluated by subjective observation as well, and in some settings this may be the only method available. Many patients will swallow reflexively with tactile stimulation around the mouth. The examiner can assess the swallowing reflex by feeling the thyroid notch for upward movement of the larynx. Swallowing can be stimulated by applying gentle upward pressure with the fingers and having the patient flex his or her head forward.

Observation of lip closure and tongue mobility will provide information about the adequacy of the oral stage of swallowing. Drooling is indicative of poor tongue control or decreased oral sensation, or both. Slurred speech or a weak voice or both are indications of impairment in the orolaryngeal musculature, which may impair swallowing ability as well.

Some patients also demonstrate primitive oral reflexes with stimulation of the oral area. These are the same reflexes that a newborn has and usually are controlled by higher brain centers by the age of 1 year. The patient's brain injury has removed the inhibitory control mechanisms of the higher brain centers, and, consequently, the primitive brain stem reflexes are released.

The most easily observed primitive oral reflexes are a suckling pattern (a repetitive forward, upward, and backward movement of the tongue usually followed by a swallow), chewing (rhythmic chewing motions without jaw closure), and biting (jaw closure and holding when the area between the teeth or the gums is stimulated). Such reflexes can be incorporated into an oral feeding program if other considerations have been met.

Respiratory Status

Another major consideration before the beginning of oral intake is the patient's respiratory status. Respiratory function should be adequate with a small metal Jackson tracheostomy tube (size 4 or below), a Kistner button, or a normal airway.

If the patient's respiratory function is such that a cuffed tracheostomy tube or a Jackson tracheostomy tube, size 5 or larger, is required, ideally the oral intake program should be postponed because a large tracheostomy gives the patient an artificial airway that alters the normal coordination of respiration and swallowing. It is impossible to cough through the vocal cords with an inflated cuff. Even with the cuff deflated, cough strength through the cords is decreased significantly owing to the large diame-

ter of the tracheostomy tube. The tracheostomy tube can limit upward and forward movement of the larynx because the tube itself anchors the trachea to the muscles and skin of the neck. Regurgitation and aspiration into the larynx may result from compression of the cervical esophagus by the tracheostomy tube.

The larger tracheostomy tubes with inflated cuffs cause even more compression of the esophagus; food or secretions may overflow and rest above the inflated cuff, and pressures from the swallow itself force liquids and even semisolids around the cuff into the trachea.

Consequently, larger tracheostomy tubes are a negative factor in attempts to reestablish swallowing function. In many settings, however, the physician prefers establishing a safe swallow before the removal of the cuffed tracheostomy tube. If this is the case, evaluation is preferred with the cuff deflated. For patients with tracheostomy tubes, a saliva test can be done at bedside to rule out aspiration. A small amount of diluted food coloring is given by mouth (blue is preferred). If colored mucus appears through the tracheostomy tube, aspiration is present and the patient cannot safely begin oral intake.

Cough Strength

The final consideration is evaluation of cough strength. The patient should demonstrate a cough reflex adequate for protection of the airway. A weak cough will not clear the airway in the event of aspiration, and thus the patient should not be started on oral intake.

Swallowing Retraining

During training for the reestablishment of oral intake, the patient is positioned best in bed or a chair from 45° to 90° upright, with the neck slightly flexed. Care should be taken not to extend the neck, because this makes upward movement of the larynx (to protect the airway from aspiration) more difficult. The ideal environment is free from distracting noises and movements for more effective concentration on the swallowing process.

Often the physician will order clear liquids for the initial oral trial. Thin liquids are affected easily by gravity, and they flow through the mouth and pharynx quickly, before the patient is able to initiate a swallow. Consequently, solids with a clear liquid base, such as gelatin and popsicles, are a better choice because they can be controlled more easily in the mouth. Small ice chips can be used to provide stimulation to the oral cavity and swallowing reflex.

Food should be chosen to provide maximum stimulation in temperature, taste, color, and texture, when possible. Bland tastes and lukewarm temperatures (eg, tepid tap water) provide minimal stimulation to the patient and should be avoided in the initial stages, especially for patients with a reduced level of awareness. Milk products should be avoided as well because they cause excess mucus production (Table 30–4).

TABLE 30–4
Stages of Swallowing Retraining

	Nursing Responsibility	Speech Responsibility	Diet
Stage "0"			
Patient dependent on tube feedings for total fluid and calorie intake	Coordinates tube feedings. Monitors intake and output.	Initiates assessment. Begins oral stimulation techniques.	NPO
Stage I			
Introduction of foods; patient on tube feedings	Coordinates tube feedings in conjunction with treatment sessions by speech therapist (ie, tube feedings after treatment sessions).	Continues oral stimulation techniques. Diet advanced in progressions as tolerated. Instruct nursing personnel in specific treatment techniques for follow through.	Ice chips Slushes Pudding Applesauce Frozen yogurt
Stage II			
Puree with supplemental tube feedings	Monitor and record calorie and fluid intake to determine supplemental feedings.	Supervise one meal daily. Evaluate patient abilities. Apply therapy techniques. Record information on patient status reports.	Puree Soft cooked egg Cooked cereal Puree meat Puree fruit Plain yogurt Puddings Custards
Stage III			
Puree food with or without supplemental tube feedings	Monitor calorie and fluid intake. Supervise meals and actually feed patient.	Apply therapy. Instruct nursing personnel in techniques for meal supervision and actual feeding.	Puree, same as stage II
Stage IV			
Soft food; all calories through oral feedings	Supervise 1 to 3 meals daily.	Supervise 1 to 3 meals daily prn. Instruct nursing personnel in therapy techniques. Reevaluate for progression to stage V. Reevaluate ability to swallow thin liquids safely.	Cooked cereals Cottage cheese Ground meat (moist) Cook vegetables Casseroles Mashed canned fruit Banana Strained cream soup Liquids, if safe
Stage V			
Advance to soft or regular diet based on evaluation of test trays	Supervise all meals.	Reevaluate patient abilities for progression of food and fluid consistency. Discharge patient from program.	*Chopped* All eggs, cereals, ground meat, bread, potatoes, chopped fruits, creamed pie *Mechanical Soft* Ground meats Soft fruits, vegetables *Regular Diet* No restrictions

Techniques used during an oral intake session depend on the patient's individual swallowing pattern, but some *general suggestions* apply to most patients. It is important to verbalize the entire process to the patient, even if understanding is questionable. The food or liquid should be described in terms of taste, smell, and appearance. The swallowing process is emphasized with comments such as "Move your tongue," "Push that food back," "Hold your breath," and "Swallow." The food is introduced as far posteriorly in the mouth as possible with firm downward pressure from the spoon. Metal spoons always should be used because plastic spoons can break and shatter easily, especially if the patient has a biting reflex. For the patient who cannot open his or her mouth voluntarily, pressure should be applied on the chin just below the lower lip. Stroking the "V-shaped" muscle under the chin (without crossing the midline) also stimulates mouth opening, as does gentle pressure with a swab or spoon inside the lower lip.

For *hemiplegic patients* with unilateral sensory or motor impairment of the face, food and liquid should be placed in the mouth on the intact side. Also, swallowing efficiency can be improved if the patient's head is tilted slightly to the intact side so gravity will direct the food or liquid to the area of normal sensory and motor function. "Pocketing" of food in the impaired side of the mouth is characteristic of hemiplegic patients, and they need to be reminded to clear food from the mouth on both sides. After a meal, it is important to check the oral cavity carefully and clear any residual food that may have lodged in the impaired side.

The *amount per swallow* initially is small, approximately 5 ml or less. Patients with poor tongue control lose food in the sides of the mouth. The food or liquid also can drop into the airway before the initiation of the swallow, causing choking. Large amounts may not be evacuated completely after the first swallow. The food remaining in the oral cavity can slide easily down the pharynx after the swallow is completed and cause choking. Many patients have greater difficulty with liquids than with solids; consequently, liquids of a thicker consistency should be given carefully in small amounts initially, with gradual progression to thin liquids.

If the introduction of food or liquid into the mouth fails to set off the reflexive swallow, *additional stimulation* is provided. Firm upward pressure under the chin, light upward stroking of the larynx, or light tactile stimulation around the mouth may provide the stimulation necessary to trigger the swallowing reflex.

Staff members who feed the severely brain-injured patient must be carefully observant of the swallowing behaviors. The staff member provides external control of the swallowing process with the introduction of food into the mouth, the amount per swallow, and the stimulation of the swallowing reflex. Too much food given too quickly greatly increases the likelihood of aspiration.

When to Discontinue Oral Intake

Oral intake should be discontinued if the patient shows evidence of aspiration pneumonia. A sudden spike in temperature, a chest roentgenogram showing right lower lobe infiltration, or increased right lower lobe sounds after feeding all are indicative of aspiration.

Aspiration pneumonia is found most frequently in the right lower lobe of the lung due to the effect of gravity and the relatively straight downward course of the right bronchus, compared to the more acute angle of the left bronchus. The oral intake program also should be discontinued if the patient has other complications that require priority treatment.

Any significant decrease in the patient's level of consciousness may indicate neurologic complications, and the oral intake program should be halted until the patient improves.

For the unconscious patient or one for whom aspiration is a hazard, nutritional support in the form of tube feeding or parenteral hyperalimentation should be started early. Enteral feedings are suitable as long as peristalsis is present. They may be given through a small nasogastric tube or surgically implanted gastrostomy or jejunostomy tubes. Whether the feedings are intermittent or continuous, the nurse should aspirate gastric–bowel contents to ensure correct tube placement, and check for excessive residual remaining. A small amount of vegetable dye food coloring added to the feeding helps the nurse assess for regurgitation and aspiration. The more acutely injured patient may need parenteral nutrition until normal bowel function returns (see Chapter 35).

Elimination Problems

Bowel Elimination

Monitoring bowel elimination and facilitating normal defecation are time-consuming nursing responsibilities. In the acute stage in the care of a severely head-injured patient, other responsibilities take priority, such as the prevention of IICP. Later, however, spending time to establish a good bowel program will enable the patient to concentrate on other aspects of the rehabilitation program.

The actual mechanism of emptying the bowel basically is a reflex activity at the spinal cord level. With brain injury, voluntary control in stimulating or inhibiting the reflex is impaired. The reflex may be stimulated by the nurse on a routine basis to establish a predictable, controlled bowel program. This may be accomplished with a gloved finger, a small-volume enema, or by a chemical irritant such as a bisacodyl (Dulcolax; Boehringer Ingelheim, Ridgefield, CT) suppository or a gentle bowel evacuant that stimulates the reflex by pressure of released carbon dioxide in the rectum (Ceo-Two suppository; Beutlich, Inc., Niles, IL).

Digital stimulation involves the insertion of a gloved, lubricated finger no further than the second knuckle into the external rectal sphincter. With a slow circular motion against the sphincter, the spinal cord reflex will be initiated. Both internal and external rectal sphincters will relax, peristalsis will increase, and bowel evacuation will occur. *This technique is to be used only on those patients who have minimal sensation in this area.* For patients who are too alert to tolerate this procedure, an enema or suppository may be preferred.

All these methods, along with attention to diet and judicious use of stool softeners and laxatives, enable the nurse to facilitate regular bowel habits for the patient. Establishing a regular routine for daily bowel movements prevents constipation and impaction as well as accidental bowel movements or continuous small stools and avoids embarrassment for the patient and family members.

Urinary Elimination

In the acutely brain-injured patient, fluid management is essential, and a Foley catheter is necessary for accurate measurement of urinary output. Too often, the Foley catheter is forgotten as a source of irritation and potential infection. Even though a brain-injured person may have lost voluntary bladder control, the reflexes for normal voiding may be intact. The bladder muscle, like other muscles in upper motor neuron disease, may become hypertonic and spastic. The patient may experience bladder spasms, frequency, incontinence, and residual collections of urine.

Management of urinary elimination without the use of an indwelling catheter is the objective of bladder management in the brain-injured patient. Once the acute phase of injury has passed and the patient's clinical condition is stable, diagnostic tests may be performed to evaluate the extent of bladder function. Such tests include an intravenous pyelogram and cystometric studies for measurement of bladder capacity and pressure. When the evaluation is complete, a decision can be made about which approaches to achieving urinary control will be of benefit. Techniques such as intermittent catheterization, frequent toileting, and the use of external collectors require skillful nursing care to be effective. For those patients who cannot be managed safely without a catheter, an indwelling suprapubic cystostomy tube may provide effective bladder drainage with less risk of infection.

Communication Problems

Dysphasia

When communicating with a dysphasic patient, it is best to use simple language with ample gestures and environmental cues. Pointing to the desired object, tone of voice, facial expression, time of day, and hospital routine all contribute to understanding. A normal tone of voice should be used. Such patients are not deaf (unless they were before the injury), but have difficulty understanding the meaning of what they hear. Short sentences should be used; the patient may forget the beginning of a long sentence by the time it is finished. Remember, one usually is communicating with an adult, so "baby-talk" is not appropriate.

Dysphasic patients quickly become adept at "filling in the blanks" when they do not understand completely. It is easy to overestimate their level of auditory comprehension and to assume that the patient understands everything being said. It is important to check this level of understanding fairly. The nurse should ask the patient to point to objects in the room, being careful not to nod or point in the correct direction. This often is difficult to do, because we all use gesture naturally. The questions that are asked patients should be modified because the patient will learn quickly what responses are expected. Getting a clear picture of the level of understanding not only is important clinically but will alleviate frustration and confusion for the staff. Patients may be labeled as uncooperative, cross, or irrational when the staff believes they understand, but they behave as if they do not.

Dysarthria is a group of speech disorders resulting from disturbances in muscular control of the speech mechanism (weakness, slowness, poor coordination, or altered muscle tone) due to damage to the central or peripheral nervous system. Motor processes of speech that may be affected include respiration, phonation, resonance, articulation, and prosody.

Patients who are difficult to understand because of slurred, dysarthric speech should be encouraged to reduce their rate of speaking and to "overemphasize" speech movements. These patients are likely to have swallowing difficulties, also because of muscle weakness or poor coordination.

Apraxia is the inability to carry out, on request, a complex or skilled movement that cannot be accounted for by muscle weakness or paralysis, sensory deficits, or lack of understanding. *Ideational apraxia* is the inability to formulate the ideational concept to perform complicated motor acts, even though the patient knows what he or she wants to do. *Ideomotor apraxia* is the state in which the patient can perform an act spontaneously or habitually but not on command. *Oral apraxia* and *verbal apraxia* refer to apraxia affecting the volitional positioning of the oral musculature to speak or perform oral movements.

Performance of an apraxic person is inconsistent and variable. In speech, the patient may be able to say words spontaneously but cannot repeat them when desired. The patient spontaneously may pick up a spoon to eat soup but cannot demonstrate its function when the soup is removed. Apraxia may be seen in any voluntary movement such as pointing, swallowing, talking, walking, or dressing.

If apraxia is present, the nurse should avoid giving the

TABLE 30–5
Cognitive Behavior of Brain-Injured Patients and Nursing Approaches

Cognitive Behavior Level	Nursing Approaches
1. *No response* to any stimuli 2. *Generalized response:* stimulus response is inconsistent, limited, nonpurposeful with random movements or incomprehensible sounds. 3. *Localized response:* responses to stimuli are specific but inconsistent. Patient may withdraw or push away, may make sounds, follow some simple commands, or respond to certain family members.	Levels 1, 2, and 3 A. Assume that patient can understand all that is said. Converse *with* the patient, not *about* him. B. Do not overwhelm the patient with talking. Leave some moments of silence between verbal stimuli. C. Manage the environment to provide only one source of stimulation at a time. If talking is taking place, the radio or TV should be off. D. Encourage the family to provide short, random periods of sensory input that is meaningful to the patient. A favorite TV program, or tape recording or 30 min of music from the patient's favorite radio station will provide more meaningful stimulation than constant radio accompaniment, which becomes as meaningless as the continual bleep of the cardiac monitor.
4. *Confused–agitated:* response is primarily to internal confusion with increased state of activity; behavior may be bizarre or aggressive; patient may attempt to remove tubes or restraints or crawl out of bed; verbalization is incoherent or inappropriate; patient shows minimal awareness of environment and absent short-term memory.	Level 4 A. Be calm and soothing in manner when handling the patient. Approach with gentle touch to decrease the occurrence of defensive emotional and motor reflexes. B. Watch for early signs that the patient is becoming agitated (eg, increased movement, vocal loudness, resistance to activity). C. When the patient becomes upset, do not try to reason with him or "talk him out of it." Talking will be an additional external stimulus that the patient cannot handle. D. If the patient remains upset, either remove him from the situation or remove the situation from him.
5. *Confused, inappropriate, nonagitated:* Patient is alert and responds consistently to simple commands; has short attention span and easily distracted memory impaired with confusion of past and present events; can perform previously learned tasks with maximal structure but is unable to learn new information; may wander off with vague intention of "going home." 5. *Confused–appropriate:* Patient shows goal-directed behavior but still requires external direction; is able to understand simple direction; is able to understand simple reasoning; follows simple directions consistently and requires less supervision for previously learned tasks; has improved past memory depth and detail and beginning immediate awareness of self and surroundings.	Levels 5 and 6 A. Present the patient with only one task at a time. Allow him to complete it before giving further instructions. B. Make sure that you have the patient's attention by placing yourself in view and touching the patient before talking. C. If the patient becomes confused or resistant, stop talking. Wait until he appears relaxed before continuing with instruction or activity. D. Use gestures, demonstrations, and only the most necessary words in giving instructions. E. Maintain the same sequence in routine activities and tasks. Describe these routines to the patient and relate them to time of day.
7. *Automatic–appropriate:* Patient is able to complete daily routines in structured environment; has increased awareness of self and surroundings but lacks insight, judgment, and problem-solving ability.	Level 7 A. Supervision is still necessary for continued learning and safety. B. Reinforce the patient's memory of routines and schedules with clocks, calendars, and a written log of activities.
8. *Purposeful–appropriate:* Patient is alert, oriented, able to recall and integrate past and recent events; responds appropriately to environment; still has decreased ability in abstract reasoning, stress tolerance, and judgment in emergencies or unusual situations.	Level 8 A. The patient should be able to function without supervision. B. Consideration should be given to job-retraining or return to school.

Reprinted with permission from Hagen C, Malkmus D, Durham P: Levels of cognitive functioning. In *Rehabilitation of the Head Injured Adult: Comprehensive Physical Management.* Downey, CA, Professional Staff Association of Rancho Los Amigos Hospital, Inc., 1979.)

patient a command to follow. Instead of saying, "Take a drink of water," the nurse simply should give the patient the glass and let him or her perform the act automatically.

Inappropriate Behavior Responses

Neurologic damage does not occur without effecting some change in a person's behavior response. The personality and entire characteristic behavior pattern will undergo some changes, either temporary or permanent, depending on the locus and severity of the injury.

Cognition involves the ability to perceive, integrate, and interpret both internal and external environmental stimuli appropriately. In this way, behavior is regulated and controlled. The brain-injured patient will perceive, integrate, and interpret the surroundings in a disorganized fashion. Consequently, behavioral response can seem inappropriate, confused, hostile, or apathetic. Nursing assessment of the patient's cognitive abilities will aid in formulating the best way to approach a brain-injured patient at various stages during recovery (Table 30–5).

During the early stages of recovery, patients may be unable to respond to any stimulation. As they progress, they may respond later in a generalized way. An example is when moving an arm to position the blood pressure cuff causes the patient to move the entire body in response to the stimulation (see Table 30–5, Cognitive Levels 1 and 2). The therapy goal during these early phases of recovery is to help increase the brain-injured patient's awareness of self and the surroundings. *Coma stimulation* or *sensory stimulation* describe the approaches used to accomplish this goal.

One of the most common results of brain injury is an inability to screen incoming sensations to concentrate only on certain ones. For this reason, a planned approach of sensory stimulation will assist the patient in learning to attend selectively to the environment. Such an approach begins with selective stimulation of the basic senses of sound, sight, touch, and smell. The senses of taste and movement also may be included (Table 30–6).

Each session of planned stimulation should last only 10 to 15 minutes. Only one sense should be stimulated at each session. Sessions should occur three to five times daily at a time when the patient is most rested, and not after a major activity (such as a bath). It is important to allow the patient to rest after each session. During the early phases of recovery, it is difficult for the brain-injured person to indicate too much stimulation is being received. Some subtle signs might include turning away from the source of the stimulation or withdrawal and decreasing responsiveness. The patient actually may go to sleep. Some patients may become more agitated and restless and have increased movements or a flushed appearance. The nurse must be alert for signs the patient has reached the tolerance limit.

The true impact of a communication disorder is that it isolates patients from their surroundings. Because the nurse has more frequent contact with the patient than any other health professional, the manner in which the nurse handles the patient's attempts at communication is a critical factor in helping the person remain in contact with the environment. The nurse should be aware that the hospitalized patient usually wants to communicate something within the following categories:

- *States of being*—pain; need for food, warmth, fluid, or rest
- *Feelings*—the patient's feelings or perception of others' feelings toward him or her
- *People*—family, friends, hospital personnel
- *Places*—inside or outside the hospital

TABLE 30–6
Sensory Stimulation:
Planned Nursing Approaches

Sound

- Explain to the patient what you are going to do.
- Play the patient's favorite television or radio program for 10–15 min. Alternatively, play a tape recording of a familiar voice of a friend or family member.
- Another approach is to clap your hands or ring a bell. Do this for 5–10 sec at a time, moving the sound to different locations around the bed.
- During the program, do not converse with others in the room or perform other activities of patient care. The goal is to minimize distractions so the patient may learn to selectively attend to the stimulus.

Sight

- Place a brightly colored object in the patient's view. Present only one object at a time.
- Alternatively, use an object that is familiar, such as a family photo or favorite poster.

Touch

- Stroke the patient's arm or leg with fabrics of various textures. Alternately, the back of a spoon can simulate smooth texture and a towel rough texture.
- Rubbing lotion over the patient's skin will also stimulate this sense. For some, firm pressure may be better tolerated than very light touch.

Smell

- Hold a container of a pleasing fragrance under the patient's nose. Use a familiar scent such as perfume, aftershave, cinnamon, or coffee.
- Present this stimulation for very short periods (1–3 min maximum).
- If a cuffed tracheostomy or endotracheal tube is in place, the patient will not be able to fully appreciate this stimulation.

Adapted from Buss PA, Chippendale JL: Sensory Stimulation: A Guide for the Family of Brain-Injured Patients. San Diego, Sharp Memorial Hospital, 1984.

Knowledge of what the patient's major concerns are and use of alternate channels of communication (eg, facial expressions, gestures, body posture, pictures) will aid in the exchange of information between nurse and patient.

Complications

Pulmonary Edema

A serious pulmonary complication of head-injured patients is pulmonary edema. It may be primarily neurogenic in origin or result from adult respiratory distress syndrome. Pulmonary edema may result from an injury to the brain that causes the Cushing reflex. An increase in systemic arterial pressure occurs as a sympathetic nervous system response to increasing ICP. This increase in general body vasoconstriction causes more blood to be shunted to the lungs. Altered permeability of the pulmonary blood vessels contributes to the process by allowing fluid to move into the alveoli. The impaired diffusion of oxygen and carbon dioxide from the blood can lead to further increases in ICP (Fig. 30–11).

Seizures

Seizures occur in approximately 10% of head-injured patients during the acute stage. The nurse should make preparations for the possibility of seizures by having a padded tongue blade or oral airway at the bedside and suction equipment close at hand. The bed side rails should be kept up; padding the rails with pillows or foam cushions may minimize the risk of secondary injury from a seizure. During a seizure, the nurse should focus attention on maintaining a patent airway while observing the progression of seizure events and preventing further injury to the patient. If there is enough time before muscle spasticity begins, and the jaws clench, a padded tongue blade, an oral airway, or a plastic bite stick should be inserted between the patient's teeth. This will prevent the patient from biting his or her tongue and will keep the airway clear. The nurse *never* must try to force *anything* between the teeth or pry the jaws open. The patient should be turned to the side to allow secretions to drain or to be suctioned more easily. The person's movements should be restrained only enough to prevent hitting objects, causing bruising or injury.

The only medical treatment for seizures is drug therapy. Diazepam is the most widely used drug and is given slowly intravenously. Because the drug depresses respirations, the patient's respiratory rate and rhythm should be monitored carefully. Once the seizure has been terminated, the physician may order phenobarbital or phenytoin (Dilantin; Parke-Davis, Morris Plains, NJ) to maintain seizure control. Because phenytoin is a cardiac depressant, the nurse should pay careful attention to the patient's cardiac rate and rhythm. This drug should be given intravenously, no faster than 50 mg/minute. See Chapter 31 for a full discussion of seizure disorders.

Cerebrospinal Fluid Leak

It is not uncommon for some head-injured patients with a skull fracture to have a leak of CSF from the ears or nose. This may result from a fracture in the anterior fossa near

(*Text continues on page 726*)

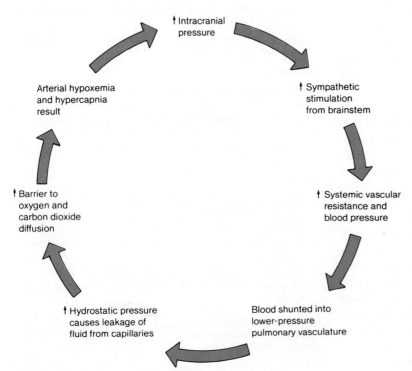

FIGURE 30–11
Mechanism of neurogenic pulmonary edema in brain-injured patients.

NURSING CARE PLAN 30-1:
The Patient With a Head Injury

NURSING DIAGNOSIS	OUTCOME CRITERIA/ PATIENT GOALS	NURSING INTERVENTIONS
Impaired gas exchange: related to loss of voluntary control of respiratory muscles and/or injury affecting rate, rhythm, depth, or automaticity of breathing.	• Patient will maintain adequate oxygenation.	1. Assess respiratory rhythm/pattern q4h and prn. 2. Assess breath sounds q2–4h. 3. Evaluate ABG results, as needed. 4. Use available oximetry to monitor oxygen saturation and end-tidal CO_2 monitors.
Ineffective airway clearance: related to retained secretions, obstructed airway, or pulmonary edema.	• Maintain patent airway.	1. Adjust patient posture with head of bed elevated or in coma position (if not contraindicated). 2. Use oral–nasal airways to maintain patent upper airway. 3. Maintain ventilator in ordered settings with operative alarm systems. 4. Suction as needed and evaluate effect.
Impaired physical mobility: related to hemiparesis, hemiplegia, abnormal posturing, spasticity, or contractures.	• Normal ROM is maintained.	1. Assess for presence of reflexive posturing and position to minimize such posturing. 2. Avoid supine position if patient demonstrates opisthotonic posturing. 3. Position in manner that decreases spasticity, if ICP permits. (trunk rotated and hips flexed). 4. Change patient position q2h. 5. Perform ROM to all limbs q4h. 6. Use splints or pillows to maintain joint alignment and prevent contractures. 7. Use hard hand cone to decrease grasp reflex and prevent contractures.
Impaired skin integrity: related to prolonged immobility.	• Sink intact over pressure areas.	1. Initiate measures to decrease pressure on body prominences. 2. Assess skin integrity and redness q2h during position changes. 3. Evaluate need for and effectiveness of special bed or mattress.

(continued)

NURSING CARE PLAN 30–1: (Continued)
The Patient With a Head Injury

NURSING DIAGNOSIS	OUTCOME CRITERIA/ PATIENT GOALS	NURSING INTERVENTIONS
		4. Change position q2h and prn.
		5. Use draw sheet or other device to manueuver patient in bed with minimal skin abrasion.
Altered nutrition, less than body requirements: related to excessive metabolic demands, inability to perform swallowing, confusion, agitation, altered level of consciousness, or depression.	• Maintain adequate body weight.	1. Assess patient's nutritional status on admission.
		2. Maintain nutritional intake with tube feedings or TPN if unable to swallow (see Chapter 35).
		3. Assess ability to swallow before feeding: assess swallowing reflex by palpating thyroid notch for upward motion; observe tongue and lip mobility.
		4. Position patient upright for reestablishment of oral intake.
		5. Assess cough reflex before reestablishment of oral intake.
		6. Begin oral intake with solid clear foods such as gelatin or popsicles.
		7. Verbalize the process to patient.
		8. Use small amounts, eg, 5 ml.
		9. After feeding, check oral cavity for pocketed food.
		10. Discontinue swallowing retraining if coughing or aspiration occur.
		11. Monitor chest x-ray results for aspiration pneumonia, especially in right lower lobe.
Colonic constipation: related to impaired voluntary control.	• Patient will have routine bowel eliminations.	1. Maintain bowel program.
		2. Empty bowel on regular basis qd.
		3. Stimulate defecation with digital stimulation if patient has minimal rectal sensation.
		4. Use enema or suppository on alert patient.
		5. Administer stool softener, as ordered.
		6. Administer laxative, as ordered.
		7. Assess and document each defecation.

(continued)

NURSING CARE PLAN 30–1: *(Continued)*
The Patient With a Head Injury

NURSING DIAGNOSIS	OUTCOME CRITERIA/ PATIENT GOALS	NURSING INTERVENTIONS
Altered urinary elimination: related to lost voluntary control of bladder, hypertonicity, or spastic bladder.	• Maintain adequate urine output, without urinary retention.	1. Assess voided urine for amount, quality, and specific gravity. 2. Check bladder residual after voiding. 3. If postvoid residual is >200 ml, maintain internal bladder catheter. 4. Record input and output. 5. If intermittent catheterization (q4–8h) is used, maintain sterile technique during procedure. 6. External urinary collectors may prevent urinary tract infection. 7. Confused or forgetful patient may benefit from frequent offering of bedpan/urinal. 8. If suprapubic catheter is used clean catheter site q8h and prn and empty drainage bag q4–8h and prn. 9. Assess temperature, elevated WBC, and turbidity of urine as signs of infection.
Impaired verbal communication: related to brain injury that resulted in dysphasia.	• Patient will be able to communicate needs to health care team and family.	1. Use simple verbal sentences. 2. Use gestures and environmental clues to communicate. 3. Allow adequate response time. 4. Establish routines for ADL. 5. Use normal voice tone. 6. Assess for communication deficits: for dysarthria and apraxia. 7. Assist family in developing communication method with the patient.
Altered thought processes: related to neurologic damage.	• Patient will respond appropriately to sensory stimulation.	1. Control stimulation in patient's environment. 2. Assess responses to controlled stimulation. 3. Avoid inappropriate labeling of responses, (eg, hostile, apathetic, angry, withdrawn.) 4. If patient is lethargic, add stimuli to environment (radio, tapes). 5. If patient is agitated, reduce environmental stimuli.

(continued)

NURSING CARE PLAN 30–1: (Continued)
The Patient With a Head Injury

NURSING DIAGNOSIS	OUTCOME CRITERIA/ PATIENT GOALS	NURSING INTERVENTIONS
High risk for injury: related to seizures, agitation, confusion, or reflexive posturing.	• Patient will not suffer injury during seizure, agitation, or reflexive posturing.	1. Assess patient for signs of trauma/bruising on the skin. 2. Apply soft restraints to wrist or vest posey if indicated. 3. Keep side rails up and bed in low position. 4. Pad side rails, headboard, and footboard if patient is agitated or potential for seizure exists. 5. If seizure activity occurs, do not restrain extremities but pad the area. Maintain patent airway but do not force jaw open. Administer muscle relaxants (diazepam), as ordered. Notify physician of seizure activity. 6. Keep patient at high risk for injury in easily visible location. 7. Check patient's environment for potentially unsafe objects.

the frontal sinuses or from a basilar skull fracture of the petrous portion of the temporal bone. In either case, the fractured bone causes damage to the thin meningeal tissues that lie adjacent, allowing CSF to escape. The presence of CSF can be detected by testing the clear, watery drainage for sugar using blood glucose test strips. Reagent strips designed to detect sugar in urine should not be used because the results may be misleading. Cerebrospinal fluid will be positive for sugar; mucus will not. Blood-tinged drainage should be collected on a sterile gauze pad and observed for the "halo" sign of blood surrounded by a clear or yellow-colored ring of spinal fluid.

When CSF rhinorrhea or otorrhea has been detected, the drainage areas should not be cleaned, irrigated, or suctioned. A sterile pad may be placed under the nose or over the ear and should be changed when damp. The nurse must instruct the awake patient not to blow the nose or sniff and not to put a finger in the nose or ear. Drainage usually slows down quickly, and the dural tear closes without any problem.

CASE STUDY

Sharon was a 17-year-old girl admitted to the critical care unit after a head-on automobile accident. She was a nonseatbelted passenger in the car driven by her boyfriend and was thrown about 40 feet from the car. The driver, who was wearing his seatbelt, was uninjured.

After skull and spine radiographs, IVP, CT scan of the head, and medical evaluation, Sharon's medical diagnoses were: severe closed head injury with moderate cerebral edema, no intracranial bleeding; probable basilar skull fracture.

The following medical orders were written:

ICP monitor

25% mannitol, $1/3$ g/kg IV prn ICP > 20 mm

Notify MD if sustained ICP > 25 mm

VS & neuro checks q30min

Foley catheter to straight drainage

NGT to suction

HOB elevated 30°

Dexamethasone 10 mg IV now, then 4 mg IV q6h

Famotidine 20 mg IV q12h

Diphenylhydantoin 100 mg IV q8h

Acetaminophen 650 mg suppository prn temperature greater than 38°C (100.4°F)

Hypothermia blanket prn temperature greater than 38.5°C (101.3°F)

Ventilator with settings of $FiO_2 = 0.5$; TV = 1200 cc; IMV = 18; CPAP = 0

End-tidal CO_2 monitor; maintain CO_2 26–30 torr

IV of D5/0.2 NS at 60 ml/hr

Total fluid limit = 1500 ml/24 hr

The following assessment data were obtained a few hours after Sharon's admission:

ABGs: pH 7.32, CO_2 42 mm Hg, PaO_2 60 mm Hg, HCO_3 20 mEq/L

BP: 180/68; P: 60; RR: 26; T: 39.2°C (102.5°F)

ICP = 32 mm Hg

Pupils equal, 4 mm, sluggishly reactive

No response to commands; assumes decerebrate posture to pain

Breath sounds = ronchi in upper lung fields, rales in both bases

An elevation of the above data by the critical care nurse demonstrated several reasons why the patient needed immediate intervention. Sharon had impaired gas exchange related to neurogenic pulmonary edema, despite a respiratory rate suggestive of hyperventilation. This contributed to CO_2 retention which, in turn, increased her ICP. The cerebral perfusion pressure is normal for now, due to systemic hypertension. Adding to the potential for secondary brain injury and increased cerebral edema is the elevated temperature and resultant increased cerebral metabolic rate.

Sharon was treated for about 1 week in the intensive care unit and then transferred to a progressive care setting specializing in the care of brain-injured patients. Approximately 3 months after injury, she was in a rehabilitation setting. Sharon was alert and able to respond to simple commands. Her speech was slow and slurred but she was able to state her needs in single words and short phrases. She recognized her immediate family but had no memory of the accident or of events several weeks before it. Sharon progressed slowly on oral feedings because aspiration was still a risk and the old tracheostomy site had not completely healed.

Nursing Care Plan

It is obvious that the care of the head-injured patient is both complex and demanding. Nursing Care Plan 30–1 outlines the major nursing diagnoses associated with this clinical problem and expected outcomes and nursing interventions.

REFERENCES

1. Frankowski RF, Annegers JF, Whitman S: The descriptive epidemiology of head trauma in the United States. Central Nervous System Trauma Status Report, 1985, pp 33–45. Bethesda, MD, National Institute of Neurological and Communicative Disorders and Stroke, National Institutes of Health, 1985
2. Landy HJ, Tucci KA: Closed head trauma. In Weiner WJ (ed): Emergent and Urgent Neurology, pp 239–259. Philadelphia, JB Lippincott, 1992
3. Walleck CA: Preventing secondary brain injury. AACN Clinical Issues in Critical Care Nursing 3(1):19–30, 1992
4. Gennarelli TA, Spielman GM, Langfitt TW: Influence of the type of intracranial lesion on outcome from severe head injury. J Neurosurg 56:26–36, 1982
5. Coburn K: Traumatic brain injury: The silent epidemic. AACN Clinical Issues in Critical Care Nursing 3(1):9–18, 1992
6. Wing D: Craniocerebral trauma. In Hickey JV, ed. Neurological and Neurosurgical Nursing, pp 351–394. Philadelphia, JB Lippincott, 1992
7. Lobato R, Rivas J, Gomez P, et al: Head-injured patients who talk and deteriorate into coma. J Neurosurg 75:256–261, 1991
8. Marshall SB, Marshall LF, et al (eds): Neuroscience Critical Care. Philadelphia, WB Saunders, 1990
9. Crosby LJ, Parsons LC: Cerebrovascular response of closed head-injured patients to a standardized endotracheal tube suctioning and manual hyperventilation procedure. Journal of Neuroscience Nursing 24:40–49, 1992
10. Godbole KB, Berbiglia VA, Goddard L: A head-injured patient: Caloric needs, clinical progress and nursing care priorities. Journal of Neuroscience Nursing 23:290–294, 1991

BIBLIOGRAPHY

Cammermeyer M, Appledorn C (eds): Core Curriculum For Neuroscience Nurses, 3rd ed. Chicago, American Association of Neuroscience Nurses, 1990

Flannery J: Famli-Rescue: A family assessment tool for use by neuroscience nurses in the acute care setting. Journal of Neuroscience Nursing 23:111–115, 1991

Mirr MP: Factors affecting decisions made by family members of patients with severe head injury. Heart Lung 20:228–235, 1991

Rudy EB, Turner BS, Baun M, et al: Endotracheal suctioning in adults with head injury. Heart Lung 20:667–674, 1991

Weiner WJ: Emergent and Urgent Neurology. Philadelphia, JB Lippincott, 1992

STUDY QUESTIONS

1. A concussion
   a. always is associated with loss of consciousness
   b. never is associated with loss of consciousness
   c. produces irreversible neurologic dysfunction
   d. produces reversible neurologic dysfunction

2. The neurophysiology of respiration includes all the following except

   a. the motor strip of the cerebral cortex
   b. the medulla oblongata in the brain stem
   c. the cranial nerves IX and X
   d. the cervical and thoracic spinal nerves

3. Cheyne–Stokes breathing is characterized by

   a. respiration with a long pause at full inspiration or full expiration
   b. the depth of each breath increasing to a peak and then decreasing to a period of apnea
   c. gasping breaths with irregular pauses
   d. totally irregular breathing with both deep and shallow breaths with irregular pauses

4. In a swallowing retraining program, all of the following interventions should be carried out except

   a. position patient from 45° to 90° upright
   b. verbalize the process to the patient regardless of his or her state of understanding
   c. slightly extend the patient's neck
   d. provide food that is stimulating in temperature, taste, and texture

5. When communicating with a dysphasic patient, all of the following techniques are recommended except

   a. use simple language punctuated with gestures
   b. do not use baby talk
   c. use longer sentences to force the patient to concentrate
   d. speak in a normal tone of voice

(continued)

CHAPTER 31

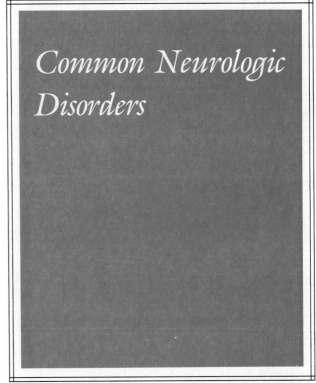

Common Neurologic Disorders

Hudak: Critical Care Nursing:
A Holistic Approach, 6th ed. © 1994
J. B. Lippincott Company.

BEHAVIORAL OBJECTIVES

Based on the content in this chapter, the reader should be able to:

1. Name three common clinical manifestations of a right hemispheric stroke.
2. Name three common clinical manifestations of a left hemispheric stroke.
3. Discuss two treatment modalities available for the patient with an arteriovenous malformation; a cerebral aneurysm.
4. Describe three appropriate nursing interventions for a patient with a cerebral aneurysm before surgery.
5. Describe four observations to be made during a seizure.
6. Discuss three important facts a patient taking phenytoin should be taught.
7. Differentiate between partial and generalized seizures.
8. Explain the pathophysiology of Guillain–Barré syndrome.
9. Formulate a teaching plan for a patient with myasthenia gravis.

Description

Common neurologic disorders may include a cerebrovascular disorder such as stroke, arteriovenous malformation or aneurysm, a seizure disorder, or a neuromuscular disorder such as Guillain–Barré syndrome or myasthenia gravis. These disorders will be addressed in this chapter.

Nurses in a critical care unit caring for patients who have acute nervous system injury or illness serve as the patient's first line of defense. To ensure superior care, a multitude of routine supportive acts must be performed in repetition.

Concomitantly, the nurse must carry out frequent neurologic and (in cases of multiple systems injuries) other evaluations with constant vigil for subtle changes in blood pressure, pulse rate and regularity, respiratory activity, sensorial status (level of consciousness), and motor and sensory function. Alterations, when they occur, may be the initial indication of impending deterioration, leading to rapid death unless immediate action is taken to alleviate the underlying pathologic condition.

Opportunity for the nurse to discover interesting and extremely important findings is ever present. Serosanguineous drainage from ears, nose, or scalp wound, even when it has been debrided and repaired but incompletely explored in the emergency unit, will represent cerebrospinal fluid (CSF) leak until proved otherwise. Progressive urinary output of abnormally high levels after injury or certain types of intracranial and facial surgery may represent diabetes insipidus. Neither of these conditions necessarily need cause concern over the immediate demise of the patient. If unobserved too long, however, they may result in unnecessary intracranial infection or hypovolemia and severe electrolyte imbalance. These in turn will lead to new problems of care and worsened condition of the patient, possibly precluding complete recovery or ultimately leading to death.

Experience aids the nurse in sharpening his or her powers of observation to recognize the slight changes that may be the precursors of the full constellation of signs of increased intracranial pressure (IICP) or brain herniation. The same holds for alterations in lower-extremity motor and sensory function after incomplete spinal cord injury. Experience also imparts confidence to the nurse, as does knowledge of the more common patterns of deterioration, in assisting him or her to determine whether additional observation is warranted or whether he or she should seek the physician's reevaluation immediately.

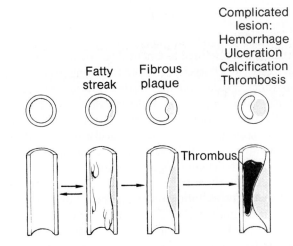

FIGURE 31–1
Vascular changes preventing blood flow (Brunner LS, Suddarth DS: Textbook of Medical-Surgical Nursing, 6th ed. Philadelphia, JB Lippincott, 1988).

Cerebrovascular Disease

Description

Cerebrovascular disease (CVD) is the most frequent neurologic disorder of adults. It is the third leading cause of morbidity and mortality in the United States, after heart disease and cancer.[1] Cerebrovascular disease includes any pathologic process that involves the blood vessels of the brain. Most CVD is due to thrombosis, embolism, or hemorrhage (Fig. 31–1). The mechanism of each of these etiologies is different, but the result is the same—ultimate ischemia or hypoxia to a focal area of the brain. Ischemia may lead to brain necrosis (infarction).

Anatomy of Brain Vasculature

The brain is supplied with blood from two major sets of vessels: the carotid, or anterior, circulation and the vertebral, or posterior, circulation (Fig. 31–2). Each system comes off the aortic arch as a pair of vessels: the left and right common carotids and the left and right vertebrals. Each carotid bifurcates to form the internal and external carotid artery. The vertebral arteries arise from the subclavian arteries. The vertebrals join to form the basilar artery, and that in turn divides to form the two posterior cerebral arteries, which supply the medial and inferior surfaces of the brain as well as the lateral portions of the temporal and occipital lobe (Fig. 31–3).

The circle of Willis is the area in which the branches of the basilar and internal carotid arteries unite. The circle of Willis is composed of the two anterior cerebral arteries, the anterior communicating artery, the two posterior cerebral arteries, and the two posterior communicating arteries (Fig. 31–4). This circular network permits blood to circulate from one hemisphere to the other and from the anterior into the posterior areas of the brain. It is a system that allows for collateral circulation if one vessel is oc-

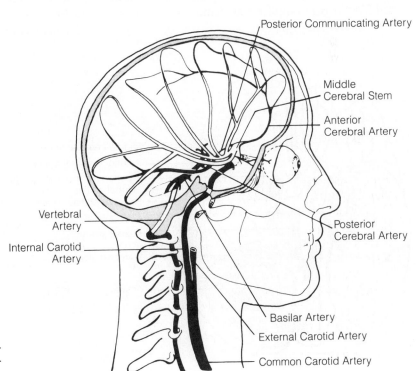

FIGURE 31–2
The major vessels to the brain. The internal carotid, anterior, and middle cerebral arteries constitute the anterior circulation. The vertebral, basilar, and posterior cerebral arteries and branches comprise the posterior circulation.

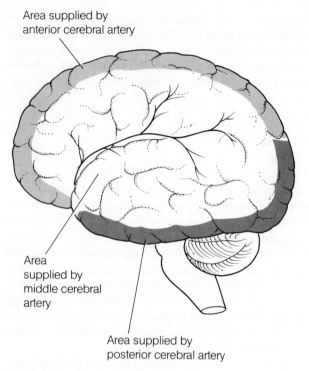

FIGURE 31–3
Arterial supply to areas in the brain.

cluded. It is not unusual, however, for some vessel within the circle of Willis to be atrophic or even absent. This accounts for different clinical presentations among patients with the same lesion. For example, an occluded carotid artery in a person with a fully patent circle of Willis may be totally asymptomatic, but a patient in whom the circle of Willis is incomplete may demonstrate a massive cerebral infarction.

Cerebrovascular Accident (Stroke)
Description

A stroke may be defined as a neurologic deficit that has a sudden onset and lasts over 24 hours resulting from CVD. Approximately three-fourths of strokes are due to vascular obstruction (thrombi or emboli), resulting in ischemia and infarction. About one-fourth of strokes are hemorrhagic, resulting from hypertensive vascular disease (which causes an intracerebral hemorrhage), a ruptured aneurysm, or an arteriovenous malformation (AVM).

Each of the three types of stroke has a fairly typical time course. Thrombotic strokes may be subdivided into transient ischemic attacks (TIAs), stroke in evolution, or completed stroke. Thrombotic strokes may occur suddenly and be complete early, or they may progress over a period of time, depending on how much blood is able to get through the vascular lumen. Both embolic and hemorrhagic strokes typically present suddenly and progress rapidly over minutes or hours. There usually is little or no warning.

Sixty percent of thrombotic strokes occur during sleep. If the stroke is not complete at the time of the initial attack, symptoms may evolve over several hours or days.

There may be some temporary improvement in clinical deficits, but then there follows a rapid progression of permanent deficits. This symptom development is referred to as stroke-in-evolution.

In principle, stroke is preventable.[2] One study suggested that 50% of cerebrovascular deaths in patients under 70 years of age might be preventable by application of existing knowledge. Stroke mortality differs in different countries. For example, Japan has a high rate of stroke and a low rate of coronary heart disease; however, men of Japanese ancestry living in the United States have a lower

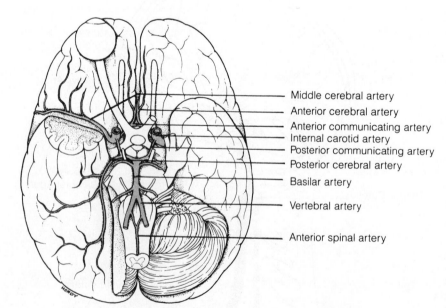

Middle cerebral artery
Anterior cerebral artery
Anterior communicating artery
Internal carotid artery
Posterior communicating artery
Posterior cerebral artery
Basilar artery
Vertebral artery
Anterior spinal artery

FIGURE 31–4
The circle of Willis seen from below the brain.

rate of stroke and a higher rate of coronary heart disease. This may indicate that international differences in mortality are not fixed.

The individual risk factors for stroke have been known for quite some time. Primary prevention may be geared toward modifying some of these risk factors, such as hypertension, serum cholesterol, smoking, obesity, impaired glucose tolerance, use of oral contraceptives in people at risk, and diet.

Pathophysiological Principles

When blood flow to any part of the brain is impeded as a result of a thrombus or embolus, oxygen deprivation of the cerebral tissue begins. Deprivation for 1 minute can lead to reversible symptoms, such as loss of consciousness. Oxygen deprivation for longer periods can produce microscopic necrosis of the neurons. The necrotic area is then said to be infarcted.

The initial oxygen deprivation may be due to general ischemia (from cardiac arrest or hypotension) or hypoxia from an anemic process or high altitude. If the neurons are only ischemic, and have not yet necrosed, there is a chance to save them. This situation is analogous to the focal injury caused by a myocardial infarction. An occluded coronary artery can produce an area of infarcted (dead) tissue. Surrounding the infarcted zone is an area of ischemic tissue, which has been marginally deprived of oxygen. This ischemic tissue, as in the brain, may either be salvaged with appropriate treatment or killed by secondary events.

Strokes due to embolus may be a result of blood clots, fragments of atheromatous plaques, lipids, or air. Emboli to the brain most often come from the heart, secondary to myocardial infarction or atrial fibrillation.

If hemorrhage is the etiology of a stroke, hypertension often is a precipitating factor. Vascular abnormalities such as AVMs and cerebral aneurysms are more prone to rupture and cause hemorrhage in the presence of hypertension.

The most frequent neurovascular syndrome seen in thrombotic and embolic strokes is due to involvement of the middle cerebral artery. This artery mainly supplies the lateral aspects of the cerebral hemisphere. Infarction to that area of the brain may cause contralateral motor and sensory deficits. If the infarcted hemisphere is dominant, speech problems result, and dysphasia may be present.

With a thrombotic or embolic stroke, the amount of brain ischemia and infarction that might occur is difficult to predict. There is a chance that the stroke will extend after the initial insult. There can be massive cerebral edema and an increase in intracranial pressure (ICP) to the point of herniation and death after a large thrombotic stroke. The prognosis is influenced by the area of the brain involved and the extent of the insult. Because thrombotic strokes often are due to atherosclerosis, there is risk of a future stroke in a patient who already has suffered one.

With embolic strokes, patients also may have subsequent episodes of stroke if the underlying cause is not treated. If the extent of brain tissue destroyed from a hemorrhagic stroke is not excessive and is in a nonvital area, the patient may recover with minimal deficits. If the hemorrhage is large or in a vital area of the brain, the patient may not recover. About 30% of intracerebral hemorrhages are less massive, making survival possible.

Assessment

History and Physical Examination

Diagnosis of a stroke is based on physical examination and history. The age of the patient is useful because strokes are more likely to occur in older people. It is helpful to know the type of onset of symptoms from the person. If the symptoms began suddenly and were severe within an hour, the most likely diagnosis is embolic ischemic brain infarction or intracranial hemorrhage. Nonvascular diseases such as tumors, abscesses, subdural hematomas, and encephalitis rarely progress that quickly.

The history will be helpful in determining what has happened to the patient. It is important to obtain a description of the neurologic event, how long it lasted, and whether the symptoms are resolving or completely gone, or the same as at the time of onset. The type of symptoms may help determine and locate a possible vascular etiology. Determination of risk factors for stroke, such as a familial history of stroke, hypertension, chronic atrial fibrillation, elevated serum cholesterol, smoking, or oral contraceptive use also will help diagnose the problem.

If atrial fibrillation or a carotid bruit is found on physical examination, it may suggest the diagnosis of stroke. It is important to note the level of consciousness (LOC) when the patient presents. Ischemic CVD usually does not cause a depression in the LOC. Nonvascular processes and intracranial hemorrhage must be considered if the person has a depressed LOC.

Clinical Manifestations

A patient with vascular disease may present with a TIA. This is a neurologic deficit that totally resolves within 24 hours. Its average duration is 10 minutes, after which the symptoms completely disappear. A patient also may present with a reversible ischemic neurologic deficit. This event may persist beyond the 24-hour duration of a TIA, but it eventually will clear completely. The third possible clinical presentation is a completed stroke, which leaves the person with a permanent deficit.

Of those people who have TIAs, one-third will have a major stroke, one third will continue to have TIAs but will not have a major stroke, and one-third will have a resolution of their TIAs.

Symptoms seen with TIAs depend a great deal on the vessels involved. When the carotid and cerebral arteries are involved, the patient may have blindness in one eye, hemiplegia, hemianesthesia, speech disturbances, and confusion. When the vertebrobasilar artery is involved, dizziness, diplopia, numbness, visual defects in one or both fields, and dysarthria can be seen. Table 31–1 is a list of common deficits seen with cerebrovascular accident and of suggested nursing interventions.

Some generalizations can be made about the probable disabilities of a patient if one knows both the side of the brain in which the stroke occurred and the "handedness" of the patient. Ninety-three percent of people are right-handed. This means that their left hemisphere is dominant. Of the 7% of the population who are left-handed, about 60% have their dominant speech center in their left hemisphere, as do right-handed people (see Display Box 31–1).

Diagnostic Studies

A computed tomography (CT) scan may be useful in differentiating between cerebrovascular lesions and non-vascular lesions. For example, a subdural hemorrhage, brain abscess, tumor, or intracerebral hemorrhage will be visible on the CT scan. An area of infarction may not show on CT scan for 48 hours.

A brain scan has limited value in the acute setting but may be helpful if it is positive. A brain scan will show major infarcted areas, but not as early as the CT scan.

Angiography was done more often before the CT scan was available to distinguish cerebrovascular lesions from nonvascular ones. Early angiography in a patient with a stroke often is performed if an intracranial hemorrhage is suspected, if the patient is rapidly deteriorating neurologically, or if the patient has a suspected acute carotid occlusion.

A lumbar puncture may be performed to look for blood in the CSF. The CT scan may not show low concentrations of blood in the CSF. It is important to know whether hemorrhage is present because this information may help the physician decide whether or not to anticoagulate the patient.

Magnetic resonance imaging (MRI) also may help in the differential diagnosis of a stroke. Ultrasound or Doppler studies are noninvasive procedures that are useful in diagnosing blocked arteries. An electrocardiogram may help determine if a dysrhythmia is present, which may have caused the stroke. Other electrocardiogram changes that might be found are an inverted T wave, ST depression, and QT elevation and prolongation.

No laboratory tests are definitive in confirming a diagnosis of stroke; however, commonly drawn blood tests include hematocrit and hemoglobin, which, when elevated, indicate a more severe occlusion; prothrombin time and partial thromboplastin time, which provide a baseline should anticoagulation therapy be initiated; and a white blood cell count, which may indicate an infection such as subacute bacterial endocarditis. In the absence of

---

DISPLAY BOX 31–1
Probable Disabilities Associated With Stroke

Left Hemispheric Stroke

- Right-sided hemiparesis or hemiplegia
- Slow and cautious behavior
- Right visual field defect
- Expressive, receptive, or global dysphasia
- High frustration

Right Hemispheric Stroke

- Left-sided hemiparesis or hemiplegia
- Spatial–perceptual deficits
- Poor judgment
- Distractibility
- Impulsive behavior
- Apparent unawareness of deficits of affected side and therefore susceptibility to falls or other injuries
- Left visual field defect

---

increased intracranial pressure, a lumbar puncture may be done. If there is blood in the CSF obtained, a subarachnoid hemorrhage usually is suspected.

In many cases the etiology of the stroke remains undetermined even with all the diagnostic tools available, and a significant proportion of patients will have evidence of more than one potential mechanism.[3]

Management

Reducing Ischemic Damage

With a cerebral infarction there is a central core of brain tissue that is irreversibly lost. Around this dead zone is an area of tissue that may be salvageable. It should be the focus of initial treatment to save as much of the ischemic area as possible. Three ingredients necessary to that area are oxygen, glucose, and adequate blood flow. The oxygen level can be monitored through arterial blood gases and oxygen can be given to the patient if indicated. Hypoglycemia can be evaluated with serial checks on blood glucose.

Cerebral perfusion pressure is a reflection of the systemic blood pressure, the ICP, the autoregulation still functioning in the brain, and the heart rate and rhythm. The parameters most easily controlled externally are the cardiac rhythm, rate, and blood pressure. Dysrhythmias usually can be corrected. Causes of tachycardia, such as fever, pain, and dehydration, can be treated.

Not widely used as yet is monitoring with a retrograde jugular catheter. Such a catheter allows for sampling of the

TABLE 31-1
*Common Deficits and Emotional Reactions to Stroke
and Related General Nursing Interventions*

Common Motor Deficits	Nursing Interventions
1. Hemiparesis or hemiplegia (side of the body opposite the cerebral episode 2. Dysarthria (muscles of speech impaired) 3. Dysphagia (muscles of swallowing impaired)	1. Position the patient in proper body alignment; use a hand roll to keep the hand in a functional position • Provide frequent passive range-of-motion exercises. • Reposition the patient every 2 hr. 2. Provide for an alternative method of communication. 3. Test the patient's palatal and pharyngeal reflexes before offering nourishment. • Elevate and turn the patient's head to the unaffected side. • If the patient is able to manage oral intake, place food on the unaffected side of the patient's mouth.

Common Sensory Deficits	Nursing Interventions

1. Visual deficits (common because the visual pathways cut through much of the cerebral hemispheres)
  a. Homonymous hemianopsia (loss of vision in half of the visual field on the same side)
 	
  b. double vision (diplopia)
  c. Decreased visual acuity
2. Absent or diminished response to superficial sensation (touch, pain, pressure, heat, cold)
	1. Be aware that variations of visual deficits may exist and compensate for them.
	  a. Approach the patient from the unaffected side; remind the patient to turn the head to compensate for visual deficits.
	  b. Apply an eye patch to the affected eye.
	  c. Provide assistance as necessary.
	2. Increase the amount of touch in administering patient care.
	• Protect the involved areas from injury.
	• Protect the involved areas from burns.
	• Examine the involved areas for signs of skin irritation and injury.
	• Provide the patient with an opportunity to handle various objects of different weight, texture, and size.
	• If pain is present, assess its location and type, as well as the duration of the pain.

3. Absent or diminished response to proprioception (knowledge of position of body parts)
4. Perceptual deficits (disturbance in correctly perceiving and interpreting self and/or environment)
  a. Body scheme disturbance (amnesia or denial for paralyzed extremities; unilateral neglect)
 	
  b. Disorientation (to time, place, and person)
 	
  c. Apraxia (loss of ability to use objects correctly)
  d. Agnosia (inability to identify the environment by means of the senses)
  e. Defects in localizing objects in space, estimating their size, and judging distance.
  f. Impaired memory for recall of spatial location of objects or places
 	
  g. Right–left disorientation
	3. Teach the patient to check the position of body parts visually.
	4. Compensate for the patient's perceptual-sensory deficits.
	
	  a. Protect the involved area.
	    • Accept the patient's self-perception.
	    • Position the patient to face the involved area.
	  b. Control the amount of change in the patient's schedule
	    • Reorient the patient as necessary
	    • Talk to the patient; tell him about the immediate environment.
	    • Provide a calendar, clock, pictures of family, and so forth.
	  c. Correct misuse of objects and demonstrate proper use.
	  d. Correct misinformation.
	
	  e. Reduce any stimuli that will distract the patient.
	
	  f. Place necessary equipment where the patient will see it, rather than telling the patient "It is in the closet" and so forth.
	  g. Phrase requests carefully, like "Lift this leg." (Point to the leg.)

(continued)

TABLE 31–1
Common Deficits and Emotional Reactions to Stroke
and Related General Nursing Interventions (Continued)

Language Deficits	Nursing Interventions
1. Expressive aphasia (difficulty in transforming sound into patterns of understandable speech)—can speak using single-word responses	1. Ask the patient to repeat the individual sounds of the alphabet as a start at retraining.
2. Receptive aphasia (impairment of comprehension of the spoken word)—able to speak, but uses words incorrectly and is unaware of these errors	2. Speak clearly and in simple sentences; use gestures as necessary.
3. Global aphasia (combination of expressive and receptive aphasia)—unable to communicate at any level	3. Evaluate what language skills are intact; speak in very simple sentences, ask the patient to repeat individual sounds, and use gestures or any other means to communicate.
4. Alexia (inability to understand the written word)	4. Point to the written names of objects and have the patient repeat the name of the object.
5. Agraphia (inability to express ideas in writing)	5. Have the patient write words and simple sentences.

Intellectual Deficits	Nursing Interventions
1. Loss of memory	1. Provide necessary information as necessary.
2. Short attention span	2. Divide activities into short steps.
3. Increased distractibility	3. Control any excessive environmental distractions.
4. Poor judgment	4. Protect the patient from injury.
5. Inability to transfer learning from one situation to another	5. Repeat instructions as necessary.
6. Inability to calculate, reason, or think abstractly	6. Do not set unrealistic expectations for the patient.

Emotional Deficits	Nursing Interventions
1. Emotional lability (exhibits reactions easily or inappropriately)	1. Disregard bursts of emotions; explain to the patient that emotional lability is part of the illness.
2. Loss of self-control and social inhibitions	2. Protect the patient as necessary so that his or her dignity is preserved.
3. Reduced tolerance to stress	3. Control the amount of stress experienced by the patient.
4. Fear, hostility, frustration, anger	4. Be accepting of the patient; be supportive.
5. Confusion and despair	5. Clarify any misconceptions; allow the patient to verbalize.
6. Withdrawal, isolation	6. Provide stimulation and a safe, comfortable environment.
7. Depression	7. Provide a supportive environment.

Bowel and Bladder Dysfunction	Nursing Interventions
Bladder: Incomplete Upper Motor Neuron Lesion	*Do not suggest insertion of an indwelling catheter immediately after the stroke.*
1. The unilateral lesion from the stroke results in partial sensation and control of the bladder, so that the patient experiences frequency, urgency, and incontinence. (Cognitive deficits affect control.)	1. Observe the patient to identify characteristics of the voiding pattern (frequency, amount, forcefulness of stream, constant dribbling, etc.).
2. If the stroke lesion is in the brain stem, there will be bilateral damage, resulting in an upper motor neuron bladder with loss of all control of micturition.	2. Maintain an accurate intake and output record. *Nursing note: Incontinence after regaining consciousness is usually attributable to urinary tract infection caused by use of an indwelling urinary catheter.*
3. Possibility of establishing normal bladder function is excellent.	3. Try to allow the patient to stay catheter-free: • Offer the bedpan or urinal frequently. • Take the patient to the commode frequently. • Assess the patient's ability to make his or her need for help with voiding known. If a catheter is necessary, remove it as soon as possible and follow a bladder training program.

(continued)

TABLE 31–1
Common Deficits and Emotional Reactions to Stroke and Related General Nursing Interventions (*Continued*)

Bowel and Bladder Dysfunction	Nursing Interventions
Bowel	
1. Impairment of bowel function in a stroke patient is attributable to: • Deterioration in the level of consciousness • Dehydration • Immobility	1. Develop a bowel training program: • Give foods known to stimulate defecation (prune juice, roughage). • Initiate a suppository and laxative regimen.
2. Constipation is the most common problem, along with potential impaction.	2. Institute a bowel program. Enemas are avoided in the presence of increased intracranial pressure.

From Hickey JV: The Clinical Practice of Neurological and Neurosurgical Nursing, 3rd ed, pp. 529–530. Philadelphia, JB Lippincott, 1992.

venous blood leaving the cerebral hemispheres, permitting calculation of venous oxygen saturation. The calculated SjO_2 (saturation of jugular oxygen) reflects what is happening at the cellular level better than ICP or cerebral perfusion pressure. Monitoring the arteriovenous difference of oxygen ($AVDO_2$) and the SjO_2 allows the physician to determine if therapies are harming or improving oxygen delivery. Normal SjO_2 is 60% to 80%.[4]

Controlling Hypertension and Increased Intracranial Pressure

Control of hypertension, ICP, and cerebral perfusion pressure may take the efforts of both nurse and physician. The nurse must assess for these problems, recognize them and their significance, and ensure that medical interventions are initiated. Later in the course of recovery explanations about the patient's deficit(s), the outcome objectives, and specifics about needs after discharge may be discussed in a collaborative effort.

Patients with moderate hypertension usually are not treated acutely. If their blood pressure is lowered after the brain is accustomed to the hypertension for adequate perfusion, the brain's perfusion pressure will fall along with the blood pressure. If the diastolic blood pressure is above about 105 mm Hg, it may need to be lowered gradually. This may be accomplished very effectively with nitroprusside.

If ICP is elevated in a stroke patient, it usually occurs after the first day. Although this is a natural response of the brain to some cerebrovascular lesions, it is destructive to the brain. The destructive response, such as edema or arterial vasospasm, sometimes can be treated or prevented. The usual methods of controlling IICP may be instituted, such as hyperventilation, fluid restriction, head elevation, avoidance of neck flexion or severe head rotation that would impede venous outflow from the head, use of osmotic diuretics such as mannitol, and perhaps administration of dexamethasone, although its use remains controversial.

Pharmacologic Therapy

Anticoagulation may be initiated if the stroke was not hemorrhagic, although heparinization of patients with an acute ischemic stroke has the potential for causing hemorrhagic complications. Low-molecular-weight heparinoids (LMWH) offer an alternative to heparin, and there is a decrease in bleeding tendency with their use. These LMWH still are in the experimental stage, but clinical trials to date are promising. These heparinoids should be initiated within 24 hours of onset of symptoms and are given intravenously, as heparin would be. They provide an antithrombotic effect, yet cause no significant change in the patient's prothrombin time and partial thromboplastin time.[5]

If the patient has not had a stroke, but a TIA, antiplatelet drugs may be indicated. Such drugs include Persantine (Boehringer Ingelheim, Ridgefield, CT), Anturane (Ciba Pharmaceutical Co., Summit, NJ), and aspirin. They reduce the platelet adhesiveness, and are given in hopes of preventing a future thrombotic or embolic event. Antiplatelet drugs are contraindicated in the presence of a hemorrhagic stroke as is heparin.

Calcium channel blockers such as nimodipine may be used to treat cerebral vasospasm. These drugs relax the smooth muscle of the vessel walls. Vasospasm is most common after rupture of a cerebral aneurysm. Trental (pentoxifylline; Hoechst-Roussel Pharmaceuticals, Somerville, NJ) may be used to increase microcirculatory capillary blood flow, thus improving perfusion and oxygenation to ischemic brain tissue.

Surgical Intervention

Transient ischemic episodes often are viewed as a warning of impending stroke due to occlusion of a vessel. Some patients with atherosclerotic disease of extracranial or intracranial vessels may be good surgical candidates. Carotid endarterectomy may be beneficial to a patient with narrowing of the vessels.

Cranial bypass surgery involves anastomosing an extracranial artery that perfuses the scalp to an intracranial artery distal to the occluded site. The procedure often used when there is intracranial involvement is the superior temporal artery anastomosis to the middle cerebral artery (STA-MCA). Collateral circulation thus is provided to areas of the brain supplied by the middle cerebral artery. Many STA-MCA anastomoses are performed with the hope of preventing a future stroke in people with unilateral focal cerebral ischemia who present with TIAs.

Preventing Complications

The nurse will play a significant role in preventing the complications associated with immobility, hemiparesis, or any neurologic deficit produced by stroke. Preventive measures are particularly important in the area of urinary tract infections, aspiration pneumonia, pressure sores, contractures, thrombophlebitis, and corneal abrasions.

Emotional and Behavioral Concerns

Victims of stroke may display emotional problems, and their behavior may be different from the prestroke baseline. Emotions may be labile; for example, the patient may cry one moment and laugh the next, without explanation or control. Tolerance to stress may be reduced. A minor stress in the prestroke state may be perceived as a major problem after the stroke. Families may not understand the behavior. Stroke victims may use loud profanity with the nursing staff or with their family members, yet the family cannot understand it because the patient may never have used any profanity before the stroke. It is the nurse's role to help the family understand these behavioral changes. There is much that the nurse can do to modify the patient's behavior, such as controlling stimuli in the environment, providing rest periods throughout the day to prevent the patient from becoming overtired, giving positive feedback for acceptable behavior or positive accomplishments, and providing repetition when the patient is trying to relearn a skill.

Communication Concerns

Stroke victims may demonstrate much frustration with their deficits. Probably no deficit produces more frustration for the patient and those trying to communicate with him or her than the one involving the production and understanding of language. Dysphasia can involve motor abilities or sensory function, or both. If the area of brain injury is in or near the left Broca's area, the memory of motor patterns of speech are affected (see Chapter 30, Figure 30–6). This results in an expressive dysphasia, in which the patient understands language but is unable to use it appropriately.

Receptive dysphasia usually is a result of injury to the left Wernicke's area, which is the control center for recognition of spoken language. The patient thus is unable to understand the significance of the spoken word. Presence of both expressive dysphasia and receptive dysphasia is referred to as global dysphasia. Display Box 31–2 summarizes differences between expressive and receptive problems.

It is important for the nursing staff to remember to tell families that just because a person has dysphasia does not mean that the patient is intellectually impaired. Communication at some level should be attempted, whether it is by writing, pointing at alphabet charts, or using gestures.

Complications

There are three primary complications of a subarachnoid hemorrhage that may result from a stroke, an AVM, or an

---

Clinical Research

Pasquarello M: Measuring the impact of an acute stroke program on patient outcomes.
Journal of Neuroscience Nursing 22(2):76–82, 1990

The purpose of this study was to evaluate the outcome of patients admitted into a nurse-managed stroke program in an acute care setting. Variables studied were length of stay, recidivism to the emergency department or ambulatory care center within 3 months after discharge, disposition on discharge, complications encountered, timeliness in initiating rehabilitation, compliance with medication regime, and compliance with follow-up appointments 3 months after discharge.

The stroke program involved inpatient care, research studies, and an outpatient program. The results of the study demonstrated a definite impact on patient outcomes. Length of hospital stay and recidivism decreased; patient medication and follow-up compliance improved; more patients were discharged home, therapy was begun sooner, and complications were decreased, compared to patients admitted before the institution of this nurse-managed unit. Development of similar acute care programs may result in further improvement of other patient outcomes.

DISPLAY BOX 31–2
Comparison of Expressive and Receptive Dysphasia

Expressive Dysphasia	*Receptive Dysphasia*
Hemiparesis is present because motor cortex is near Broca's area.	Hemiparesis is mild or absent because lesion is not near motor cortex.
	Hemianopsia or quadrantanopsia may be present.
Speech is slow, nonfluent; articulation is poor; speaking requires much effort. Total speech is reduced in quantity. Patient may use telegraphic speech, omitting small words.	Speech is fluent; articulation and rhythm are normal. Content of speech is impaired; wrong words are used.
Patient understands written and verbal speech.	Patient does not understand written and verbal speech.
Patient writes dysphasically.	Content of writing is abnormal. Penmanship may be good.
Patient may be able to repeat single words with effort. Phrase repetition is poor.	Repetition is poor.
Object naming is often poor, but it may be better than attempts to use spontaneous speech.	Object naming is poor.
Patient is aware of deficit, often experiencing frustration and depression.	Patient is often unaware of deficit.
Curses or other ejaculatory speech may be well articulated and automatic. Patient may be able to hum normally.	Patient may use wrong words and sounds.

---

aneurysm. They are vasospasm, hydrocephalus, and dysrhythmias. See pages 747 and 748 for a discussion of these problems.

In addition, patients with stroke who are on anticoagulation therapy are at risk for bleeding from other sites, and vigilance and early intervention is required to prevent serious complications.

Nursing Care Plan

Nursing Care Plan 31–1 outlines the salient features of care for the patient who has experienced a stroke.

Arteriovenous Malformations

Description

Most AVMs occur in patients younger than 30 years of age. Each AVM is a tangled mass of arterial and venous blood vessels that shunt blood directly from the arterial system into the venous system, bypassing the capillary system.

These congenital developmental defects in the capillaries may occur at any site in the central nervous system (CNS) but frequently are found in the area of the middle cerebral artery. The capillaries in an AVM have failed to develop normally between the arterial and venous blood supplies, so the channels of the two blood supplies are connected by abnormally thin vessels.

Arteriovenous malformations are not confined to the cerebral circulation. They may be seen in the spinal cord, the gastrointestinal tract, under the skin, or in the renal system. Small, superficial AVMs may be detected by port wine stains of the skin.

Pathophysiological Principles

There is degeneration of the brain parenchyma around and within the malformation. Blood is shunted directly from the arterial to the venous system. This pathway offers less resistance to blood flow than the normal capillary bed, so the AVM consequently receives a large blood flow. Arteries dilate to handle the increased perfusion of the AVM, and veins enlarge to drain the additional blood away. Collateral vessels may dilate in an attempt to carry the additional load, adding to the mass of the lesion.

Large AVMs may cause an "intracerebral steal" situation whereby arterial blood is diverted away from one area of the brain because of lowered vascular resistance in

(*Text continues on page 743*)

NURSING CARE PLAN 31–1:
The Patient With a Stroke

NURSING DIAGNOSIS	OUTCOME CRITERIA/ PATIENT GOALS	NURSING INTERVENTIONS
Altered thought process: related to left hemispheric stroke manifested by possible speech involvement, right hemiplegia, dysphasia (expressive or receptive); slow, cautious disorganized behavior, right visual field cut, high level of frustration.	• Patient will be able to cope with the deficit, as demonstrated by interacting with others without evidence of prolonged or frequent frustration.	1. Initiate neurologic rehabilitation, including occupational therapy, physical therapy, speech therapy, cognitive therapy, and others as indicated. 2. Encourage use of facilitative equipment to improve speech or communication (eg, writing board, picture board, alphabet board). 3. Speak slowly to patient and allow adequate time for response, and avoid speaking to patient as if a child. 4. Help patient establish a daily routine schedule to follow to help organize behavior. 5. Provide orientation to environment through use of clock, calendar, pictures, and verbalization. 6. Organize care to occur within visual field on left, when possible.
Altered thought process: related to right hemispheric stroke manifested by possible left hemiplegia, spatial perceptual deficits, memory deficits, emotional lability, left hemianopsia, apraxia, or poor judgment.	• Patient will be able to cope with the deficit, as demonstrated by use of pencil and paper to augment memory, compensation for unilateral neglect, and absence of frequent emotional outbursts.	1. Participate in neurologic rehabilitation consultation. 2. Promote awareness of body and environment on the affected side. 3. Divide tasks into simple steps; elicit return demonstration of skills. 4. Use nonverbal clues to enhance patient understanding. 5. Use slow minimal movements and avoid clutter around the patient. 6. Provide emotional support to patient/family. Allow ventilation. Explain to family the reason for patient's emotional lability. 7. Position patient in bed to prevent falls. Consider posey restraints and side rails.

(continued)

NURSING CARE PLAN 31–1: *(Continued)*
The Patient With a Stroke

NURSING DIAGNOSIS	OUTCOME CRITERIA/ PATIENT GOALS	NURSING INTERVENTIONS
		8. Reorient patient to environment frequently through use of clock, calendar, radio, etc.
		9. Encourage use of notebook to write down things patient needs to remember, and to carry the notebook with him or her.
		10. Use brief periods of teaching, because attention span is limited, and divide tasks into multiple simple steps.
		11. Assure that medications will be given under supervision at home so patient does not forget to take them and takes the correct dose.
High risk for altered tissue perfusion: related to interruption in cerebral blood flow, cerebral hemorrhaging, increased ICP.	• Patient will maintain cerebral perfusion pressure of at least 60 mm Hg and ICP of less than 20 mm Hg.	1. Enhance venous outflow from the head by keeping head of bed elevated without neck flexion or severe head rotation.
		2. Avoid or minimize frequency and duration of nursing care which may increase intra-abdominal or intrathoracic pressure (eg, suctioning).
		3. Check tape around endotracheal tube or tracheostomy to ensure ties are not tight enough to impede cerebral blood flow.
		4. Maintain normothermia.
		5. Avoid use of restraints if possible, because the ICP will increase and CPP will decrease if patient fights against them.
		6. Report increased systolic BP, widening pulse pressure, bradycardia, headache, vomiting, and papilledema, all of which might indicate herniation.
		7. Prevent constipation. Record all bowel movements.
		8. Document neurologic status using Glasgow Coma Scale and compare with baseline.
		9. Report changes in level of consciousness.

(continued)

NURSING CARE PLAN 31–1: (Continued)
The Patient With a Stroke

NURSING DIAGNOSIS	OUTCOME CRITERIA/ PATIENT GOALS	NURSING INTERVENTIONS
High risk for injury: related to seizure activity, altered thought processes, immobility, impaired self-protective mechanisms, motor weakness, impulsiveness, decreased level of responsiveness, or dysphagia/aspiration.	• Level of consciousness will be maintained or improved. • Patient will be free from physical injury.	1. Use seizure precautions: side rails up and padded, bed in low position, tongue blade or airway available, oxygen and suction at bedside. 2. Accurately observe and record seizure. 3. Assist unsteady or ataxic patient to ambulate. 4. Teach self-protective actions (eg, teach patient to scan total environment with head to make up for visual field cut on one side). 5. Assure adequate swallow, gag, and cough reflexes before offering oral fluids and food. 6. Teach family to assess home environment for hazards (eg, throw rugs, stairs without railings, bathroom without grab bars, etc.). 7. Teach family what to do if patient seizes after discharge from the hospital.
High risk for altered nutrition, less than body requirements: related to muscle weakness during swallowing, confusion, depression, critical illness, or inability to feed self.	• Patient will take in adequate calories to meet body's metabolic demands, as measured by calorie count and calculation of metabolic requirements.	1. Document calorie count daily. 2. Initiate dietary consultation. 3. Administer tube feedings, total parenteral nutrition, or assist with oral feeding based on patient's condition. 4. Assess serum albumin, total protein, and WBC. 5. Maintain daily weight record.
High risk for impaired physical mobility: related to hemiparesis, hemiplegia, contractures, foot drop, muscle atrophy, pain, altered level of consciousness, or fatigue.	• Patient will be free of preventable complications of immobility such as atelectasis, pressure sores, and deep vein thrombosis.	1. Initiate rehabilitation consultation. 2. Perform passive/active ROM tid and record. 3. Provide space boots or high-top tennis shoes. 4. Apply splints if needed, as directed by physical therapy. 5. Mobilize patient to chair as soon as possible. 6. Position patient correctly with pillows while in bed.

(continued)

NURSING CARE PLAN 31-1: *(Continued)*
The Patient With a Stroke

NURSING DIAGNOSIS	OUTCOME CRITERIA/ PATIENT GOALS	NURSING INTERVENTIONS
		7. Turn patient q2h.
		8. Provide egg-crate mattress, sheep skin, or consider kinetic bed as indicated.
		9. Provide heel and elbow protectors.
		10. Ensure adequate nutrition.
		11. Teach patient to use spirometry or to cough/deep breathe frequently, or suction as needed to keep lungs clear.
		12. Assess lower extremities frequently for redness, tenderness, warmth, or pain.
		13. Apply elastic stockings or pneumatic stockings while immobile.

another. It is thought that AVMs can steal enough blood from adjacent areas of the brain to cause ischemic damage in the otherwise normal area. The neurologic signs and symptoms seen in the patient correlate with the area of the brain that is deprived of blood flow. The size, shape, and location of the AVM also determine the deficits seen.

Assessment

Initial assessment of the patient depends on the presenting symptoms. The patient may or may not be able to provide a history of what happened. A history of headache or seizures may cause the patient to seek medical attention, but may not be very helpful in pinpointing the diagnosis of AVM.

Clinical Manifestations

The onset of symptoms may occur in childhood or early adult life. In many patients, the chief complaint is headache, which often is unilateral. Seizures may be another initial symptom: first focal, then developing to generalized. Hemorrhage occurs in about 50% of patients before they are admitted to the hospital. An AVM that has bled once has a one in four chance of bleeding again within 4 years. An AVM that has bled more than once has a one in four chance of bleeding again within 1 year. Hemorrhage associated with an AVM can be intracerebral, subdural, or subarachnoid.

Alteration of brain tissue within the AVM and deple-

tion of blood perfusion to adjacent areas may cause the patient to exhibit paresis or mental deterioration. There may be transient episodes of dizziness, syncope, sensory deficits or tingling, visual deficits (usually hemianopsia), and confusion. If the bleeding is severe, there may be elevation of intracranial pressure with brain stem compression and unconsciousness.

A few patients report a constant swishing sound in the head with each heartbeat, representing a bruit which may be auscultated occasionally by placing a stethoscope over the skull.

Diagnostic Studies

If an AVM is suspected from the clinical manifestations or from a noncontrast scan, a CT with contrast usually is done to visualize better the cerebral vasculature. An electroencephalogram (EEG) may be done to localize the focus of any seizure activity or to demonstrate areas of cerebral ischemia or atrophy. For confirmation of the diagnosis, an angiogram is performed to identify the arteries feeding the AVM and the veins that are draining it.

Management

Embolization and Surgery

Two available management techniques for AVMs are artificial embolization and surgical excision. The embolization technique involves the introduction of small Silastic beads into the internal carotid artery, where they subsequently enter the AVM. This results in thrombosis and destruction of the lesion (Fig. 31–5). This technique is useful when the AVM is not in a surgically accessible area and excision is impossible. It is effective for AVMs supplied by the middle cerebral artery because the Silastic beads tend to follow the flow pattern of the middle cerebral artery.

The primary danger of this procedure is that a bead may dislodge from the AVM and migrate to the capillaries of the lung. Sometimes the AVM may appear occluded after the procedure, but collateral circulation redevelops, providing a new vascular supply to the area and reactivating the AVM.

Complete surgical excision eliminates the possibility of recurrent bleeding. Surgery usually is performed after the patient has stabilized from the hemorrhage—about 2 to 3 weeks. Sometimes the artificial embolization procedure is performed first, followed by surgical excision 4 weeks later.

Balloon Occlusion

A third treatment modality involves use of an intravascular detachable balloon. Carotid–cavernous sinus fistulas and vertebrovertebral fistulas have had the best results. Specific vascular anatomy with large feeding vessels deep to the nidus or aneurysms within feeding arteries favor the use of the detachable balloon over other embolic agents. Preoperative use of balloon occlusion may reduce the difficulty of surgical resection of the malformation. There usually is marked reduction of flow into the AVM by occlusion of major arterial fistula feeders. This procedure is used most often as an adjunct surgical intervention.

Pharmacologic Therapy

Propranolol hydrochloride (Inderal; Ayerst Laboratories, New York, NY) may be prescribed before and after surgery to reduce risk of postoperative hemorrhage. Because an AVM can cause an increase of blood flow by 50% to 100% above normal, cerebral autoregulation may be disrupted. After excision of the AVM, the increased blood flow gets rerouted into the brain's normal circulation, which was accustomed to minimal flow. Hyperperfusion is the result, and a hemorrhage may develop in adjacent parts of the brain. Propranolol will reduce cerebral blood flow and cardiac output.[6]

Irradiation

A noninvasive treatment for AVM that is available in only two centers in this country is the proton beam, which uses radiation energy given off by protons in a cyclotron. This shrinks the AVM, and is very useful in treating deep-seated intraparenchymal AVMs that are not accessible to surgical management.

The nursing care of patients with an AVM or a cerebral aneurysm is similar. See the discussion under Nursing Management.

Complications

Complications for patients with an AVM and subsequent subarachnoid bleed are similar to those seen in the setting of an aneurysm (see pages 747 and 748).

Cerebral Aneurysms

Description

An aneurysm is a round, saccular dilation of the arterial wall that develops as a result of weakness of the wall. Concern arises if the outpouching in the vessel wall ruptures or becomes large enough to exert pressure on surrounding brain structures.

Between 20% to 40% of victims die at the time of the initial bleed of their aneurysms. Rebleeding is the leading cause of death in patients with a history of ruptured aneurysm. Of those who survive the first hemorrhage, 35% to 40% bleed again, with a mortality rate of about 42% at that time. Rebleeding most often occurs around the seventh day after the original bleed.

Pathophysiological Principles

Arterial vessels are composed of three layers: the endothelial lining, the smooth muscle, and the connective tissue. A defect in the smooth muscle layer allows the endothelial lining to bulge through, creating an aneurysm.

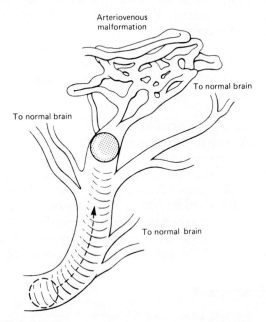

FIGURE 31–5
Small silastic beads or spheres are introduced into artery to block blood flow to the AVM (Hickey J: The Clinical Practice of Neurological and Neurosurgical Nursing, 2nd ed, p 536. Philadelphia, JB Lippincott, 1986).

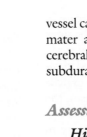

Saccular   Berry

FIGURE 31–6
Saccular and berry aneurysms (Hickey J: Clinical Practice of Neurological and Neurosurgical Nursing, 3rd ed, p 542. Philadelphia, JB Lippincott, 1992).

Some aneurysms are called "berry aneurysms" because they look like a berry, having a stem and neck. Saccular aneurysms do not have a neck but resemble a ballooning of the vessel (Fig. 31–6).

Most aneurysms arise from larger arteries around the anterior section of the circle of Willis. The most frequent site of occurrence is the juncture of the posterior communicating artery and the internal carotid artery. Other common aneurysm sites include the basilar artery, anterior cerebral artery, anterior communicating artery, and middle cerebral artery. Only about 15% of aneurysms occur within the vertebrobasilar system. Aneurysms most often form at the bifurcation of arteries.

Because aneurysm-forming vessels usually lie in the space between the arachnoid and the brain, hemorrhage from an aneurysm usually occurs in the subarachnoid space. Sometimes, however, the force of the rupturing vessel can be so great that it pushes blood through the pia mater and into the brain substance, causing an intracerebral hemorrhage, or through the arachnoid into the subdural space, causing a subdural hemorrhage.

Assessment

History

The nursing history should include identification of risk factors such as familial predisposition, hypertension, cigarette smoking, or use of over-the-counter medications (eg, nasal sprays or antihistamines that have vasoconstrictive properties). Occupational history may be relevant, because if the patient has an occupation involving strenuous activity, there may be a significant delay in going back to work or the need to change occupations entirely.

Clinical Manifestations

Many aneurysms are silent and never cause a problem but may be discovered on postmortem examination. If an aneurysm does cause problems, they usually will occur in the 35- to 60-year age group. Aneurysms are graded according to their severity, and a classification system is shown in Display Box 31–3.

Before an aneurysm bleeds or ruptures, about half the patients will have some warning signs. These may include headaches, lethargy, neck pain, a "noise in the head" (a bruit), and optic, oculomotor, or trigeminal cranial nerve dysfunction.

After an aneurysm has bled or ruptured, the patient usually complains of an explosive headache. There is a decrease in the LOC, cranial nerve dysfunction, visual disturbances, perhaps hemiparesis or hemiplegia, and of-

---

DISPLAY BOX 31–3
Botterell Classification of Aneurysms

Grade	Criteria
Grade I (minimal bleed)	Patient alert, with no focal neurologic signs and no signs of meningeal irritation.
Grade II (mild bleed)	Patient alert with minimal deficits and usually signs of meningeal irritation.
Grade III (moderate bleed)	Patient lethargic, confused, with or without neurologic deficits and signs of meningeal irritation.
Grade IV (moderate to severe bleed)	Patient stuporous or comatose with some purposeful movements. Major neurologic deficits may or may not be evident.
Grade V (severe bleed)	Patient comatose and often decerebrate. Appears moribund.

From Mitchell M: Neuroscience Nursing: A Nursing Diagnosis Approach, p 72. Baltimore, Williams & Wilkins, 1989

ten vomiting. All these signs are related to an increase in ICP. With a subarachnoid hemorrhage, there will be signs of meningeal irritation, such as a stiff and painful neck, photophobia, blurred vision, irritability, fever, and positive Kernig's and Brudzinski's signs. Exactly which deficits are present depends on the location of the aneurysm, the subsequent hemorrhage, and the severity of the bleeding.

The actual amount of blood loss through an aneurysm usually is quite small because of the severe vasoconstriction of vessels in the area of the aneurysm. This vasospasm may help stop the bleeding, but it also can cause ischemia to parts of the brain, resulting in localized neurologic deficits.

When there is blood in the subarachnoid space, it irritates the brain stem, causing abnormal activity in the autonomic nervous system centers, often with cardiac dysrhythmias and hypertension. Another complication of blood in the subarachnoid space is hydrocephalus. This may occur as the result of obstruction of the narrow channels through which the CSF flows (eg, the aqueduct of Sylvius) by red cells in the CSF. The blood in the subarachnoid space also may impede reabsorption of the CSF from the arachnoid villi. Both these situations will cause hydrocephalus, with enlargement of the lateral and third ventricles.

Diagnostic Studies

The diagnosis of a cerebral aneurysm usually is made on the basis of the history, physical examination, lumbar puncture, cerebral arteriogram, and often a CT scan.

Transcranial Doppler ultrasonography may be used in patients to diagnose and help treat vasospasm, a common complication of subarachnoid hemorrhage. This is a non-invasive, low-cost procedure that may be performed at the bedside. Daily serial correlations can be made to the patient's neurologic status, as measured by the Glasgow Coma Scale. Trends can be established over time, and it also is a predictor of impending vasospasm. Transcranial Doppler ultrasonography monitors the velocity of red blood cells as they flow through the circle of Willis, the anterior cerebral artery, the middle cerebral artery, and posterior communicating artery. The readings are obtained through the thin-walled temporal bony structure. The middle cerebral artery seems to be the most reliable vessel for detecting vasospasm, due to its limited collateral circulation.[7]

Management

General Measures

Management of a patient with a ruptured or leaking aneurysm before surgical repair includes bed rest in a dark environment to minimize the photophobia, often sedation, and a quiet room with minimal stimulation to reduce meningeal irritation. Visitors may need to be limited. Sometimes hot or cold beverages and caffeine products are not allowed. Constipation should be prevented, as well as straining or vigorous coughing.

Pharmacologic Treatment

Some physicians include the use of aminocaproic acid (Amicar; Lederle Laboratories, Pearl River, NY) in their management of the patient with an aneurysm. This is an antifibrinolytic agent that delays the lysis of blood clots. At the time of hemorrhage from an aneurysm, about 10 to 20 ml of blood escapes from the vessel. Loss of 30 to 50 ml of blood would be a massive hemorrhage, and the person probably would not survive. A blood clot normally forms over the bleeding vessel, then dissolves several days later. Aminocaproic acid may be used to prevent the breakdown of the clot over the aneurysm.

A calcium antagonist such as nimodipine may be used to reduce cerebral ischemia and vasospasm. Plasma volume should not be allowed to fall. Hyponatremia must be anticipated, which may result from hemodilution as a result of inappropriate secretion of antidiuretic hormone.

Stool softeners often are used in the management of the aneurysm patient to prevent straining. Mild analgesics may be used for relief of headache; acetaminophen or codeine can be used without masking neurologic signs. If hypertension is present, a drug that can control it is used, such as hydralazine hydrochloride (Apresoline; Ciba Pharmaceutical Co., Summit, NJ) or methyldopa (Aldomet; Merck Sharp & Dohme, West Point, PA).

Blood in the subarachnoid space will cause an elevated temperature. An antipyretic, usually acetaminophen, and hypothermia blankets are used if necessary. Steroids are controversial, but if used, dexamethasone (Decadron; Merck Sharp & Dohme) is the steroid of choice. Fluids often are restricted to prevent cerebral edema.

Surgical Intervention

Surgical excision of the aneurysm may be considered if it is in an accessible area. Aneurysms of the vertebrobasilar system often present a problem of surgical inaccessibility. Some aneurysms may be wrapped in a gauzelike material and coated with an acrylic substance that gives the aneurysm support. There is some controversy about when to surgically intervene in an aneurysm. Some physicians believe in stabilizing the patient after the hemorrhage for 7 to 10 days. Others believe that surgery should be performed immediately after the hemorrhage.

The current trend is to operate sooner rather than later. Some of the past hesitation to operate quickly was due to the increased risk of postoperative brain ischemia, but with improved techniques of microsurgery and anesthesia, operating early is less risky.[8]

Balloon angioplasty still is an experimental procedure under study at a few centers for treatment of ruptured aneurysm. A small silicone balloon is inserted at the end of a catheter and inflated in a major artery where blood flow to the brain has been reduced by vasoconstriction. Its success rate to date is about 50%, but the complication rate is 10% to 20%, and the complications can be fatal. Papaverine also has been injected directly into the cerebral artery that is in spasm, but still is considered experimental.

After AVM excision or aneurysm clipping, the patient may be intubated and on mechanical ventilation to minimize postoperative cerebral swelling. The hyperventilation will keep the PCO_2 low, causing vasoconstriction of cerebral vasculature, reducing the volume of blood flow to the head, and thus reducing the ICP. Maintenance of an adequate airway is vital. If suctioning is necessary, it is important that the suction catheter go in and out quickly so that a PCO_2 build-up is avoided and sustained coughing by the patient is prevented.

Signs of vasospasm, such as hemiparesis, visual disturbance, seizures, or a decreasing LOC, should be noted and reported so that rapid medical interventions may be initiated (see discussion under Complications).

Control of IICP is a collaborative effort. Nurses should be aware of keeping the head elevated without neck flexion or severe head rotation. Osmotics may be used as necessary based on the assessments made.

Control of temperature is important, because fever increases the metabolic demands in the brain. Whenever blood gets into the subarachnoid space, whether from a leaking AVM or a ruptured aneurysm, the patient will be febrile. Control usually is by acetaminophen suppositories and a cooling blanket.

Nursing Management

The severity and duration of any postoperative disability will depend largely on the location and extent of the vascular lesion and the resultant ischemia. Immediately after surgery, the patient should be watched for a change in neurologic status, especially a change in LOC. The nurse must be alert for the development of new deficits or for a worsening of those present before surgery. Cerebral edema may develop after surgery, causing a change in neurologic status.

Obviously, a patent airway is required, and mechanical hyperventilation may be necessary to reduce ICP. Management of fluids and electrolytes is very important, with a careful watch for hyponatremia, which can cause an increase in cerebral edema. Accurate intake and output records are important.

Monitoring of vital signs is crucial. The goal is to avoid any significant change, especially in blood pressure. Hypotension must be treated immediately to prevent a drop in cerebral perfusion. Cardiac dysrhythmias may be present, especially if there was bleeding into the subarachnoid space. Many dysrhythmias cause a drop in cardiac output, and consequently the cerebral perfusion falls. For this reason, dysrhythmias should be treated.

The critical care nurse may help awaken an unconscious patient by talking directly to the person. Research, however, indicates that even in an unconscious person, talking *about* that person around the bed causes a rise in ICP. Conversation over the unconscious person's bed should be limited to what would be said if the patient were fully awake. One can never be sure when the patient's brain

stem is intact and conversation is being perceived, regardless of whether there is motor response to demonstrate this. The critical care nurse should talk to the patient about what is going to be done, even if the LOC is impaired. This applies to all patients with a neurologic problem that affects the LOC.

Preoperative education of patient and family will make the postoperative period less stressful. Rehabilitation for specific deficits should begin early, and family participation in the rehabilitation program should be encouraged.

Nurses caring for a patient with a subarachnoid hemorrhage should be aware of the person's baseline neurologic status and be alert to changes. Patients sometimes are difficult to assess clinically when they are receiving sedation. A change in LOC is probably the first clinical sign that will be seen if the patient is deteriorating, unless an intracranial monitoring device is in place, in which case IICP may be recognized immediately. Size and reactivity of the patient's pupils are important to document, along with changes in motor and sensory function. Sudden appearance of a cranial nerve defect or increasing severity of headache should be reported immediately. Blurred vision and dysphasia also may be present, along with other neurologic deficits.

Complications

Vasospasm

Vasospasm can occur after as well as before surgery in the person with an aneurysm. In fact, 30% to 50% of patients have preoperative vasospasm, whereas 65% have postoperative vasospasm. The aneurysm may have been clipped successfully, but owing to this challenging complication, the patient may end up with a large area of ischemic or infarcted brain and severe deficits.

Vasospasm usually occurs from 3 to 12 days after subarachnoid hemorrhage. The peak incidence is between days 4 through 8, although there is some variation. Vasospasm is of clinical significance because it decreases cerebral blood flow, depriving brain tissue of oxygen, and promoting accumulation of metabolic waste products such as lactic acid.

The etiology of vasospasm is not clear. There does seem to be a positive correlation between the size of the hemorrhage seen on CT scan and subsequent development of spasm. There is a release of calcium ions from lysed red blood cells, and it is believed that calcium ions are mediators for spasm. There has been some success with use of nimodipine after subarachnoid hemorrhage, improving patient outcomes after the bleed. There may be an inflammatory response to subarachnoid hemorrhage, and this may stimulate release of vasoactive mediators. Some drugs are being tested that act to protect the cell membrane from this reaction.

Hypervolemic hemodilution therapy has gained popularity in recent years as a treatment for vasospasm. This "triple-H" therapy consists of hypervolemic expansion, hemodilution, and induced hypertension in postoperative patients. The unique nature of this therapy dictates that the critical care nurse be knowledgeable about the relationship between subarachnoid hemorrhage and cerebral blood flow as well as the potential complications of this form of treatment.

Hypervolemia is accomplished by volume expansion, using both colloid and crystalloid solutions. Objectives of hypervolemia are to have a pulmonary capillary wedge pressure approximately 14 mm Hg (usual base is 6–8) and a cardiac output of 6.5 to 8 L/minute (4.5–5.0 L/minute is normal). Hemodilution decreases blood viscosity, increases regional cerebral blood flow, and may decrease infarction size and increase oxygen transport. The goal for hemodilution is to reduce the hematocrit by 15% to 20%. Pressor agents are used to induce hypertension; the combination of dobutamine and dopamine is used frequently. The objective is to maintain systolic blood pressure at greater than 20 mm Hg over normal.

For this therapy to be effective against vasospasm, the nurse must monitor hemodynamic parameters closely and assess frequently for signs of acute pulmonary edema.

Hydrocephalus

Hydrocephalus indicates an imbalance between the production and absorption of the CSF. It occurs in 15% to 20% of patients with subarachnoid hemorrhage.[8] When there is blood in the subarachnoid space, the red blood cells can occlude the very small channels leading from one ventricle to another. If that occurs, an obstructive hydrocephalus develops in the patient—that is, there is an obstruction to the normal flow of CSF, very often between the third and fourth ventricle or at the exits from the fourth ventricle. There also is potential for a reabsorption problem when there is blood in the subarachnoid space. The red blood cells occlude the arachnoid villi, impeding reabsorption and resulting in a communicating hydrocephalus. A shunt may be placed, often between one of the lateral ventricles and the peritoneal cavity (a V-P shunt) to drain the CSF and relieve the hydrocephalus.

Dysrhythmias

Dysrhythmias of any type may occur in patients with subarachnoid hemorrhage, perhaps because blood in the CSF that bathes the brain stem is irritating to that area. The brain stem influences heart rate, so the presence of a chemical irritation can result in irregular rhythms.

Rebleeding

Another complication in patients with subarachnoid hemorrhage can be a rebleeding if the AVM or aneurysm is not repaired. At least 10% of all patients with subarachnoid hemorrhage have another bleed within hours of the initial hemorrhage. Without intervention, the risk of rebleeding in the remaining patients is a least 30% over the subsequent 4 weeks. The immediate mortality of rebleeding is 50%.[8]

Increased Intracranial Pressure

In CNS injury, IICP is a potential complication. It may be the result of ischemia after a stroke, or a hemorrhagic stroke where the blood causes a mass lesion effect. It may result from a leaking AVM or aneurysm, or may be postoperative after manipulation of the brain during a craniotomy.

There are many nursing interventions that can minimize this potentially fatal complication (see Nursing Care Plan 31–2). Early medical interventions such as hyperventilation, use of osmotics, steroids, barbiturate coma, hypothermia, and fluid restriction also are valuable in treating this complication. (Osmotics are not used when there is an active cerebral hemorrhage, however, because they may increase the bleeding by shrinking the brain and releasing the tamponade effect of the leaking vessel.)

CASE STUDY

Mrs. B was a 50-year-old woman who, while playing with her dog, collapsed, grabbing her head. She was rushed to the hospital where she was diagnosed as having a small ruptured cerebral aneurysm. She was awake on entering the ICU, but complained of a severe headache and a stiff neck. She was taken to surgery within 4 hours, where the aneurysm was clipped successfully. Postoperative angiogram demonstrated no evidence of vasospasm. On day 5, Mrs. B became confused, disoriented, weak in one arm, and wanted to sleep more than usual. She was sent to radiology for an emergent CT scan, where hydrocephalus and rebleeding were ruled out. Transcranial Doppler ultrasonography was done, which confirmed vasospasm.

"Triple-H" therapy (hypervolemia, hemodilution, and induced hypertension) was initiated, and follow-up transcranial Doppler ultrasonography showed normal lumen diameter of the vessels. By the next day, Mrs. B was oriented and following commands, had normal strength in all extremities, and was neurologically intact. She was discharged home 2 weeks later, doing well.

Nursing Care Plan

Nursing Care Plan 31–2 details the important aspects of nursing care for the patient with an aneurysm or AVM.

Seizure Disorders

Description

A seizure is a sudden discharge of a group of neurons resulting in a transient impairment of consciousness, movement, sensation, or memory. The term *epilepsy* usually is reserved for a chronic disorder involving recurrent seizures. The term *seizure disorder* may refer to one isolated occurrence or to a recurrent situation. There seems to be less social stigma associated with the term *seizure disorder* than with *epilepsy*.

Seizures may be caused by a variety of pathologic conditions, including brain tumors, trauma, blood clots,

NURSING CARE PLAN 31–2:
The Patient With Cerebral Aneurysm or AVM

NURSING DIAGNOSIS	OUTCOME CRITERIA/ PATIENT GOALS	NURSING INTERVENTIONS
Altered tissue perfusion: related to interruption in cerebral blood flow or increased intracranial pressure.	• Patient will maintain cerebral perfusion pressure of at least 50 mm Hg. • Patient will maintain ICP less than 15 mm Hg. • LOC will not deteriorate below that of baseline.	1. Report cerebral perfusion pressure less than 50 mm Hg. 2. Report ICP rises over 15 mm Hg. 3. Report decrease in Glasgow Coma Scale. 4. Keep head of bed elevated 30° with no neck flexion or hip flexion greater than 90° and no severe head rotation. 5. Minimize frequency and duration of suctioning if it is necessary. Hyperventilate and hyperoxygenate before suctioning, and limit procedure to 10 seconds at a time. 6. Base nursing care activities on ICP. Allow ICP to drop between activities. 7. Coordinate activities with other departments to avoid ICP elevation (eg, x-rays, therapies, etc.), allowing adequate rest periods. 8. Report changes in patient's condition before a critical change in vital signs may alter cerebral perfusion. 9. Provide sedation or analgesia as ordered. 10. Tell patient what is about to be done to him or her before the activity (the brain stem may be intact even though the patient appears nonresponsive). 11. Avoid conversations over the patient's bed that you would not have if he or she were fully awake. 12. Use restraints only when absolutely necessary, because fighting restraints will raise intrathoracic and intra-abdominal pressure, thus impeding venous outflow from the head. 13. Allow only passive ROM exercises when ICP is labile.

(continued)

NURSING CARE PLAN 31–2: *(Continued)*
The Patient With Cerebral Aneurysm or AVM

NURSING DIAGNOSIS	OUTCOME CRITERIA/ PATIENT GOALS	NURSING INTERVENTIONS
		14. Calculate CPP if an ICP monitor and an arterial line are in place (CPP = mean systemic arterial pressure minus ICP).
		15. Minimize activity preoperatively, providing a quiet environment.
High risk for sensory–perceptual alteration: related to altered LOC, disorientation, impaired communication skills, restricted and/or unfamiliar environment.	• Patient will interpret environmental stimuli appropriately.	1. Provide frequent orientation; clock, calendar etc.
		2. Explain unfamiliar machinery, noises, and role of people in patient's environment.
		3. Converse with unconscious patient as if he or she were awake.
		4. Label bedside with patient's perceptual deficit so all caregivers are aware (eg, "patient cannot speak").
		5. Allow for adequate sleep and rest. Alter lighting and reduce auditory stimuli to promote normal circadian sleep patterns.
		6. Provide alternate communication method if unable to verbalize (eg, alphabet chart).
		7. Apply coma stimulation techniques to awaken patient from coma.
		8. Encourage family visits and verbalization to patient and suggest they bring in personal items, such as pictures, to help reorient patient.
High risk for pain: related to meningeal signs (stiff neck, headache, photophobia) from subarachnoid hemorrhage.	• Patient will rate discomfort less than 4 on a scale of 1–10 (1 being minimal pain and 10 being excruciating).	1. Teach patient to use a pain rating scale before administration of analgesics and 30 min after administration.
		2. Position to prevent neck flexion or hip flexion over 90°.
		3. Keep room dark to minimize photophobia.
		4. Keep environment quiet.
		5. Administer analgesics around the clock, as ordered, to prevent pain from getting out of control.

(continued)

NURSING CARE PLAN 31–2: (Continued)
The Patient With Cerebral Aneurysm or AVM

NURSING DIAGNOSIS	OUTCOME CRITERIA/ PATIENT GOALS	NURSING INTERVENTIONS
High risk for fluid volume excess: related to neuro/hormonal dysfunction of hypervolemia used to treat vasospasm or deficit related to fluid restriction and use of osmotics to control ICP.	• Patient will maintain adequate hydration.	1. Record intake and output, vital signs, and hemodynamic parameters at least q4h. 2. Report signs of fluid overload: tachypnea, tachycardia, neck vein distention, edema, gallop rhythm. 3. Report signs of fluid volume deficit: hypotension, oliguria, dry mucous membranes, poor skin turgor, complaints of thirst. 4. Auscultate and record breath sounds frequently. 5. Calculate fluid balance at least q24h. 6. Use an IV pump for accurate administration of fluids. 7. Report signs of increased ICP or change in LOC. 8. Monitor serum electrolyte values.

meningitis, encephalitis, electrolyte disorders, alcohol and drug overdose and withdrawal, metabolic disorders, uremia, overhydration, toxic substances, and cerebral anoxia. Some seizures are idiopathic (ie, of unknown etiology).

Between 5% and 50% of patients with head trauma have post-traumatic seizures. When trauma is the cause, the seizures occur within 2 years of the injury in 90% of the cases. Craniotomies may leave scar tissue, which can be a future site for seizure activity.

Seizures develop in 10% to 20% of patients with strokes. Central nervous system infections result in 17% to 34% of those people having seizures. Lesions of the brain can be produced by degenerative CNS diseases, such as multiple sclerosis, Alzheimer's disease, and Huntington's chorea, and these can be a site for seizure activity. Seizures usually are a symptom of some cerebral pathologic condition, and not a disease entity in themselves.

Pathophysiological Principles

The exact mechanism that causes seizure activity in the brain is not fully understood. Some trigger causes a sudden abnormal burst of electrical stimulation, disrupting the brain's normal nerve conduction. In a non–seizure-prone brain, there is a balance between excitatory and inhibitory synaptic influences on postsynaptic neurons. In a seizure-prone brain, this balance somehow is disrupted, causing an imbalanced pattern of electrical conduction called paroxysmal depolarization shifts. These shifts may be seen either when there is excessive excitatory influence or insufficient inhibitory influence.

The pathophysiological process is a bit different with different types of seizures, leading to a variety of clinical manifestations (see Clinical Manifestations, under Assessment).

Classification of Seizures

Seizures are classified according to clinical and EEG criteria established by the Commission on Classification and Terminology of the International League Against Epilepsy (see Display Box 31–4). The two main categories are generalized and focal, or partial, seizures. Generalized seizures are those that show synchronous involvement of all regions of the brain in both hemispheres. Partial seizures are those that show clinical or EEG evidence of a focal onset, involving one particular part of the brain.

DISPLAY BOX 31–4
*International Classification
of Epileptic Seizures*

I. Partial seizures
   A. Simple partial (consciousness retained)
      1. Motor
      2. Sensory
      3. Autonomic
      4. Psychic
   B. Complex partial (consciousness impaired)
      1. Simple partial, followed by impaired
         consciousness
      2. Consciousness impaired at onset
   C. Partial seizures with secondary generaliza-
      tion
II. Generalized seizures
   A. Absences
      1. Typical
      2. Atypical
   B. Generalized tonic-clonic
   C. Tonic
   D. Clonic
   E. Myoclonic
   F. Atonic
III. Unclassified seizures

From International League Against Epilepsy: Proposal for
revised clinical and electroencephalographic classification of
epileptic seizures. Epilepsia 22:489, 1981. New York, Raven
Press. Reprinted with permission

Partial Seizures

There are two types of partial seizures: simple and complex. Partial seizures of either type may progress to a
generalized seizure if the abnormal electrical discharges
spread from the initial focus to involve the remainder of
the brain.

Differentiation of the two types of partial seizures is
based on whether consciousness is retained or impaired.
When there is no impairment of consciousness, the attack
is termed a simple partial seizure, which may be motor,
sensory, autonomic, or psychic in nature, depending on
the seizure focus. If the focus is in the posterior frontal
lobe near the motor cortex, there will be motor involvement of the contralateral side of the body.

The old term, "Jacksonian seizure," is an example of a
simple partial seizure with motor involvement. Clinically,
there are repetitive, usually unilateral involuntary contractions of a specific muscle group, such as thumb flexors.
Adjacent muscle groups are affected progressively, often
until one entire side of the body is involved. In the individual patient, the seizure almost always begins in the same
area and migrates in the same pattern, called the Jacksonian march.

If the focus is in the anterior parietal lobe, which is
involved with the sensory cortex, no clinical evidence of
seizure may appear. The patient may describe sensory
phenomena related to the focus in the contralateral side of
the brain. Partial seizures with psychic symptoms are rare.

Complex partial seizures (also known as temporal
lobe, psychomotor seizures, or automatisms) often have
their focus in or near the temporal lobe, although sometimes the focus is in the frontal lobe. There always is an
impairment in the LOC. Clinical manifestations with this
type of seizure are varied, and the behavior exhibited may
be quite bizarre. There may be visual, auditory, or olfactory hallucinations (eg, seeing things not really in the
environment, hearing voices telling the patient to do something, or smelling an odor, such as that of brewing coffee).
A visceral sensation such as nausea, vomiting, or profuse
sweating may precede the seizure.

The patient may demonstrate automatisms, or automatic behaviors, such as playing with buttons on clothing
or becoming preoccupied with some other motor activity.
During the seizure, the person usually is not combative,
but if provoked or if someone attempts restraint, the
person may become agitated and asocial. After the seizure
episode, the patient has no recall of the behavior that was
displayed. Such a person may be misdiagnosed as having a
psychiatric problem because behaviors often are similar in
both situations.

Generalized Seizures

In a generalized seizure, the entire brain is activated at
once, synchronously, without a focal onset (Fig. 31–7).
There is no aura or prodromal warning unless it is a partial
seizure that has generalized.

Typical absence seizures, formerly called petit mal, are
diagnosed by 3-second spike wave activity on EEG (ie, 3
cycles/second [Hz]). These seizures usually occur in children and often are outgrown by puberty. After puberty, the
person may not have any further seizure activity, or the type
of seizure may change to a generalized type of activity.

Clinically, a typical absence seizure does not involve
any violent involuntary movements or incontinence. There
may be minor motor manifestations such as eyeblinking.
There is a transient, often unnoticed loss of consciousness
or contact with the environment. The behavior, with vacant staring, may resemble daydreaming and is over within a
few seconds. Teachers may report to parents that their
child daydreams when in fact the child may be having
several typical absence seizures during the day. There are
no postictal symptoms.

Atypical absence seizures clinically resemble the typical
absence seizures. The primary difference is demonstrated on
EEG; only the typical absence seizure demonstrates 3-sec-
ond spike wave activity. Atypical absence seizures may be
seen in both children and adults. There may be minor
automatisms, and the patient usually has other types of
seizures as well, which often are refractory to medical

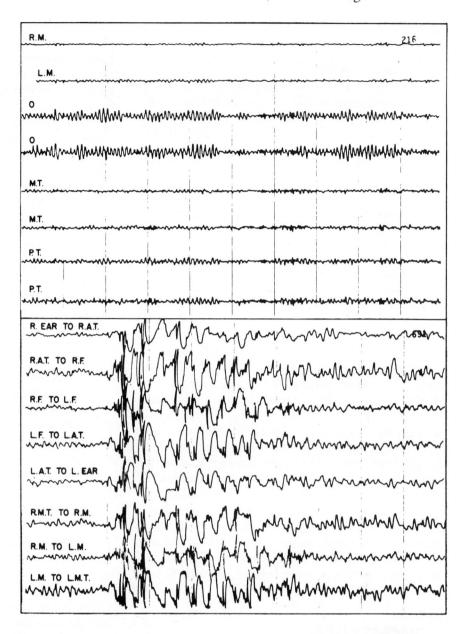

FIGURE 31–7
Contrast of a normal EEG (*top*) with that of an epileptic patient during a tonic–clonic seizure (*bottom*). Note the sharp, spiky waves recorded during the seizure (Hickey J: The Clinical Practice of Neurological and Neurosurgical Nursing, 3rd ed, p. 584. Philadelphia, JB Lippincott, 1992).

therapy. Atypical absence seizures frequently are associated with mental retardation.

In the old classification, generalized tonic–clonic seizures were called grand mal, or major motor, seizures. These seizures involve a bilateral tonic extension of the extremities followed by synchronous bilateral jerking movements. There may be a cry, incontinence of stool or urine, or both, tongue-biting, and foaming at the mouth. There is a sudden loss of consciousness. The seizure is followed by a postictal period, during which the patient is exhausted and extremely difficult to arouse. As the person awakens, diffuse muscle soreness and initial confusion may be experienced.

Tonic or clonic generalized seizures exhibit only one phase of the previously described tonic–clonic activity.

Myoclonic seizures are typified by synchronous, asymmetrical rapid jerking of one or more extremity, the trunk,

or a specific muscle group. They may be seen with metabolic encephalopathies such as hepatic failure, with infectious processes, and with degenerative processes. There is no loss of consciousness associated with myoclonic seizures.

Atonic seizures, previously classified as "drop attacks," or akinetic seizures, are another type of generalized seizure. There usually is loss of consciousness, but the episode may be so brief that the patient is unaware of the blackout. The patient is aware of the sudden loss of muscle tone as he or she falls to the ground.

Unclassified Seizures

Some seizures do not fit any of the aforementioned classifications, perhaps because clinically or electrographically they do not meet the criteria of the established categories. Sometimes the diagnosis of a seizure disorder needs to be confirmed with observation and inhospital monitoring, rather than on an outpatient basis.

Status Epilepticus

Status epilepticus is a medical emergency characterized by a series of seizures without recovery of the baseline neurologic status between the seizures. Most authorities agree that clinical, or EEG, seizure activity that lasts 30 minutes or more constitutes status epilepticus. The newer classification of status epilepticus is shown in Display Box 31–5.

Convulsive status includes muscle twitching, generalized tonic–clonic seizures, simple partial seizures, and myoclonic seizures. The nonconvulsive category includes absence seizures and complex partial seizures.

Pseudoseizures

Pseudoseizures are psychologically based. They have no associated abnormal discharges from the brain. They may resemble epileptic seizures closely, thus making the diagnosis difficult. Some patients may have both disorders present, pseudoseizures and a real seizure disorder.

Pseudoseizures are frequent in children and adolescents (the mean age range is 18.5 to 27.5 years), and the incidence is twice as high in women as in men. The onset of a pseudoseizure may be gradual or sudden, and it usually is longer than an epileptic seizure. Pseudoseizures occur more often around witnesses. Environmental influences can affect the course of a pseudoseizure and may precipitate it. Patients may follow commands and focus their eye contact on a witness. When one woman was asked if she would allow her seizure to be filmed, she immediately began seizing. The investigator asked her to wait until he got his camera, and she stopped the seizure immediately.

There is abnormal motor activity with pseudoseizures. One unusual type is opisthotonus, in which the head and legs are bent backward and the trunk arches forward. The protective mechanisms we have to prevent us from harming ourselves, such as breaking a fall with our arms and protecting our head from hitting the ground, are present in patients who have pseudoseizures but not in those who have real seizures.

With pseudoseizures, there is no tongue-biting, incontinence, or dilated pupils, the corneal reflex is present, and there is response to painful stimulation. Confusion after the pseudoseizure usually is absent.

Display Box 31–6 distinguishes epileptic seizures from pseudoseizures.

Because the nurse spends more time with a patient than most other personnel do, it is important that he or she develop skills in differentiating pseudoseizures from true seizures through clinical observations. Once the patient is diagnosed, the nurse should be aware of the stigma that family and society may associate with the condition. The nurse can help by promoting use of the more objective term *pseudoseizure* rather than the judgmental term *hysterical seizure*, which some people use to describe the condition.

The treatment plan usually involves the use of psychotherapy. Hypnosis also has been a helpful intervention, especially in determining the precipitating cause of the pseudoseizure. Often, the cause can be abolished by hypnotic suggestion.

Assessment

History and Physical Examination

A complete neurologic examination should be performed in a seizure work-up because a focal finding may help determine the origin of some seizure activity. Along with the neurologic examination, a history should be elicited. Often the history will reveal precipitating factors that may have provoked the seizure, even in usually well controlled patients. Some common precipitating factors may be fever, injury, menses, sleep deprivation, drug use, physical exhaustion, and hyperventilation. Emotional stress from the home or work environment also is a possible precipitating factor.

An often invaluable piece of information in the assessment of seizure disorders is a description of the attack by an eyewitness. The patient also may be able to help in the description of the event, especially if an aura was felt before the attack.

Seizure activity charts are very helpful for describing seizures of hospitalized patients. An example is shown in Figure 31–8.

The critical care nurse who witnesses an actual seizure can help the physician diagnose the type of seizure and localize the focus. A specific description of the seizure should include the following, whether from a witness or by history:

DISPLAY BOX 31–5
Classification of Status Epilepticus

I. Convulsive status
    A. Generalized tonic-clonic status
    B. Partial motor status ("epilepsia partialis continua")
II. Nonconvulsive status
    A. Absence status (petit mal status)
    B. Complex partial status (psychomotor status)
    C. Partial sensory status

From Earnest M: Neurologic Emergencies. New York, Churchill-Livingstone (modified from International League Against Epilepsy: Proposal for revised clinical and electroencephalographic classification of epileptic seizures. Epilepsia 22:489, 1981. New York, Raven Press. Reprinted with permission).

DISPLAY BOX 31-6
Criteria for Distinguishing Epileptic Seizures from Pseudoseizures

	Epileptic	*Pseudoseizure*
Apparent cause	Absent	Emotional disturbance
Warning	Varies, but more commonly unilateral or epigastric aura	Palpitation, malaise, choking, bilateral foot aura
Onset	Commonly sudden	Often gradual
Scream	At onset	During course
Convulsion	Rigidity followed by "jerking"; rarely rigidity alone	Rigidity or "struggling"; throwing limbs and head about
Biting	Tongue	Lips, hands, or more often other people and things
Micturition	Frequent	Never
Defecation	Occasional	Never
Duration	A few minutes	Often half an hour or several hours
Restraint needed	To prevent self-injury	To control violence
Termination	Spontaneous	Spontaneous or artificially induced (water, etc.)

From Konikow N: Hysterical seizures or pseudoseizures. Journal of Neuroscience Nursing 15:22–26.

- *Onset.* The nurse should determine whether the seizure had a sudden onset or whether it was preceded by a warning aura.
- *Duration.* Timing of the seizure from onset to end is important. What was the frequency of seizures?
- *Motor activity.* The nurse should note the parts of the body involved and determine whether both left and right sides were involved. In what part of the body did the seizure begin, and how did it progress? Was rigidity, jerking, or twitching observed?
- *Eyes and tongue.* The nurse should notice whether there was any deviation of the eyes or tongue to one side or the other.
- *State of consciousness.* Arousability is important. Was the patient arousable during the seizure or immediately after it? If there was unconsciousness, the duration of that period should be timed. Was there confusion or awareness and clear memory of the event after the seizure?
- *Distractibility.* The nurse should determine whether the patient responds to the environment during the seizure, such as when his or her name is called. Some patients, often drug abusers, may try to feign seizures, which will be revealed when they respond to their names.
- *Pupils.* The nurse should note any change in size,

shape, or equality of the pupils and their reaction to light or any deviation to one side.
- *Teeth.* The nurse should observe whether the teeth were clenched or open.
- *Respirations.* The rate, quality, or absence of respiration and the presence of cyanosis should be observed.
- *Body activities.* Incontinence, vomiting, salivation, and bleeding from the mouth or tongue should be reported.
- *After the seizure.* Sometimes after a seizure there can be a transient paralysis, weakness, numbness, tingling, dysphasia, other injuries, a postictal period, or amnesia regarding the seizure and events before and after it.
- *Precipitating factors.* By talking to the patient, the nurse may uncover a precipitating factor. Fever, emotional or physical stress, and anticonvulsant noncompliance all may precipitate a seizure.

Diagnostic Studies

A CT scan usually is part of the seizure diagnostic work-up. Such pathologic conditions as tumor, edema, infarct, congenital lesion, hemorrhage, AVM, or ventricular enlargement can be seen on CT scan.

Skull x-rays usually are not of much help in the diag-

SEIZURE ACTIVITY SHEET

Patient's Name _____

Room No. _____ Age _____

Physician _____

Date	Time	Before		During								After				Nurse's Initials
		Warning Signs	Part of Body Where Seizure Began	General or Localized	Type of Movement	Duration of each Phase Tonic	Clonic	Level of Conscious- ness	Pupils	Other	Behav- ior	Paral- ysis	Loca- tion of Paral- ysis	Sleep		

FIGURE 31–8
An example of a seizure activity chart (Hickey J: The Clinical Practice of Neurological and Neurosurgical Nursing, 3rd ed, p. 600. Philadelphia, JB Lippincott, 1992).

nostic work-up of seizures, except perhaps to rule out a fracture. The CT scan is more inclusive.

An MRI also may be done to determine the presence of pathologic CNS changes.

A metabolic work-up may be useful. Tests for blood glucose, electrolytes, calcium, and hepatic and renal function often are obtained. Presence of infection may be searched for. Platelet count, sedimentation rate, and serologic or immunologic tests also may be ordered. A lumbar puncture may help determine presence of an infection, such as meningitis. The CSF also is examined for cells, protein, glucose, and cultures. In the presence of a CNS infection, there may be an elevation of white blood cells and protein and a decrease in the glucose level, compared to the serum values. Normally, the serum glucose is one half to two thirds the serum value.

An EEG often is beneficial in confirming the seizure diagnosis and in localizing a lesion if one exists. Electroencephalograms show neurologic function, whereas CT scans demonstrate anatomy. Most EEGs are done during a time when the patient is not actively seizing, however, so it may not be too informative unless the person happened to be seizing during the EEG recording. Sometimes, photic stimulation and hyperventilation can provoke a generalized seizure of the absence type. These stimuli usually are included during the routine EEG recording. If a patient appears to be clinically seizing and the concurrent EEG is normal, the possibility of hysterical seizures or pseudoseizures should be considered.

Management

Pharmacologic Treatment

Drug management of any seizure activity, whether status epilepticus or other types, should be systematic (see Display Box 31–7). Patients may be admitted to the critical care unit having received a little diazepam, some phenytoin, and some phenobarbital in the emergency depart-

---

```
┌─────────────────────────────────────────┐
│ DISPLAY BOX 31–7                          │
│ Principles of Treatment of Seizures       │
└─────────────────────────────────────────┘
```

    I. Establish the diagnosis and rule out underlying cerebral pathologic condition.

    II. Classify seizure type, using clinical and EEG criteria.

    III. Select drug of first choice for seizure type.

    IV. Increase dose slowly until end point is reached:
        A. Complete seizure control,
        B. Optimum plasma drug level, or
        C. Toxic side effects appear

    V. If poor seizure control, gradually withdraw first drug while replacing with second drug of choice for seizure type; monotherapy is preferable to polypharmacy.

    VI. If improvement is only partial, other drugs may be necessary.

    VII. Adjust dose gradually according to plasma levels, keeping in mind:
        A. Pharamacokinetics of each drug
        B. Potential drug interactions

    VIII. If best medical therapy is unsuccessful, refer to specialized epilepsy center for intensive monitoring and possible surgical therapy

From Earnest M: Neurologic Emergencies. New York, Churchill-Livingstone (modified after Meinardi H, Rowan AJ (eds): Advances in Epileptology, p 211. Amsterdam, Swets and Zeitlinger).

---

ment. No drug is therapeutic, and it is difficult to know how to treat the patient.

Typically, a patient should be started on one drug, and it should be pushed until it reaches a therapeutic blood level. If the person continues to seize, a second drug should be added to the regimen until it is at therapeutic levels, and so on until the seizures are controlled.

Different types of seizures respond better to specific drugs. Partial seizures (simple or complex) and generalized seizures of the tonic–clonic type respond to carbamazepine, phenytoin, primidone, and phenobarbital. Some studies suggest that valproate, chlorazepate, clonazepam, and methsuximide are useful in some refractory cases of complex partial seizures.

Ethosuximide is the drug of choice for simple absences, and phenobarbital usually is the second choice. Valproate or clonazepam is useful in atypical absences, atonic seizures, and myoclonic seizures. Myoclonic seizures may be treated with adrenocorticotropic hormone or a ketogenic diet, or both.

Therapeutic blood levels should be checked periodically. Drug screens can identify patients who are not compliant with their treatment, those who may metabolize the drugs at different rates, or those who are not absorbing it. It generally is agreed that most anticonvulsive drugs may be taken once or twice daily, and still maintain therapeutic levels, because of the long half-life of these drugs.

Baclofen recently has had some success as an adjunct to conventional anticonvulsant therapy to control complex partial seizures. Animal studies indicate that baclofen increases the threshold for induced seizures.

No new antiepileptic drug has been marketed in the United States since the Food and Drug Administration approved the use of valproate in 1978. At least three new antiepileptic drugs, nitrazepam, clobazam, and vigabatrin, currently used in Europe are not yet available in this country. They may be approved within the next few years.

Treatment of status epilepticus usually involves the use of diazepam, phenytoin, phenobarbital, or any combination of these drugs. Diazepam, a rapid-acting drug with short duration, may stop all types of status epilepticus activity immediately. Because of the rapid onset of action, it can be dose-regulated according to the effects it has. The dosage of diazepam is 5 to 20 mg, injected intravenously at a rate of 5 mg or less per minute, while the nurse watches for respiratory depression. Because the duration of action of diazepam is short, 10% to 50% of patients treated with this drug alone experience recurrent seizure activity.

It is recommended that diazepam be accompanied by another drug, such as phenytoin. Phenytoin provides long-term control in about 80% of cases of status epilepticus. The dose of phenytoin is 12 to 18 mg/kg. A loading dose of 1 to 1.5 g is given to most adults. The drug should be administered at a rate of 40 to 50 mg/minute while the patient is on a cardiac monitor. If the drug is given too rapidly, there may be a widening of the QRS complexes, cardiac conduction disturbances, bradycardia, hypotension, and cardiac arrest.

Phenytoin is highly alkaline and will precipitate easily in any intravenous solution that contains dextrose. It should be given in normal saline or lactated Ringer's solution. The onset of action is 10 to 20 minutes. When given with diazepam, which acts immediately, the phenytoin will be effective by the time the diazepam is beginning to wear off. Phenytoin usually is not effective against typical absence seizures.

Phenobarbital may be given intravenously to stop status epilepticus, or the drug may be administered to treat seizures on a long-term basis. The dose is 5 to 8 mg/kg, and the effects are seen in 5 to 25 minutes. The rate of injection is 40 to 60 mg/minute. When phenobarbital is given along with diazepam, the respiratory depression effect of each may be compounded, so respirations should be monitored carefully.

Once the status epilepticus is under control, the etiology should be searched for because seizures often are a sign of an underlying pathologic process and not the disease entity in itself.

Surgical Intervention

Recent advances in diagnostic and microsurgical techniques have made surgical intervention more possible for selected patients who are resistant to drug therapy. Technology now exists to map electrical activity from deep within the brain.

Temporal lobectomy is a surgical treatment for selected patients with some refractory partial-type epilepsy. The epileptogenic focus is localized with extensive evaluation and tests. If the site is in a surgically accessible area, it is resected. Eighty percent of patients with medically intractable seizures have localized pathologic regions in the anterior temporal cortex. Temporal lobectomy usually involves resection of the anterior 4 to 6 cm of the temporal lobe, medial temporal structures including the amygdala, and the anterior portion of the pes hippocampus.[9]

Complications of the procedure may include cerebral edema, intracranial hemorrhage, hydrocephalus, cerebral infarction, or increased seizures. Reasons for surgical failure include epileptogenicity in the unresected hemisphere or cortical scarring, which forms a new site for seizure activity.

Some patients with multifocal intractable seizures who do not meet criteria for resection may benefit from a callosotomy. This is a palliative procedure that helps stop the spread of seizures from one hemisphere to the other. If a total callosotomy is performed, the patient is at risk for split-brain syndrome, in which one half of the brain may be unaware of the other half's activities—for example, while one hand is reaching for a door handle, the other may be pushing it away. Patients in whom this syndrome develops must learn to compensate after the surgery.

Studies on vagal nerve stimulation are underway. This treatment involves an implantable neurocybernetic prosthesis (NCP), which is similar in construction to a cardiac pacemaker. The NCP stimulates the vagus nerve with intermittent electrical impulses to prevent or reduce some complex partial seizures. An electronic device is implanted under the skin between the clavicle and the nipple. It is programmable from outside the skin, so changes can be made in its initial program. The NCP delivers a stimulation every 5 to 20 minutes, with a duration of 30 to 90 seconds. It is hypothesized that stimulation of the vagus nerve desynchronizes cerebral electrical activity, giving an antiepileptic effect. Preliminary reports on the effectiveness of NCP are favorable.[10]

Patient Education

Teaching the patient and family about the importance of anticonvulsant medications is a vital part of the nurse's role. Side effects should be taught, as well as toxic effects. The nurse may suggest interventions that can minimize side effects (eg, good oral hygiene for patients taking phenytoin may help minimize gum hyperplasia and infection). Patients can be taught to look for early signs of drug toxicity that they should report to the physician (eg, nystagmus, which a patient can identify in the mirror, or ataxia, may be early signs of phenytoin toxicity). The importance of not suddenly stopping an anticonvulsant should be stressed, for fear the abrupt withdrawal will trigger a seizure. With this in mind, the patient needs to plan ahead to be sure the prescription is renewed, for example before a holiday weekend, when he may not be able to get the needed medication.

Information on what to do if a seizure occurs may help alleviate some anxiety in the patient and family as well. This information empowers the patient and family to control the unpredictability of seizure activity to some extent. A battle plan of sorts can be established and put into use if a seizure occurs.

If one particular trigger, such as flashing lights, is identified as the precipitating event to a seizure, this trigger can be avoided. When the stimulus is not clear, general advice may include avoidance of getting overtired, tackling too many stressful activities at once, and avoidance of alcohol and excessive caffeine. Patients should be advised to wear a MedicAlert bracelet or necklace and stay hydrated.

Complications

Physical and Dental Injury

Some common complications after seizures are physical injury and broken teeth if someone tries to insert a tongue blade or oral airway after the teeth already are clenched tight. Sometimes teeth also can be aspirated into the lungs.

Another complication of seizure activity may be rhabdomyolysis and myoglobinuria. Myoglobin is an iron-containing pigment found in skeletal muscle, especially in those specialized for sustained contraction. There is muscle damage with seizure activity, as with many other activities. Severe exercise, such as jogging, performing military calisthenics, marathon running, and riding mechanical bulls, can cause the same type of muscle breakdown. Patients who are found after lying unconscious for a period of time, those who present with amphetamine or heroin overdoses (with the accompanying shaking chills), and those who demonstrate phencyclidine (PCP, angel dust) abuse when there is unusual muscular hyperactivity may have profound rhabdomyolysis.

The protein from the destroyed tissue turns the patient's urine red or cola-colored. The muscle cell breakdown releases myoglobin into the bloodstream, which is rapidly filtered by the kidneys, producing the dark red or brown urine. The myoglobin can occlude the kidneys, and renal failure may result. The critical care nurse may be the first to recognize the signs of this serious complication.

Treatment of rhabdomyolysis involves flushing the kidneys. Extensive skeletal muscle necrosis may be associated with massive loss of arterial volume into necrotic muscle and subsequent shock. The large volume replacement necessary for these patients approximates that seen in extensively burned patients. Furosemide or mannitol, or both, are used sometimes for diuresis, along with volume replacement. The hyperkalemia due to the cellular breakdown and renal dysfunction also may require treatment.

Psychological Aberrations

The psychological reaction of a patient with a known seizure disorder is varied. One response to the feelings of dependency and loss of self-esteem that seizures may precipitate is social withdrawal. This may seem to the patient to be an adequate coping mechanism, but it can foster feelings of depression.

People with long histories of seizures may have personality disorders. They may be manipulative, hostile, and aggressive. Children may demonstrate personality disorders through temper tantrums, hyperactivity, or antisocial behavior. The reaction of others to people with seizure disorders must be one of acceptance and support. Therapeutic interaction can help the patient achieve resocialization.

Denial is another psychological coping mechanism that may be displayed by patient or family. If the interval between seizures is long, this mechanism is easier to use. When a patient uses denial, there may be concurrent noncompliance with medical therapy.

Family members, especially parents, often feel guilty about the seizure disorder. This can result in overprotection and prevent the person from developing independence. Conversely, the person with the seizure disorder may become the scapegoat for the family, and all the family troubles may be attributed to him or her.

Epilepsy has had a negative connotation throughout history. At one time it was thought that people with "fits" were controlled by evil spirits. Insanity and mental deficiency also have been linked with this disorder.

Today, although people are better informed, many still avoid a person with epilepsy. A seizure is viewed as a form of deviant behavior and can be very frightening to onlookers because of the unexpectedness and unpredictability of the episodes. Much of the social stigma of seizures could be alleviated by improvement of society's understanding of the problem. Public education is very important because general reaction to the disorder can influence how a person copes with his or her disorder.

CASE STUDY

The patient, a 12-year-old girl, was sent home from school one hot day by the school nurse. It was thought that the girl had become overheated while playing volleyball during gym class.

Her behavior was described as "weird" by her classmates all day. She had had several episodes of staring out the classroom window that morning, with a vacant look on her face. During a later class she was responsive only intermittently, answering a few questions with "yes" or "no." Her answers were somewhat delayed. Occasionally, she played with the buttons on her dress and exhibited brief periods of lip-smacking.

The patient did not recall the behavior when questioned by her mother. The girl's mother took her to a physician, where an EEG showed somewhat irregular, generalized spike waves at 3 Hz. The EEG became normal after intravenous injection of 5 mg diazepam. Also, the girl immediately became more responsive.

This history and the physical findings, along with the girl's response to treatment are consistent with a diagnosis of absence status seizure.

Nursing Care Plan

If a nurse encounters a person who is seizing, he or she should stay with the patient to offer protection from the environment. A seizing patient never should be restrained. Any tight or restrictive clothing can be loosened. If the patient already has the teeth clenched, the nurse should not attempt to insert an oral airway or tongue blade because such action may break off teeth, which the patient may aspirate. A patent airway should be maintained during the seizure. It may help to turn the patient on the side to prevent aspiration. The nurse should reassure and reorient the patient if the seizure has caused fright and disorientation.

Details are presented in Nursing Care Plan 31–3.

Guillain–Barré Syndrome

Description

Guillain–Barré syndrome (GBS) is a clinical syndrome characterized by an acute onset of symptoms involving the peripheral and cranial nerves. The disease process involves demyelination and degeneration of the myelin sheath of peripheral and cranial nerves. The etiology is unknown, but an allergic response or an autoimmune response is strongly suspected. Some researchers believe the syndrome has a viral origin, but no virus has been isolated thus far.

Guillain–Barré occurs with equal frequency in both sexes and in all races. A slight peak seems to occur in the 16- to 25-year age group, but it may develop at any age. About half the victims have a mild febrile illness 2 to 3 weeks before onset of symptoms. The febrile infection usually is of respiratory or gastrointestinal origin.

Pathophysiological Principles

In GBS, the myelin sheath surrounding the axon is lost. The myelin sheath is quite susceptible to injury by many agents and conditions, including physical trauma, hypoxemia, toxic chemicals, vascular insufficiency, and immunologic reactions. Demyelination is a common response of neural tissue to any of these adverse conditions.

Myelinated axons conduct nerve impulses more rap-

NURSING CARE PLAN 31–3:
The Patient With a Seizure Disorder

NURSING DIAGNOSIS	OUTCOME CRITERIA/ PATIENT GOALS	NURSING INTERVENTIONS
Knowledge deficit: related to need for self-management of chronic condition.	• Patient will verbalize understanding of diagnosis, medications, treatment plan, and safety measures. • Patient/family will verbalize what to do if patient has a seizure. • Patient will be aware of resources from which further information and support may be obtained.	1. Provide information (verbal and written) about patient's condition and medical regime. 2. Encourage questions about all content presented. 3. Evaluate discharge needs and attempt to meet them before discharge. 4. Provide written information about community resources and support groups. 5. Correct misconceptions and misunderstandings. 6. Validate patient/family understanding of content presented.

High risk for injury: related to altered consciousness, cognitive impairment during a seizure, or impaired self-protective mechanisms.	• Patient will be free of physical injury.	1. Pad bed rails and keep bed in low position.
		2. If patient has an aura, teach patient to lie down before the seizure begins to prevent falling down.
		3. Maintain patent airway with plastic airway or padded tongue blade during seizure if able to safely insert it before jaws clench shut.
		4. Administer supplemental O_2 as ordered during and after seizures.
		5. Maintain lines and tubes during seizure activity because IV access is critical.
		6. Observe for aspiration during seizure; turn patient on side.
		7. Document motor activity and state of consciousness during seizure.
		8. Given phenytoin as ordered:
		  • causes ↓ BP, bradycardia, and widens QRS complex
		  • given 50 mg/min or slower
		  • dilute in NS because dextrose causes precipitation

(continued)

NURSING CARE PLAN 31–3: (Continued)
The Patient With a Seizure Disorder

NURSING DIAGNOSIS	OUTCOME CRITERIA/ PATIENT GOALS	NURSING INTERVENTIONS
High risk for ineffective individual coping: related to fear of the diagnosis, myths, and public stigma.	• Patient will demonstrate effective and adaptive coping strategies.	1. Assess patient's ability to understand the condition and the medical regimen necessary for seizure control. 2. Encourage active participation in self-care and in recreational and social activities of interest to maintain dignity and feelings of self-worth and prevent social isolation. 3. Provide information to decrease fear of the unknown and to dispel myths about seizures. 4. Encourage patient and family to discuss feelings or questions. 5. Encourage use of coping mechanisms that have worked for the patient in the past. 6. Help patient identify problems that can be controlled directly or immediately. 7. Refer to available hospital support systems. 8. Involve support of family or significant others in helping patient cope.

idly than nonmyelinated axons. Along the course of a myelinated fiber are interruptions in the sheath (nodes of Ranvier) where there is direct contact between the cell membrane of the axon and the extracellular fluid. The membrane is highly permeable at these nodes, thus making conduction good. The movement of ions into and out of the axon can occur rapidly only at the nodes of Ranvier (Fig. 31–9); thus, a nerve impulse along a myelinated fiber may jump from node to node (saltatory conduction) quite rapidly. Loss of the myelin sheath in Guillain–Barré syndrome makes saltatory conduction impossible, and nerve impulse transmission is aborted.

Assessment

History

The history often is one of an upper respiratory or gastrointestinal disorder occurring 1 to 4 weeks before onset of neurologic manifestations. The history of the onset of symptoms may be revealing, because those of GBS usually begin with weakness or paresthesias (numbness and tingling) of the lower extremities and ascends in a symmetrical pattern.

Clinical Manifestations

A flaccid, symmetrical, ascending paralysis quickly develops. The trunk and cranial nerves may become involved. Respiratory muscles may become affected, resulting in respiratory insufficiency.

Autonomic disturbances such as urinary retention and postural hypotension sometimes occur. Superficial and deep tendon reflexes may be lost. Usually no muscle wasting is noted because the flaccid paralysis develops so rapidly. Some patients experience tenderness and pain on deep pressure or movement of some muscles.

Sensory symptoms of paresthesias including tingling "pins and needles" and numbness may occur transiently. If cranial nerves are involved, the facial (VII) nerve is af-

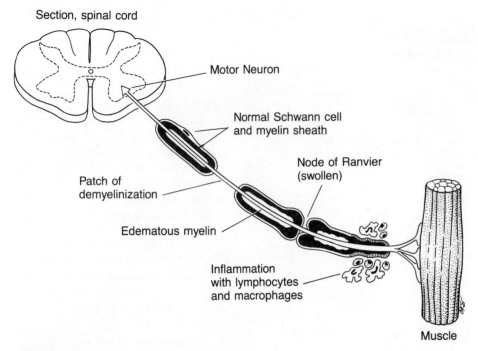

FIGURE 31–9
Pathologic changes with Guillain–Barré syndrome. Note the patchy demyelination and loss of the Schwann cell.

fected most often. Signs and symptoms of facial nerve dysfunction include inability to smile, whistle, or frown. Guillain–Barré does not affect LOC, pupillary signs, or cerebral function.

Symptoms usually peak within a week, but may progress for several weeks. The level of paralysis may stop at any point. Motor function returns in a descending fashion. Demyelination occurs rapidly, but the rate of remyelination is only about 1 to 2 mm per day.

Diagnostic Studies

Diagnosis of GBS depends a great deal on the history and the clinical progression of symptoms. There is no one test available that will confirm the diagnosis of GBS; it is a "rule out" disorder. Lumbar puncture may reveal a normal protein level initially, with an elevation in the 4th to 6th week.

Nerve conduction studies record impulse transmission along the nerve fiber, and in a patient with GBS the velocity of conduction will be reduced.

About 25% of people with this disease have antibodies to either cytomegalovirus or Epstein–Barr virus. It has been suggested that an altered immune response to peripheral nerve antigens may contribute to development of the disorder.

Pulmonary function tests may be done when GBS is suspected, so a baseline is established for comparison as the disease progresses. Declining pulmonary function capacity may indicate the need for mechanical ventilation.

Management

The major goals in caring for a patient with GBS are to provide functional maintenance of the body systems, promptly treat life-threatening crises, prevent infections and complications of immobility, and provide psychological support for the patient and family.

Respiratory and Cardiovascular Support

If the respiratory musculature is involved, mechanical ventilation will be necessary. Tracheostomy may be needed if the patient cannot be weaned from the ventilator in a couple of weeks. Respiratory failure should be anticipated until the progress of the disorder plateaus, because it never is clear how far the paralysis will ascend.

If there is autonomic nervous system involvement, drastic changes in blood pressure (hypotension or hypertension) and heart rate can occur and the patient should be monitored closely. Cardiac monitoring will allow dysrhythmias to be identified and treated quickly. An autonomic nervous system disturbance may be triggered by the Valsalva maneuver, coughing, suctioning, and position changes, so these activities should be performed very carefully.

Plasmapheresis

Plasmapheresis may be used both for GBS or myasthenia gravis to remove the offending antibodies from plasma.

The patient's plasma is separated selectively from whole blood, and its abnormal constituents are washed out or the plasma is exchanged with normal plasma or a colloidal substitute. Many centers begin this plasma exchange if it appears the patient is worsening and will be unable to return home within about 2 weeks, approximately the time it would take to complete a course of plasma exchanges.[11] If plasmapheresis is started 3 weeks or longer after the onset of symptoms, it does not appear to be very effective.

Corticosteroids may be used, although this still is controversial.

Pain Management

Pain management may be a part of the concern in a patient with GBS. Severe muscle pain usually subsides as muscle strength improves. Transcutaneous electrical stimulation units are helpful for some. Later, pain commonly is hyperesthetic. Some drugs may provide temporary relief. Pain usually is worse between 10 PM and 4 AM, preventing sleep, and narcotics may be used liberally at night if the patient is not so marginally compensated that narcotics will cause respiratory failure. In that case, the patient usually is intubated and then given narcotics.[11]

Nutrition

Adequate nutrition must be maintained. If the patient is unable to take oral feedings, tube feedings may be initiated. Tube feedings, however, may cause diarrhea and a resultant electrolyte imbalance, so careful monitoring by physician and nurse is required.

Sleep Deprivation

Sleep deprivation can become a severe problem for a patient with this disorder, especially because the pain seems to accelerate at night. Comfort measures, analgesics and careful control of the environment (eg, turning out lights and providing a quiet room) may help to promote sleep and rest. It also should be kept in mind that a patient who is paralyzed and perhaps on mechanical ventilation may be very frightened to be alone at night, for fear of being unable to summon help if he or she gets into trouble. A call light or some mechanism should be available so the patient knows he or she can call for help. Setting up a routine schedule of checking on the patient also may help overcome the fear.

Emotional Support

Fright, hopelessness, and helplessness all may be seen in patients and families over the often long course of this disorder. Frequent explanations of the interventions and the progress may be very useful. The patient should be allowed to make as many decisions as possible over the course of recovery.

Sometimes these patients are very difficult to care for because they require much nursing time. They may use the call light excessively if insecure about being alone. The nurse should consider allowing the family to spend more time with the patient. Having a primary nurse may give the patient and family more security, knowing there is one person from whom they can get consistent information. Team conferences with the patient and family should be held on a routine basis to discuss progress and plans.

Complications

Respiratory Failure

The most severe complication of GBS and myasthenia gravis is respiratory failure. Weakened respiratory muscles put patients with these disorders at great risk for hypoventilation and repeated pulmonary infections. Dysphagia also may be present, leading to aspiration. There may be the same complications of immobility as in the stroke victim.

Cardiovascular Aberrations

There may be a disturbance of the autonomic nervous system with GBS that could result in a fatal cardiac dysrhythmia or drastic life-threatening changes in vital signs.

Plasmapheresis Complications

A patient with GBS or myasthenia gravis receiving plasmapheresis is at risk for potential complications with that procedure. An infection may develop at the site of vascular access. Hypovolemia may result in hypotension, tachycardia, dizziness, and diaphoresis. Hypokalemia and hypocalcemia may lead to cardiac dysrhythmias. The patient may experience temporary circumoral and distal extremity paresthesias, muscle twitching, and nausea and vomiting related to administration of citrated plasma. Careful observation and assessment are necessary to prevent these problems.

CASE STUDY

Tom Adams was a 32-year-old businessman who presented in the physician's office with a chief complaint of weakness and numbness in both feet that had been developing over the past 4 days. At first only the bottoms of his feet were involved. Now the numbness was up to his ankles. Two weeks before this, he stated he had had a "mild case of the stomach flu."

The physician admitted him to the hospital and ruled out many disorders with extensive laboratory tests. Over the next 6 days, the patient lost his ability to walk. His feet and legs felt like "pins and needles" up to groin level, and he had no motor ability in his legs. The symptoms were ascending in a symmetrical pattern. The symptom progression and history made the physician highly suspicious that this was Guillain–Barré syndrome.

Mr. Adam's symptoms plateaued after 6 days and did not ascend further than his hips. He went to a rehabilitation center, where over the next 4 months he gradually regained the strength in his lower extremities. The symptom onset was rapid, but the recovery much slower. After the disease was explained to him, Mr. Adams considered himself extremely lucky the disease plateaued where it did, and did not involve his upper extremities or his respiratory muscles.

Nursing Care Plan

Careful nursing intervention can prevent many of the complications related to immobility in the patient with GBS. Nursing Care Plan 31–4 provides further details.

Myasthenia Gravis

Description

Myasthenia gravis is a neuromuscular transmission disorder thought possibly to be caused by an autoimmune response. The name "myasthenia gravis" means "grave muscle weakness," which is the primary clinical feature, along with abnormal fatigability. It is seen more often in women than men. Symptoms most commonly show up in the third decade of life, although any age group may be affected. The incidence of myasthenia gravis is 1 in 10,000 to 1 in 50,000.

Pathophysiological Principles

Most researchers believe that the autoimmune response in myasthenia gravis occurs at the neuromuscular junction, specifically on the postsynaptic membrane of the muscles, where antibodies destroy acetylcholine receptor sites. By reducing the number of functioning acetylcholine receptor sites, complete depolarization of the muscle is difficult or impossible. This causes striated voluntary muscle weakness, which characteristically is greater after activity, and improves after rest.

There are several other theories about the exact nature of the transmission deficit at the neuromuscular junction. Some researchers think there is a deficient amount of acetylcholine released from the presynaptic membranes into the synapse. This deficiency may be in the synthesis of the enzyme choline acetylase, impaired transport of the acetylcholine into the synapse, or other possible defects.

Abnormalities in the thymus gland are frequent in patients with myasthenia gravis. The thymus is involved intimately in the immune responses of the body. Eighty percent of victims of myasthenia gravis have structural

changes of the thymus, such as thymic hyperplasia. These data support the pathogenic role of the immune system in myasthenia gravis.

Assessment

History

Diagnosis of myasthenia gravis is based on the history and clinical presentation. A history of muscle weakness after activity and partial strength restoration after rest is highly suspect for myasthenia gravis. The patient may complain of weakness after simple physical tasks. A history of drooping eyelids on upward gaze also may be significant, as well as evidence of other cranial muscle weakness.

Clinical Manifestations

There may be extraocular muscle weakness causing ocular palsy, drooping eyelid, or intermittent diplopia. Facial expression may be masklike when facial muscles are affected. The patient may have dysphagia and difficulty chewing. Speech may be dysarthric.

If muscular involvement of the trunk and extremities is present, the proximal muscles usually are affected more severely than the distal ones. This disorder may produce signs such as mild ocular involvement to severe muscular involvement involving the diaphragm, intercostal muscles, and abdominal and external sphincters. Dyspnea and dysphagia are two life-threatening symptoms that may result in aspiration and acute respiratory failure.

Pupillary signs and cerebral function remain intact. There may be remissions and relapses.

Diagnostic Studies

The Tensilon (edrophonium chloride; Roche Laboratories, Nutley, NJ) test is the classic diagnostic tool for this disorder. Tensilon is a short-acting anticholinesterase, and when injected, transiently inhibits the breakdown of acetylcholine at the neuromuscular junction. The patient shows marked improvement of muscle strength within 30 seconds that lasts up to 5 minutes.

Electromyography also may help to confirm the diagnosis. This involves repetitive nerve stimulation at a slow rate, which in a normal person produces very little decrease in muscle action potential. In the patient with myasthenia gravis, this repetitive slow stimulation produces a rapid decline in muscle action potential because of the deficient number of acetylcholine receptors available.

Because myasthenia gravis often is seen along with other conditions, other studies that might be performed are a CT scan of the thymus, thyroid studies, serum creatine phosphokinase, sedimentation rate, antinuclear antibody levels, and immunologic studies.

NURSING CARE PLAN 31–4:
The Patient With Guillain–Barré Syndrome

NURSING DIAGNOSIS	OUTCOME CRITERIA/ PATIENT GOALS	NURSING INTERVENTIONS
Impaired physical mobility: related to muscle paralysis, bed rest, or pain.	• Patient will be free of preventable complications of immobility (eg, contractures, skin breakdown, atelectasis, footdrop, DVT).	1. Maintain joint range of motion. 2. Position correctly in bed. 3. Obtain rehabilitation or PT and OT consultation. 4. Provide space boots or high-top tennis shoes to prevent footdrop. 5. Use pneumatic stockings on lower extremities. 6. Turn at least q2h. 7. Consider kinetic bed. 8. Avoid exercising patient's muscles during time of tenderness or pain, because it may increase demyelination. 9. Assess for signs of redness, heat, swelling or pain or Homan's sign in lower extremities each shift. 10. Provide analgesia before therapy sessions or prn as ordered. 11. Begin teaching family exercises for ROM.
High risk for ineffective breathing pattern: related to skeletal muscle and diaphragm weakness/paralysis.	• Adequate gas exchange will be maintained.	1. Auscultate breath sounds frequently. 2. Monitor O_2 saturation with oximetry. 3. Report subjective complaints of muscle weakness or difficulty breathing. 4. Remain with patient complaining of SOB. 5. Suction as necessary to keep airway patent. 6. Position patient to facilitate adequate gas exchange (↑ HOB). 7. Document respiratory parameters (rate, volume, work of breathing). 8. Record ABGs and note trend. 9. Explain to patient and family about intubation and ventilator if it appears this will be needed. 10. Keep ventilator alarms on.

(continued)

NURSING CARE PLAN 31–4: (Continued)
The Patient With Guillain–Barré Syndrome

NURSING DIAGNOSIS	OUTCOME CRITERIA/ PATIENT GOALS	NURSING INTERVENTIONS
High risk for constipation: related to change in diet, bed rest, immobility, or use of narcotics.	• Patient's bowel routine will remain the same as before hospitalization.	1. Ensure adequate hydration; record intake and output. 2. Administer stool softeners or suppositories as indicated. 3. Provide digital stimulation as ordered. 4. Time performance of bowel program to make use of gastrocolic reflex after meals. 5. Position patient in upright position to perform elimination.
High risk for fear and anxiety: related to critical illness, paralysis, inability to communicate, and unknown future.	• Patient and family will verbalize concerns to health care team.	1. Allow for ventilation of feelings and fear. 2. Encourage questions and be available to answer them. 3. Develop a communication system such as eye blinks if respiratory system and upper extremities are involved. 4. Set up schedule so patient knows nurse will check frequently on needs. 5. Keep call light within reach, using system patient can activate. 6. Reduce sensory deprivation by talking to patient and involving family.

Management

Medical

Medical management includes medication therapy with anticholinesterases and steroids. Drugs such as neostigmine (Prostigmin; Roche Laboratories) inactivate or destroy cholinesterase so the acetylcholine is not immediately destroyed. Steroids, by reducing the amount of antibodies produced via the immune response, block the immune mechanism and restore chemical reaction at the myoneural junction. Azathioprine (Imuran; Burroughs Wellcome Co., Research Triangle Park, NC) or other immunosuppressive drugs may be useful. Thymectomy (surgical excision of the thymus gland) may be indicated. It is thought that this procedure removes a source of antigen and reduces the immune response. Plasmapheresis or plasma exchange may be initiated to remove circulating anti-acetylcholine receptor antibodies from the plasma, resulting in some clinical improvement. As with GBS, respiratory failure may occur and mechanical ventilatory support may be necessary.

Nursing Care Plan

Details of nursing care are given in Nursing Care Plan 31–5.

Emotional Support

Like GBS, myasthenia gravis can be a very frightening disease. Unlike GBS, it is a chronic disorder in that once an

NURSING CARE PLAN 31–5:
The Patient With Myasthenia Gravis

NURSING DIAGNOSIS	OUTCOME CRITERIA/ PATIENT GOALS	NURSING INTERVENTIONS
Impaired gas exchange: related to muscle weakness or poor airway clearance.	• Patient will maintain adequate gas exchange.	1. Document O_2 saturation with oximetry, especially with activity. 2. Measure respiratory parameters frequently. 3. Suction as necessary (anticholinesterase drugs increase bronchial secretions). 4. Auscultate breath sounds q4h. 5. Cough and deep breathe q2h. 6. Administer anticholinesterase drugs on time if ordered. 7. Keep call light close to patient. 8. Record ABGs, noting trend over time. 9. Establish alternate communication system if patient is ventilated. 10. Assure patient you know it is difficult to breathe and will not leave him or her alone.
Self-care deficits: related to muscle weakness, generalized fatigue.	• Patient will be able to perform at least 25% of self-care and grooming activities.	1. Schedule self-care at intervals, not consecutively. 2. Allow for rest periods between activities. 3. Perform self-care for patient during periods of extreme muscle weakness or enlist family's participation. 4. Demonstrate energy-saving techniques.
Altered nutrition, less than body requirements: related to dysphagia, intubation, or muscle paralysis.	• Caloric intake will be adequate to meet metabolic demands.	1. Assess gag, swallow, and cough reflex before oral feedings. 2. Stop oral feedings if patient is unable to handle oral secretions, or in case of depressed gag, swallow, or cough reflex. 3. Stay with patient as he or she eats, in case suctioning is necessary. 4. Provide small supplemental feedings. 5. Avoid milk products if there is increase in secretions.

(continued)

NURSING CARE PLAN 31–5: (Continued)
The Patient With Myasthenia Gravis

NURSING DIAGNOSIS	OUTCOME CRITERIA/ PATIENT GOALS	NURSING INTERVENTIONS
		6. Position patient upright and allow plenty of time to swallow oral feedings.
		7. Pass a small feeding tube and provide tube feedings if dysphagia is present.
		8. Administer total parenteral nutrition if oral/tube feeding is contraindicated.
		9. Record intake and output.
		10. Initiate dietary consultation for caloric evaluation.
		11. Weigh patient daily.

---

exacerbation is treated, it does not reverse itself and go away. Chronic management is indicated for myasthenia gravis. Keeping the patient and family informed and giving honest information will help them make decisions about options for care.

Complications

There are two types of crises a patient may experience: myasthenic crisis and cholinergic crisis. *Myasthenic crisis* is a condition in which the symptoms of myasthenia gravis are exaggerated and the patient requires more anticholinesterase drugs. This crisis usually is precipitated by stress, such as infection, emotional turmoil, pregnancy, alcohol ingestion, or cold, but in some cases the cause cannot be identified readily. Myasthenic crisis is not distinguished easily from *cholinergic crisis*, in which the patient has received too much anticholinesterase drug. Cholinergic crisis often involves nausea, vomiting, pallor, diarrhea, diaphoresis, bradycardia, and salivation.

To determine the type of crisis, Tensilon may be used. With its administration, there will be marked improvement of symptoms in myasthenic crisis. There will be a transient exacerbation of symptoms if the patient is having a cholinergic crisis. Atropine, a cholinergic reactivator, may be given for cholinergic crisis. Neostigmine may be given for myasthenic crisis, because the Tensilon quickly wears off. Because there often is a narrow range of therapeutic control, the patient must understand the importance of taking the correct amount of medication, and not skipping doses or doubling up on a dose if a previous dose was missed.

Some of the complications experienced by the patient with GBS are similar to those experienced by the patient with myasthenia gravis. Refer to the section on Complications of Guillain–Barré syndrome for further information.

REFERENCES

1. Bonita R: Epidemiology of stroke. Lancet 339(8789): 342–347, Feb. 18, 1992
2. Marmot M, Poulter N: Primary prevention of stroke. Lancet 339:344–347, 1992
3. Bamford J: Clinical examination in diagnosis and subclassification of stroke. Lancet 339(8790):400–402, Feb. 15, 1992
4. Sheinberg M, Kanter M, Robertson C, Constant C, Narayan R, Grossman R: Continuous monitoring of jugular venous oxygen saturation in head injured patients. J Neurosurg 76:212–217, 1992
5. Massey E, Biller J, Davis J, Davis J, Adams H Jr, Marler J, Goldstein L, Alberts M, Bruno A: Large-dose infusions of heparinoid ORG 10172 in ischemic stroke. Stroke 21: 1289–1293, 1990
6. Mitchell M: Neuroscience Nursing: A Nursing Diagnosis. Baltimore, Williams & Wilkins, 1989
7. Manifold S: Aneurysmal subarachnoid hemorrhage: Cerebral vasospasm and early repair. Critical Care 10(8):62–69, 1990
8. Van Gijn J: Subarachnoid haemorrhage. Lancet 339(8794): 653–655, March 14, 1992
9. Rusy K: Temporal lobectomy: A promising alternative. Journal of Neuroscience Nursing 23:320–324, 1991

10. Michael J: Vagal nerve stimulation in treatment of intractable partial seizures: Nursing implications. Journal of Neuroscience Nursing 24:19–23, 1992
11. Ropper A, Wijdicks E, Truax B: Guillain–Barré Syndrome. Philadelphia, FA Davis Co., 1991

BIBLIOGRAPHY

Anderson S: Guillain–Barré syndrome: Giving the patient control. Journal of Neuroscience Nursing 24:158–163, 1992
George M: Neuromuscular respiratory failure: What the nurse knows may make the difference. Journal of Neuroscience Nursing 20:110–117, 1988
Hickey JV: The Clinical Practice of Neurological and Neurosurgical Nursing, 3rd ed. Philadelphia, JB Lippincott, 1992
Leonard A, Newburg S: Cardioembolic stroke. Journal of Neuroscience Nursing 24:69–76, 1992
McIntyre K, Elesha-Adams M: Sexual limitations caused by stroke. Journal of Sex Education and Therapy 16:57–60, 1990
Stewart-Amidei C: Hypervolemic hemodilution: A new approach to subarachnoid hemorrhage. Heart Lung 181: 590–598, 1989
Willis D, Harbit M: Transcatheter arterial embolization of cerebral arteriovenous malformations. Journal of Neuroscience Nursing 22:280–284, 1990

STUDY QUESTIONS

1. Which cerebrovascular problem may present with a chief complaint of unilateral headache?

   a. stroke
   b. arteriovenous malformation
   c. hydrocephalus
   d. Guillain–Barré syndrome

2. Hemorrhage from an aneurysm most often occurs in which space in the brain?

   a. subdural space
   b. epidural space
   c. subarachnoid space
   d. intracerebral space

3. The most serious and most common type of status epilepticus is

   a. absence status
   b. partial motor seizures
   c. generalized tonic–clonic status
   d. complex partial status

4. Patients with which type of seizure may follow commands and maintain eye contact with an observer?

   a. absence seizures
   b. pseudoseizures
   c. complex partial seizures
   d. simple partial seizures

5. What complication is possible with both Guillain–Barré syndrome and myasthenia gravis?

   a. respiratory failure
   b. seizures
   c. bleeding
   d. nuchal rigidity

6. How can a myasthenic crisis be distinguished from a cholinergic crisis?

   a. the clinical manifestations are different
   b. atropine will cause improved muscle strength in myasthenic crisis
   c. neostigmine will cause improved muscle strength in cholinergic crisis
   d. Tensilon will cause improved muscle strength in myasthenic crisis

CHAPTER 32

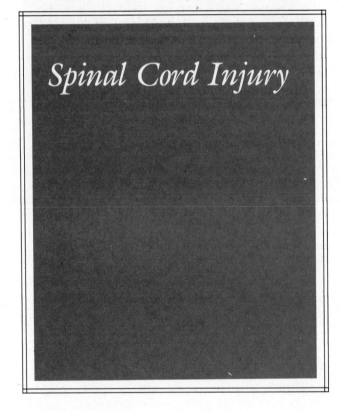

Spinal Cord Injury

Hudak: Critical Care Nursing:
A Holistic Approach, 6th ed. © 1994
J. B. Lippincott Company.

BEHAVIORAL OBJECTIVES

Based on the content in this chapter, the reader should be able to:

1. Differentiate between a complete and an incomplete spinal cord injury (SCI).
2. Explain the pathophysiological processes involved with a Brown–Séquard syndrome, a central cord syndrome, and an anterior cord syndrome.
3. Describe three clinical features of spinal shock.
4. Describe two immediate nursing actions to take after autonomic dysreflexia is recognized.
5. Develop a holistic care plan for a patient with an acute SCI.

Description

Every year there are 8,000 to 10,000 new spinal cord injuries (SCI) in the United States. This catastrophic injury has been documented throughout history, beginning with the ancient Greeks and Egyptians. Historical figures, such as Lord Nelson, are described as having a spinal injury. The prognosis for anyone with a SCI before World War II was dim. After 1945, a team approach to management was implemented. Improved acute and long-term care facilities with social and vocational counseling became available. Today, the person with a SCI is perceived as physically disabled, but also a healthy individual with potential for a productive future in society.

Spinal cord injury is most common in young adults ages 16 to 30. Most are men (82% men versus 18% women). Almost 50% of SCIs result from motor vehicle accidents. Falls account for approximately 20.8% of SCIs, acts of violence 14.6%, and sports 14.2%. Etiology varies in different groups depending on age of onset, sex, and racial or ethnic background. Motor vehicle accidents occur

most in 15- to 30-year-olds, but those over age 60 have more spinal injuries due to falls. Violence as an etiology of SCI is increasing in the 16- to 30-year-old group, and primarily in nonwhites. Motor vehicle accidents account for most SCIs among whites.

Slightly more than one half of all new injuries involve the cervical spine; thoracic vertebral injuries account for more than one-third of all new injuries, and lumbar and sacral injuries account for the remainder. Motor vehicle accidents cause an equal number of quadriplegias and paraplegias. Quadriplegia results more from sports injuries, especially diving accidents and contact sports. Paraplegia results more from penetrating wounds.[1]

Statistics have been compiled on SCI over the past several decades. The National SCI Database is located in Birmingham, Alabama. Profiles have been developed that describe the demographics of spinal injury. The typical profile is a young, single man between ages 16 and 30 with a high school education, whose injury occurs in July.

The combination of early onset of spinal injury, which results in severe disability, coupled with advances in health care that allow almost a full life expectancy, can result in a catastrophe in terms of human disability and social economics. Economic consequences of this type of injury, especially if there are repeated hospitalizations, may be staggering. Analysis of SCI statistics has helped to direct efforts to prevent spinal cord injury through education.

Primary prevention has been addressed through attempts to change high-risk behavior that may result in a SCI. Drug and alcohol education in schools and in television, radio, and newspaper advertisements is common. Because most victims of SCI are young, it seems reasonable to focus primary prevention programs at the middle school and high school populations. In these age groups, there is a sense of invulnerability and peer pressure for risk-taking behavior, especially in men.

Secondary prevention measures aim to reduce the severity of the injury once it has happened. Most of the injury to the spinal cord occurs at the time of the accident. Secondary injury may occur from movement of an unstable spine, which causes further cord compression or cord damage from bony fragments. It is vitally important that the rescue crew at the scene of the accident and the emergency department personnel have as their primary goal prevention of further neurologic damage.

Because elapsed time from injury significantly affects prognosis, the patient with SCI should be transported as rapidly as possible to a specialized unit or a hospital with adequate diagnostic and treatment facilities to handle such trauma. Some sort of neck immobilization is necessary before transport is possible. A long back board may be used effectively to keep the spine rigid, and sandbags and tape will secure the head.

If there will be some delay in removing the injured person from the accident scene, a soft collar may be applied temporarily. It still allows some movement of the head, so should be used only until a more stable device can be applied.

Four-poster braces also are used in the field. If rescuers have good access to the victim, this brace provides better immobilization than a soft collar. The Stifneck collar (California Medical Products, Long Beach, CA) is used frequently, and manufacturer's guidelines include directions for quickly measuring the victim's neck to determine correct size (Fig. 32–1).

Paramedic and emergency medical technician (EMT) training in how to immobilize and extricate a victim from the scene of an accident would be an example of secondary prevention.

Tertiary prevention occurs throughout the trauma care the patient receives. It may be carried out by nurses and others in the rehabilitative phase, teaching the patient to do weight shifts or catheterizations to prevent complications such as pressure sores or urinary tract infections.

Pathophysiological Principles

Complete Versus Incomplete Lesions

The level of SCI is defined by the number of the most distal uninvolved segment of the cord. Functional abilities at the different levels of SCI are not completely determined for every patient. Functional performance may vary among patients depending on whether the lesion is complete or incomplete. An incomplete lesion implies preservation of the motor or sensory fibers (or both) below the level of the lesion, whereas a complete lesion implies total loss of voluntary muscle control and sensation below the injury. When a SCI is incomplete, segments distal to the lesion still may be intact, although the orthopedic level of injury is higher. For instance, the orthopedic level of injury may be a C5 fracture, but the patient may be neurologically intact to C6. Because it is important to know what level of performance a patient can achieve, the neuro-

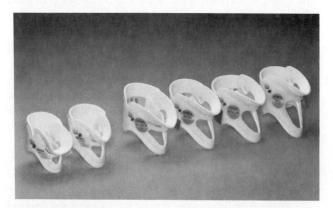

FIGURE 32–1
The Stifneck collar is available in a variety of sizes. (Photo courtesy of Laerdal Medical Corp., One Labriola Court, Armonk, NY 10504.)

logic level to which he or she can perform is more significant than knowledge of the location of orthopedic injury.

When speaking of a complete cord injury, the orthopedic level of injury may be the same as the neurologic level of injury. No segments distal to the injury are preserved. A person with complete cord injury will follow closely the dermatome chart for the level of sensory loss (Fig. 32–2).

Cervical Injuries

C1–C4 Lesions

With a C1–C4 lesion, the trapezius, sternomastoid, and platysma muscles remain functional. Intercostal muscles and the diaphragm are paralyzed, and there is no voluntary movement (physiologic or functional) below the spinal transection. Sensory loss for levels C1 through C3 includes the occipital region, the ears, and some regions of the face. Sensory loss is illustrated by a diagram of the dermatomes of the body (see Figure 32–2).

A patient with a C1, C2, or C3 quadriplegia requires full-time attendance because of dependency on a mechanical ventilator. This person also is dependent in all daily living skills, such as feeding, bathing, and dressing. A person with this level of injury is able to operate an electric wheelchair (which should have a high back for head support) with chin or breath control. A mouthstick can be used to operate a typewriter or a telephone.

A C4 quadriplegic usually also needs a mechanical ventilator, but may be removed from it intermittently. The patient usually is dependent on others in daily living skills, although he or she may be able to self-feed with the aid of feeding devices. This patient still needs an electric wheelchair, although because of better head control, a high-backed chair is not essential.

C5 Lesions

When the C5 segment of the cord is damaged, the function of the diaphragm is impaired secondary to posttraumatic edema in the acute phase. Intestinal paralysis and gastric dilation may compound the respiratory distress. The upper extremities are rotated outwardly from impairment of the supraspinous and infraspinous muscles. The shoulders may be elevated markedly due to uninhibited action of the levator scapulae and trapezius muscles. After the acute phase, reflexes below the level of the lesion are exaggerated. Sensation is present in the neck and the triangular area of the anterior aspect of the upper arms.

A C5 quadriplegic usually is dependent in activities such as bathing, shaving, and combing of hair, but the patient has better hand-to-mouth coordination, allowing self-feeding with the aid of a feeder or brace. These aids permit the patient to brush teeth and to dress upper extremities. With the use of mechanical aids, this patient usually can write.

Assistance is needed, as with higher-level quadriplegia, in transfers from wheelchair to bed or *vice versa*. An electric

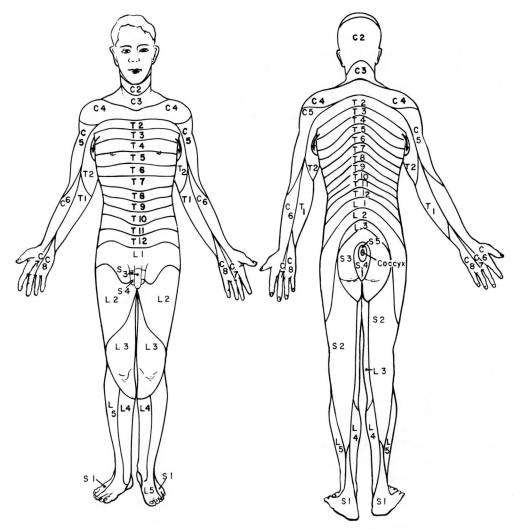

FIGURE 32-2
Sensory dermatomes. (Barr, M: The Human Nervous System, p. 85. New York, Harper & Row, 1993.)

wheelchair still is preferable with a C5 quadriplegic, although a manual wheelchair may be managed if it has quad pegs (projections on the hand rim that allow for greater ease of movement of the wheelchair). A person with this level of injury may find that manual manipulation of a wheelchair is very tiring.

C6 Lesions

In a C6 segment lesion, respiratory distress may occur because of intestinal paralysis and ascending edema of the spinal cord. The shoulders usually are elevated, with arms abducted and forearms flexed. This is due to the uninhibited action of the deltoid, biceps, and brachioradialis muscles. Functional recovery of the triceps depends on correct positioning of the arms (forearm in extension, arm in adduction). Sensation remains over the lateral aspect of the arms and dorsolateral aspect of the forearm.

A C6 quadriplegic is independent in most hygiene requirements and sometimes is successful in lower extremity dressing and undressing. This patient is independent in

feeding with or without mechanical aids. Light housework can be accomplished, and the person is able to drive a car with hand controls.

C7 Lesions

Cord lesions at the level of C7 allow the diaphragm and accessory muscles to compensate for the affected abdominal and intercostal muscles. The upper extremities assume the same position as in C6 lesions. Finger flexion usually is exaggerated when the reflex action returns.

A C7 quadriplegic has the potential for independent living without the care of an attendant. Transfers are independent, as are upper and lower extremity dressing and undressing, feeding, bathing, light housework, and cooking.

C8 Lesions

The abnormal position of the upper extremities is not present in C8 lesions because the adductors and internal rotators are able to counteract the antagonists. The latissimus dorsi and trapezius muscles are strong enough to support a sitting position. Postural hypotension may occur when the patient is raised to the sitting position owing to the loss of vasomotor control. This postural hypotension can be minimized by having the patient make a gradual change from the lying to the sitting position. The patient's fingers usually assume a claw position.

A C8 quadriplegic should be able to live independently. This person is independent in dressing, undressing, driving a car, homemaking, and self-care.

Thoracic Injuries

T1–T5 Lesions

Lesions in the T1–T5 region may cause diaphragmatic breathing. The inspiratory function of the lungs increases as the level of the thoracic lesion descends. Postural hypotension usually is present. A partial paralysis of the adductor pollicis, interosseous, and lumbrical muscles of the hands is present, as is sensory loss for touch, pain, and temperature.

T6–T12 Lesions

Lesions at the T6 level abolish all abdominal reflexes. From the level of T6 down, individual segments are functioning, and at the level of T12, all abdominal reflexes are present. There is spastic paralysis of the lower limbs. Patients with lesions at a thoracic level should be functionally independent.

The upper limits of sensory loss in thoracic lesions are:

T2	Entire body to inner side of the upper arm
T3	Axilla
T5	Nipple
T6	Xiphoid process
T7, T8	Lower costal margin
T10	Umbilicus
T12	Groin

Bowel and bladder function may return with the reflex automatism.

Lumbar Injuries

L1–L5 Lesions

The sensory loss involved in L1–L5 lesions is:

L1	All areas of the lower limbs, extending to the groin and back of the buttocks
L2	Lower limbs, except the upper third of the anterior aspect of the thigh
L3	Lower limbs and saddle area
L4	Same as in L3 lesions, except the anterior aspect of the thigh
L5	Outer aspects of the legs and ankles and the lower limbs and saddle area

Patients with lesions should attain total independance.

Sacral Injuries

S1–S6 Lesions

With lesions involving S1–S5, there may be some displacement of the foot. From S3 through S5, there is no paralysis of the leg muscles. The loss of sensation involves the saddle area, scrotum, glans penis, perineum, anal area, and the upper third of the posterior aspect of the thigh.

Incomplete Cord Transections

Incomplete cord transections often fit into recognizable neurologic syndromes.

Central Cord Syndrome

Damage to the spinal cord in this syndrome is centrally located. Hyperextension of the cervical spine often is the mechanism of injury, and the damage is greatest to the cervical tracts supplying the arms. Clinically, the patient may present with paralyzed arms but with no deficit in the legs or bladder (Fig. 32–3).

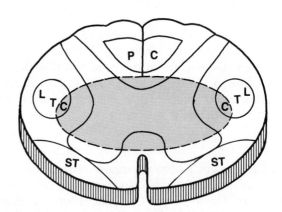

FIGURE 32–3
Cross-section of the spinal cord to show the area involved in the central cord syndrome. Sensory loss typically is slight, and weakness is greater in the arms and hands than in the legs because of the distribution of nerve fibers in the corticospinal tracts. L, descending lumbar nerve fibers; T, thoracic nerve fibers; C, cervical nerve fibers. (Redrawn from Ernest, MP: Neurologic Emergencies. New York, Churchill-Livingstone, 1983)

Brown–Séquard Syndrome

The damage in this syndrome is located on one side of the spinal cord, such as a hemisection from a stab wound. The clinical presentation is one in which the patient has either increased or decreased cutaneous sensation of pain, temperature, and touch on the same side at the level of the lesion. Below the level of the lesion on the same side, there is complete motor paralysis. On the patient's opposite side, below the level of the lesion, there is loss of pain, temperature, and touch because the spinothalamic tracts cross soon after entering the cord. The posterior columns will be interrupted ipsilaterally, but this does not cause a major deficit because some fibers cross instead of running ipsilaterally. Clinically, the patient's limb with the best motor strength has the poorest sensation. Conversely, the limb with the best sensation has the poorest motor strength (Fig. 32–4).

Anterior Cord Syndrome

The area of damage in this syndrome is, as the name suggests, the anterior aspect of the spinal cord. Clinically, the patient usually has complete motor paralysis below the level of injury (corticospinal tracts) and loss of pain, temperature, and touch sensation (spinothalamic tracts), with preservation of light touch, proprioception, and position sense (posterior columns; Fig. 32–5).

Assessment

Initial Assessment

A primary survey done at the scene of an accident includes a rapid assessment of airway, breathing, and circulation—

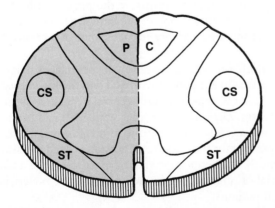

FIGURE 32–4
Cross-section of the spinal cord to show the area involved in the Brown–Séquard syndrome. There are hemiparesis and loss of position and vibratory sense on the side of the lesion, with contralateral loss of pain and temperature. PC, posterior columns; CS, corticospinal tract; ST, anterolateral spinothalamic tract. (Redrawn from Ernest MP: Neurologic Emergencies. New York, Churchill-Livingstone, 1983)

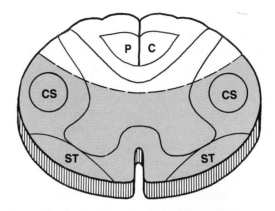

FIGURE 32–5
Cross-section of the spinal cord to show the area involved in the anterior cord syndrome. There are motor paralysis and loss of pain and temperature to the level of the lesion (or just below it), but position and vibratory sense are relatively spared. (Redrawn from Ernest MP: Neurologic Emergencies. New York, Churchill-Livingstone, 1983)

the so-called ABCs. Along with checking for airway patency, the cervical spine is immobilized. The patient is assessed for presence of spontaneous respirations, and breath sounds are auscultated. Circulation is checked by presence or absence of a pulse. The patient also is assessed for external hemorrhage or signs of shock. The primary survey also includes a brief neurologic assessment to see if the patient is alert, responds to verbal or painful stimuli, of if he or she is unresponsive. Clothing is removed to assess for hidden injuries.

Secondary survey includes obtaining a history of what happened, vital signs, noting any odors such as alcohol, fuel, urine, or feces, and also a more thorough neurologic examination, including pupil check and head-to-toe survey (inspection and palpation; see Chapter 28).

Assessing Concomitant Injuries

From 25% to 65% of patients with SCI have other injuries associated with the spinal cord trauma. Head injuries are the most common and usually accompany a cervical cord injury. Chest injury often accompanies a thoracic SCI. A complete neurologic examination should be performed, with special attention given to ventilatory status. The chest, head, and abdomen should be examined. Appropriate radiographs of the chest, skull, abdomen, and long bones may be indicated. Placement of a nasogastric tube and urinary catheter also can help to evaluate the patient for other injuries.

Assessing Complete Versus Incomplete Injury

During the initial assessment of a SCI patient, a digital rectal examination is important in determining whether the injury is incomplete or complete. The lesion is incomplete if the patient can feel the palpating finger or can contract the perianal muscles around the finger voluntarily. Sensation may be present in the absence of voluntary motor activity. Sensation seldom is absent when voluntary perianal muscle contraction is present. In either case, the prognosis for further motor and sensory return is good. Preservation of sacral function might be the only finding that indicates an incomplete lesion, and significant neurologic recovery may occur in the patient with an incomplete cord injury.

Rectal tone by itself, without the criteria of voluntary perianal muscle contraction or rectal sensation, is not evidence of an incomplete cord injury. Some rectal tone may be accounted for by local reflexes.

Clinical Manifestations

Clinical manifestations other than those associated with concomitant injuries may include hypoventilation or respiratory failure, particularly with high cervical injuries. *Hypoventilation* from inadequate innervation of respiratory muscles is a common problem after SCI. It is important to assess whether the intercostal muscles are functioning or whether the patient has only diaphragmatic breathing. The diaphragm, the major respiratory muscle, is innervated by the phrenic nerve, which travels through the third, fourth, and fifth cervical segments of the cord.

Any time a person has a cervical cord injury, *respiratory failure* should be anticipated. Although the patient initially may have what appears to be adequate diaphragmatic breathing (the intercostals would not be functioning because they are innervated from the thoracic region of the cord), cord edema can act like an ascending lesion and may compromise function of the diaphragm. Frequent checks of tidal volume and vital capacity and frequent auscultation of breath sounds should be routine.

The SCI patient may have further respiratory compromise because of preexisting pulmonary disease or coexistent chest injuries. Alveolar ventilation may be affected directly by the pulmonary collapse or by consolidation from *retained secretions* or aspiration of vomitus. *Pulmonary edema* also may result from incorrect management of intravenous fluids. Paralytic ileus and gastric dilation may increase the pressure on the diaphragm and cause further respiratory embarrassment. Interference with the cough reflex and fluid imbalance may combine to obstruct the airways.

The patient with SCI demonstrates a surprisingly florid metabolic response to an injury that usually is associated with little tissue damage. If the injury is uncomplicated, the metabolic derangement reaches a peak within 48 to 72 hours postinjury. A return to normal may be anticipated between 10 and 14 days postinjury.

When the spinal injury is complicated by other factors such as surgical intervention or other medical problems, the metabolic response is greater and more prolonged. This metabolic response is characterized by a marked retention of sodium and water, increased potassium excretion, breakdown of body protein, and an oliguric period followed by diuresis. A reduced glomerular filtration rate secondary to hypotension compounds the sodium and water retention.

Starvation also is a factor in the metabolic disturbance because most cord-injured patients are unable to tolerate oral food or fluid for at least a week after the injury. This can lead to a negative nitrogen balance in the body.

Because it may be difficult to ascertain the patient's state of hydration on admission due to the vasodilation, *monitoring of fluid intake and output* is necessary for prevention of pulmonary edema, tubular necrosis, electrolyte imbalance, and congestive heart failure.

The intravenous caloric intake should be approximately 2,000 calories/24 hour. It may be necessary to give the patient total parenteral nutrition to accomplish this. Patients with SCI tend to lose weight easily because of the increased catabolic activity.

Research on metabolic and endocrine changes in patients with SCIs has provided some interesting data. Apparently, body areas that have become insensitive as a result of the cord injury do not secrete anti-inflammatory steroids in adequate amounts. This lack of secretion may play a role in the genesis of pressure sores in the patient with SCI. This attenuation of the normally expected rise in corticosteroid levels also is seen during surgical procedures. Because excessive inflammation of the surgical site may occur as a result of the minimal cortisol release, this must be kept in mind if the patient undergoes surgery.

Cord-injured patients also have a decrease in testosterone levels that is significant enough to contribute to the *negative nitrogen balance* seen in these patients. Thus, careful positioning and turning of the patient with SCI are necessary for prevention of pressure sores, and exercising and sitting are necessary for avoidance of excessive bone loss.

Both the sudden absence of muscular activity and sensations in the patient with SCI and the mental state of helplessness appear to alter central nervous system metabolism. *Depression* coincides with a fall in a brain metabolite excreted in the urine as tryptamine. Thus, it is important for the nurse to understand that depression in some SCI patients might have a metabolic basis and that a trial of pharmacologic therapy might be beneficial to such patients.

During the *spinal shock* phase, vasomotor tone is lost and blood pools in the periphery, lowering blood pressure because of the decreased circulating volume. *Orthostatic hypotension* also may occur because the patient is unable to compensate for changes in position. The vasoconstricting message from the medulla cannot reach the blood vessels because of the cord lesion. Thus, hypotension is a common manifestation following spinal cord injury. *Bradycardia* also frequently is present owing to reflex vagal activity. The effects of the vagus nerve (parasympathetic innervation to the heart) are unopposed by sympathetic response (Fig. 32–6).

There also may be *flaccid paralysis* and *loss of reflex activity* below the level of the injury, along with *loss of sensation. Hypothermia* often results from vasodilation and excessive loss of body heat. The patient tends to take on the temperature of the environment.

Incontinence of urine and possibly feces may have occurred at the scene of the accident. *Urine incontinence* or *retention* may result from injury to the spinal cord. There may be an imbalance between parasympathetic and sympathetic innervation to the bowel, and thus a loss of voluntary control (Display Box 32–1).

Spinal shock may last from weeks to months. The vasodilation usually resolves within a few days, but it may be months before deep tendon reflexes reappear.

DISPLAY BOX 32–1
Clinical Manifestations of Spinal Shock

- Flaccid paralysis below the level of injury
- Absence of cutaneous and proprioceptive sensation
- Hypotension and bradycardia
- Absence of reflex activity below the level of injury; this may cause urinary retention, bowel paralysis and ileus
- Loss of temperature control; vasodilation and inability to shiver make it difficult for the patient to conserve heat in a cool environment, and the inability to perspire prevents normal cooling in a hot environment
- Reappearance of a reflex that has been depressed after injury is a sign that spinal shock is resolving

---

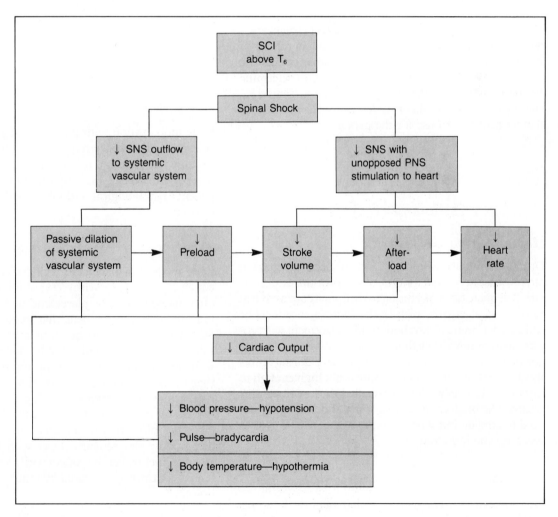

FIGURE 32–6
Mechanisms involved in spinal shock (Zejdlik C: Management of Spinal Cord Injury. Boston, Jones and Bartlett Publishers, 1992. Reprinted by permission. Based on L. Belange, SCI Unit, Shaughnessy Site, Vancouver, BC, unpublished material).

Diagnostic Studies

Diagnostic tests common for patients with SCI include radiographic assessment of spine fractures and possible cord compression. Magnetic resonance imaging also may be used to assess the amount of cord compression and the type of injury that the spinal cord has sustained (ie, either hemorrhage or edema). Computed tomography (CT) scanning will outline the spine and perispinal structures.

Tomography or polytomography is being replaced by CT scanning in many areas, but still may be useful to assess the extent of bony injury. Somatosensory evoked potentials may be recorded to establish a prognosis more clearly. A peripheral nerve below the level of injury is stimulated and the neurologic response (evoked potential) is recorded from the cerebral cortex through scalp electrodes.

There are several important diagnostic examinations done to determine bladder function. One of these is the intravenous pyelogram, which is a series of radiographs that demonstrate the size, location and configuration of the kidneys, and outline the ureters and bladder. Cystoscopy is an examination that allows for direct visualization of the bladder and urethra. Calculi, infection, or tumors of the bladder can be diagnosed. Urodynamic studies are very helpful in patients with SCI. These studies determine the mechanics of bladder filling, storing, and emptying. The results of these studies may determine the best type of bladder program to use for the patient.

Management

Medical Management

Hemodynamic Stability

During the initial postinjury period, medical management often focuses on regulation of blood pressure and heart rate. Adequate tissue perfusion to the spinal cord as well as to other vital organs, such as the kidneys, needs to be addressed. Careful intravenous fluid replacement will provide hydration without fluid overload. Vasopressors may not be needed to maintain blood pressure during spinal shock, but when the blood pressure is not high enough to sustain vital organ perfusion, usually low-dose dopamine is used. The bradycardia during spinal shock also may not need treatment, but if necessary, atropine may be used to speed up the heart rate.

Cord Decompression and Immobilization

Decompression of the cord by realignment of the spinal canal is of concern initially. Closed reduction of a cervical fracture often may be accomplished with skeletal traction. Surgical reduction may be indicated for other spinal fractures. Surgical stabilization is accomplished by placement of Harrington rods, by laminectomy and fusion, or by anterior fusion. Bone for fusion usually is taken from the iliac crest, tibia, or ribs.

Respiratory Management

Respiratory management may include tracheostomy, mechanical ventilation, or frequent respiratory treatment and assistive coughing, depending on the level of injury.

Nutrition

Nutrition is of significant concern even during the acute phase of injury, and must not be overlooked while hemodynamic stability is being addressed. Optimal nutrition is necessary for this stability to to be achieved. Once the patient is in negative nitrogen balance, this contributes to skin breakdown, poor wound healing, and lack of energy for rehabilitative efforts. The stress of this type of injury increases caloric requirements. Caloric requirements should be calculated to ensure adequate, but not excessive, nutritional support.

Until bowel sounds return, nutritional intake may need to be parenteral. Once the gastrointestinal tract is usable, it is the preferred route for intake.

Early Mobilization

Early mobilization with position and posture changes is an early medical concern to prevent complications such as postural hypotension, urinary stasis, and other complications of immobility. Early mobilization also improves the patient's psychological outlook toward rehabilitation and recovery.

Treatment of Paralytic Ileus

Early medical management includes NPO status for the patient, particularly with cervical-injured patients, and often nasogastric tube placement, with intermittent suction, for the paralytic ileus that frequently accompanies SCI. Peristalsis should be stimulated as soon as bowel sounds are present. This may be done safely with stool softeners, mild laxatives, or suppositories. Enemas, other than the oil-retention type, should be avoided because the risk of intestinal perforation is high.

Bowel training is based on a fixed time pattern that takes the place of the cerebrally monitored urge. The defecation reflex remains intact with lesions above the sacral segments. For the patient with a lower motor neuron lesion, continence is assured by regular evacuation of the bowel.

Urinary Management

Acute tubular necrosis may occur during the first 48 hours postinjury as a result of hypotension. An indwelling urinary catheter is necessary to allow for hourly measurement of urinary output during this phase, with a goal of keeping it at least 30 ml/hour. Fluid and electrolyte balance should be monitored closely. Removal of the indwelling catheter as soon as spinal shock has resolved will reduce risk of infection.

Early establishment of an appropriate bladder program will help promote independence. A suprapubic catheter may be indicated for high-level quadriplegics without the motor coordination to do intermittent catheterization.

Medications

Trauma to the spinal cord seems to result in an auto-destructive process that progressively slows spinal cord blood flow. Recent research seems to indicate that meth-ylprednisolone (Solu-Medrol; The Upjohn Company, Kalamazoo, MI), in large doses begun within 8 hours of injury, improves motor and sensory function in patients with acute SCI.[2] The exact mechanisms of action are not clear, although they are thought to be threefold: facilitation of spinal cord impulse generation, enhancement of spinal cord blood flow, and decreased spinal lipid peroxidation.

Low-dose heparin may be used prophylactically against venous thrombosis, although there still is controversy over its effectiveness.

Medications may be necessary in establishing a bladder program. For example, α-blockers may be indicated for patients with tight or spastic internal sphincters, cholinergics for patients with urinary retention, antispastic drugs for those with a tight or spastic external urinary sphincter, or detrusor relaxants for those with bladder spasms.

Collaborative Management

Spinal Immobilization

Care must be taken when moving the patient to prevent damaging an unstable spine and spinal cord. The patient may be log-rolled as a unit to keep the spine aligned. When a patient is in a halo device, care must be taken not to use the hardware of the vest to move him or her (Fig. 32–7).

Temperature Control

A spinal cord injury above the thoracolumbar outflow of the sympathetic nervous system disconnects the thalamic thermoregulatory mechanisms. As a result, the patient fails to sweat to get rid of body heat and there is an absence of vasoconstriction, resulting in the patient's inability to shiver to increase body heat. The degree of thermal control and dysfunction is directly proportional to the extent of body area with loss of thermal regulation. Hence, a quadriplegic has a more difficult time with thermoregulation than a paraplegic.

Hypothermia usually is manageable using warmed

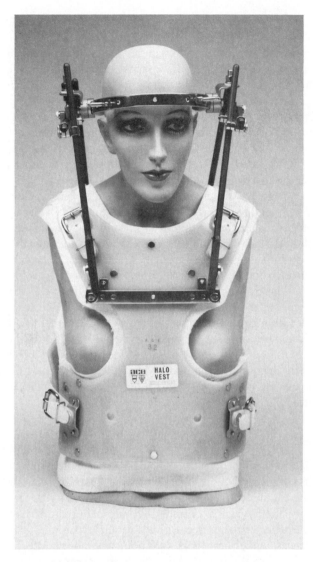

FIGURE 32–7
Halo vest.

blankets. Electric heating blankets or hot water bottles may present a danger for body parts with no sensation. An attempt is made to stabilize the patient's temperature above 96.5°F (35.8°C). Over the long term, thermal control can be facilitated by use of clothing appropriate for the weather conditions.

Prevention of Deep Venous Thrombosis

Measures to prevent deep venous thrombosis (DVT) may include antiembolic stockings. During the acute phase, devices that sequentially compress the lower extremities may be used. Some SCI centers use prophylactic anticoagulation; others rely on passive range-of-motion exercises and early mobilization. The RotoRest bed also is available for use in preventing this complication; it keeps the patient in continuous motion. Functional electrical stimulation is a technology that, with the help of computers, provides electrical neuromuscular stimulation that causes muscle contractions and movement and functional activities of paralyzed extremities. It still is considered an experimental therapy, and requires a great deal of patient energy to use, but may have some future application in helping prevent DVT formation.

Hypercoagulability of a patient's blood may be minimized by ensuring adequate hydration, and if a female SCI patient is taking birth control pills, they should be discontinued. The patient should be educated about the hazards of birth control pills, and another form of birth control can be investigated with the patient.

Leg veins should not be used as sites from which to draw blood for fear that the trauma to the vessel wall may enhance platelet aggregation and clot formation. Smokers should be encouraged to quit, because it is thought that nicotine causes vasoconstriction, thus slowing blood flow through the periphery.

There is some controversy over the effectiveness of serial leg measurements in monitoring for DVT. If leg measurements are used, a standard measurement protocol should be established and followed by all staff. For example, there should be use of special measuring tape rather than sewing tape, there should be independent measurements by two nurses, and running averages should be used.[3]

Urinary Management

The long-range objective of bladder management, regardless of the level of the lesion, is to achieve a means whereby the bladder consistently empties, the urine is sterile, and the patient remains continent. The ultimate goal is to have the patient catheter free, with consistent low residual urine checks, no urinary tract infection, and no evidence of damage to the upper urinary tract structures.

One method of bladder management is accomplished by intermittent catheterization, and it may begin in the early recovery phase after spinal shock has resolved. The purpose of this program is to exercise the detrusor muscle, with the goal again being to have the patient catheter free. The advantage of this method is that no irritant remains in the bladder; consequently, the risk of urinary tract infec-

tion, periurethral abscess, and epididymitis is reduced (Display Box 32–2).

With this method, the patient initially is catheterized every 4 hours. A record is kept of voided amounts and residual amounts. If there is a residual of over 500 ml, the frequency of catheterization should be increased until residuals are under that amount. A urine specimen is obtained for culture and sensitivity at the start of the program. The fluid intake between catheterizations is limited to 600 to 800 ml. The number of catheterizations can be decreased as voided amounts increase or as residual amounts decrease. When a male patient begins to void between catheterizations, an external collector can be used to maintain continence.

Before the catheterization procedure, the patient should be assisted in emptying the bladder by Credé and Valsalva maneuvers and dilation, or any other method that will trigger voiding. These methods stimulate the sacral reflex arc. The objective is to achieve a repeatable residual urine volume of 10% of the voided volume. The catheterizations may be stopped when the residuals become less than 150 ml.

Factors that may hinder efforts to achieve urinary continence include bowel impactions, cystitis, bladder stones, pressure sores, systemic infections, and anxiety.

Psychological Support

The psychological adjustment to the loss of previous physical abilities is unique to each person. The rate at which a person works through this process varies, and none of the stages is static. A person can move back and forth between stages. The emotions felt and displayed by someone with a cord injury are no different from the emotions felt by all of us at one time or another, and recognition of that fact may help one empathize with the patient.

Whatever names are given to the stages of grief, there are certain emotions that are felt after a cord injury.

Stage I—Shock and Disbelief. During this phase, the patient does not request an explanation of what has happened. The patient is overwhelmed by the injury. There may be more concern with whether

---

Clinical Research

Moore KN: Intermittent catheterization: Sterile or clean? Rehabilitation Nursing 16(1):15–18, 1991

Summation of current research on bacteriuria in patients requiring intermittent catheterization is given in this article. Research generally supports the idea that urinary tract infection in patients with a neurogenic bladder most often is the result of residual urine, bladder overdistention, and ischemia of the bladder wall instead of introduction of organisms during the catheterization procedure. Most researchers endorse treatment of the catheter as clean, rather than sterile.

Catheterization done every 4 hours may be more important in reducing infection than catheter sterility or catheterization done less often.

DISPLAY BOX 32–2
Steps in an Intermittent Catheterization Protocol

Goal of intermittent catheterization: To eliminate the need for an indwelling urethral or suprapubic catheter, consequently reducing the incidence of urinary tract complications, for example, infections, periurethral abscess, and epididymitis, and to establish and maintain a safe, catheter-free state for patients with neurogenic bladders.

1. Limit fluid intake to 600–800 ml between catheterizations.
2. Catheterize patient every 4 hours initially. When residual urine volumes are consistently less than 400 ml/2 days, decrease catheterizations to every 6 hours.
3. Record voided amounts and residuals on intake and output record.
4. Decrease number of catheterizations as voiding amounts increase or residuals decrease.
5. Catheterize patient every 8 hours when residual urine volumes are consistently less than 300 ml/2 days.
6. Catheterize patient every 12 hours when residual urine volumes are consistently less than 200 ml/2 days.
7. Catheterize patient every 24 hours when residual urine volumes are consistently less than 150 ml/2 days.
8. Catheterize postvoiding every other day for 1 week when residuals are consistently less than 100 ml/2 days.
9. Catheterize postvoiding to measure residual urine volume every third day for 1 week, then once the next week, and then once a month for 3 months. As long as the patient is in the hospital, catheterize postvoiding to measure residual urine volume any time urine infection is demonstrated.
10. Obtain urine culture at start of the program and every 7 days thereafter.
11. When patient begins to void between catheterizations, use an external collector to maintain continence with men. Spiral it around the penis but do not overlap it.
12. Before catheterization procedure, assist patient to empty bladder by Credé or Valsalva maneuvers, anal dilation, or any other method that will trigger voiding for the particular patient. Sometimes tapping or percussing the bladder with one or two fingers will initiate voiding.
13. Notify physician of difficulty with catheterization, increased sediment or mucus in urine, hematuria, or continuous high residuals (over 500 ml).

With permission, from Mitchell M: Neuroscience Nursing: A Nursing Diagnosis Approach, p 202. Baltimore, Williams & Wilkins, 1989.

he or she will live than with whether he or she will walk again. This period may result in extreme dependence on the staff members. Staff members at the same time may feel that the patient does not understand the ramifications of the injury. The staff may identify with the feelings of being overwhelmed because they themselves often are overwhelmed with the acute medical management of this catastrophic illness.

Stage II—Denial. The process of denial is an escape mechanism. Generally, the whole disability is not denied, but particular aspects of it are. For instance, the patient may say he or she cannot walk now, but in 6 months will be able to. Bargaining, instead of being a separate stage, can be considered a form of denial. Bargains with God may be in the form of offering Him the legs if He will

just return function of the arms. Staff often find it difficult to deal with patients in this stage.

A helpful approach is to focus on the here and now instead of trying to break down the denial. For instance, when a patient refuses to go to physical therapy or refuses certain aspects of care because this is not a permanent disability, the staff can say that *today* he or she cannot walk; therefore, these treatments are necessary.

Focus on the present problems. This is not the stage to discuss long-term changes, such as ordering a wheelchair or making modifications to the home. More appropriate matters to deal with would be bladder training, skin care, and range-of-motion exercises.

Stage III—Reaction. During this stage, instead of denying the impact of the injury, the patient expresses this impact. There may be severe depression and loss of motivation and involvement. Previous hobbies or interests lose their meaning. There is great helplessness during this period, and there may be suicidal statements.

Staff members can help at this stage by listening to the patient as feelings are verbalized. The staff should avoid setting up failure situations, which could happen if they push the patient too fast. Because the patient tends to withdraw during this stage, staff may help by introducing diversional activities.

Another type of reaction seen is *acting out*, which may include anger or sexual, drug, or alcohol abuse. Anger may be expressed verbally or physically. The patient feels no one can do anything right—including family and staff. This kind of behavior makes staff want to avoid contact with the patient. Some limits do need to be set to protect the patient and the staff from truly abusive actions.

Stage IV—Mobilization. Problem-solving behavior can be seen during this stage. The patient is looking toward the future and wants to learn about self-care. In fact, the patient may become very possessive of the therapist or nurse and resent the time spent with other patients. This is a time of sharing and planning between patient and staff.

Stage V—Coping. It is thought by some in the field of rehabilitation that people do not accept the disability *per se* but instead learn to cope with it. Disability still is an inconvenience, but it is no longer the center of their lives. Life is again meaningful to the person, and the patient is again involved with others.

All staff should have an understanding of the types of feelings and reactions the patient with SCI may exhibit. This process of recovery can be shared with family members in helping them to support the injured person and participate in the rehabilitation. Psychological support should be provided for family members as well. They no doubt have many concerns, such as finances, role changes, long-term outcomes, and more. It is important to be supportive of them and help them, as well as the patient, with coping strategies.

Nursing Management

Respiratory Management

Although a patient with an injury below C4 will have the diaphragm intact, during the initial period after a cervical SCI there may be ascending cord edema that will impair the function of the diaphragm temporarily. During the time of the edema the patient may require mechanical ventilation.

Anyone with a cervical cord injury should have respiratory parameters such as tidal volume and vital capacity measured frequently, along with frequent auscultation of breath sounds. Respiratory failure should be anticipated.

Normally, ventilation is accomplished through a complex interaction between muscles of the chest, the abdominal wall, and the diaphragm. A SCI results in paralysis of inspiratory and expiratory muscles. Dysfunction of intercostal and accessory muscles decreases ventilation and predisposes the patient to atelectasis. Dysfunction of abdominal muscles and expiratory intercostal muscles diminishes the patient's ability to generate a cough to clear secretions. The intercostal muscles also normally provide support to the lateral chest wall. When the intercostals are impaired, this part of the chest wall collapses during inspiration as the abdomen expands. This breathing pattern is discernible easily, and results in ineffective ventilation.

The degree of respiratory compromise is determined primarily by the level of the injury, although not entirely. For example, a 28-year-old C5 quadriplegic with no lung disease may have better ventilation than a 65-year-old C8 quadriplegic with a long history or smoking and chronic obstructive pulmonary disease.[4]

Respiratory complications are a major cause of death in the acute and chronic phases of SCI, especially among quadriplegics. Therefore, careful respiratory assessment and early intervention are important.

Assisting the patient with the quad coughing technique may help clear airways more effectively despite weakness or loss of the respiratory muscles that produce the automatic cough reflex. With this quad coughing technique, the sides of the patient's chest (if patient is on side or abdomen) or the diaphragm (if supine) are compressed during exhalation. This technique often is most helpful after postural drainage or clapping of the chest.

Suctioning may be necessary if the patient's airway cannot be cleared effectively with other techniques. Nurses should remember that suctioning (or nasogastric tube insertion) may trigger an abnormal vasovagal response, which can cause bradycardia. Patients being suctioned should be hyperoxygenated before and after the procedure.[5] The duration of each suctioning pass should not exceed 10 seconds to help prevent hypoxia and possible cardiac dysrhythmias.

When turning a patient to a prone position on a Stryker frame, the nurse needs to remain at the bedside for the first few turns to evaluate the patient's respiratory tolerance of the turn. High-level quadriplegics can experience respiratory arrest in the prone position because movement of the diaphragm is compromised. Bradycardia in the prone position also is common.

Bowel Training

Smooth muscle peristalsis begins as soon as the paralytic ileus secondary to spinal shock resolves. The nurse must keep in mind that bowel impaction occurs frequently during the period of ileus. In patients with injuries above the sacral segments of the cord, the defecation reflex will be intact. The reflex is interrupted with lower motor neuron lesions, but the autonomous bowel has an intrinsic contractile response.

Upper motor neuron (above S2) injuries result in a spastic or automatic bowel. Fecal incontinence, due to the intact sacral arc that results in reflex defecation, is the primary problem. Lower motor neuron injuries (S2–S4) are characterized by a flaccid bowel, and the primary problem may be fecal retention due to involvement of the sacral arc.

The actual bowel program may be based on bowel habits before the injury. The time of day should be established in relation to the patient's future social needs. A bowel program can be used in conjunction with digital stimulation (Display Box 32–3).

DISPLAY BOX 32-3
Steps in a Bowel Training Program

Goal: to attain and maintain bowel continence.

1. Determine bowel habits preinjury if possible.
2. Follow established bowel program. An example of a bowel program is:
   For patients who are being fed (tube feedings or regular food):
   • Colace 100 mg orally or per nasogastric tube three times a day.
   • Dulcolax suppository every night unless the patient has had a bowel movement that day.
   • Milk of magnesia 30 ml orally or per nasogastric tube every other night or even dates unless patient has had a bowel movement that day.
   For patients who are NPO:
   • Dulcolax suppository every other night on even dates.
3. Slush enema may be given every day until peristalsis is present. This consists of giving approximately a liter tap water enema, then holding the container below the level of the bed, allowing the water to return, and repeating the procedure several times.
4. Use bowel program in conjunction with digital stimulation. Digital stimulation consists of inserting a lubricated, gloved index finger into the anal sphincter, using a rotating motion of the finger around the sphincter. The sphincter will slowly dilate as the stimulation occurs. The finger is inserted to about half its length, and the circular rotation is continued for 15–20 minutes until stool passes into the rectum and is then evacuated from the rectum.
5. Once a pattern of evacuation is established, use only digital stimulation if possible, eliminating the suppository. Use only the bowel program on individuals unable to tolerate digital stimulation.
6. Use digital stimulation after each involuntary bowel movement while the bowel pattern is being established.
7. Modify the bowel program according to individual needs as determined by stool consistency.
8. Use Nupercainal ointment or Xylocaine jelly to insert suppository or for digital stimulation if patient is prone to episodes of autonomic dysreflexia. The ointment or jelly may be used in the rectum and around the anal sphincter before insertion of the suppository or finger.
9. Maintain high fluid intake when not contraindicated—for example, in cases of fluid restriction or increased intracranial pressure.
10. Use incontinence pads rather than a bedpan when giving routine bowel care. A bedpan does not work well for these reasons: it is hard and can cause pressure areas over the coccyx; it does not allow access to the anus for digital stimulation; and it can upset the spinal alignment necessary for proper healing in spinal cord-injury patients.
11. Notify physician of prolonged or severe diarrhea, impaction, rectal bleeding, or hemorrhoids.

With permission, from Mitchell M: Neuroscience Nursing: A Nursing Diagnosis Approach, p 201. Baltimore, Williams & Wilkins, 1989.

Once a pattern is established, digital stimulation may be used alone. While the pattern of evacuation is being established, digital stimulation should be used after any involuntary bowel movement so that complete evacuation of the rectum is ensured. There may be patients who will not tolerate digital stimulation without having an episode of autonomic dysreflexia. Dibucaine (Nupercainal; Ciba Pharmaceutical Co., Summit, NJ) can be used for insertion of the suppository or for digital stimulation in those patients prone to this phenomenon.

A bowel program may be modified according to individual need, as determined by stool consistency. A high fluid intake should be maintained unless the patient is on an intermittent catheterization protocol.

Patients with injuries at C4 and above will be dependent in their bowel program, whereas those with injuries at C8 and below should be able to be independent in their bowel program. With appropriate teaching, patients, regardless of the level of injury, should be able to direct their own bowel program. When considering who will help a patient with toileting, nurses should not automatically assume that it will be the spouse or significant other. Assisting with toileting may deter from sexual appeal, so the patient or spouse may prefer another caregiver to help with the bowel and bladder program. This should be a matter for discussion before teaching.

In determining if the patient should be taught to do the bowel program on the toilet or in bed, several considerations must be made: the stability of the spine with or without orthosis, the patient's tolerance for sitting at 90°, skin integrity over the sacrum and perineal area, and how the program will be done at home. The program established in the hospital or rehabilitation center should be the one the patient plans to follow at home.

The nurse should instruct the patient about the four areas affecting the bowel that could influence the success of the program: diet, fluids, activity, and medications. The importance of maintaining the bowel program to prevent autonomic dysreflexia needs to be stressed.

There are several nonmedication techniques for facilitating defecation that may be useful for patients to know. Advantage should be taken of the gastrocolic reflex, which is an automatic response that increases peristaltic movement of the bowel after eating. It often is strongest after the first meal of the day. Sometimes a hot drink may stimulate the reflex for some patients. Timing of the bowel program to take advantage of this increased bowel motility should be considered.

Abdominal massage may increase bowel peristalsis. This is done by massaging the abdomen from right to left in a circular downward motion, which follows the direction of peristalsis.

In patients with intact abdominal musculature, the Valsalva maneuver may be taught. This will increase intrathoracic pressure when the patient forcibly exhales against a closed glottis.

The sitting position should be recommended for patients who are able to accomplish this. If the program is done in bed, the patient should lie on the left side.

Skin Care

Pressure is a common cause of structural damage to a muscle and its peripheral nerve supply. There is a definite time–pressure relationship in the development of pressure sores. Skin can tolerate minute pressure indefinitely, but great pressure for a short time is disruptive. Microscopic tissue changes secondary to local ischemia occur in less than 30 minutes. Pressure interferes with arteriolar and capillary blood flow.

When the pressure is prolonged, there is definite damage to superficial circulation and tissue. The damage may be associated with congestion and induration of the area or blistering and loss of superficial epidermal layers of skin. As the pressure continues, the deeper skin layers are lost, leading to necrosis and ulceration. Serous drainage from such an ulceration can constitute a continuous protein loss of as much as 50 g/day. Prolongation of the pressure results in deep penetrating necrosis of the skin, subcutaneous tissue, fascia, and muscle. The destruction may progress to gangrene of the underlying bony structure. Pressure necrosis can begin from within the tissue over a bony prominence, where the body weight is greatest per square inch.

A turn schedule for the patient obviously is important. Turning should be carried out at least every 2 hours. Use of an air or egg-crate mattress does not preclude the need to turn. The condition of the skin should be checked before and after the position change. Patients should be encouraged to check their own skin condition with a mirror, when possible, and to recognize their skin's tolerance to pressure—that is, the amount of time they can lie or sit in the same position without redness that does not fade within 15 minutes.

Numerous kinetic beds that are in continuous motion are available. They slowly turn from side to side, but may be stopped in any position. They are helpful for mobilizing pulmonary secretions, improving gas exchange, and for preventing skin breakdown. These beds are useful both for preventing and treating complications of immobility.

Patients also should be taught how to do weight shifts, especially when they are getting up in the wheelchair for long periods during the day. A weight shift is a means of relieving pressure from any bony prominence. When the patient is in the sitting position, the main bony prominences are the ischial tuberosities and the sacrum.

There are several methods of accomplishing a weight shift. There is a full recline, in which the patient is reclined in the wheelchair to relieve the ischial pressure, and the weight thereby is distributed throughout the entire dorsal surface. The patient accomplishes the side-to-side weight shift by hooking the forearm around one push-handle of the wheelchair and then leaning sideways over the opposite wheelchair tire. The half push-up weight shift to relieve pressure from one ischium is accomplished by leaning on one elbow and pushing off the opposite wheelchair tire or arm rest. This process is repeated in the other direction to relieve pressure from the opposite ischium. With the full push-up weight shift, the patient relieves ischial pressure by pushing up with the arms from the tires or arm rests of the wheelchair. Which of these weight shifts a patient can accomplish will depend of course on the motor ability.

Use of incontinence pads tends to hold the perspiration next to the skin and thus should be avoided. A bedpan does not work well with an SCI patient. It is so hard that it can cause a pressure area over the coccyx, it does not allow access to the anus for digital stimulation, and it can upset the spinal alignment necessary for proper healing.

As the largest organ of the body, the skin also is perhaps the most vulnerable to injury as a result of SCI. Skin breakdown slows the progress of rehabilitation, puts the patient at risk for infection, makes sitting in a wheelchair difficult or impossible, and adds greatly to the patient's cost and suffering if surgical repair is required. Skin breakdown is a preventable complication of SCI, and nurses have a challenging role in ensuring it does not happen in the hospital or rehabilitation setting, as well as educating the patient in how to prevent it at home. Display Box

32–4 outlines some common-sense instructions regarding skin care.

Medication Administration

Nurses administering medications to patients with SCI should recognize several special considerations for this population.

Subcutaneous and intramuscular injections are not absorbed well because of the lack of muscle tone. Sterile abscesses may result, causing autonomic dysreflexia or an increase in spasms. *Injection sites* are the deltoid area, the anterior thigh, and the abdominal area. These sites should be rotated, and the volume injected should not exceed 1 ml at any one site.

As a rule, sensation in the cord-injured patient is limited. Intractable pain may be present after spinal shock and is due to nerve root damage. Abnormal sensation may occur at the level of the lesion in injuries causing diverse nerve root damage, such as with gunshot or knife wounds. Narcotics are not favored because of the high probability of addiction. Attention to position and other comfort measures, along with the use of mild analgesics such as aspirin or acetaminophen, is a more acceptable approach.

Nurses often start peripheral intravenous lines. The intravenous site of choice, however, is the subclavian vein, because in this area of high blood flow, there is less chance

---

DISPLAY BOX 32–4
Skin Care Instructions for the SCI Patient

1. Wear your braces in the car, if you have them, because they will keep your feet where you want them and help maintain balance.
2. When traveling in a van, be sure the wheelchair is secured to the floor and that safety belts are used.
3. Apply elastic stockings or Ace wraps or abdominal binder evenly to prevent skin pressure.
4. Check hands, feet, and legs for swelling. Elevate swollen extremity above the level of the heart. If the swelling does not decrease within 6–8 hours, notify your physician.
5. Use lotion or other lubricating cream if you have dry skin.
6. Protect skin from perspiration, stool, and urine.
7. Wear properly fitting belts, shoes, and socks. Tug at the toes of socks after putting them on to prevent ingrown toenails. Be sure clothing is not tight-fitting.
8. Avoid use of a rubber air ring, because it can cause pressure to the skin and block off the blood supply to the area of skin inside the ring.
9. Avoid nylon underwear, because it retains moisture.
10. Carry coins, billfold, or keys in a place other than a pocket.
11. Items such as a thin metal ashtray should not be rested on your lap, because the heat from the metal may be undetected and cause a burn.
12. Avoid sitting on a vinyl car seat that has been sitting in the sun without covering it with a towel or blanket.
13. Hot water bottles, heating pads, and electric blankets should be avoided.
14. Wear shoes when in a wheelchair to avoid bumping and scraping your feet or toes.

of thrombosis secondary to vasomotor paralysis, especially during spinal shock. For these reason, the veins of the lower extremities never should be used for intravenous administration.

Bladder Training

Establishing a bladder training program is discussed in the section on Collaborative Management. Specific steps are outlined for an intermittent catheterization protocol in Display Box 32–2. It is important for nurses to recognize that an alteration in urinary elimination has profound physiological and psychological significance. Urinary incontinence can cause a patient to become socially isolated for fear of "an accident."

Patients with injuries at C8 and below should be independent in bladder management. Those with injuries above C5 usually are dependent in bladder care, but should be able to direct the care. Urodynamic studies should be done to determine the best bladder program for each patient. There are some techniques that can be taught to patients to help stimulate voiding, as part of the program, based on the level of injury.

For patients with an injury above the sacral segments resulting in an automatic reflex bladder, the anal stretch may inhibit urethral sphincter contraction. Anal stretch also can be a helpful technique to insert a catheter in patients with urethral sphincter spasms. Other techniques to trigger voiding are tapping the suprapubic area, stroking the inner thigh, pulling pubic hair, massaging the penoscrotal area, or pinching the posterior aspect of the glans penis. In patients with a lower motor neuron injury with an atonic bladder, Valsalva or Credé maneuvers may be used to help empty the bladder.

Nurses also need to instruct patients on the administration and side effects of drugs they may be taking as part of their bladder management program. For example, a patient should be aware that abrupt withdrawal of baclofen (an external sphincter antispasmodic) may result in hallucinations. Written instructions about medications, as well as other protocols or teaching, can be given to patients before discharge.

Sexuality and Self-Concept

People have different interpretations of what sex is or what a sexual loss may represent, so it is impossible to organize a sexual health care service with the universal application of a bowel or bladder program. The diversity of beliefs and practices makes this a difficult area to approach with a constant body of information. It is important to find out from each patient what is and is not acceptable sexual activity, the patient's beliefs about birth control and fertility issues, and an assessment of sexual beliefs and practices. With this information, the nurse will be able to give the patient and his or her partner specific information that will allow for a healthy sex life, regardless of the SCI disability.

It is important for patients to recognize that sexuality involves more than intercourse. Sexuality also is what one thinks about oneself, how one views oneself in relationships, how one communicates. It involves the total person, not just sexual behavior. It has been said that "sex is something we do. Sexuality is something we are." So although the specific sexual behaviors or practices may need to change or be modified, a SCI patient still can be a sexual person.

After a cord injury, patients are concerned about their ability to function sexually, although many may not verbalize this concern for quite a time. When the questions do come, it is helpful if the nurse can respond in an informed way instead of telling the patient to ask the physician. Failure of professionals to inquire about the patient's sexual concerns tends to confirm fears that sexual life is over.

Most cord-injured men believe that their total sexuality is tied to erection and ejaculation. There are three general types of erection in men: psychogenic, reflexogenic, and spontaneous.

A psychogenic erection can result from sexual thoughts. The area of the cord responsible for this type of erection is between T11 and L2. Therefore, if the lesion is above this level, the message from the brain cannot get through the damaged area.

Reflexogenic erections are a direct result of stimulation to the penis. Some patients may get this type of erection when changing their catheter or pulling the pubic hairs. The length of time the erection can be maintained is variable; thus, its usefulness for sexual activity is variable. Reflexogenic erections are better with higher cervical and thoracic lesions. Damage to lumbar and sacral regions may destroy the reflex arc.

The third type of erection is spontaneous. This may occur when the bladder is full, and it comes from some internal stimulation. How long the spontaneous erection lasts will determine its usefulness for sexual activity. The ability to achieve a reflexogenic or spontaneous erection comes from nerves in the S2, S3, and S4 segments of the cord.

There are medical interventions that may be prescribed to enhance a man's erection. One method is injection of the spongy tissue of the penis with a vasodilating medication such as papaverine, either alone or in combination with phentolamine mesylate, or prostaglandin E1. The motor skills necessary to draw up the medication in a syringe and to inject it may not be available to all quadriplegics. Test doses of the medication usually are given by the physician to determine the appropriate dosage.

An external method of assisting with erection is a vacuum-principle device, Erectaid, which involves placing a firm cylinder over the flaccid penis. Air is pumped out of the cylinder with a small hand pump. The penis becomes engorged with blood and becomes erect, at which time a rubber ring is placed on the base of the penis to retain the blood inside the penis. Then the cylinder is removed. Most recommend that the ring not be kept on longer than 30 minutes.

Dildos, which are rubbery casings that fit over the soft penis and are held on with suction, adhesive, or straps, may provide stimulation inside the vagina. Another external device is the vibrator, which may be used on a patient with a SCI or an able-bodied partner over areas of the body with intact sensation. In patients with high-level injuries, the stimulus of the vibrator to the genitalia may cause tachycardia, hypertension, tachypnea, and headache, so the use of a vibrator in these people is not recommended.

Surgically, insertion of internal penile prostheses is available. Some of these fluid-filled rods require pumping up when an erection is desired. The pump usually is located inside the scrotum and some motor agility is required to pump up the prosthesis and to release it.

Not many men with a complete cord injury have ejaculations. Sometimes retrograde ejaculation into the bladder will occur. Some male patients remove their urethral catheter before intercourse. Others leave their catheter in place and fold it back over the penis. Despite the physical side effects of the SCI, the patient's sex drive should not change from what it was before the injury.

Lack of sexual interest may be related to chronic pain or fatigue related to complications of SCI. Other causes may be medication, especially sedatives, psychotherapeutic drugs, or antispasmodics. Worry or stress also can cause a patient to lose sexual interest, such as concern about finances, a job, a housing situation, feelings of powerlessness and depression, and relationship and role conflicts.

Women with SCI may find they need to use a lubricating jelly such as K-Y jelly (water soluble) before intercourse. If the woman was practicing birth control before the injury, it should still be a concern after the injury.

When considering the method for birth control, some considerations need to be made specific to the spinal injury. Oral contraceptives containing estrogen pose a thromboembolic hazard that is intensified for a woman who spends much time in a wheelchair. Those oral contraceptives containing progesterone may cause weight gain, making transfers more difficult. Women with SCI may not recognize complications with an intrauterine device (IUD), such as perforation of the uterus or pelvic inflammatory disease. The IUD can increase menstrual flow, which may be difficult to deal with. Tubal ligation, which has little or no complications, is another possibility for a woman with SCI.

The menstrual pattern usually is interrupted for approximately 6 months after injury, but then is reestablished. Women with SCI are able to become pregnant and seem to have no increase in rate of miscarriage. There are potential complications for the pregnant spinal-injured woman, such as urinary tract infection, pressure sores, and anemia,

but with careful medical attention, they usually can be avoided or minimized.

Labor may be painless, or the woman may experience other signs that indicate labor is occurring (eg, abdominal or leg spasms, back pain, difficulty breathing). Autonomic dysreflexia is a complication of labor in women with injuries above T4–T6, and should be anticipated so it can be controlled. Women with SCI can breast-feed their baby if desired.

Fertility in men is influenced by the ability or inability to ejaculate, the sperm count, and motility of the sperm. Fertility is not based on the ability to have an erection or the ability for genital sensation. Recently there have been new techniques developed to recover sperm from men with SCI for artificial insemination. The electroejaculation procedure is one in which electrodes are applied to the posterior surface of the prostate gland. The patient usually is anesthetized briefly while an electric shock is applied, which causes ejaculation. This technique may be used in patients regardless of the level of their injury. For those with an injury at T10 or above, there is a vibratory procedure available in which an electrical vibrator is applied to the glans penis for 1 to 5 minutes, resulting in ejaculation in over half the patients. Some researchers also have used intrathecal injection of neostigmine and subcutaneous physostigmine to elicit an ejaculation, but less than half the patients responded with ejaculation.[6]

The SCI patient needs to be instructed in how to plan for sexual activity. Spontaneous sex often is not possible because the patient often prefers to prepare in advance for the bowel program, bladder status, disconnection of urinary drainage devices, transferring to a suitable area like the bed, positioning, and undressing. Frequently there is concern about bowel or bladder accidents. To minimize this risk, fluid intake may be restricted for several hours, and the bladder can be emptied. Women often have more risk for a bowel accident during intercourse, because it is thought that the penis inside the vagina activates bowel reflexes. Patients may plan for sexual activity after their bowel program.

When educating patients for a return to sexual activity, the nurse should encourage open communication with the partner. The patient should feel comfortable giving verbal guidance to the partner, letting the partner know the areas of the injured person's body that have sensation and whether that sensation is pleasant or not. Some areas may be hypersensitive or even painful to caressing. Preferred ways of stimulation and flexibility in trying new positions or techniques need to be communicated.

A SCI may create many technical problems, but with good communication and information from professionals, they can be adapted to and the patient can have a healthy sexual life. Sometimes ongoing sexual counseling is appropriate. Sometimes relationships improve because more time is spent and there is more communication between partners.

It is essential that nurses address this area of concern for patients with SCI. By avoiding discussion of this important area of a patient's life, professionals validate the patient's fear that there can be no sex with a SCI, and that certainly is not true.

Complications

Pulmonary Problems

Pulmonary complications are the ones most commonly associated with death in people with SCI, both in the acute and chronic phases. These pulmonary complications are especially prevalent in people injured above T10. If there is concomitant chest trauma or preexisting pulmonary disease, a history of smoking, or older age, there is higher risk for these complications.

Atelectasis is possible in any immobilized patient. Early mobilization and ensuring the airways are clear of secretions, as well as bronchial hygiene, may be useful in minimizing or preventing atelectasis. Pneumonia also may result from hypoventilation and inability to keep airways clear. Adequate hydration helps keep secretions liquefied for ease of removal, and bronchoscopy may be necessary to remove mucus plugs. Supplemental oxygen administration is used to treat hypoxia. Ventilator-dependent patients need exquisite pulmonary care (see Chapter 19).

Especially during the acute phase of SCI, pulmonary embolus is a potential problem. Many emboli break off a DVT and lodge in the lung. Patients particularly at risk for a fat embolus are those with long bone fractures. Signs of chest or neck petechiae and low-grade fever may be early indications.

Stress Ulcers

During the spinal shock period of SCI, acute stress ulcers may occur and may be seen as an acute gastrointestinal bleed. If the patient has a nasogastric tube in place, the gastric acidity may be monitored, and an antacid given to maintain a gastric pH above 4.5. Histamine receptor antagonists also may be used. As long as the patient is on steroids, gastrointestinal bleeding is a possibility. Often when a gastric bleed develops in a patient, the pain is referred to the back between the scapulae, so particular attention should be paid to this complaint.

Autonomic Dysreflexia

Autonomic dysreflexia, or hyperreflexia, is a syndrome that sometimes occurs after the acute phase in patients with a spinal cord lesion at T7 or above, and constitutes a medical emergency. The syndrome presents quickly and can precipitate a seizure or a stroke. Death can occur if the cause is not relieved.

The syndrome can be triggered by bladder or intestinal distention, spasticity, decubitus ulcers, or stimulation of the skin below the level of the injury. Ejaculation in the man can initiate the reflex, as can strong uterine contractions in the pregnant woman (Display Box 32–5).

These stimuli produce a sympathetic discharge that causes a reflex vasoconstriction of the blood vessels in the skin and splanchnic bed below the level of the injury. The vasoconstriction produces extreme hypertension and a throbbing headache.

Vasoconstriction of the splanchnic bed distends the baroreceptors in the carotid sinus and aortic arch. They in turn stimulate the vagus nerve, resulting in a bradycardia, which is the body's attempt to lower the blood pressure. The body also attempts to reduce the hypertension by superficial vasodilation of vessels above the SCI. As a result, there is flushing, blurred vision, and nasal congestion. Because the SCI interrupts transmission of the vasodilation message below the level of the lesion, the vasoconstriction continues below the level of the lesion until the stimulus is identified and interrupted. The vasoconstriction results in pallor below the level of the lesion, whereas flushing occurs above the lesion (Display Box 32–6).

When autonomic dysreflexia is recognized, there are several things the alert nurse can do quickly and can teach the patient to do. The head of the bed should be elevated, and frequent checks of the blood pressure should be made. The bladder drainage system can be checked quickly for kinks in the tubing. The urine collection bag should not be

---

DISPLAY BOX 32–5
Potential Precipitating Factors of Autonomic Dysreflexia

- Bladder distention or urinary tract infection
- Bladder/kidney stones
- Distended bowel
- Pressure areas or decubiti
- Thrombophlebitis
- Acute abdominal problems such as ulcers, gastritis
- Pulmonary emboli
- Menstruation
- Second stage of labor
- Constrictive clothing
- Heterotopic bone
- Pain
- Sexual activity; ejaculation by a man
- Manipulation/instrumentation of bladder or bowel
- Spasticity
- Exposure to hot or cold stimuli

DISPLAY BOX 32–6
Manifestations of Autonomic Dysreflexia

- Paroxysmal hypertension
- Pounding headache
- Blurred vision
- Bradycardia
- Profuse sweating above the level of the injury
- Flushing or splotching of the face and neck
- Piloerection
- Nasal congestion
- Nausea
- Pupil dilation

---

overly full. Some protocols for checking the patency of the urinary drainage system include irrigation of the catheter with 10 to 30 ml of irrigating solution. The nurse should make sure that absolutely no more than that amount is used because the addition of the fluid may aggravate the massive sympathetic outflow already present. If the symptoms persist after these checks are made, the catheter should be changed so that the bladder can empty. If the patient did not have a catheter in place when the hyperreflexia began, one should be inserted.

If the urinary system does not seem to be the cause of the stimulus, the patient should be checked for bowel impaction. The impaction should not be removed until the symptoms subside. Dibucaine or lidocaine ointment can be applied to the rectum to anesthetize the area until symptoms subside. Patients prone to autonomic dysreflexia use these ointments routinely with their bowel program.

If the patient's blood pressure does not return to normal, the use of a sympathetic ganglionic blocking agent such as atropine sulfate, guanethidine sulfate (Ismelin; Ciba Pharmaceutical Co.), reserpine (Serpasil; Ciba Pharmaceutical Co.), or methyldopa (Aldomet; Merck Sharp & Dohme, West Point, PA) may be used. Hydralazine (Apresoline; Ciba Pharmaceutical Co.) and diazoxide (Hyperstat; Schering Corporation, Kenilworth, NJ) also sometimes are used (Display Box 32–7).

Hypercalcemia

Immobilization hypercalcemia occurs most often in adolescent male quadriplegics who have prolonged enforced immobilization and sometimes dehydration. These two factors cause decreased bone formation, yet calcium reabsorption is elevated, which leads to this problem. The etiology of this endocrine complication is not clear. Treatment usually includes steroids, hydration, and lowering of serum calcium levels.

Bone, Joint, and Muscle Problems

Fifteen percent to 20% of patients with SCI have heterotopic ossification or excessive bone formation around joints. It occurs most often in quadriplegics, but the cause is unknown. Joint calcification results in joint swelling, stiffness, and limited joint functioning. There will be an elevated serum phosphatase level and erythrocyte sedimentation rate. Risk factors seem to include older age, presence of decubitus ulcers and spasticity, and completeness of the injury. There is prophylactic treatment available with disodium editronate diphosphonate, but once the bony formation is mature, it may require surgery for removal. Early mobilization and weight-bearing and range-of-motion exercises help in prevention of this complication. Radiographs and bone scans are diagnostic.

Osteoporosis may occur after SCI. There is increased porosity and bone softening from immobility, which may result in a bone fracture after minimal trauma to an extremity. Signs include localized swelling, a change in alignment of an extremity, hematoma, crepitus, or significant increase in spasticity. The patient may have heard a snap or crack at the time the bone broke. Long bone fractures often require surgical fixation.

Contractures may be another complication of SCI that can impede functional recovery and rehabilitation. Correct positioning of paralyzed extremities, as well as regular turning and range-of-motion exercises all are very important in prevention of contractures. Foot-drop may be prevented by space boots or high-top tennis shoes.

Spasticity is a state of exaggerated muscular tone with increased tendon reflexes, associated with an upper motor neuron lesion that may appear after spinal shock has resolved. In mild cases, spasticity actually may be helpful in promoting blood flow from the periphery back to the heart. Again, proper positioning and range-of-motion exercise are important, and the use of heat and cold may help in treatment of spasticity. Functional electrical stimulation is used in some centers to induce contraction of spastic muscles by electrical stimulation of a peripheral nerve. This seems to reduce spasticity in some patients, perhaps through muscle fatigue.

There are drugs that can help control this complication, the main three being baclofen, dantrolene, and diazepam. Patient education should include the fact that spasticity cannot be eliminated completely with these drugs, so their use should be based on the functional goals the patient is trying to achieve. Baclofen and morphine have been used experimentally with an implanted intrathecal drug delivery system. By delivering the drugs intrathecally, some of the systemic side effects may be minimized. Further trials are under way.

Surgical intervention also may be used to manage spasticity, including rhizotomy, myelotomy and localized cordectomy, ablative neurologic procedures, epidural stimulation, and tendon lengthening.

DISPLAY BOX 32–7
Nursing Treatment Checklist for Autonomic Dysreflexia

1. Elevate head of bed.
2. Apply blood pressure cuff and check blood pressure every 1 to 2 minutes.
   A. If BP is above 180/90, proceed to step 5.
   B. If BP is below 180/90, proceed as follows.
3. Quickly insert bladder catheter or check bladder drainage system in place to detect possible obstruction.
   A. Check to make sure plug or clamp is not in catheter or on tubing.
   B. Check for kinks in catheter or drainage tubing.
   C. Check inlet to leg bag to make sure it is not corroded.
   D. Check to make sure leg bag is not overfull.
   E. If none of these are evident, proceed to step 4.
4. Determine if catheter is plugged by irrigating the bladder slowly with no more than 30 ml of irrigation solution. Use of more solution may increase the massive sympathetic outflow already present. If symptoms have not subsided, proceed to step 5.
5. Change the catheter and empty the bladder.
6. When you are sure the bladder is empty and if BP is:
   A. Above 180/90, call physician immediately.
   B. Below 180/90, proceed as follows:
      Atropine given according to physician's order. If BP rises or fails to subside, call physician immediately. Ismelin, Apresoline, or inhaled amyl nitrate may then be ordered by the physician. Dibenzylene may be used for chronic dysreflexia.
7. Ideally, this procedure requires three people: one to check the BP, one to check the drainage system, and one to notify the physician.

If bladder overdistention does not seem to be the cause of the dysreflexia,

1. Check for bowel impaction. Do not attempt to remove it, if present. Apply Nupercainal ointment or Xylocaine jelly to the rectum and anal area. As the area is anesthetized, the BP should fall. After the BP is again stable, using a generous amount of anesthetizing ointment or jelly, manually remove impaction.
2. Change patient's position. Pressure areas may be the source of dysreflexia.

With permission, from Mitchell M: Neuroscience Nursing: A Nursing Diagnosis Approach, p 199. Baltimore, Williams & Wilkins, 1989.

Chronic Pain Syndromes

Chronic pain syndromes develop in a significant number of patients with SCI, with most occurring within 6 months of the injury. The type and nature of the pain varies depending on the level of injury. Patients with a cauda equina injury have the highest probability of having a pain syndrome, and those with a cervical injury are the least likely to have one. Careful evaluation of the pain must be made. There are psychological, social, emotional, and cultural factors associated with any pain syndrome, and all these should be assessed before determining a management program for the pain.

Substance Abuse

Chemical (drug or alcohol) dependency is a complication that may be seen in response to an overwhelming injury like a SCI. A patient may feel powerless, dependent, and depressed, and turn to self-destructive behaviors as a way to cope. The disabled are vulnerable to substance abuse, and this must be kept in mind by those who care for the SCI patient.

Spinal Cord Ischemia

Post-traumatic spinal cord ischemia is the loss of adequate blood flow to the spinal cord. This phenomenon is common after SCI, and the exact etiology is not clear. It may be due to vasospasm or vascular thrombosis from biochemical changes after injury. Methods to counteract this poor perfusion to the cord are being researched. Some drugs, such as calcium channel blockers combined with dextran, have resulted in improved blood flow and restored function as demonstrated by evoked potentials in research animals.

Surgical decompression of the spinal cord is controversial, but some studies indicate that early surgical intervention may improve recovery. Internal decompression also has been studied, whereby the dead, hemorrhagic tissue from the cord is removed in the hope of preserving the viable surrounding tracts of the cord.

Recently, there has been experimentation with methods to promote axonal recovery or regeneration in SCI. Specific hormones such as thyroid hormones have been shown to influence growth of normal axons. Other agents, such as nerve factors, accelerate the rate of axonal growth. Both biologic and nonbiologic bridges have been implanted into the space at the site of spinal cord transection. Some growth of axons into the bridging material has been demonstrated. Peripheral nerves that have been used as bridges in the spinal cord have shown some promising results in carrying the axons across the lesion.

Other researchers are studying fetal brain or spinal cord tissue transplants or grafts into injured spinal cords.

CASE STUDY

Adam Davis is a 19-year-old college student who fell 30 feet to the ground while rock climbing. He was picked up at the scene of the accident by paramedics who found him lying in a supine position, unable to move any extremities and complaining of some neck pain. He appeared awake, alert, and oriented to his current location, the date and day of the week, and details of the fall. His pupils were equal and reactive to light. He showed no other signs of injury except for several scrapes on his arms. Vital signs were BP 110/72, HR 86, respirations 18, unlabored and regular. The paramedic applied a cervical collar, placed him on a backboard, and he was transported to the medical center by helicopter.

On initial exam, his vital signs were BP 100/60, HR 68, respirations 24 and somewhat shallow, temperature 99.8°F (37.7°C). His color was dusky, skin warm and dry, and his arm veins were quite distended. He had no motor function or sensation past a couple of inches below midaxillary level. He could tighten his biceps but could not overcome gravity to raise his arms. There were no deep tendon reflexes.

DISPLAY BOX 32–8
Care of a Patient in a Halo Brace

1. Keep wrench taped to front cross-bar so anterior vest can be removed should the need arise to do CPR (some models bend up to give access to the chest).
2. Move patient as a unit. Never use upright bars to move or roll patient.
3. Check skull pins for tightness every day. If loose to finger tightness, report to physician. Pins should not be painful to patient once in place, unless loose.
4. Clean pin sites twice a day as prescribed to prevent infection (usually with Betadine and cotton-tipped applicators).
5. Place rubber cork over tips of halo pins to diminish magnification of sound and for protection of those caring for patient.
6. Avoid placing pillow directly under halo ring. A rolled towel may be used to support the neck.
7. Check edges of vest for comfort and fit by inserting finger between the jacket and the patient's skin. If jacket is too tight, skin breakdown, edema, and possible nerve damage can occur.
8. Check all nuts and bolts for finger tightness daily.
9. Slide pillowcase between vest and patient's skin daily to check for evidence of skin breakdown (serosanguineous drainage).
10. Encourage patient to sleep prone, using pillows under hips and chest and a towel or small pillow to support head.
11. Complaints of difficulty swallowing should be assessed closely. This symptom often indicates an over-hyperextension of the neck and adjustments must be made to the halo immediately to reestablish proper alignment.

A rather new psychological phenomenon has been observed in patients who are having their halo brace removed for the first time, after 12 to 16 weeks. Although patients may have been told repeatedly during the period preceding removal of the brace that their deficits are permanent, many patients seem to attribute the deficits to their halo brace. Perhaps unconsciously, they believe that after the halo is removed, they will improve. When removal of the halo brace does not improve their deficits, they may experience significant depression and begin to grieve for a loss that actually occurred several months earlier. This has been termed *post-halo depression*, and it can be a significant problem. Intervention with psychological support may be necessary at this time.

Full spine, skull, and chest radiographs were done. Intravenous lactated Ringer's solution was started and a Foley catheter was inserted into his bladder. A nasogastric tube was inserted and connected to low intermittent suction.

The radiographs revealed that Adam had a dislocated fracture of C5 and C6. The chest film showed a lack of full lung field expansion. Blood work was normal with the exception of arterial blood gases, which showed respiratory acidosis (pH 7.30).

The treatment plan for his spinal shock included careful IV fluid replacement to avoid overhydration, the use of dopamine or a similar drug if his hypotension compromised adequate perfusion of vital organs, atropine to correct the bradycardia if he became symptomatic, and careful monitoring of his respiratory function. Although an injury at C5–C6 would spare his diaphragm, mechanical ventilation might become necessary owing to ascending edema around the cord. The respiratory acidosis probably reflected hypoventilation with resultant CO_2 retention.

During the spinal shock phase, it is important to measure urine output to ensure adequate renal perfusion. Because he likely had an atonic bladder, to ensure emptying with no retention, and to monitor output accurately, the indwelling catheter was inserted. The nasogastric tube will decompress a possible distended stomach and prevent aspiration, and if an ileus is present, nasogastric drainage will facilitate its resolution.

Neurosurgeons stabilized Adam's neck by the use of traction to reduce the fracture. Once the spine was in proper alignment, a halo vest was applied that he would wear for 13 weeks to allow healing to occur. See Display Box 32–8 for nursing management of Adam while he wore the halo vest.

Once past the acute phase of his injury, Adam was transferred to a rehabilitation facility for further recovery and adaptation to his injury.

Nursing Care Plan

Nursing Care Plan 32–1 details care of the patient with a spinal cord injury.

(*Text continues on page 798*)

NURSING CARE PLAN 32–1:
The Patient With Spinal Cord Injury

NURSING DIAGNOSIS	OUTCOME CRITERIA/ PATIENT GOALS	NURSING INTERVENTIONS
Altered tissue perfusion, cardiopulmonary, renal, peripheral, cerebral: related to vasomotor paralysis and pooling of blood during spinal shock.	• BP is adequate to allow urine output of 30 ml/hr and clear mental status (no confusion).	1. Monitor vital signs and other assessment parameters. 2. Report cardiac dysrhythmias. 3. Administer vasopressors as ordered for hypotension. 4. Administer atropine for bradycardia as ordered. 5. Administer anticoagulants as ordered. 6. Document intake and output. 7. Weigh patient daily. 8. Apply pneumatic leg stockings. Elevate feet and legs frequently during the day. 9. Promote blood flow in paralyzed limbs with regular turning; position to prevent gravitational edema. Teach ankle-pumping exercises. 10. Instruct patient not to massage legs. 11. Encourage range-of-motion exercises (active or passive). 12. Document trend in ABGs. 13. Avoid sudden changes in patient position that may produce orthostatic hypotension.

(*continued*)

NURSING DIAGNOSIS	OUTCOME CRITERIA/ PATIENT GOALS	NURSING INTERVENTIONS
Constipation: related to paralytic ileus and gastric dilation during spinal shock.	• Patient will be able to tolerate or perform own bowel program or to direct own program.	14. Consider need for kinetic bed. 1. Encourage fluid intake and high-fiber diet. 2. Administer bowel program daily (mild laxative prn, stool softener, suppository followed by digital stimulation). 3. Establish bowel program timing based on social needs of patient. 4. Provide privacy and optimal positioning to enhance elimination. 5. Begin bowel program soon after injury to prevent impaction during period of ileus. 6. Test stools for occult blood, which may be a side effect of steroids or anticoagulant administration or stress ulcer. 7. Teach patient or caregiver to do bowel program, depending on level of motor ability. 8. Teach patient signs of autonomic dysreflexia (if injury is T6 or above) and how to prevent/treat it.
Altered urinary elimination: related to loss of innervation to bladder and loss of reflex arc.	• Urinary continence will be maintained.	1. Remove indwelling catheter as soon as spinal shock is resolved and begin intermittent catheterization program. 2. Limit fluid intake if on intermittent catheterization program. Force fluids with indwelling (Foley or suprapubic) catheter. Fluid restriction is 600–800 ml between catheterizations. 3. Teach patient methods of triggering micturition. 4. Teach patient about autonomic dysreflexia and what to do if it occurs as a result of a suspected overfull bladder. 5. Based on type of bladder (neurogenic, flaccid, etc.) discuss options of urinary management (eg, suprapubic catheter, external devices, intermittent catheterization).

(*continued*)

NURSING CARE PLAN 32–1: (Continued)
The Patient With Spinal Cord Injury

NURSING DIAGNOSIS	OUTCOME CRITERIA/ PATIENT GOALS	NURSING INTERVENTIONS
		6. Teach management of option chosen and have patient return to demonstrate.
		7. Teach patient signs and symptoms of urinary tract infection and when physician should be notified.
		8. Document and trend BUN, creatinine, WBC as ordered.
		9. Note clarity, color, odor of urine to identify presence of UTI.
		10. Never clamp an indwelling catheter.
Impaired physical mobility: related to motor and sensory deficits, spinal immobility, decreased strength and endurance, pain.	• Patient will be free from complications of immobility.	1. Begin range-of-motion exercises as soon as possible.
		2. Mobilize as soon as possible (eg, tilt table).
		3. Apply pneumatic leg stockings.
		4. Measure circumference of thigh and calf size daily and report increase of 2 cm from one day to the next.
		5. Place patient in Trendelenburg position 1 hour every 8 hours if no concomitant head injury is present.
		6. Use space boots or high-top tennis shoes to prevent footdrop.
		7. Maintain proper spinal alignment.
		8. Initiate deep-breathing exercises, use of incentive spirometry, and teach quadriplegic coughing technique.
		9. Logroll patient after surgery. Ensure position change of all patients at least every 2 hours.
		10. Initiate bleeding precautions if on anticoagulants (eg, electric razor, Hematest stools).
		11. Consider use of kinetic bed.
		12. Report signs of pulmonary infection, inability to handle secretions, pulmonary embolus, and respiratory fatigue.

(continued)

NURSING CARE PLAN 32–1: *(Continued)*
The Patient With Spinal Cord Injury

NURSING DIAGNOSIS	OUTCOME CRITERIA/ PATIENT GOALS	NURSING INTERVENTIONS
		13. Begin rehabilitation program as soon as patient is medically stable.
		14. Report signs of local redness, heat, swelling in an extremity with stiffness of a joint, which may indicate heterotropic ossification.
Hypothermia: related to lack of vasomotor tone, disruption of autonomic nervous system.	• Patient will maintain core body temperature greater than 35°C (95°F).	1. Initially monitor temperature continuously with probe.
		2. Apply layered warming blankets as needed.
		3. Regulate environmental temperature to patient's comfort.
		4. Encourage warm fluids when hypothermic.
		5. Educate patient about need for dressing warmly in cold weather and dressing lightly in hot weather because patient's body will tend to take on the temperature of the environment.
Body image disturbance: related to change in body structure, function, and appearance.	• Patient participates in care and rehabilitation.	1. Allow emotional communication.
		2. Assign unit workload with continuity of care as a priority.
		3. Provide accurate information based on patient's readiness to learn, to help patient adapt to changes.
		4. Encourage and praise patient's willingness to learn new tasks or activities.
		5. Discuss with patient his or her strengths and capabilities.
		6. Create positive outlets for anger and frustration.
		7. To help reentry into society, role play with patient what might occur when a new situation arises.
		8. Provide vocational rehabilitation.
High risk for impaired skin integrity: related to loss of sensation, immobility, bowel and bladder incontinence, altered nutritional status.	• Skin will remain intact.	1. Establish turn schedule.
		2. Consider use of kinetic bed in acute phase.

(continued)

NURSING CARE PLAN 32–1: (Continued)
The Patient With Spinal Cord Injury

NURSING DIAGNOSIS	OUTCOME CRITERIA/ PATIENT GOALS	NURSING INTERVENTIONS
		3. Teach patient or caregiver how to do weight shifts and how to do skin checks.
		4. Protect skin from perspiration, stool, urine, and adhesive tape.
		5. Avoid use of incontinence pads except during bowel program.
		6. Observe patient for signs of skin irritation.
		7. Monitor and teach patient to monitor temperature of bath water, heating devices, etc.
		8. Ensure adequate fluid and caloric intake.
		9. Use mild soap without alcohol for cleansing skin.
		10. Massage bony prominences.
		11. Instruct patient in proper transfer techniques (eg, avoid scraping buttocks on slide board).
		12. Clean pin sites if patient is in halo, per hospital protocol, and check skin condition under halo vest daily (see Display Box 32–8: Care of a Patient in a Halo Brace).
		13. Teach positioning and padding techniques for use in bed. Elbow and heel protectors may be indicated, especially if patient has severe spasms.
		14. Instruct patient on types of clothing to be avoided (tight clothing with seams) and danger of carrying wallet or keys in pocket.
High risk for ineffective breathing pattern: related to reduced muscular innervation.	• Patient will maintain adequate ventilation and oxygenation.	1. Ensure patent airway.
		2. Document respiratory rate and report significant deviation from norm.
		3. Measure respiratory parameters.
		4. Perform appropriate pulmonary hygiene and assess for ability to handle own secretions.
		5. Suction as necessary. Auscultate breath sounds before and after procedure.

(continued)

NURSING CARE PLAN 32-1: *(Continued)*
The Patient With Spinal Cord Injury

NURSING DIAGNOSIS	OUTCOME CRITERIA/ PATIENT GOALS	NURSING INTERVENTIONS
		6. Monitor arterial blood gases as ordered.
		7. Stay with patient who is on Stryker frame being turned prone to assess tolerance of the turn.
		8. Provide method for patient to call for nurse at all times.
		9. Elevate HOB for means and coughing exercises.
		10. Assist with quadriplegic coughing technique as necessary and teach to patient and caregiver.
		11. Consider kinetic bed as necessary to clear or prevent pulmonary complications.
		12. Discourage smoking.
		13. Teach patient to do deep-breathing exercises or to use spirometer to prevent pulmonary stasis, especially if quadriplegic.
High risk for altered nutrition, less than body requirements: related to interruption of bowel innervation, oral intake restrictions, GI dysfunction, limited ability to feed self, anorexia from lack of taste sensation or depression.	• Patient will maintain preinjury weight ± 1–5 pounds.	1. Document calorie count.
		2. Weigh patient daily.
		3. Measure intake and output.
		4. Administer TPN as ordered.
		5. Auscultate bowel sounds q shift.
		6. Maintain patency of NG tube.
		7. Check pH of gastric aspirate while NG tube is in place, and administer antacids or histamine blockers as ordered.
		8. Assess gag and swallow reflexes before initiating oral feedings. Videofluoroscopy may diagnose dysphagia.
		9. Feed patient if unable to assist self.
High risk for sexual dysfunction: related to loss of nerve innervation distal to level of spinal cord lesion and misinformation/lack of knowledge about sexual options.	• Patient will feel comfortable asking questions about sexual functioning.	1. Encourage patient to express feelings concerning sexuality.
		2. Foster open communication between patient and significant other (eg, provide for privacy but be available to answer questions).

(continued)

NURSING CARE PLAN 32–1: (Continued)
The Patient With Spinal Cord Injury

NURSING DIAGNOSIS	OUTCOME CRITERIA/ PATIENT GOALS	NURSING INTERVENTIONS
		3. Provide answers or resources for patient questions. Offer information on sexual techniques using books, manuals, movies, etc. Resource also may be another SCI patient.
		4. Discuss birth control and fertility as possible issues of concern to patient.
		5. Encourage counseling as indicated.
High risk for ineffective individual coping: related to loss of physical mobility, altered lifestyle necessary after injury, unrealistic perception of self or disability, inadequate or ineffective support system or coping abilities.	• Patient will demonstrate effective coping mechanisms.	1. Demonstrate acceptance of patient behavior and emotions in different stages of grief.
		2. Provide information about community resources and support groups.
		3. Listen to patient and provide atmosphere of trust.
		4. Encourage independence within functional abilities.
		5. Use available hospital resources.

REFERENCES

1. Stover SL, Fine P: Spinal Cord Injury: The Facts and Figures. Birmingham, AL, National Spinal Cord Injury Research Data Center, University of Alabama, 1986
2. Hilton G, Frei J: High-dose methylprednisolone in the treatment of spinal cord injuries. Heart Lung 20:675–680, 1991
3. Swarczinski C, Dijkers M: The value of serial leg measurements for monitoring deep vein thrombosis in spinal cord injury. Journal of Neuroscience Nursing 23:306–317, 1991
4. Gausch P, Linder S, Williams T, Ryan S: A functional classification of respiratory compromise in spinal cord injury. Spinal Cord Injury Nursing 8(1):4–10, 1991
5. Mitchell M: Neuroscience Nursing: A Nursing Diagnosis Approach. Baltimore, Williams & Wilkins, 1989
6. Zejdlik C: Management of Spinal Cord Injury. Boston, Jones & Bartlett, 1992

BIBLIOGRAPHY

Hickey JV: The Clinical Practice of Neurosurgical and Neurological Nursing, 3rd ed. Philadelphia, JB Lippincott, 1992
Mackenzie E: The Cost of Injury: A Report to Congress. Baltimore, Johns Hopkins Research and Development Center, 1990

STUDY QUESTIONS

1. Clinical signs of autonomic dysreflexia include

   a. tachycardia and hypotension
   b. hypertension and headache
   c. sweating and fever
   d. bradycardia and pupil constriction

2. Which would most likely describe a patient in spinal shock as he or she would present initially?

   a. pink, warm, dry skin; vasodilation
   b. pale, cool, wet skin; vasoconstriction
   c. bradycardia and hypertension
   d. pounding headache and blurred vision

3. At what level of quadriplegia can a patient usually be ventilator independent?

   a. C3
   b. C4
   c. C5
   d. C7

4. In teaching a patient about a bowel program, which statement is true?

   a. the bowel program should begin as soon as spinal shock is resolved
   b. a bowel program is necessary only for quadriplegics
   c. laxatives will need to be used daily
   d. autonomic dysreflexia may be triggered in some patients with each bowel program

5. What level of the spinal cord is responsible for psychogenic erection in men?

   a. C1–C8
   b. T1–T6
   c. T11–L2
   d. L3–S2

6. Factors precipitating an episode of autonomic dysreflexia might include all of the following except

   a. pain
   b. spasticity
   c. decubitus
   d. hyperventilation

7. Which statement holds true for bladder training?

   a. force fluids with an intermittent catheterization program
   b. restrict fluids with an intermittent catheterization program
   c. clamp indwelling catheter several hours before discontinuing it
   d. restrict fluids with a suprapubic catheter

UNIT V

Gastrointestinal Disorders

CHAPTER 33

Anatomy and Physiology of the Gastrointestinal System

BEHAVIORAL OBJECTIVES

Based on the content in this chapter, the reader should be able to:

1. List three major functions of the gastrointestinal system.
2. Outline the result of each digestive organ's secretion and processing of substrates.
3. Describe the breakdown of carbohydrates, proteins, fats, and vitamins.
4. Outline the events that occur during emesis.
5. Identify three steps in the process of defecation.
6. List five important functions of the liver.

Hudak: Critical Care Nursing:
A Holistic Approach, 6th ed. © 1994
J. B. Lippincott Company.

Introduction

All body cells require proteins, carbohydrates, fats, minerals, vitamins, and water. These nutrients provide an energy source for life functions. After they are broken into smaller components, they also provide substrates for the manufacture of new cell structures, contents, and secretions. Most nutrients are present in the external environment in forms that cannot enter the bloodstream to reach tissue cells (eg, complex large molecules). The functions of the digestive system are to:

- receive these nutrients (ingestion);
- break them down into molecules that are small enough to reach and enter the bloodstream (digestion);
- enable these molecules to enter the bloodstream (absorption) so that they can be delivered to all tissues.

Accessory operations include the movement of ingested food along the digestive system, the recycling of materials used in digestion (colonic reabsorption of water, bicarbonate, potassium, bile salts), and the elimination of the undigested food residue from the body (defecation).

Structure

Macrostructure

Alimentary Canal

The general structure of the digestive system is shown in Figure 33–1. It is composed of the alimentary canal, which is a tube about 8 m (25 ft) long that begins at the oral cavity and ends at the anus. The accessory glands (eg, salivary glands) and organs (eg, liver and pancreas) empty their products into this tube at certain points.

The oral cavity opens into the pharynx, a structure that allows the passage of both nutrients and air. The anterior pharynx is divided into an oropharynx and nasopharynx, connecting to the oral and nasal cavities, respectively. The posteroinferior end of the pharynx (at about the level of the sixth cervical vertebra) connects to the esophagus and larynx. A thin cartilaginous flap covered by soft tissue, the epiglottis, reflexively covers the larynx during swallowing and the passing of food and water to the esophagus.

The esophagus is a 25-cm (10-in) tube that leads to the stomach. The walls of the upper one-third of this tube are composed of skeletal muscle, as are the walls of the mouth and pharynx. The remaining esophageal walls contain smooth muscle, as does the remainder of the alimentary canal until the external anal sphincter, which again is composed of skeletal muscle. The lower esophageal sphincter (LES), which is the muscle between the stomach

and esophagus, is thickened and has more tonus than other esophageal muscle, and it prevents reflux of gastric contents up into the esophagus. The other end of the stomach opens into the small intestine. This opening is surrounded by the pyloric sphincter, a structure that minimizes intestinal reflux.

The first 25 to 30 cm (10–12 in) of the small intestine is called the duodenum. The next 2.6 m (8.5 ft) comprises the jejunum and ileum, and the last 1.1 m (3.6 ft) the colon. The opening of the ileum into the first part of the colon (cecum) is guarded by the ileocecal valve, which prevents reflux of colonic contents back into the ileum. Protruding inferiorly from the cecum is a blind-ended 2.5- to 20-cm (1–8 in) tube called the vermiform appendix. The ascending colon extends superiorly from the cecum to a point just inferior to the lower border of the liver. The colon then flexes transversely and crosses to the left side of the abdominal cavity to a point just inferior to the stomach, where it curves again to become the descending colon. This part of the colon passes down on the left side of the abdomen to the level of the iliac crest, where it becomes the sigmoid colon. This **S**-shaped portion of colon bends first toward the right side of the abdomen, but almost immediately it sharply bends posteriorly and upward toward the sacrum. Just as abruptly it curves anteriorly again, completing its **S** shape, and then continues downward to the pelvic floor as the rectum. The last 2.5 cm (1 in) or so of the rectum, the anal canal, passes between the levator and muscles of the pelvic floor and opens to the exterior body surface as the anal orifice. Two sphincters guard this orifice: an internal one composed of smooth muscle and an external one composed of skeletal muscle.

Innervation

The gastrointestinal tract is supplied with both somatic motor and autonomic motor fibers. The former innervate the skeletal muscles of the oropharyngeal cavity, the first few centimeters of the esophagus, and the external anal sphincter. This enables voluntary control of such activities as chewing, initiation of swallowing, and defecation. Autonomic fibers supply the remainder of the digestive system, including salivary glands, pancreas, and liver (Fig. 33–2).

Autonomic fibers function in the regulation of:

the secretions from the exocrine cells of the salivary glands, pancreas, stomach, and intestines;

tonicity of sphincter muscles; and

motility of the gastrointestinal tract in general.

The operations are not usually voluntarily controlled, although they can be reflexively altered by psychoemotional stimuli mediated by higher brain centers. Fear can decrease the volume and increase the viscosity of salivary gland secretions, resulting in the sensation of a dry mouth.

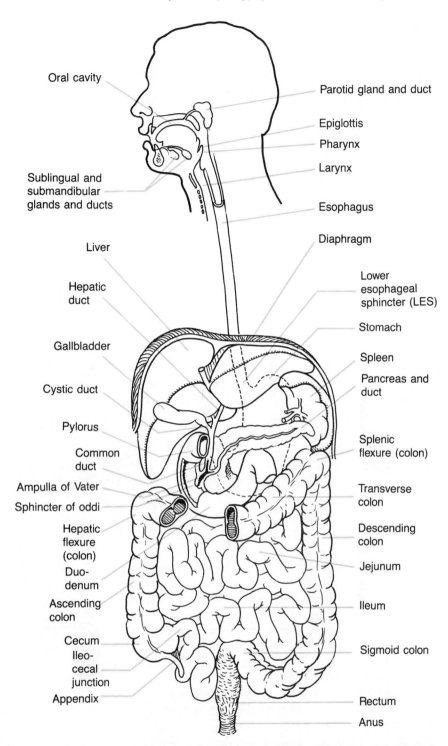

FIGURE 33–1
Diagram of the digestive tract.

Merely the sight or smell of a meal can trigger gastric and pancreatic secretions. Emotions can increase or decrease gastrointestinal motility, thereby promoting diarrhea or constipation.

Most parts of the gastrointestinal tract receive both sympathetic and parasympathetic fibers (see Figure 33–2). In general, these two types of autonomic fibers have contrasting influences. Sympathetic stimulation results in decreased motility, increased sphincter tonicity (closure), and decreased exocrine secretions. Parasympathetic stimu-

lation results in increased motility, opening of sphincters, and increased exocrine secretions. Note also that a cranial nerve (vagus) carries parasympathetic fibers to most of the gastrointestinal tract.

Circulation

The upper esophagus receives blood from the esophageal artery, branching from the thoracic aorta. The celiac artery, branching from the abdominal aorta, supplies blood

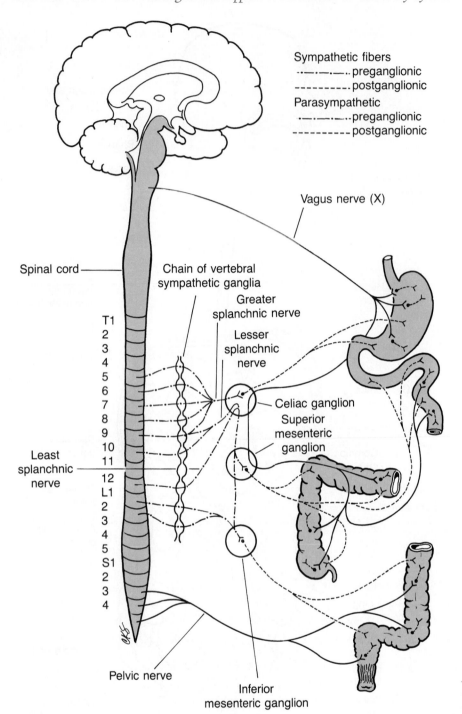

Sympathetic fibers
·—·—·—·· preganglionic
---------- postganglionic
Parasympathetic
·—·—·—·· preganglionic
---------- postganglionic

Vagus nerve (X)

Spinal cord

Chain of vertebral sympathetic ganglia

Greater splanchnic nerve

Lesser splanchnic nerve

T1
2
3
4
5
6
7
8
9
10
11
12
L1
2
3
4
5
S1
2
3
4

Celiac ganglion

Superior mesenteric ganglion

Least splanchnic nerve

Pelvic nerve

Inferior mesenteric ganglion

FIGURE 33–2
Diagram showing the autonomic innervation of the gastrointestinal tract.

to the lower esophagus, stomach, duodenum, gallbladder, and pancreas. The next aortic branch, the superior mesenteric, supplies blood to the intestine from the jejunum to the transverse colon. The next branch from the abdominal aorta, the inferior mesenteric artery, supplies blood to the descending and sigmoid colon and rectum.

Venous drainage of the majority of the gastrointestinal tract is illustrated in Figure 33–3. Two points bear mention. First, almost all blood from the alimentary canal, from the stomach to and including the upper portion of the rectum, drains into the hepatic portal vein. This blood contains all absorbed nutrients, reabsorbed water, electrolytes, bile salts, and any products from commensal colonic bacteria. This material from the gastrointestinal tract is subject to "hepatic processing" before being mixed with blood in the general circulation. This hepatic processing removes potentially harmful materials before they can reach the rest of the body. For example, ammonia produced by the protein catabolizing action of colonic bacteria can (within limitations) be hepatically removed, thereby preventing ammonium encephalopathy. The second important point is that blood from the lower two-thirds of

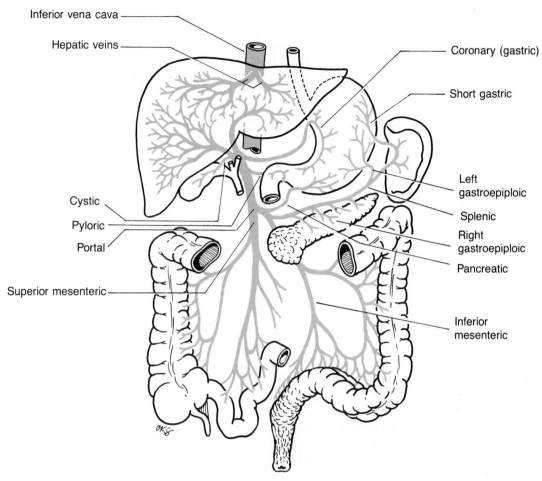

Inferior vena cava

Hepatic veins

Coronary (gastric)

Short gastric

Left gastroepiploic

Splenic

Right gastroepiploic

Pancreatic

Cystic

Pyloric

Portal

Superior mesenteric

Inferior mesenteric

FIGURE 33–3

The portal circulation. Blood from the gastrointestinal tract, spleen, and pancreas travels to the liver by way of the portal vein before moving into the vena cava for return to the heart. (Chaffee EE, Lytle IM: Basic Physiology and Anatomy, 4th ed. Philadelphia: JB Lippincott)

the rectum and from the lower esophagus bypasses the hepatic portal system. Instead, blood from the lower rectum drains by the middle and inferior rectal veins and the external iliac vein into the inferior vena cava. Blood from the lower esophagus is drained by way of the hemizygous and azygous veins directly into the inferior vena cava.

Microstructure

The alimentary tract is basically composed of a central hollow tube, the lumen, through which food passes. It is surrounded by five layers of tissue. Proceeding from the lumen outward, they are the mucosa, submucosa, circular smooth muscle, longitudinal smooth muscle, and serosa. The mucosal layer contains cells responsible for gastrointestinal secretions and those sensitive to chemical and mechanical stimuli. In parts of the gastrointestinal tract in which absorption occurs, this layer is more convoluted or possesses fingerlike projections (villi). Such structural modifications increase the surface area per unit volume,

thereby facilitating absorption. The submucosa contains blood vessels, nerve networks, and connective tissue. The submucosa of the small intestine contains aggregates of lymphatic tissue (Peyer's patches), which are especially numerous within the ileum. In the process of absorption, molecules in the lumen of the gastrointestinal tract must pass through the mucosa and connective tissue before they enter the capillaries of the submucosa. Viral and bacterial antigens are absorbed by specialized mucosal cells that lie above the patches of lymphatic tissue in the small intestine. These specialized cells pass on the antigens together with a chemical that sensitizes the lymphatic cells to manufacture and secrete antibodies of immunoglobulin class A (IgA) against this particular antigen the next time (or times) this antigen enters the small intestine.

The two smooth muscle layers function in the two major types of gastrointestinal motility: propulsive motion and mixing movements. The stomach has an additional layer of smooth muscle to facilitate its food-mixing movements. The outer serosa layer is continuous with the mesenteries and forms part of the visceral peritoneum.

There are two nerve networks that extend the length of the gastrointestinal tract: the submucosal plexus and the myenteric plexus. The submucosal network is composed of sensory neurons that receive stimulation from the sensory cells in the mucosal layer. The myenteric plexus, located between the two smooth muscle layers, is a network of motor neurons that stimulate the smooth muscles of the gastrointestinal tract. The myenteric plexus receives sensory input from the submucosal plexus. Together, these two plexuses function in locally coordinated regulation of gastrointestinal motility (eg, peristalsis) and secretion (eg, certain gastric secretions). These networks are often called "intrinsic" because their operations can proceed even if autonomic nerves to the gut are severed.

Functions

Oropharyngeal Cavity

Secretions

The majority of saliva is produced by three pairs of salivary glands: submaxillary, sublingual, and parotid. Saliva (Table 33–1) is composed of mucus, which serves primarily as a lubricant to facilitate swallowing, lingual lipase (a fat-digesting enzyme secreted by tongue glands), salivary amylase (a starch-digesting enzyme), class A antibodies (IgA) that provide a first line defense against bacteria and viruses, and bacteriostatic and anticariogenic chemicals. Lingual lipase is estimated to digest about 30% of the dietary fat while it is in the stomach. About one-half of digestive amylase is secreted by the salivary glands, the other 50% from the pancreas.

Stimuli eliciting salivation include sight, smell, and thoughts of food, as well as a pleasant taste and smooth texture of food in the mouth. Rough, bad-tasting, unpleasant-smelling foods reduce salivary gland secretions. These stimuli are received by the two salivary centers in the medulla of the brain stem. These centers then send "autonomic motor impulses" to the salivary glands by the seventh and ninth cranial nerves (parasympathetic fibers) and branches from the first and second thoracic nerves (sympathetic fibers). Parasympathetic stimulation, or the administration of drugs that mimic such stimulation (cholinergics) or enhance it (neostigmine), promote a copious secretion of watery saliva. Sympathetic stimulation or sympathomimetic drug administration produces a scanty output of thick saliva. Cholinergic blockers (eg, atropine) also produce scanty salivation.

Motility

Food in the mouth is initially subject to mechanical breakdown by the act of chewing. This produces a bolus of food held together and lubricated by saliva that then can be swallowed. Swallowing has two phases: (1) an initial voluntary phase, described here and including the first third of the esophagus, and (2) an involuntary phase, described under the discussion of the esophagus.

Swallowing is triggered by the presence of food or fluid in the pharynx. This presence mechanically stimulates pharyngeal sensory receptors that cause impulses to be sent along sensory fibers in the fifth cranial nerve to the swallowing center in the medulla. The arrangement of neurons in this center is such that the arrival of "sensory impulses" reflexively triggers the outflow of impulses down motor fibers in the ninth and tenth cranial nerves to pharyngeal and laryngeal structures. This causes the following coordinated events, which propel the solid or fluid substance into the esophagus:

> pull of the soft palate upward to seal off the nasopharyngeal area;
>
> closure of the epiglottis down over the opening into the larynx;
>
> relaxation of the muscles of the upper esophagus; and
>
> contraction of pharyngeal muscles, which moves the food or fluid into the opened esophagus.

Damage to sensory or motor fibers (in cranial nerves V, IX, or X) or to the swallowing center in the brain stem can weaken or eliminate the ability to swallow or can produce poorly coordinated swallowing wherein food or fluid enters the nasopharynx or larynx or both.

Esophagus

Secretions

Cells of the mucosal layers in the esophagus secrete only mucus (see Table 33–1). This protects the esophageal lining from damage by gastric secretions or food substances and acts as a lubricant to facilitate the passage of food.

Motility

Once food or fluid enters the esophagus, it continues to be propelled through the first third of the lumen by reflexes involving the swallowing center and the ninth and tenth cranial nerves. In these reflexes, food or fluid stimulates pressure or stretch receptors in the wall of the esophagus. Stimulation of these receptors causes impulses to be conducted along sensory fibers to the swallowing center. Reflex output from the swallowing center to the muscle (down motor fibers in the ninth and tenth cranial nerves) produces a pattern of esophageal relaxation ahead of the food or fluid and esophageal muscle contraction behind it, thereby propelling the matter being swallowed through this first part of the esophagus.

In contrast, propulsion of food or fluid along the remainder of the esophagus is accomplished by local reflexes involving sensory receptors and the two nerve plex-

TABLE 33–1
Major Gastrointestinal Secretions Related to Digestion and Absorption

Organ	Cell Type	Substance Secreted	Target of Secretion	Result of Secretion
Tongue Salivary glands	Ebner's glands	Lingual lipase α Amylase Mucus	Ingested triglycerides Ingested carbohydrate (CHO) Ingested food	Free fatty acids and glycerol CHO changed to simple sugars Binding of food, lumen protection
Esophagus	Mucosal	Mucus	Ingested food	Lumen protection
Stomach	Parietal	HCl Intrinsic factor	Pepsinogen, ingested food Small intestine lumen cells	Pepsinogen changed to pepsin, other food bonds broken Vitamin B_{12} absorption
	Chief	Pepsinogen	Ingested proteins	Proteins changed to amino acids
	G cells (in antrum only)	Gastrin, into bloodstream	Chief and parietal cells Gastric mucosa	Chief and parietal cells begin and maintain secretion Gastric mucosa grows and repairs itself

Pancreas	Exocrine acinar	H_2O
		
		HCO_3^-
		
		Enzymes:
		  Trypsinogen
		  Chymotrypsin
		  Elastase
		  Carboxypeptidase
		
		  Lipase
		  Colipase
		  Esterase
		  Phospholipase
		  Nucleases
			Chyme
			
			HCl
			
			Proteins and connective tissue; other enzymes
			
			Fats
			
			Cell membranes, DNA and RNA
				Dilution of chyme increases absorption of nutrients
				Neutralization of acid protects intestinal lumen
				Proteins and amino acids further reduced, connective tissue reduced; trypsin converts many other pancreatic enzymes to their active form
				Fats changed to free fatty acids and triglycerides
				Cell membranes and nuclear acids changed to lipids, phosphates, amino acids, and small peptides

Gallbladder		Holds and concentrates bile from liver	Ingested fats	Fats emulsified and formed into micelles; with fat-soluble vitamins are now absorbable across intestinal lumen
Duodenum	Brunner's glands	H_2O HCO_3^-	Chyme Acidic chyme	Dilution of chyme increases absorption of nutrients Neutralization of acid protects intestinal lumen
Duodenum and Jejunum	Mucosal	Mucus Enteropeptidase Peptidases Nucleases Maltase, lactase, and sucrase Secretion, into bloodstream	Chyme Trypsinogen Polypeptides Gallbladder Nucleic acids Ingested CHO Pancreas	Lumen protection Trypsinogen converted to trypsin Gallbladder empties bile into duodenum Pentoses, purines, pyrimidines, and bases CHO changed to simple sugars and absorbed Pancreas secretes H_2O and HCO_3^- into duodenum

(continued)

TABLE 33–1
Major Gastrointestinal Secretions Related to Digestion and Absorption (Continued)

Organ	Cell Type	Substance Secreted	Target of Secretion	Result of Secretion
		Cholecystokinin (CCK), into bloodstream	Pancreas	Pancreas secretes enzymes into duodenum
			Gallbladder	Gallbladder empties bile into duodenum
		GIP (glucose-dependent insulinotropic peptide), into bloodstream	Beta cells of the islets of Langerhans	Insulin secretion
			Stomach	Decreased gastric secretions and motility
Colon	Mucosal	Mucus	Feces	Lubrication of fecal material to ease passage
				Lumen protection

uses in the wall of the esophagus. This process, peristalsis, occurs as food or fluid distends the esophageal area. The distention stimulates stretch receptors that reflexively (by the two plexuses) promote both relaxation of the esophageal muscles ahead of the area of distention and contraction of the esophageal muscles in and behind it. This squeezes the food or fluid ahead into the newly relaxed area, which then becomes the distended one. The peristalsis reflex repeatedly recurs until the food or fluid arrives at the LES. The LES is the last centimeter (0.5 in) or so of the esophagus, in which smooth muscles remain normally in a contracted state. This prevents the reflux of gastric contents into the esophagus and subsequent damage to the esophageal lining by gastric acid and enzymes. The wave of peristalsis causes the LES to relax, thereby allowing food to enter the stomach. Tonus of the LES can be altered by a variety of agents (Table 33–2). Some people suffer from a hypertensive LES that impedes esophageal emptying (and can lead to overdistention of the lower esophagus), whereas others have a hypotensive LES that results in repeated episodes of gastric reflux

(which can lead to lower esophageal strictures). In addition, the LES is a modified portion of the esophagus, not a true sphincter. Its autonomic stimuli alter the motility and normal tone of the smooth muscles in the wall of the gastrointestinal tract.

Stomach

Secretions

In addition to mucus-secreting cells, three types of secretory cells are contained in the gastric mucosa: parietal cells, which secrete hydrochloric acid (HCl) and intrinsic factor; chief cells, which secrete digestive enzymes; and G cells (in antrum only), which secrete the hormone gastrin (see Table 33–1). The luminal surface membranes of the gastric mucosal cells and their tight fit against one another provide a protective barrier against damage caused by the HCl. This barrier can be disrupted by a variety of agents, including bile salts, alcohol, aspirin, and steroids.

The digestive enzymes are secreted as an inactive precursor, pepsinogen, which is activated by HCl in the gastric lumen to provide three pepsins that digest the ingested proteins. The chemical action of HCl also breaks down food molecules. Intrinsic factor is necessary for the intestinal absorption of vitamin B_{12}. Gastrin stimulates secretion by the chief and parietal cells and promotes the growth of the gastric mucosa.

Stomach secretions are regulated in three phases: cephalic, gastric, and intestinal. These phases are controlled by neural and hormonal mechanisms.

In the cephalic phase, sight, smell, and thoughts of food—as well as the presence of food in the mouth—act on brain stem centers, reflexively prompting parasympathetic (vagal) stimulation of salivation, pancreatic secretion, bile release, and gastric secretions by the chief and parietal cells. Although G cells also are innervated by vagal fibers, such parasympathetic influences are not important in the regulation of human gastrin secretion. The stomach

TABLE 33–2
Factors Influencing Lower Esophageal Sphincter (LES) Tonus

Increased Tonus	Decreased Tonus
Gastrin	Secretin
Proteins in chyme	CCK-PZ
Prostaglandin F_2	Glucagon
Moclepramide	Fats in chyme
	Nicotine
	Alcohol
	Prostaglandins E, E_2, A_2
	Anticholinergic drugs

also receives sympathetic stimulation in the cephalic phase, in response to emotional and situational events. Such neural pathways provide the mechanisms whereby emotions can influence gastrointestinal secretions. Fear and depression seem to decrease secretions, whereas anger and hostility increase them.

The gastric phase refers to the stimulation of gastric secretions by the presence of food (chyme) in the stomach. Distention of the stomach wall by the food stimulates stretch receptors in the wall of the stomach. Chemicals, mainly proteins, in the chyme stimulate chemoreceptors in the mucosa. The stretch receptors and chemoreceptors in turn activate neurons in the submucosal plexus, which then stimulate neurons in the myenteric plexus, which in turn stimulate secretion by the parietal and chief cells. Proteins in the chyme also directly promote gastrin secretion by G cells; the gastrin provides an additional stimulus for parietal and chief cell secretion. The gastric phase is eventually halted by a combination of events. The stretch receptors and chemoreceptors in the wall of the stomach become refractory to stimulation, the acidity of the chyme inhibits further gastrin secretion, and GIP (glucose-dependent insulinotrophic peptide) decreases HCl secretions and gastric motility.

The intestinal phase begins after chyme reaches the duodenum. The acidity of this mixture stimulates duodenal mucosal cells to release secretin into the bloodstream, proteins trigger the release of cholecystokinin (CCK) into the blood from similar cells, and glucose and fat stimulate the secretion of GIP. Secretin and CCK cause pancreatic secretion and release of gallbladder contents into the duodenum. GIP stimulates the release of insulin from the islets of Langerhans and decreases gastric motility and secretions. Stretch receptors in the duodenum trigger peristalsis, so that chyme is degraded, mixed with enzymes and diluents, and moved past the highly absorbent small intestine lumen.

The surfaces of parietal cells contain receptors for acetylcholine, histamine and gastrin. The stimulation of one or more of these receptors prompts the parietal cell to secrete HCl. Likewise, acid secretion is inhibited by chemicals that block the histamine receptor (eg, H_2 antagonists such as cimetidine [Tagamet] and ranitidine [Zantac]) or the acetylcholine receptor (eg, atropine). Excess HCl secretion can cause duodenal ulcers. Some prostaglandins inhibit HCl secretion. Therefore, drugs that inhibit prostaglandin secretion (eg, nonsteroidal anti-inflammatory medications such as Motrin) can be ulcerogenic. Another drug, omeprazole (Prilosec), inhibits an intracellular step in the HCl secretion process in parietal cells. Other factors that stimulate gastric secretions are alcohol, caffeine, and hypoglycemia. The first two factors act directly by way of gastric chemoreceptors and the intramural nerve plexuses in the stomach wall. Hypoglycemia acts by way of the brain stem and vagal fibers.

Motility

The passage of food from the esophagus into the stomach reflexively initiates receptive relaxation. After the stomach has thereby filled with food, peristaltic contractions mix the food and repeatedly squirt small amounts of it at a controlled rate into the duodenum. The pyloric sphincter plays only a minor role in gastric emptying. Its main function is to prevent duodenal reflux. The bile acids in chyme that re-enters the stomach through duodenal reflux damage the chemical barrier that coats the surfaces of gastric mucosal cells. Because this barrier normally prevents the HCl which has been secreted from damaging the cells, duodenal reflux plays a major role in the pathogenesis of gastric ulcers. Mild peristaltic contractions that persist after the stomach has completely emptied are called hunger contractions. They play no obligatory role in appetite regulation. Gastric emptying can be retarded by vagotomy; by the presence of fats, proteins, or HCl in the duodenal chyme; by duodenal distention; and by intestinal hormones.

Vomiting (Emesis)

Vomiting results from the relaxation of the LES and the rest of the esophagus combined with simultaneous strong contractions of abdominal muscles and diaphragm and closure of the epiglottis over the airway. The contractions squeeze the stomach and force its contents up the esophagus and out the mouth. In addition, irritation of the small intestine (by materials in the chyme, by inflammation, or by disease process) can cause special movements that constitute reverse peristalsis. These movements, identical with peristaltic movement, move chyme toward the pyloric valve. They can be sufficiently strong to force open the pylorus and enter the stomach. This is how intestinal contents are vomited. If golden yellow bile from the duodenum spends any appreciable time in the stomach, acids turn it green. Occasionally, vomiting of intestinal contents can be so rapid that bile spends hardly any time in the stomach and the vomitus contains golden yellow bile. If blood is allowed time in the stomach, acids turn it brownish black (coffee-ground color). If vomiting does not allow sufficient time for this acid action to occur, blood in the vomitus has its normal red color.

Pancreas

This organ contains both exocrine tissue and endocrine tissue. The latter constitutes the islets of Langerhans, which is discussed in a later section on endocrine metabolism. The exocrine (acinar) cells are arranged in lobules and empty their secretions into an internal pancreatic ductal system (see Figure 33–1). These internal ducts drain into an external pancreatic duct (duct of Wirsung) that joins the common bile duct to form a shared short duct called the ampulla of Vater. This ampulla, carrying both bile and pancreatic secretions, opens into the duodenum. It is encircled by a smooth muscle ring, the sphincter of Oddi. Because of the anatomical arrangements between the common bile duct and the duct of Wirsung, a gallstone that obstructs the ampulla of Vater can obstruct both the normal flow of bile and pancreatic secretions. (Such obstruction, although rare, can lead to a stasis of pancreatic secretion resulting in acute pancreatitis.) Some persons have a second external pancreatic duct (duct of Santorini) that opens into the duodenum near the pylorus.

Secretions

The large amount of water secreted by the pancreas is instrumental in diluting chyme before absorption. The exocrine acinar cells secrete both a watery alkaline solution (sodium bicarbonate and potassium bicarbonate) and digestive enzymes (see Table 33–1). The bicarbonate neutralizes the highly acidic chyme just recently arrived in the duodenum from the stomach. The pancreatic enzymes digest proteins (trypsin, chymotrypsin, elastase, and carboxypeptidase), fats (lipase, calipase, and esterase), phospholipase and nucleic acids (nucleases), and starch (amylase). These are secreted from the pancreas in inactive forms. Once the pancreatic secretions arrive in the duodenum, inactive trypsin (trypsinogen) is activated by an intestinal mucosal enzyme, enteropeptidase. Active trypsin then activates the other pancreatic enzymes. Regulation of pancreatic secretion occurs by neural and hormonal means. Vagal stimulation results in the secretion of pancreatic enzymes. Hormonal regulation occurs as a result of duodenal mucosal responses to chyme and is discussed later.

Gallbladder

In the duodenum, chyme mixed with pancreatic secretions is watery. The fat in chyme is not water soluble, and requires a solvent–enzyme mixture from the liver to render it absorbable by intestinal human cells.

Hepatocytes, among many other metabolic functions, also make bile (see Table 33–1). Bile is a mixture of bile salts, cholesterol, bilirubin, and acids suspended in water. This solution emulsifies the fat in chyme, breaking the fat into very small globules that can be absorbed across the intestinal lumen. Fat-soluble vitamins are ionized into absorbable forms by the action of bile. Bile also acts to suspend cholesterol, triglycerides, and multiple-density lipoproteins in the bloodstream, preventing precipitation and deposition of these molecules in the vasculature, until they can be catabolized.

Bile is stored and concentrated in the gallbladder. Under the influence of vagal activity, or CCK, the gallbladder contracts, emptying bile into the duodenum, to mix with chyme.

Small Intestine

Secretions

Chyme in the duodenum is mixed with digestive enzymes, alkaline substances, water, mucus, and bile from the stomach, pancreas, and gallbladder. Intestinal enzymes are added to this mixture.

Secretin, CCK, and enteropeptidase, which converts trypsinogen from the pancreas into trypsin, have already been discussed. The small intestine contributes mucus, and Brunner's glands in the duodenal mucosa contribute more bicarbonate and water to chyme, in response to acid, secretin, and gastrin.

Motility

The small intestine has two types of movement: mixing and peristaltic contraction. The intramural plexuses are primarily responsible for these movements, but they can be enhanced or retarded by extrinsic autonomic stimulation, as discussed previously. Peristalsis operates here, just as it did in the esophagus and stomach, to propel food along. During mixing movement, intestinal distention provokes (by the intramural reflex arcs) constrictions at intervals along its length. This makes the distended area resemble links of sausage. These constrictions then relax, and new areas become constricted. Repetition of this process continually kneads the chyme, thereby eventually exposing all molecules of this material to the absorptive surfaces of the intestinal mucosa.

Emptying of the small intestine into the colon occurs in the same way as gastric emptying. Peristaltic waves build up pressure in the ileum behind the ileocecal valve and push the chyme through the valve into the colon. The valve then acts to prevent backflow. Ileal emptying can be retarded by intramural reflexes, which are initiated by a full (distended) colon.

Absorption

The mucosal layer of the small intestine has many folds covered with numerous fingerlike projections (villi). The luminal surface of each villus is covered with microvilli. These vastly increase the absorptive area of the small intestine.

Carbohydrates. Breakdown of carbohydrates (CHO) begins in the mouth, through the action of salivary amylase, and continues in the duodenum. Conversion to very simple sugars continues in the small intestine by intestinal enzymes. Both active and passive transport are used to absorb sugars across the intestinal lumen into the bloodstream.

Proteins. Protein degradation begins in the stomach by HCl and pepsin. Polypeptides in the small intestine are degraded into peptide fragments and amino acids by trypsin, chymotrypsin, and carboxypeptidase. Amino acids are absorbed into the blood by active and passive diffusion.

Fats. Triglycerides, lipids, and phospholipids are first degraded in the small intestine. Bile salts, in a process called emulsification, encourage the creation of small droplets of fats from larger globules of fat. Pancreatic enzymes then contact the fats and degrade them into fatty acid chains and monoglycerides. These smaller molecules form into even smaller globules, called micelles. Fatty acids and monosaccharides are transported across the intestinal mucosa from a micelle passively, leaving bile behind.

In the submucosa, free fatty acids are passed into the blood directly, if small enough. If too large for this direct but passive diffusion, the free fatty acid is reorganized into a triglyceride, coupled with lipoproteins and cholesterol, and passed into the lymph fluid as chylomicron.

The bile left behind in the intestine after absorption of fats from a micelle is reabsorbed in the ileum. If bile salts enter the colon, they decrease the reabsorption of sodium and water, thereby increasing the liquidity of the undigested food residues in the colon. Most fat is absorbed by the time chyme reaches the middle of the jejunum.

Vitamins, Minerals, and Water. Most vitamins, whether they are fat- or water-soluble, diffuse across the intestinal mucosa and submucosa into the blood. Fat-soluble vitamins do, however, require bile salt emulsification. Vitamin B_{12} couples with intrinsic factor, forming an extremely large molecule. In this form, B_{12} is absorbed; it is unusual for a molecule to increase, rather than decrease, in size in order to be absorbed.

Minerals and electrolytes vary in their absorption. Sodium and iron require active transport, whereas other minerals and electrolytes diffuse passively.

Water is absorbed passively throughout the stomach and small and large intestines. The gastrointestinal tract is highly permeable, in *both* directions, to water. Should a hypertonic solution enter the duodenum, osmosis occurs in the lumen. The converse is true: a hypotonic chyme in the stomach and duodenum causes an extremely rapid movement of water into the bloodstream.

Large Intestine

Secretions

The mucosal cells of the colon secrete mucus, which lubricates the passage of chyme (see Table 33–1).

Motility

Colonic movements include mixing and peristaltic movements. These operate as described for the small intestine. A third movement, which only the colon possesses, is mass movement. This consists of simultaneous contractions of colonic smooth muscle over large portions of the descending and sigmoid portions of the colon. Mass movement rapidly moves the undigested food residue (feces) from these areas into the rectum.

Humans cannot digest the cellulose, hemicellulose, or lignin in plant tissues. These plant materials form a large portion of the undigested food residue. They are usually termed "vegetable fiber" or "dietary bulk." These fibers attract and "hold" water, causing a larger, softer stool. Low quantities of bulk result in a relatively inactive colon, leading to bowel movements that are relatively infrequent and feces that are relatively smaller, dryer, and more difficult to pass. Epidemiological reports suggest that high-fiber diets are associated with a decreased incidence of diverticulitis and colon cancer.

Defecation. Filling of the rectum triggers the defecation reflex by stimulating stretch receptors in the rectal wall. Stimulation of the stretch receptors causes sensory (afferent) nerve fibers to transmit impulses to the lower part of the spinal cord. Because of anatomical arrangements of neurons in this part of the cord, these afferent impulses reflexively cause nerve impulses to travel out of the cord along parasympathetic motor fibers that innervate the smooth muscles of the descending and sigmoid colon, the rectum, and the internal anal sphincter. The afferent impulses also reflexively cause nerve impulses to be sent out of the cord along somatic motor neurons that innervate the skeletal muscle of the external anal sphincter. The total effect of these events is to produce (1) coordinated expulsive contractions of the colon and rectum, (2) relaxation (opening) of the sphincters, and (3) output of feces from the anus.

The urge to defecate begins after the pressure within the rectum reaches 18 torr. After intrarectal pressure reaches 55 torr, reflex bowel evacuation occurs. This defecation reflex is inhibited in a "continent" person by sending nerve impulses down descending cord fibers from higher brain centers to inhibit the actions of the somatic motor neurons that innervate the external sphincter. Such inhibition keeps the external anal sphincter closed, thereby averting inappropriate defecation. After a few minutes, the defecation reflex subsides; but it usually becomes active again a few hours later. Defecation is a spinal cord reflex that does not require intact pathways between the sacral cord and the brain. The event of a complete cord transection above the sacral cord segments affects defecation in two ways. During spinal cord shock, the hyperpolarization of cord internuncials prevents the operation of the reflex for defecation. After cord shock is ended, reflex defecation occurs once again, but voluntary inhibition is not possible (neurogenic bowel).

Absorption

It is in the large intestine that most of the water and potassium are absorbed from the chyme. This produces a semisolid residue of undigested food (feces) that can be eliminated from the body. Diarrhea can reduce the transit time for chyme, thereby limiting such potassium and water reabsorption. This can result in hypokalemia and dehydration. Diarrhea also can be caused by materials that "hold" water in the chyme (eg, MgSO₄), resulting in semiliquid, fast-moving stool.

Commensal Bacteria

At birth, the colon is sterile, but large colonic bacterial populations become established soon afterward. Some of these organisms manufacture vitamin K and a number of B vitamins. For a long time, such bacterially produced vitamins were thought to be absorbed by the colonic mucosa. This is now known to be untrue for vitamin K and most of the B vitamins. Only bacterially produced folic acid is colonically absorbed. Other bacteria produce ammonia, which is colonically absorbed. Normally, this is removed from the blood once it reaches the liver. However, in persons with seriously impaired liver function or with collateral circulatory routes that bypass the liver (usually the result of portal hypertension), such ammonia can remain in the circulation and lead to encephalopathy.

Liver

Macroscopic Structure

This organ has two lobes (right and left) and lies just below the diaphragm, with its greatest portion located to the right side of the body. Its superior (rounded) surface fits into the curve of the diaphragm and is in contact with the anterior wall of the abdominal cavity. The inferior surface is molded over the stomach, the duodenum, the pancreas, the hepatic flexure of the colon, the right kidney, and the right adrenal gland.

The *portal vein* is formed behind the head of the pancreas by the union of the superior mesenteric and the splenic veins. At its entrance to the liver, the portal vein divides into two trunks, which supply the two lobes of the liver. The branches of the portal vein then disperse throughout the tissue of the liver and become the interlobular veins as they encircle each lobule. The blood sinusoids then pass toward the center of each lobule, where they unite and form the central veins, which in turn form the sublobular veins, which then become the hepatic veins. The two hepatic veins drain into the inferior vena cava.

The *hepatic artery* supplies the liver with nutrients. This artery, along with the left gastric and splenic arteries, is the terminal branch of the celiac artery. The branches of the hepatic artery within the lobule of the liver form capillaries that communicate with the sinusoids from the interlobular veins.

Microscopic Structure

The functional unit of the liver is a cylindrically shaped lobule that measures approximately 1.5 mm in diameter and 8 mm in length. Each lobe of the liver contains between 50,000 and 100,000 lobules. Microanatomy of the lobules is shown in Figure 33–4. Rows of liver cells (hepatocytes) radiate from a central venule like spokes of a wheel. Branches of the hepatic artery and the hepatic

portal vein lie at the periphery of the wheel. Blood from these branches is poured into open channels (hepatic sinuses) that run between alternate rows of hepatocytes. Kupffer cells, specialized white cells of the reticuloendothelial system, phagocytize bacteria, debris, and other foreign matter in the sinus blood. The sinuses drain into the central venule, which in turn carries blood to the hepatic vein. Approximately 400 ml of blood, held within the venous sinuses, can be made available in emergencies to compensate for hypovolemia. Blind-ended bile canaliculi arise between the other rows of hepatocytes. They carry newly secreted bile to larger ducts located at the periphery. These smaller ducts eventually drain into the common bile duct. Bile that is leaving the liver is concentrated and stored in the gallbladder. Fluid and electrolyte reabsorption in the gallbladder can increase the concentration of bile salts, cholesterol, and bilirubin twelve-fold. Thus the gallbladder, with a maximum capacity of 50 ml, can hold a 24-hour output of bile (600 ml) from the liver. The intestinal hormone CCK and vagus nerve activity stimulate gallbladder contraction. CCK and local reflexes initiated by duodenal peristalsis open the sphincter of Oddi. These events permit an outflow of bile down the common bile duct into the duodenum.

The common bile duct and the main duct from the pancreas usually unite just before the duct enters the lumen of the duodenum. There is often a dilation of the tube after this junction (the ampulla of Vater). The opening of the common bile duct in the duodenum is about 8 to 10 cm from the pylorus.

Function of Hepatocytes

The liver cells perform many functions (Table 33–3). Liver function is essential to life.

Liver cells degrade steroid hormones, thereby preventing excess blood levels of estrogen, testosterone, progesterone, aldosterone, and glucocorticosteroids.

Another hepatic function concerns protein metabolism. Hepatocytes deaminate proteins and synthesize nitrogenous wastes (eg, uric acid). They also convert ammonia manufactured by colonic bacteria into another waste, urea. They also synthesize plasma proteins (eg, albumins and globulins). The albumins maintain normal plasma colloid osmotic pressure. A fall in this pressure leads to edema and contributes to ascites. The globulins bind to a certain portion of the daily hormonal output from the thyroid and adrenal cortex glands. Binding inactivates these hormones, thereby keeping blood levels low. Bound hormones can be released slowly to maintain normal plasma levels of those hormones. Decreased hepatic protein levels can lead to a clinical excess of these hormones.

Hepatocytes also make bile, which contains water, bile salts, cholesterol, bilirubin, gluconate, and inorganic acids. Bile salts aid digestion by emulsifying dietary fats and fostering their absorption and the absorption of fat-soluble vitamins through the intestinal mucosa. They also

Cross section of liver lobule

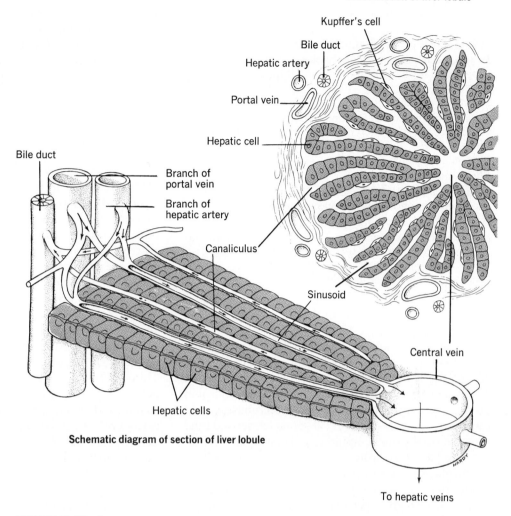

FIGURE 33–4

A section of liver lobule showing the location of the hepatic veins, hepatic cells, liver sinusoids, and branches of the portal vein and hepatic artery. (Chaffee EE, Lytle IM: Basic Physiology and Anatomy, 4th ed. Philadelphia, JB Lippincott)

prevent the cholesterol in the bile from precipitating out of solution and forming calculi. More than 90% of the daily output of bile is reabsorbed for recycling by an active transport process of the ileal mucosa.

The liver contributes to adipose stores through the metabolism of triglycerides, fatty acids, and cholesterol. During fasting, triglycerides from adipose tissue are catabolized by the liver into fatty acids and glycerols. The free fatty acids in prolonged fasting are further catabolized into acetyl coenzyme-A and then into ketone bodies. Ketone bodies provide an important source of energy to tissues that can use them in the Krebs cycle, which excludes the nervous system.

Fat-soluble vitamins and many minerals are stored in the liver. These vitamins and minerals are released under the influence of hormones and serum concentrations of inorganic elements.

Another hepatic function is elimination of bilirubin

from the body. Old or defective erythrocytes are phagocytosed by large reticuloendothelial cells lining the large veins and the sinuses of the liver and spleen. These phagocytes degrade the hemoglobin of these cells into biliverdin, iron, and globulin molecules. The last two components are recycled by the body in future erythropoiesis. The biliverdin is almost immediately converted to free bilirubin. Because this is an insoluble compound, it is transported bound to plasma albumin molecules. The hepatocytes convert this insoluble bilirubin into a soluble (and thus excretable) form by conjugating it with glucuronic acid to form bilirubin gluconate. This soluble form of bilirubin is then added to the bile and is eliminated from the body by the feces. Bilirubin gluconate gives the bile its normal golden yellow color. Commensal organisms in the intestines convert most of the bilirubin gluconate into a darker brown compound, urobilinogen, which gives the feces its natural brown color. Because it is

TABLE 33–3
Hepatocyte Functions

Steroid (hormone and drug) catabolism

Protein metabolism, including synthesis of plasma proteins, conversion of ammonia to urea, deamination, and transamination

Production of bile

Fat metabolism, including lipoprotein synthesis, cholesterol synthesis, and conversion of protein and carbohydrates into fat

Mineral and vitamin storage

Elimination of bilirubin

Carbohydrate metabolism, including glycogen storage, gluconeogenesis, and release of glucose into plasma

Degradation of certain drugs

Synthesis of coagulation factors I (fibrinogen), II (prothrombin), V (proaccelerin), VII (proconvertin), IX (plasma thromboplastin component), X (Stuart factor)

Synthesis of complement proteins

soluble in water, urobilinogen can also be absorbed from the colon back into the bloodstream and be excreted by way of the kidneys. Excess plasma levels of either the conjugated (direct) or unconjugated (indirect) bilirubin produce jaundice. Excess unconjugated bilirubin can cross the immature or damaged blood–brain barrier and bind with the basal ganglia, resulting in kernicterus.

The liver participates in carbohydrate metabolism. Serum glucose levels are maintained by "hepatic glucostatic function," involving two mechanisms. If plasma glucose levels are high, hepatocytes remove glucose from the plasma. This glucose is stored in polymer form as glycogen. As plasma glucose levels decline, the hepatocytes convert the glycogen back into glucose molecules (glycogenolysis) and release them into the bloodstream. Although many body tissues have the requisite cellular enzymes for glycogenolysis, hepatocytes are one of the few cell types that can release this intracellular glucose into the bloodstream. Hepatocytes do not simply respond directly to plasma glucose. These glucostatic functions are mediated by several hormones; some (eg, insulin) promote hepatic glucose uptake, and others (eg, glucagon, growth hormone, and epinephrine) stimulate glycogenolysis and the release of glucose from liver cells.

The liver does not contain enough glycogen reserves to be able to buffer plasma glucose during prolonged fasting or severe exercise. During these times, low plasma glucose levels stimulate the secretion of one or more hormones (glucagon, glucocorticoids, or thyroxine) that trigger the biochemical conversion of intracellular fatty and amino acids into glucose (gluconeogenesis), which the liver cell can then release into the bloodstream or store as glycogen. Only hepatocytes possess the enzyme that is critical for gluconeogenesis. Glycogen storage is important for other functions of liver cells. A glycogen-rich hepatocyte conjugates bilirubin at a faster rate and is more resistant to toxins and infectious agents.

Hepatocytes possess a "mixed-function–oxidase system" (MFOS) of enzymes that degrade certain drugs, among which are alcohol, benzodiazepines, tranquilizers, phenobarbital, phenytoin (Dilantin), and sodium warfarin (Coumadin). This system operates in addition to other intracellular systems that also degrade some of these drugs. Its clinical significance lies in the nature of the drugs that this system catabolizes and in the fact that MFOS activity can be either inhibited or augmented ("induced") by these same drugs, depending on *when* they are taken. Administration of two MFOS-catabolized drugs within a few hours of one another or together causes each agent to act competitively, slowing down the degradation of the other. For example, simultaneous ingestion of diazepam (Valium) and alcohol can result in slower degradation of each drug. The outcome is higher blood levels of both chemicals for a longer time after administration. The repeated administration of one MFOS-catabolized drug for several days causes the MFOS system to enlarge physically and to possess more enzymes. This is called "induction." Once induced, the MFOS degrades drugs more rapidly (including the drug that initiated the induction). If administration of a second MFOS-catabolized drug is begun after MFOS induction, a larger dose of this drug will be required to produce a given effect. For example, induction of the MFOS by diazepam increases the dosage of Coumadin needed to produce a given therapeutic effect. Other drugs are degraded by various hepatic systems.

Many elements that constitute the coagulation cascade are synthesized in the liver. Fibrinogen, prothrombin, proaccelerin, proconvertin, plasma, thromboplastin component, and Stuart factor are all made in the liver. Coagulation is therefore delayed in patients with deficient liver function. Also, several complement proteins are synthesized here.

BIBLIOGRAPHY

Ganong WF: Review of Medical Physiology, 15th ed. Norwalk, CT, Appleton & Lange, 1991

Guyton AC: Textbook of Medical Physiology, 8th ed. Philadelphia, WB Saunders, 1991

McCance KL, Huether SE: Pathophysiology: The Biologic Basis for Disease in Adults and Children. St Louis, CV Mosby, 1990

Prezbindowski KS, Tortora GJ: Learning Guide to Accompany Principles of Anatomy and Physiology. New York, Harper & Row, 1990

Tortora GJ, Anagnostakos NP: Principles of Anatomy and Physiology. New York, Harper & Row, 1990

**STUDY
QUESTIONS**

1. The pancreas secretes

    1. amylase
    2. bicarbonate
    3. hydrochloric acid
    4. secretin

        a) 1 & 2
        b) 3 & 4
        c) 1 & 3
        d) 2 & 4

2. The colon is a major site for

    a) digestion
    b) absorption of digested foodstuffs
    c) reabsorption of water and electrolytes
    d) manufacture of certain vitamins

3. The liver does NOT function in

    a) manufacture of clotting factors
    b) lipid digestion
    c) synthesize nitrogenous wastes
    d) convert bilirubin from an insoluble to a soluble form

4. Defecation

    1. is initiated by pressure of feces on the internal anal sphincter
    2. is initiated by stretching of the rectal wall
    3. cannot occur after recovery from a complete transection of the spinal cord in the lumbar region
    4. is a cord reflex that can be voluntarily inhibited providing CNS pathways between the cerebral cortex and the sacral cord are intact

        a) 1 & 2
        b) 3 & 4
        c) 1 & 3
        d) 2 & 4

CHAPTER 34

Assessment: Gastrointestinal System

BEHAVIORAL OBJECTIVES

Based on the content of this chapter, the reader should be able to:

1. Identify the basic components of a nursing history in assessing the gastrointestinal (GI) system.
2. Name the five features assessed in a review of the gastrointestinal system.
3. Describe a basic examination of the oral cavity using inspection and palpation.
4. Describe a physical examination of the abdomen and specific modifications used during inspection, auscultation, percussion, and palpation.
5. Describe two nursing interventions for patients undergoing endoscopic and radiographic studies of the gastrointestinal tract.

Hudak: Critical Care Nursing:
A Holistic Approach, 6th ed. © 1994
J. B. Lippincott Company.

Description

Differentiation of the signs and symptoms of a gastrointestinal disorder is a challenging part of the nursing process. One must determine whether the assessment findings are related to a known condition or whether they herald a new complication. Is the comatose patient's respiratory distress caused by a pulmonary disorder or by a mucus plug lodged in the nasopharynx? Is the bright red blood in the stool a result of a gastrointestinal bleed or of bleeding from external hemorrhoids? Is the complaint of abdominal pain due to the trauma of recent bowel surgery or to a distended stomach? Assessment of the gastrointestinal system is important to determine causes of nutritional disorders, acid–base imbalances, bleeding episodes, and pain within the system. It is also performed to monitor therapy, to determine the necessity of preventive health teaching, and to monitor an abnormality in another system that is reflected in the gastrointestinal system. Careful assessment of the gastrointestinal system provides the nurse with information that clarifies specific problems.

History

Excluding emergency conditions that require immediate action to preserve life, an assessment of the gastrointestinal system begins with the history. The patient should be questioned about any past problems with anorexia, indigestion, dysphagia, nausea, vomiting, pain, jaundice, constipation, gas, diarrhea, bleeding, or hemorrhoids. It is necessary to follow through and expand on positive responses to determine when the problem appeared, whether medical treatment was sought, what precipitated the symptom, what relieved it, what made it worse, and whether the problem is current. A nutritional history is important and should include dietary intake, food allergies, food intolerances, special diets, difficulty swallowing (dysphagia), and alcohol and caffeine intake. A thorough medication history is also necessary. The patient should be asked about recent weight gain or loss, bowel habits, recent surgeries (including dental work), and any family history of ulcers, colitis, or cancer.

Pain originating in the gastrointestinal (GI) system varies depending on the underlying cause and origin. The pain should be described by type, location, quality, duration, character, mode of onset, aggravating and/or relieving factors, and relation to respiration. Associated signs and symptoms (eg, hyperventilation, guarding, and tachycardia) should also be described. Table 34–1 lists some conditions that produce abdominal pain. The most common complaints about the GI system are pain, dysphagia, nausea, vomiting, diarrhea, and constipation. A review of the GI system focuses on the following five features:

- *General appearance*: Motor activity, body position,

TABLE 34–1
Conditions that Produce Intra-Abdominal Pain and Tenderness

1. Perforated peptic ulcer
2. Dissecting or ruptured aneurysm
3. Pancreatitis
4. Cholecystitis
5. Regional enteritis
6. Ulcerative colitis
7. Diverticulitis
8. Appendicitis
9. Occlusion of mesenteric artery
10. Ruptured ectopic pregnancy
11. Acute renal infections
12. Pelvic inflammatory disease
13. Hepatitis
14. Extra-abdominal causes
    (a) Myocardial disease
    (b) Respiratory disease
    (c) Diabetic or thyroid crisis
    (d) Spinal cord lesion
    (e) Acute intermittent porphyria
    (f) Pneumonia
    (g) Acute glaucoma

nutritional state recent changes in weight, eating habits, and apparent state of health
- *Skin*: Color (jaundice, cyanosis, pallor), turgor, edema, texture (oily, dry), and dermatological conditions
- *Head*: Color of sclerae, sunken eyes, breath odor, condition of teeth, tongue, and buccal mucosa
- *Abdomen*: Size, shape, skin coloration, visible protrusions, scars, fistulas, limited respiratory excursion, and excessive skin folds (indicates muscle wasting)
- *Psychological factors*: Recent emotional upsets, depression, and anxiety

Examination

Oral Cavity

Examination of the oral cavity is accomplished by inspection and palpation. A good light source, a tongue depressor, an examining glove, and a mask are needed. The patient should be placed in a comfortable position, preferably sitting upright. The nurse should explain the procedure and obtain the patient's cooperation. The first step is inspection of the lips and jaw for abnormal color, texture, lesions, symmetry, and swellings. The temporomandibular joint is palpated bilaterally for mobility, tenderness, and crepitus. The lips should be retracted to allow adequate visualization during the inspection. If the patient has dentures, the nurse should inspect how well they fit, then remove them for the oral exam. The inside of the mouth should be inspected with a good light source. Missing, broken, loose, and decayed teeth should be identified. Redness, pallor, white patches, plaques, ulcers, bleeding, and masses of the gums and entire buccal mucosa should be noted. The parotid ducts and the submaxillary ducts should be located.

Any suspicious area should be palpated with a gloved finger for tenderness or induration. The patient should be asked to stick out his or her tongue, which is checked for symmetry of movement, swellings, lesions, and an abnormal coating. The tongue blade is used to depress the tongue, and the movement of the soft palate and uvula is observed as the patient says "Ah"; these structures should rise symmetrically. The hard and soft palates, the uvula, the tonsils, the pillars, and the posterior pharynx are inspected for redness, pallor, patches, lesions, and petechiae. Any unusual breath odor should be described. Mouth odors are characteristic of gastrointestinal disease such as peptic ulcer disease, severe bowel obstruction, hepatic failure, and neoplasms of the esophagus.

Abdominal Examination

Physical examination of the patient should be performed with the patient's comfort in mind.

The patient should be instructed to empty the bladder, and then should be placed in the supine position with arms down and knees slightly bent. This position relieves tension on the abdominal wall.

The need for an abdominal examination should be evaluated if the patient is experiencing pain. An abdominal examination is not performed if the patient has appendicitis, dissecting abdominal aortic aneurysm, polycystic kidneys, or previous organ transplantation. The abdominal examination must be stopped if the procedure becomes too uncomfortable for the patient, if it increases the intensity of the pain, or if findings indicate one of the aforementioned diagnoses.

The abdominal examination is performed by inspection, auscultation, percussion, and palpation, in that order. Auscultation precedes percussion and palpation because they can alter the frequency and quality of bowel sounds. The patient should be draped in a manner that exposes the abdomen but protects the patient's modesty. The abdomen is divided into its four quadrants (RUQ, LUQ, LLQ, RLQ). The underlying structures are visualized in Figure 34–1). Signs and symptoms elicited during the exam are evaluated with this anatomy in mind.

Observation

Begin the examination by standing at the foot of the patient and inspecting for symmetry of the abdomen, visible masses, and visible pulsations. Then move to the

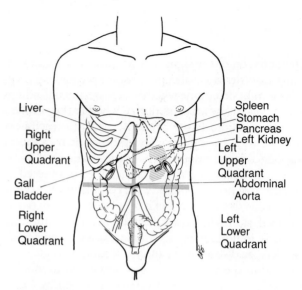

FIGURE 34–1
A map of abdominal organs.

patient's side, position yourself to obtain an eye-level view across the abdomen, and inspect for any asymmetry, any abdominal movement from respirations, peristalsis, or pulsations, any exaggerated movement, and eversion of the umbilicus. Pulsation of the aorta is normally seen in the epigastric area. In a thin person, the femoral pulses may be visible. The color of the skin should be observed. Signs of edema (eg, tense, shiny skin) or the presence of a hernia that becomes visible with a cough should be recorded. The presence of any rashes, striae, ecchymoses, lesions, scars, or dilated veins should be noted. A blue-tinged umbilicus is known as "Cullen's sign" and can be an indication of intra-abdominal bleeding.

Auscultation

Next, the four quadrants of the abdomen are auscultated with the diaphragm of the stethoscope. To prevent contraction of the abdominal muscles (which obscures other sounds), the examiner lifts the stethoscope completely off the abdominal wall when changing its location. Use only light pressure on the diaphragm, and listen for a full 3 to 5 minutes in each quadrant to confirm the absence of bowel sounds. The frequency and character of sounds heard should be described. Normal bowel sounds are irregular, bubbly sounds and occur every 5 to 15 seconds. Hyperactive bowel sounds are rapid, high-pitched (tinkling), and loud. Edema of the abdominal wall can be detected by observation of any imprint of the diaphragm. The bell of the stethoscope is used to auscultate over the abdominal aorta, the renal arteries, and the femoral arteries for bruits (continuous purring, blowing, or humming sounds). If a bruit is heard, neither percussion nor palpation should be performed. The physician must be notified of this finding if it was not previously heard.

Percussion

Following auscultation, percussion should be performed in all four quadrants, for identification of air, gas, and fluid in the abdominal cavity and to determine organ size. The sound that is percussed depends on the underlying structure. A dull sound is heard over solid organs, such as the liver or a stool-filled colon. A tympanic sound is heard over air, as in the gastric bubble. Percussion for determining the size of the liver should be performed along the right midclavicular line. One method is to begin at the iliac crest and work upward. The point at which the sound becomes dull is marked, and then percussion is performed from the clavicle down. A dull sound represents a rib, which must not be mistaken for the superior edge of the liver. The superior edge is marked and is measured in centimeters. The normal liver measures 6 to 12 cm in height at the midclavicular line (Fig. 34–2).

Palpation

Light palpation should be done first to identify muscular resistance and areas of tenderness. One or two fingers are used to depress the abdominal wall 1 cm (0.5 in). Skin temperature, muscle resistance, tender areas, and masses are recorded. The femoral artery is palpated bilaterally. Always palpate a symptomatic area last to assure patient cooperation and relaxed muscles.

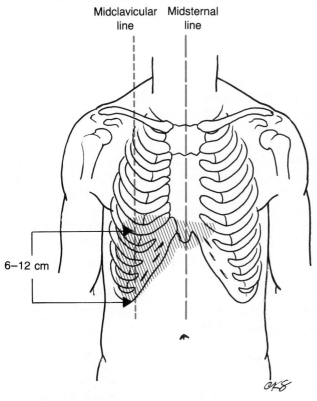

Midclavicular line   Midsternal line

6–12 cm

FIGURE 34–2
Location of the liver for percussion.

TABLE 34–2
Clinical Recording of Gastrointestinal Assessment

Wears upper and lower dentures. Lips are cyanotic; no ulcers or cracking. Buccal mucosa bright red; no ulcers or nodules. Tongue, gums, and floor of mouth cyanotic. Unable to identify parotid and submaxillary ducts. Tonsils absent. No lesions, plaques, or exudates.

No complaints of abdominal pain. Appetite good. No difficulty swallowing; no nausea or vomiting. Has indigestion when eating while stressed. Bowel movement every day. No diarrhea or constipation. No history of jaundice, gallbladder, or liver disorders.

Abdomen is flat and symmetrical with good muscle tone and without visible pulsations or peristalsis. Frequent borborygmi in all quadrants. Renal and femoral arteries not auscultated because of overriding bowel sounds. No palpable areas of tenderness or masses. Liver span percussed at 4 cm. Spleen not palpable. Pole of right and left kidney palpated in respective upper outer quadrants approximately 2 cm below costal margin. Aortic and femoral pulses 4+.

Deep palpation is used for localization of organs (enlarged spleen, liver edge, poles of right and left kidney) and large masses. The tips of the fingers are used to depress the abdominal wall firmly to a depth of 7.5 cm (3 in). Palpation is performed in the epigastric area for the pulse of the aorta. If an area of tenderness is found with light palpation, rebound tenderness should be checked by quickly withdrawing the fingertips following depression. Rebound tenderness usually indicates an inflammation of the peritoneum.

Rectal Examination

The rectum is assessed by inspection and palpation. The skin around the rectum is normally darker than the surrounding area. One should inspect for inflammation, lesions, fissures, and hemorrhoids. Palpate with a well-lubricated rubber-gloved finger for outpouching, nodules, tenderness, irregularities, and fecal impaction.

Documentation

The final step in an assessment of the GI system is the documentation of findings. The documentation should be concise and informative. Pertinent negative findings should be indicated. Table 34–2 is an example of documentation of an assessment.

Diagnostic Tests

A variety of diagnostic tests can be used to help in the diagnosis of gastrointestinal and abdominal abnormalities in the critical care setting.

X-rays

The abdominal series, or three-way view of the abdomen, consists of films of the flat abdomen, films of the upper abdomen and upper chest with the patient erect, and films obtained with the patient lying on one side (decubitus). Radiographs help delineate free air in the abdomen caused by problems such as a perforated viscus or a ruptured abscess. Bowel obstructions, as indicated by dilated loops of bowel with air fluid levels or intestinal volvulus, can be seen on these films. Decubitus films help determine the presence of ascites.

Gastrointestinal Endoscopy

This procedure is an important adjunct to the barium studies because it allows direct observation of portions of the intestinal tract. The instrument used is a flexible fiberoptic endoscope. It is designed with a movable tip so that it can be manipulated through the intestinal tract by the operator. It also includes an instrument channel that allows for biopsy of lesions, such as tumors, ulcers, or inflammation. Fluids can be aspirated from the lumen of the intestinal tract, and air can be insufflated to distend the intestinal tract for better observation. Cytology brushes and electrocautery snares can also be passed through the scope. The basic upper intestinal endoscope and the colonoscope are designed in a similar fashion and differ only in their diameter and their length. A side-viewing upper intestinal endoscope has also been designed for special studies on the common bile duct and the pancreatic duct. This is called endoscopic retrograde cholangiopancreatography (ERCP).

The indications for upper intestinal endoscopy are multiple. In the critical care setting the most common indication is acute gastrointestinal hemorrhage, which can be caused by ulcers, gastritis, or esophageal varices. Endoscopy is helpful in diagnosing neoplasms of the upper intestinal tract. Biopsies or brushings of these abnormal areas can be done to obtain diagnostic material.

Specific therapies can be performed through the upper gastrointestinal endoscope, including sclerosis of esophageal varices. In this procedure a sclerosing agent, such as sodium morrhuate, is injected into the dilated veins in the esophagus in hopes that scarring will occur within the vein to prevent further spontaneous bleeding.

Colonoscopy

Colonoscopy is used to evaluate for the presence of tumors, inflammation, or polyps within the colon. It is also used to evaluate a surgical anastomotic site from a previous surgery and to assess the degree of stricture from either previous surgeries or inflammation.

The colonoscope can be passed from the rectum through the full length of the colon into the cecum. From here the ileocecal valve can be assessed as well as other abnormalities, such as early carcinomas or polyps of the right side of the colon. These polyps can be removed through the endoscope, or they can be fulgurated and cauterized. Specific sites of bleeding, such as occurs in colitis, polyps, tumors, or angiodysplasia (a collection of abnormal blood vessels that can bleed extensively) can be observed.

Because patients are usually sedated for endoscopic procedures, it is important to guard their airways to prevent respiratory depression or aspiration and to monitor vital signs.

Barium Contrast Studies

These studies are extremely important to define abnormalities within the intestinal tract. The upper gastrointestinal x-ray or barium swallow is performed by having the patient drink a radiopaque barium meal while the radiologist observes the coating of this material within the esophagus, stomach, and small intestine. The barium outlines structural defects such as tumors or ulcers and can define inflammation or strictures. The barium enema is performed by instilling barium through the rectum in a retrograde fashion into the entire colon. A thin coat of barium helps to outline tumors, polyps, diverticula, or inflammation such as Crohn's disease or ulcerative colitis.

Ultrasonography

This noninvasive test uses echowaves to detect abnormalities in the abdominal cavity. Dilation of the common bile duct, distended gallbladder with gallstones, and pancreatic abnormalities such as tumors, pseudocysts, or abscesses can be defined. Abdominal aortic aneurysms can be quantitated to help decide if surgical excision is required. Thickening of the descending colon and sigmoid colon with pericolonic abscesses caused by such conditions as diverticulosis can be identified. This is a procedure that is usually performed in the radiology department of a hospital but can be performed in the critical care setting.

Computed Axial Tomography (CT) and Magnetic Resonance Imaging (MRI)

Tumors of the liver, pancreas, esophagus, stomach, and colon can be identified using these scans. Retroperitoneal tumors or lymph nodes can be seen as well. Through the use of the CT scan, needle biopsies of these structures can be performed to determine the tumor cell type. A needle is passed through the abdominal wall using local anesthesia.

The needle is then directed into the desired structure with the aid of the CT scan. Fluid can be aspirated and subsequently evaluated by a pathologist for the presence of neoplastic cells.

Nuclear medicine techniques are often used to help diagnose abnormalities of the hepatogastrointestinal systems. Radionuclide liver scans can help determine hepatic cell dysfunction. CT scanning can be used to define tumors or abscesses within the liver or upper abdomen.

Cholescintograms can be performed to determine the functional capacity of the biliary system and the patency of the bile ducts and the cystic duct. In recurrent intestinal bleeding, if the source has not been found, technetium scans can be helpful. In this technique the blood is labeled with technetium, and if the patient is actively bleeding a "hot spot" can show up on the scan of the abdomen. It is a very nonspecific test for locating the exact site of the bleeding but can help in directing the surgeon to the general site. Angiodysplasia and a bleeding Meckel's diverticulum can be diagnosed with this procedure.

Arteriography

This procedure is useful in defining the sites of bleeding that are otherwise difficult to determine. The catheter is placed in either the superior or inferior mesenteric artery, and contrast is injected. Arteriography is also extremely helpful in defining aneurysms of the aorta.

Paracentesis

Peritoneal tap with lavage of the peritoneal cavity can be most useful in trauma cases in which intra-abdominal hemorrhage must be defined. It can also help determine whether pancreatitis is present by measurement of the amylase and lipase in the fluid aspirated and whether tumors are present by cytology studies.

Management

Many diagnostic tests, especially those involving the use of contrast media, require preparation of the gastrointestinal tract before the procedure to provide a clear field for study. Many of these tests are time consuming and place the patient in uncomfortable positions. Therefore, every effort should be made to be sure the protocol for preparing the tract is followed and that the area to be studied is emptied of food and stool. This prevents the need to repeat a test owing to poor preparation.

Preprocedure Care

Studies of the upper gastrointestinal tract require withholding all oral intake (food, liquids, oral medications) for a period of 8 to 10 hours before the test is performed. Studies of the lower intestinal tract require a low-residue diet and the administration of a potent laxative the evening before the test. Enemas can be given the morning of the test to make certain the rectum and colon are completely empty. No more than three enemas should be necessary.

Endoscopic studies require an empty stomach for good visualization. It may be necessary to lavage the stomach with a wide-bore gastric tube before beginning these tests. Because of the size of these tubes (Ewald, Edlich, or Levacuator), they are passed into the stomach orally and left in place only as long as necessary to empty the stomach of food or blood clots. Before passage of the endoscope, the patient is placed on the left side, three-fourths prone. This position provides easy access to the pylorus and improves viewing of the greater curvature of the stomach. A local anesthetic is applied to the throat and a sedative such as diazepam (Valium) or midazolam hydrochloride (Versed) is administered intravenously.

During the procedure, the patient must be observed closely for condition changes and untoward reactions to the test. A thorough nursing history assists in anticipating reactions, and nursing intervention can prevent unfavorable responses such as a drug reaction or pain and discomfort due to positional limitations. Patient education in all aspects of the test promotes cooperation and allays many fears.

Paracentesis and peritoneal lavage are accomplished using a local anesthetic and strict sterile technique. The patient's bladder must be empty at the time of the tap to prevent accidental puncture of the bladder. The patient is positioned according to the physician's preference. Emotional support is provided during the procedure, and condition changes are monitored.

Postprocedure Care

After a barium study, stools should be observed to be sure barium is expelled. The protocol may call for administration of a laxative to promote barium excretion. Following an endoscopic procedure, the patient must be observed for signs of bleeding (hematemesis, melena, tachycardia, hypotension), perforation (pain on swallowing, epigastric substernal pain increased with breathing and movement, shoulder pain, abdominal pain, back pain, dyspnea, tachycardia, hypotension), and adverse drug reactions (anxiety, erythema, fever, angioedema, wheezing, dyspnea, cyanosis, palpitations, hypotension, vomiting, diarrhea). If an ERCP has been performed, watch for signs of cholangitis (fever, chills, hyperbilirubinemia) or pancreatitis (see Chapter 38). Following paracentesis, the patient must be observed for signs and symptoms of internal bleeding due to laceration of a blood vessel or peritonitis due to perforated viscus.

BIBLIOGRAPHY

Ahern H, Rice K: How do you measure gastric pH? Am J Nurs 91(5):70, 1991

Balthazar EJ, Chako AC: CT tomography in acute gastrointestinal disorders. Am J Gastroenterol 85(11):144–152, 1990

Bryant G: When the bowel is blocked. RN 55(1):56–58, 1992

Hahn PF: Advances in contrast-enhanced magnetic resonance imaging. Gastrointestinal contrast agents. Am J Roent 156(2):252–254, 1991

Holmgren C: Abdominal assessment. RN 55(3):28–34,1992

Malasonos L, Barkauskas V, Stotenberg-Allen K: Health Assessment, 4th ed. St Louis, CV Mosby, 1990

Nemcek AA: CT of acute GI disorders. Radiol Clin North Am 27(4):773–789, 1989

O'Toole MT: Advanced assessment of the abdomen and gastrointestinal problems. Nurs Clin North Am 25(4):771–775, 1990

Sleisenger MH: Gastrointestinal Disease: Pathophysiology, Diagnosis and Management, 4th ed. Philadelphia, WB Saunders, 1989

STUDY QUESTIONS

1. Auscultation of the abdomen

   a. is best done with the bell of the stethoscope
   b. should be performed before palpation
   c. is only done to evaluate bowel sounds
   d. should reveal continuous bubbling sounds

2. During percussion of the abdomen, a dull sound is heard over

   a. solid organs
   b. hollow organs
   c. the gastric air bubble
   d. an empty colon

3. The diagnostic study that allows for direct visual observation of the intestinal tract is the

   a. abdominal x-ray
   b. endoscopy
   c. ultrasonography
   d. computed axial tomography

4. Signs of perforation of the bowel following a barium study include

   a. pain on swallowing
   b. dyspnea
   c. hypotension
   d. all of the above

CHAPTER 35

*Management
Modalities:
Gastrointestinal
System*

BEHAVIORAL OBJECTIVES

Based on the content of this chapter, the reader should be able to:

1. Describe the body's metabolic response to a traumatic event.
2. State three parameters used to assess nutritional status.
3. Describe appropriate measures for treatment of malnutrition.
4. State two complications of enteral hyperalimentation and two complications of central hyperalimentation.
5. Identify three nursing interventions for a patient receiving enteral hyperalimentation.
6. Identify three nursing interventions for a patient receiving central hyperalimentation.

Hudak: Critical Care Nursing:
A Holistic Approach, 6th ed. © 1994
J. B. Lippincott Company.

Nutritional Support for the Critically Ill Patient

Description

Adequate nutritional support of the critically ill patient is one of the most important advances in patient care since the development of antibiotics.

Historically, it has long been recognized that health and nutrition go hand in hand. As the fund of knowledge of normal metabolism has increased, the effects of stress (eg, injury and infection) have also been investigated. More than 50 years ago it was found that among patients who were undergoing surgical treatment for peptic ulcer, there was a 33% mortality rate in those with a preoperative loss of more than 20% of their body weight. This compared with a 3.5% mortality rate for those who were in a better nutritional state. Similarly, almost 20 years ago Cahill noted that a loss of one-third of total body protein by a previously normal person was fatal. It became readily obvious that significant stress increases mortality and morbidity by reducing body mass, delaying wound healing, and altering the normal immune responses.

This chapter presents a basic overview of energy requirements and the effects of stress on the nutritional state of the patient. After this, assessment, procedure, and interventions for nutritional support are discussed.

Physiological Principles

For homeostasis, there must be a balance between energy supply and energy expenditure. The total expenditure of energy by the body is the sum of physical activity, growth, and basal metabolic rate (BMR). The BMR is the energy that a person requires to perform the essential physiological processes at rest. The resting metabolic rate (RME) is very similar to BMR except that it takes into account the energy required for minimal physical activity. RME is often used because the conditions for measurement are not as strict as those for BMR measurement.

The effect of stress on energy balance is illustrated by the following considerations. Fever increases the RME by 7% for each degree Fahrenheit; the postoperative state increases the RME by 10% to 15%; infection increases the RME by 20% to 50%; and thermal burns raise the RME by as much as 125%. It is evident that maintenance of an energy balance in these states requires a tremendous number of calories.

Beside requiring energy balance, the body must also maintain nitrogen balance. This is crucial because nitrogen represents the building blocks of protein. If the body is building protein, a state of anabolism exists and protein balance is said to be positive. If, however, the body is breaking down protein, a state of catabolism exists and negative nitrogen balance is present.

The catabolic state is seen in trauma, sepsis, and many disease states. It represents the breakdown of protein for energy purposes. Protein loss impacts on body functions, because protein is necessary for enzymes, cell membranes, contractile protein in muscle, and blood proteins. Proteins are also important in maintaining cellular osmotic pressure.

Metabolic Response to Injury

A traumatic event, regardless of its cause, triggers a complex series of hormonal responses that significantly alter the body's metabolism. The major effect is an increase in protein and fat catabolism, with a retention of water and sodium and a loss of potassium. Antidiuretic hormone (ADH) is released from the pituitary in response to such factors as hypovolemia, pain, stress, and drugs. By acting on the collecting ducts of the kidney, ADH reduces free water excretion, thus correcting the hypovolemic state. Corticotropin (ACTH) also is released from the pituitary and stimulates the adrenal gland to secrete mineralocorticoids and glucocorticoids. The mineralocorticoid aldosterone causes sodium retention and potassium excretion by its action on the kidney. This function, along with the action of ADH, is the major volume regulatory system by which the body maintains blood pressure in the face of trauma.

The glucocorticoids, of which cortisol is the most important, act in several ways to produce energy substrate for the body during stress. They act on the liver to stimulate gluconeogenesis but also are catabolic in that they cause muscle protein breakdown to amino acids as well as decreased protein synthesis. They also release free fatty acids from lipid stores. Fatty acids meet the requirements of all organs with the exception of those that specifically require glucose (eg, the brain and nervous system).

The catecholamines, epinephrine and norepinephrine, are released from the adrenal medulla during stress. They also set into motion a series of reactions aimed at increasing energy substrate for the body.

Lipolysis results from increased catecholamine secretion. Free fatty acids are then available for use as an energy source by the liver, kidney, lung, heart, and skeletal muscle. Ketone bodies are formed from fatty acids by the liver. These also are used as an energy source.

Catecholamines cause hyperglycemia to develop during stress; this is called "stress diabetes." This clinical state arises through a variety of mechanisms. Liver glycogen and muscle glycogen are converted to glucose. Insulin released from the pancreas is suppressed, and glucagon is released. Uptake of glucose in the peripheral tissues also is reduced.

Both ACTH and catecholamines act to release glucagon. Glucagon then acts on the liver to promote gluconeogenesis. It also helps break down skeletal muscle glycogen to glucose and aids in oxidation of fat.

ACTH, catecholamines, glucagon, insulin, and growth hormone act in synergism to supply the body with energy substrate and to control blood volume to help ensure survival during stress. This stress can be either starvation or trauma. However, in starvation, the levels of cortisol and catecholamines are not elevated to the magnitude seen in severe trauma. This can account for the fact that there is a rise in metabolic rate in the posttraumatic state rather than the fall that occurs in starvation. In starvation, the body tends to preserve lean body mass and protein, but in trauma, protein becomes the major source of calories. The mechanisms for this are not well understood.

During the initial phase of stress, the body uses carbohydrates in the form of glycogen. These stores can last as long as 8 to 12 hours. After this, amino acids from protein, and to some degree fatty acids, make up the bulk of energy substrate.

Nitrogen, a major component of amino acids, helps form the building blocks of protein. One gram of nitrogen equals 6.25 g of protein, which is equal to about 30 g of lean body mass. If losses of 15 to 25 g/day occur, as is often seen in major trauma (ie, burns, major fractures, and sepsis), as much as 7.5 kg (16 lb) of lean body mass can be lost.

Although these drastic losses cannot be avoided, they can be offset by an adequate supply of calories and amino acids. If the nutritional substrate is supplied and other factors of support such as blood pressure and respiratory status are maintained, the body enters a phase of "available opportunity." During this time, the levels of catecholamines, cortisol, and glucagon drop and that of insulin rises. Protein breakdown is curtailed, and protein resynthesis is favored.

If catabolism is allowed to continue without the support of calories and amino acids, wound healing, immune function, and muscular strength are compromised. At this point, there is direct competition for the necessary substrate by the rest of the body. If this situation continues, malnutrition can occur.

There are two major classifications of malnutrition: protein and protein–calorie. Either can occur in critically ill patients. Protein malnutrition is characterized by general apathy, decreased visceral protein synthesis as indicated by decreased plasma albumin and transferrin, edema, muscular wasting, and a decreased total lymphocyte count.

Protein–calorie malnutrition is accompanied by a recent unplanned loss of 10% or more of body weight, decreased subcutaneous fat stores, muscle mass atrophy, diarrhea, and anorexia. Assessing for malnutrition and identifying high risk patients is important because there is a significant difference in morbidity and mortality rates between groups of malnourished and well-nourished patients. High risk patients include those with chronic disease, severe catabolism, inability to use the gastrointestinal tract, intravenous support with intravenous fluid for more than 5 days, and those with beginning signs or symptoms of malnutrition.

Nutritional Assessment

The assessment of the patient who needs nutritional assistance is multifaceted and includes dietary history, anthropometric measurements, measurement of visceral proteins, immunologic studies, nitrogen balance studies, and nutritional requirement determinations.

Dietary History

The dietary history should be obtained as soon as possible. This history should include a description of the patient's type of diet, any changes in weight, appetite changes, or difficulty in eating. Knowledge of food preferences and cultural influences is helpful in planning nutritional therapies. Behavioral changes such as listlessness, increased fatigue, or apathy should be noted. A complete medication history also is important.

Anthropometric Measurements

These measurements involve physical measures of the body and provide an estimate of fat content of subcutaneous tissue. They can be used to determine body fat stores. Skin fold measurements of the arms (triceps) are most often used; however, other measurements (biceps, subscapular, thigh, periumbilical) can be taken to improve accuracy. Estimates of muscle mass are determined from mid-arm muscle circumference and mid-arm muscle area. These are compared with standard tables.

Measurement of Visceral Proteins

Low serum protein concentrations with malnutrition reflect the protein mass of the internal organs. The visceral proteins most often measured are albumin, transferrin, prealbumin, and fibronectin. They can be used to determine degree of malnutrition. Albumin may not be a good marker for acute nutritional deficiency because of the large concentrations stored in the body and its long half-life, and because underhydration affects serum levels without reflecting body stores. Transferrin can be more sensitive to acute malnutrition because of its shorter half-life. However, a disadvantage is that serum levels can be affected by non-nutritional factors. Fibronectin has recently been proposed as an acute marker of malnutrition and is still being studied.

Immunological Studies

Malnutrition, stress, and disease negatively affect the body's defenses against infection. Evaluation of recall antigens to TB, mumps, and *Candida* are used to measure cellular immunity. These are applied as skin tests, and if there is no cutaneous reaction a state of altered immunocompetence may exist. This can be caused by malnutrition. It has been documented that normal lymphocyte response to skin tests is not seen in malnourished people. Reduced lymphocyte counts may also be found. Total lymphocyte count (percentage of lymphocytes × white blood cell count) of less than $1,500/mm^3$ is associated with impaired immune function.

Nitrogen Balance Studies

One very important parameter of protein synthesis and metabolism is the measure of nitrogen balance. This balance is calculated from the amount of nitrogen intake versus that which is excreted in the urine as urea. The normal adult turns over about 300 g of protein in 24 hours and excretes the equivalent 50 to 65 g of protein during that time.

Nitrogen balance is calculated with the following equation:

$$\frac{\text{Protein intake}}{6.25} - \text{Urinary urea nitrogen} + 4 = \text{Nitrogen balance.}$$

If the number derived is zero, nitrogen balance is present. If the number is positive, protein synthesis is occurring. A negative number indicates that protein catabolism exists. The amino acid and nitrogen needs of the patient can be calculated by this measurement.

Determining Nutritional Requirement

Determining individual nutritional requirements is the final step in a nutritional assessment. Rather than measure the RME, the energy requirements are estimated to determine nutritional needs. Estimates of energy requirements at rest (basal energy expenditure, BEE) are most often done using the Harris–Benedict equation. A correction factor is used to determine energy requirements in states of stress (see Table 35–1).

Once malnutrition is recognized as an actual or potential problem, nutrients should be provided early in the course of treatment. Patients with a long-term postoperative course, those with multiple trauma, those receiving chemotherapy, and those being treated with hemodialysis are examples of candidates for hyperalimentation, as indicated in Table 35–2. The increased energy required by the body to handle the stresses imposed by these conditions leads to the starvation state without nutritional support. With the use of nutritional therapies, sufficient calories and nitrogen to sustain life and promote healing can be supplied to the body.

Methods of Nutritional Support

Enteral Feeding

It is not uncommon to find patients in the intensive care unit whose intestinal tracts are fully operational. In these patients it is preferable to use the functioning gastrointestinal tract as the route of nutritional support. It is the least complicated, the least costly, and the least dangerous

---

TABLE 35–1
Basal Energy Expenditure

BEE: Men

$66.47 + (13.75 \times \text{weight in kg}) + (5.0 \times \text{height in cm}) - (6.76 \times \text{age in yr})$

BEE: Women

$655.10 + (9.56 \times \text{weight in kg}) + (1.7 \times \text{height in cm}) - (4.68 \times \text{age in yr})$

Correction Factors

Low stress: 1.3 × BEE	Severe stress: 2.0 × BEE
Moderate stress: 1.5 × BEE	Cancer: 1.6 × BEE

Adapted from Young ME: Malnutrition and wound healing. Heart Lung 17:1, 60–69, 1988

TABLE 35–2
Indications for Hyperalimentation

Malabsorption

Ulcer disease	Pancreatitis
Chronic diarrhea	Diverticulitis
Chronic vomiting	Alimentary tract fistula
Failure to thrive	Alimentary tract anomalies
Gastrointestinal obstruction	Hepatic failure
Granulomatous enterocolitis	Biliary disease
Ulcerative colitis	Short bowel syndrome
Protein-losing gastroenteropathy	

Inability to Take in Nutrients

Difficulty swallowing	Coma
Neurological weakness	Unable to afford
Malignant disease	NPO 5 or more days
Anorexia nervosa	

Hypermetabolic States

Indolent wounds and decubitus ulcers
Complicated trauma or surgery
Sepsis
Burns

way of providing nutrients. The introduction of the small-bore silastic feeding tube (Fig. 35–1) has made this method of providing nutrition more comfortable for the patient. The tube's flexibility, coating, size (8 mm), and tungsten tip create a less irritating and safer tube for long-term placement.

Procedure

The tube is passed into the stomach using the same procedure for passing any nasogastric tube. An x-ray of the abdomen is taken after insertion to confirm placement of the tube. Tube placement should then be verified every 4 hours by aspirating gastric contents from the tube and by injecting air into the tube and auscultating the gastric bubble. However, it should be noted that it is difficult to assure placement of this type of tube through the auscultation method. Although an air bubble may be heard in the esophagus, the sound can be transmitted to the epigastrium leading to false verification. Any time the exact location of the tube is in question, the tube should be removed and reinserted.

Commercially prepared elemental nutritional solutions (eg, Sustacal, Ensure, and Isocal) are usually used, because they deliver 1 to 2 calories per ml (carbohydrate, fat, protein, and vitamins). Special formulas for specific patient populations (patients with respiratory disease, liver failure, or renal failure) or patients who are hypermetabolic (those with sepsis or trauma) are also available.

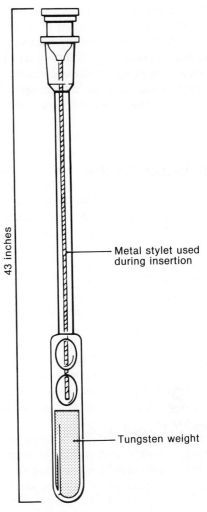

43 inches

Metal stylet used during insertion

Tungsten weight

FIGURE 35–1
Characteristics of small-bore feeding tube.

The patient's tolerance to enteral feeding depends on the rate of flow and the osmolarity of the formula. Feedings are generally diluted initially and gradually increased to full strength.

Feedings can be administered by bolus, intermittent infusion, or continuous infusion. Bolus feedings are generally not well tolerated, because they are often accompanied by nausea, bloating, cramping, diarrhea, or aspiration. Intermittent slow-gravity drip feedings are administered 4 to 6 times a day over a period of 30 to 60 minutes. Continuous infusion can used with the aid of a feeding pump to assure a constant flow rate. The continuous method is best suited to the critically ill patient, because it allows greater time for absorption of nutrients in the intestine.

Complications

Nursing care is aimed at monitoring the patient's response to enteral feedings, including the complications associated with this nutritional therapy.

Diarrhea is the most frequent problem and can be caused by too rapid an infusion rate or by intolerance of lactose, fat, or osmolarity. Generally, adjusting the rate or type of feeding can reduce this complication. The administration of an absorbing product (Metamucil) or antidiarrheal medication may also be necessary. To prevent diarrhea resulting from bacterial contamination of the solution and administration sets, the open solution should be used within 24 hours, and administration sets should be changed daily. Administration sets should be rinsed between feedings, and personnel should use good handwashing technique when handling the equipment. *High gastric residuals* can also be problematic. A high residual is defined as a return of at least half the amount given over an hour. The initial intervention is to hold the feeding for 1 hour and recheck the residual. This procedure is repeated every 1 to 2 hours until feedings can be resumed. Nausea and vomiting can be the result of too rapid infusion or lactulose intolerance.

Fluid and electrolyte alteration can be caused by *dehydration* occurring from lack of adequate fluid intake and *hyperglycemia* if the body does not tolerate the glucose load, resulting in osmotic diuresis. An accurate intake and output record, daily weights, assessment of urinary output, and determination of blood glucose and other serum electrolytes assists in early recognition of fluid and electrolyte imbalances.

A potential for impaired gas exchange can be caused by *aspirating the feeding* solution into the lung. This complication can be prevented by maintaining the person in a Fowler's position of at least 30 degrees, and by checking for gastric residuals (already discussed). Feedings should be discontinued at least 30 minutes before any procedure that requires the patient to remain flat. Feedings can also be colored with food coloring to allow for early detection of aspiration.

Peripheral Parenteral Nutrition

Indications

Generally, intravenous nutrition is used for patients with functional impairment of the gastrointestinal tract and for those who need short-term nutritional support. It can also be used when placement of a central venous catheter is difficult or poses a danger to the patient.

It can be used to supply calories to early postoperative patients who are expected to start eating within several days to a week after surgery. It can also be used as a supplement for patients whose nutritional and caloric intake is marginal.

Solutions

In this setting, protein-sparing calories are supplied by a solution of D5–10%/3.5% amino acids and lipids which are isotonic. The dextrose and amino acids are given as routine intravenous solutions, and flow rates depend on fluid needs. A 20% lipid emulsion by peripheral vein provides almost 2,000 kcal per day. Phlebitis is the most frequent complication. The lipid solution should be given over a 24-hour period, and the frequency should vary from daily to twice weekly depending on caloric needs or the philosophy of the ordering physician. The peripheral lipids must be administered alone or in conjunction with the amino acid solutions. They should not be mixed with dextrose solutions.

This particular approach preserves body protein by supplying amino acids for normal protein synthesis but does not assist in tissue repair. Calories for energy are supplied by the D5–10% solution and fat emulsion. Up to 2,000 kcal a day can be provided. If the patient requires long-term nutritional support or progresses to protein–calorie malnutrition, as in hypermetabolic states, total parenteral nutrition should be instituted.

Central Hyperalimentation (Total Parenteral Nutrition)

Solution Admixture

Total parenteral nutrition (TPN) begins with a solution containing a final concentration of 15% to 35% glucose and 3.5% to 5% amino acids. Protein needs are influenced by illness. During critical illness, 2.0 to 3.5 g of protein per kg of body weight is needed. Specialized amino acid preparations for renal failure and hepatic failure are also available. Fat, in the form of lipid emulsions, is included in the nutritional regime to prevent essential fatty acid deficiency.

Glucose–Amino Acid Ratio

The ratio of the calories (glucose) to nitrogen (amino acid) should be 200:1. This ratio preserves the nitrogen balance of the body; the hypertonic glucose is used for calories, allowing the amino acids to be used for protein synthesis. If this ratio is not preserved, excess amino acids are lost in the urine if adequate glucose is present, or amino acids are used for calories if adequate glucose is not present. Optimal therapy requires 200 kilocalories to each 1 gram of nitrogen.

Electrolytes

Daily additions to the TPN solution to meet daily requirements include potassium, sodium, chloride, magnesium, acetate, and phosphorous. Additional electrolyte supplements may be needed in patients who experience unusual electrolyte loss or have increased requirements.

Vitamins

A multiple vitamin preparation is added to TPN solutions daily, including fat-soluble and water-soluble vitamins.

Adult products do not contain Vitamin K, and if this is needed it can be provided by intravenous or intramuscular injection to prevent development of prolonged prothrombin time.

Trace Minerals

Trace elements are also routinely added to solutions including zinc, copper, chromium, and magnesium. Certain patients may also require iron.

Decisions concerning the amount of additives necessary to maintain the patient's electrolyte balance are based on serial blood tests. Positive nitrogen balance is monitored by serial blood urea nitrogen (BUN) and creatinine levels. A hyperalimentation panel (Table 35–3) is done daily until the electrolytes are stabilized. After stabilization is achieved, the serum levels can be checked every other day to once a week.

Insulin

Glucose intolerance can occur at the onset of treatment if the pancreas does not respond to the increased glucose load. Blood glucose levels can be easily monitored with a finger stick and a blood glucose reagent strip. Parenteral insulin, either by continuous intravenous infusion, by the addition of insulin to the base solution, or by intermittent subcutaneous or intravenous injection, should be administered when necessary to maintain blood glucose levels within normal values.

Fat Emulsion

A percentage of the required calories is provided with a fat emulsion. This is done not only to prevent an essential fatty acid deficiency but also to help control hyperglycemia and the production of carbon dioxide. Calories obtained from fat do not require the use of insulin for metabolism. Therefore, patients prone to glucose intolerance can be more easily controlled. The metabolism of glucose results in a much higher production of carbon dioxide than does the metabolism of fat. Therefore, patients with respiratory impairment benefit from less glucose metabolism.

These fat emulsions are available in a 10% or 20% solution. The 10% solution delivers 1.1 kcal/ml and the 20% solution delivers 2 kcal/ml. The percent of calories provided by fat versus glucose is dependent on the patient's condition but should never exceed 60% of total caloric intake.

The fat emulsion is an isotonic solution and, therefore, can be administered by way of a peripheral vein or given through a "Y" connector in the main intravenous line. Fat emulsions are administered without a filter because the large fat molecule cannot pass through most filters. During initial infusion, the patient must be closely monitored for complications such as nausea, fever, chills, muscle aches, pain in chest or back, and urticaria.

There are several disadvantages to the use of fat emulsion. The instability of the emulsion requires that fluid and electrolyte needs be met separately, thereby losing the ability to tailor the solution to the patient. The risk of infection is increased due to the inability to use a filter during administration and the inability to check the solution for particulate matter due to its milky appearance.

Total Nutrient Admixture

In this system, lipid emulsions are mixed with the amino acid and dextrose solution and administered in a single container. This system has the potential for reducing infection rates, personnel time, and cost.

Procedure

Flow Rate and Volume

The rate of infusion of the hypertonic solution must be constant over a 24-hour period to achieve maximum assimilation of the nutrients and to prevent hyperglycemia or hypoglycemia. The flow rate cannot be increased to compensate for interruptions or slowing of the infusion, because glycosuria with osmotic diuresis (diuresis from body compartments and cells leading to dehydration) can occur. Headache, nausea, and lassitude are early symptoms of too rapid an infusion. Too slow an infusion results in the administration of fewer nutrients, and hypoglycemia with a rebound of insulin can occur.

The aim of treatment is a continuous infusion that meets the caloric requirements of the patient by allowing maximum use of the carbohydrate and protein substrates with minimal renal excretion. The flow rate must be maintained. An infusion pump helps ensure continuous accurate infusion. However, because such pumps are mechanical devices subject to malfunctions, the nurse must keep a close watch on the flow rate. It is recommended that infusions that have fallen behind schedule **not** be accelerated to "catch up." TPN is never discontinued abruptly, and solutions containing at least 5% dextrose are infused to prevent rebound hypoglycemia in this situation.

TABLE 35–3
Possible Tests on a Hyperalimentation Panel

Chemistry	Normal Ranges
pH	7.35–7.45
Sodium	135–145 mEq/L
Potassium	3.5–5.3 mEq/L
Chlorides	100–109 mEq/L
Calcium	4.5–5.7 mEq/L
Phosphorus	1.45–2.76 mEq/L
Magnesium	1.4–2.1 mEq/L
Glucose	70–115 mg/dl
BUN	8–22 mg/dl
Creatinine	0.8–1.6 mg/dl
Bicarbonate	22–26 mEq/L
Total protein	5.5–8.0 g/dl

Volume is given according to established water metabolism levels (2,500 ml/24 hr in adults and 100 ml/kg/24 hr in infants) and carbohydrate metabolism (0.5 g/kg/hr). The initial intake is 1,000 to 2,000 ml/24 hr, with a gradual increase according to the patient's tolerance, as established by careful clinical and chemical monitoring. Generally, the maximum daily volume is 3 liters. However, patients undergoing massive catabolism, such as that occurring in severe or extensive burns or severe traumatic injuries, often require 4 to 5 L/day.

If there is a problem with the integrity of the kidneys or heart, carefully calculate fluid volume to prevent cardiopulmonary overload. A special hypertonic solution, nephramine, can be used in this setting. This solution provides the eight essential amino acids in 250 ml and, diluted with the 500 ml of the hypertonic glucose solution, provides the necessary calories and proteins for 24 hours without an excess of water.

If the patient is receiving adequate nutrition, the weight gain should be 100 to 300 g/day (0.25–0.5 lb/day). If the patient is gaining much more, it is probably due to water retention and not tissue gain, and the volume infused needs to be adjusted downward.

Infusion Sites

Knowing the nature of the hyperalimentation solution, one can easily understand that the usual normal intravenous routes are not used because this hypertonic solution would rapidly cause thrombosis at the tip of the intravenous catheter. Because this high caloric nitrogen solution must be rapidly diluted and dispersed within the blood vessels, the superior vena cava is an excellent site. Figure 35–2 indicates the different routes that can be used. Passage of the intravenous catheter into the superior vena cava by way of the subclavian vein is the route of choice, because it allows the patient the greatest freedom of movement without disturbing the injection site, and because the incidence of infection at this level of the body is lower. Jugular veins can be used, but it is not as comfortable for the patient. Basilic vein routes are too susceptible to irritation and infection for long-term therapy. The femoral vein as a route to the inferior vena cava is rarely selected, because it is highly susceptible to contamination from body pathogens, such as abdominal wound drainage, urine, and stool.

Complications

Infection

Two key factors are involved in the success of hyperalimentation therapy: (1) the long-term presence of the indwelling catheter directly in the superior vena cava, and (2) the hypertonic solution. Both are prime sites for the source of infection.

Insertion Site and Catheter. The puncture site is a potential portal of entry of organisms, and the solution is an excellent culture medium for many species of bacteria and fungi. Meticulous asepsis in the care of the line and in the preparation of the solution cannot be overstressed.

Asepsis starts with the insertion of the indwelling catheter. This is performed under strict sterile technique.

TPN should be administered through a catheter that is reserved solely for nutritional therapy.

A sterile transparent dressing is applied to the site of insertion and is changed every 24 to 72 hours. At the time of the dressing change, the site should be examined for

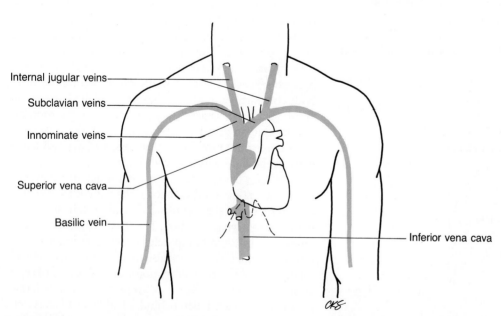

Internal jugular veins

Subclavian veins

Innominate veins

Superior vena cava

Basilic vein

Inferior vena cava

FIGURE 35–2
Venous anatomy for hyperalimentation routes.

signs of leakage, edema, and inflammation, and the catheter should be checked for any kinking of the tube. Clean the skin with a solvent such as acetone to remove surface skin fat that harbors pathogenic organisms and adhesive tape that, if allowed to accumulate, causes irritation and skin breakdown. A large area surrounding the catheter is cleaned with an antibacterial solution (eg, an iodine preparation). A transparent or gauze dressing is applied over the area. The presence of a tracheostomy or open and draining wounds near the insertion site requires special precautions to maintain sterility of the site.

Vital signs, including temperature, are also monitored. A rise in blood or urine sugar levels in a patient who was previously tolerating the glucose in TPN can indicate catheter sepsis. If there is a suspicion of catheter sepsis, the line is removed and the tip is cultured. Antibiotic therapy may also be necessary.

Solution Sterility. Maintaining sterility of the solution is mandatory. As already stated, the solution is an excellent culture medium for pathogens. It should be prepared by a pharmacist under a laminar air-flow hood to assure a particle-free environment. All of the intravenous tubing should be changed every 24 hours, at the time a new solution is hung.

The new tubing, the new solution, and the dressing change should be correlated to take place at the same time. If dressings are changed every 48 to 72 hours and the tubing is changed daily, the indwelling catheter and tubing connection sites should be situated so that a change of tubing does not interfere with the integrity of the dressing. The tubing change is made with the patient in a low Fowler's position or flat in bed to prevent an air embolism from occurring with a deep inspiration.

Connections and tubing are closely inspected for cracks and leaks. If a tubing separation occurs, the tubing should be reconnected immediately to stop the flow of air into the patient's circulation. If air embolism is suspected, the patient is positioned on his left side, with the head down. This allows the air bubbles to rise to the upper part of the right atrium of the heart where they are less likely to obstruct blood flow to the pulmonary artery.

Drug Administration Precautions

No intravenous push or piggyback medications should be given in the same line as the hyperalimentation solution. No steroids, pressor drugs, antibiotics, or other parenteral drugs are ever added to the base solution, because they can interact with the fibrin hydrolysate or with one another, forming a precipitate that would not be visible to the naked eye. In addition, the mixing of drugs (other than the electrolytes) in the solution could necessitate adjusting the flow rate according to their requirements rather than those of the nutritional hypertonic solution. If any intravenous medication or blood transfusions are necessary, an alternate route should be started for their administration. Only the hyperalimentation solution with its electrolyte

additives added under aseptic conditions should be administered through the central line. The subclavian catheter should not be used to draw blood samples, either. Any break in the system is an entrance for infection; maintenance of the sterility is of the utmost importance.

The introduction of the three-way subclavian (Fig. 35–3) and Hickman catheters has greatly facilitated the care of patients who are receiving hyperalimentation therapy. These catheters provide three separate infusion channels with exits in three different sites in the central vein. Therefore, one channel can be used for the hyperalimentation solution, one for intravenous antibiotics and other medications, and one for the infusion or withdrawal of blood. Ideally, TPN should be administered through a single lumen catheter reserved for nutritional therapy.

Glucose Intolerance. Blood sugar levels of patients receiving TPN must be closely monitored. As already mentioned, insulin can be administered using a sliding

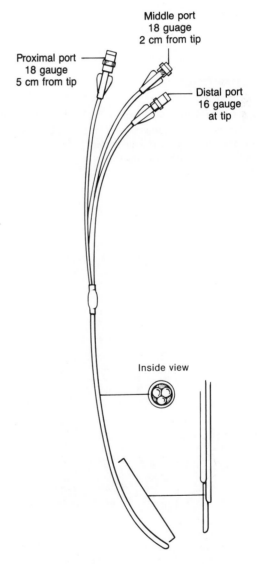

FIGURE 35–3
Characteristics of three-way intravenous catheter.

scale. Uncontrolled hyperglycemia can lead to an osmotic diuresis, which is life-threatening.

Hepatic Dysfunction. Liver dysfunction is common with TPN and reverses with discontinuation of the therapy. The cause of this dysfunction is not well understood, but it is thought to be related to imbalance in nutrients administered intravenously.

Respiratory Distress. Carbohydrate metabolism produces carbon dioxide and water. In patients with respiratory disease, the increase in CO_2 production from the metabolism of the hypertonic glucose solutions in TPN may not be tolerated. More calories can be administered using fat emulsion, and fewer from carbohydrates, to control this problem.

Assessment and Management

The goals of care are to provide adequate nutrition for anabolism, maintain fluid balance, and prevent infection and other complications associated with hyperalimentation therapy. This requires a multidisciplinary approach involving the nurse, physician, dietitian, and pharmacist. Care also includes providing information and emotional support. Examples are explaining the procedure, what to expect, risks, and expected outcomes to the patient and family and informing them that although TPN provides all nutrients necessary to maintain body processes, the patient may experience hunger and food cravings. Nursing care is outlined in Nursing Care Plan 35–1.

NURSING CARE PLAN 35–1:
The Patient Undergoing Parenteral Hyperalimentation

NURSING DIAGNOSIS	OUTCOME CRITERIA/ PATIENT GOALS	NURSING INTERVENTIONS
Altered nutrition less than body requirements: related to inability to maintain adequate nutritional status by oral intake or tube feedings.	• Nutritional needs of patient will be met.	1. Administer TPN solution, as ordered, by infusion pump. 2. Monitor flow rate by marking IV bag with hourly calibrations. 3. Maintain accurate intake and output records. 4. Weigh patient daily with same scale at same time. 5. Monitor nutrition parameters of assessment including albumin, transferrin, BUN, creatinine, total lymphocyte count. 6. Monitor serum glucose as ordered; administer insulin according to sliding scale protocol. 7. Monitor serum electrolytes for abnormalities; replace as ordered. 8. Encourage exercise (eg, ROM, isotonic exercises, ambulation) as tolerated to promote protein synthesis; physical therapy consult. 9. Administer 5% to 10% dextrose solution if TPN is interrupted and it is unable to be administered as ordered.

(continued)

NURSING CARE PLAN 35–1: (Continued)
The Patient Undergoing Parenteral Hyperalimentation

NURSING DIAGNOSIS	OUTCOME CRITERIA/ PATIENT GOALS	NURSING INTERVENTIONS
High risk for infection: related to central venous access and use of a hypertonic glucose solution.	• Patient will not acquire a nosocomial infection.	1. Maintain asepsis in line care, in dressing changes, and in solution preparation. 2. Change solution q24h. 3. Change intravenous tubing using aseptic technique q24–48h, according to institutional policy. 4. Change dressing over insertion site q24–72h, according to protocol. 5. Inspect insertion site for signs of inflammation, edema, tenderness, and leakage. 6. Monitor temperature, vital signs, and WBCs. 7. Monitor blood glucose. 8. Report and record any signs of infection. 9. If any sign of infection occurs, follow protocol for obtaining cultures. This may require removal and culture of catheter tip. 10. Maintain TPN line as a dedicated nutritional therapy. Do not administer other medications through the line.
High risk for fluid volume deficit: related to high glucose load.	• Patient will remain uvolemic without weight fluctuations.	1. Administer fluids as ordered. 2. Maintain accurate intake and output records; calculate fluid balance. 3. Weigh patient daily on same scale at same time. 4. Monitor serum glucose; administer insulin per sliding scale order. 5. Monitor urine specific gravity. 6. Monitor for signs of dehydration, excessive thirst, decreased skin turgor, headache, fatigue, nausea and vomiting, dry skin, pale and dry mucous membranes, weakness, dizziness, concentration of serum electrolytes, decreased CVP or PCWP.

(continued)

NURSING CARE PLAN 35–1: (Continued)
The Patient Undergoing Parenteral Hyperalimentation

NURSING DIAGNOSIS	OUTCOME CRITERIA/ PATIENT GOALS	NURSING INTERVENTIONS
Fluid volume excess: related to high glucose level, large fluid volumes.	• Patient will remain uvolemic without weight fluctuations.	1. Monitor for signs of fluid overload, lung congestion, jugular vein distention, weight gain, increased CVP or PCWP. 2. Administer diuretics, as ordered. 3. Maintain accurate intake and output records. 4. Weigh patient daily on same scale, same time.

BIBLIOGRAPHY

Bockus S: Troubleshooting your tube feedings. Am J Nurs 91(5):24–29, 1991

Bowman M, Eisenberg P, Katz B et al: Effect of tube feeding osmolality on serum sodium levels. Crit Care Nurse 9(1):22–28, 1989

Curtas S, Chapman G, Meguid M: Evaluation of nutritional status. Nurs Clin North Am 24(2):301–313, 1989

Davidson LJ, Belknap DC, Flournoy DJ: Flow characteristics of enteral feeding with psyllium hydrophilic mucilloid added. Heart Lung 20(4):404–413, 1991

Eisenberg P: Enteral nutrition. Nurs Clin North Am 24(2):311–337, 1989

Evans M: Hyperglycemia during nutrition support. Crit Care Nurse 12(1):64–69, 1992

Kemper M, Weissman C, Hyman A: Caloric requirements and supply in critically ill surgical patients. Crit Care Med 20(3):344–348, 1992

Kohn CL, Heithley JK: Enteral nutrition: Potential complications and patient monitoring. Nurs Clin North Am 24(2):339–351, 1989

Kuhn MM: Nutritional support for the shock patient. Crit Care Nurs Clin North Am, 2(2):201–220, 1990

Worthington PH, Wagner BA: Total parenteral nutrition. Nurs Clin North Am 24(2):355–369, 1989

Young ME: Malnutrition and wound healing. Heart Lung 17(1):60–69, 1988

STUDY QUESTIONS

1. One mechanism that explains hyperglycemia during the stress response is
   a. increased insulin release from the pancreas
   b. glucagon suppression
   c. increased uptake of glucose in the peripheral tissues
   d. catecholamine release

2. A diagnostic test that reflects low protein mass of internal organs is
   a. serum albumin
   b. anthropometric measurements
   c. immunological studies
   d. nitrogen balance

3. A nursing intervention to prevent aspiration of enteral feedings is
   a. Trendelenburg position
   b. bolus feedings
   c. gastric residual checks
   d. insertion of large bore feeding tube

4. The most common complication of TPN therapy is
   a. hypomagnesemia
   b. hypoglycemia
   c. sepsis
   d. hypovolemia

CHAPTER 36

Acute Gastrointestinal Bleeding

BEHAVIORAL OBJECTIVES

Based on the content of this chapter, the reader should be able to:

1. Describe presenting signs and symptoms of acute gastrointestinal bleeding.
2. Identify the four steps in management of a patient with a gastrointestinal bleed.
3. Describe two treatments to control upper gastrointestinal bleeding.
4. Identify five nursing diagnoses and related nursing interventions for a patient experiencing an upper gastrointestinal bleed.
5. Describe the nursing management of a patient with a Sengstaken–Blakemore tube.

Hudak: Critical Care Nursing:
A Holistic Approach, 6th ed. © 1994
J. B. Lippincott Company.

Description

Bleeding in the gastrointestinal tract is caused primarily by gastric ulcers or gastritis. However, esophageal varices, Mallory-Weiss tears of the gastroesophageal junction, carcinoma of the esophagus or stomach, duodenal ulcers, ulcerative colitis, polyps, diverticula, hemorrhoids, and hypocoagulable states can erupt in a bleeding episode. Bleeding that occurs from the lower gastrointestinal tract is rarely life-threatening and usually does not warrant admission to a critical care unit or is treated surgically (Table 36–1).

The appearance of the person presenting with upper gastrointestinal tract bleeding varies considerably, depending on the amount and rapidity of blood loss. Gastrointestinal bleeding that is the result of an erosion through an artery is profuse and does not stop with medical management. Bleeding that is caused by gastritis or oozing from granulation tissue at the base of an ulcer is smaller in quantity, transient in nature, and usually responds to medical management.

Pathophysiology

Peptic ulcer disease is the most common cause of upper gastrointestinal bleeding. These ulcers are characterized

TABLE 36–1
Causes of Gastrointestinal Bleeding

Upper Gastrointestinal Bleeding

Esophageal
    Varices
    Inflammation
    Ulcers
    Tumors
    Mallory-Weiss tears
Gastric
    Ulcers
    Gastritis
    Tumors
    Angiodysplasia
Small intestine
    Peptic ulcers
    Angiodysplasia
    Crohn's disease
    Meckel's diverticulum

Lower Gastrointestinal Bleeding

    Malignant tumors
    Polyps
    Ulcerative colitis
    Crohn's disease
    Angiodysplasia
    Diverticula
    Hemorrhoids
    Rectal fissures
    Massive upper gastrointestinal hemorrhage

by a break in the mucosa extending through the muscularis mucosae. It is usually surrounded by inflamed cells which over time are replaced by granulation and finally scar tissue.

Excess secretion of acid is important to the pathogenesis of ulcer disease. Impaired ability of the mucosa to secrete mucus for protection is also thought to contribute to the development of the ulcer. Known risk factors for the development of peptic ulcer disease include aspirin and nonsteroidal anti-inflammatory drugs, both of which can cause mucosal damage. Cigarette smoking is also linked to this disease and, in addition, it significantly impairs ulcer healing. A family history of ulcer disease is also known to be a risk factor.

Stress ulcers are found in critically ill patients and are characterized by mucosal erosion. The lesions are associated with patients who have sustained severe trauma; patients who have sepsis, severe burns, cranial or central nervous system disease; and patients on long-term ventilatory support. Abnormalities range from small surface hemorrhages to deep ulcerations with massive hemorrhage. Hypoperfusion to the stomach mucosa is thought to be the main mechanism. Decreased perfusion is thought to contribute to impaired mucus secretion, lowered the mucosal pH, and decreased mucosal cell regeneration. All of these factors contribute to the development of the ulcer.

In chronic cirrhotic liver failure, cell death in the liver results in increased portal venous pressure. As a result, collateral channels develop in the submucosa of the esophagus and rectum and the anterior abdominal wall to divert blood from the splanchnic circulation away from the liver. As pressure rises in these veins, they become distended with blood and enlarge. These dilated vessels are called varices and can rupture, resulting in massive gastrointestinal hemorrhage.

Upper gastrointestinal hemorrhage results in a sudden loss of blood volume, decreased venous return to the heart, and decreased cardiac output. If the bleeding is significant, it results in decreased tissue perfusion. In response to the decreased cardiac output, the body initiates compensatory mechanisms to attempt to maintain perfusion. These mechanisms account for the major signs and symptoms seen in patients on initial assessment. If blood volume is not replaced, decreased tissue perfusion results in cellular dysfunction. The cells shift to anaerobic metabolism, and lactic acid is formed. Decreased blood flow affects all of the body systems, and without sufficient oxygen supply they begin to fail.

History and Clinical Manifestations

The history includes asking about the signs and symptoms and the presence of precipitating factors. Patients exhibit blood loss from the gastrointestinal tract in several ways, including hematemesis and melena.

Hematemesis

The patient who is vomiting blood is usually bleeding from a source above the ligament of Treitz (at the duodenojejunal junction). Reverse peristalsis is seldom sufficient to cause hematemesis if the bleeding point is below this area. The vomitus can be bright red or coffee-ground in appearance, depending on the amount of gastric contents at the time of the bleed and the length of time the blood has been in contact with gastric secretions. Gastric acid converts bright red hemoglobin to brown hematin, accounting for the coffee-ground appearance of the drainage. Maroon or bright red blood results from profuse bleeding and little contact with gastric juices.

Melena

Tarry stools consistently occur in all persons who accumulate 500 ml of blood in their stomachs. A tarry stool may be passed if as little as 60 ml of blood has entered the intestinal tract. Massive hemorrhage from the upper gastrointestinal tract, along with the increased intestinal motility that occurs, can result in stools containing bright red blood. It takes several days after the bleeding has stopped for melena stools to clear. Gastrointestinal blood loss can also be occult, detected by testing the secretions (nasogastric drainage or stool) with a chemical reagent (guaiac).

Assessment of Blood Loss

To evaluate the severity of blood loss and to prevent or correct clinical deterioration into hypovolemic shock, the nurse must assess the patient frequently. In the first stage of bleeding—less than 800 ml of blood loss—the person may show signs only of weakness, anxiety, and perspiration. With a significant bleed, the body temperature elevates to 38.4° to 39°C (101° to 102°F) in response to the bleeding, and bowel sounds are hyperactive due to the sensitivity of the bowel to the blood.

If blood loss is moderate to severe (>800 ml loss), a sympathetic nervous system response causes a release of the catecholamines, epinephrine and norepinephrine. These initially cause an increase in heart rate and peripheral vascular vasoconstriction in an attempt to maintain an adequate blood pressure. With moderate to severe blood loss, signs and symptoms of shock are present.

As the shock syndrome progresses, the release of catecholamines triggers the blood vessels in the skin, lungs, intestines, liver, and kidneys to constrict, thereby increasing the volume of blood flow to the brain and heart. Because of the decreased flow of blood in the skin, the person's skin is cool to the touch. With decreased blood flow to the lungs, hyperventilation occurs to maintain adequate gas exchange.

As blood flow to the liver decreases, metabolic waste products accumulate in the blood. This, combined with the absorption of decomposed blood from the intestinal tract and a decrease of blood flow through the kidneys, causes an increase in the blood urea level. The blood urea nitrogen (BUN) can be used to follow the course of a gastrointestinal bleed. A BUN above 40—in the setting of a gastrointestinal bleed and a normal creatinine level—indicates a major bleed. The BUN will return to normal approximately 12 hours after the bleeding has stopped.

Urinary output is a very sensitive measure of intravascular volume which *must* be measured hourly. As the intravascular volume decreases, urine output decreases, owing to the reabsorption of water by the kidneys in response to the release of antidiuretic hormone (ADH) by the posterior lobe of the pituitary gland. The effects of hypovolemic shock on the kidneys are discussed in more detail in Chapter 25.

A change in blood pressure greater than 10 mm Hg, with a corresponding heart rate increase of 20 beats per minute in sitting or standing position, indicates blood loss of greater than 1,000 ml. The patient's response to blood loss depends on the amount and rate of blood loss, age, degree of compensation, and rapidity of treatment.

The patient may report pain with the GI bleed, and this is thought to arise from gastric acid eating the ulcer crater. Epigastric tenderness is an uncommon sign. The abdomen can be soft or distended. Bowel sounds are most often hyperactive due to the sensitivity of the bowel to blood.

Diagnostic Studies

Common diagnostic studies ordered for the patient with acute gastrointestinal bleeding are listed in Table 36–2. A hematocrit and hemoglobin are ordered with the complete blood count. It is important to consider that the

TABLE 36–2
Diagnostic Findings for Acute GI Bleeding

Complete Blood Count
   Decreased Hemoglobin
   Decreased Hematocrit
   Elevated WBC Count
Electrolyte Panel
   Decreased Serum Potassium
   Elevated Serum Sodium
   Elevated Serum Glucose
   Elevated Lactate (severe bleed)
Hematology Profile
   Prolonged Prothrombin Time
   Prolonged Partial Thromboplastin Time
Arterial Blood Gases
   Respiratory Alkalosis
   Hypoxemia

hematocrit generally does not change substantially during the first few hours after an acute gastrointestinal bleed because of compensatory mechanisms. Fluids that are administered on admission also can affect the blood count. The white blood cell count and glucose may be increased, reflecting the body's response to stress. Decreases in potassium and sodium may be found due to the accompanying vomiting. Liver function tests are used to evaluate the patient's hematological integrity. A prolonged prothrombin time can indicate liver disease or concurrent long-term anticoagulant therapy. Respiratory alkalosis is common due to activation of the sympathetic nervous system from the loss of blood. If large amounts of blood are lost, metabolic acidosis occurs as a result of anaerobic metabolism, as described above. Hypoxemia may also be present because of decreased circulating hemoglobin levels and resultant impairment in oxygen transport to cells.

Endoscopy is the procedure of choice to diagnose the exact site of the bleed, because direct mucosal inspection is possible with use of a fiberoptic scope (Fig. 36–1). Flexible endoscopes allow this test to be performed at the bedside, and the test is routinely ordered by the physician after the patient has become hemodynamically stabilized. Diagnostic accuracy of this test ranges from 60% to 90%.

Management
Collaborative Management

Management of the patient with acute gastrointestinal bleeding is a collaborative endeavor. Initial interventions include four steps:

1. Assess the severity of blood loss.
2. Replace a sufficient amount of fluids and blood products to counteract shock.
3. Diagnose the cause of bleeding.
4. Plan and implement a definitive treatment.

Fluid and Blood Product Resuscitation

The patient with an acute gastrointestinal bleed requires immediate intravenous access with a large-caliber intracatheter or cannula. To prevent progression of hypovolemic shock, fluid replacement is begun using intravenous solution such as Ringer's lactate or normal saline. Vital signs are assessed continuously as fluids are replaced. Blood losses of greater than 1,500 ml require blood replacement in addition to fluids. The patient's blood is typed and crossmatched, and packed red blood cells are usually infused to re-establish oxygen-carrying capacity of the blood. Other blood products such as platelets, clotting factors, and calcium may also be ordered according to results of lab tests and the patient's underlying condition.

Rarely, vasoactive drugs are used until fluid balance is restored to maintain blood pressure and perfusion to vital body organs. Dopamine, epinephrine, and norepinephrine are drugs that can be ordered to stabilize the patient until definitive treatment can be undertaken.

Diagnosing the Cause of Bleeding

As mentioned earlier, flexible endoscopy is the diagnostic procedure of choice to determine the cause of the bleed. A nasogastric tube can be inserted to assess the rate of bleeding, but this is a controversial intervention. Barium studies also can be done, although they are often not conclusive if there are clots in the stomach or if there is superficial bleeding. Angiography is used only if the source of bleeding is not accessible by the endoscope.

Definitive Treatments
Endoscopic Therapies

Sclerotherapy is the treatment of choice if the site of the bleed can be found using endoscopy. The bleeding sites are most often sclerosed using a sclerosing agent such as

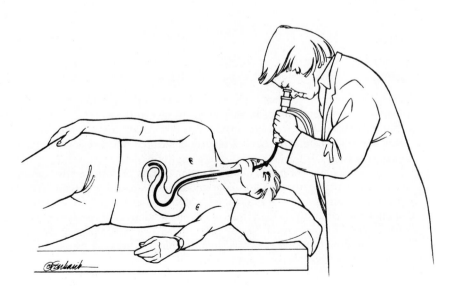

FIGURE 36–1
Patient undergoing gastric endoscopy. (From Smeltzer S, Bare B: Brunner and Suddarth's Textbook of Medical-Surgical Nursing, 7th ed. Philadelphia, JB Lippincott, 1992)

sodium morrhuate or sodium tetradecyl sulfate. These agents traumatize the endothelium, causing necrosis and eventual sclerosis of the bleeding vessel. Thermal methods of endoscopic tamponade include the heater probe, laser photocoagulation, and electrocoagulation.

Gastric Lavage

Gastric lavage may be ordered during acute bleeding episodes, but it is a controversial treatment modality. Some clinicians believe that lavage disrupts the normal body clotting mechanism over the bleeding site. Other clinicians believe it can help to clear blood from the stomach, assisting diagnosis of the cause of the bleed during endoscopy. If lavage is ordered, 1,000 to 2,000 ml of room temperature sterile normal saline or water is instilled by nasogastric tube. It is then removed by hand with a syringe or placed to intermittent suction until gastric secretions are clear. Ice lavage is not recommended, because research indicates that it causes increased bleeding. Continuous irrigation of the stomach with saline containing levarterenol is used in some institutions. The principal action of this drug is vasoconstriction. After absorption of the drug in the stomach, it is immediately sent through the portal system to the liver, where metabolism takes place. A systemic reaction is thereby prevented. The usual dilution is two ampules of levarterenol per 1,000 ml of solution.

Patients are at risk for aspiration of gastric contents related to the nasogastric tube and increased intragastric pressure from blood or gastric lavage fluid in the stomach. Monitoring for gastric distention and positioning of the patient with head elevation are nursing priorities to prevent gastric reflux. If head elevation is contraindicated, a right lateral decubitus position facilitates passage of gastric contents across the pylorus.

Administration of Pitressin

If the bleeding is due to esophageal varices or gastritis that cannot be controlled with stomach lavage or sclerotherapy, intravenous vasopressin (Pitressin) may be instituted. This drug lowers portal hypertension and therefore decreases the flow of blood at the site of bleeding. Pitressin is administered in a dose of 0.2 to 0.6 units per minute. Because it is a vasoconstrictor, it should be infused through a central line. Pitressin must be used with caution because it can cause a hypertensive state. It can also affect the urinary output because of its antidiuretic properties.

Reducing Gastric Acid

Because gastric acid is extremely irritating to bleeding sites in the upper gastrointestinal tract, it is necessary to decrease the acidity of the gastric secretions. This is accomplished by the use of the histamine (H_2)-antagonistic drugs. Examples include cimetidine (Tagamet), ranitidine hydrochloride (Zantac), and famotidine (Pepcid). These drugs decrease the production of gastric acid by inhibiting the action of histamine. A single dose decreases acid secretion for up to 5 hours. The intravenous dose of ranitidine is 50 mg diluted in 50 ml D5W every 6 hours. Intravenous cimetidine can be administered in intermittent doses of 300 mg diluted in 50 ml D5W every 6 hours or as a continuous intravenous infusion of 50 mg/hr. Best therapeutic results are achieved when a gastric pH of 4 is maintained.

Antacids are also usually ordered. Antacids act as a direct alkaline buffer and are administered to control gastric pH. The nurse is responsible for correctly aspirating gastric contents for pH and monitoring for side effects of therapy. Sucralfate, a basic aluminum salt of sucrose octasulfate, acts locally as a mucosa-protective drug and can also be ordered for stress bleeding prophylaxis.

Correcting a Hypocoagulable State

It is not unusual to find a patient with severe gastrointestinal bleeding who is having a hypocoagulable state that is due to a variety of clotting factor deficiencies. One of the foremost problems in this category is liver failure in a patient who is unable to manufacture the factors. Another common clinical situation is one of prolonged intravenous

---

Clinical Research

Rosen HR, Vlahakes GJ, Rattner DW: Fulminant peptic ulcer disease in cardiac surgery patients: Pathogenesis, prevention and management. Critical Care Medicine 20:3, 354–358, 1992

The purpose of this research study was to identify pathologic factors associated with the development of peptic ulcers in patients following cardiac surgery. A total of 9,199 patients were studied after cardiac surgery. Life-threatening complications of peptic ulcers were defined as hemorrhage of >2 units of packed red blood cells requiring therapeutic intervention.

The development of peptic ulcers as a complication of postoperative cardiac surgery correlated with age, the need for reoperation, and decreased perfusion. The use of prophylactic treatments such as histamine H_2 blockers and antacids to suppress acid secretion did not correlate with the development of complications. This study suggests that factors which directly impair blood flow to gastric mucosa and the ability of the mucosal defense systems to prevent hydrochloric acid from reaching the mucosa are most important in the development of postoperative peptic ulcers.

feedings in patients who have been on multiple antibiotics and who are subsequently vitamin K deficient. Regardless of the cause, one must correct this situation to try to reduce the amount of bleeding. Vitamin K can be given in the form of phytonadione (AquaMEPHYTON), 10 mg intramuscularly or, very slowly, intravenously, in an attempt to restore the prothrombin time to normal. If other major factor deficiencies are thought to exist, fresh frozen plasma is ordered to correct the abnormality.

Balloon Tamponade

Esophageal varices should be suspected in the patient who has been addicted to alcohol and who presents with upper gastrointestinal bleeding. To control the hemorrhage from the varices, if it is not responsive to other therapy, pressure is exerted on the cardia of the stomach and against the bleeding varices by a double-balloon tamponade (the Sengstaken–Blakemore tube; Fig. 36–2).

After the tube is positioned in the stomach, the stomach balloon is inflated with no more than 50 ml of air. The tube is then slowly withdrawn until the gastric balloon fits snugly against the cardia of the stomach. After it is determined by radiograph examination that the gastric balloon is in the right place, at the cardia and not in the esophagus, the gastric balloon can be further inflated—up to the desired amount without surpassing the balloon's capacity. Traction is then placed on the tube where it enters the patient. This can be achieved by means of a piece of sponge rubber, as shown in Figure 36–2, or by traction fixed to a head helmet device or foot of bed.

If bleeding continues, the esophageal balloon is inflated to a pressure of 25 to 40 mm Hg and maintained at this pressure for 24 to 48 hours. Pressure for longer than 24 hours can cause edema, esophagitis, ulcerations, or perforation of the esophagus.

SENGSTAKEN-BLAKEMORE TUBE

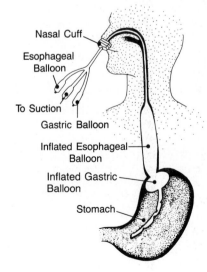

Nasal Cuff
Esophageal Balloon
To Suction
Gastric Balloon
Inflated Esophageal Balloon
Inflated Gastric Balloon
Stomach

FIGURE 36–2
Sengstaken-Blakemore tube.

The potential dangers of this treatment require constant observation and intelligent care. It is essential that the three tube openings be identified, correctly labeled, and checked for patency before insertion. The pressures in the balloons must be maintained, and the balloons must be kept in their proper positions. If the gastric balloon ruptures, the entire tube could rise into the nasopharynx and completely obstruct the airway. A pair of scissors should be readily available at the bedside. The tube should be cut immediately to deflate the balloons rapidly, and the entire tube should be removed whenever a question of respiratory insufficiency or aspiration occurs. If the patient is agitated and restless, it is wise to restrain his or her arms prophylactically to prevent dislodging the tube.

Nursing Care. Nursing care of a patient with a Sengstaken–Blakemore tube in place involves skillful application of knowledge:

> The person is kept at complete rest, because exertion, such as coughing or straining, tends to increase intra-abdominal pressure, which predisposes to further bleeding.
>
> The head of the bed is kept elevated to reduce the flow of blood into the portal system and to prevent reflux into the esophagus.
>
> Because the person is unable to swallow, saliva must be suctioned frequently from the upper esophagus.
>
> The nasopharynx also needs frequent suctioning due to the increased secretions resulting from irritation by the tube. A nasogastric tube can be inserted into the esophagus to the top of the esophageal balloon to control these secretions and to prevent their aspiration into the lungs.
>
> The nasogastric tube should be irrigated every 2 hours to ensure its patency and to keep the stomach empty.
>
> The nostrils are checked frequently, cleansed, and lubricated to prevent tube-caused pressure areas.

Persons with liver damage tolerate the breakdown products of blood in the intestinal tract very poorly. Therefore, it is imperative that blood *not be* allowed to remain in the person's stomach, because it will migrate into the intestinal tract. Bacterial action on the blood in the intestinal tract produces ammonia, which is absorbed into the bloodstream. The ability of the liver to convert ammonia to urea is impaired, and ammonia intoxication ensues (see Chapter 37).

Surgical Therapies

Surgery is considered for patients who have massive bleeding that is immediately life-threatening, and for patients who continue to bleed despite aggressive medical therapies. Surgical therapies for peptic ulcer disease or stress

(*Text continues on page 846*)

NURSING CARE PLAN 36–1:
The Patient With Gastrointestinal Bleeding

NURSING DIAGNOSIS	OUTCOME CRITERIA/ PATIENT GOALS	NURSING INTERVENTIONS
Fluid volume deficit: related to acute blood loss, rapid volume replacement with crystalloid fluids.	• Patient will remain hemodynamically stable.	1. Monitor vital signs q h and prn. 2. Monitor hemodynamic values (ie, PAS, PAD, PCWP, CI, CO, SVR, CVP). 3. Measure urine output q1h. 4. Measure intake and output and assess balance. 5. Administer replacement fluids and blood products as ordered. Monitor for adverse reactions to component therapy (eg, transfusion reaction). 6. Complete bedrest. Place patient in supine position with legs elevated to increase preload if patient is hypotensive. If normotensive, place HOB at 45 degrees to prevent aspiration of gastric contents. 7. Minimize blood taken for laboratory analysis. 8. Monitor hemoglobin and hematocrit. 9. Monitor electrolytes which may be lost with fluids or altered due to fluid loss or shift. 10. Test stool for blood for 72 hours after acute episode.
Impaired gas exchange: related to decreased oxygen carrying capacity and to aspiration risk factors.	• Patient will maintain adequate oxygenation and gas exchange.	1. Monitor SaO_2 with oximetry or ABGs. 2. Monitor breath sounds and pulmonary symptoms. 3. Use supplemental O_2, as ordered. 4. Monitor temperature. 5. Monitor for abdominal distention. 6. Position patient with head of bed up if at all possible. 7. Maintain functioning and patency of nasogastric catheter as appropriate. 8. Treat nausea promptly.

(continued)

NURSING CARE PLAN 36–1: (Continued)
The Patient With Gastrointestinal Bleeding

NURSING DIAGNOSIS	OUTCOME CRITERIA/ PATIENT GOALS	NURSING INTERVENTIONS
High risk for infection: related to intravenous lines(s).	• Patient will not acquire a nosocomial infection.	1. Maintain stable intravenous line. Anchor intravenous appliance and tubing securely. 2. Assess temperature q4h. 3. Monitor intravenous system for patency, infiltration, and signs of infection (localized pain, inflammation, fever, sepsis). 4. Change intravenous site q48–72h and prn. 5. Change intravenous solution at least q24h. 6. Monitor insertion site every shift. 7. Document tubing, dressing changes, and appearance of insertion site. 8. Use aseptic technique when changing dressings and tubings. Maintain an occlusive, transparent, sterile dressing. 9. Assess WBC for elevation. 10. Remove and culture all catheters if signs and symptoms of infection occur.
Anxiety: related to critical illness, fear of death or disfigurement, role changes within social setting, or permanent disability.	• Patient will express anxieties to appropriate resource person. • Patient will begin to identify source of anxiety.	1. Provide environment that encourages open discussion of emotional issues. 2. Mobilize patient's support system and involve these resources as appropriate. 3. Allow time for patient to express self. Actively listen. 4. Provide simple explanations of events and environmental stimuli. 5. Identify possible hospital resources for patient/family support. 6. Encourage open family-to-nurse communications regarding emotional issues. 7. Validate patient and family knowledge base regarding the critical illness. 8. Involve religious support systems as appropriate.

BILLROTH I & II PROCEDURES

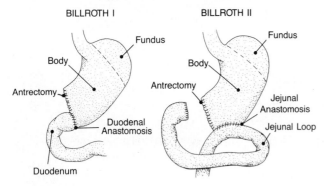

FIGURE 36–3
Billroth I & II Procedures.

ulcers include gastric resection (antrectomy), gastrectomy, gastroenterostomy, or combined surgeries to restore gastrointestinal continuity. A vagotomy decreases gastric acid secretion. An antrectomy removes acid-producing cells in the stomach. Billroth I is a procedure that includes a vagotomy and antrectomy with anastomosis of the stomach to the duodenum. A Billroth II involves a vagotomy, a resection of the antrum, and anastomosis of the stomach to the jejunum (Fig. 36–3). A gastric perforation can be surgically treated by simple closure or use of a patch to cover the mucosal hole.

Surgical decompression of portal hypertension can be used in patients with esophageal or gastric varices. In this surgery, called a portal caval shunt, a connection is made between the portal vein and the inferior vena cava that diverts blood flow into the vena cava to decrease pressure.

Nursing Management

Nurses coordinate the multidisciplinary team efforts for the patient with acute gastrointestinal bleeding. Nursing priorities include performing assessments, monitoring activities to detect changes in the patient's condition, reporting activities, and carrying out of orders for treatment. Nursing is also specifically concerned with the patient's psychosocial response to the bleeding episode. Common patient responses during the acute phase include fear and anxiety. These responses to the disease need to be incorporated into the nursing plan of care along with physiological problems. The patient's need for information is also especially high during this time.

A case study describing Mr. Lane's gastrointestinal bleed follows. Next, a plan of care is presented in Nursing Care Plan 36–1 as an example of the nursing management of a patient, such as Mr. Lane, who has an acute gastrointestinal bleed.

CASE STUDY

Mr. Lane is a 45-year-old male admitted from the emergency room to the ICU with an admitting diagnosis of upper gastroin-

testinal bleeding. Earlier in the day he had vomited what he described as a large amount of coffee-ground emesis. He also reported passing one to two maroon-colored stools per rectum. He reported nausea and weakness accompanied by a dull pain in the epigastric region on admission. Mr. Lane reports a previous history of peptic ulcer disease and has been hospitalized twice in the past 18 months for active GI bleeding. A duodenal ulcer near the pylorus was diagnosed by endoscopy at that time. Both episodes required blood transfusions and were controlled with medical management. Significant risk factors include a family history of peptic ulcers disease, social alcohol use, and a 20-year, one pack per day smoking history.

His admission assessment revealed the following:

BP lying 90/60, sitting 78/50; HR 120, sinus tachycardia with rare PVC's; no S3,S4; RR 25/min deep; scattered rhonchi with wheezing anteriorly; Temp 96.6 R. Alert; oriented × 3; anxious.

Skin: diaphoretic, pale mucous membranes. No edema. Peripheral pulses present, equal, thready.

GI: abdomen distended with hyperactive bowel sound in all 4 quadrants. Very tender RUQ; liver border WNL.

Significant admission laboratory results were as follows:

Hct 25, Hgb 7, WBC 17,000;

Coag panel and Liver function tests WNL;

Na 145, K 2, Creat 0.8, BUN 40, Glucose 210;

pH 7.48, PaCO₂ 32, PaO₂ 58, Sat 89%.

Three 16-gauge peripheral IVs were inserted, and lactated Ringer's solution was infused at 200 ml/hr. A Salem sump nasogastric tube was inserted with an immediate return of 800 ml of coffee-ground, guaiac-positive drainage. Mr. Lane was typed and crossmatched for 8 units of packed red blood cells (PRBC). Oxygen was delivered at 2 liters through a nasal cannula. A 16 Fr indwelling bladder catheter was inserted with an immediate return of 50 ml of dark amber urine. The GI service was consulted for an emergency endoscopy.

BIBLIOGRAPHY

Doglio G et al: Gastric mucosal pH as a prognostic index of mortality in critically ill patients. Crit Care Med 19(8): 1037–1040, 1991

Eisenberg P: Monitoring gastric pH to prevent stress ulcer syndrome. Focus Crit Care 17(4):316–322, 1990

Konopad E, Noseworthy T: Stress ulceration: A serious complication in critically ill patients. Heart Lung 17(4):339–348, 1988

Peterson WL: GI bleeding. In Sleisenger MH, Fordtran JS (eds): Gastrointestinal Disease: Pathophysiology, Diagnosis and Management vol. 1, 4th ed, pp 397–427. Philadelphia, PA, WB Saunders, 1989

Rosen H, Vlahakes G, Rattner D: Fulminant peptic ulcer disease in cardiac surgery patients: Pathogenesis, prevention and management. Crit Care Med 20(3):354–359, 1992

Wardell TL: Assessing and managing a gastric ulcer. Nursing 21(3):34–41, 1991

STUDY QUESTIONS

1. Which of the following patient assessment parameters most accurately help the nurse to estimate the volume loss in a patient who is actively bleeding from the gastrointestinal tract?

    a. vital signs
    b. hematocrit
    c. urine output
    d. amount of hematemesis

2. The most important goal in the initial management of an active upper gastrointestinal bleed is

    a. preparing the patient for surgery
    b. administering intra-arterial vasopressin to decrease blood flow to the area
    c. replacing volume losses to stabilize hemodynamics
    d. administering intravenous histamine antagonists to decrease bleeding from the initiating site

3. The greatest danger from rupture or sudden deflation of the gastric balloon of the Sengstaken–Blakemore tube is

    a. tearing of the cardiac sphincter
    b. upward movement of the tube with obstruction of the airway
    c. excessive pressure on the nares with necrosis
    d. damage to the esophagus with formation of tracheoesophageal fistula

CHAPTER 37

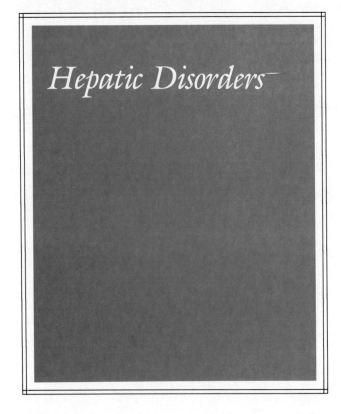

Hepatic Disorders

BEHAVIORAL OBJECTIVES

Based on the content of this chapter, the reader should be able to:

1. Identify four types of hepatitis.
2. Describe two liver disorders and their respective symptoms.
3. Identify five nursing diagnoses for the patient with liver failure.
4. Identify five nursing interventions for each nursing diagnosis.

Hudak: Critical Care Nursing:
A Holistic Approach, 6th ed. © 1994
J. B. Lippincott Company.

Description

Disease processes in the liver can affect the parenchyma, Kupffer's cells, bile ducts, and blood vessels. If severe, disease can lead to fulminant liver failure. Causes of liver failure include hepatitis and cirrhotic liver disease. Pathophysiology, assessment, and collaborative management of each of these diseases are discussed. The nursing plan of care for patients with liver failure is also presented.

Hepatitis

Pathophysiology

Diffuse inflammation of the liver (hepatitis) can be caused by infections from viruses and by toxic reactions to drugs and chemicals. The basic functional unit of the liver is called a lobule, and it is unique in that it has its own blood supply (see Chapter 33). As inflammation in the liver progresses, the normal pattern of the liver is disturbed. This interrupts the normal blood supply to liver cells, causing necrosis and breakdown of cells. Over time, liver cells that become damaged are removed from the body by the immune system response and replaced with healthy liver cells. Therefore, most patients with hepatitis do recover with normal liver function. The viral infections of liver parenchyma have been classified according to their specific infecting agent. There are four types of acute viral hepatitis: A, B, non-A non-B (C), and delta (D).

Hepatitis A

Type A, formerly known as infectious hepatitis, is transmitted by the fecal–oral route. The organism is also foodborne and waterborne; hence shellfish are also associated with transmission. Type A hepatitis can be epidemic in nature. The clinical course usually runs 1 to 3 months. Recovery is usually complete and does not lead to chronic hepatitis or cirrhosis. In rare instances, type A hepatitis can lead to fulminating liver failure.

Hepatitis B

Type B hepatitis is spread by contact with blood or blood products. Some of the more common mechanisms of transmission are through the parenteral route, such as through blood transfusions, needle-stick injuries in medical personnel, and the use of contaminated needles by drug addicts. However, a significant number of patients contract type B hepatitis through non-parenteral routes. The antigen has been identified in body secretions such as semen, mucus, and saliva; therefore, sexual exposure to a person with type B hepatitis can result in infection. Maternal perinatal exposure also occurs. It appears that a break in the skin or the mucous membrane is necessary for the transmission to occur.

Chronic active hepatitis is seen in 10% of the patients who have type B hepatitis. They continue to have high levels of surface antigen and can be infective to others. The degree of liver impairment in chronic active hepatitis is variable from mild to serious and can progress to cirrhosis. This type of hepatitis is the leading cause of fulminant liver failure.

Non-A Non-B Hepatitis

The transmission and clinical course of non-A non-B hepatitis are similar to those for type B hepatitis. These patients, however, tend to develop chronic hepatitis with a greater frequency than patients with type B hepatitis. A significant percentage of patients with non-A non-B hepatitis develop fulminant hepatic failure, but the percentage is less than that of patients with type B hepatitis.

Clinical Research

McMahon BJ, Helminiak C, Wainwright RB, Bulkow L: Frequency of adverse reactions to hepatitis B vaccine in 43,618 persons. Am J Med 92:254–256, 1992

The purpose of this study was to determine the incidence of adverse reactions to hepatitis B plasma derived vaccine. Subjects were 43,618 native Alaskans who worked for the Indian Health Service and received 101,360 doses of the vaccine. Thirty-nine adverse reactions to Hepatovax (Merck, Sharp & Dohme) were reported to healthcare providers—an incidence of less than 1 in 1,000. The most frequent reactions were myalgia and arthralgia lasting for more than 3 days, dizziness, and rash. The incidence of adverse reactions might have been slightly underestimated because subjects were not contacted after each injection but rather were to report symptoms.

A serious adverse reaction, Guillain–Barré syndrome, occurred slightly less often than in the general unvaccinated population. This low incidence should allay fears that the hepatitis B vaccine causes a disporportionate number of serious adverse reactions.

Delta Hepatitis

Hepatitis D (delta hepatitis) always occurs in the presence of hepatitis B and relies on this virus to spread. This type of hepatitis is transmitted in the same way as hepatitis B.

Drug-Induced Hepatitis

The picture of viral hepatitis can be mimicked both clinically and pathologically by a drug-induced hepatitis. This actually results from a toxic reaction to the liver cells from either the drug itself or one of its metabolites.

The major drugs involved in toxic reactions include the halogenated anesthetic agents such as halothane, the antihypertensive medication methyldopa, the antituberculosis medication isoniazid, and the phenytoins such as phenytoin (Dilantin). Most of these medications cause their toxicity through intermediate metabolites of the drug and rarely by their direct effect on the hepatocytes. There also can be a hypersensitivity reaction to the drug or to one of its metabolites. Acetaminophen and aspirin are other medications that can cause some degree of hepatic toxicity. The acetaminophen toxicity can be overwhelming and fatal because of the toxic effect of its metabolites on the liver cells (see Chapter 46).

Assessment

Hepatitis A

Hepatitis A (HA) is diagnosed by the presence of hepatitis A antibodies (anti-HAV) in the blood. These antibodies occur within 2 to 6 weeks and remain in the blood serum indefinitely. These initial antibodies are of the IgM class of immunoglobulins and indicate a current active infection. Later, these are replaced by the IgG class, and this indicates immunity to HA. As parenchymal cells are injured, various intracellular enzymes called transaminases are released into the blood. The most common of these transaminases are the serum glutamic-oxaloacetic transaminase (SGOT) and serum glutamic-pyruvic transaminase (SGPT). Therefore, high transaminase levels are found in hepatitis A. Liver function tests are listed in Table 37–1.

Other signs and symptoms of HA are listed in Table 37–2. Early in the course of the disease, there is an incubation period during which the patient is asymptomatic but highly contagious. After symptoms are apparent, the virus can be misdiagnosed because many of the symptoms are similar to those of the flu. Some patients seek medical attention because they become jaundiced. Acute symptoms can progress or disappear once jaundice is present. It is important to note that by the time the patient presents with symptoms of hepatitis, he or she is no longer shedding the virus in the stool and is generally not infectious. Recovery is signaled by liver function tests returning to normal.

Hepatitis B

There are three antigens identified with type B hepatitis: surface antigen, core antigen, and "e" antigen. Hepatitis B surface antigen (HBsAg) is the first to rise in the patient's blood and is usually present at the time the SGOT and SGPT are rising. As the patient improves, the transaminase levels and the level of HBsAg decrease. Usually as the patient's clinical condition improves, the surface antibody (anti-HBs) rises. Core antigen and core antibody titers are useful in determining a previous infection with type B hepatitis after the surface antigen is negative. "E" antigen (HBeAg) is useful in determining patients who are the most infectious. Patients with "e" antigens usually have very active liver disease which can be either acute or chronic. Those with high antibody to "e" antigen have a tendency to be carriers for long time.

Clinical signs and symptoms for hepatitis B (HB) during the acute phase are the same as for HA. There is, however, a greater risk of patients with HB developing fulminant hepatic failure, which is characterized by sudden degeneration of the liver and loss of all normal liver functions. The most important clinical sign is a decrease in liver size.

Prophylactic measures for hepatitis A and B virus are available both before and after exposure to the virus. Preexposure prophylaxis is recommended to persons traveling to countries where hepatitis A is prevalent. Hepatitis B vaccine is recommended for all medical personnel at risk for exposure to blood and body fluids.

Non-A Non-B Hepatitis

There are no specific tests for non-A non-B hepatitis, and the diagnosis is one of exclusion (eg, type A and type B hepatitis have been ruled out by blood tests, and the patient has an acute episode of hepatitis). Clinical signs and symptoms are similar to those listed for hepatitis A.

Management

There is no specific treatment for the viral hepatitis infections. Treatment is primarily supportive and includes providing rest and adequate nutrition and preventing further stress on the liver through avoiding hepatotoxic medications and substances. Hospitalization is rarely required. Maintaining adequate nutrition is a priority. A high carbohydrate diet is recommended in order to supply enough calories.

Intravenous feedings are needed only if oral intake is limited by nausea and vomiting. Patients with severe fatigue require frequent rest and spacing of activities. If jaundice becomes excessive and subsequent pruritus becomes unbearable, a bile salt sequestering agent, cholestyramine, can be used to help alleviate this symptom. Toxic hepatitis is treated primarily by avoidance of the offending agent.

TABLE 37–1
Liver Function Tests

Tests	Normal Values	Comments
Protein Studies	**(g/100 ml)**	
Total (Serum)	6.5–8	
Albumin	4–5.5	Albumin is a major part of total blood proteins. It is important in the maintenance of osmotic pressure between blood and tissue.
Globulins	2–3	Globulins are needed for the production of antibodies and to help maintain osmotic pressure.
Fibrinogen	0.2–0.4	Fibrinogen is necessary in the coagulation process.
Electrophoresis	*(percent of 100% total protein)*	
Albumin	53%	Electrophoresis separates the various protein fractions by an electric current. In parenchymal liver cell disease, the amounts of serum proteins is depressed or the ratio of the proteins to each other is altered.
α globulins	14%	
β globulins	12%	
γ globulins	20%	
Prothrombin Time	12–15 seconds	Prothrombin is synthesized to thrombin (in the absence of vitamin K) by the liver. This test is a good index of prognosis, because a prolonged prothrombin time is indicative of severe function loss.
Enzyme Studies		
SGOT	10–40 units	Transaminases are catalysts in the breakdown of amino acids. SGPT is the specific enzyme released by damaged liver cells. LDH is present in large amounts in liver tissue.
SGPT	5–35 units	
LDH	165–300 units	
Alkaline phosphatase	2–5 Bodansky units	This enzyme hydrolyzes phosphate esters and is useful in differential diagnosis if jaundice is present. It is excreted through the biliary tract. If it is elevated, nucleotidase and leucine amino peptidase will determine whether elevation is due to biliary obstruction.
Gamma glutamyle transferase	0–30 IU	This endothelia enzyme is found in the liver and closely follows elevations in alkaline phosphatase.
Bilirubin		
Total	0.9–2.2 mg/100 ml (0.8 mg/dl)	This test measures the ability of the liver to conjugate and excrete bilirubin. If the conjugated bilirubin is low and the unconjugated high, a preliver block is indicated. If the conjugated bilirubin is high and the unconjugated normal or low, a postliver block is indicated.
Conjugated (direct)	0.5–1.4 mg/100 ml (0.6 mg/dl)	
Unconjugated (indirect)	0.4–0.8 mg/100 ml (0.2 mg/dl)	
Isotope Liver Scans		Radionuclide scanning of the liver helps define liver cell function and replacement of active liver cells with nonfunctioning tissue, such as scar tissue secondary to cirrhosis, tumors, and abscesses.
CT Liver Scanning		CT scanning is an adjunct that helps define space-occupying lesions within the liver, such as tumors and abscesses. It may be more specific for the finding of tumors and less helpful than the nuclide scanning in the determination of liver cell function.

After exposure to *hepatitis A virus*, passive immunization can be achieved through the use of immune serum globulin. Most preparations of immune serum globulin contain adequate quantities of anti-HAV. The immune serum globulin may not entirely abort an infection, but it significantly ameliorates the symptoms. It is usually given to intimate contacts of patients with hepatitis A.

Hepatitis B exposure carries a much greater risk to the exposed person. After accidental exposure, such as an inadvertent needle stick, passive immunoprophylaxis can be achieved by using high anti-HBs titer hepatitis B immune globulin (HBIG). This is a pooled serum containing high titers of the antihepatitis B immune globulin. It is recommended only for postexposure inoculations of high-risk patients.

Fortunately a vaccine exists for active immunization

TABLE 37–2
Common Signs and Symptoms
of Type A Hepatitis

Brown urine
Depression
Loss of appetite
Nausea and vomiting
Fever
Weakness
Chills
Headache
Right upper quadrant pain
Irritability
Clay-colored feces

against hepatitis B (Recombivax-HB, Engerix-B). This vaccine, administered prophylactically over a 6-month period, provides active immunization against hepatitis B. It is highly recommended for health care personnel whose risk of infection with hepatitis B is substantial. It is also recommended for persons who have had intimate contacts with persons already infected with hepatitis B. All nursing personnel who have the potential of needle sticks should be immunized against hepatitis B. Precautions to protect against exposure to bloodborne pathogens must be followed.

Alcoholic Cirrhosis of the Liver

Pathophysiology

The toxic effects of alcohol on the liver cause severe alterations in the structure and function of liver cells. These changes are characterized by inflammation and liver cell necrosis which can be focal or diffuse. Fatty deposits within the parenchymal cells may be seen initially. The cause of the fatty changes is unclear, but it may be a response to alterations in enzymatic function responsible for normal fat metabolism.

The enlarged liver cells cause compression of the liver lobule, leading to increased resistance to blood flow. Hypertension in the portal system results. With sufficient back pressure on the portal system, collateral circulation develops and allows blood to flow from the intestines directly to the vena cava. The increased blood flow to the veins of the esophagus leads to esophageal varices; of the gastric veins, gastric varices; of the spleen, splenomegaly; and of the hemorrhoidal veins, hemorrhoids.

Necrosis is followed by regeneration of liver tissue, but not in a normal fashion. Fibrous tissue is laid down over time which distorts the normal architecture of the liver lobule. These fibrotic changes are irreversible, resulting in chronic liver dysfunction and eventual liver failure.

Assessment

Portal hypertension associated with liver failure results in high cardiac output failure. Clinical signs and symptoms of this disorder are identical to those of heart failure and include jugular vein distention, lung congestion, and decreased perfusion to organs. Initially, the patient may have hypertension, flushed skin, and bounding pulses. As perfusion to organs falls, hypotension and dysrhythmias are common. Increased portal venous pressure causes the formation of varices which are problematic because they can rupture and cause massive upper gastrointestinal bleeding (see Chapter 36).

Liver dysfunction results in disruption of its metabolic processes. Altered carbohydrate, fat, and protein metabolism results. Clinical signs include decreased synthesis of blood clotting factors, decreased removal of activated clotting components, decreased metabolism of vitamins and iron, and decreased ability of the liver to detoxify substances. Loss of the ability to convert ammonia to urea results in impaired ammonia metabolism. Altered carbohydrate metabolism can result in unstable blood sugars. Altered fat metabolism can cause fatigue and decreased activity tolerance. Protein metabolism is also decreased. Albumin synthesis is decreased. Albumin is necessary for colloid osmotic pressure to hold fluid in the intravascular space. Globulin, another protein, is essential for normal blood clotting. This, coupled with a decreased synthesis of many blood clotting factors, predisposes the patient to hematological complications. Clinical signs and symptoms can range from bruising to frank hemorrhage. The patient can also develop disseminated intravascular coagulation (see Chapter 43).

The liver's inability to metabolize bile is reflected clinically in an elevated serum bilirubin and staining of tissue by bilirubin (jaundice). Jaundice can occur from the liver cells' inability to excrete bile or from obstruction of the bile ducts. Generally, jaundice is present with any bilirubin greater than 3 mg/dl.

Management

Management of the patient in liver failure is aimed at supportive therapies and early recognition and treatment of complications associated with the disease. Treatment of these patients consists of:

- supporting cardiopulmonary status
- intervening if assistance is required to maintain specific function (ie, fluid balance)
- supporting hematologic and nutritional functions of the liver

The patient in liver failure often arrives in ICU in some state of unconsciousness with jaundiced skin and sclera. Coagulation times are prolonged, so bleeding is apt to occur from many sources. Mild sores, if not present, can develop because of the debilitated state of the patient.

Nursing care is determined by a careful assessment that includes a nursing history, a physical examination, laboratory results, and the medical regimen. The plan of care must consider fluid and dietary requirements, replacement therapy, prevention of infection, caution in drug administration, potential for bleeding disorders and for neurological changes, possible bowel cleansing requirements, and prevention of respiratory, circulatory, and skin complications.

Maintaining fluid and electrolyte balance requires constant nursing consideration. Imbalance can result from replacement therapy, malnutrition, gastric suction, diuretics, vomiting, diaphoresis, ascites, diarrhea (which many times is induced), inadequate fluid intake, and elevated aldosterone levels. The patient may complain of headache, weakness, numbness and tingling of extremities, muscle twitching, thirst, nausea, or muscle cramps, and may become confused. The nurse should frequently assess all systems for changes. Observe for an increase or decrease in urinary output, cardiac dysrhythmias, changes in mental status including stupor or coma, prolonged vomiting or frequent liquid stools, muscle tremors, spasms, edema, or poor skin turgor.

By continuously evaluating the effectiveness of the nursing interventions, the plan of care can be changed whenever interventions are no longer necessary or effective or if new problems arise requiring new interventions (see Nursing Care Plan 37–1).

Complications

Ascites

Impaired handling of salt and water by the kidney and other abnormalities in fluid homeostasis predispose the patient to an accumulation of fluid in the peritoneum (ie, ascites). This complication can be problematic because it can impair movement of the diaphragm, causing impairment of the patient's breathing pattern. Vigilant assessment of respiratory status is critical. Ascites is medically managed through bedrest, a low sodium diet, fluid restriction, and diuretic therapy. Careful monitoring of electrolyte balance is important with diuretic administration. Paracentesis is another medical therapy to treat ascites; in this procedure, ascitic fluid is withdrawn from the abdomen through a percutaneous needle aspiration. Close monitoring of vital signs is important during this procedure because sudden loss of intravascular pressure and tachycardia can occur.

Peritoneal–venous shunt is a surgical procedure used to relieve ascites that is resistant to other therapies. The Leveen shunt is inserted by placing the distal end of a tube under the peritoneum and tunneling the other end into a central vein (eg, superior vena cava). This allows for ascitic fluid to flow into the central vein (Fig. 37–1).

Hepatic Encephalopathy

Patients with severe liver disease can progress to hepatic encephalopathy. Clinically, they start with a quiet delirium or stupor and then can progress to profound coma. Sometimes, they become very agitated and difficult to manage. Often, they have a characteristic hyperventilation syndrome with a respiratory alkalosis.

The cause of the hepatic encephalopathy and the hyperventilation syndrome is probably related to toxic agents absorbed from the intestinal tract. Elevated serum ammonia and some amino acids have been implicated as these agents. The amino acids can act as false neurotransmitters and contribute to the encephalopathic state.

Those with portal systemic shunts can develop hepatic encephalopathy quite rapidly, and they often hemorrhage from esophageal varices or other sites in the gastrointestinal tract. The hemorrhage produces a significant nitrogenous load to the intestinal tract in the form of blood, from which bacterial deamination produces the ammonia. Normally, this ammonia is detoxified to urea by the liver. If the liver is unable to perform this detoxification or if a good portion of the portal blood is shunted around the liver, the circulating level of ammonia rises. If ammonia and the other toxic agents can be reduced through effective therapy, the encephalopathy gradually clears.

Measures to decrease ammonia production are necessary in the treatment of this disorder. Protein intake is limited to 20 to 40 g/day. Neomycin and lactulose are two drugs that can be administered to reduce bacterial breakdown of protein in the bowel. Nursing measures to pro-

(*Text continues on page 857*)

THE LeVEEN SHUNT

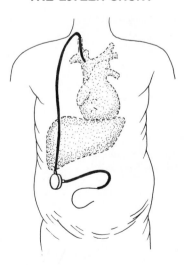

FIGURE 37–1
The Leveen shunt.

NURSING CARE PLAN 37–1:
The Patient With Hepatic Failure

NURSING DIAGNOSIS	OUTCOME CRITERIA/ PATIENT GOALS	NURSING INTERVENTIONS
Altered nutrition less than body requirements: related to altered liver metabolism of food nutrients, impaired absorption of fat-soluble vitamins, decreased appetite.	• Nutritional needs of patient will be met.	1. Limit protein intake; provide calories with carbohydrates and fats. 2. Offer small, frequent feedings. 3. Provide oral hygiene, especially before eating. 4. Administer vitamins synthesized by liver. 5. Consider enteral nutrition if oral intake is insufficient. 6. Monitor parameters of nutritional status (ie, albumin, nitrogen balance, BUN).
Altered thought processes: related to impaired medication metabolism, impaired ammonia metabolism, aggressive diuretic therapy.	• Patient will remain alert and oriented.	1. Administer cleansing enemas and cathartics to keep bowel empty. 2. Observe for changes in mentation (eg, confusion, lethargy, hallucination). 3. Administer oral non-absorbant antibiotics (neomycin) to decrease bacteria in colon. 4. Administer lactulose to decrease intestinal pH and increase ammonia excretion. 5. Monitor patient response to diuretic therapy. 6. Monitor patient response to therapy by monitoring serum ammonia levels and through neurologic assessments. 7. Observe for asterixis. 8. Judicious use of medications metabolized by the liver. 9. Provide for safety of patient during periods of mental status changes. 10. Re-orient patient.
Fluid volume excess: related to sodium excess and hypo-albuminemia.	• Patient will remain uvolemic and will not experience weight gain.	1. Monitor daily weight. 2. Monitor and evaluate intake and output. 3. Monitor vital signs for overload (eg, heart sounds for gallop, breath sounds for crackles).

(continued)

NURSING CARE PLAN 37–1: *(Continued)*
The Patient With Hepatic Failure

NURSING DIAGNOSIS	OUTCOME CRITERIA/ PATIENT GOALS	NURSING INTERVENTIONS
		4. Observe external jugular vein for distention.
		5. Check for signs of dyspnea or orthopnea.
		6. Assess edema.
		7. Assess, instruct, encourage regarding fluid, sodium, and protein restrictions.
		8. Monitor patient response to diuretics if ordered.
		9. Monitor chest x-ray for signs of vascular congestion.
Altered comfort: related to excessive bilirubin pigments in blood that infiltrate and irritate the skin, abdominal distention.	• Skin will remain intact. • Skin will remain moist. • Patient will experience decreased puritus.	1. Bathe skin with cool water; blot dry. 2. Maintain a cool environment. 3. Maintain fluid intake. 4. Lubricate skin. 5. Apply antipruritic medication prn. 6. Use light covers, possibly over a bed cradle. 7. Turn q2h. Position for comfort. 8. Observe skin for areas of potential breakdown. 9. Medicate with analgesics, as ordered.
High risk for impaired skin integrity: related to altered nutrition, mobility, mental status, and fluid balance.	• Patient will maintain intact skin.	1. Assess risk for skin breakdown and intervene to reduce contributing factors. 2. Establish a repositioning schedule, position as flat as possible to relieve key pressure points without interfering with breathing. 3. Teach/assist patient to shift weight or reposition as scheduled. When moving/turning patient, use technique and assistance to lift rather than slide. Avoid wrinkles in bed clothes. 4. Gently massage areas not reddened or edematous with each position change.

(continued)

NURSING CARE PLAN 37–1: (Continued)
The Patient With Hepatic Failure

NURSING DIAGNOSIS	OUTCOME CRITERIA/ PATIENT GOALS	NURSING INTERVENTIONS
		5. Inspect pressure points for erythema, blanching, warmth, texture, and other evidence of pressure shearing.
		6. Consider footboard and use of pressure relief overlay, mattress or bed, depending upon risk for breakdown.
		7. Perform or oversee passive or active movement (eg, ROM, ambulation) depending on patient condition.
High risk for infection: related to loss of function of Kupffer's cells in fighting infection.	• Patient will not exhibit signs or symptoms of infection. • WBCs, will remain within normal limits.	1. Maintain aseptic technique when performing procedures. 2. Maintain sterility of invasive lines and tubes. 3. Observe invasive sites for signs of infection. 4. Change invasive lines q72h. 5. Monitor temperature, WBC count, and chest x-ray results. 6. Culture all suspicious drainage. 7. Administer antibiotics as ordered.
Impaired gas exchange: related to prolonged bedrest and immobility, changes in mentation, ascites.	• Patient will have adequate gas exchange and oxygenation.	1. Monitor respiratory status through physical assessment and correlate with arterial blood gas results. 2. Assist patient with coughing, deep breathing. 3. Administer O_2 as ordered. 4. Administer sedatives and analgesics cautiously. 5. Monitor fluid status. 6. Monitor abdominal girth with ascites. 7. Use SaO_2 monitor (ie, oximeter). 8. Monitor chest x-ray results.
High risk for injury: related to complications of cirrhosis, variceal bleeding, coagulation disturbances, hepatorenal syndrome.	• Patient will expect complications to be prevented or minimized.	1. Inspect for signs of bleeding (eg, gastric contents, stools, urine) and test for occult blood. Observe for petechiae, bruising. 2. Monitor vital signs and hemodynamic pressures.

(continued)

NURSING CARE PLAN 37–1: *(Continued)*
The Patient With Hepatic Failure

NURSING DIAGNOSIS	OUTCOME CRITERIA/ PATIENT GOALS	NURSING INTERVENTIONS
		3. Assess intake and output, observing for a decrease in urinary output without changes in intake. *4.* Monitor HCT, HGB, clotting factors, and tests for renal function (eg, BUN, creatinine). *5.* Administer blood and blood products as ordered. *6.* Assist with treatments such as paracentesis, insertion of Sengstaken-Blakemore tube. Provide gastric lavage as ordered.

tect the patient with mental status changes from harm are a priority.

Hepatorenal Syndrome

Acute renal failure that occurs with liver failure is called hepatorenal syndrome. The pathophysiology of this disorder is not well understood. Decreased urine output and elevated serum creatinine are clinical signs. The prognosis for the patient is generally poor once renal failure is evident. Management goals include therapies to support liver and kidney functions.

BIBLIOGRAPHY

Aach R: Update on viral hepatitis. Patient Care 24(19):14–18, 26–30, 33, 1990

Chmielewski C: Case study: End stage liver failure patient managed with CAVH pretransplant. ANNA J 18(6):583–584, 1991

Diehl A: Alcoholic liver disease. Med Clin North Am 73(4): 815–827, 1989

Gammal SH: Hepatic encephalopathy. Med Clin North Am 73(4):793–807, 1989

Gibson G: Hepatitis B infection and prevention. US Pharmacist 9:H-1-H-26, 1989

Heeg JM, Coleman DA: Hepatitis kills. RN 55(4):60–66, 1992

Katelaris PH, Jones, DB: Fulminant hepatic failure. Med Clin North Am 73(4):955–970, 1989

Lancaster S, Stockbridge J: PV shunts relieve ascites. RN 55(8): 58–60, 1990

Lisanti P: Hepatitis update: The delta virus. AORN J 55(3): 790–7, 793–4, 796–7, 1992

Maddrey WC: Viral hepatitis today. Emerg Med 21(16):126–5, 131, 135–6, 1989

Martin FL: When the liver breaks down. RN 55(8):52–57, 1992

McMahon BH, Helminiak C, Wainwright RB, Bulkow L: Frequency of adverse reactions to hepatitis B vaccine in 43,618 persons. Am J Med 92(3):254–256, 1992

Rhoads J: Cirrhosis of the liver. Emerg Med Serv 19(3):44,46–7, 1990

Sleisenger D, Fordtran S: Gastrointestinal Disease (4th ed). Philadelphia, WB Saunders, 1989

Stewart C: The liver: An overview. Emerg Med Serv 19(3): 22,24–5, 1990

Van de Linder J: Hepatitis B: The disease, the risk, the answer. J Post Anesth Nurs 4(6):416–419, 1989

STUDY QUESTIONS

1. In a patient with liver failure, which of the following laboratory values is (are) the most specific to hepatocellular damage?

   a. PT, PTT
   b. alkaline phosphate
   c. SGOT, SGPT
   d. amylase

2. The clinical sign of jaundice indicates that the patient has a problem conjugating

   a. bilirubin
   b. iron
   c. cholesterol
   d. bile

3. A complication of liver failure related to ammonia metabolism is

   a. hepatorenal syndrome
   b. hepatic insufficiency
   c. hepatic encephalopathy
   d. hepatitis

4. The intervention(s) used to specifically decrease serum ammonia levels in the patient with liver failure include

   a. administration of enteral neomycin
   b. administration of lactulose
   c. restriction of protein intake
   d. all of above

BEHAVIORAL OBJECTIVES

Based on the content of this chapter, the reader should be able to:

1. Identify three major causes of acute pancreatitis.
2. Describe the pathophysiology of acute pancreatitis.
3. Name two presenting symptoms associated with acute pancreatitis.
4. List three diagnostic tests used to evaluate the patient for acute pancreatitis.
5. Name four major complications of acute pancreatitis.
6. Describe the multidisciplinary management of the patient with acute pancreatitis.
7. Develop a nursing care plan for the patient with acute pancreatitis.

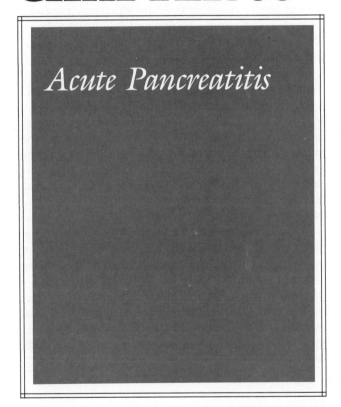

CHAPTER 38

Acute Pancreatitis

Description

Acute pancreatitis is characterized by an acute inflammatory process within the pancreas. The pancreas has both exocrine functions (production of digestive enzymes) and endocrine functions (production of insulin and glucagon). The cells of the pancreas called acini secrete the major pancreatic exocrine enzymes essential for normal digestion of fats, carbohydrates, and proteins. Some of these are trypsin, chymotrypsin, phospholipase A, elastase, and carboxypeptidase. These enzymes are normally secreted in an inactive form to prevent autodigestion of the gland. In acute pancreatitis, these enzymes are prematurely activated, initiating an inflammatory process in and around the pancreatic gland.

Depending on degree and extent of pancreatic inflammatory involvement, the intensity of the disease ranges from mild to severe. In 85% to 90% of patients, the disease is self-limiting (mild acute pancreatitis) and the patient generally recovers rapidly. However, with severe cases, multiple system organ failure is characteristic and is associated with significant mortality rates.[1] Management of the severe form of the disease requires intensive nursing and medical care.

Acute pancreatitis has many causes, but the most common are gallstone disease and alcohol abuse, which together account for more than 70% of all cases. Alcohol is known to change the composition of pancreatic juice by increasing the amount of trypsinogen. Biliary stones and biliary sludge (cholesterol crystals or calcium bilirubinate granules) are other causes.[2] Many drugs can initiate acute pancreatitis if taken in toxic doses or as a result of a drug reaction. High triglyceride levels is another important cause of pancreatitis that can be prevented in susceptible persons. Idiopathic pancreatitis is associated with pregnancy, the administration of total parenteral nutrition, or major surgery. Pancreatitis due to blunt or penetrating abdominal trauma or following endoscopic exploration of the biliary tree has also been reported. Infectious processes such as mumps, staphylococcus, scarlet fever, and viral processes have also been implicated as precipitating factors.[3,4] Table 38–1 summarizes major causes of acute pancreatitis.

Pathophysiology

The exact mechanism by which enzymes made by the pancreas become activated to initiate autodigestion of the gland has been widely studied but remains unknown. Some theories propose that a toxic agent, such as alcohol or drugs, alters the way in which the pancreas secretes enzymes, causing premature activation. Another theory proposes that reflux of duodenal contents containing activated enzymes enters the pancreatic duct and causes inflammation. Obstruction of biliary ducts can lead to increased pressure and rupture of the pancreatic duct,

TABLE 38–1
Major Causes of Acute Pancreatitis

Biliary Disease
Gallstones
Common bile duct obstruction
Biliary sludge
Alcohol Abuse
Drugs
Thiazide diuretics
Furosemide
Procainamide
Tetracycline
Sulfonamides
Hypertriglyceridemia
Hypercalcemia
Idiopathic
Postoperative
Ectopic pregnancy
Ovarian cyst
Total parenteral nutrition
Abdominal Trauma
Endoscopic Retrograde Cholangiopancreatography
Infectious Processes

activation of pancreatic exocrine enzymes, or reflux of bile and duodenal juice into the pancreas. Regardless of how the enzymes are activated, enzymatic damage to pancreatic cells (acinar cells) is the outcome of the disease process. As more pancreatic cells are damaged, more digestive enzymes are released, causing a repeatable cycle of more pancreatic damage. Trypsinogen, phospholipase A and elastase have been proposed as the primary enzymes responsible for the autodigestive process.[5]

Acute pancreatitis has been classified by the gradation of the lesions found in the pancreas. In the mild form, there are areas of fat necrosis in and around pancreatic cells along with interstitial edema; frank pancreatic necrosis is absent. This mild form can progress to a more severe form with extensive fat necrosis in and around the pancreas, pancreatic cellular necrosis, and hemorrhage within the pancreas.

In a great majority of patients, acute pancreatitis resolves spontaneously within 5 to 7 days, with return of normal pancreatic endocrine and exocrine function. Conversely, severe pancreatitis can affect every organ system in the body.

Assessment

A diagnosis of acute pancreatitis can only be made based on history, careful clinical examination, and diagnostic studies. Because history and clinical examination findings can mimic those of other diseases, laboratory and radiographic studies are particularly important in the assessment and diagnosis of the patient with acute pancreatitis. Nurses are responsible for initial and ongoing clinical assessments and for the monitoring, recording, and reporting of physical and laboratory data.

History

If acute pancreatitis is suspected, the possible causes should be evaluated, particularly biliary tract disease and excessive alcohol intake. In rare cases, acute pancreatitis is hereditary. The patient may report steatorrhea (fatty stools), as well as weight loss, nausea, vomiting, and abdominal distention. Ascertain the characteristics and frequency of bowel movements. The history should also include a complete assessment of pain: location, duration, precipitating factors, and relation of pain to meals, posture, alcohol ingestion, anorexia, and food intolerances. The urine should be observed for discoloration associated with obstructive jaundice.

Clinical Manifestations

In 95% of cases, patients with acute pancreatitis present with complaints of severe abdominal pain.[6] The pain is believed to be caused by edema and distention of the pancreatic capsule, a chemical burn caused by activated pancreatic enzymes, or obstruction of the biliary tree. The pain is most often midepigastric, but can be generalized or localized in the left upper quadrant, often radiating to the back. It usually begins abruptly, and commonly after a large meal or alcohol binge. The pain associated with acute pancreatitis is often steady and severe, but it can increase gradually for several hours. Vomiting due to reflux irritation of the inflamed pancreas does not relieve the pain and can be persistent. The vomitus consists of gastric and duodenal contents. The patient characteristically curls up with both arms over the abdomen to relieve the pain.

Fever is also a common symptom, but it is usually less than 39°C. Persistent fever can indicate gastrointestinal complications of the disease such as peritonitis, cholecystitis, or intra-abdominal abscess. Slight jaundice may be present owing to edema of the pancreas.

On physical examination, abdominal tenderness or guarding may be present. Distention of the upper abdomen and tympany may also be present. Hypoactive or absent bowel sounds are common due to the effect of the inflammatory process and enzyme activation on gut motility. There may be a paralytic ileus with its sequelae, including loss of fluid into the bowel lumen. This further complicates fluid imbalances common to this disorder.

In severe acute hemorrhagic pancreatitis, the patient exhibits overt signs of dehydration and hypovolemic shock. Patients with more severe pancreatic disease can also have ascites, jaundice, or palpable abdominal masses. A bluish discoloration of the lower abdominal flanks (Grey Turner's sign) or around the umbilical area (Cullen's sign) indicates the presence of hemorrhagic pancreatitis and accumulation of blood in these areas. These signs usually do not appear for 1 to 2 weeks as more of the pancreatic gland is destroyed. The abdominal girth should be measured at least every 4 hours if hemorrhagic pancreatitis is suspected in order to detect internal bleeding.

Diagnostic Studies

Serum lipase and amylase tests are the most specific to acute pancreatitis, because these enzymes are released as the pancreatic cells and ducts are destroyed. However, there are problems in using these values as pure indicators of the disease. Serum amylase and lipase levels are usually elevated during the first 24 to 48 hours after the onset of symptoms. In mild pancreatitis, these levels can be close to normal, and if a few days have elapsed since the beginning of symptoms, enzymes can be completely normal even with acute inflammatory processes in the pancreas.[7] The clinical diagnosis is complicated because amylase is present in other body tissues. Therefore, other diseases cause an elevation of serum amylase, including biliary tract disease, tumors, salivary gland lesions, cerebral trauma, gynecological disorders, and renal failure.

Serum amylase measurement is much more specific if isoenzymes are elevated (isoamylase) or if urinary amylase is also measured. Serum amylase can be falsely lowered in patients with elevated blood serum triglycerides. Amylase values of pleural fluid and paracentesis drainage are used in diagnosing pancreatitis. Other pancreatic enzymes such as lipase, trypsin, elastase, and phospholipase are being studied for use in laboratory diagnosis but are not yet more accurate than the amylase which is currently the most widely used.

Other common laboratory abnormalities associated with acute pancreatitis include an elevated white blood cell (WBC) count due to the inflammatory process and an elevated serum glucose due to beta cell damage. Hypokalemia may be present because of associated vomiting. Hypocalcemia is common with severe disease and usually indicates pancreatic fat necrosis. Elevations in serum bilirubin, LDH, SGOT, and prothrombin time are common in the presence of concurrent liver disease. Alkaline phosphatase is elevated with biliary tract disease. Triglycerides can be extremely elevated and may be a causative factor in the premature activation of pancreatic enzymes. A low serum calcium level is found in the more severe forms of the disease.

Arterial blood gas (ABG) analysis may show hypoxemia and retained CO_2 levels, which would indicate associated respiratory failure. Both endocrine and exocrine functions of the pancreas can be impaired in mild and severe manifestations of the disease. Therefore, hyperglycemia, hypoglycemia, and nutritional depletion are common effects of all forms of acute pancreatitis.

Advances in the diagnosis of acute pancreatitis have been made as a result of improved imaging modalities such as ultrasound, computed tomography (CT), and magnetic resonance imaging (MRI).[8] The size of the pancreas, collections of fluid around the pancreas, abscesses, and masses can be seen using these technologies. Contrast enhancement allows for more detailed imaging of the gland. Of importance is the fact that gastrointestinal complications of acute pancreatitis such as pancreatic pseudocyst, abscess, perforation, or obstruction of the biliary tree are distinguishable, allowing for early detection. If the patient presents with acute abdominal pain, radiographs of the chest and abdomen are also done to rule out intestinal ileus, perforation, pericardial diffusion, and pulmonary disease. Abdominal films can also reveal intestinal gas-filled loops, which are signs of paralytic ileus. Table 38–2 summarizes assessment parameters in the patient presenting with acute pancreatitis.

Management

There are no known therapies that stop the cycle of pancreatic enzyme activation with inflammation and necrosis of the gland. Definitive therapies are aimed at the cause of the disorder. Medical and nursing priorities for the supportive management of acute pancreatitis include the following:

- fluid resuscitation and electrolyte replacement to maintain or replenish vascular volume and electrolyte balance;
- supportive therapies aimed at preventing the release of pancreatic secretions (resting the pancreas) while maintaining the nutritional status of the patient; and
- analgesics for pain control.[9]

Collaborative management of the patient with acute pancreatitis is summarized in Table 38–3.

Fluid and Electrolyte Replacement

In all forms of acute pancreatitis, fluid collects in the retroperitoneal space and peritoneal cavity. Initially, most patients present with some degree of dehydration, and in severe cases with overt hypovolemic shock. They may have sequestered up to 12 liters of fluid on admission. Hypovolemia and shock are major causes of death early in the disease process. In some cases, aggressive fluid resuscitation fails to reverse the shock process. Fluid replacement then becomes a high priority in the treatment of acute pancreatitis.

The solution ordered by the physician for fluid resuscitation is usually colloids or Ringer's lactate; however, fresh frozen plasma and albumin can also be used. Some

TABLE 38–2
Assessment Parameters in Acute Pancreatitis

History

Alcohol disease
Biliary disease
Nausea and vomiting
Steatorrhea
Urinary discoloration
Hereditary disposition

Clinical Manifestations

Abdominal pain
Abdominal guarding, distention
Paralytic ileus
Fever
Grey Turner's sign
Cullen's sign

Laboratory Findings

Elevated serum and urine amylase
Elevated serum lipase
Elevated WBC count
Hyperglycemia
Elevated bilirubin, SGOT, LDH (with liver disease)
Elevated alkaline phosphatase (with biliary disease)
Hypertryglyceridemia
Hypocalcemia
Hypoxemia

Diagnostic Studies

Ultrasound
Computer tomography
Magnetic resonance imaging

research has been done on the advantage of using one solution over the other, but none proved to be more effective. Regardless of which solution is used, fluid replacement serves to perfuse the pancreas, which is thought to decrease the severity of the progression of the disease. Also, the kidneys remain perfused, and this can prevent the development of acute renal failure. Patients with acute hemorrhagic pancreatitis may also need packed red blood cells in addition to fluid therapy to restore volume.

Critical assessments to evaluate fluid replacement include accurate monitoring of intake and output and daily weights. Patients with more severe manifestations of the disease may require hemodynamic monitoring to help evaluate fluid status and response to intervention. The pulmonary capillary wedge pressure (PCWP) is the most sensitive measure of volume status and left ventricular filling pressure. A PCWP of 11 to 14 mm Hg is a realistic goal for most patients.

Patients with severe disease whose hypotension fails to respond to fluid therapy may need medications to support blood pressure. The drug of choice is dopamine, which can be started at a low dose (2–5 µg/kg/min). An

TABLE 38–3
Management of Acute Pancreatitis

Fluid Replacement

Colloids
Crystalloids
Blood products

Electrolyte Replacement

Calcium
Magnesium
Potassium

Resting the Pancreas

NG tube to intermittent suction
NPO
Bedrest

Nutritional Support

Pain Management

Non-opiate analgesics
Patient positioning

---

advantage of this drug is that at low doses it maintains renal perfusion while supporting blood pressure.

Urinary output is a sensitive measure of the adequacy of fluid replacement, and it should be maintained at greater than 30 ml per hour. Blood pressure and heart rate are also sensitive measures of volume status. Expected outcomes need to be customized for each patient, but reasonable goals are to maintain mean arterial pressure (MAP) at greater than 60 mm Hg, BP without an orthostatic drop, and HR less than 100 beats per minute. The presence of warm extremities is one indicator of adequate peripheral circulation.

Hypocalcemia (< 8 mg/dl) is a common electrolyte imbalance occurring in about one-third of patients with acute pancreatitis.[10] The exact mechanism for this metabolic complication is not completely understood, but it is thought to be related to decreased binding with proteins in the plasma. Patients with severe hypocalcemia should be placed on seizure precautions with respiratory support equipment on hand. The nurse is responsible for monitoring calcium levels, for administering replacement solutions, and for evaluating the patient's response to any calcium given. Calcium replacements should be infused through a central line, because peripheral infiltration can cause tissue necrosis. The patient also needs to be monitored for calcium toxicity; symptoms include lethargy, nausea, shortening of the Q-T interval, and decreased excitability of nerves and muscles. Hypomagnesemia may also be present with hypocalcemia and so magnesium may need to be replaced as well. Correction of serum magnesium levels is usually required before calcium levels can return to normal.

Potassium is another electrolyte that may need to be replaced early in the treatment regimen owing to the

vomiting associated with acute pancreatitis. Potassium is also abundant in pancreatic juices. Hypokalemia is associated with cardiac dysrhythmias, muscle weakness, hypotension, and irritability. Potassium should be administered slowly over 1 hour using an infusion pump.

Hyperglycemia is surprisingly a less common complication of acute pancreatitis and is related to impaired secretion of insulin by islet cells in the pancreas or release of glucagon by alpha cells. In some cases, hyperglycemia can be associated with dehydration or other electrolyte imbalances. Sliding scale regular insulin may be ordered; it needs to be administered very cautiously, because glucagon levels are only transiently elevated in acute pancreatitis.

Resting the Pancreas

Nasogastric suction is used in most patients with acute pancreatitis to suppress pancreatic exocrine secretion by preventing the release of secretin from the duodenum. Normally secretin, which stimulates production of pancreatic secretions, is released whenever there is acid in the duodenum. Nausea, vomiting and abdominal pain may also be decreased when a nasogastric (NG) tube is placed to suction early in treatment.[11] An NG tube is also necessary in patients with ileus, severe gastric distention, or decreased level of consciousness to prevent complications resulting from pulmonary aspiration. Strict NPO (nothing by mouth) status should be maintained until the abdominal pain subsides and serum amylase levels have returned to normal. Starting oral intake sooner can cause the abdominal pain to return and can induce further inflammation of the pancreas by stimulating the autodigestive disease process.

Total parenteral nutrition is recommended for patients with fulminant pancreatitis who are being kept on prolonged NPO status with NG suction because of paralytic ileus, persistent abdominal pain, or pancreatic complications. Lipids should not be administered, because this can further increase triglyceride levels and exacerbate the inflammatory process. In the patient with mild pancreatitis, oral fluids can usually be restarted within 3 to 7 days with slow advancement of solids as tolerated.

Prolonged NPO status is difficult for patients. Frequent mouth care and proper positioning and lubrication of the NG tube are important to maintain skin integrity and maximize patient comfort. bed rest is prescribed to decrease the patient's basal metabolic rate; this, in turn, decreases the stimulation of pancreatic secretions.

Pain Management

Pain control is a nursing priority in patients with acute pancreatitis, not only because of the extreme discomfort but also because pain increases pancreatic enzyme secretion. The pain of pancreatitis is a result of the edema and distention of the pancreatic capsule, obstruction of the biliary system, and peritoneal inflammation from pancreatic enzymes. Pain is related to the degree of pancreatic inflammation, and it can be severe, constant, and last for many days.

Careful pain assessments during the patient's admission history should include information on the onset, intensity, duration, and location (local or diffuse) of the pain. Analgesics will be needed to control discomfort. Some analgesics cause spasm of the sphincter of Oddi which holds the duodenum in place and can thus exacerbate the pain associated with acute pancreatitis. Morphine is one such drug, and therefore, non–opiate-containing analgesics such as Levo-Dromoran and Demerol have been considered the drugs of choice. Fentynl citrate (Sublimaze), although it is an opiate, has also been used successfully to control this type of pain.

Analgesia should be routinely administered at least every 3 to 4 hours to prevent uncontrollable abdominal pain. Use of a pain rating scale is recommended for evaluating the patient's response to medication. An NG tube attached to low intermittent suction can help ease pain considerably. Patient positioning can also relieve some of the discomfort.

Predicting the Severity of Acute Pancreatitis

After a diagnosis of acute pancreatitis is confirmed, criteria for predicting the prognosis of patients can be reviewed. Ranson's criteria are used most often in this country.[12] These criteria have been widely studied, and the number of signs present during the first 48 hours of admission directly relate to the patient's chance of significant morbidity and mortality.[13] These signs are summarized in Table 38–4.

In Ranson's research, the mortality rate is 1% for patients with fewer than three signs, 15% for those with three to four signs, 40% if five to six signs are present, and 100% if 7 or more signs are positive. The scale has a 96% accuracy rate and is useful clinically in identifying high risk patients and those who need early aggressive treatment to prevent complications. The APACHE (Acute Physiology, Age, Chronic Health Evaluation) II score has also been studied and found to be useful in predicting severity. The advantage of these scoring systems is that a patient's risk can be identified within hours of admission.

Complications

Multisystem complications of acute pancreatitis are related to the pancreas' ability to produce many vasoactive substances that affect organs throughout the body.[14] These are reviewed in Table 38–5.

TABLE 38–4
Ranson Severity Criteria

Evaluate on Admission or on Diagnosis:

Age > 55 years
Leukocyte count > 16,000/μl
Serum Glucose > 200 mg/dl
Serum lactic dehydrogenase > 350 IU/ml
Serum aspartate aminotransferase > 250 IU/dl

During Initial 48 Hours:

Fall in hematocrit > 10%
Blood Urea Nitrogen level rise > 5 mg/dl
Serum Calcium < 8 mg/dl
Base deficit > 4 mEq/L
Estimated fluid sequestration > 6 liters
Arterial PaO_2 < 60 torr

It appears that as pancreatic cells are damaged, more digestive enzymes are released, which in turn causes more pancreatic damage. Local effects of pancreatitis include inflammation of the pancreas, inflammation of the peritoneum around the pancreas, and fluid accumulation in the peritoneal cavity. Hemodynamically significant fluid sequestration is characteristic of the disease in the fulminant form. Another major systemic effect of enzyme release into the circulatory system is peripheral vasodilation, which in turn can cause hypotension and shock.

Decreased perfusion to the pancreas itself can result in the release of myocardial depressant factor (MDF). Myo-

TABLE 38–5
Major Complications of Acute Pancreatitis

Pulmonary

Atelectasis
Acute Respiratory Distress Syndrome

Cardiovascular

Hypotensive shock
Myocardial depression (MDF)

Renal

Acute renal failure

Hematologic

Disseminated intravascular coagulation

Metabolic

Hypocalcemia
Metabolic acidosis

Gastrointestinal

Pancreatic pseudocyst
Pancreatic abscess
Gastrointestinal bleed

cardial depressant factor is known to decrease heart contractility and therefore to affect cardiac output. Perfusion of all body organs can then become compromised. Early and aggressive fluid resuscitation is thought to prevent the release of MDF. Trypsin activation is known to cause abnormalities in blood coagulation and clot lysis. Disseminated intravascular coagulation with the associated bleeding disorder can further impact on fluid balance.

The release of other enzymes (eg, phospholipase) is thought to cause the many pulmonary complications associated with acute pancreatitis. These include arterial hypoxemia, atelectasis, pleural effusions, pneumonia, acute respiratory failure, and acute respiratory distress syndrome. Ranson found evidence of arterial hypoxemia in patients with mild disease without clinical or x-ray findings to support the pulmonary dysfunction.[15] Arterial blood gases should be drawn every 8 hours for the first few days to monitor for this complication. Treatment for hypoxemia includes vigorous pulmonary care (eg, deep breathing and coughing) and frequent position changes. Oxygen therapy can also be used to improve overall oxygenation status. Careful fluid administration is also necessary to prevent fluid overload and pulmonary congestion. Patients with acute respiratory compromise require mechanical ventilatory support.

Acute renal failure is thought to be a consequence of hypovolemia and associated decreased renal perfusion. Death during the first 2 weeks of acute pancreatitis usually results from pulmonary or renal complications.

Metabolic complications of acute pancreatitis include hypocalcemia and hyperlipidemia, which are thought to be related to areas of fat necrosis around the inflamed pancreas. Hyperglycemia can be present and is most commonly caused by the stress response. Damage to the cells of the islets of Langerhans causes refractory hyperglycemia. Metabolic acidosis can result from hypoperfusion and activation of anaerobic metabolism.

Gastrointestinal complications of acute pancreatitis include pancreatic pseudocyst, pancreatic abscess, and acute gastrointestinal hemorrhage. Pancreatic pseudocysts occur in up to 20% of all cases of acute pancreatitis and are a part of the necrotizing process. A pseudocyst is a collection of inflammatory debris and pancreatic secretions. The pseudocyst can rupture and hemorrhage or become infected causing bacterial translocation and sepsis. A pseudocyst should be suspected in any patient who has persistent abdominal pain with nausea and vomiting, a prolonged fever, and elevated serum amylase. A CT scan can be helpful in diagnosing the location and size of the pseudocyst.

Pancreatic abscess is a walled-off collection of purulent material in or around the pancreas. There is 100% mortality associated with this complication without surgical intervention. Signs and symptoms of an abdominal abscess include increased WBC count, fever, abdominal pain, and vomiting. Sources of gastrointestinal hemorrhage include peptic ulcer bleeds, hemorrhagic gastroduodenitis, stress ulcer, and Mallory–Weiss Syndrome.

Management of Systemic Complications

In addition to medical interventions to support organ function, peritoneal lavage and surgical therapies have been used in the treatment of acute pancreatitis.

Peritoneal lavage has been used since the 1960s for the treatment of systemic complications. The rationale for this therapy is that it removes the toxic substances released by the damaged pancreas into the peritoneal fluid before systemic effects can be initiated. Lavage is usually used if standard therapies have not been effective during the first few days of hospitalization.

The procedure for peritoneal lavage involves placement of a peritoneal dialysis catheter. Isotonic solutions with dextrose, heparin, and potassium are added. An antibiotic may also be used in the solution. Two liters of solution are infused over 15 to 20 minutes and then are

---

Clinical Research

Ranson JH, Berman RS: Long peritoneal lavage decreases pancreatic sepsis in acute pancreatitis. Ann Surg 211(6):708–717, 1990

The purpose of this study was to determine the effect of long peritoneal lavage on the incidence of pancreatic sepsis, a severe complication of acute pancreatitis. Late infection of devitalized pancreatic tissue can be a significant cause of death in this patient population. Twenty-nine patients with severe pancreatitis (three of more prognostic signs) were assigned to short peritoneal lavage for 2 days (15 patients) or to long peritoneal lavage for 7 days (14 patients). Longer lavage dramatically reduced the frequency of pancreatic sepsis as well as death from sepsis. These findings indicate that lavage of the peritoneal cavity for 7 days can significantly reduce both the frequency and mortality rate of pancreatic sepsis in severe acute pancreatitis.

drained by gravity. This cycle is repeated every 1 to 2 hours for 48 to 72 hours. If peritoneal lavage is effective, the hemodynamic response by the patient is usually immediate.

Respiratory status must be closely monitored during peritoneal lavage, because accumulation of fluid in the peritoneum causes restricted movement of the diaphragm. Hyperglycemia can be another effect of this therapy, because dextrose can be absorbed from the fluid into the bloodstream.

A pancreatic resection for acute necrotizing pancreatitis can be performed to prevent systemic complications of the disease process.[16] In this procedure, dead or infected pancreatic tissue is surgically removed. In some cases, the entire pancreas is removed.

Surgery may also be indicated for pseudocysts; however, it is usually delayed, because some pseudocysts have been known to resolve spontaneously. Surgical treatment of the pseudocyst can be done through internal or external drainage or needle aspiration. Acute surgical intervention may be required if the pseudocyst becomes infected or perforates.

Surgery may also be performed if gallstones are thought to be the cause of the acute pancreatitis. A cholecystectomy or endoscopic retrograde cholangiopancreatography (ERCP) and endoscopic sphincterotomy are performed.

CASE STUDY

Mr. Jackson, a 52-year-old adult male, was admitted to the emergency room reporting agonizing, knife-like pain in the midepigastrium, radiating to his back. His pain began suddenly, about 1 hour after he returned home with his wife from a dinner party. His wife, concerned he was suffering a heart attack, called the ambulance for emergency transport. En route, he became nauseated and vomited several times. This did not relieve the relentless pain.

Admission assessment findings:

BP 96/40 with 15 mm Hg orthostatic drop

Sinus tachycardia (135) with ST segment depression

T 100.3°F

Respiratory rate 34, diminished breath sound in bases; pulse oximetry 87%

Alert, oriented to time place and person; anxious

Extremities cool, pulses present and equal

Abdomen soft, distended with hypoactive bowel sounds, tender to palpation

Mr. Jackson denied a history of cardiovascular disease, diabetes, or renal disease. He reported a history of cholecystitis with two acute episodes within the last 2 years which were medically managed. He states he does not smoke and drinks socially.

Intravenous lines were placed and normal saline was infused to maintain MAP greater than 60. A bladder catheter was placed to assist with fluid assessments. Supplemental oxygen was administered to improve oxygenation, and an ABG was drawn. Serum blood counts, chemistries, and cardiac enzymes were also sent to the lab. Levo-Dromoran was administered for abdominal pain. The nurse helped Mr. Jackson assume a knee-to-chest position which relieved some of his pain. A chest x-ray and 12-lead ECG were obtained. The patient was scheduled for admission to the ICU.

The initial medical and nursing goals were to assess vital signs and respiratory status. Fluid resuscitation was immediately begun and assessments initiated to monitor hemodynamic status. Serum tests and radiographic studies were done to enable the physician to make a definitive diagnosis. Analgesia was administered and the patient was positioned to promote optimal comfort. See Nursing Care Plan 38–1.

NURSING CARE PLAN 38–1:
The Patient With Acute Pancreatitis

NURSING DIAGNOSIS	OUTCOME CRITERIA/ PATIENT GOALS	NURSING INTERVENTIONS
Fluid volume deficit: related to fluid sequestration due to activated pancreatic enzymes in peritoneum; vomiting; prolonged NG suction; potential hemorrhage into the pancreas.	• Patient will remain hemodynamically stable.	1. Monitor vital signs and urine output q1h and prn; skin turgor capillary refill, peripheral pulses, q4h and prn.
		2. Monitor hemodynamic values if pulmonary artery catheter is placed; PCWP, CVP, SVR, cardiac output, and cardiac index.
		3. Maintain patent IV line; central line preferred.

(continued)

NURSING CARE PLAN 38–1: (Continued)
The Patient With Acute Pancreatitis

NURSING DIAGNOSIS	OUTCOME CRITERIA/ PATIENT GOALS	NURSING INTERVENTIONS
		4. Administer fluid replacements (eg, colloids, crystalloids, blood or blood products) and monitor patient response.
		5. Maintain and evaluate intake and output records.
		6. Weigh patient daily on same scale at same time.
		7. Monitor of signs and symptoms of hemorrhage: hematocrit and hemoglobin q2h; Cullen or Turner's sign.
		8. Measure abdominal girth q4h.
		9. Monitor electrolytes, CBC, and coagulation factors; replace electrolytes as prescribed.
		10. Monitor renal function studies (eg, BUN, creatinine, urinary Na, osmolality).
		11. Place patient on bed rest.
		12. Maintain NPO status.
Pain: related to interruption of blood supply to the pancreas; edema and distention of the pancreas; peritoneal irritation from activated pancreatic exocrine enzymes.	• Patient reports pain is within tolerable limits.	1. Perform a pain assessment noting onset, duration, intensity, and location.
		2. Instruct patient on use of a 0–10 pain rating scale.
		3. Assess patient anxiety.
		4. Administer non-opiate analgesic; schedule pain medication regulary to prevent severe pain episodes.
		4. Keep activities at a minimum. Maintain bed rest restriction. Position patient to optimize comfort.
		5. Provide comfort measures; mouth care, positioning; control fever.
Altered nutrition, less than body requirements: related to prolonged NPO status; nausea and vomiting; depressed appetite; impaired nutrient metabolism due to pancreatic injury and altered production of digestive enzymes.	• Nutritional needs of patient will be adequately met.	1. Assess nutritional status through clinical exam and laboratory analysis.
		2. Calculate caloric needs and compare to actual intake.
		3. Administer TPN as ordered. Avoid lipid therapy.

(continued)

NURSING CARE PLAN 38–1: (Continued)
The Patient With Acute Pancreatitis

NURSING DIAGNOSIS	OUTCOME CRITERIA/ PATIENT GOALS	NURSING INTERVENTIONS
		4. Prevent complications by attention to aseptic technique in the handling and administration of TPN and catheter care.
		5. Monitor for signs and symptoms of infection.
		6. Monitor glucose, albumin, and electrolytes to detect complications of therapy.
		7. Assess acid–base balance with ABGs.
Impaired gas exchange: related to atelectasis; pleural effusions; ARDS; fluid overload during fluid administration; pulmonary emboli; splinting from pain.	• Patient will have adequate breathing pattern and gas exchange.	1. Monitor pulmonary status closely. Auscultate breath sounds q2–4h and prn; monitor respiratory rate, chest excursion and symmetry; assess for signs of respiratory distress.
		2. Administer vigorous pulmonary hygiene; coughing and deep breathing; humidification therapy.
		3. Note secretions for amount, color, consistency, and odor.
		4. Administer oxygen as prescribed.
		5. Monitor with oximetry for SaO_2.
		6. Administer analgesia to prevent splinting due to pain.
		7. Reposition patient frequently to maximize ventilation and perfusion and to prevent pooling of secretions.
		8. Assist with paracentesis as ordered when ascites compromises respiratory status.

REFERENCES

1. Singh M, Simsek H: Ethanol and the pancreas. Gastroenterology 98(14):1051–1062, 1990
2. Lee SP, Nicholis JF, Park HZ: Biliary sludge as a cause of acute pancreatitis. New Engl J Med 326(9):589–593, 1992
3. Carter DC: Pancreatitis and the biliary tree: The continuing problem. Am J Surg 155(1):10–17, 1988
4. Levelle-Jones M, Neoptolemos JP: Recent advances in the treatment of acute pancreatitis. Surg Annual 22:235–261, 1990
5. Levelle-Jones M, Neoptolemos JP: Recent advances in the treatment of acute pancreatitis. Surg Annual 22:235–261, 1990
6. Brown A: Acute pancreatitis. Focus Crit Care 18(2):121–130, 1991
7. Agarwal N, Pitchumoni CS, Sivasprasad AV: Evaluating tests for acute pancreatitis. Am J Gastroenterol 85(4):356–365, 1990
8. Clavien PA, Hauser H, Meyer P, Rohner A: Value of contrast-enhanced computerized tomography in the early diagnosis and prognosis of acute pancreatitis. Am J Surg 155(1):457–466, 1988

9. Levelle-Jones M, Neoptolemos JP: Recent advances in the treatment of acute pancreatitis. Surg Annual 22:235–261, 1990
10. Sleisenger M, Fordtran J: Gastrointestinal Disease, 4th ed. Philadelphia: WB Saunders, 1989
11. Brown A: Acute pancreatitis. Focus Crit Care 18(2): 121–130, 1991
12. Ranson JH: Risk factors in acute pancreatitis. Hosp Pract 20(4):69–73, 1985
13. Agarwal N, Pitchumoni CS: Assessment of severity in acute pancreatitis. Am J Gastroenterol 86(10):1385–1391, 1991
14. Pitchumoni CS, Agarwal J, Jain NK: Systemic complications of acute pancreatitis. Am J Gastroenterol 83(6): 597–605, 1988
15. Ranson JH: Risk factors in acute pancreatitis. Hosp Pract 20(4):69–73, 1985
16. Pitchumoni CS, Agarwal J, Jain NK: Systemic complications of acute pancreatitis. Am J Gastroenterol 83(6): 597–605, 1988

BIBLIOGRAPHY

D'Egidio A, Schein M: Surgical strategies in the treatment of pancreatic necrosis and infection. Br J Surg 78:133–137, 1991
Jeffres C: Complications of acute pancreatitis. Crit Care Nurse 9(4):38–50, 1989
Latifi R, McIntosh K, Dudrick S: Nutritional management of acute and chronic pancreatitis. Surg Clin North Am 71(3): 579–595, 1991
Loos F: Acute pancreatitis. Can Crit Care Nurse J 6(4):5–11, 1989
Meehan M: Nursing Dx: Potential for aspiration. RN 55:1 30–34, 1992
Smith A: When the pancreas self-destructs. Am J Nurs 91(9): 38–52, 1991
Stewart C: Acute pancreatitis. Emerg Care Q 5(3):71–83, 1989
Thompson C: Managing acute pancreatitis. RN 55(3):52–57, 1992

STUDY QUESTIONS

1. The most helpful laboratory test for the diagnosis of acute pancreatitis is the serum

   a. SGOT
   b. amylase
   c. bilirubin
   d. acid phosphatase

2. In acute pancreatitis, the major pathophysiologic process that explains the fluid shift from the vascular space into the interstitium is

   a. pancreatic enzymes that are toxic to blood capillaries cause the vessels to rupture and fluid to escape
   b. lipase is prematurely released into the duodenum causing increased capillary permeability
   c. chemical mediators released into the duodenum cause the fluid shift
   d. pancreatic enzymes are absorbed into the blood where they activate vasoactive substances which then increase permeability

3. The primary goal in the collaborative management of acute pancreatitis is to

   a. conserve nutritional reserves
   b. prevent gastrointestinal complications
   c. prevent proteolytic enzyme secretion
   d. facilitate diagnostic evaluation

4. Initial treatment of acute pancreatitis includes

   a. invasive monitoring, IV antibiotics, and rest
   b. oxygen, fluid replacement, and surgical exploration
   c. volume and electrolyte replacement, analgesia, and monitoring for systemic effects
   d. needle aspiration of pancreatic enzymes, TPN, and positive inotropic support

5. Complications of acute pancreatitis amenable to surgical intervention include

   a. abscess
   b. pseudocyst
   c. hemorrhage
   d. all of above

UNIT VI

Endocrine System

CHAPTER 39

Anatomy and Physiology of the Endocrine System

(continued)

Hudak: Critical Care Nursing:
A Holistic Approach, 6th ed. © 1994
J. B. Lippincott Company.

BEHAVIORAL OBJECTIVES

Based on the content in this chapter, the reader should be able to:

1. Describe the production, actions, and regulation of ADH, growth and thyroid hormones, insulin, and glucagon.
2. Identify how activated vitamin D, parathormone, and calcitonin each influence calcium metabolism.
3. Explain how glucocorticoids are secreted.
4. Summarize the renin–angiotensin mechanism for regulating mineralocorticoid secretion.
5. List three effects of pharmacologic dosages of glucocorticoid medications.
6. Describe the site of manufacture, stimulus for secretion, and action(s) of natriuretic hormone and erythropoietin.

Description

Communications between subsystems in the body are accomplished by way of three modalities. One is the nervous system, and another is the cellular secretions of chemicals that are locally contributed in interstitial fluid. Examples of such chemicals include those that trigger a local inflammatory response, such as histamine, complement, and prostaglandins. The third modality is the cellular secretion of chemicals that are circulated through the bloodstream. This last modality of communication is known more commonly as the *endocrine system*. The secretions of endocrine cells are termed *hormones*.

Until the mid-1950s, the boundary between the endocrine and nervous systems was quite clear. Then, with the discovery of hypothalamic neurons that secreted blood-borne chemicals, the line of demarcation blurred. Now, hormones identical with those produced by established endocrine glands (eg, insulin, adrenocorticotropic hormone [ACTH], and cholecystokinin pancreozymin [CCK-PZ]) are known to be secreted by various parts of the brain, where it is postulated they function as neurotransmitters. Table 39–1 lists the more commonly recognized endocrine glands and their secretions. This chapter, however, considers only those major glands whose pathology can provoke crisis situations relevant to critical care nursing (eg, water intoxication, hypertensive crises, hypocalcemic tetany, thyroid storm, addisonian crisis, and diabetic ketoacidosis).

As a preface to the discussion of the separate glands, let us review commonalities regarding hormone production, secretion, transport, metabolism, and modality of action. Basic principles concerning all but the last of these are illustrated in Figure 39–1. From this we see that the level of hormonal activity in the body depends on the relation between production and degradation. In the case of a protein-bound hormone (eg, the thyroid hormones and cortisol), the level of activity also depends on the level of free as opposed to bound plasma hormone. Hormones act on target cells in one of three ways. Some act to increase intracellular levels of cyclic adenosine monophosphate (AMP), which in turn acts as a second messenger within the cell to produce the hormonally triggered response of the target cell. Examples of hormones that increase cyclic AMP are calcitonin, ACTH, glucagon, catecholamines bound to β-receptors, parathormone, vasopressin, and thyroid-stimulating hormone (TSH). Other hormones, such as epinephrine and norepinephrine, when bound to receptors, act by increasing calcium influx into cells. Steroid hormones from the adrenal cortex, testes, and ovaries act by entering the nucleus of the target cell and binding to the genetic material, deoxyribonucleic acid (DNA). This binding triggers the target cell to produce certain enzymes, which in turn cause the typical hormonally induced response of the target tissue.

TABLE 39–1
Endocrine System in Summary

Endocrine Gland and Hormone	Principal Site of Action	Principal Results
Hypothalamus		
Corticotropin-releasing factor	Anterior pituitary	Release of adrenocorticotropin
Thyrotropin-releasing factor	Anterior pituitary	Release of thyrotropin
Luteinizing hormone-releasing factor	Anterior pituitary	Release of luteinizing hormone
Follicle-stimulating hormone-releasing factor	Anterior pituitary	Release of follicle-stimulating hormone
Growth hormone-releasing factor	Anterior pituitary	Release of growth hormone
Growth hormone-release inhibiting factor	Anterior pituitary	Inhibition of release of growth hormone
Prolactin-releasing factor	Anterior pituitary	Release of prolactin
Prolactin-release inhibiting hormone	Anterior pituitary	Inhibition of release of prolactin
Pituitary Gland		
Anterior Lobe		
Growth hormone	General	Growth of bones, muscles, and other organs
	Liver	Somatomedin
Thyrotropin	Thyroid	Growth and secretory activity of thyroid gland
Adrenocorticotropin	Adrenal cortex	Growth and secretory activity of adrenal cortex
Follicle-stimulating	Ovaries	Development of follicles and secretion of estrogen
	Testes	Development of seminiferous tubules, spermatogenesis
Luteinizing or interstitial cell-stimulating	Ovaries	Ovulation, formation of corpus luteum, secretion of progesterone
	Testes	Secretion of testosterone
Prolactin or lactogenic	Mammary glands	Secretion of milk
Melanocyte-stimulating	Skin	Pigmentation (?)
Posterior Lobe		
Antidiuretic (vasopressin)	Kidney	Reabsorption of water; water balance
Oxytocin	Arterioles	Blood pressure (?)
	Uterus	Contraction
	Breast	Expression of milk
Pineal Gland		
Melatonin	Gonads	Sexual maturation
Thyroid Gland		
Thyroxine and tri-iodothyronine	General	Metabolic rate; growth and development; intermediate metabolism
Thyrocalcitonin	Bone	Inhibits bone resorption; lowers blood level of calcium
Parathyroid Glands		
Parathormone	Bone, kidney, intestine	Promotes bone resorption; increased absorption of calcium; raises blood calcium level
Adrenal Glands		
Cortex		
Mineralocorticoids (eg, aldosterone)	Kidney	Reabsorption of sodium; elimination of potassium
Glucocorticoids (eg, cortisol)	General	Metabolism of carbohydrate, protein, and fat; response to stress; anti-inflammatory
Sex hormones	General (?)	Preadolescent growth spurt (?)

(continued)

TABLE 39–1
Endocrine System in Summary (Continued)

Endocrine Gland and Hormone	Principal Site of Action	Principal Results
Medulla		
Epinephrine	Cardiac muscle, smooth muscle, glands	Emergency functions: same as stimulation of sympathetic system
Norepinephrine	Organs innervated by sympathetic system	Chemical transmitter substance; increases peripheral resistance
Islet Cells of Pancreas		
Insulin	General	Lowers blood sugar; utilization and storage of carbohydrate; decreased gluconeogenesis; increased lipogenesis
Somatostatin	Other islet cells	Inhibits secretion of insulin and glucagon
Glucagon	Liver	Raises blood sugar; glucogenolysis and gluconeogenesis
Testes		
Testosterone	General	Development of secondary sex characteristics
	Reproductive organs	Development and maintenance; normal function
Ovaries		
Estrogens	General	Development of secondary sex characteristics
	Mammary glands	Development of duct system
	Reproductive organs	Maturation and normal cyclic function
Progesterone	Mammary glands	Development of secretory tissue
	Uterus	Preparation for implantation; maintenance of pregnancy
Prostaglandins	General smooth muscle, cell membranes	Contraction–relaxation, enzyme activation
Kidney and Liver		
Calcitrol	Intestine	Calcium absorption
Erythropoietin	Bone marrow	Erythropoiesis
Renin	Vascular smooth muscle	Vasoconstriction
	Adrenal cortex	Aldosterone secretion
Gastrointestinal Tract		
Gastrin	Stomach	Production of gastric juice
Enterogastrone	Stomach	Inhibits secretion and motility
Secretin	Liver and pancreas	Production of bile; production of watery pancreatic juice (rich in $NaHCO_3$)
CCK-PZ	Pancreas	Production of pancreatic juice rich in enzymes
	Gallbladder	Contraction and emptying
Cardiac Atria		
Natriuretic hormone	Kidney	Increased excretion of sodium and water

Adapted from Chaffee EE, Lytle IM: Basic Physiology and Anatomy, 4th ed. Philadelphia: JB Lippincott, 1980

Hypothalamus

This inferior portion of the diencephalon of the brain has many functions. Our concern here is limited to two of these: (1) the production of antidiuretic hormone and oxytocin, which are stored in the posterior pituitary, and (2) the regulation of anterior pituitary hormone secretion. The anatomic interrelation between the hypothalamus and pituitary is depicted in Figure 39–2.

Antidiuretic Hormone (ADH or Vasopressin) and Oxytocin

Production

These hormones are produced by nerve cells originating from areas (nuclei) in the hypothalamus that lie just above the optic chiasma and lateral to the third ventricle (ie, they are supraoptic and paraventricular). Antidiuretic hormone

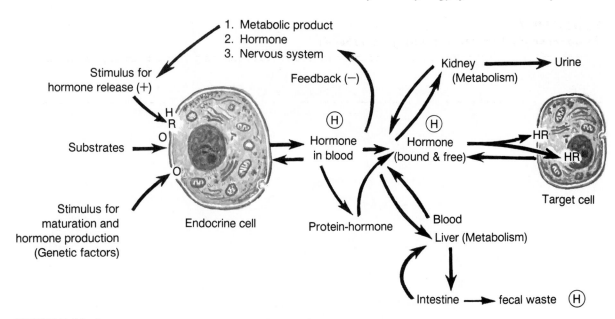

FIGURE 39-1
Diagram of the complex cellular interactions required to maintain an effective balance of hormones within the blood to regulate cellular functions. Specific cell receptors (R) react to hormones (H) or other substances (O) in the blood that can act as stimuli for cellular mechanisms. (Chaffee EE, Lytle IM: Basic Physiology and Anatomy, 4th ed. Philadelphia, JB Lippincott)

(ADH) and oxytocin "drip" from the axonal ends of these nerve cells into the tissue of the posterior pituitary, where they are stored. Neural impulses from the same hypothalamic cells cause the posterior pituitary to release these hormones into the bloodstream. Because of their production in neural tissue, ADH and oxytocin are sometimes termed *neurosecretory materials*.

Metabolic Fate

The half-life of ADH is 18 minutes. It is degraded principally by the liver and kidneys.

Actions

Antidiuretic hormone acts on the cells of the renal collecting ducts to increase their permeability to water. This results in increased water reabsorption unaccompanied by and independent of any electrolyte reabsorption. This reabsorbed water increases the volume of and decreases the osmolarity of the extracellular fluid (ECF). At the same time, it decreases the volume of and increases the concentration of the urine excreted. The term *vasopressin* originated from the observation that large, supraphysiological dosages of ADH act on arteriole smooth muscle to elevate blood pressure. Although this pressor action of ADH does not appear to play a role in the normal homeostasis of blood pressure, some researchers think that it helps counteract the fall in blood pressure that results from hemorrhagic or other drastic hypovolemic states.

Regulation of ADH

There are three major stimuli for the regulation of ADH secretion. The first is plasma osmolality, which is monitored by osmoreceptors in the anterior hypothalamus. An increase above the normal osmolality of plasma (290 mOsm/kg) results in neural stimuli from these receptors to the ADH-secreting cells, increasing ADH secretion. This in turn increases water retention, thereby diluting the ECF and lowering the plasma osmolality back to normal. Similarly, a fall in plasma osmolality triggers a decrease or cessation in ADH secretion. This allows more water excretion, thereby raising the ECF osmolality again. Antidiuretic hormone secretion can be altered by changes in osmolality of less than 1%. This osmoreceptor-mediated reflex arc functions in maintaining normal osmotic homeostasis of the ECF.

The second stimulus consists of changes in ECF volume. Stretch receptors in the low pressure portion of the cardiovascular system (eg, vena cavae, right side of the heart, and pulmonary vessels) monitor blood volume. Stimuli from these receptors are conducted by afferent fibers to the hypothalamus (by way of the brain stem). A decrease in blood volume stimulates ADH secretion. The resultant increase in water retention elevates the blood volume without affecting arterial blood pressure. A rise in blood volume stops ADH secretion. This halts water retention, thereby restoring the normal volume of the ECF compartment. This mechanism operates to alter ADH secretion in response to changes in body position. Move-

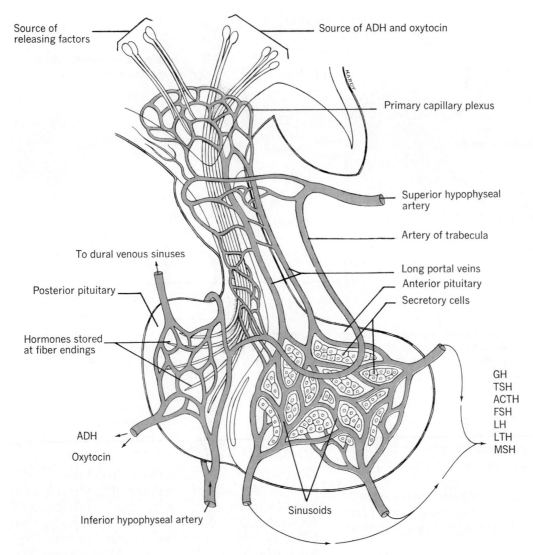

Source of releasing factors

Source of ADH and oxytocin

Primary capillary plexus

Superior hypophyseal artery

Artery of trabecula

To dural venous sinuses

Long portal veins
Anterior pituitary
Secretory cells

Posterior pituitary

Hormones stored at fiber endings

GH
TSH
ACTH
FSH
LH
LTH
MSH

ADH
Oxytocin

Inferior hypophyseal artery

Sinusoids

FIGURE 39-2
Highly diagrammatic and schematic representation of hypophyseal nerve fiber tracts and portal system. Releasing factors produced by cell bodies in hypothalamus trickle down axons to proximal part of stalk, where they enter the primary capillary plexus and are transported via portal vessels to sinusoids in adenohypophysis for control of secretions. ADH and oxytocin, produced by other cell bodies in hypothalamus, trickle down axons for storage in neurohypophysis until needed. (Chaffee EE, Lytle IM: Basic Physiology and Anatomy, 4th ed. Philadelphia, JB Lippincott)

ment from the recumbent to the upright position causes a temporary decrease in the stimulation of volume receptors because blood pools in the legs. This results in an increase in ADH secretion. Recumbency increases venous return from the legs. The increased volume triggers a decrease in ADH secretion, thereby increasing the volume of urine excreted. Such recumbent diuresis is especially notable in persons with edema of the lower extremities.

The third stimulus, changes in arterial blood pressure, also can regulate ADH secretion. The hypothalamus receives information from pressure receptors located in the carotid sinuses and aorta. A fall in arterial pressure in-

creases ADH secretion. The water retention thereby produced increases the plasma volume and pressure. A rise in arterial pressure produces the opposite effect. This mechanism may be more important in compensating for large changes in arterial blood pressure (eg, impending or actual shock).

Various other stimuli have been shown to influence ADH secretion. Increased ADH secretion can be prompted by angiotensin II, pain, "stress," opiates, nicotine, clofibrate (Atromid S), chlorpropamide (Diabinese), and barbiturates. Secretion of ADH is inhibited by alcohol and certain opiate antagonists.

Actions and Regulation of Oxytocin Secretion

This hormone stimulates contraction of the myoepithelial cells that line the milk ducts of the breast. This causes milk to be squeezed into the sinuses leading to the nipple surface (ie, milk ejection, or "let-down"). Oxytocin secretion is triggered by the hypothalamic receipt of afferent impulses from touch receptors around the nipples and also by receipt of afferent optical and aural stimuli. Therefore, suckling by the infant, manual stimulation of the nipples, or the sight or sound of a crying infant can trigger milk let-down. Ocytocin also causes contraction of the smooth muscles of the uterus. Such contractions play a role in labor and may facilitate the transport of sperm from the cervix to the fallopian tubes. During pregnancy, oxytocin secretion is stimulated by cervical dilation and estrogen and inhibited by progesterone and alcohol.

Hypophysiotropic Hormones

Other hypothalamic neurons produce "hypophysiotropic" hormones that stimulate or inhibit hormonal secretion by the anterior pituitary (adenohypophysis). These hormones are secreted into a capillary plexus near the median eminence that supplies blood to the anterior pituitary. A given hypophysiotropic hormone regulates the secretion of one or two anterior pituitary hormones. Both growth hormone (somatotropin) and prolactin are dually controlled by a stimulatory and an inhibiting hypophysiotropic hormone. Figure 39–3 illustrates the hypophysiotropic regulation of adenohypophyseal secretions.

Such hypothalamic regulation of pituitary functioning can be disrupted by hypothalamic lesions. This can lead to over- or undersecretion of one or more hormones released from the anterior or posterior pituitary. The hypothalamus also receives input from various higher and lower brain centers. These neural connections, together with the influence of the hypothalamus on the pituitary,

provide a beginning biologic basis for the construction of conceptual models that describe how stress, emotions, environmental stimuli, and perceptions affect endocrine functions.

Anterior Pituitary (Adenohypophysis)

This organ contains five morphologically different types of cells that secrete polypeptide hormones:

1. somatotrops, which secrete growth hormone (GH, somatotropin)
2. mammotrops, which secrete prolactin (luteotropic hormone, or LTH)
3. thyrotrops, which secrete TSH
4. corticotrops, which secrete ACTH, β-lipotrophin (BLPH), β-endorphin, and Γ-melanophore-stimulating hormone (MSH)
5. gonadotrops, which secrete luteinizing hormone (LH) and follicle-stimulating hormone (FSH)

Each type of cell is separately regulated by hypophysiotropic hormones (see Figure 39–3). LTH, LH, and FSH act on cells of the gonads (ovaries and testes) to regulate gamete (sperm and egg) and hormone production.

TSH stimulates cells of the thyroid gland to produce and secrete the two thyroid hormones. This and the manner by which these hormones alter TSH output are discussed later in this chapter. The corticotrops manufacture a long polypeptide chain, 265 amino acids long, called *proopiomelanocortin (POMC)*. Before secretion, POMC is separated into shorter fragments. Three of these are readily identified as ACTH, Γ-MSH, and BLPH. Part of the BLPH molecule can be further split off to form an endogenous opiate called β-*endorphin*. Endogenous opiates are further discussed in Chapter 27. The role of this opiate from the pituitary is not yet known.

Melanin is a dark pigment contained in special struc-

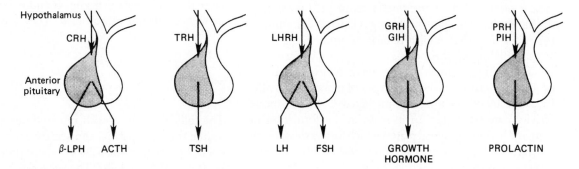

FIGURE 39–3
Effects of hypophysiotropic hormones on the secretion of anterior pituitary hormones. (Ganong WF: Review of Medical Physiology, 13th ed. Norwalk, CT, Appleton & Lange, 1987)

tures called *melanophores* within the cells of the skin of lower vertebrates (eg, fish, amphibians, and reptiles). MSH stimulates the dispersion of the melanin granules within these melanophores. This darkens the animal temporarily. Birds and mammals (including humans) have melanin, but it cannot be dispersed and is not contained within melanophores. The normal function of MSH in humans is not known, although there is some evidence that it can cause a darkening of certain areas of skin in humans with Addison's disease. In this condition, excess corticotropin (ACTH)-releasing hormone (CRH) stimulates corticotrops to secrete ACTH. Along with this, the other fragments of POMC, including MSH, are released. The role and regulation of ACTH is discussed in the section on the adrenal cortex. This leaves only growth hormone to be discussed here.

Growth Hormone (Somatotropin)

The production and secretion of growth hormone (GH) occurs in the anterior pituitary.

Metabolic Fate

Growth hormone is degraded primarily in the liver. Other metabolic sites have yet to be uncovered. The half-life of plasma GH is approximately 25 minutes.

Actions

This hormone acts both directly on target cells and indirectly by stimulating the liver and other as yet unidentified tissues to secrete various growth factors termed *somatomedins*. These growth factors are structurally similar to insulin. Human beings possess two such insulin-like growth factors (IGFs): IGF-I and IGF-II.

Direct actions of GH include (1) increasing the breakdown of fats (lipolysis) in adipose cells and the release of the fatty acids produced by lipolysis into the bloodstream (this is termed its *ketogenic effect*); (2) increasing hepatic glycolysis and thereby increasing plasma glucose levels (this is often called an *anti-insulin action*); (3) increasing the sensitivity of insulin-producing cells to certain stimuli; (4) increasing the cellular uptake of amino acids; and (5) stimulating erythropoiesis.

The various somatomedins seem to exert growth-promoting activity in different types of tissues. Normally, the net result of somatomedin-mediated growth hormone activity consists of (1) an increase in the formation of cartilage in the epiphyseal plates, which fosters the growth in length of long bones; (2) an increase in other skeletal growth; and (3) the growth of all other parts of the body (eg, soft tissue and viscera).

All growth hormone actions operate together to produce growth (eg, by cell division) and to provide the materials needed for this growth (ie, amino acids for synthesis of protein cell structure, fatty acids and glucose to provide energy, and erythrocytes to increase the availability of oxygen).

Regulation

Plasma concentrations of GH are controlled by the release of GH-releasing factor and GH release-inhibiting factor from the hypothalamus. Several stimuli influence the secretion of GH. Age is the most important overriding variable, and the actions of many of these other stimuli are influenced by it.

In general, factors that, at the appropriate age, can stimulate the secretion of GH include hypoglycemia, fasting, exercise, protein meal, glucagon, stress (both physiological and psychological), deeper stages of sleep, and drugs that bind to dopamine receptors. Major stimuli that decrease the output of GH include rapid eye movement sleep (dreaming), elevated plasma levels of glucose or fatty acids, and cortisol. Fluctuations in the levels of GH are dramatic; the *average* serum level, however, is remarkably similar at all ages. Growth is facilitated by GH, but other factors direct the rate of growth and the organs targeted for growth.

Thyroid

This gland is a bilobed, richly vascularized structure. The lobes lie lateral to the trachea just beneath the larynx and are connected by a bridge of thyroid tissue, called the *isthmus*, that runs across the anterior surface of the trachea. Microscopically, the thyroid is composed primarily of spheroid follicles, each of which stores a colloid material in its center. The follicles produce, store, and secrete the two major hormones: T_3 (triiodothyronine) and T_4 (thyroxine). If the gland is actively secreting, the follicles are small and contain little colloid. Inactive thyroid tissue contains large follicles, each of which possesses a large quantity of stored colloid. Other cells, the parafollicular cells (C cells), are scattered between the follicles. Parafollicular cells secrete the hormone calcitonin. It and two other hormones influence calcium metabolism. They are discussed later.

Thyroid Hormones

Manufacture and Secretion

The follicular cells absorb tyrosine (an amino acid) and iodide from the plasma and secrete them into the central colloid portion of the follicle, where they are used in the synthesis of T_3 and T_4. (The subscript refers to the number of iodide molecules that each substance contains.) Two iodide molecules are attached, first one and then the other, to each tyrosine molecule. Two such doubly iodinated tyrosines are combined to form T_4. T_3, which is much more biologically active than T_4 and is the predominant form of thyroid hormone produced, is formed by the combination of a doubly iodinated tyrosine with a singly iodinated one. These hormones are then stored in the colloid until they are needed. When they are to be secreted, the follicle cells transport them from the colloid to the plasma. Because of the role of iodine in the manufacture of thyroid hormones, the active uptake (from the plasma), storage, and release of small amounts of radioactive iodine by the thyroid can be used to measure the activity of this gland. Because the thyroid gland is virtually the only tissue of the body that absorbs and stores iodine, larger amounts of radioactive iodine can be used to destroy portions of the thyroid gland as a treatment for hyperthyroidism.

Transport and Metabolic Fate

Less than 1% of the secreted T_3 and T_4 remains free and physiologically active in the plasma. The remainder is bound to plasma proteins. Most is bound to thyroxine-binding globulin (TBG), a molecule manufactured by the liver, and the remainder is bound to two types of plasma albumin. Such protein-bound hormone serves as a reservoir to replace free T_3 and T_4 that has been degraded, thereby maintaining stable blood levels of thyroid hormones. The plasma proteins involved in transporting T_3 and T_4 are manufactured in the liver. Consequently, liver damage that decreases the plasma levels of these proteins can produce a condition resembling thyroid hormone excess (ie, hyperthyroidism). Plasma levels of these proteins also can be depressed by glucocorticoids, androgens, and L-asparaginase (an antineoplastic drug). They are elevated during pregnancy, and by estrogens, opiates, clofibrate, and major tranquilizers.

Thyroid hormones are deiodinated and catabolized by the liver, kidneys, and various other tissues. A small amount of degraded hormone is added to the bile secreted by the liver and is excreted in the stool.

An earlier index of thyroid secretion, the protein-bound iodine (PBI) index, used the protein-bound fraction of secreted thyroid hormones. It measured the iodide contained in the T_3 and T_4 attached to plasma proteins. This index is still used occasionally, although now plasma T_3 and T_4 are measured directly by radioimmunoassay.

Actions

T_3 directly crosses target cell membranes, whereas T_4 is changed into T_3 by target cell membranes before crossing. T_3 binds with receptors on the cell nucleus. Through this interaction with the nucleus, these hormones can alter the cellular synthesis of various enzymes and thereby modify cellular operations. Interestingly enough, the iodine in these hormones does not seem requisite for their actions:

several synthetic non–iodine-containing thyroid hormone analogues exist.

The actions of thyroid hormones are widespread and apparently stem from their stimulation of the basal metabolic rate (BMR) of most tissues (excluding brain, anterior pituitary, spleen, lymph nodes, testes, and lungs). The exact manner by which these hormones act on cell metabolism is not yet clear. Evidently, T_3 and, to a lesser extent, T_4 act to increase the mitochondrial enzyme systems involved in the oxidation of foodstuffs. The energy released by such oxidation is not efficiently stored in the high-energy bonds of ATP. Much is lost in the form of heat. This increases O_2 consumption of and heat production by these tissues (ie, the BMR). This is also termed the *calorigenic action*.

Effects secondary to calorigenesis include an increased cellular need for vitamins, increased nitrogen excretion, catabolism of protein and fat stores if the supply of carbohydrates is insufficient, and weight loss. The hepatic conversion of carotene to Vitamin A requires thyroid hormone.

T_3 and T_4 have other effects that are independent of their calorigenic ones. The ways in which these effects are produced are even less well understood than calorigenesis. Thyroid hormones are essential for the normal growth and development of many body systems, notably the skeletal and nervous systems. These hormones may stimulate the secretion of growth hormone and potentiate its effect on various tissues. The effect of thyroid hormones on the nervous system is best illustrated by the cretinism resulting from congenital thyroid insufficiency. Thyroid hormones are also necessary for normal levels of neuronal functioning. Thyroid insufficiency leads to slowed reflexes, slowed mentation, and decreases in level of consciousness (by way of decreased levels of reticular-activating system activity). Hyperthyroidism lowers synaptic thresholds within the central nervous system, causing hyperreflexia and a silky skeletal muscle tremor. Thyroid hormone increases the number of β_1 and β_2 adrenergic receptors in various tissues and the affinity of these receptors for catecholamine. This is why an increased heart rate and sweating often occur in hyperthyroidism. The catabolism of skeletal muscle proteins is increased by thyroid hormones to such a degree that pronounced muscle weakness results from prolonged hyperthyroidism (thyrotoxic myopathy). Thyroid hormones increase the rate of carbohydrate absorption from the small intestine and decrease circulating levels of cholesterol.

Regulation

The secretion of T_3 and T_4 by the thyroid gland is primarily regulated by the secretion of TSH from the anterior pituitary gland. TSH stimulates the manufacture and secretion of T_3 and T_4. A negative-feedback regulatory loop exists whereby increased levels of free (unbound) T_3 and T_4 suppress TSH secretion. Decreased plasma TSH results in decreased thyroid function, which causes a fall in free plasma T_3 and T_4. Low T_3 and T_4 levels act to stimulate TSH secretion. If, for some reason, a TSH-induced increase in thyroid activity does not raise the plasma levels of free T_3 and T_4, the continued high levels of TSH eventually cause an increase in the size of the thyroid gland (nontoxic goiter). In this case, an enlarged thyroid is not associated with overproduction of hormone.

This feedback loop maintains homeostasis of the daily secretion of TSH and thyroid hormones. In addition to being influenced by circulatory T_3 and T_4 levels, TSH secretion is regulated by a hypothalamic neurosecretory material termed *thyrotropin-releasing hormone* (TRH). The hypothalamic regulation of TSH and, consequently, of thyroid function seems to function in infant thermoregulation. In this process, TRH output is increased in response to cold and decreased in response to heat. The elevated thyroid hormone production presumably increases calorigenesis, which raises the body temperature of the "cold" infant. Similarly, a heat-provoked decrease in TRH causes a decrease in TSH and thyroid activity. This is thought to decrease calorigenesis, thereby decreasing the temperature of the "hot" infant. The effect of TRH in thermoregulation of adults is negligible.

Hormonal Influences on Calcium Metabolism

Three hormones exert a major influence on calcium metabolism. Two of these, activated vitamin D, or 1,25-dihydroxycholecalciferol, and parathormone, elevate plasma calcium levels; one, calcitonin, decreases blood levels of calcium.

1,25-Dihydroxycholecalciferol

Manufacture

This hormone is produced by the action of the liver and the kidneys on vitamin D. Ultraviolet light changes certain provitamins in the skin to a group of compounds, collectively referred to as *vitamin D*. One of these, D_3, can also be obtained from vitamin D-enriched and other foods. The liver converts D_3 to 25-hydroxycholecalciferol, which is then altered by kidney cells to a more active form, 1,25-dihydroxycholecalciferol.

Transport and Metabolic Fate

Details are not known.

Actions

Activated vitamin D acts on intracellular enzymes of intestinal mucosal cells to increase calcium absorption. To a lesser extent, it also increases the active transport of calcium out of osteoblasts into the bloodstream. Both these actions elevate plasma calcium levels. In vitamin deficiency states, the effect of decreased intestinal absorption outweighs any decrease in the mobilization of calcium from bone to produce an overall hypocalcia and poor mineralization of bone.

Regulation

Plasma calcium and phosphate levels operate in a negative-feedback loop to influence the activity of the renal enzyme system, which catalyzes the conversion of metabolically inactive vitamin D to the metabolically active 1,25-dihydroxycholecalciferol. High plasma calcium levels decrease this activation process, whereas low levels increase it. The formation of activated vitamin D is also facilitated by parathormone and decreased by metabolic acidosis and hypoinsulinemia (diabetes mellitus). The hypocalcemia seen in chronic renal disease results from an activated vitamin D deficiency.

Parathormone

This hormone is produced by the parathyroid glands. Each lobe of the thyroid gland typically contains two parathyroid glands: one in its superior pole and one in its inferior pole. Individual variation exists with respect to the number and distribution of parathyroid glands. Some persons have more or fewer than four. Others have parathyroid tissue in the mediastinum.

Manufacture and Secretion

Parathormone is a polypeptide produced and secreted by the chief cells of the parathyroid glands.

Transport and Metabolic Fate

Parathormone is transported free (unbound) in the plasma, has a half-life of less than 20 minutes, and is metabolically degraded by cells in the liver.

Actions

Parathormone acts on two target tissues: bone cells and kidney tubules. In bone, it stimulates osteoclast activity and inhibits osteoblast activity. This results in bone reabsorption with consequent mobilization of calcium and phosphate from the bony matrix into the bloodstream. In the kidney, parathormone increases the reabsorption of calcium by distal tubule cells and decreases the reabsorption of phosphate by proximal tubule cells. The net effect of these multiple actions is elevation of plasma calcium levels and lowering of plasma phosphate levels. At the cellular level, parathormone produces these effects by activating adenyl cyclase, thereby increasing the intracellular levels of cyclic AMP in the target tissues.

Regulation

Plasma calcium levels alter parathormone secretion by way of a negative-feedback loop. Secretion is inhibited by high plasma calcium levels and stimulated by low blood levels of calcium. The activated vitamin B deficiency-induced hypocalcemia, which occurs in chronic renal failure, typically produces a secondary hyperparathyroidism. Parathyroid gland secretion also is stimulated by hypomagnesemia.

Calcitonin

Manufacture and Secretion

This polypeptide hormone is produced by the parafollicular cells (C cells) of the thyroid gland. It can also be secreted by nonthyroidal tissue (eg, lung, intestine, pituitary, and bladder).

Transport and Metabolic Fate

Calcitonin seems to be transported unbound in the plasma. It has a half-life of less than 10 minutes.

Actions

Calcitonin lowers plasma calcium and phosphate levels by (1) inhibiting osteoclastic bone reabsorption, and (2) increasing urinary phosphate and calcium excretion. Calcitonin levels are elevated during pregnancy and lactation. This suggests that it may help to protect the mother's skeleton from excess calcium loss during these periods of calcium drain.

Regulation

Calcitonin does not seem to function in the normal daily homeostasis of plasma calcium levels. It appears to serve more of an "emergency function" in that it is secreted only if the plasma calcium level exceeds 9.3 mg/dl. At high blood calcium levels, calcitonin secretion is stimulated by increased levels of plasma calcium.

Other Hormones That Influence Calcium Metabolism

Four hormones bear mention here. T_3 and T_4 are thought by some to produce hypercalcemia, but the mechanism of action is unknown. Estrogens prevent parathormone from raising plasma calcium by mobilizing calcium from bone. Growth hormone increases urinary calcium excretion while also increasing intestinal calcium absorption. These two effects counterbalance each other, thereby producing

no net change in plasma calcium levels. Glucocorticoids tend to lower plasma calcium levels by decreasing intestinal absorption of calcium and increasing renal calcium excretion.

Islets of Langerhans

This name refers to the more than one million ovoid islands (clusters) of cells that are scattered throughout the pancreas, predominantly in the tail. Because of this distribution of islet cells, acute attacks of pancreatitis, which generally spare the tail, usually spare the islets. Episodes of chronic recurrent pancreatitis, however, typically involve all of the pancreas. Consequently, these episodes cause islet cell destruction and diabetes mellitus. Each cell cluster is richly supplied with capillaries, into which its hormones are secreted. The islets are composed of four types of cells: (1) alpha cells, which secrete glucagon; (2) beta cells, which secrete insulin; (3) delta cells, which secrete somatostatin; and (4) F cells, which secrete pancreatic polypeptide.

Insulin

Manufacture and Secretion

The precursor of insulin, proinsulin, is manufactured in the granular endoplasmic reticulum, as are all cell proteins. Proinsulin is a "necklace" of amino acid beads that has one end folded over the other, so that it resembles a squashed figure nine. It leaves the reticulum and is stored as secretory granules in another cell structure. Here, two ends of the folded proinsulin necklace become attached to one another (by way of disulfide bonds) to form two parallel chains resembling railroad tracks. The two ends are then separated from the center of the necklace. This center chain of amino acids is termed *C-peptide*. Proinsulin can be found in the plasma as a result of certain islet tumors or overstimulation of the beta cells. C-peptide is secreted into the bloodstream along with insulin. Because there is a 1:1 ratio between C-peptide and insulin, plasma C-peptide levels can be used to measure endogenous insulin secretion or degree of beta cell activity.

Metabolic Fate

Insulin is currently known to act only on a few types of tissues. However, the membranes of nearly all types of body cells possess insulin receptors. The possession of insulin receptors by cells on which insulin does not act may be explained by the discovery of the growth factors (IGF-I and IGF-II). The insulin receptors serve as receptors for these growth factors as well as for insulin.

Binding of insulin to the insulin receptors initiates the physiological action of insulin on the cell. After a molecule of insulin binds to a receptor, the insulin-receptor complex is taken into the cytoplasm of the cell by endocytosis and is destroyed within 14 to 15 hours by lysosomal enzymes. New receptors replace the destroyed one in the cell membranes. Plasma insulin has a half-life of approximately 5 minutes. About 80% of all circulating insulin is catabolized by liver and kidney cells.

Actions

The mechanism by which insulin exerts its action is currently unknown. It is known only that insulin does not activate adenyl cyclase. The actions of insulin are summarized in Table 39–2.

In addition, insulin is known to facilitate glucose uptake by connective tissue, leukocytes, mammary glands, lens of eye, aorta, pituitary, and alpha islet cells. In general, insulin enables glucose to be readily available for aerobic oxidation by the Krebs citric acid cycle in muscle, adipose, and connective tissue cells. Facilitation of the preferential use of glucose as cellular fuel means that the cells do not need to oxidize (burn) fatty or amino acids. Instead, these can be conserved. Protein synthesis and fat storage are increased in liver, muscle, and adipose tissue. Breakdown of fats and proteins is decreased. Hepatic gluconeogenesis also is decreased or halted, and glycogen synthesis is increased.

Regulation

Insulin secretion is influenced by a variety of factors (Table 39–3). Monosaccharides serve as the primary regulatory mechanism for insulin secretion. Elevated plasma levels of glucose, fructose, and mannose act in a negative-feedback loop to increase the secretion of insulin. Lower levels of these sugars decrease insulin output. Other monosaccharides (eg, galactose, xylose, and arabinose) have no effect on insulin secretion. Glucagon and β-adrenergic-stimulating chemicals increase insulin secretion by stimulating adenyl cyclase, an enzyme that elevates levels of cyclic

AMP within beta cells. Theophylline, which inhibits the degradation of beta cell cyclic AMP, also promotes production. Beta cells are also stimulated to secrete insulin by tolbutamide and other sulfonylurea derivatives, acetylcholine, impulses from vagal nerve branches to the islets, selected amino acids such as arginine, and beta ketoacids. The mechanisms of action of these stimuli are currently unclear. Insulin production is inhibited by the following: (1) α-adrenergic-stimulating agents, (2) β-adrenergic-blocking agents, (3) diazoxide (Proglycem), (4) thiazide diuretics, (5) phenytoin (Dilantin), (6) alloxan, (7) agents that prevent glucose metabolism (2-deoxyglucose or mannoheptulose), (8) somatostatin, and (9) insulin itself. See Table 39–3.

Chronic stimulation of beta cells, such as by a high carbohydrate diet for several weeks, can cause a limited amount of hypertrophy and subsequent increase in the insulin-producing capacity. Overstimulation, however, produces beta cell exhaustion. Stimulation of these exhausted cells produces beta cell death and a depletion in the beta cell reserve. Beta cell activity is also decreased by the administration of exogenous insulin. Such decreased activity enables the cells to "rest" and results in their being temporarily hyperproductive after the withdrawal of exogenous insulin. The quantity and activity of insulin receptors also can be regulated by various factors. Increased amounts of insulin, obesity, acromegaly, and excess glucocorticoids decrease the receptors' number or activity or both. Exercise and decreased circulating levels of insulin increase the activity of insulin receptors.

Glucagon

Secretion

This polypeptide hormone is manufactured and secreted by the alpha islet cells.

Metabolic Fate

The half-life of plasma glucagon is 5 to 10 minutes. This hormone is degraded mainly by the liver.

Actions

The major function of glucagon is to elevate blood sugar levels by influencing enzyme systems within liver, fat, and muscle cells and then to enable this plasma glucose to enter and be used by body cells (eg, muscle) by stimulating the secretion of insulin. By this function, glucagon prevents hypoglycemia between meals, during exercise, during the first few days of fasting, and after a high-protein meal (dietary protein stimulates an increase in plasma insulin, which causes a rapid cellular uptake of absorbed dietary carbohydrates).

TABLE 39–2
Major Actions of Insulin Upon Fat and Muscle Cells

Muscle Cells	Adipose Cells
Increased glucose entry	Increased glucose entry
Increased K$^+$ uptake	Increased K$^+$ uptake
Increased glycogen synthesis	Increased fatty acid entry and synthesis
Increased amino acid entry	Increased fat deposition
Increased protein synthesis	Increased conversion of glucose to fatty acids
Decreased protein catabolism	Inhibition of lipolysis
Increased ketone entry into cells	

TABLE 39–3
Factors Affecting Insulin Secretion

Stimulators	Inhibitors
Glucose	Somatostatin
Mannose	2-Deoxyglucose
Amino acids (leucine, arginine, others)	Mannoheptulose
Intestinal hormones (GIP, gastrin, secretin, CCK, glucagon, others?)	α-Adrenergic-stimulating agents (norepinephrine, epinephrine)
β-Keto acids	β-Adrenergic-blocking agents (propranolol)
Acetylcholine	Diazoxide
Glucagon	Thiazide diuretics
Cyclic AMP and various cyclic AMP-generating substances	Phenytoin
	Alloxan
β-Adrenergic-stimulating agents	Microtubule inhibitors
Theophylline	Insulin
Sulfonylureas	

(Reproduced, with permission, from Ganong WF: Review of Medical Physiology, 13th ed., Norwalk, CT, Appleton & Lange Medical Publications, 1987)

To perform this function, glucagon stimulates liver cells to perform glycogenolysis and gluconeogenesis. This increases the glucose concentration within liver cells, and, because these cells can dephosphorylate intracellular glucose, this glucose can be released from the liver into the bloodstream. The fatty acids and amino acids needed for gluconeogenesis are supplied by the glucagon-stimulated breakdown of fats in adipose cells and the release of fatty acids into the bloodstream. If the supply of fatty acids is not sufficient, glucagon also stimulates the breakdown of proteins into amino acids in muscle cells and the release of amino acids into the plasma. These fatty acids and amino acids are then taken up by hepatocytes and used as raw materials in gluconeogenesis. Glucagon also elevates plasma ketone levels by increasing hepatic ketone production and promotes the secretion of somatostatin and GH.

Although glucagon opposes the effects of insulin on blood sugar levels, it also stimulates the secretion of insulin. This apparent contradiction is actually a logical "second step" in the biologic function of this hormone. It enables the increased plasma glucose to enter and be used by various tissues. An elevated plasma glucose level itself stimulates insulin secretion, but this takes a while. The direct action of glucagon on beta cells simply is faster.

At the cellular level, the actions of glucagon on cell enzyme systems are mediated by glucagon-induced elevations in intracellular cyclic AMP. This chemical then acts as a "second messenger" to alter the enzyme activity of the cell to produce the "actions of glucagon." Because of this effect on intracellular cyclic AMP, large amounts of exogenous glucagon act to increase the inotropic capacity of myocardial tissue. However, lower levels of endogenous glucagon do not seem to have this effect.

Regulation

As is the case with beta cells, alpha cells are stimulated by β-adrenergic agonists, theophylline, elevated plasma levels of dietary amino acids (primarily those used in gluconeogenesis), and vagal (cholinergic) stimulation. Glucagon secretion is also prompted by glucocorticoids (eg, cortisol, CCK, and gastrin). Exercise, physical stress, and infections also increase alpha cell activity. Whereas the effects of exercise on glucagon secretion seem to be mediated by increased β-adrenergic activity, stress and infection probably operate by increasing plasma glucocorticoid levels. Dietary amino acids are believed to enhance glucagon secretion by their effects on CCK or gastrin or both, because intravenous amino acids exert little or no effect on alpha cells.

Elevated plasma glucose operates by a negative-feedback loop to retard or halt the output of glucagon; however, plasma insulin must be present for this mechanism to operate. Like beta cell secretion, alpha cell secretion is inhibited by α-adrenergic agonists, phenytoin, and somatostatin. Fatty acids and ketone bodies in the plasma can inhibit glucagon secretion, but this inhibition must be weak, because plasma glucagon levels can be quite elevated during diabetic ketoacidosis.

Somatostatin

Manufacture and Secretion

This tetradecapeptide is produced not only by the delta cells of the pancreas but also by (1) the hypothalamus, where it functions as an inhibitor of anterior pituitary growth hormone secretion; (2) neurons of the CNS, where it probably functions as a synaptic neurotransmitter agent; and (3) delta cells in the gastric mucosa, where it inhibits the secretion of gastrin and other lesser known gastrointestinal hormones. Islet cell somatostatin is secreted into the bloodstream and therefore functions as a hormone.

Metabolic Fate

This is currently not known.

Actions

Pancreatic somatostatin inhibits the activity of all other islet cells. The biologic significance of this action is not yet known. The only current clinical data of relevance concern delta cell tumors. These produce a clinical picture that resembles diabetes mellitus but that is reversible with tumor ablation.

Regulation

The secretion of somatostatin from islet cells is increased by glucose, certain amino acids, and CCK. Factors that inhibit islet somatostatin secretion are currently unknown.

Pancreatic Polypeptide

Not much is known about this islet hormone in humans. Its secretion in humans is enhanced by dietary protein, exercise, acute hypoglycemia, and fasting. Somatostatin and elevated plasma glucose levels decrease the secretion of this polypeptide. No definite actions of this hormone have been established for humans.

Adrenal Glands

An adrenal gland lies at the superior pole of each kidney. Each gland is composed of an inner core, the medulla, surrounded by an outer layer, the cortex. Although they are structurally related, the medulla and cortex are derived from different embryologic tissues and function as separate entities.

Adrenal Medulla

This gland is basically a modified sympathetic ganglion. The axons of preganglionic sympathetic neurons arrive from the thoracic cord by way of splanchnic nerves (see Figure 27–11 and Table 27–1). They synapse in the adrenal medulla with modified postganglionic cells that have lost their axons and secrete chemicals directly into the bloodstream. Therefore, the adrenal medullas may appro-

priately be viewed as endocrine extensions of the sympathetic arm of the autonomic nervous system.

Manufacture and Secretion

Four chemicals are produced and secreted by two morphologically different cell types: (1) dopamine, a precursor of norepinephrine; (2) norepinephrine, the typical product of postganglionic sympathetic neurons; (3) epinephrine, a methylated version of norepinephrine; and (4) opioid peptides (enkephalins). The first three chemicals are collectively termed *catecholamines*. They are stored in granules within the medulla cells. Their secretion is triggered by stimulation of the preganglionic neurons that innervate the medulla. This causes the neurons to release acetylcholine, which in turn prompts the formerly postganglionic medulla cells to secrete. The stimulus for the secretion of opioid peptides has not yet been identified.

Metabolic Fate

The half-life of plasma catecholamines is approximately 2 minutes. These compounds are rapidly degraded by plasma renal and hepatic catechol O-methyl transferase enzymes into vanillylmandelic acid (VMA), metanephrine, and normetanephrine, which are excreted in the urine. Only small quantities of nondegraded catecholamines are found in the normal urine. The metabolism and fate of the medullary enkephalins are unknown.

Actions

Predictably, the epinephrine and norepinephrine secreted by the adrenal medulla mimic the effects of mass discharge from sympathetic neurons (see Table 27–1). Apart from this, however, they produce several metabolic actions. First, they elevate blood sugar levels by activating an enzyme, phosphorylase, that promotes hepatic glycogenolysis. Because liver cells possess the enzyme glucose-6-phosphatase, the glucose produced by this glycogen breakdown is able to diffuse out of hepatocytes and into the bloodstream. These hormones also induce muscle cells to participate in elevating blood sugar levels, although this process is less direct. Phosphorylase in muscle cells also is activated by these catecholamines. However, the intracellular glucose thereby produced is unable to exit the muscle cells, because they do not possess glucose-6-phosphatase. Instead, this glucose is catabolized to lactate, which can leave the muscle cells. Lactate then circulates to the liver, where it is converted to glucose that can enter the bloodstream. These hormones can also elevate plasma glucose levels by stimulating the secretion of glucagon and increase the uptake of glucose into body tissues by stimulating the secretion of insulin. Epinephrine and norepinephrine can also produce the opposite effects by stimulating α-adrenergic receptors on islet cells. Because of differential effects of both hormones on α- and β-adrenergic receptors, the net result is that epinephrine elevates plasma glucose much more than does norepinephrine.

A second metabolic effect of catecholamines is promotion of lipolysis in adipose tissue. This elevates plasma free fatty acid levels and provides an alternative energy source for many body cells. Circulating catecholamines also increase alertness by stimulating the reticular activating system (see Chapter 27).

Lastly, these hormones produce an increase in the metabolic rate of the body and a cutaneous vasoconstriction, both of which result in an elevation in body temperature. However, the accelerated metabolism requires the presence of the thyroid and adrenal cortex hormones.

The physiological actions of both adrenal medullary dopamine and the enkephalins are currently unknown. Exogenous dopamine is useful in combating certain shocks because it has a positive inotropic effect on the heart (by way of β_1 receptors) and produces renal vasodilation and peripheral vasoconstriction. The overall effect of moderate dosages is elevation of systolic blood pressure (without an appreciable increase in diastolic blood pressure) together with retention or restoration of renal output. To understand and compare the actions of drugs that mimic adrenal medullary hormones, one must learn which receptors are stimulated by these agents (α_1, α_2, β_1, β_2) and determine what effects these receptors mediate (see Table 27–1).

Regulation

Stimulation of the adrenal medulla glands is part of a general sympathetic-adrenal medulla (SAM) response to exercise and to perceived threats to one's biopsychological integrity and survival (Cannon termed the latter the "fight or flight" response). Hypoglycemia also stimulates increased adrenal medulla secretion.

The results of the SAM response enable the body to perform vigorous physical exertion optimally. The heart rate and blood pressure are increased (increasing perfusion), and blood flow is shunted away from the skin and gastrointestinal tract to more "vital" organs for exertion, such as skeletal muscles, brain, and heart. The reticular activating system is stimulated, fostering alertness. Blood glucose and fatty acid levels are raised, thereby increasing the available energy sources for cells. Pupils are dilated, increasing the field of peripheral vision and the amount of light entering the eyes. Sweat glands are stimulated, providing cooling of the body in advance of and during the time that the body temperature is elevated as the result of the physical exertion. The majority of this SAM response is mediated by sympathetic nerve fibers to various body structures; circulating catecholamines play only a minor role. Furthermore, many tissue responses (eg, those of muscle cells) to such sympathetic demands require the presence of glucocorticoids to enable the tissues to meet the demands of the SAM response, and indeed the SAM

response often accompanies the stress-induced secretion of adrenal steroids discovered by Seyle (this and the endocrine response to both physical and psychological stress are discussed in the section on the adrenal cortex).

The SAM response is initiated by the perception of a stimulus or situation that a person evaluates on the basis of past experience and current resources to be a threat to his well-being. This response involves the cerebral cortex. Impulses from the cortex travel by way of nerve fibers to the limbic system, where they are involved in generating an emotional response. Additional impulses from both the cortex and the limbic system stimulate sympathetic centers in the diencephalon. These centers in turn discharge a specific pattern of impulses down descending fibers to various sympathetic neurons in the cord, bringing about the SAM response.

Adrenal Cortex

This gland is composed of three histologically different layers. Its exterior is covered by a capsule. The outermost layer, the zona glomerulosa, lies just beneath the capsule. It produces and secretes primarily mineralocorticoids, such as aldosterone. The inner two layers, the zona fasciculata and zona reticularis, manufacture and secrete glucocorticoids (cortisol and corticosterone) and adrenal androgens and estrogens. If these inner cortical layers are destroyed, they can be regenerated from zona glomerulosa cells. Because the biosynthetic pathways and metabolic fates for all adrenocortical hormones are interrelated, these are discussed together for all hormones. Actions and regulation are considered separately for mineralocorticoids, glucocorticoids, and sex steroids.

Manufacture and Secretion

Figure 39–4 depicts the metabolic pathways for synthesis of all adrenocortical hormones. Each of these metabolic steps is governed by a specific enzyme. Genetic deficiencies in one or more of these enzymes produce syndromes involving the underproduction or overproduction of various cortical hormones. Drugs that act to inhibit specific enzymes are used clinically to assess cortical function. One such drug is metyrapone, which inhibits cortisol synthesis.

Metabolic Fate

After secretion, plasma cortisol and, to a lesser extent, corticosterone are bound to a plasma globulin called *corticosteroid-binding globulin (CBG)*, or *transcortin*. Only the unbound hormones are physiologically active. The bound glucocorticoids serve as a hormone reservoir that is used to replace degraded unbound hormone. The half-lives of plasma corticosterone and cortisol are roughly 50 and 80 minutes, respectively. CBG is manufactured by liver cells. Therefore, decreased hepatic function (eg, cirrhosis)

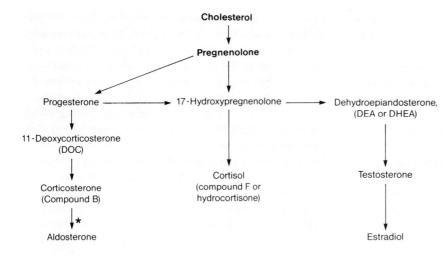

FIGURE 39–4
Biosynthetic pathways for adrenal cortical hormones. Cells in all three layers contain all pathways except that from corticosterone to aldosterone: only cells of zona glomerulosa can perform this step (*).

can lead to subnormal quantities of plasma CBG, which in turn results in excess quantities of circulating unbound, active glucocorticoids.

Only a small amount of aldosterone is bound to plasma proteins. Its half-life is approximately 20 minutes.

Adrenal steroids are degraded by the liver. Their metabolites are converted to a soluble form by the same enzyme system that conjugates bilirubin (ie, the glucuronyltransferase system). The adrenal steroids and bilirubin compete for this system, and an excess of one type of substance can potentially inhibit the degradation of the others. Depressed hepatic function also can retard the degradation of adrenal steroids, thereby producing a clinical picture of hormone excess. The soluble degraded steroid metabolites are excreted by the kidneys.

Actions of Glucocorticoids

The effects of pharmacologic dosages of these hormones are considered separately from those of normal physiological levels. As the name "glucocorticoid" suggests, cortisol and corticosterone influence glucose metabolism. They elevate plasma glucose levels by promoting hepatic gluconeogenesis and glycogenolysis. To facilitate gluconeogenesis, these hormones cause the breakdown of fat and proteins and the release of fatty and amino acids into the bloodstream, which carries them to the liver.

Glucocorticosteroids enable tissues to respond to glucagon and catecholamines; they also prevent rapid fatigue of skeletal muscle. The mode by which glucocorticoids produce these effects is not currently understood, and they go unnoticed in the normal person. One can best appreciate them by observing the result of their absence in adrenalectomized patients and in untreated people who are exposed to perceived threat or stress. These "enabling" and metabolic effects possibly constitute a major portion of the "stress resistance" provided by the glucocorticosteroids.

Cortisol and corticosterone also act on the kidneys to permit the excretion of a normal water load in one of three

ways: (1) glucocorticoids make distal or collecting tubules more permeable to the reabsorption of water independently of sodium reabsorption; (2) glucocorticoids increase the glomerular filtration rate; or (3) glucocorticoids reduce the output of ADH.

The effects of glucocorticosteroids on plasma components are mixed. They decrease the number of plasma eosinophils and basophils but increase the number of circulating neutrophils, platelets, and erythrocytes. By both suppressing production and increasing destruction, glucocorticoids decrease the number of lymphocytes. They also decrease the size of lymph nodes. A major function of lymphocytes is to provide either humoral immunity (with antibodies) or cell-mediated immunity. Stress-induced elevations in glucocorticoid secretion and the resulting decrease in lymphocytes may explain the decrease in immunocompetence that so often occurs in people who are under psychological or physical stress.

Other effects of physiological levels of glucocorticoids include decreasing olfactory and gustatory sensitivity. People with adrenal insufficiency can detect various chemicals (eg, sugar, salt, urea, and KCl) by either taste or smell with a sensitivity that is 40 to 120 times greater than normal.

In pharmacologic dosages, glucocorticoids possess immunosuppressive anti-inflammatory and antihistaminic activity. Glucocorticoids suppress the immune system by inhibiting the production of interleukin-II by T4 (helper) lymphocytes. Decreases in Interleukin-II reduce the proliferation of T8 (suppressor, cytotoxic) and B lymphocytes. Glucocorticoids act in several ways to suppress the inflammatory response, including the influx of phagocytes and the activation of complement and kinins. First, they inhibit the formation of the raw material (arachidonic acid) needed for the manufacture of chemicals that trigger the inflammatory response (eg, leukotrienes, prostaglandins). Second, they inhibit the release of interleukin-I from granulocytes. Third, glucocorticoids prevent fibroblasts from acting to wall off an infectious areas from the rest of the body. This can be very dangerous to patients with infections, because the inflammatory response destroys invading microorganisms and facilitates both the immune system and normal wound healing. Conversely, glucocorticoids can be of great benefit in the treatment of certain noninfective inflammatory conditions (eg, rheumatoid arthritis and systemic lupus erythematosus). Inhibition of fibroblasts can prevents the formation of keloids and postsurgical adhesions. Glucocorticoids can also be beneficial in the treatment of certain allergies (eg, asthma, hives, and minimal change glomerular disease) because they prevent the release of histamines from mast cells. Their use as immunosuppressives enables patients to receive organ transplants. In any case, the potentially deleterious side effects of glucocorticoids usually require that they be used only after other treatments (eg, non-steroidal anti-inflammatory drugs or antihistamines) have failed or if the benefits clearly outweigh the risks (eg, in renal disease or with organ transplants). In addition to immunosuppression, glucocorticoids trigger the development of all or part of Cushing's syndrome (eg, diabetes, hypertension, protein-wasting, and osteoporosis) and inhibit growth in infants and children.

Regulation of Glucocorticoid Secretion

The secretion of glucocorticoids is triggered by the release of corticotropin-releasing factor (CRF), a neurosecretory material released by the hypothalamus. CRF stimulates the cells of the anterior pituitary to secrete ACTH. Without the stimulus of ACTH, the cells of the zona fasciculata and zona reticularis do not secrete glucocorticoids. Elevated plasma glucocorticoid levels function in a negative-feedback loop to decrease or halt the secretion of CRF and thereby indirectly ACTH as well.

There is a diurnal rhythm to the secretion of CRF that causes a similar rhythm in the output of ACTH and glucocorticoids. The net result is that maximal glucocorticoid secretion occurs between 6:00 and 8:00 AM in persons sleeping from midnight to 8:00 AM in a 24-hour day. Tumors that secrete CRF, ACTH, or glucocorticoids do not demonstrate such a rhythm, a fact that is useful in their diagnosis. The "biologic clock" that regulates this and other diurnal, or circadian, rhythms is located in the hypothalamus, just above the area where the optic nerves cross (optic chiasma). Presumably, fibers from this area send impulses to the CRF-secreting area of the hypothalamus to regulate this neurosecretion.

The hypothalamic neurosecretion of CRF is also triggered by neural impulses from higher brain centers (eg, cerebral cortex) in response to psychological stress. This type of stress is defined according to Lazarus' cognitive-phenomenological theory as a situation in which demands exceed coping resources. This can occur slowly and deliberately or instantaneously and without the person's being precisely aware that such a phenomenon has occurred. Before the mid-1970s, Seyle's proposed general adaptation syndrome was the only existing model for physiological responses to stress. According to this theory, any type of stress, physical or psychological, triggers the release of glucocorticoids by the CRF–ACTH mechanism. Then, in an elegant series of experiments on monkeys that separated psychological from purely physical stressors, Mason and coworkers discovered that glucocorticosteroids were typically released only in response to psychological stress. These researchers found that physical stressors (eg, cold, starvation) each induced a different pattern of responses from almost all the endocrine glands. Each type of stressor studied produced a different profile of endocrine responses that continued to change over several days after exposure of the animal to the stress-provoking agent. This work was later confirmed in humans. Thus, the physiological responses to stress can no longer be attributed only to the glucocorticoids.

Now we can conceptualize the perception of a potential physical or psychological threat to one's well-being as triggering a SAM response. If the demands of this or any other situation are evaluated as exceeding one's current resources, the CRF–ACTH–glucocorticosteroid mechanism is activated. The beneficial functions of normal levels of glucocorticoids in enabling tissues to respond to glucagon and catecholamines are more than adequate to meet the needs of the SAM mechanism for a short time. If these needs continue, additional stress-induced glucocorticoid secretion is required. Eventually, if the stress continues unameliorated, exhaustion of the adrenal cortex occurs, glucocorticoid levels drop, tissues are no longer able to meet the demands of the SAM mechanism, muscle fatigue occurs, readily available cell energy sources (eg, plasma glucose and fatty acid) are depleted, and vascular collapse and death result.

Actions of Mineralocorticoids

Aldosterone and glucocorticoids that have some mineralocorticoid function (eg, DOCA) increase sodium reabsorption by the cells of the collecting ducts and distal tubules of the nephrons. Because of the cation exchange system in the distal tubule cells (see Chapter 22), such sodium reabsorption can increase potassium secretion, thereby fostering potential hypokalemia. The reabsorption of sodium osmotically causes water reabsorption. This expands the volume of ECF. The increase in blood volume causes an elevation in blood pressure. Edema does not usually result, however, because above a certain level of aldosterone-induced sodium reabsorption, the expansion of the ECF compartment can trigger (1) the secretion of natriuretic hormone, or (2) decreased sodium reabsorption in the proximal tubule. Either of these effects opposes the action of aldosterone and sodium excretion.

Regulation of Mineralocorticoid Secretion

The primary mechanism for this is the renin–angiotensin system. Pituitary ACTH does not stimulate zona glomerulosa cells under normal conditions. Cells of the juxtaglomerular apparatus (JGA) are wedged between the renal afferent arteriole as it enters the glomerulus and the distal tubule as it passes by this area. The JGA contains baroceptor cells that monitor the afferent arteriole blood pressure and other cells that monitor the sodium and chloride concentration in the urine within the distal tubule (the lower the concentration, the slower the formation of filtrate, if all other factors are equal). A fall either in blood pressure or in the concentration of electrolytes stimulates the JGA to secrete the glycoprotein hormone renin. The major classes of stimuli that trigger renin secretion are (1) decreased renal perfusion (eg, cardiac failure, dehydration, and hemorrhage), and (2) low ECF salt concentrations (eg, from excessive use of diuretics).

Renin converts a circulating plasma globulin into angiotensin I. As the blood passes through the lungs (and to a lesser extent in other parts of the circulatory system), angiotensin I is converted to angiotensin II. This physiologically active chemical acts on (1) the zona glomerulosa to promote aldosterone secretion, which leads to retention of salt and water, and (2) vascular smooth muscle, thereby stimulating profound vasoconstriction. The net result of both actions of angiotensin II is elevation of systemic blood pressure, which, among other things, improves renal perfusion.

The JGA contains β_2 receptors and can also be stimulated by sympathetic fibers. Prostaglandins also stimulate the JGA. All three stimulate the secretion of renin. Therefore, the secretion of renin can be pharmacologically decreased by β_2-blockers (eg, propranolol [Inderal]). Prostaglandin inhibitors (aspirin, non-steroidal anti-inflammatory agents, or indomethacin [Indocin]) can exert a similar action. Captopril (Capoten) prevents the conversion of angiotensin I to angiotensin II. These effects have made captopril and β_2-blockers useful as antihypertensive agents.

Aldosterone secretion is also stimulated by an increase in plasma potassium levels, but not by increased sodium levels. The potassium seems to act by facilitating the conversion of cholesterol to aldosterone in zona glomerulosa cells. Another regulating factor for aldosterone secretion is posture. An upright body position increases aldosterone levels by increasing production and decreasing degradation. How this works is unclear, but because of this, aldosterone levels of bedridden patients are slightly subnormal. There also is a poorly understood diurnal rhythm of aldosterone secretion, with highest levels occurring in the early morning hours just prior to the person's awakening. This rhythm is not due to the diurnal CRF-ACTH rhythm because that affects only glucocorticoid secretion.

Other Hormones

Natriuretic Hormone

Manufacture and Secretion

Natriuretic hormone is manufactured by cells in the walls of the atria of the heart. For this reason, its other name is atrial natriuretic peptide (ANP).

Metabolic Fate

This is currently unknown.

Actions

ANP increases renal excretion of salt and water. The mechanism of this action is currently debated. Some evidence suggests that ANP acts by increasing glomerular filtration. Other evidence indicates ANP inhibits the "membrane active transport mechanism" responsible for the reabsorption of sodium by renal tubule cells. Decreased sodium reabsorption decreases the movement of water from the urine in the nephron back into the blood of the peritubular capillaries, thereby increasing the elimination of water and salt from the body. Natriuretic hormone also inhibits the secretion of renin by the juxtaglomerular apparatus of the kidney, thereby lowering plasma angiotensin levels.

ANP also acts to inhibit the "membrane active transport mechanism" responsible for "pumping" sodium out of vascular smooth muscle cells. The consequent rise in intracellular sodium acts to inhibit the entry of calcium ions, thereby lowering the intracellular concentration of calcium ions. The decrease in the intracellular free calcium promotes vasodilation and a lowering of the systemic blood pressure.

Regulation

Natriuretic hormone is secreted in response to a rise in ECF volume caused by the ingestion of salt and water. The exact stimulus appears to be a stretch of the muscle fibers in the atrial walls which results from the increased venous return that is caused by the rise in extracellular fluid volume. As the natriuresis causes the extracellular fluid volume to fall back to normal, the secretion of natriuretic hormone stops.

Erythropoietin

Manufacture and Secretion

Erythropoietin is formed and secreted by Kupffer cells and hepatocytes in the liver and by the endothelial cells of the peritubular capillaries in the renal cortex.

Metabolic Fate

The half-life of circulating erythropoietin is 5 hours. It is degraded by hepatocytes.

Action

Erythropoietin increases the manufacture of erythrocytes (red blood cells) in the bone marrow by stimulating stem cells to be converted to erythrocyte precursors. The circulating level of red blood cells increases within 3 to 4 days after stimulation of the marrow by erythropoietin.

Regulation

Tissue oxygen levels regulate the secretion of erythropoietin. Secretion of erythropoietin is stimulated by hypoxia of the liver and kidneys. As the increase in circulating erythrocytes supplies more oxygen to these tissues, the disappearance of hypoxia halts the secretion of this hormone. Cobalt salts, catecholamines, and androgens also can stimulate the secretion of erythropoietin.

BIBLIOGRAPHY

Ganong WF: Review of Medical Physiology, 15th ed. Norwalk, CT, Appleton & Lange, 1991

Guyton AC: Textbook of Medical Physiology, 8th ed. Philadelphia, WB Saunders, 1991

McCance KL, Huether SE: Pathophysiology, The Biologic Basis for Disease in Adults and Children. St Louis, CV Mosby, 1990

Prezbindowski KS, Tortora GJ: Learning Guide to Accompany Principles of Anatomy and Physiology. New York, Harper & Row, 1990

Tortora GJ, Anagnostakos NP: Principles of Anatomy and Physiology. New York, Harper & Row, 1990

STUDY QUESTIONS

1. Excess secretions of anterior pituitary hormones could cause

   a. Addison's disease
   b. acromegaly
   c. Cushing's disease
   d. two of the above

2. Side effects of steroid medications include

   1. osteoporosis
   2. nervousness and insomnia
   3. peptic ulcer
   4. hypoglycemia

      a. 1 and 2
      b. 3 and 4
      c. 1 and 3
      d. 2 and 4

3. Growth hormone secretion is decreased by

   a. increased plasma glucose levels
   b. insulin
   c. exercise
   d. two of the above

4. Blood glucose levels are NOT affected by

   a. aldosterone
   b. insulin
   c. glucagon
   d. norepinephrine

5. Thyroid hormones cause

1. increased basal metabolism
2. decreased TSH secretion
3. hyperglycemia
4. poor wound healing

   a. 1 and 2
   b. 3 and 4
   c. 1 and 3
   d. 2 and 4

(continued)

CHAPTER 40

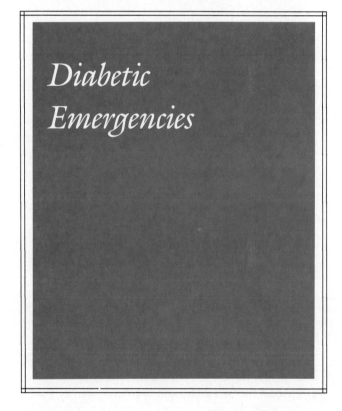

Diabetic Emergencies

Hudak: Critical Care Nursing:
A Holistic Approach, 6th ed. © 1994
J. B. Lippincott Company.

893

BEHAVIORAL OBJECTIVES

Based on the content in this chapter, the reader should be able to:

1. Identify the two basic nutritional tasks of feeding and fasting.
2. Describe the brain's dependence on glucose.
3. Discuss the metabolic and hormonal activity that occurs in the four phases of nutrition—fed state, postabsorptive state, short fasting state, and prolonged fasting state.
4. Differentiate the two forms of diabetes—type I or insulin-dependent diabetes (IDDM) and type II or non–insulin-dependent diabetes (NIDDM).
5. Identify the precipitating factors of diabetic ketoacidosis.
6. Describe the three major physiological disturbances of diabetic ketoacidosis—hyperosmolality, metabolic acidosis, and volume depletion.

7. Identify the clinical manifestations of diabetic ketoacidosis and concomitant complications.
8. Demonstrate knowledge of the principles underlying biochemical therapy for diabetic ketoacidosis—volume replacement, potassium and phosphorus replacement, and bicarbonate replacement.
9. Using a nursing diagnosis format, formulate a nursing care plan for patients with diabetic ketoacidosis.
10. Differentiate between the major physiological disturbances of diabetic ketoacidosis and hyperosmolar hyperglycemic nonketotic coma.
11. Describe the neurologic responses to a hypoglycemic episode.

Description

Critically ill patients with diabetes present a bewildering array of signs and symptoms: stupor, hyperventilation, vomiting, decreasing urine output, and unstable blood pressure all may be present and require attention. The number and complexity of laboratory measurements can be intimidating. Understanding diabetes requires understanding the physiology of nutrition, because diabetes is a disease of disordered nutrition.

Physiology of Nutrition

Feeding and Fasting

The body faces two different nutritional challenges every day: nutrient storage and the release of nutrients from storage depots. Nutrient storage occurs because ingested nutrients are absorbed from the gastrointestinal tract over a relatively brief period of time. Under the usual circumstances of daily living, glucose absorption occupies roughly a 3-hour period following each meal, or about one-third of the 24 hours. Most tissues, however, use nutrients fairly constantly, particularly for energy, over the 24 hours. The body must therefore jealously guard the excess nutrient being absorbed, storing it away for use between feeding times, in order to maintain a relatively constant internal environment. Preventing waste of ingested nutrient must have been extremely important for survival during evolution because it led to extraordinarily efficient storage mechanisms. Nutrient storage in the feeding phase of nutrition is referred to as an *anabolic* state.

After storing incoming nutrients, the body faces an entirely different nutritional task: feeding the tissues from stored reserves. This is a delicate task. Nutrients must be released from storage depots at exactly the right rate. If release is too slow, other tissues may "starve in the midst of plenty." If release exceeds consumption by even a small amount, nutrients are lost, primarily in urine. This leads to accelerated depletion of body reserves. If release becomes totally uncontrolled, both consumption and excretion mechanisms become swamped; nutrients accumulate in extracellular fluid, distorting the physiochemical environment that bathes every cell, leading to physiological malfunction, symptoms, and ultimately death.

A key concept in understanding the physiology of the fasting state is the dynamic balance that regulates the release of nutrients. In general, nutrient release from tissue storage sites does not depend on a positive signal, such as a hormonal trigger, to call it into action. Rather, the storage tissues, when deprived of both nutrient substrate and hormonal signals, spontaneously break down and release their stored nutrients. They are in a *catabolic* state, almost as if it were their fundamental condition to sacrifice their own constituents for "more important" functions elsewhere. This process is further controlled by a second, negative hormonal signal, which restrains the rate of nutrient release, setting it precisely to meet the required rate of nutrient demand. This dynamic balance between spontaneous tissue nutrient release and hormonally controlled damping of this release in the fasting phase of nutrition is sometimes referred to as an *anticatabolic* state.

It is apparent from this discussion of nutritional physiology that at any one moment in the course of a normal 24-hour day, the human body can almost never be said to be in nutrient balance. Rather, balance shifts from hour to hour, from moderately positive to moderately negative, and it is only over the course of the entire day that the sum of these positives and negatives begins to approach balance (zero). Indeed, in healthy adults, energy balance probably approximates zero only in the course of 1 to 2 weeks.

pounded by the fact that the adult brain stores almost no glucose (as glycogen). As a result, normal brain function depends from minute to minute on a supply of glucose from the bloodstream, as evidenced by the rapid appearance of cerebral dysfunction when blood sugar falls below normal levels. Equally dramatic is restoration of cerebral function to normal when blood sugar rises again. The brain also needs its glucose-derived energy at the same rate day and night, waking and sleeping, working and resting, at a rate of about 5 g (1 tsp) per hour, which represents about half of the average daily adult glucose intake.

A number of other tissues also are either relatively dependent (eg, white blood cells, renal medulla) or totally dependent (eg, red blood cells) on glucose-derived energy. Glucose deprivation, however, does not have such immediate, obvious, or potentially harmful consequences for these tissues as it does for the brain. Feeding the brain is a primary task in human nutritional physiology. In the course of evolution, preservation of brain function has emerged as a development of highest priority, as indicated by the number and importance of the physiological mechanisms directed at providing energy to the brain, sometimes at the expense of other organs.

The brain can use one other major energy source, namely *ketone bodies*. These are not a normal dietary constituent but are generated within the body from its own fat stores as a kind of emergency fuel. This is especially true in the fasting state. An understanding of the changing tissue fuel requirements and fuel sources over time (including feeding and prolonged fasting) provides a view of the physiological mechanisms involved in the maintenance of normal nutrition and facilitates the understanding of diabetes.

The two basic nutritional tasks are

- storage of excess nutrient during food absorption
- re-release of nutrient from storage tissues between meals

The Brain and Glucose

- In humans the brain is disproportionately large.
- The brain requires glucose continuously for energy, at 5 g/h.
- Without its energy supply, brain function deteriorates in minutes.

The Brain and Glucose

Apart from understanding the feeding–fasting duality and its control, one must have a knowledge of another major concept to understand diabetes and diabetic catastrophes, namely, the unique metabolic role of the brain. In humans, the brain is not only disproportionately large but also almost completely dependent on glucose for its energy supplies. This is different from most other large organs, which can easily switch to long-chain free fatty acids and in fact do so in preference to glucose when both substrates are presented together.

The large size of the human brain and its continuous dependence on glucose as an energy source are com-

The Four Phases of Nutrition

The Fed State

From the first mouthful of a meal through the absorption of the last of the ingested nutrients from the gastrointestinal tract, the fed state is characterized by a condition of metabolic plenty. Most meals contain a mixture of the three macronutrients (carbohydrate, protein, and fat), with carbohydrate usually predominating. Three different physiological mechanisms are required to store these nutrients, which enter the body in excess of need. A limited fraction of carbohydrate not burned immediately is stored as glycogen in the liver and in muscle. The remainder is promptly converted to fatty acids and glycerol and ultimately stored as triglyceride in adipose tissue. Feeding the brain its needed ration of glucose is no problem under these circumstances.

Dietary fat enters the circulation as chylomicrons, a complex microdroplet fat emulsion, which is cleared primarily for storage directly into adipose tissue. Amino acids are taken up into most tissues in proportion to their need, and amino acids in excess of immediate need are probably stored temporarily in a depot of skeletal muscle proteins.

If the meal contains even small quantities of carbohydrate, the metabolic storage response to feeding results in a shutting down of nutrient release from storage depots and an almost complete switch to primary dependence on glucose for the energy needs of nearly all tissues. This nutrient influx appears to end about 3 hours after the meal is started.

The Postabsorptive State

The term *postabsorptive* describes the timing of this nutritional phase and clearly marks this condition as a normal, physiological, daily event; a condition of "non-input" of nutrients. This state can be distinguished from the rigorous and stressful condition of more prolonged fasting. After glucose ceases to enter the circulation from the gastrointestinal tract, the brain must be fed from glucose stored in tissues that can release it into the circulation for use elsewhere in the body. Liver glycogen is the only such store, and because the glycogen content of the whole liver amounts to only about 75 g, at a utilization rate that decreases slowly from its initial 5 g/hour, this source lasts only about 18 hours. This production of glucose in the liver from the breakdown of glycogen is termed *glycogenolysis*. Defined in terms of reliance on liver glycogen, the 15-hour period, from 3 to 18 hours after the last meal, constitutes postabsorptive metabolism.

During these 15 hours, long-chain free fatty acids are released at an increasing rate from adipose tissue and, when presented to most tissues (other than brain, red cells, renal medulla, etc.), are metabolized for energy in preference to glucose. Over the period of the postabsorptive state, the body progressively makes the switch from a predominantly carbohydrate to a primarily fat economy. Although this change is in part brought about by the decrease in available glucose supplies, it also has the secondary effect of "sparing" glucose from use by most tissues other than the brain.

The Short Fasting State

Gluconeogenesis

As fasting progresses beyond the point of liver glycogen depletion, the brain must rely on an alternative glucose supply, one in which new glucose is created from precursor substances. The details of this process of *gluconeogenesis* (*neo* = new; *genesis* = creation) and its regulation are extraordinarily complex, but the essentials can be outlined fairly briefly. Glucose, a 6-carbon molecule, can be created anew only from 3-carbon fragments. In mammalian metabolism, this structural constraint has important nutritional and physiological consequences, because such 3-carbon compounds can be supplied only from sources other than fatty acids. The 2-carbon units that form the basic structure of fatty acids cannot be combined or rearranged to make new glucose.

Therefore, despite the abundant fat stores in fasting humans, gluconeogenesis must depend on three non-fat sources for these 3-carbon building blocks: (1) lactate, from partial breakdown of glucose in several peripheral tissues; (2) glycerol, from the degradation of triglyceride stored in adipose tissue; and (3) certain amino acids derived ultimately from tissue proteins. All these are brought centrally to the liver, the only organ capable of converting these smaller precursors back into glucose for re-release into the bloodstream.

Gluconeogenesis from the first two of the 3-carbon precursors, lactate and glycerol, represents a strict recycling of carbons without a net loss to the body, because these 3-carbon molecules are derived in the first place from peripheral glucose metabolism. In contrast, that portion of gluconeogenesis that uses amino acids puts a net drain on body protein stores, because the nitrogen is not reused for the most part but converted to urea in the liver and excreted in the urine. The overall result of the amino acid-to-glucose conversion is the sacrifice of structural and functional tissue proteins for the primary purpose of providing the brain with its obligatory glucose substrate.

Ketogenesis

The reassembly of 3-carbon fragments to glucose within the liver requires energy, which the liver, like the other tissues, at this point finds most available by oxidizing fatty acids from the abundant supply present in the circulation. During fasting, however, the liver alters its fatty acid metabolizing mechanism. It no longer oxidizes fatty acids all the way to CO_2 and water, but to their constituent 2-carbon fragment, acetate. These acetate molecules recombine, while still in the liver, into 4-carbon fatty "by-products," the ketone bodies, acetoacetate and hydroxybutyrate. The ketones then leave the liver and enter the circulation, representing a kind of water-soluble fat, which is used very efficiently for energy by most peripheral tissues. The rate of ketone body consumption by most tissues, particularly the brain, increases in proportion to the level in the circulation.

Ketogenesis and gluconeogenesis are critically important physiological adaptations to the metabolic stress of fasting; under the usual conditions of fasting the two processes are closely related. The net result of these adaptations is the increasing flow of lactate, glycerol, amino acids, and long-chain fatty acids into the liver and the net release from the liver of glucose, ketone bodies, and urea.

As fasting progresses beyond 18 hours, the time at which liver glycogen is depleted, the rates of both gluconeogenesis and ketogenesis increase rapidly, reaching a maximum at 48 to 72 hours after the meal. The circulating level of ketone bodies at this point has risen 10- to 20-fold, from its "fed state" level of about 0.1 mEq/L to a level of about 1 to 2 mEq/L. This level is high enough to exceed the renal threshold and produce the characteristic *ketonuria* of fasting. Beyond this time, ketogenesis continues at a steady, rapid rate in the liver, as the consumption of ketone bodies by muscle and adipose tissues diminishes slowly and progressively. As a result, the circulating ketone level continues to rise, reaching 6 to 7 mEq/L if fasting is prolonged to 3 weeks, a rise of some 50- to 75-fold above its initial fed level.

The Prolonged Fasting State

After 3 weeks of total fasting, the level of circulating ketone bodies plateaus and remains relatively constant thereafter. Metabolism then enters the phase of prolonged fasting, a more or less steady state of adaptation to the most serious metabolic challenge of all, starvation. This adaptation is characterized by its extremely tight regulation, directing itself to maximal preservation of body stores while not permitting the composition of nutrients circulating in blood to become too greatly displaced from normal.

The most important result of the great increase in circulating ketones is that an energy alternative to glucose is made available to the brain. After 3 to 4 weeks of complete fasting, ketones provide 60% of the brain's energy supply. The demand for glucose production in the liver is thus lessened by at least this amount, which in turn reduces the drain on body protein stores. As a result, urinary nitrogen excretion drops progressively from 10 g/day in the postabsorptive state to about 3 g/day after prolonged fasting. This spares about 42 g of tissue protein or 150 g of lean tissue weight per day, an adaptation that is critical to prolonged survival. In addition to this drop in gluconeogenic requirement, the body adapts to fasting in a general way by lowering its overall resting metabolic energy requirement 20%, further sparing endogenous energy and protein reserves.

The circulating level of free fatty acids, which rises to a maximum during the period of short fasting, remains constant thereafter, supplying a high proportion of energy needs in muscle and most visceral tissues other than the brain. Blood glucose levels, in contrast, fall during the first 3 to 4 days of fasting and then remain constant thereafter. The blood sugar levels may go extremely low during fasting, generally lower in women than in men, sometimes as low as 25 to 30 mg/dl, without any accompanying symptoms of cerebral disturbance. This is presumed to occur

because ketone bodies have partially replaced glucose as the energy supply to the brain.

The Four Phases of Nutrition

- *Fed.* Glucose is available for tissue energy needs.
- *Postabsorptive.* Liver glycogen provides limited glucose supplies.
- *Short fasting.* Fatty acids provide most tissue energy; glucose for the brain comes from gluconeogenesis; ketogenesis develops; ketonuria occurs.
- *Prolonged fasting.* Tightly regulated gluconeogenesis and ketogenesis provide brain nutrient, sparing body protein breakdown; maximal switch to a "fat economy."

Hormonal Control of Nutritional Physiology

Insulin

Understanding the control of nutritional balance is simplified by the realization that both feeding and fasting metabolism are primarily regulated by a single hormone, *insulin*. After a meal, insulin levels rise rapidly into the anabolic range of 50 to 100 μU/ml, then decline as entering nutrients are stored (Fig. 40–1). At its tissue target sites, these large amounts of insulin directly stimulate a variety of important biochemical storage steps, including the rate of glucose entry into insulin-sensitive cells across the plasma membrane and the rate of glycogen, fatty acid, and protein synthesis.

As the postabsorptive state draws on, insulin levels fall into their anticatabolic range of 5 to 10 μU/ml, about tenfold below the anabolic range, passing through a "null point" poised between these two different insulin actions. In the anticatabolic range, insulin no longer stimulates storage mechanisms but provides the negative signal that suppresses the otherwise self-sustaining breakdown of glycogen, triglycerides, and proteins in a variety of tissues and gluconeogenesis in the liver. Of course, insulin in its higher, anabolic range maximally suppresses these catabolic events at the same time it triggers storage mechanisms.

Other Hormones

Besides insulin, there are other hormones that play some role in the "fine tuning" or modulation and smoothing of metabolic control. In particular, *glucagon* provides a counterregulatory "pull" to insulin's "push" because glucagon directly stimulates the breakdown of glucose stored as glycogen (glycogenolysis), and of fat stored as triglyceride (lipolysis), and the synthesis of new glucose (gluconeogenesis) in the liver. On a minute-to-minute basis, the rates of the major opposing nutrient storage and release

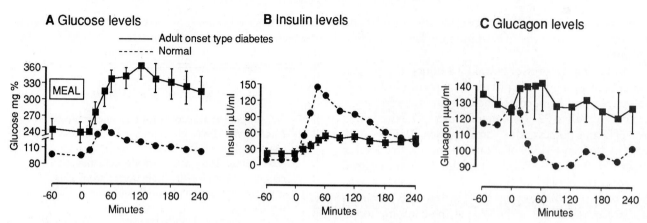

FIGURE 40–1

Patterns of (**A**) glucose, (**B**) insulin, and (**C**) glucagon levels that occur at specific time intervals after ingestion of a large carbohydrate meal. Normal subject levels are compared with diabetic subject levels. For normal subjects, note the large, early, rapidly rising increase in insulin level, the simultaneous drop in glucagon level, and the moderate, well-damped excursion of blood glucose level. For diabetic subjects, the insulin level rises late, sluggishly, and relatively little; the glucagon level increases paradoxically, and blood glucose remains at abnormally high levels for a long time. (Adapted from Muüller W et al: Abnormal alpha cell function in diabetes. N Engl J Med 283:109–115, 1970)

processes are regulated by the balance between insulin and glucagon levels. Moreover, glucocorticoids from the adrenal cortex, catecholamines from the adrenal medulla and peripheral adrenergic neurons, and growth hormone (somatotropin) from the anterior pituitary provide "permissive" control of metabolism by both direct effects on tissues and indirect effects on insulin/glucagon release. As a group, these other hormones, like glucagon, all work to stimulate tissue breakdown and nutrient release, in essence, a part of the "stress response."

Despite the importance of these catabolic, or counter-regulatory, hormones in normal physiology, the absence of one or another of them seems to be well tolerated, apparently because the presence of the others can compensate for the loss. In contrast, insulin emerges as the only "storage hormone" and thus is uniquely important as the prime regulator of metabolism. Insufficient insulin produces a series of disruptions in metabolism collectively referred to as *diabetes mellitus*.

Hormonal Control of Nutritional Physiology

- Insulin is the "storage hormone."
- High insulin levels cause nutrient storage (anabolism).
- Low insulin levels regulate release of stored nutrients (anticatabolism).
- Glucagon promotes nutrient release, gluconeogenesis, and ketogenesis.
- The "stress hormones" cortisol, catecholamines, and growth hormone all oppose insulin action.

Pathophysiology

Type I (IDDM) and Type II (NIDDM) Diabetes

An estimated 14 million Americans have diabetes today. Of these, 10% to 20% are diagnosed as Type I, and 80% to 90% are diagnosed as Type II.

Type I diabetes, or insulin-dependent diabetes (IDDM), can show presentation ranging from mild, nonspecific symptoms to frank coma. It generally affects persons under the age of 30 years, who frequently display the classic signs of diabetes: polyuria, polydipsia, and polyphagia. Persons with Type I diabetes are insulinopenic (possess an absolute deficiency of insulin resulting from destruction of pancreatic beta cells); therefore they require exogenous insulin administration to prevent ketoacidosis and sustain life.

Type II, or non–insulin-dependent diabetes (NIDDM), can present with few or none of the classic symptoms of diabetes mellitus. It typically occurs in persons over the age of 30 who have a relative lack of insulin due to insulin resistance or decreased tissue sensitivity or responsiveness to exogenous and endogenous insulin. Persons with Type II diabetes can have normal, mildly depressed, or elevated levels of insulin and usually do not require exogenous insulin for survival although it may be necessary for control of hyperglycemia. These individuals are generally not prone to the development of diabetic ketoacidosis but are at risk for hyperosmolar hyperglycemic nonketotic coma. Both persons with Type I and Type II diabetes are subject to the same devastating, long-term vascular and neuropathic complications of the disease.

The Basic Disturbance

If insulin secretion becomes slightly impaired, the insulin-secreting beta cells of the pancreatic islets have no difficulty providing the low levels of insulin required to regulate fasting metabolism. It is only when the challenge of feeding calls for anabolic levels of insulin that the insulin secretory mechanism of the beta cells is insufficient. The rate of storage of glucose (and other macronutrients) therefore is diminished, and it is this lag in storage that permits glucose to rise to *higher* levels and to return to baseline levels more *slowly* than normal.

These alterations characterize an abnormal glucose tolerance test, the major diagnostic tool for detecting diabetes, standing in sharp contrast to the brief, tightly damped excursions of blood sugar in nondiabetic subjects (see Figure 40–1). In some forms of diabetes such as Type II, all these nutrients are retained within the body and ultimately taken up into tissues. Overall glucose utilization rates may remain normal, and many of these patients therefore continue to gain weight.

As insulin secretory capacity declines further, the beta cells cannot supply even the small amounts required in the postabsorptive or fasting states. Fasting metabolism becomes progressively unregulated, resulting not only in loss of nutrient storage capacity but also in uncontrolled catabolism. Thus, even in the absence of any ingested food, blood sugar rises above normal due to inappropriately accelerated glycogenolysis and gluconeogenesis. Concomitantly, the rates of lipolysis and ketogenesis become uncontrolled, leading to spiraling levels of ketones in the circulation. As the concentrations of glucose and ketones rise above the renal threshold, these nutrients are excreted in the urine, imposing a calorie drain on the body and giving rise first to glycosuria and ultimately to ketonuria.

In uncontrolled Type I diabetes, body weight may not be maintained, despite large calorie and protein intakes, and the flesh can be literally melted down and lost through the siphon of the urine. The word *diabetes*, from the Greek word meaning "siphon," was first applied to the disease several thousand years ago.

In summary, insulin possesses both anabolic and anti-catabolic functions. The anabolic functions of insulin seem to be widely appreciated because a storage regulator would be needed to control nutritional physiology during the feeding phase. In contrast, the anticatabolic effects of insulin, which prevent excessive mobilization of stored glucose, fat, and protein as well as excessive glucose and ketone production during fasting, are generally more difficult to conceptualize. It is therefore somewhat ironic that a defect in secretion of feeding phase insulin produces relatively minimal disruptions in metabolism, whereas loss of the basal, fasting insulin levels permits the intrinsic catabolic processes of the body to become so unregulated that body substance is lost, distorting the amount and composition of body fluids to the point at which serious illness or even death results. This most extreme form of diabetic abnormality, ketoacidosis, represents a major diabetic emergency.

Type I vs Type II Diabetes

- Type I (IDDM) diabetes occurs when even the low levels of insulin needed to regulate fasting metabolism are not maintained.
- Type II (NIDDM) diabetes represents insufficient insulin for nutrient storage.

Diabetic Ketoacidosis

Description

Diabetic ketoacidosis results from severe insulin deficiency and the accompanying disordered metabolism of proteins, carbohydrates, and fats. It is sometimes referred to as a state of "accelerated fasting" and is the most serious metabolic disturbance in insulin-dependent diabetics. Diabetic ketoacidosis is responsible for more than 160,000 hospitalizations and is associated with mortality rates between 6% and 10%.

Assessment

History

Diabetic ketoacidosis can occur in patients who have completely lost their capacity to secrete insulin without obvious precipitating factors. However, it is very common for stressful events—usually infections, sometimes emotional turmoil—to be precipitating factors. The hormonal responses to stress drive catabolic processes at accelerated rates and this can provide the "last straw" that sets the process in motion. Therefore, look for physiological stressors such as influenza, pneumonia, gastroenteritis, trauma, and myocardial infarction. Interview for emotional stressors as well.

Another precipitating event occurs when diabetics who are completely dependent on insulin stop or skip insulin injections, particularly in the presence of infection or stress. Mismanagement of sick days—improper food intake or insulin administration and failure to report symptoms—is also a precipitating factor. A precipitating cause can be found in approximately 80% of the cases of diabetic ketoacidosis.

Diabetic ketoacidosis is often precipitated by one of the following:

- infection
- physiological or emotional stress
- withdrawal of insulin therapy

Clinical Manifestations and Diagnostic Findings

The clinical hallmarks of diabetic ketoacidosis are

- hyperosmolarity
- acidosis
- volume depletion

The pathophysiological events that result in these three disturbances interact with one another. The severity of each disturbance can vary from slight to very severe, however, and some patients can have a severe abnormality in one area but none at all in the others. Figure 40–2 outlines these mechanisms and their interrelations.

Hyperglycemia and Hyperosmolarity

The first major consequence of diabetic ketoacidosis is hyperosmolarity due to hyperglycemia. Patients in diabetic ketoacidosis often have blood sugars of 300 to 800 mg/dl or higher. It is clear that the mechanisms that usually protect the body from such catastrophic rises in blood sugar must have broken down in such patients. The central

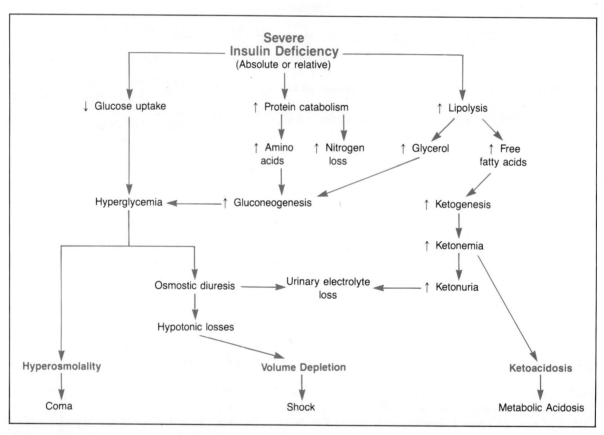

FIGURE 40–2
The metabolic consequences of severe insulin deficiency and their interrelations leading to diabetic ketoacidosis. (Adapted from Davidson MD: Diabetic ketoacidosis and hyperosmolar nonketotic syndrome. In Diabetes Mellitus: Diagnosis and Treatment, 3rd ed, pp 175–212. New York, Churchill Livingstone, 1991)

mechanism that protects against hyperosmolarity or hyperosmolality is renal glucose excretion, the very same mechanism that causes the second type of abnormality in diabetic ketoacidosis, volume depletion (see Figure 40–2).

As long as the circulating blood volume remains relatively normal, glucose is filtered at the kidney glomerulus into the renal tubules. As long as the filtered glucose load remains relatively small, all of this glucose is reabsorbed into the bloodstream. However, when the filtered load increases above a certain level, such as when the blood sugar exceeds the normal threshold of about 180 mg/dl, glucose begins to escape into the urine because the reabsorption capacity of the tubules is exceeded. As the filtered load increases further, urinary glucose loss increases very rapidly. After this nearly all extra glucose put into the circulation is lost into the urine. This renal "escape valve" serves as a very powerful protective device to prevent extreme accumulation of glucose in blood. Indeed, in people with diabetes whose circulating blood volume is well maintained, it is extremely unusual to find blood sugar levels in excess of 500 mg/dl because of the intense glucose diuresis. Conversely, *any patient whose blood sugar is higher than this level must be suspected of having either a severely reduced circulating blood volume, renal damage, or both.*

It is glycosuria that is largely responsible for volume depletion. In a patient whose diabetes is badly out of control and in whom oral replacement of sodium and water has been sufficient to compensate for urinary losses, a vicious cycle is set up in which hyperglycemia leads to volume depletion, which, uncompensated, in turn reduces urinary glucose losses, which again permits the blood sugar to rise even higher.

It appears to be the hyperosmolality of body fluids resulting from this upward spiral in blood sugar, rather than ketosis, acidosis, or volume depletion, that primarily accounts for the lethargy, stupor, and, ultimately, coma that occur as diabetic ketoacidosis worsens. The evidence for this conclusion rests on the general correlation between degree of hyperosmolarity and degree of coma, in contrast to preserved mental function in states in which pure ketoacidosis exists without hyperosmolarity.

The development of hyperglycemia, hyperosmolality, and coma in diabetic ketoacidosis is schematically outlined in Figure 40–2.

Possible findings:

- hyperglycemia
- glycosuria (↑ glucose duiresis)
- volume depletion
- hyperosmolality
- lethargy → stupor → coma

Ketosis and Acidosis

The second major consequence of severe insulin deficiency is uncontrolled ketogenesis. As ketoacids enter the extracellular fluid, the hydrogen ion is stripped from the molecule (see Equation 1) and neutralized by combining with bicarbonate ion buffer, thus protecting the pH of extracellular fluids and leaving behind ketoacid anion residues. The resultant carbonic acid (see Equation 2) breaks down into water and CO_2 gas, which literally "fizzes" out through the lungs.

$$\left. \begin{array}{l} \text{Equation 1:} \\ \quad H^+\text{-acetoacetic acid} \\ \quad H^+\text{-}\beta\text{-hydroxybutyric acid} \end{array} \right\}$$
$$+ HCO^-_3 \rightarrow H_2CO_3^- \left\{ \begin{array}{l} \text{acetoacetate}^- \\ \beta\text{-hydroxybutyrate}^- \end{array} \right.$$
$$\text{Equation 2:}$$
$$H_2CO_3 \rightarrow H_2O + CO_2 \text{ gas}(\uparrow)$$

As ketoacid anions accumulate, they progressively displace bicarbonate from extracellular fluid. The usual laboratory determination of electrolytes does not measure ketoacid concentrations directly. However, an excess of total measured cations (sodium plus potassium) over total measured anions (chloride plus bicarbonate) provides a clue to the presence of these so-called unmeasured anions. This excess, sometimes referred to as the *anion gap*, can serve as an indirect measure of the quantity of ketoacids present.

A total of 6 to 7 mEq/L of ketoacids, which would reduce serum bicarbonate from its usual 25 mEq/L to 18 to 19 mEq/L, seems to be well tolerated by most diabetic patients. Because prolonged fasting (without diabetes) can cause a physiological starvation ketosis of this degree, it seems logical to consider this a *mild* degree of ketoacidosis when it is produced by uncontrolled diabetes rather than by starvation.

In the range of 6 to 15 mEq/L of ketone bodies, with corresponding bicarbonate levels of 10 to 19 mEq/L, the buffering and acid-compensating mechanisms of the body become more seriously stressed, but in this range pH usually remains at least partially protected. Ketoacidosis of this degree is never physiological, and when due to diabetes it can therefore be considered to be *moderate* in degree. Once the bicarbonate level falls below 10 mEq/L because of ketoacid accumulations greater than 15 mEq/L, the protection against acidosis rapidly reaches its outer limit. Then, even slight interference with compensating mechanisms can send body pH plummeting to very low levels. Ketoacidosis of this degree (15 mEq/L of ketoacid accumulation) is obviously severe and life-threatening.

Hyperventilation, A Compensatory Mechanism

The neutrality of body fluids is primarily protected by the bicarbonate buffering system, which determines the pH at all times by the ratio of bicarbonate anion to CO_2 gas in plasma. If bicarbonate anion is lost owing to its displacement by ketoacid anions, extra CO_2 gas must be driven off at the lung by hyperventilation in order to keep the ratio at or close to its usual value of 20 : 1 and to maintain pH close to its physiological value of 7.4. Hyperventilation, gradual at first, then rapidly more vigorous and more obvious as arterial pH drops below 7.2, is therefore a characteristic physical finding in diabetic ketoacidosis. This dramatic increase in ventilation, which occurs more by an increase in the *depth* than in the *frequency* of breathing, is known as *Kussmaul breathing*. It is associated with the classic "fruity" odor of the breath in diabetic ketoacidosis. The presence of clear-cut Kussmaul breathing is a signal that extracellular fluid pH is at or below 7.2, a relatively severe degree of acidosis.

The outer limit of compensation for a declining bicarbonate buffer reserve is imposed by the maximal rate of hyperventilation that the lungs can achieve. At the usual rates of total CO_2 production by the body, the lungs breathe fast enough to drive the total CO_2 gas level in blood down to about one-fourth its normal value but not lower. Hyperventilation can therefore compensate, at least partially, for bicarbonate levels as low as 6 to 8 mEq/L, one-fourth of the normal range of 24 to 32 mEq/L. As bicarbonate drops below that level, however, CO_2 gas remains disproportionately high relative to bicarbonate, and pH then drops at an alarming rate. It is for this reason that bicarbonate levels below 10 mEq/L are taken as an indicator of severe acidosis and call for more aggressive therapy.

Testing For Serum Ketones

Serum ketones can be measured semiquantitatively at the bedside by testing progressive dilutions of serum with *nitroprusside reagent* (powder or crushed tablets). This maneuver serves several important purposes.

1. It rapidly helps confirm the diagnosis of diabetic ketoacidosis once it has been suggested by history, physical examination, and urine testing.
2. It is possible to make a rough assessment of degree of ketoacidosis, at least to the extent of categorizing it as mild, moderate, or severe.
3. A major discrepancy between the amount of ketones estimated by the serum nitroprusside procedure and the total anion gap calculated from the

electrolytes determined in the laboratory suggests that a second unmeasured anion, usually lactate, is contributing to the acidosis in addition to keto-acids.

Kidney Action

Finally, because ketoacids are excreted in the urine largely as their sodium, potassium, and ammonium salts, the loss of ketones through the kidneys contributes to the problems of water and electrolyte losses, the third important category of physiological damage in diabetic ketoacidosis. The development of metabolic acidosis in diabetic keto-acidosis is outlined on the right side of Figure 40–2.

Fluid and Electrolyte Losses: Volume Depletion

Osmotic Diuresis

Although glucose loss through the kidneys helps protect against the ravages of extreme hyperosmolality, the diabetic patient developing ketoacidosis pays a price for this glycosuria. Glucose remaining in the glomerular filtrate, after the renal tubules have reabsorbed all they can, forces water to remain in the tubules. This glucose-rich filtrate then sweeps out of the body, carrying with it water, sodium, potassium, ammonium, phosphate, and other salts. The resulting rapid urine flow and obligate loss of water and electrolytes that would otherwise be reabsorbed is known as an *osmotic diuresis*. Salts of ketone bodies, as well as the urea resulting from rapid protein breakdown and accelerated gluconeogenesis, also contribute to the solute load in the renal tubule, further aggravating the diuresis.

Salt and Water Loss

The average amounts of salts and water lost to the body through osmotic diuresis during the development of diabetic ketoacidosis have been measured directly. These numbers serve as important markers for understanding the degree of physiological damage done to the patient. Overall water loss in a 70 kg adult patient presenting in diabetic ketoacidosis amounts to about 6 to 7 liters, or 15% of total body water.

One can determine that of this amount, about 3 liters are derived from the extracellular compartment, judging from the accompanying average loss of 420 mEq of *sodium* and assuming that the sodium concentration of normal extracellular fluid is 140 mEq/L. This represents a loss of at least 20% of extracellular water, which is a very major insult to the integrity of the body fluids. Another 3 liters is derived from the intracellular space, as indicated by the loss of 300 mEq of *potassium*, the major intracellular cation, because the potassium concentration within cells is normally about 100 mEq/L.

The fluid lost to the body is slightly hypotonic, meaning that it contains a slight excess of water as compared with the volume of salts, as would be expected from an osmotic diuresis due to glucose and urea. These figures, as

---

Possible findings:

- hyperventilation
- Kussmaul breathing and "fruity" breath
- increased anion gap (> 7 mEq/L)
- decreased bicarbonate (< 10 mEq/L)
- decreased pH (< 7.4)

noted, represent averages. The *net* losses found in any particular patient result from the combination of many different factors, among them the intensity and duration of the hyperglycemia and thus the intensity of osmotic diuresis; the amount of water and electrolyte replaced by mouth during this time; the presence of other fluid and electrolyte losses such as vomiting, diarrhea, or sweating; and the integrity of renal function.

Compensatory Mechanisms

Sodium and water make up the central structure of the extracellular fluid, including the vascular volume. Removal of these large quantities of sodium and water from the body is therefore perceived as a serious threat to the maintenance of the circulation, and a variety of compensatory mechanisms are called into play to prevent vascular collapse and shock. For example, an increase in pulse rate usually occurs that helps maintain cardiac output in the face of shrinking intravascular volume.

At least as important, however, is a protective shift in body fluid brought about by the hyperglycemia itself. Because free glucose is limited almost entirely to the extracellular water, an osmotic pressure gradient is set up across the cell membrane, between the extracellular compartment and the interior of the cells. Therefore, the higher the blood sugar, the more water is drawn out of cells and into the extracellular space. Thus, as sodium and water are lost into the urine, shrinking the extracellular fluid, they are, in effect, "replaced" (at least as to their osmotic effect) by glucose entering from the liver and by water entering from all cells, which reexpands the extracellular fluid.

The very hyperosmolality that produces damaging central nervous system (CNS) effects and osmotic diuresis therefore provides at least a partial and temporary mechanism for preventing vascular collapse, an important "prop" to the structure of the extracellular fluid in ketoacidosis. It is, however, rather shaky because of its rapid reversal when blood glucose is lowered again.

Adverse Effects

Despite these efforts at compensation, circulatory integrity is progressively compromised as diabetic ketoacidosis progresses, leading ultimately to a series of secondary pathological changes, some of which in turn develop into self-perpetuating, vicious spirals.

Decrease in Glomerular Filtration.

First, loss of vascular volume produces a fall in glomerular filtration, which is why the usual measures of renal function, including BUN and creatinine levels, are characteristically elevated in ketoacidotic patients. Not only does decreasing renal function permits blood glucose levels to spiral to extreme values, but other consequences, particularly difficulty in controlling potassium excretion, also result from this change. Because the excretion of potassium by the kidney occurs by the exchange of potassium for sodium, adequate sodium must be present at the exchange site in the kidney for the rate of potassium excretion to keep pace with the need for excretion. If vascular volume is diminished and renal perfusion is consequently reduced, not enough sodium may be available for this exchange. Despite a total body depletion of potassium, the serum potassium level may therefore rise above normal, even to dangerous or lethal levels.

Decreased glomerular filtration leads to

↑ BUN
↑ serum creatinine
↑ blood glucose
↑ serum potassium

Decrease In Tissue Perfusion.

A second major consequence of diminished vascular volume is a generalized decrease in tissue perfusion. Well before the drop in volume has reached the point at which blood pressure actually falls and full-blown shock is said to be present, blood is shunted away from many tissues, and the perfusion of nearly all tissues suffers. The resultant decrease in oxygen delivery causes those tissues to shift to some degree of anaerobic glucose metabolism, resulting in the increased production of lactic acid. The release of this second organic acid into the circulation simply lowers the bicarbonate further, aggravating the already existing metabolic acidosis. A combined lactic acidosis and ketoacidosis is not an uncommon finding, therefore, in patients with diabetic ketoacidosis.

Decreased tissue perfusion leads to

↑ production of lactic acid
↓ bicarbonate
↑ metabolic acidosis

Phosphate Loss.

Tissue hypoxia due to decreased tissue perfusion may be aggravated indirectly in ketoacidosis as the result of urinary loss of another electrolyte, phosphate. As body phosphate stores are depleted, circulating phosphate levels fall quite low in plasma, depriving the red cells of an essential reactant used to form a variety of organic phosphate compounds. Under these circumstances, red cells become depleted of certain key phosphate derivatives, which in turn increases the tightness of oxygen binding to the hemoglobin within those cells. As these cells pass through the poorly perfused tissues, less oxygen is given up than from red cells with a normal complement of phosphate compounds, and tissue hypoxia is worsened.

Shock. Finally, if vascular volume falls low enough, compensation mechanisms fail, blood pressure drops, and true shock supervenes. A rapidly worsening cycle of acidosis, tissue damage, and deepening shock may then occur, leading ultimately to irreversible vascular collapse and death.

The full-blown syndrome of diabetic ketoacidosis is characterized by major contributions from all three major pathophysiological disruptions, each of which is primarily responsible for one of the major clinical features: coma, shock, and metabolic acidosis (see Figure 40–2).

The three major disturbances of physiology in diabetic ketoacidosis are

- Hyperosmolality, due to hyperglycemia
- Metabolic acidosis, due to accumulation of keto-acids
- Volume depletion, due to osmotic diuresis

Each of these three disturbances

- May be more or less severe in any single patient
- May interact to aggravate or compensate for the other disturbances

---

Management

Therapy for diabetic ketoacidosis is based on an understanding of the primary and secondary mechanisms of metabolic damage, just described. Each therapeutic maneuver is directed primarily at one of the three areas of physiological disruption: hyperosmolality caused by hyperglycemia, ketoacidosis, and volume depletion. None of these disruptions exists completely separate from the others. Therapy that reverses one abnormality can also have important *benefits and risks* in other areas because of their interlocking nature.

Volume: Salt and Water Replacement

The most immediate threat to life in a critically ill ketoacidotic patient is *volume depletion*. Once the diagnosis is even seriously considered, the first priority is always to get a large, secure intravenous line in place. A cutdown may be necessary in a severely dehydrated patient almost in shock, because veins may be collapsed and hard to find. As soon as this line is established, 0.9% (normal) saline is rapidly infused with consideration given to heart or renal failure. The goal is to reverse the worst of the extracellular volume depletion as soon as possible. Infusing the first liter in 1 hour is not too fast a rate in patients with normal cardiac function, because this will replace only one-third of the extracellular loss in the average patient and even less in others who are more dehydrated.

Fluid replacement should continue at roughly 1 liter per hour until the heart rate, blood pressure, and urine flow indicate depletion is alleviated. Hypotonic solutions, such as 0.45% normal saline, can be administered at a rate of 150 to 250 ml per hour after the intravascular volume has been restored, or if the serum sodium level is greater than 155 mg/dl. Other plasma expanders, such as albumin and plasma concentrates, may be necessary if low blood pressure and other clinical signs of vascular collapse do not respond properly to saline alone.

Rapid infusion of saline in diabetic ketoacidosis is not without its own complications. The rapid dilution of plasma proteins during saline infusion lowers the oncotic (osmotic) pressure of plasma. The lowered oncotic pressure in turn allows fluid to leak out of the vascular space through the capillary walls and is suspected of contributing to the development of pulmonary edema or cerebral edema in some patients during therapy, particularly children and the elderly. Even though they are improving biochemically, patients should therefore be carefully observed during the first 24 to 36 hours for the clinical signs of pulmonary edema: increasing cough, frothy sputum, dyspnea, cyanosis and rales, and failure to awaken from stupor or coma, which could represent the development of cerebral edema.

Further Replacement

After volume replacement has been initiated, there is time to plan the remainder of therapy in a somewhat more considered fashion. At this point, review findings to determine the severity of total volume depletion. The history, intensity, and duration of symptoms; amount of oral intake; presence of other fluid losses (eg, through vomiting); and documentation of the amount of weight actually lost all will provide important clues to the seriousness of volume depletion. The physical examination provides additional information. Decreased tissue turgor (sometimes even to the extent of softened consistency of the eyeballs in severely dehydrated patients), tachycardia, decreased sweating, oliguria or anuria, and postural or supine hypotension all help confirm the extent of volume loss. A numerical estimate of total body fluid loss is extremely valuable in planning phased therapy (eg, the fraction of loss to be replaced over each time interval).

Goals

Volume replacement is critical in

- preserving the integrity of the circulation
- treating hyperglycemia
- preventing hyperkalemia
- reducing lactic acidosis

Because any patient with a blood sugar significantly above 450 to 500 mg/dl became that way in large part because of volume depletion severe enough to prevent compensatory renal glucose loss, it makes physiological sense to rely on volume replacement for restoration of that glucose excretory mechanism. About 80% of the fall in blood sugar during treatment of diabetic ketoacidosis is attributable to glucose loss into the urine, rather than being primarily the result of insulin-induced changes in glucose production and consumption. Therefore, in the earliest phases of treatment, insulin therapy *complements* proper fluid and electrolyte replacement.

Finally, remember that volume losses will continue throughout the first several hours of therapy as long as glycosuria and the osmotic diuresis are not completely controlled. Volume replacement must therefore restore not only the deficits that *exist* at the time of the patient's arrival but also those that continue to be *created* during therapy, before full metabolic control is achieved.

Insulin

Because the primary deficit leading to diabetic ketoacidosis is severe insulin deficiency, insulin obviously stands as a key component of successful therapy. Indeed, until the advent of insulin, diabetic ketoacidosis was almost never fully reversible and was usually fatal.

Several metabolic effects of insulin are of special importance in the treatment of ketoacidosis. First, insulin promptly shuts off the supply of free fatty acids emerging from adipose tissue, thereby restricting the production of ketones at its source. Second, insulin directly inhibits hepatic gluconeogenesis, preventing further addition of glucose to an already overburdened extracellular fluid. Simultaneously, hepatic ketogenesis is further reduced, which assures the ultimate reversal of the ketoacidosis itself. Third, insulin restores cellular protein synthesis. Although this effect occurs more slowly, it in turn permits the restoration of normal potassium, magnesium, and phosphate stores within tissues.

Insulin induces a relatively limited increase in tissue glucose uptake during the therapy of diabetic ketoacidosis. It is therefore primarily the *anticatabolic* effects of insulin, the reduction of glucose and ketone *inflow*, that are important in the early part of therapy. After glucose and ketones are no longer entering the extracellular fluid, the body is in a position to reduce hyperglycemia and ketonemia by both urine losses and continuing tissue consumption. The *anabolic* effects of insulin have little role early in the therapy of ketoacidosis, becoming much more important in later phases.

Cautions

The extremely high glucose values found initially in patients with diabetic ketoacidosis are psychologically distressing to contemplate. It is always tempting, therefore, to choose a course of therapy that will reduce the blood sugar as quickly as possible. However, there are two good reasons to avoid dropping the blood sugar too fast or too far, particularly if the approach to its lowering is primarily to rely on insulin without sufficient simultaneous volume replacement.

In the first instance, recall that large quantities of glucose in the extracellular space draw water out of cells; glucose and water together partially reexpand the volume lost from osmotic diuresis of sodium and water. Sudden and rapid lowering of the blood sugar with insulin, through a combination of increased tissue uptake plus decreased gluconeogenesis, allows water to move very rapidly back into cells, withdrawing the prop to extracellular volume and provoking potentially catastrophic vascular collapse. The sequence of events highlights in yet another way *the importance of early volume replacement with sodium and water*, preceding or concurrent with insulin therapy.

The second problem arises in patients with prolonged, severe hyperglycemia, in whom large quantities of glucose (or glucose-derived compounds) accumulate slowly within the brain. Compared with water, these compounds are only poorly permeating. If the blood sugar is lowered too fast and too far (below about 250 mg/dl), particularly without sufficient electrolyte replacement in extracellular fluid, water is freed up to move into the brain, drawn by the accumulated intracerebral glucose metabolites. The result may be cerebral edema, with a worsening of coma instead of the expected improvement as the blood sugar falls.

High vs. Low Dosage

In the past, insulin was used in relatively large doses, such as 200 to 400 U in the first 24 hours, usually in intravenous bolus doses, in treating diabetic ketoacidosis; this was based on the theory that "insulin resistance" was present. Although some work[1] indicates that all ketoacidotic patients are indeed insulin-resistant and although such high-dose insulin therapy was generally quite successful, further experience indicates that lower doses are often equally effective. Low doses also reduce the risks of hypoglycemia and hypokalemia because decreases in glucose and potassium are more predictable.[2] Preferably, low-dose insulin is given by continuous intravenous infusion rather than by the conventional intravenous bolus or subcutaneous doses. Intramuscular insulin injections are an alternative to intravenous insulin; however, they should be avoided in hypotensive patients because absorption is unpredictable.

As the trend toward ever lower doses has grown, considerable controversy has developed concerning the optimal dose and route of insulin therapy. Whether to give an initial loading dose of insulin has also become a controversial issue. Some studies indicate that there is no clinical evidence to support administration of an initial insulin loading dose.[3,4] Other experts, however, still advocate beginning insulin therapy with a bolus of regular insulin.[5] The most useful position at this point is to be aware of the pitfalls of both high- and low-dose insulin treatment.

The following principles can guide insulin administration.

1. Administer insulin intravenously to the patient with diabetic ketoacidosis to minimize the trauma of repeated injections.
2. Use only human regular insulin in intravenous insulin infusions, because it is less antigenic than animal (beef, pork) insulins.
3. The adsorption of insulin to intravenous containers and tubing has been demonstrated, although there is disagreement about the extent to which it effects insulin delivery. Therefore, to saturate all insulin adsorption sites, the insulin infusion should contain at least 25 units of insulin in every 500 ml of saline, and the entire apparatus should be flushed with at least 50 ml of solution before patient infusion.[6]
4. Administer the insulin infusion through an intravenous infusion pump.
5. When the serum glucose level reaches 250 mg/dl, the intravenous fluids should be changed to contain glucose.
6. Changes in blood sugar and clinical state should indicate a clear-cut, beneficial response to insulin and fluid replacement. If blood sugar does not drop and blood pressure and urine output do not stabilize, insulin and/or fluid replacement may not be adequate.

Potassium and Phosphate Replacement

All patients in diabetic ketoacidosis are deficient in total body potassium stores to some degree. Many other factors conspire to affect the circulating plasma potassium level in patients with diabetic ketoacidosis, however, and most of these factors tend to raise the plasma level. Insulin deficiency, hyperchloremic acidosis,[7] and hyperosmolality all allow potassium to shift out of cells and into the extracellular space. Moreover, the renal excretion of potassium, which usually serves as the major minute-to-minute regulator of plasma potassium, also is impaired in diabetic ketoacidosis because hypovolemia reduces renal perfusion, and intrinsic kidney function is often reduced due to diabetic renal disease. These last two factors prevent potassium excretion from the plasma. Depending on the balance between total body potassium losses and rises in plasma potassium, the initial plasma potassium in patients with ketoacidosis can range from very low to very high. Therefore, potassium replacement must be withheld until an accurate measurement is reported back from the laboratory.

Beginning intravenous K^+ therapy in the presence of unrecognized hyperkalemia and inadequate renal mechanisms for handling potassium loads can rapidly lead to a fatal outcome. Although the electrocardiogram (ECG) can provide bedside clues to the presence of high or low K^+ levels, there is enough room for error in its interpretation to discourage a decision about K^+ therapy based on the ECG alone.

If the initial serum potassium level is low, intravenous K^+ is generally begun right away. This is particularly important because both insulin and saline can be predicted to drive the K^+ even lower, possibly to dangerously low levels at which skeletal muscle paralysis and cardiac arrest may occur. If the initial K^+ is normal or high, intravenous K^+ is generally withheld until it is clear that the level has begun to drop *and* that urine flow is established. Potassium is usually replaced at concentrations of 20 to 40 mEq/L, depending on the serum potassium level.

Failure of the K^+ to fall can occur because of

- persistent, uncorrected acidosis (which drives K^+ out of cells and into extracellular fluid)
- hyperosmolality itself
- intrinsically impaired renal function; or, perhaps most importantly
- insufficient restoration of circulating volume

Phosphate levels generally also drop during therapy, aggravating any preexisting tendency of red cells to bind oxygen more tightly. Therefore, many patients receive phosphate in the middle and later phases of therapy, usually combined with K^+ replacement, in the form of potassium phosphate salts added to the intravenous infusion. Patients who are receiving phosphate therapy intravenously should be watched carefully for signs of tetany: tingling around the mouth or in the hands, neuromuscular irritability, carpopedal spasm, or even seizures. Tetany can occur because the phosphate lowers the level of circulating calcium.

Bicarbonate Replacement

Patients with mild or moderate ketoacidosis who are properly and promptly treated with salt, water, and insulin will eventually excrete and metabolize the ketone bodies remaining in extracellular fluid. As this process continues, bicarbonate anions are increasingly reabsorbed from the renal tubules to replace the disappearing unmeasured anions, and the bicarbonate deficit is slowly repaired. Sometimes, the large amounts of chloride administered along with the sodium in intravenous saline can produce a confusing but transient hyperchloremia and delay for several days the full return of the bicarbonate level to normal.

For patients with the most severe degrees of acidosis, as indicated by an arterial pH of 7.0 or less, whose bicarbonate levels are initially 5 mEq/L or lower, concern arises about a relatively sudden decompensation of buffering capacity when CO_2 gas cannot be driven any faster from the body by hyperventilation, with resultant rapid worsening of the acidosis. These patients should have bicarbonate infused intravenously early in the course of therapy. The deficit in bicarbonate can be calculated and an appropriate amount given intravenously over several hours to raise the level at least to the 10 to 12 mEq/L range. If used, sodium bicarbonate should be administered by slow intravenous infusion over several hours. It is only administered as a bolus injection in the case of cardiac arrest. Accelerated reduction in plasma potassium concentration and sodium overload are other potential harmful effects of sodium bicarbonate therapy.

Possible Central Nervous System Acidosis

The major risk to rapid correction of the acidosis by bicarbonate replacement arises from an imbalance between the extracellular fluids of the body and those surrounding the brain. This results from unequal rates of movement of certain molecules across the blood–brain barrier. In this instance, bicarbonate moves into the brain-associated fluids much more slowly than CO_2 gas (plus H_2CO_3). As a result, the desired parallel rise of both HCO_3^- and CO_2 that occurs elsewhere in the body during treatment does not occur in the cerebral compartment. Instead CO_2 (and H_2CO_3) rises more quickly than HCO_3^-. The net result is a shift in the $HCO_3^- : CO_2$ ratio that drives the cerebral fluid pH down, producing a paradoxical, although again transient, worsening of cerebral acidosis.

This CNS acidosis can then be manifested clinically by deepening stupor or coma in a patient whose arterial pH seems to be improving. Fortunately, a major degree of cerebral impairment due to this pH disequilibrium is unusual, and the central acidosis corrects itself with time if the patient is otherwise managed.

Principal Concerns in Biochemical Therapy for Diabetic Ketoacidosis

- Volume replacement, primarily sodium and water
- Insulin
- Potassium and phosphate replacement
- Bicarbonate

Abdominal Symptoms

Gastric motility is greatly impaired as diabetic ketoacidosis develops. Gastric distention with stagnant, dark, heme-positive "crankcase oil" fluid is therefore quite common. Vomiting, with the ever-present threat of aspiration, par-

ticularly in the stuporous patient, can be a significant problem. Nasogastric intubation for decompression may be necessary both to reduce discomfort and to minimize the risk of aspiration.

Conscious patients are often *extremely* thirsty, but avoid giving them water to drink, because adding fluid to an already distended stomach inevitably leads to worsening abdominal distress and usually to vomiting. Instead, reassure that the thirst will pass as therapy progresses and provide ice chips to minimize the sensation of thirst.

Severe abdominal pain, tenderness, and ileus frequently prove to be due to the ketoacidosis itself. But, these symptoms initially may be difficult to distinguish from an intra-abdominal catastrophe, such as perforated viscus, which may have precipitated the ketoacidosis.

Interpreting Coma

A similar problem arises in interpreting stupor or coma: did intracerebral bleeding or infection precipitate both the acidosis and the coma, or did the acidosis produce coma? Lumbar puncture may be necessary to look for evidence of infection (eg, meningitis, encephalitis, or brain abscess).

Obtaining Urine Samples

Early access to bladder urine samples is important

- in determining whether a urinary tract infection is the precipitating event
- in assessing circulatory status and the need for potassium replacement
- for monitoring urine flow, sugar, and acetone levels
- in complementing the measurements of plasma metabolites and fluid balance.

A catheter is not necessary for conscious patients who can void voluntarily. An indwelling catheter or repeated straight catheterizations may be necessary for patients who are unable to void voluntarily due to lethargy or coma, or who have longstanding diabetes with neurogenic bladder and incomplete emptying.

Phases of Management

Although there are no sharp lines between them, the course of management of diabetic ketoacidosis naturally divides itself into several phases.

First Phase

The first phase consists of the immediate effort to establish the diagnosis and, if ketoacidosis is even strongly suspected, to ensure that life-preserving therapy is begun. An abbreviated history from family or friends of an unconscious patient, a search for a diabetic identification card or jewelry, a rapid assessment for clinical clues of volume depletion and Kussmaul respiration, and blood drawing for initial chemistries should not take more than a few moments. Blood glucose levels by means of capillary blood (obtained by a finger stick and using a blood glucose meter) and serum ketone measurements at the bedside may be all that is needed to clinch the diagnosis. While these preliminaries are being performed, the best possible intravenous line is established, and volume replacement is begun.

Second Phase

After the first phase is completed, a second phase of more considered assessment and therapy begins. Details of the history and physical examination, including the careful search for precipitating causes, should be obtained while the more complete laboratory assessment is awaited. Cultures (blood, urine, and throat), ECG, and appropriate radiologic studies are performed at this point. Decisions are made about coma care, intubation, and catheterization.

Third Phase

A third phase is then entered in which the worst of the metabolic damage is repaired. This phase lasts roughly 8 to 24 hours, depending on how sick the patient is on admission and how responsive he or she proves to be to therapy. The goal during this phase is *not* to achieve complete correction of all the abnormalities. Indeed, as we have seen, excessive speed of correction can be hazardous, particularly in patients in whom ketoacidosis has been developing gradually over a long period of time, because the body's adaptations to the metabolic insults are not all immediately reversible, and overly aggressive therapy can actually make some problems worse.

The key difficulties to be watched for during this phase are as follows.

Worsening stupor or coma. Aside from the possibility of CNS infection or stroke, the major concerns are for osmotic or pH disequilibrium from excessively rapid correction of blood sugar or bicarbonate. The most important clue here is clinical worsening of mental state in the face of "chemical" improvement.

Hypotension. Certainly sepsis, myocardial infarction, and other causes of shock must be looked for, but again, rapid reduction of blood sugar without sufficient sodium and water replacement may be responsible.

Hyperkalemia. Early occlusion of the arterial supply to a limb (not rare in diabetics with severe periph-

eral vascular disease and easily overlooked in a comatose, hypotensive patient) can permit leakage of large amounts of potassium into the circulation, producing or aggravating hyperkalemia. The limbs should therefore be monitored for asymmetric pallor, coldness, rubor, and so forth. More often, hyperkalemia results from premature K^+ infusion, persistent acidosis, and insufficient volume replacement.

Fourth Phase

Finally, a fourth phase arrives in which the patient's clinical state is stable or improving and the majority of the metabolic abnormalities are reversed. The completion or recovery then occurs over a period of about 12 days and includes replenishment of body stores of many nutrients (eg, magnesium, protein, phosphate) as cell constituents are resynthesized.

Once it is clear that gastrointestinal tract function has been restored, oral replacement is not only desirable but also necessary to provide all of the complex nutrition required for recovery; however, oral feedings should be withheld until gastric distention is gone and intestinal motility is clearly present. It is during this phase that attention should be directed at *preventing* future recurrences of diabetic ketoacidosis.

Preventing Recurrence

Often overlooked, prevention is one of the most important aspects of diabetic ketoacidosis management. It can be argued that diabetic ketoacidosis is not only unpleasant, dangerous, and expensive but also unnecessary because, in theory, it should always be preventable. In practical terms, of course, there is probably no way in which all episodes can be prevented, particularly for undiagnosed diabetics in whom the disease is not even suspected. In many other patients, however, the recurrence of ketoacidosis represents a failure in management.

It is the responsibility of the health professional to teach the patient and family the skills and information they need to manage diabetes.

Patient Education and Self-Management Issues

Patients and their families should understand enough about the mechanism and meaning of ketoacidosis to avoid things that are likely to bring it about; to recognize its approach; to slow down or minimize its development; and to seek help fast, if it does begin to happen.

The most common management problem patients have is understanding the importance of insulin's *anticatabolic effects*. Although most ketosis-prone patients easily and intuitively accept the need for insulin injections when they are hungry and eating well, they may have considerable difficulty recognizing their need for insulin when they are ill, anorectic, not eating, or vomiting.

To achieve self-management, every such patient needs to know the following information.

The body of a diabetic person, like that of any person, must have insulin, even if no food is being taken in.

The amount of insulin required in the postabsorptive or fasting state alone is about half of the total needed when eating; when fasting, it must be spread out as an insulin "trickle" rather than given in insulin "bursts."

Illness generally increases insulin need, so that even if not eating, the diabetic person may actually require more than 50% of the usual daily dose.

Each patient should have an "illness" regimen planned, discussed, and rehearsed ahead of time. It should include the following:

- religious injection of usual daily dose of insulin or administration of oral hypoglycemic agent
- an early call to the patient's nurse and physician to inform them of symptoms and actions
- frequent self-monitoring of blood glucose every 4 hours or a minimum of 4 times a day
- urine testing for ketones every 4 hours if blood glucose is 240 mg/dl or greater
- injections of small, supplemental doses of short-acting insulin several times daily, if necessary, according to the results of the blood glucose tests, until glucose levels come under control
- a sick day diet which includes liberal intake of fluids such as water, tea, bouillon, and food sources of carbohydrate that may be more easily digested during a period of illness such as apple juice, grape juice, popsicles, custard, pudding, cream soup, saltine crackers, and toast

The second most frequent management problems patients report are obtaining insulin refills on a timely basis and obtaining advice about crisis management. A patient may miss several days of insulin therapy and explain that the situation occurred because of any of various pitfalls: "I ran out and my doctor's appointment was only a few days away"; "In the excitement of the . . . , I skipped a few doses"; or "I did not have enough money to purchase my insulin." Similarly, difficulty reaching a medical person for advice by phone or limited access to a medical care facility can interfere with timely therapy and foster unnecessary episodes of ketoacidosis. Instructing the patient to call a diabetes hotline such as the local American Diabetes Association in this situation can dramatically reduce the number of episodes.

Barriers To Effective Self-Management

Beyond these general causes, certain diabetic patients seem to develop their own individual patterns for recurrent episodes of ketoacidosis: the patient who is mentally incompetent and without an adequate caretaker network; the alcoholic patient who develops ketoacidosis during sprees; the adolescent patient in whose battle with parents neglect of diabetes has become the "ultimate weapon"; the patient who has denied the existence of diabetes so firmly that its care is viewed with utmost lack of concern. These patients challenge the ingenuity, persistence, and professionalism of the entire health care team, but many patients will eventually respond.

Inpatient Settings

Prevention of diabetic ketoacidosis in inpatient settings is a different matter entirely. Here the keys are close monitoring, by professionals, of patients known to be ketosis-prone and maintaining a high index of suspicion in patients not previously known to be diabetic. Regular blood glucose and urine ketone testing in known diabetics always permits prevention of ketoacidosis, as long as the materials used for testing of strips and meter are known to be fresh and accurate, the testing is properly done, and abnormal results are promptly reported. Of course, not all urinary ketosis is diabetic ketosis, because fasting regularly produces ketonuria. The main differential clue is, of course, the absence of concurrent hyperglycemia with fasting ketonuria.

In hospitalized patients not known to be diabetic who develop unexplained extreme thirst, negative fluid balance, stupor, or hyperventilation, diabetic ketoacidosis is a part of the differential diagnosis, particularly in those with obvious triggering stresses such as severe infection, trauma, or CNS bleeding. A high index of suspicion and proper testing will exclude or make the diagnosis, and in the latter instance may be lifesaving.

Concerns in the Management of Diabetic Ketoacidosis

- Help in the search for precipitating causes
- Manage thirst and vomiting, and prevent aspiration
- Care for coma and bladder function
- Monitor intake, output, and medications
- Prevent recurrence by education and early recognition of high-risk inpatients

Hyperosmolar Hyperglycemic Nonketotic Coma

Description

Not infrequently, patients develop the marked hyperglycemia and hyperosmolarity of diabetic ketoacidosis but without the ketoacidosis. This is the syndrome of hyperosmolar hyperglycemic nonketotic coma. This syndrome is important because of

- its similarities to and differences from full blown diabetic ketoacidosis
- the differential diagnosis
- the differences in management

Table 40–1 compares hyperosmolar hyperglycemic nonketotic coma and diabetic ketoacidosis.

Assessment

History

Although the reason that some patients develop hyperosmolar coma without acidosis is very intriguing, it is usually not known. In experimental animals, a combination of mild diabetes, large doses of glucocorticoids, and extreme water deprivation is required to produce a model of the disease. The model may have important similarities to the human situation, because the patient's history frequently includes extremely poor water intake in the face of continuing insensible and urinary water loss and because on recovery the patient's diabetes is usually mild and does not require insulin.

TABLE 40–1
Comparison of Usual Clinical Manifestations of Hyperosmolar Hyperglycemic Nonketotic Coma and Diabetic Ketoacidosis

Hyperosmolar Coma	Diabetic Ketoacidosis
1. Patient has Type II diabetes and may be treated by diet alone, diet and an oral hypoglycemic agent, or diet and insulin therapy	1. Patient has type I, insulin-dependent diabetes
2. Patient usually more than 40 years of age	2. Patient usually less than 40 years of age
3. Insidious onset	3. Usually rapid onset
4. Symptoms include	4. Symptoms include
a. Slight drowsiness, insidious stupor or frequent coma	a. Drowsiness, stupor, coma
b. Polyuria for 2 days to 2 weeks before clinical presentation	b. Polyuria for 1 to 3 days prior to clinical presentation
c. Absence of hyperventilation, no breath odor	c. Hyperventilation with possible Kussmaul breathing pattern, "fruity" breath odor
d. Extreme volume depletion (dehydration, hypovolemia)	d. Extreme volume depletion (dehydration, hypovolemia)
e. Serum glucose 600 mg/dl to 2400 mg/dl	e. Serum glucose 300 mg/dl to 1000 mg/dl
f. Occasional gastrointestinal symptoms	f. Abdominal pain, nausea, vomiting, and diarrhea
g. Hypernatremia	g. Mild hyponatremia
h. Failure of thirst mechanism leading to inadequate water ingestion	h. Polydipsia for 1 to 3 days
i. High serum osmolarity with minimal CNS symptoms (disorientation, focal seizures)	i. High serum osmolarity
j. Impaired renal function	j. Impaired renal function
k. HCO_3 level greater than 16 mEq/L	k. HCO_3 level less than 10 mEq/L
l. CO_2 level normal	l. CO_2 level less than 10 mEq/L
m. Anion gap less than 7 mEq/L	m. Anion gap greater than 7 mEq/L
n. Usually normal serum potassium	n. Extreme hypokalemia
o. Ketonemia absent	o. Ketonemia present
p. Lack of acidosis	p. Moderate to severe acidosis
q. High mortality rate	q. High recovery rate

In some patients, it is clear that the syndrome is iatrogenic, induced by one of a variety of medications (eg, glucocorticoids, diazoxide [Proglycem], and diuretics), by dialysis against hyperosmolar glucose solutions, or by prolonged intravenous hypertonic glucose infusion (eg, in central hyperalimentation regimens).

Clinical Manifestations

Characteristically, these patients are middle age or elderly with type II diabetes sometimes not yet diagnosed. They become a bit drowsy, take in less and less by mouth, are noted over several days to slip ever deeper into stupor, and are finally brought to the hospital in a state of extreme volume depletion. Hyperglycemia in these patients may be extreme and is by definition over 600 mg/dl. In addition to the total extracellular sodium and water losses, a large additional "free water" deficit exists, probably because of failure of the thirst mechanism and consequent lack of oral intake. These patients therefore often have very high serum levels of both sodium and glucose, with the latter sometimes in excess of 2,000 mg/dl, and extraordinarily high serum osmolarities.

From our discussion of the mechanism of extreme hyperglycemia, one might expect that poor renal function must contribute even more greatly to the development of the hyperosmolar hyperglycemic nonketotic syndrome than to diabetic ketoacidosis itself and, indeed, renal function is generally much worse in the former. As in most things related to diabetes, the hyperosmolar syndrome is not always "pure." Some patients have a degree of ketosis as well. However, it seems logical to consider the diagnosis to be the hyperosmolar syndrome only if the anion gap attributable to ketoacids is less than 7 mEq/L and to diagnose full-blown ketoacidosis if this anion gap is greater than 7 mEq/L (see Table 40–1).

Management

In a general way, therapy for the hyperosmolar syndrome is very similar to those aspects of therapy for diabetic ketoacidosis that are directed at the hyperglycemia and volume depletion. The major difference is the extent or degree of the volume depletion, which is, on the whole, considerably greater in the hyperosmolar syndrome and which calls for extremely vigorous replacement. Moreover, these patients not only seem to require less insulin to control their hyperosmolar state but also are even more vulnerable to sudden loss of circulating blood volume with rapid, insulin-induced blood sugar reduction than are ketoacidotic patients. Therefore, low doses of insulin are generally given.

Patients who develop the hyperosmolar hyperglycemic nonketotic coma syndrome do not do very well. Complications are frequent, and mortality rates can be 25% to 50%. The multiplicity of associated diseases in what is mostly an elderly population, the inability of the cardiovascular system to handle the rapid volume shifts during the development and treatment of the syndrome, and the intravascular thrombosis and focal seizures (presumably due to extreme hyperconcentration of blood and poor local blood flow) all seem to contribute to this rather bleak outlook.

> Hyperosmolar coma is a complication of diabetes characterized by
> - Extreme hyperosmolality and water losses
> - Lack of acidosis
> - Frequent coma and focal seizures
> - Occurrence primarily in the elderly
> - High mortality rate

Hypoglycemia

Description

Although it may be apparent to health professionals that of the two diabetic emergencies ketoacidosis is actually far more life-threatening than hypoglycemia, the patient usually perceives even mild hypoglycemia as a much greater problem.

Pathophysiology

The minute-to-minute dependence of the brain on glucose supplied by the circulation results from the inability of the brain to burn long-chain free fatty acids, the lack of

glucose stored as glycogen within the adult brain, and the unavailability of ketones under fed or postabsorptive conditions.

There is little doubt that when blood sugar falls abruptly, the brain recognizes its energy deficiency after the serum level goes much below about 45 mg/dl. The exact level at which symptoms occur varies widely from person to person, however, and it is not uncommon for levels as low as 30 to 35 mg/dl to occur (eg, during glucose tolerance tests) with no symptoms whatsoever.

More controversial is the question of whether symptoms develop in response to a rapidly falling blood sugar even before it has gone below the usual lower limit of normal. Because certain physiological responses, such as growth hormone release, occur with declining but still normal blood sugars, it is likely that symptoms can occur on this basis, but the stimulus of a falling level is probably less strong and consistent than reduction below an absolute threshold. However, the brain seems to adapt at least partially to lowered blood sugar levels, particularly if the decline is slow and chronic. It is not unusual for patients with extremely low blood sugars, as occurs in patients with insulin-secreting tumors, to exhibit perfectly normal cerebral function in the face of blood sugars that are persistently below the normal range.

Assessment

History

Occasional insulin reactions can and do happen in even the most stable insulin-requiring diabetic. As long as they are mild, they can usually be tolerated without difficulty and are not cause for alarm or for changes in regimen. Frequently, the precipitating event is clear (eg, a skipped meal or an unusually strenuous bout of exercise).

When reactions are relatively frequent, recurrent, or severe, however, it is a different matter entirely. Unless the cause of the reactions is identified and prevented, the patient can become functionally disabled—always terrified that one is about to occur, unwilling or unable to drive a car, overeating to prevent them from happening, and so forth.

The search for causes and for corrective measures is a complex and individual matter for each patient, but usually the underlying mechanism can be discovered. Inadequate nutrient intake and exercise often contribute to hypoglycemia; however, a common and important mechanism is an atypical response to the usual insulin therapy. Such "early" and "late" responders are quite common and frequently not recognized as such. When the nature of their response pattern is properly defined, some relatively simple adjustments in insulin regimen often virtually eliminate both insulin reactions and excessive hyperglycemia.

A related problem is the patient whose blood glucose appears to be getting progressively worse, particularly in the morning, despite higher and higher insulin doses. Such a paradoxical response can be a clue to undetected nocturnal insulin reactions, followed by a counterregulatory response of such intensity that the blood sugar overshoots, leading to hyperglycemia by the next day. This is called Somogyi effect.

A second mechanism must be sought when a previously stable, reaction-free patient begins to experience hypoglycemic episodes. Certain biological explanations must, of course, be excluded, such as increased insulin sensitivity due to weight loss or the onset of azotemia. More often than not, such a physiological phenomenon is not discovered, and a meticulous search for problems with insulin dosage or administration should then be undertaken.

Thoroughly investigate every detail of insulin therapy, including insulin purchase, appearance, species, units, and syringes; injection sites, injection technique, and especially any recent change in any part of the regimen. Explore in detective fashion, looking for flaws and inconsistencies. Prescription errors, mismatched syringe and insulin unitages, use of new injection sites, and other errors may well emerge.

Finally, the administration or withdrawal of other drugs may be the precipitating event for recurrent insulin reactions.

Alcohol is by far the worst offender. Not only do patients often eat less when they have a few drinks, but also alcohol shuts off gluconeogenesis by interfering with intermediate biochemical steps within the liver. When combined with injected insulin, this combination not infrequently leads to hypoglycemia, which can be difficult to distinguish clinically because of concurrent inebriation.

Salicylates in large doses can reduce blood sugar and again, in combination with insulin, can produce hypoglycemia when either drug alone would not do so in the doses used.

Because *glucocorticoids* used therapeutically cause insulin resistance, insulin doses are often raised to meet the increased insulin demand. If the steroids are then tapered without appropriate downward adjustments in insulin dose, frequent reactions can supervene.

These are the major but by no means the only examples of drug–insulin interactions relevant to hypoglycemic episodes. It must not be forgotten, moreover, that oral hypoglycemic agents (sulfonylureas), which are still used in a great many patients, also can produce severe and long-lasting hypoglycemia.

Typically, patients who experience such episodes tend to be elderly and undernourished with impaired renal or hepatic function. Virtually any patient on oral agents can become hypoglycemic, especially in the presence of another potentiating agent such as phenylbutazone (Azolid), salicylates, or, above all, alcohol.

Clinical Manifestations

First, hypoglycemia in diabetics, although most prevalent in the insulin-dependent group, is much more common than ketoacidosis. Second, the onset of hypoglycemia is much more rapid, and its manifestations are much more variable, often occurring in such subtle ways as to evade the person's notice until he or she is unaware of what is happening and unable to seek the proper remedy. Insulin-induced hypoglycemia reactions therefore often occur in the midst of the patient's daily life, which can be, at the very least, embarrassing and, at worst, highly dangerous. Third, even though measurable recovery from hypoglycemia is rapid and complete within minutes after proper treatment, many patients remain emotionally (and possibly physiologically) shaken for hours or even days following insulin reactions. Finally, in extreme, severe situations, prolonged or recurrent hypoglycemia, although uncommon, does have the potential to cause permanent brain damage and can even be fatal.

Central Nervous System Response

As blood sugar falls below normal, the CNS responds in two distinct fashions: first, with impairment of higher cerebral functions, and soon thereafter with an "alarm" response in vegetative functions.

Cerebral Responses

Patients most commonly describe the symptoms of mild or early insulin reactions as fuzziness in the head, trouble with thinking or concentrating, shakiness, lightheadedness, or giddiness. These changes occur when the cerebral cortex is deprived of its main energy supply, usually when the blood glucose has fallen to 50 mg/dl or less, or is rapidly declining. This part of the brain is apparently the most sensitive to the loss of glucose.

Changes in personality and behavior may not be apparent to the patient during an insulin reaction. As with alcohol and other agents that affect cerebral function, these changes in personality vary with the person, the situation, the rapidity of onset, and other unknown factors. They range from silly, manic, inappropriate behavior through withdrawal, sullenness, or truculence, to grumpy, irritable, suspicious, or, in the extreme, paranoid and even, rarely, violent behavior. It is no wonder that, particularly when combined with difficulties in motor function such as trouble walking and slurred speech, patients who are well into insulin reactions may closely resemble people who have been drinking alcohol. It is for this reason that diabetic identification cards and jewelry indicate that such findings in the bearer may represent hypoglycemia rather than drunkenness.

The major lesson to be learned from this discussion is that *any patient taking insulin whose behavior or personality becomes inappropriate or uncharacteristic should be suspected of having an insulin reaction and treated accordingly.* The index of suspicion should be particularly high if such changes are episodic, occur at a time when the particular type of insulin used is expected to have its peak activity, and are accompanied by blood glucose levels consistently below normal.

A major source of anxiety for many diabetics who are taking insulin is concern for unrecognized hypoglycemia during sleep, leading to possible brain damage, such that they may "never wake up." Many patients who are having insulin reactions are wakened by the reaction, so it is possible to be realistically reassuring about this. However, some patients seem not to waken consistently and must rely on the presence or availability of a family member or partner to detect and treat nocturnal reactions.

Although the manifestations of cerebral cortical dysfunction from hypoglycemia are usually diffuse rather than focal, some patients develop focal signs or symptoms such as aphasia, vertigo, localized weakness, and even focal seizures with their insulin reactions. Such focal changes usually occur when there is prior focal damage to the specific area of the cortex, as from a previous stroke or head injury. Occasionally, these focal symptoms occur without any obvious predisposing factor, which makes for an extremely confusing diagnostic puzzle.

Vegetative Responses

Closely following the cortical changes is a series of vegetative neurologic responses. The primary response is discharge from the centers that control adrenergic autonomic impulses, with the resultant release of norepinephrine throughout the body and epinephrine from the adrenals. The resultant tachycardia, pallor, sweating, and tremor are characteristic of hypoglycemia and usually serve as important early warning signs by which many patients recognize an oncoming reaction. This adrenergic discharge is part of a larger stress response that includes release of large quantities of the "counterregulatory" hormones, such as glucocorticoids, growth hormone, and glucagon, which attempt to drive the blood sugar back up, primarily by stimulating hepatic glycogen breakdown.

Other vegetative signs and symptoms can occur during hypoglycemic reactions but are less constant. Despite myths to the contrary, hunger is not a prominent feature of insulin reactions in most patients (although it does sometimes occur), headache can occur, and the stress response can on occasion trigger secondary sequences of symptoms, including angina or pulmonary edema in patients with fragile cardiovascular disease.

Ultimately, as hypoglycemia persists and worsens, consciousness is progressively impaired, leading to stupor, seizure, or coma. This is characteristic of severe hypoglycemia. The vegetative centers controlling fundamental systems such as respiration and blood pressure maintenance are the most resistant to hypoglycemia and continue to function even when most other cerebral functions are lost.

The more profound the hypoglycemia and the longer it lasts, the greater the chance of transient or even permanent cerebral damage after blood sugar is restored. There does not seem to be a clear duration threshold for such damage, but severe hypoglycemia lasting more than 15 to 30 minutes can result in at least some symptoms that persist for a time after glucose is given.

Diagnosis

In principle, the diagnosis of hypoglycemia should be relatively simple and clear-cut. Because of the extreme *nonspecificity* of its manifestations and the extraordinary *biological variation* in response to low blood sugar, the diagnosis, in actual practice, is often subtle and complex. A serum sugar found to be below 25 mg/dl may always be held responsible for accompanying symptoms. Even in the range from 25 to 45 mg/dl, however, symptoms may not always be attributable to the hypoglycemia (particularly in spontaneous or reactive hypoglycemia), and between 45 to 65 mg/dl the relation becomes even more difficult to prove.

Making a reasonably secure diagnosis of *symptomatic hypoglycemia* therefore depends on three elements:

- documentation by an independent observer that symptoms are occurring, at a time when the blood sugar can be determined
- correlation of the symptoms with a blood sugar level that is either absolutely low or declining very rapidly
- prompt reversal of the symptoms on administration of glucose, with a correlated rise in blood sugar level

In the absence of any of these three criteria, the diagnosis, although it may be strongly suspected, is less certain. It is therefore of prime importance that a blood sugar level be drawn (or determined by capillary glucose testing) if at all possible *before* administration of glucose. Although blood sugar is easily measured in the hospital, it may be less feasible at home if there is not immediate access to a glucometer or the ability to perform the test during a hypoglycemic episode.

Urine sugars are not a reliable indicator of hypoglycemia because the bladder urine represents an "integral" sample of blood sugar levels over time. The sample voided just before or after an insulin reaction may well contain glucose from a glucose peak several hours earlier, thus giving a *false–positive* impression. Even uniformly negative urine tests are not diagnostic for hypoglycemia.

Management

The treatment of insulin reactions is always glucose. If the patient can swallow, the glucose is most conveniently given as a glucose- or sucrose-containing drink, because in this form it probably gets through the stomach and into the absorbing intestine in the fastest possible time. If the patient is too groggy, stuporous, or uncooperative to drink, a bolus of Δ50w is given intravenously over several minutes. If this route or dosage is unavailable, 1 mg of glucagon given subcutaneously or intramuscularly reverses the symptoms by inducing a rapid breakdown and release of glucose into the bloodstream from hepatic glycogen stores.

The amount of glucose needed to reverse an insulin reaction acutely is not large. The blood sugar can be raised from 20 to 120 mg/dl with less than 15 g (3 tsp) of glucose in an average sized adult. Glucose in almost any oral form will serve. Typical treatments for hypoglycemia include 3 glucose tablets, 6 ounces of regular cola, 6 ounces of

orange juice, 4 ounces of 2% or skim milk, or 6 to 8 lifesavers. Starch, as in crackers and cookies, is broken down to free glucose once through the stomach and absorbed so rapidly that blood sugar rises virtually as fast as with free glucose or sucrose.

As an extension of their fears that they might "never wake up" from nocturnal insulin reaction, patients are frequently concerned about what to do if they do not respond to the initial therapy. They must be reassured that if the first bolus of glucose consumed does not seem to work, the sensible thing to do is to take in more. Insulin reactions are *always* reversible with enough glucose. The response to oral glucose, of course, takes time, perhaps 5 to 15 minutes, whereas the response to intravenous glucose should occur within 1 or 2 minutes at most.

Failure to respond fully in the appropriate time indicates that not enough glucose has been given, that the diagnosis is incorrect, or that the hypoglycemia has been long and severe enough to produce persistent, although not necessarily permanent, cerebral dysfunction.

Hypoglycemia in diabetics

- Is frequently confused with ketoacidosis by patients and their families
- Can be precipitated in insulin-dependent patients by many factors, including inappropriate insulin regimen, errors in insulin administration, exercise, inadequate nutrient intake, and ingestion of alcohol and other drugs
- Produces a wide range of signs and symptoms, from personality change to confusion to coma
- Should be documented by correlation of blood sugar with symptoms whenever possible
- Responds promptly to glucose administration

Case Study: Diabetic Ketoacidosis

Mr. Oliver, age 31, was admitted to the hospital with the chief complaints of fatigue, cough, nausea, and vomiting for 4 days.

He had been diagnosed as having diabetes mellitus 1½ years before admission. Since that time, he had been maintained without incident on 24 units of NPH and 9 units of regular insulin in the morning and 11 units of NPH and 6 units of regular insulin in the evening. Four days before admission, Mr. Oliver began to cough, raising first clear, then brownish, sputum. He soon became fatigued, then experienced some nausea and intermittent vomiting. Two days before admission, he omitted his evening insulin, then took no further insulin the day before and day of admission, "because he was not eating anything." On the day of admission, the patient's wife

Clinical Research

Kresevic DM, Slavin SM: Incidence of hypoglycemia and nutritional intake in patients on a general medical unit. Nursing Connections 2(4):33–40, 1989

The purpose of this study was to examine the occurrence of complications in hospitalized patients with diabetes. Subjects included 47 medical patients, who were all the diabetes patients admitted to one general medical unit over a 3-month period. The following information was reviewed for each patient during the course of hospitalization: (1) demographic data, (2) admission weight, desirable body weight, and serum albumin level, (3) food intake, (4) hypoglycemic episodes, (5) hypoglycemia treatment, and (6) blood glucose values. This preliminary study found that hypoglycemia occurred in 28% of the study population and that reduced carbohydrate intake coupled with a low serum albumin level was found to be a more accurate clinical indicator of patients at risk for hypoglycemia than low calories and carbohydrate intake. Areas to improve care, such as the need to standardize treatment for hypoglycemia, were also identified.

noted that he had become "less responsive and was breathing fast and deeply" and brought him to the emergency room.

On admission, the patient's rectal temperature was 36.1°C (97°F), pulse was 132, respirations were 28 and deep, and blood pressure was 108/72. He was oriented but lethargic, with coarse rales at both lung bases.

Admission laboratory work revealed a hematocrit of 51.6, white blood cell count of 36,400, and 4+ glucose and ketones on urinalysis. Admission laboratory work included glucose 910 mg/dl, Na^+ 128, K^+ 6.7, Cl^- 90, HCO_3^- 4, BUN 43, creatinine 2.3 mg/dl, serum ketones 4+ at 1:2 dilution, and trace to 1:32 dilution. Arterial blood pH was 7.06, PO_2 112, PCO_2 13, and HCO_3^- 2.5. The admission chest film was negative, but sputum cultured on admission ultimately grew out *Haemophilus influenzae* and *Streptococcus pneumoniae*.

Initial therapy consisted of an intravenous infusion of normal saline and 20 U regular insulin by intravenous push, followed by an infusion of insulin at 5 U/hour during the first 9 hours. The patient's mental status and sense of well-being improved rapidly. The flow sheet below summarizes the biochemical changes over the first 15 hours.

Mr. Oliver remained afebrile and was not treated with antibiotics. By the time of discharge 4 days later, he was eating well, his blood sugars were controlled on his usual doses of NPH insulin, and his cough had improved.

Case Analysis of Clinical Findings

Hyperglycemia and Hyperosmolality

Mr. Oliver presented with the chemical findings of extreme hyperglycemia. As expected in this situation, the BUN and creatinine were elevated, indicating that renal perfusion was reduced, permitting less glucose to escape into the urine and allowing the blood sugar to reach these high levels. The patient's lethargic mental state was the result of the moderately severe hyperosmolality.

Ketosis and Acidosis

For Mr. Oliver, the extremely low initial serum bicarbonate concentration of 2.5 to 4 signalled the consumption of nearly all the available buffering capacity of plasma, indicating the presence of *severe* metabolic acidosis. This con-

Biochemical Flow Sheet Indicating Diabetic Ketoacidosis in Mr. Oliver

Time	Sugar	pH	Na^+	K^+	Cl^-	HCO_3^-	BUN/ Creatinine
1:00 PM	710	7.06	128	6.9	90	4	43/2.3
3:00 PM	492		132	6.8	101	6	41/1.7
5:15 PM	375	7.25	137	4.1	106	8	45/1.4
10:00 PM	303		139	4.7	114	15	27/1.2
4:00 AM	304		143	4.3	113	22	22/1.1

clusion was reinforced by the anion gap of $(128 + 7) - (90 + 3) = 42$, about 27 mEq above the usual anion gap upper limit of 15, indicating the presence of 27 mEq of "unmeasured anions." The semiquantitative serum ketones were strongly positive at a dilution of $1:2$, confirming the presence of a large quantity of ketone bodies, which could account for most of the unmeasured anions. The diagnosis of diabetic ketoacidosis of severe degree was thus firmly established.

The patient's deep, rapid respirations represented Kussmaul breathing, a critically important compensating mechanism that had reduced his arterial CO_2 level (P_{CO_2}) to about one-fourth its usual level and had helped keep his blood pH from falling below its already very low level of 7.06.

Fluid and Electrolyte Losses: Volume Depletion

Mr. Oliver's history of increasing symptoms over at least 4 days suggested that this episode of ketoacidosis had been developing for a substantial period of time, sufficient for osmotic diuresis to produce extensive salt and water losses. Nausea prevented volume replacement by mouth, and vomiting further aggravated the losses. Mr. Oliver failed to realize the need to initiate sick day measures to control his serum glucose level or the need to consult his physician immediately.

The rapid pulse and low blood pressure on admission were further clues to the presence of significant hypovolemia, which was confirmed by the elevated BUN and creatinine, reflecting inadequate circulating blood volume to maintain renal perfusion. Finally, the elevated serum potassium ($K^+ = 6.7$ mEq/L, normal = 3.5–4.8 mEq/L) indicated that not enough sodium was being filtered in the kidney to permit adequate potassium exchange and potassium excretion.

Response to Treatment

Despite evidence of severe hyperglycemia, metabolic acidosis, and volume depletion, Mr. Oliver responded promptly to standard and fairly conservative therapy that included volume replacement with saline and low-dose intravenous insulin. Clinical and chemical signs indicated steady and progressive improvement over the first 15 hours of treatment:

The falling blood sugar from 710 to 304 mg/dl over this time reflected continued renal glucose loss with concomitant insulin-induced decrease in hepatic glucose production.

The falling BUN and creatinine indicated that volume replacement had restored renal perfusion.

Without the use of intravenous bicarbonate, the serum bicarbonate level rose from 4 to 22 mEq/L

as the production of ketones was turned off by insulin and ketones were metabolized to bicarbonate, which was then reabsorbed by the kidney.

Arterial blood pH was restored from its initial very low level of 7.06 to 7.25 as the bicarbonate buffer reappeared in plasma.

Serum potassium fell from 6.9 into the normal range as insulin drove potassium back into cells, pH improved, osmolality returned to normal, and improved renal perfusion permitted exchange of potassium for sodium.

Finally, the rise in serum chloride from the low initial value of 90 mEq/L (normal range: 96–103 mEq/L) to the abnormally high level of 114 mEq/L is not entirely understood but reflects in part the intravenous infusion of large amounts of chloride.

Fortunately, despite Mr. Oliver's severe chemical abnormalities, he was lethargic rather than comatose. This may have been because he was young and otherwise healthy, and the ketoacidosis had developed over a short time. He did not need to be intubated or catheterized, and he tolerated the rapid shifts in volume, pH, and osmolality induced by therapy very well. His rapid response resulted in a brief hospitalization. The slow replenishment of body constituents and readjustment of diabetic regime—the fourth phase of therapy—could be safely carried out at home with nurse and physician supervision.

Preventing Recurrence

The precipitating causes of the episode of ketoacidosis in Mr. Oliver were classic: (1) the onset of an episode of respiratory infection and possibly some initial gastroenteritis; and (2) failure of this totally insulin-dependent patient to understand the continuing need for insulin even in the absence of food intake. This episode of ketoacidosis could probably have been prevented if Mr. Oliver had continued to take insulin, at perhaps one-half to two-thirds his usual dose, with supplemental short-acting insulin as needed. If the nausea and vomiting had been controlled early, he might also have been able to continue oral fluid and sodium replacement. This situation points out the value of a "diabetes illness plan" and of early contact during an acute illness with a physician or a nurse familiar with diabetes management.

Care Planning

The two nursing diagnoses identified for Mr. Oliver are fluid volume deficit and knowledge deficit. There is also a potential complication of respiratory insufficiency related to chest infection. Nursing Care Plan 40–1 describes the nursing interventions and outcome criteria for Mr. Oliver.

NURSING CARE PLAN 40–1:
The Patient With Diabetic Ketoacidosis

NURSING DIAGNOSIS	OUTCOME CRITERIA/ PATIENT GOALS	NURSING INTERVENTIONS
Fluid volume deficit: related to hyper-glycemia secondary to diabetes keto-acidosis (DKA).	• Restore fluid and electrolyte balance.	1. Administer intravenous fluids, insulin, and, as needed, electrolyte replacements, per physician's order.
		2. Monitor laboratory reports (ie, Hct, Hgb, sodium, chloride, magnesium, BUN, creatinine, phosphate, CO_2, HCO_3^-, and pH).
		3. Monitor hydration $q\frac{1}{2}h$ to q1h initially: intake and output, urine specific gravity, skin moisture, and turgor.
		4. Monitor blood pressure, temperature, and pulse q1h initially, then q4h.
		5. Monitor ECG strips for indications of electrolyte changes q1h.
	• Slowly bring serum glucose within normal limits.	6. Monitor blood glucose $q\frac{1}{2}h$ until stable, also urine ketones.
		7. Observe for signs of electrolyte and acid–base imbalance (ie, "fruity" odor of breath, cherry red color of skin and mucous membranes, tetany, carpopedal spasm, neuromuscular irritability, and seizures).
		8. Evaluate mental status q1h until crises subside, and q4h thereafter.
	• Resolution of nausea and vomiting, abdominal pain, tenderness, and rigidity.	1. Provide care measures for nasogastric intubation.
		2. Maintain gastric decompression.
		3. Monitor bowel sounds q2h.
		4. Assist with oral hygiene q2h.
		5. Withhold food and fluids, per physician's order.
		6. Provide ice chips, per physician's order. Fluid restriction as ordered.
		7. Record color, amount, and frequency of vomiting.
	• Promote normal nutrition as appetite improves and symptoms decrease.	1. Provide calm atmosphere during meals.
		2. Involve patient in diet plan.

(continued)

NURSING DIAGNOSIS	OUTCOME CRITERIA/ PATIENT GOALS	NURSING INTERVENTIONS
		3. Identify factors (eg, depression, acid–base imbalance) that may contribute to loss of appetite.
		4. Minimize unpleasant sights and odors in immediate environment.
High risk for impaired gas exchange: related to pneumonia, DKA Kussmal respirations.	• Resolve infectious process.	1. Identify factors contributing to decreased resistance to infection.
		2. Monitor temperature q4h.
		3. Observe for signs and symptoms of infection (eg, fatigue, elevated WBC, elevated temperature).
		4. Promote rest.
	• Promote natural gas exchanges and breathing pattern.	1. Monitor results of chest film.
		2. Auscultate lungs q1h until stable, then q4h.
		3. Elevate head of bed to facilitate breathing comfort.
		4. Assess respiratory rate and depth q4h.
		5. Perform pulmonary toilet, per physician's order.
Knowledge deficit: related to inability to manage episode of diabetic crisis.	• Patient can explain physiological stressors that may precipitate diabetic ketoacidosis.	1. Assess patient's knowledge of precipitating factors and sick day guidelines.
		2. Instruct on events that could precipitate diabetic ketoacidosis (eg, infection, injury, or emotional stress).
	• Patient and family can state 5 sick day guidelines.	3. Instruct or review sick day guidelines concerning
		administering insulin;
		food and fluid intake;
		testing blood or urine for glucose and urine for ketones; notifying health provider to inform and receive further direction;
		emergency resources.
	• Patient and family can identify symptoms requiring medical/nursing intervention.	4. Instruct patient and family in signs and symptoms of diabetic emergencies.
		5. Instruct on importance of having sufficient insulin on hand.
		6. Provide names and telephone numbers of resource persons to contact if problems arise.
		7. Instruct patient to wear medical identification bracelet.

REFERENCES

Diabetic Ketoacidosis

1. Barrett EJ, DeFronzo RA, Bevilacqua A et al: Insulin resistance in diabetic ketoacidosis. Diabetes 31:932–938, 1982
2. Carroll P, Matz R: Uncontrolled diabetes mellitus in adults: Experience in treating diabetic ketoacidosis and hyperosmolar nonketotic coma with low-dose insulin and a uniform treatment regimen. Diabetes Care 6:579–585, 1983
3. Davidson MB: Diabetes Mellitus: Diagnosis and Treatment, 3rd ed, p 190. New York, Churchill-Livingstone, 1991
4. Lindsay R, Bolte RG: The use of an insulin bolus in low-dose insulin infusion for pediatric diabetic ketoacidosis. Pediatr Emerg Care 5:77–79, 1989
5. White NH, Henry DN: Special issues in diabetes management. In Haire-Joshu D (ed.) Management of Diabetes Mellitus, p 254. St Louis, Mosby Year Book, 1992
6. Peterson L, Caldwell J, Hoffman J: Insulin adsorbance to polyvinylchloride surfaces with implications for constant infusion therapy. Diabetes 25:72–74, 1976
7. Androgue HJ, Madias NE: Changes in plasma potassium concentration during acute acid–base disturbances. Am J Med 71:456–469, 1981

BIBLIOGRAPHY

Brody GM: Diabetic ketoacidosis and hyperosmolar hyperglycemic nonketotic coma. Top Emerg Med 14(1):12–22, 1992

Cefalu WT: Diabetic ketoacidosis. Crit Care Clin 7(1):89–108, 1991

Ellis EN: Concepts of fluid therapy in diabetic ketoacidosis and hyperosmolar hyperglycemic nonketotic coma. Pediatr Clin North Am 37:313–321, 1990

Graves L: Diabetic ketoacidosis and hyperosmolar hyperglycemia nonketotic coma. Crit Care Nurs Q 13(3):50–61, 1990

Kresevic DM, Slavin SM: Incidence of hypoglycemia and nutritional intake in patients on a general medical unit. NursingConnections 2:33–40, 1989

Mulcahy K: Hypoglycemic emergencies. AACN Clin Issues Crit Care Nurs 3(2):361–369, 1992

Peterson A, Drass J: Managing acute complications of diabetes. Nursing 21(2):34–40, 1991

Rothenberg MA: Diabetic Emergencies. Emerg Med Serv 29(10): 18, 20, 23, 1991

Sauve DO, Kessler CA: Hyperglycemic emergencies. AACN Clin Issues Crit Care Nurs 3(2):350–360, 1992

STUDY QUESTIONS

1. During the short fasting phase of nutrition, the body relies primarily on which of these substances to provide most of the tissue energy?

   a. glucose
   b. fatty acids
   c. liver glycogen
   d. ketones

2. Type I diabetes is characterized by

   a. insulin resistance
   b. onset after 40 years of age
   c. insulinopenia
   d. elevated levels of circulating insulin

3. During diabetic ketoacidosis

   a. insulin is present in sufficient amounts and utilized appropriately
   b. counterregulatory hormones increase lipolysis and glycogenolysis
   c. there is fluid retention
   d. counterregulatory hormones are suppressed

4. Diabetic ketoacidosis is often precipitated by all of the following except

   a. overinsulinization
   b. stress
   c. illness
   d. mismanagement of sick days

5. Traditional therapy for diabetic ketoacidosis consists of

   a. fluid replacement with isotonic or hypotonic saline
   b. a bolus of sodium bicarbonate
   c. a tracheostomy to assist respirations
   d. hemodialysis to correct underlying fluid and electrolyte

6. A person with diabetes should be instructed to do the following during a sick day episode:

   a. omit insulin if unable to eat
   b. maintain strict bed rest
   c. follow a fluid restriction plan
   d. check urine for presence of ketones

7. During hyperosmolar hyperglycemic nonketotic coma

   a. the anion gap is usually 8 mEq/L or greater
   b. ketonemia is present
   c. serum glucose levels may be 600 mg/dl to 2,400 mg/dl
   d. serum bicarbonate level is less than 10 mEq/L

8. The initial treatment goal of hyperosmolar hyperglycemic nonketotic coma is

   a. to bring the blood glucose level to a normal range
   b. to alleviate ketosis
   c. to diurese the patient
   d. to rehydrate the patient

9. A patient with mild hypoglycemia may best self-treat by ingesting

   a. 8 lifesavers
   b. 6 glucose tablets
   c. 8 ounces of orange juice
   d. 4 ounces of orange juice with 2 teaspoons of sugar

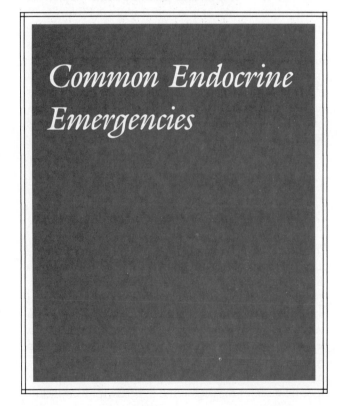

CHAPTER 41

Common Endocrine Emergencies

BEHAVIORAL OBJECTIVES

Based on the content in this chapter, the reader should be able to:

1. Describe the pathophysiological principles of thyroid crises, myxedema coma, adrenal crises, and SIADH
2. Identify key precipitating factors, laboratory findings, and clinical manifestations for each of these disorders.
3. Discuss nursing diagnoses and interventions for the acute phase of each of these disorders.

Hudak: Critical Care Nursing:
A Holistic Approach, 6th ed. © 1994
J. B. Lippincott Company.

Description

Understanding the derangements of the hypothalamic–pituitary axis, both posterior and anterior, requires knowledge of normal function (see Chapter 39). The presenting clinical manifestation of these derangements range from asymptomatic to acute and life-threatening. Generally, these conditions can be divided into two sections, the hypothalamic-anterior, which includes thyroid, adrenal and other endocrine illnesses, and hypothalamic-posterior dysfunction, which primarily includes disorders of antidiuretic hormone (ADH) secretion.

Chronic or acute disease conditions may have significant affects on normal endocrine function, leading to hypofunction and, less commonly, hyperfunction of the neuroendocrine system. This is becoming more apparent in multisystem organ failure. Patients at risk may have a known preexisting endocrine disorder (Table 41–1). A significant group of patients who also are at risk, but have no known endocrine history, include patients with multisystem organ failure or prolonged illness (Table 41–2). Therefore, dysfunction should be a consideration in the assessment and management of all critically ill patients. Subtle clinical parameters may provide the initial clues that dysfunction is occurring. This chapter presents an overview of the etiologies, as well as guidelines for assessing and managing hypothyroid and hyperthyroid dysfunction, hypofunction of the adrenal glands, and excessive ADH secretion.

Thyroid Crisis

Pathophysiological Principles

Thyrotoxic crisis is a severe form of hyperthyroidism that often is associated with physiological or psychological stress. Thyroid crisis is a critical worsening of the thyrotoxic state. Rapid deterioration and death can occur if untreated. The condition may develop spontaneously, but it occurs most frequently in people who have undiagnosed or partially treated severe hyperthyroidism. By definition, hyperthyroidism is a condition in which thyroid hormones actions result in greater-than-normal responses. Specific diseases that can cause hyperthyroidism include Graves' disease, exogenous hyperthyroidism, thyroiditis, toxic nodular goiter, toxic multinodular goiter, and thyroid cancer. Certain drugs, such as contrast material for radiographic procedures or amiodarone (an antidysrhythmic drug), may precipitate the thyrotoxic state owing to their high iodine content. Recognizing clinical signs and symptoms of hyperthyroidism is the key to recognizing thyroid crisis.

The etiology of thyroid crisis, often referred to as thyroid storm or thyrotoxicosis, is poorly understood.

TABLE 41–1
Patients at Risk for Development of Endocrine Crisis for Whom the Preexisting Endocrine Disorder is Known

Precipitating factors
  Infection
  Trauma
  Coexistent medical illness (ie, myocardial infarction, pulmonary disease)
  Pregnancy
  Exposure to cold
Medications
  Chronic steroid therapy
  β-blockers
  Narcotics, anesthetics
  Alcohol, tricyclic antidepressants
  Glucocorticoid therapy
  Insulin therapy
  Thiazide diuretics
  Phenytoin
  Chemotherapy agents
  Nonsteroidal anti-inflammatory agents

Adapted from Halloran T: Nursing responsibilities in endocrine emergencies. Critical Care Nursing Quarterly 13:(3):74–81, 1990.

There are three physiological mechanisms thought to induce thyroid crisis:

1. The sudden release of large quantities of thyroid hormone
2. Adrenergic hyperactivity
3. Excessive lipolysis and fatty acid production

The abrupt release of large quantities of thyroid hormone is thought to produce the hypermetabolic manifestations seen during thyroid crisis. Laboratory analyses of triiodothyronine (T_3) or thyroxine (T_4) may not verify

TABLE 41–2
Patients at Risk for Development of Endocrine Crisis for Whom the Preexisting Condition is Unknown

Precipitating factors
  Pituitary tumors
  Radiation therapy of the head and neck
  Autoimmune disease
  Neurosurgical procedures
  Metastatic malignancies (eg, lung, breast)
  Surgery
  Long-term illness
  Shock
  Postpartum
  Trauma

Adapted from Halloran T: Nursing responsibilities in endocrine emergencies. Critical Care Nursing Quarterly 13:(3):74–81, 1990.

this phenomenon and may only reflect values similar to the known hyperthyroid state of the patient.

Adrenergic hyperactivity is considered a possible link to thyroid crisis. Although thyroid hormone and catecholamines potentiate each other, studies have shown the catecholamine levels during thyroid crisis are within the normal range. It is uncertain whether the effects of hypersecretion of thyroid hormone or increased catecholamine levels are causing heightened sensitivity and effector organ function. Thyroid–catecholamine interactions result in an increased rate of chemical reactions, increased nutrient and oxygen consumption, increased heat production, alterations in fluid and electrolyte balance, and a catabolic state.

The third mechanism is excessive lipolysis and fatty acid production. With excessive lipolysis, increased fatty acids will oxidize and produce an overabundance of thermal energy that is difficult to dissipate through vasodilation. The thermal energy is not in the form of adenosine triphosphate at the molecular level, and cannot be used by the cell as such.[1]

Assessment

In general, hyperthyroidism has a range of endocrine, reproductive, gastrointestinal, integumentary, and ocular manifestations. These are caused by increased circulating levels of thyroid hormone and by stimulation of the sympathetic nervous system.

Identifying the underlying precipitating factor for thyroid storm so that treatment can be initiated is an important assessment factor. Precipitating factors include insufficient antithyroid therapy and, rarely, excessive exogenous administration of thyroid hormone. Trauma, stress, or infection also may precipitate a crisis.

Signs and symptoms of hyperthyroidism include sweating, heat intolerance, nervousness, tremors, palpitations, hyperkinesis, and increased bowel sounds. Extremes of these clinical signs and symptoms, specifically fever greater than 100°F, tachycardia out of proportion to the fever, and central nervous system (CNS) dysfunction, are indicative of thyroid storm (Table 41–3). Central nervous system abnormalities include agitation, seizures, or coma. The elderly patient may not present with the classic signs and symptoms, and thyroid crisis therefore may be overlooked and untreated. Frequently, however, they have suggestive clinical signs and symptoms. In these circumstances, ask if the patient has heart disease, because β-blocker therapy may mask the classic cardiovascular clues. The predominance of cardiac abnormalities in the elderly may draw attention away from clues to the hyperthyroid state.

The diagnosis of thyroid crisis is based on clinical findings. Diagnostic studies may reveal an elevated total and free T_3 and T_4 and an elevated T_3 resin uptake. Non-

TABLE 41–3
Clinical Manifestations of Thyroid Emergencies

Thyroid Storm	Myxedema Coma
Tachycardia	Bradycardia
Hyperthermia	Hypothermia
Tachypnea	Hypoventilation
Hypercalcemia	Hyponatremia
Hyperglycemia	Hypoglycemia
Metabolic acidosis	Respiratory and metabolic acidosis
Cardiovascular collapse due to cardiogenic shock hypovolemia cardiac arrhythmias	Cardiovascular collapse due to decreased vascular tone
Depressed LOC	Depressed LOC
Emotional lability	Seizures, coma
Psychosis	
Tremors, restlessness	Hyporeflexia

LOC, level of consciousness.
From Halloran T: Nursing responsibilities in endocrine emergencies. Critical Care Nursing Quarterly 13:(3):74–81, 1990.

endocrine laboratory tests are not diagnostic; however, serum electrolytes, liver function tests, and complete blood count may reveal clinical abnormalities that require treatment. Laboratory studies also may assist in identifying the precipitating cause. Electrolyte imbalances due to dehydration, excessive bone resorption, and increased insulin degradation often occur.

Management

Medical management goals of thyroid crisis are fourfold: treating the precipitating factor(s), controlling excessive thyroid hormone release, inhibiting thyroid hormone release, and antagonizing the peripheral effects of thyroid hormone. Nursing management goals include recognizing these effects, monitoring for the appropriate clinical outcomes, and providing supportive care to the patient and family.

Antithyroid drugs are used to control thyroid release or biosynthesis. Propylthiouracil is the preferred agent, although it can be given only orally. Propylthiouracil is preferred because it blocks the conversion of T_4 to T_3 in peripheral tissues and binds iodine to prevent synthesis of the hormone. If the oral route is not possible, methimazole can be given rectally.

Inhibiting or blocking thyroid hormone release is achieved with iodide solutions such as potassium iodide, or sodium iodide intravenously or orally (Lugol's solution). These agents should not be given until 1 hour after

NURSING CARE PLAN 41–1:
The Patient in Thyroid Crisis

NURSING DIAGNOSIS	OUTCOME CRITERIA/ PATIENT GOALS	NURSING INTERVENTIONS
Fluid volume deficit: related to hyper-metabolic state.	• Patient will be normovolemic.	1. Assess volume status (BP, HR, RR, temperature, heart sounds) q1h and prn. 2. Administer IV fluids, as ordered. 3. Assess all laboratory data. Report abnormal electrolyte values. 4. Monitor cardiac rhythm. 5. Give medications and electrolytes, as ordered. 6. Give β-adrenergic medications, as ordered.
Hyperthermia: related to hyper-metabolic state.	• Body temperature will return to patient's normal range.	1. Monitor temperature q1h. 2. Institute measures to lower body temperature (medications, tepid baths, cooling blanket). 3. Prevent shivering.
Altered tissue perfusion, cerebral: related to hyperthyroidism.	• Patient will return to usual wakeful state.	1. Assess neurologic status q1h and prn. 2. Implement seizure precautions. 3. Assess restlessness, airway patency, and safety, if level of consciousness decreases. 4. Institute safety measures to prevent injury.
Decreased cardiac output: related to heart failure and hypermetabolic state.	• Patient will remain hemodynamically stable.	1. See Nursing Care Plan 14–1: The Patient With Heart Failure.

the administration of antithyroid medications. Lithium is the drug of choice for patients who are iodine sensitive. Glucocorticoids may be ordered because they also inhibit thyroid hormone release.

The peripheral effects of excessive thyroid hormone include hyperthermia, increased metabolic rate, and tachycardia. Cardiovascular decompensation, secondary to decreased stroke volume and reduced cardiac output, may be life threatening. The use of β-adrenergic blockers, specifically propranolol, is directed not against the underlying disease of hyperthyroidism but rather against its symptoms. This therapy may be ordered to restore cardiac function by decreasing the catecholamine-mediated symptoms. The goal of therapy is to decrease myocardial oxygen consumption, decrease the heart rate (ideally below 100 beats per minute), and increase cardiac output. Intrinsic cardiac disease may worsen if the negative inotropic effect of this drug is not monitored carefully. Those patients with lung disease may require a cardiac specific β-blocker. Propranolol also blocks the conversion of T_4 to T_3. Digoxin may be considered for the treatment of congestive heart failure or supraventricular tachydysrhythmias.

Antipyretic agents, particularly acetaminophen, are recommended for fever control. Aspirin is not recommended because it increases free T_3 and T_4 levels. External cooling devices may be helpful. Cooling to the extent of shivering and piloerection may have a rebound effect of raising body temperature even higher and increasing metabolic activity. Other supportive care requirements focus on meeting the metabolic demands of the hypermetabolic state; these includes administering glucose-containing solutions and nutrient therapy.

Nursing interventions focus on the hypermetabolism, which may cause decompensation of organ systems, electrolyte and fluid imbalances, and a worsening neurologic status. These include decreasing unnecessary external stimuli, decreasing overall oxygen consumption by maintaining appropriate activity levels, and monitoring for outcome criteria. After the crisis period, interventions are directed to patient teaching and prevention of a worsened disease process (see Nursing Care Plan 41–1).

Complications

Even without preexisting coronary artery disease, untreated thyroid crisis can cause angina pectoris and myocardial infarction, congestive heart failure, cardiovascular collapse, coma, and death.

Myxedema Coma

Pathophysiological Principles

Hypothyroidism is caused by a deficiency in production of thyroid hormone by the thyroid gland. This condition may be primary or secondary. Deficient production of thyroid hormone results in the clinical state termed *hypothyroidism*. Myxedema coma is a rare, life-threatening emergency brought on by extreme hypothyroidism. It usually is seen in elderly patients during the winter months.

Hypothyroidism is a chronic disease that is 10 times more common in women than in men, and occurs in all age groups, most commonly in those older than the age of 50 years; it is less common than hyperthyroidism. Hypothyroidism can be primary or secondary. Primary causes include congenital defects, loss of thyroid tissue after treatment for hyperthyroidism, defective hormone synthesis due to an autoimmune process, and antithyroid drug administration or iodine deficiency. Secondary causes include peripheral resistance to thyroid hormone, pituitary tumors or infarction, and hypothalamic disorders. Transient hypothyroidism can occur after withdrawal of prolonged T_4 or T_3 treatment.

Hypothyroidism generally affects all body systems; a low basal metabolic rate and decreased energy metabolism and heat production are characteristic. Myxedema results from an alteration in the composition of the dermis and other tissues. The connective fibers are separated by an increased amount of protein and mucopolysaccharides; this binds water, producing nonpitting, boggy edema, especially around the eyes, hands, and feet, and also is responsible for thickening of the tongue and the laryngeal and pharyngeal mucous membranes, resulting in slurred speech and hoarseness. In addition to the clinical symptoms of hypothyroidism, a decrease in T_4 and free T_4 is a common finding.

Assessment

Signs and symptoms of hypothyroidism include fatigue, weakness, decreased bowel sounds, decreased appetite, weight gain, and electrocardiographic changes. Myxedema coma is a rare manifestation of hypothyroidism, characterized by severe depression of the sensorium, hypothermia, hypoventilation, hyponatremia, hyporeflexia, hypotension, and bradycardia. Myxedema coma patients do not shiver, although temperatures have been reported below 80°F. The diagnosis of myxedema coma depends on recognizing the clinical symptoms and identifying the underlying precipitating factor. The most common precipitating factor is pulmonary infection; others include trauma, stress, infections, drugs such as narcotics or barbiturates, surgery, and metabolic disturbances. Symptoms of thyroid emergencies are compared in Table 41–3.

Management

The most serious complication of hypothyroidism is a progression to myxedema coma and death, if untreated. A multiple-systems approach must be used in treating this emergency. Mechanical ventilation is used to control hypoventilation, hypercapnea, and respiratory arrest. Intravenous hypertonic normal saline and glucose will correct the dilutional hyponatremia and hypoglycemia. Fluid administration plus vasopressor therapy may be necessary to correct hypotension.

Pharmacologic therapy includes the administration of thyroid hormone and corticosteroids. There are several approaches to this aspect of medical management. Initial drug therapy will include 300 to 500 μg of L-T_4 intravenously to saturate all protein binding sites and establish a relatively normal T_4 level. Subsequent doses may include 100 μg daily. The ideal preparation is T_3 because severely ill hypothyroid patients will have a block in converting T_4 to T_3; however, a T_3 intravenous preparation is not commercially available in the United States.[2]

Additional interventions include managing hypothermia by gradual warming and treating abdominal distention or fecal impaction. When the patient is comatose, care includes preventing complications related to aspiration, immobility, skin breakdown, and infection. An important aspect of care is to detect early signs of complications. As the patient recovers, interventions will focus on patient self-care and education.

In addition to coma, complications include pericardial and pleural effusions, megacolon with paralytic ileus, and seizures (see Nursing Care Plan 41–2).

NURSING CARE PLAN 41–2:
The Patient With Myxedema Coma

NURSING DIAGNOSIS	OUTCOME CRITERIA/ PATIENT GOALS	NURSING INTERVENTIONS
Altered tissue perfusion, cerebral: related to hypothyroidism.	• Patient will return to usual wakeful state.	1. Implement seizure precautions. 2. Closely monitor patient's neurological status for changes in LOC. 3. Monitor patient's ability to protect airway, effectively cough and gag. 4. Administer thyroid replacement therapy (thyroxine), and glucocorticoids, as ordered.
Hypothermia: related to decreased metabolic state.	• Body temperature will return to patient's norm.	1. Assess temperature q1h. 2. Implement measures to raise body temperature; gradual warming is recommended.
High risk for injury: related to decreased level of consciousness and hypothyroid state.	• Patient will be injury and infection free.	1. Prevent infection. Monitor clinical signs and symptoms. A normothermic patient may indicate an infectious process. 2. Provide skin and other supportive care required for an immobile patient.
Cardiac output: related to decreased inotropic state.	• Hemodynamic stability will be maintained.	1. Administer fluid therapy that is dependent on patient's clinical status. 2. Monitor therapy to prevent fluid overload. 3. Assess PB, HR, T, and rhythm q15min until stable.

Adrenal Crisis

Pathophysiological Principles

Adrenal insufficiency is a major life-threatening dysfunction of the adrenal cortex. It also is known as hypoadrenalism or hypocorticism. Adrenal hormone insufficiency can occur with direct involvement of the adrenal gland (primary), or because of lack of stimulation by adrenocorticotropic hormone (ACTH) due to hypothalamic–pituitary disease (secondary).

Primary adrenal insufficiency is termed *Addison's disease*. The most common cause of primary hypoadrenalism is autoimmune adrenalitis, whereas the second leading cause is destruction of the gland secondary to *Mycobacterium tuberculosis* infection. Other causes include bilateral hemorrhage of the glands secondary to bacterial infection with sepsis and shock, metastatic malignancies, and acquired immunodeficiency syndrome.

CASE STUDY

Mr. Cerelo, age 55, was seen in the emergency room with initial symptoms of generalized weakness, fever, orthostatic hypotension, tachycardia, and gastrointestinal complaints. The patient has Addison's disease. A chest radiograph revealed multiple infiltrates. Laboratory values indicated decreased serum sodium and increased serum potassium. The initial diagnosis was impending adrenal crisis precipitated by a lung infection.

The most common cause of secondary adrenal insufficiency is iatrogenic. Other causes include metastatic carcinomas of the lung or breast, pituitary infarction, surgery or irradiation, and CNS disturbances such as basilar skull fractures or infections.

Acute adrenal insufficiency or adrenal crisis occurs when there is a change in the chronic condition. In addition to the chronic disease, an infection, trauma, surgical procedure, or some extra stress occurs, precipitating acute adrenal crisis in the patient.

Assessment

Anorexia, nausea, vomiting, diarrhea, and abdominal pain may be initial clues to adrenal crisis. These findings are nonspecific until linked with the history of a chronic condition requiring past or present corticosteroid use. Specifically, use of more than 20 mg of hydrocortisone or its equivalent, taken for longer than 7 to 10 days, has the potential for suppressing the hypothalamic–pituitary–adrenal axis. Hyperpigmentation on areas of the elbows, knees, hands, or buccal mucosa is seen in primary adrenal insufficiency. Its presence strengthens the clinical picture of adrenal crisis. The most common physical changes include weight loss and orthostatic hypotension. Clinical signs and symptoms are listed in Table 41–4.

Laboratory evaluation of patients with suspected adrenal insufficiency is essential. Laboratory values in acute

TABLE 41–4
Clinical Signs and Symptoms of Adrenal Crisis

Aldosterone deficiency
  Hyperkalemia
  Hyponatremia
  Hypovolemia
  Elevated BUN
Cortisol deficiency
  Hypoglycemia
  Decreased gastric motility
  Decreased vascular tone
  Hypercalcemia
Generalized signs and symptoms
  Anorexia
  Nausea and vomiting
  Abdominal cramping
  Diarrhea
  Tachycardia
  Orthostatic hypotension
  Headache, lethargy
  Fatigue, weakness
  Hyperkalemic ECG changes
  Hyperpigmentation

BUN, blood urea nitrogen; ECG, electrocardiograph.
Adapted from Halloran T: Nursing responsibilities in endocrine emergencies. Critical Care Nursing Quarterly 13:(3):74–81, 1990.

conditions with combined glucocorticoid and mineralocorticoid deficiency commonly will show evidence of hyponatremia, hyperkalemia, decreased serum bicarbonate levels, and elevated blood urea nitrogen. Dehydration also is present and can lead to a metabolic acidosis. Hypoglycemia generally is present. Other abnormal laboratory findings include anemia and a relative lymphocytosis with eosinophilia. Hormonal testing, such as serum cortisol levels and an ACTH stimulation test, are necessary to confirm the diagnosis.

Management

The immediate goal of therapy is to administer the needed hormones and restore fluid and electrolyte balance. Hydrocortisone, 100 mg intravenously, is administered immediately. Fluid resuscitation is begun immediately with normal saline and 5% dextrose solutions. The rate of fluid and electrolyte replacements is dictated by the degree of volume depletion, serum electrolyte levels, and clinical response to therapy. Associated medical or surgical problems may indicate the need for invasive blood pressure and hemodynamic monitoring. Preventing complications is another management goal.

Emotional support, simple explanations, and a quiet environment are effective in assisting the patient emotionally through the physiological crisis. Once the acute crisis is over, patient education is a goal of care. Patient education is necessary because the ultimate prognosis depends on the patient's ability to understand and follow through with self-care. This includes knowing the medication regime, stress factors and their effect on the disease, and signs of impending crisis; wearing a Medic-Alert tag, bracelet, or carrying a wallet card; and taking medication as prescribed (see Nursing Care Plan 41–3).

Complications

Loss of bilateral adrenal function is fatal if not treated. Death is preceded by dysrhythmias, hypovolemia leading to circulatory collapse, loss of oxygen transport to the tissues, and seizures progressing to coma.

Syndrome of Inappropriate Antidiuretic Hormone Secretion (SIADH)

Pathophysiological Principles

There are two disorders involving ADH, an excess or a deficiency of hormone; SIADH is the former, whereas diabetes insipidus is the latter. In SIADH, there is either

NURSING CARE PLAN 41-3:
The Patient in Adrenal Crisis

NURSING DIAGNOSIS	OUTCOME CRITERIA/ PATIENT GOALS	NURSING INTERVENTIONS
Fluid volume deficit: related to loss of sodium and water associated with adrenal insufficiency.	• Fluid volume and electrolytes will return to normal.	1. Administer intravenous fluids (usually D5%/NS) with electrolyte replacements, as ordered. Initial volume replacement may be rapid to restore intravascular volume.
		2. Administer scheduled doses of intravenous hydrocortisone, as ordered.
		3. Monitor serum electrolyte levels; assess for signs and symptoms of hyponatremia and hyperkalemia.
		4. Assess cardiovascular function: BP, HR, rhythm (ie, dysthrythmias, bradycardia).
		5. Monitor urinary specific gravity q4h.
		6. Assess neuromuscular status; weakness, twitching, hyperreflexia, paresthesia.
		7. Conserve energy stores initially by providing rest periods, and assist with ADLs.
Decreased cardiac output: related to hypovolemic vascular shock associated with adrenal insufficiency.	• Hemodynamic stability will be maintained.	1. Assess cardiac workload q15min: BP, orthostatic hypotension, central venous pressure, skin color and temperature, capillary refills, and presence of subjective symptoms.
		2. Monitor urinary output q1h.
		3. Administer vasoconstrictive agents, as ordered.

increased secretion or increased production of ADH. This increase in ADH is unrelated to osmolality, and therefore causes an increase in total body water. SIADH is considered whenever there is a condition of hypotonic hyponatremia.

CASE STUDY

A 65-year-old woman, Mrs. Perez, was admitted to the ICU with an initial diagnosis of acute mental status changes and severe hyponatremia. Past medical history included recent treatment for pneumonia and a history of congestive heart failure related to coronary artery disease. Drug therapy included an antibiotic and

a thiazide diuretic. No structural defect was found on the CT scan. An evaluation of the patient's fluid status revealed a hyponatremic state. The initial clinical findings were depressed level of consciousness and decreased deep tendon reflexes. ABGs were normal, heart and lung sounds normal; distal perfusion was adequate without generalized edema. On admission to the ICU, Mrs. Perez had a grand mal seizure. Laboratory values were:

Na: 115 mEq/L

K: 4.5 mEq/L

Cl: 90 mEq/L

Plasma osmolality: 260 mOsm

Urinary sodium levels were elevated.

NURSING CARE PLAN 41–4:
The Patient With SIADH

NURSING DIAGNOSIS	OUTCOME CRITERIA/ PATIENT GOALS	NURSING INTERVENTIONS
Fluid volume excess: related to increased production of ADH.	• Fluid volume and electrolytes will return to normal limits.	1. Restrict water intake. 2. Monitor intake and output and signs of volume overload (crackles) q1–2h. 3. Monitor serum electrolytes/ osomolality. Risk of neurologic sequelae is significant if serum Na < 125 mEq/L. 4. Assist with identification and treatment of underlying cause. 5. Administer fluids, depending on fluid volume status, as ordered. (Isotonic saline is the initial fluid of choice.) 6. Administer hypertonic chloride, as ordered. 7. Lasix (furosemide) may be ordered to facilitate free water clearance. 8. Monitor neurologic status q1–2h and prn. 9. Initiate safety measures for potential seizure activity.
Altered thought process: related to electrolyte imbalance secondary to intravascular hypervolemia.	• Patient's mental status will improve.	1. Monitor for orientation to person, place, and time. 2. Reinforce appropriate behavior. 3. Explain all procedures to patient and family. 4. Maintain safe environment. 5. Apply soft restraints if necessary. 6. Reorient patient to person, place, and time.

The secretion of ADH is considered "inappropriate" in that it continues despite the decreased osmolality of the plasma. Other reasons for increased ADH also are lacking. There is absence of hypokalemia and edema; cardiac, renal, and adrenal function is normal; and there is either normal or expanded plasma and extracellular fluid volumes.

SIADH occasionally is caused by a pituitary tumor but more commonly caused by a bronchogenic (oat cell) or pancreatic carcinoma. These tumors actually secrete ADH, but are independent of normal physiologic controls. Other possible causes of SIADH include head injuries, other endocrine disorders, pulmonary diseases such as pneumonia, lung abscesses, CNS infections and tumors, and drugs such as tricyclics, oral hypoglycemic agents, diuretics, and cytotoxic agents.

Assessment

The symptoms of SIADH basically are those of water retention and eventually water intoxication secondary to sustained ADH effect. The hyponatremia in SIADH has two components, an early dilutional component due to increased water, and a later, clinically undetectable component, caused by the increased urinary sodium excretion.

Symptoms produced by SIADH are predominantly neurologic and gastrointestinal. The most common symptoms are personality changes, headache, decreased mentation, lethargy, nausea, vomiting, diarrhea, anorexia, decreased tendon reflexes, and, finally, seizures and coma. The clinical focus and probable cause of hospital admission is hyponatremia. When the serum sodium falls to less that 120 to 125 mEq/L, nausea, vomiting, muscular irritability, and seizures often result. If the condition develops acutely (ie, within 24 hours), a mortality rate of 50% has been reported.[2]

The cardinal laboratory abnormality in SIADH is plasma hyponatremia and hypoosmolality, which occurs simultaneously with inappropriate hyperosmolality of the urine. By definition, any patient with a normal serum sodium does not have SIADH. Another laboratory feature is the inappropriately high urinary sodium excretion. Specific diagnosis may be made by radioimmunoassay of plasma ADH. Other laboratory findings include low blood urea nitrogen, creatinine, and uric acid levels, decreased hemoglobin and hematocrit, and hypocalcemia and hypokalemia (see Chapter 30, Table 30-3, which compares SIADH with diabetes insipidus).

Management

Management of SIADH may be divided into three categories: treatment of the underlying disease, alleviation of the excessive water retention, and all of the care needed when the patient has a depressed level of consciousness.

The first step in managing SIADH is to restrict fluid intake. In mild cases, fluid restriction is sufficient. A general guideline is that until the serum sodium concentration normalizes and symptoms abate, water intake should not exceed urinary output. In severely symptomatic patients, the administration of 3% hypertonic saline and furosemide is the treatment of choice. Newer approaches that include demeclocycline and lithium carbonate have been shown to be effective by interfering with the normal ADH effect.

Nursing interventions include monitoring serum electrolytes, especially sodium; rapid changes in sodium levels can result in worsening neurologic symptoms. Complications of SIADH include neurologic deterioration leading to seizures, coma, and death. Careful monitoring of intake and output is necessary. The patient's nutritional needs must be met without increasing fluid intake. Because patients may find it difficult to limit their fluid intake, emotional support is needed to foster cooperation during fluid restriction (see Nursing Care Plan 41–4).

REFERENCES

1. Evangelisti JT, Thorpe CJ: Thyroid storm: A nursing crisis. Heart Lung 12:184–193, 1983
2. Isley W: Thyroid disease. In Civetta JM, Taylor RW, Kirby RR (eds): Critical Care, 2nd ed, pp 1653–1664. Philadelphia, JB Lippincott, 1992

BIBLIOGRAPHY

Batcheller J: Disorders of antidiuretic hormone secretion. Clinical Issues in Critical Care Nursing 3(2):370–378, 1992

Chin R: Adrenal crises. Critical Care Clinics 7(1):23–42, 1991

Epstein CD: Adrenocortical insufficiency in the critically ill patient. Clinical Issues in Critical Care Nursing 3(3): 705–713, 1992

Gavin LA: Thyroid crises. Med Clin North Am 75:179–193, 1991

Lee L: Adrenocortical insufficiency: A medical emergency. Clinical Issues in Critical Care Nursing 3(2):319–330, 1992

McMorrow ME: The elderly and thyrotoxicosis. Clinical Issues in Critical Care Nursing 3(1):114–119, 1992

Reasner C: Adrenal disorders. Critical Care Nursing Quarterly 13(3):67–73, 1990

Sikes PJ: Endocrine responses to the stress of critical care illness. Clinical Issues in Critical Care Nursing 3(2):379–391, 1992

Spittle L: Diagnoses in opposition: Thyroid storm and myxedema coma. Clinical Issues in Critical Care Nursing 3(2): 300–308, 1992

STUDY QUESTIONS

1. Which of the following pharmacologic agents is *not* recommended for treating thyroid disease?

   a. aspirin
   b. propranolol
   c. glucocorticoids
   d. propylthiouracil

2. Myxedema coma is characterized by all but which one of the following symptoms?

   a. hypotension
   b. tachycardia
   c. hypothermia
   d. hypoventilation

3. Which of the following symptoms should the nurse recognize as a good indicator of thyroid crisis?

   a. tachycardia
   b. neurologic dysfunction
   c. fever
   d. all of the above

PART IV

Multisystem Organ Failure Conditions

BEHAVIORAL OBJECTIVES

Based on the content in this chapter, the reader should be able to:

1. Define septic shock.
2. Identify risk factors associated with the development of septic shock.
3. Describe the pathophysiologic processes implicated in septic shock.
4. Explain the anticipated medical management and rationale for the treatment of septic shock.
5. Identify four nursing diagnoses and interventions for the patient in septic shock.

CHAPTER 42

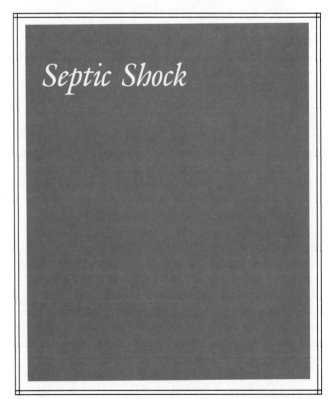

Septic Shock

Description

Septic shock is a complex clinical problem occurring frequently in critically ill patients. Sepsis develops in approximately 1 in every 100 hospitalized patients, and septic shock develops in 40% of these.[1] The mortality rate with septic shock is in the range of 50%.[2] This high mortality rate necessitates prompt recognition and early treatment. The critical care nurse, with a thorough understanding of sepsis and septic shock, can play a pivotal role in the detection and clinical management of these patients.

Sepsis often is defined as the presence of pathogenic microorganisms or their toxins in the bloodstream. The term *sepsis syndrome* is defined as the systemic response to sepsis, manifested as tachycardia, fever or hypothermia, tachypnea, and evidence of inadequate organ perfusion.[3] Signs of inadequate organ perfusion include decreased mental status, hypoxemia, decreased urine output, or increased serum lactate. When sepsis syndrome is accompanied by hypotension, it is called *septic shock*.[4]

Septic shock is a form of distributive or vasogenic shock characterized by a decrease in systemic vascular resistance and an abnormal distribution of the vascular volume.[5] Other types of distributive shock include neurogenic and anaphylactic shock.

Etiology

Septic shock results from a series of hemodynamic and metabolic events triggered in part by the invading microbe, and, more importantly, by the body's defense system.[6] Sepsis and septic shock may be caused by any invading microorganism; however, these conditions are associated most commonly with aerobic and anaerobic bacterial infections, in particular those caused by gram-negative bacteria (ie, *Escherichia coli*, *Klebsiella* sp, *Pseudomonas* sp, *Bacteroides* sp, and *Proteus* sp). Gram-negative bacteria contain a lipopolysaccharide in their cell walls called *endotoxin*. When released in the bloodstream, endotoxin produces a variety of adverse biochemical changes and activates immune and other biologic mediators that contribute to the development of septic shock.

Gram-positive organisms (staphylococci, streptococci, and pneumococci) also are implicated in the development of sepsis. Gram-positive organisms release *exotoxins*, which have the ability to trigger immune mediators in a way similar to that of endotoxins. In addition, viral, fungal, and rickettsial infections can lead to the development of sepsis and septic shock. In 20% to 30% of patients, multiple causative microorganisms have been identified, making it difficult to control the septic process effectively.[1]

The usual sites of infection are the genitourinary (GU), gastrointestinal (GI), and pulmonary systems; however, in 10% to 20% of cases, no site of infection is established

definitively.[7] Positive blood cultures may not always be obtained in the presence of sepsis or septic shock.

Risk Factors

Certain host factors and the use of certain therapies increase the risk for development of septic shock (Table 42–1). The high incidence of sepsis may reflect an increased number of chronically ill or immunocompromised patients who are alive longer owing to improved medical therapy, and yet are at greater risk for sepsis because of invasive medical procedures and devices.[2]

Prevention

Because the diagnosis of sepsis is so complex and the mortality rate from septic shock is so high, it is imperative that preventative infection control measures be in place.[8] The critically ill patient with impaired defense mechanisms must be protected from hospital-acquired (nosocomial) infections (see Chapter 47). Nosocomial infections have two sources: (1) the hospital environment itself, due to unwashed hands of personnel, use of contaminated equipment, or the sharing of equipment between patients; and (2) the patient's own normal flora of the skin and GI, GU, and pulmonary tracts. Nosocomial infection rates among critically ill patients range from 15% to 25%, and range in severity from mild cellulitis to life-threatening conditions involving sepsis and shock.[8] A critical aspect of nursing care involves adherence to aseptic techniques, thorough handwashing, and a continuing awareness of the multiple sites and causes of infection in the critically ill patient (Table 42–2).

Pathophysiological Principles

The series of events leading from sepsis to septic shock are triggered by complex hormonal and chemical substances

TABLE 42–1
Risk Factors for Septic Shock

Host Factors	Treatment-Related Factors
Extremes of age	Use of invasive catheters
Malnutrition	Surgical procedures
General debilitation	Traumatic or thermal wounds
Chronic illness	Invasive diagnostic procedures
Drug or alcohol abuse	Drugs (antibiotics, cytotoxic agents, steroids)
Neutropenia	
Spleenectomy	
Multiple organ failure	

TABLE 42–2
Equipment-Related Sources for Infection

Intravascular catheters
Endotracheal/tracheostomy tubes
Indwelling urinary catheters
Surgical wound drains
Intracranial bolts, catheters
Orthopedic hardware
Nasogastric tubes
Gastrointestinal tubes

produced directly and indirectly by the body's immune system in response to the adverse effects of bacterial toxins. Toxin-induced activation of cellular, humoral, and immunologic defense systems results in a generalized inflammatory response. This inflammatory response generates a variety of chemical mediators (Table 42–3) that may be responsible for the multisystem derangements associated with septic shock.[9]

Assessment

History

Patients with septic shock will have some form of infection, frequently noted to be gram-negative bacterial, and often located in the GI, GU, or pulmonary system. Patients may or may not have risk factors that predispose them to sepsis (see Table 42–1), but they often have multiple problems that can be attributed to the development of sepsis. Having a high index of suspicion and

TABLE 42–3
Mediators Associated With Septic Shock

Cellular mediators
  Granulocytes
  Lymphocytes
  Macrophages
  Monocytes
Humoral mediators
  Cytokines (lymphokines, tumor necrosis factor,
    interleukins)
  Endotoxin/exotoxin
  Oxygen free radicals
  Platelet activation factor
  Prostaglandins
  Proteases
  Thromboxanes
Other mediators
  Endorphins
  Histamine
  Myocardial depressant factor

identifying who is at risk for development of sepsis is of great importance when assessing critically ill patients.

Clinical Manifestations

Cardiovascular Manifestations

Circulatory Alterations

The major hemodynamic characteristic of septic shock is a low systemic vascular resistance (SVR), due in large part to vasodilation that occurs secondary to the effects of various mediators (ie, prostaglandins, kinins, histamine, and endorphins). These same mediators also may cause increased capillary permeability, resulting in loss of intravascular volume across leaky membranes, thereby reducing the effective circulatory volume.[9] In response to a decreased SVR and circulating volume, the cardiac output (CO) usually is high but inadequate to maintain tissue and organ perfusion. Inadequate blood flow is manifested in part by the development of lactic acidemia.

In conjunction with vasodilation and low SVR, there is a maldistribution of blood flow. Systemic release of vasoactive mediators produces selective vasodilation and vasoconstriction of certain vascular beds, leading to inadequate flow to some tissues while other tissues receive excessive flow. In addition, a massive inflammatory response occurs in the tissues, resulting in capillary occlusion due to leukocyte aggregation and fibrin deposits, with resultant irreversible endothelial and organ damage.[2]

Myocardial Alterations

Although maldistribution of blood flow is certainly one of the major abnormalities associated with septic shock, there is evidence that depressed myocardial performance, in the form of decreased ventricular ejection fraction and impaired contractility, also is involved.[10] Myocardial depressant factor, thought to originate from ischemic pancreatic tissue, is one proposed causative agent.[2] Other studies suggest that impaired coronary perfusion is at fault.[9] A final explanation for cardiac dysfunction is the abnormal metabolic state that results from shock, namely, the presence of lactic acidosis, which decreases the myocardial responsiveness to catecholamines.[9] Whatever the mechanism, the heart demonstrates impaired contractility and ventricular performance in the presence of septic shock. Figure 42–1 summarizes the cardiovascular pathophysiologic events known to occur in the presence of septic shock.

Two different patterns of cardiac dysfunction are evident in septic shock. One form is characterized by high CO and low SVR, and has been termed *hyperdynamic shock*. The second form is characterized by low CO and increased SVR, and is termed *hypodynamic shock*. It is appropriate to view these processes as a continuum rather than distinct forms, with the hyperdynamic response de-

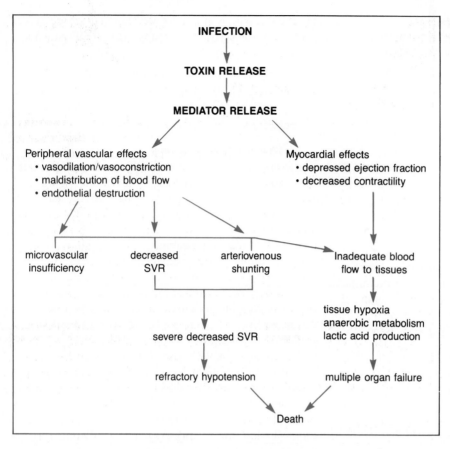

INFECTION

TOXIN RELEASE

MEDIATOR RELEASE

Peripheral vascular effects
• vasodilation/vasoconstriction
• maldistribution of blood flow
• endothelial destruction

Myocardial effects
• depressed ejection fraction
• decreased contractility

microvascular insufficiency

decreased SVR

arteriovenous shunting

Inadequate blood flow to tissues

severe decreased SVR

tissue hypoxia
anaerobic metabolism
lactic acid production

refractory hypotension

multiple organ failure

Death

FIGURE 42–1
Pathophysiological cardiovascular events that occur in the presence of septic shock. (Reproduced with permission from Parillo JE [moderator]: Septic shock in humans: Advances in understanding of pathogenesis, cardiovascular dysfunction, and therapy. Ann Intern Med 113:227–242, 1990)

noting early shock and the hypodynamic phase indicative of late or preterminal shock.[9, 11]

Pulmonary Manifestations

Endotoxin affects the lung both directly and indirectly. The initial pulmonary response is bronchoconstriction, resulting in pulmonary hypertension and increased respiratory work. Neutrophils are activated and infiltrate the pulmonary tissue and vasculature, causing an accumulation of extravascular lung water. Activated neutrophils are known to produce other substances that alter the integrity of pulmonary parenchymal cells, resulting in increased permeability.[9] As fluid collects in the interstitium, pulmonary compliance is reduced, gas exchange is impaired, and hypoxemia results.

Adult respiratory distress syndrome (ARDS) frequently is associated with septic shock, with the risk for development of ARDS from septic shock being 40% to 60%. The various vasoactive mediators discussed previously all have been implicated in the development of ARDS secondary to increased capillary permeability, resulting in pulmonary edema.

Hematologic Manifestations

Bacteria or their toxins cause complement activation. Because sepsis involves a global inflammatory response, complement activation may contribute to responses that eventually become detrimental rather than protective.[9]

Complement causes mast cells to release histamine. Histamine stimulates vasodilation and increases capillary permeability. These actions further contribute to the circulatory alterations in volume distribution and the development of interstitial edema.

Platelet abnormalities also occur in septic shock because endotoxin indirectly causes platelet aggregation and the subsequent release of more vasoactive substances (ie, serotonin and thromboxane A). Circulating platelet aggregates have been identified in the microvasculature, causing blood flow obstruction and compromised cellular metabolism. In addition, endotoxin or the bacterial infectious process itself activates the coagulation system and, over time, as clotting factors are depleted, a coagulopathy, potentially progressing to disseminated intravascular coagulation, results.[6]

Metabolic Manifestations

Widespread metabolic disturbances are seen with septic shock. The body manifests a progressive inability to use glucose, protein, and fat as energy sources. Hyperglycemia is a frequent finding in early shock due to increased gluconeogenesis and insulin resistance, which prevents the uptake of glucose into the cell. As shock progresses, hypoglycemia results as glycogen stores are depleted and peripheral supplies of proteins and fats are insufficient to meet the body's metabolic demands.

Protein breakdown occurs in septic shock and is evidenced by high urinary nitrogen excretion. Muscle protein is broken down to amino acids, some of which are used for oxidation, whereas others are transported to the liver for use in gluconeogenesis. In the later stages of shock, the liver is unable to use the amino acids owing to its own metabolic dysfunction, and the amino acids then accumulate in the bloodstream.

As the shock state progresses, adipose tissue is broken down (lipolysis) to furnish the liver with lipids for energy production. Lipid metabolism produces ketones, which then are used in the Krebs cycle. As liver function decreases, however, triglycerides begin forming that collect in the mitochondria and inhibit the Krebs cycle (oxidative metabolism), thereby causing increased lactate production.

The net effect of these metabolic derangements is that the cell becomes energy starved. This energy deficit is implicated in the emergence of multiple organ failure that frequently develops regardless of the ability to support the circulatory and organ systems.

Table 42–4 lists the symptoms and clinical findings of septic shock and contrasts the clinical pictures seen with hyperdynamic and hypodynamic shock. It is important to remember that these are phases of a continuum in the progression of shock, and not separate entities.

Some of the earliest signs of shock include changes in mental status—confusion or agitation, increased respiratory rate with respiratory alkalosis, and either fever or hypothermia. Although fever usually is evident in the body's response to infection, it is not always present. Some patients, for example the elderly, alcoholics, immunocompromised, or chronically debilitated, may not be able to generate a febrile response to infection.[6] Because early recognition and prompt treatment of sepsis is essential, it is crucial to identify these early clinical signs.

Diagnostic Studies

The diagnostic studies that may be helpful in the diagnosis of sepsis are summarized in Display Box 42–1. Despite the use of such diagnostic testing, the *early* diagnosis of sepsis and septic shock usually is made on the basis of clinical findings.

Management

Patients with septic shock require prompt and aggressive monitoring and management in a critical care unit. Because septic shock is a complex and generalized process, its management involves all organ systems and requires a multidisciplinary team approach.

Identification and Treatment of Infection

Identifying and eradicating the source of infection is of utmost concern. It is essential to initiate empiric antibiotic therapy before the source or type of organism has been ascertained. Patients will require multiple antibiotics to provide broad-spectrum coverage against gram-negative and gram-positive bacteria and anaerobes. Many clinicians empirically will use a broad-spectrum, third-generation cephalosporin, such as cefotaxime or ceftazidime, and

---

TABLE 42–4
Clinical Manifestations of Septic Shock

Hyperdynamic Shock	Hypodynamic Shock
Hypotension	Hypotension
Tachycardia	Tachycardia
Tachypnea	Tachypnea
Respiratory alkalosis	Metabolic acidosis
High cardiac output with low SVR	Low CO with high SVR
Warm, flushed skin	Cool, pale skin
Hyperthermia/hypothermia	Hypothermia
Altered mental status	Worsening mental status
Polyuria	Other organ and cellular dysfunction (eg, oliguria, DIC, ARDS)
Increased WBCs	Decreased WBCs
Hyperglycemia	Hypoglycemia

SVR, systemic vascular resistance; WBCs, white blood cells; CO, cardiac output; DIC, disseminated intravascular coagulation; ARDS, adult respiratory distress syndrome.

DISPLAY BOX 42–1
Physiologic Data Helpful in Diagnosing Sepsis

1. Cultures: from blood, sputum, urine, surgical or nonsurgical wounds, sinuses, and invasive lines. Positive results are not necessary for diagnosis
2. CBC: WBCs usually will be elevated, may decrease with progression of shock
3. SMA-7: hyperglycemia may be evident, followed by hypoglycemia in later stages
4. Arterial blood gases: respiratory alkalosis present in sepsis (pH >7.45, pCO_2 <35), with mild hypoxemia (PO_2 <80)
5. CT Scan: may be needed to identify sites of potential abscesses
6. Chest and abdominal radiographs: may reveal infectious processes

an aminoglycoside, such as gentamycin or amikacin.[12] Other definitive measures to isolate and alleviate the cause of sepsis include resection or drainage of purulent tissues or secretions.

Removing the cause of sepsis is not sufficient to treat the generalized systemic reactions seen with septic shock. The patient needs supportive measures to establish and maintain adequate tissue perfusion in addition to other therapies aimed at blocking or interfering with the action of the various mediators implicated in the shock process. Aspects of supportive care include (1) restoring intravascular volume, (2) maintaining an adequate cardiac output, (3) ensuring adequate ventilation and oxygenation, and (4) providing an appropriate metabolic environment.[1]

Restoration of Intravascular Volume

Adequate volume replacement is important for reversing hypotension, and patients may require several liters or more of fluid. Fluid replacement should be guided by hemodynamic parameters; therefore, patients will require pulmonary artery and arterial catheterization for close monitoring. There is some controversy as to whether crystalloid or colloid fluids should be used for volume replacement[11]; the patient's underlying condition and response will guide this decision. Administering the fluid and closely monitoring the patient's response to fluid therapy (see Nursing Care Plan 42–1) is an important nursing responsibility.

Maintenance of Adequate Cardiac Output

In the hyperdynamic phase of septic shock, cardiac output is either normal or elevated, yet because of decreased SVR and peripheral vasodilation, it is not adequate to maintain tissue oxygenation and perfusion. In the later hypodynamic phase, the cardiac output begins to drop owing to cardiac dysfunction. Therefore, in both phases, enhancing cardiac output is a therapeutic goal. If adequate volume replacement does not improve tissue perfusion, vasoactive drugs will be administered to support circulation. Dopamine, which increases SVR and improves renal and mesenteric blood flow, is one preferred agent, with dobutamine occasionally added for its inotropic effects on the heart. Other vasoactive drugs frequently used include levarterenol (Levophed), epinephrine, phenephrine, and the vasodilator, nitroprusside (Nipride). Some patients with a low cardiac output and high SVR may benefit from the use of vasodilators to redistribute blood flow and improve perfusion.[5]

Many times, no single drug can achieve the desired hemodynamic effects, so various combinations of drugs that are individualized to the patient's response must be tried. The nurse's role in this therapy is to administer the drugs, usually titrating the dosage to a desired response or effect, and closely monitoring the patient for response and potentially harmful side effects to the drugs (see Nursing Care Plan 42–1).

Maintenance of Adequate Ventilation and Oxygenation

Maintaining a patent airway, augmenting ventilation, and ensuring adequate oxygenation in the patient with septic shock usually necessitates endotracheal intubation and mechanical ventilation. Positive end-expiratory pressure (PEEP) frequently is needed to aid oxygenation (for nursing management issues, see Chapter 19).

Maintenance of Appropriate Metabolic Environment

The many and varied metabolic derangements associated with septic shock necessitate frequent monitoring of hematologic, renal, and liver function. Concurrently, nutritional stores are depleted in shock and the patient will need supplemental nutrition (usually total parenteral nutrition) to prevent malnutrition and to optimize cellular function (see Chapter 35 for a discussion of total parenteral nutrition).

Investigational Therapies

Although antibiotics and supportive therapy are the mainstays of treatment for septic shock, certain investigational drugs and therapies may be used in treatment (Table 42–5). These drugs are aimed directly at the bacterial

TABLE 42–5
Management Highlights for Septic Shock

Definitive therapies
    Identify and eliminate the source of infection
    Multiple broad-spectrum antibiotics
Supportive therapies
    Restore intravascular volume
    Maintain adequate cardiac output
    Ensure adequate ventilation and oxygenation
    Provide appropriate metabolic environment
Investigational therapies
    Antihistamines
    Monoclonal antibodies to:
        Endotoxin and exotoxin
        Tumor necrosis factor
        Complement factors
    Naloxone
    Neutrophil inhibitors
    Prostaglandin inhibitors (nonsteroidal anti-inflammatory
        drugs)
    Steroids

Clinical Research

Franzoni G, Leech J, Jensen G, Brotman S: Tumor necrosis factor α: What role in sepsis and organ failure? Journal of Critical Illness 6:796–805, 1991

This article investigated the role of tumor necrosis factor α (TNFα) as a mediator of sepsis, and the roles it plays in the complications associated with septic shock. Several studies (human) cited in this article appear to confirm that levels of TNFα correlate with degree of illness. In addition, other studies suggest modalities that may reduce TNFα, including dietary fish-oil supplements, dexamethasone, ibuprofen, and antibodies to TNFα and endotoxins.

Because the mortality with sepsis and multiorgan failure is so high, critical care nurses must stay informed about new therapies and early indicators of septic shock.

toxins and the mediators implicated in the immunologic response seen with sepsis. The complexity of this response leads many investigators to believe that it is unlikely that any one agent will prove to be effective, and that multiple therapies, tailored to individual circumstances, most likely will be needed.[4]

Complications

Display Box 42–2 summarizes the potential complications from septic shock. Refer to the earlier discussion under Pathophysiological Principles for an understanding of how these complications may evolve.

Multiple Organ Failure

Multiple organ failure, defined as the failure of two or more organs, has a 75% to 90% mortality rate when associated with surgical sepsis.[13] Multiple organ failure, as a cause for late mortality after major multiple trauma, is discussed in Chapter 44. Multiple organ failure occurring as a result of sepsis has a similar clinical course but a different initiating event. Sepsis-induced multiple organ failure is heralded by hypermetabolism, which, in the face of inadequate organ perfusion, results in progressive cellular damage and eventual organ failure. It usually is manifested 7 to 14 days after the infection and is associated with ARDS, jaundice, hyperbilirubinemia, and renal failure.[13] Therapy is targeted at controlling the source (ie,

treat the sepsis), maintaining oxygenation, and providing general supportive measures such as adequate nutrition and renal dialysis.

CASE STUDY

Mrs. Cox, a 50-year-old woman, presented to the clinic with complaints of abdominal pain with nausea and vomiting for 3 days, and one episode of lower GI bleeding. Past medical history includes chronic renal failure, on dialysis three times/ week, kidney transplant 1.5 years ago, with rejection and transplant nephrectomy 2 months ago. She reported feeling weak and tired.

On physical exam, Mrs. Cox was an obese woman with abdominal tenderness in the epigastric region, with no rebound or guarding. She had a peritoneal dialysis catheter in place with redness and swelling noted at the insertion site. Her vital signs were: HR 116, RR 30, BP 140/90, T 38.5°C.

Lab Values:

Hgb 5 g/dl

Hct 15%

WBC 19.4

Glucose 140 mg/dl

Sodium 135 mEq/L

Potassium 4.1 mEq/L

Chloride 102 mEq/L

CO_2 19 mEq/L

BUN 24 mg/dl

Creatinine 6.0 mg/dl

Amylase 140 U/L

SGOT and SGPT within normal limits

Mrs. Cox was admitted to the hospital for abdominal pain work-up and anemia. She was transfused with 2 units of packed red blood cells, her hematocrit increased to 26%, her skin color was improved, and she reported less weakness. Two days after admission, she had an increase in WBCs to 26.1, her temperature was 39.8°C, and colonoscopy findings suggested ischemic bowel versus intra-abdominal infection (perhaps secondary to an infected peritoneal dialysis catheter). Surgery was scheduled for later that day. Blood cultures were drawn and Mrs. Cox received

---

DISPLAY BOX 42–2
Complications of Septic Shock

Adult respiratory distress syndrome
Disseminated intravascular coagulation
Multiple organ failure

preoperative antibiotics. She had an arterial line and pulmonary artery catheter inserted. Initial parameters were: cardiac output (CO) 8.0 L/minute, cardiac index (CI) 5.2 L/minute/m², pulmonary capillary wedge pressure (PCWP) 6 mm Hg, SVR 800 dynes/second/cm⁻⁵, BP 100/60, mean arterial pressure (MAP) 50 mm Hg, HR 132. Arterial blood gases (ABGs) revealed respiratory alkalosis with pH 7.50, pCO_2 20 mm Hg, pO_2 68 mm Hg, HCO_3 17 mEq/L. Mrs. Cox received 4 L of IV fluid and was started on dopamine to maintain her MAP > 60 mm Hg.

O.R. findings: Mrs. Cox had pancreatitis with a collection of inflamed tissue and pus drained, and 6 feet of necrotic small bowel resected. Her abdominal incision was only partially closed; she was hemodynamically unstable, remained intubated and on the ventilator, and was transported to the Surgical Intensive Care Unit (SICU).

On postop day 1, Mrs. Cox remained hemodynamically unstable: T 39.3°C, HR 140–150, BP 110/90 on 12 μg/kg/minute of dopamine and 6 μg/kg/minute of dobutamine. Pulmonary artery readings were hyperdynamic: CO 9.2 L/minute, CI 5.8 L/minute/m², PCW 18 mm Hg, SVR 480 dynes/second/cm⁻⁵. She required large amounts of fluid resuscitation (6–8 L in the first 24 hours postop), and was given 0.9% normal saline and blood products for a persistently low hematocrit (25%). Her ABGs revealed a metabolic acidosis, and a serum lactate level of 5.8 mmol/L. WBCs dropped to 8.6 and her preop blood cultures were positive for *Proteus*. Mrs. Cox was responsive to pain, unable to follow commands, and was being medicated with intermittent doses of midazolam and morphine.

On postop day 2, the patient's hemodynamic status was not improved. Epinephrine at 12 μg/kg/minute was added to help maintain her MAP greater than 60 mm Hg. Her lactate level was 9.0 mmol/L, WBCs dropped to 2.3, and her coagulation parameters were showing evidence of a coagulopathy: PT > 15 seconds, PTT 40 seconds, platelets 60,000. Liver function tests were elevated and Mrs. Cox was showing signs of scleral jaun-

dice. She remained on the ventilator with PEEP at 12 cm H_2O to improve oxygenation. Her mental status fluctuated between being obtunded yet responsive to pain, to awake and agitated. The SICU care was focused on supportive and monitoring issues. Triple antibiotics were being administered (metronidazole, vancomycin, gentamycin) and she had no change in blood culture results. Her wound remained open without any signs of infection and she was started on total parenteral nutrition.

The large fluid requirements combined with her chronic renal failure and septic shock produced significant peripheral edema, especially in her face and extremities. Because of the potential for skin breakdown, the nurses placed her on a specialty bed designed to prevent skin breakdown and improve pulmonary status.

By postop day 5, Mrs. Cox began showing signs of improvement. Her BP was stabilizing and the vasoactive drugs were being weaned; her hemodynamic parameters were normalizing (CO 7.7 L/minute, CI 5.0 L/minute/m², PCW 11–16 mm Hg, SVR 1,100 dynes/second/cm⁻⁵); her lactate levels were decreasing; coagulation parameters were WNL; WBCs remained low but were improving, and her blood cultures were negative. Mrs. Cox's mental status was clearing and although she had brief episodes of confusion, she was able to communicate and interact with her family. Her skin remained intact, and her wound was showing signs of granulation.

By postop day 8, Mrs. Cox was extubated, off all vasoactive drugs, and had only a central line in place for central venous pressure monitoring. Over the next 2 weeks she continued to improve, resumed dialysis, and eventually was transferred to the Med/Surg unit, with eventual discharge home.

Nursing Care Plan

Nursing Care Plan 42–1 summarizes the significant nursing care points for the patient with septic shock.

NURSING CARE PLAN 42–1:
The Patient in Septic Shock

NURSING DIAGNOSIS	OUTCOME CRITERIA/ PATIENT GOALS	NURSING INTERVENTIONS
Decreased cardiac output: related to vasodilation, impaired cardiac function, and fluid volume deficit.	• Maintain cardiac output to ensure adequate tissue perfusion.	1. Assess and monitor cardiovascular status q1–4h, or as indicated: skin color, pulse, BP, hemodynamic parameters, peripheral pulses, cardiac rhythm. 2. Administer IV fluids, as ordered. 3. Administer dopamine, dobutamine, or epinephrine as ordered to maintain adequate BP (>90 mm Hg systolic) and U/O >30 ml/h.

(continued)

NURSING CARE PLAN 42–1: (*Continued*)
The Patient in Septic Shock

NURSING DIAGNOSIS	OUTCOME CRITERIA/ PATIENT GOALS	NURSING INTERVENTIONS
		4. Administer Nipride, as ordered.
		5. Monitor Hgb and Hct as ordered.
		6. Monitor acidosis with ABG's, qd and prn.
Impaired gas exchange: related to pulmonary hypertension, edema, and ARDS.	• Patient will maintain adequate oxygenation and ventilation.	1. Monitor RR, work of breathing q1–2h.
		2. Assess breath sounds, skin color, mental status q1–2h.
		3. Prevent atelectasis with T, C, DB as indicated.
		4. Consider low-air-loss kinetic bed to improve pulmonary status.
		5. Monitor ABGs as indicated.
		6. Monitor oxygenation status with pulse oximetry.
		7. Correct acid–base imbalance with ventilator changes and/or $NaHCO_3$ as ordered.
		8. If patient is intubated, see Nursing Care Plan 19–1: The Mechanically Ventilated Patient.
		9. See Nursing Care Plan 21–1: The Patient With Adult Respiratory Distress Syndrome.
High risk for infection: related to shock, debilitated state.	• Prevent nosocomial infection and manage identified microorganisms.	1. Obtain blood cultures as ordered.
		2. Obtain urine, sputum, and wound or drainage cultures as indicated.
		3. Accompany patient for diagnostic radiology tests.
		4. Monitor T, VS, and WBCs.
		5. Administer antibiotics, as ordered.
		6. Monitor antibiotic drug levels, as ordered. Report serum levels.
		7. Administer other drugs as ordered, (ie, antihistamines, NSAIDs, monoclonal antibodies, steroids).
		8. Use strict aseptic technique when dealing with invasive lines, catheters, tubes, etc.
Altered tissue perfusion: related to inadequate cardiac output.	• Patient will maintain systemic perfusion.	1. Monitor neurologic status.
		2. Monitor hemodynamic function (PAP, PCWP, CI) q1–4h.

(continued)

NURSING CARE PLAN 42–1: (Continued)
The Patient in Septic Shock

NURSING DIAGNOSIS	OUTCOME CRITERIA/ PATIENT GOALS	NURSING INTERVENTIONS
		3. Assess oxygenation with pulse oximeter.
		4. Report urine output <30 ml/h.
		5. Assess abdomen q4h for bowel sounds, pain.
		6. Monitor laboratory values daily: liver function, bilirubin, BUN, creatinine.
		7. Assess skin color, temperature and presence/absence of diaphoresis q4h and prn.
		8. Monitor cardiac rhythm.
Altered nutrition, less than body requirements: related to response to sepsis, critical illness.	• Patient's nutritional needs will be met.	1. Record daily weight.
		2. Administer TPN or enteral feedings as ordered. See Nursing Care Plan 35–1: The Patient Undergoing Parenteral Hyperalimentation.
		3. Monitor laboratory values: albumin, urine urea nitrogen, blood sugar, electrolytes.
		4. Monitor serum glucose with fingerstick or lab draw q6h.
		5. Administer supplemental insulin as ordered.
High risk for altered tissue perfusion: related to development of DIC.	• Patient will have no evidence of bleeding.	1. Assess for signs of bleeding (ie, urine, sputum, gums, wounds, venipunctures, or invasive line sites).
		2. Monitor PT, PTT, and platelets qd.
		3. Assess body surface for ecchymosis q shift.
		4. If evidence of DIC, see Nursing Care Plan 43–1: The Patient With Disseminated Intravascular Coagulation.
High risk for impaired skin integrity: related to decreased tissue perfusion and edema.	• Patient will maintain intact skin, without bruises, open wounds, or decubitus ulcers.	1. Turn q2h.
		2. Prevent pressure with use of specialty bed.
		3. Massage areas of redness caused by pressure.
		4. Avoid shearing effect of linen on skin by using lift sheets.
		5. Maticulously clean all wound edges, line insertion sites.

REFERENCES

1. Rice V: Shock, a clinical syndrome: An update. Part One: An overview of shock. Part Three: Therapeutic management Critical Care Nurse 11:20–27, 34–39, 1991
2. Dal Nogare AR: Southwestern Internal Medicine Conference: Septic shock. Am J Med Sci 302:50–65, 1991
3. Balk RA, Bone RC: The septic syndrome: Definition and clinical implications. Critical Care Clinics 5:1–8, 1989
4. Bone RC: Gram negative sepsis. Chest 100:802–808, 1991
5. Parrillo JE (moderator): Septic shock in humans: Advances in the understanding of pathogenesis, cardiovascular dysfunction, and therapy. Ann Intern Med 113:227–242, 1990
6. Brown KA, Sheagren JN: Recognition and emergent treatment of septic shock/multiple organ systems failure. Internal Medicine 11:3–11, 1990
7. Houston MC: Pathophysiology of shock. Critical Care Nursing Clinics of North America 2:143–150, 1990
8. Hoyt NJ: Preventing septic shock: Infection control in the intensive care unit. Critical Care Nursing Clinics of North America 2:287–298, 1990
9. Littleton MT: Pathophysiology and assessment of sepsis and septic shock. Critical Care Nursing Quarterly 11:30–38, 1988
10. Parker MM: Cardiac dysfunction in human septic shock. In Parrillo JE (moderator): Septic shock in humans: Advances in the understanding of pathogenesis, cardiovascular dysfunction, and therapy, pp 229–230. Ann Intern Med 113: 227–242, 1990.
11. Parrillo JE: Septic shock in humans: Clinical evaluation, pathogenesis, and therapeutic approach. In Shoemaker WC (ed): Textbook of Critical Care, pp 1006–1024. Philadelphia, WB Saunders, 1989
12. Roach AC: Antibiotic therapy in septic shock. Critical Care Nursing Clinics of North America 2:179–186, 1990
13. Lekander BJ, Cerra FB: The syndrome of multiple organ failure. Critical Care Nursing Clinics of North America 2:331–342, 1990

BIBLIOGRAPHY

Bone RC: A critical evaluation of new agents for the treatment of sepsis. JAMA 266:1686–1691, 1991
Guyton AC: Textbook of medical physiology, 8th ed. Philadelphia, WB Saunders, 1991
Moore EE, Mattox KL, Feliciano DV (eds): Trauma, 2nd ed. Norwalk, CT, Appleton & Lange, 1991
Shoemaker WC (ed): Textbook of Critical Care. Philadelphia, WB Saunders, 1989

STUDY QUESTIONS

1. Patients at greater risk for development of sepsis and septic shock include those with

   a. diabetes
   b. cancer
   c. multiple trauma
   d. all of the above

2. The patient in the early stages of septic shock may have the following hemodynamic parameters

   a. MAP 80 mm Hg, CO 4.2 L/minute, CI 1.6 L/minute/m², PCW 10 mm Hg, SVR 1,600 dynes/second/cm^{-5}
   b. MAP 60 mm Hg, CO 2.5 L/minute, CI 1.0 L/minute/m², PCW 18 mm Hg, SVR 400 dynes/second/cm^{-5}
   c. MAP 50 mm Hg, CO 9.4 L/minute, CI 4.8 L/minute/m², PCW 10 mm Hg, SVR 500 dynes/second/cm^{-5}
   d. MAP 50 mm Hg, CO 9.0 L/minute, CI 4.0 L/minute/m², PCW 11 mm Hg, SVR 1,900 dynes/second/cm^{-5}

3. During the initial treatment for septic shock, the nurse would expect to

   a. limit IV fluids to keep open rate, give antibiotics pending culture results, administer vasopressors to increase the blood pressure
   b. administer many liters of IV fluid, give antibiotics before culture results, titrate vasopressors according to BP response
   c. closely monitor the patient, pending treatment until definitive culture results are obtained
   d. assist with intubation and ventilation, monitor vital signs, and prepare the patient for surgery

4. Which signs and symptoms best describe the patient in early septic shock?

   a. confused, hypothermic, hypotensive, respiratory alkalosis
   b. obtunded, hyperthermic, hypotensive, metabolic alkalosis
   c. agitated, normothermic, hypotensive, respiratory acidosis
   d. confused, hyperthermic, hypotensive, metabolic acidosis

5. The initial priority for care of the patient in septic shock is

   a. identifying and treating the infection
   b. maintaining adequate nutrition
   c. restoring intravascular volume
   d. preventing the development of disseminated intravascular coagulation

6. As septic shock progresses, a variety of treatment modalities may be tried, including

   a. steroids, multiple antibiotics, vasopressors/vasodilators, endotoxin
   b. monoclonal antibodies, antibiotics, vasopressors, NSAIDs
   c. monoclonal antibodies, steroids, exotoxin, vasopressors
   d. antihistamines, steroids, antibiotics, tumor necrosis factor

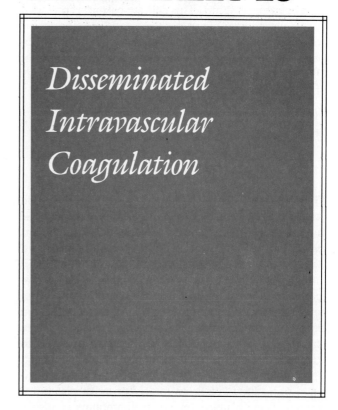

CHAPTER 43

Disseminated Intravascular Coagulation

BEHAVIORAL OBJECTIVES

Based on the content in this chapter, the reader should be able to:

1. Describe the pathophysiological process of disseminated intravascular coagulation (DIC).
2. List the abnormal laboratory findings associated with DIC.
3. Explain the anticipated medical management and rationale for the treatment of DIC.
4. Describe four nursing diagnoses and interventions for DIC.

Hudak: Critical Care Nursing:
A Holistic Approach, 6th ed. © 1994
J. B. Lippincott Company.

Description

Disseminated intravascular coagulation (DIC) syndrome has the distinction of being the oldest universally accepted hypercoagulable clinical state known. The veins, venules, capillaries, arterioles, and arteries constitute an intricate network of conduits for the transportation of blood to and from the body tissue. The patency of the conduits and the containment of blood within the vasculature depend on the maintenance of the integrity of the transporting conduits. States of physiological disequilibrium that increase permeability or weakening of the vessel walls may lead to leaking of blood outside the vasculature, resulting in hemorrhage. If the response of the hemostatic system to this threat to vascular integrity is too great, thrombus formation that occludes the vasculature may result, inhibiting the transportation of blood.

It is clear that a delicate balance must be maintained in the vasculature to ensure the patency of the vasculature and liquid state of the blood, so that neither thrombosis nor hemorrhage occurs. This delicate balance is provided by the interrelationship of the hemostatic and fibrinolytic systems working in concert. To understand the pathogenesis and the diagnostic and therapeutic modalities of DIC, the nurse must first be familiar with the physiology of these two systems.

Physiological Principles

Hemostatic System

The components of the hemostatic system are the blood vessels, platelets, and blood clotting factors of the intrinsic and extrinsic systems. These interdependent components are responsible for maintaining hemostatic homeostasis.

In the course of normal wear and tear, the endothelial lining of blood vessels is subject to numerous insults that require local repair to prevent leakage of the blood. Damage to the endothelium or sloughing of the endothelium exposes the underlying collagen. This exposed collagen attracts and activates platelets to adhere to the exposed collagen; that begins the formation of platelet plugging.

With the attraction of platelets to the exposed collagen of a blood vessel, an initial barrier of platelets is formed. These platelets release small amounts of adenosine diphosphate, which causes additional platelets to be attracted and to stick to each other. Last, there is a release of platelet factor 3 from the platelet membrane, which interacts with various blood coagulation proteins and accelerates clotting. Platelets play two major roles in the clotting process. First, the platelet plug temporarily plugs the leak in the blood vessel. This plug provides the architectural foundation for the building of the fibrin clot. The second role is to initiate clotting via the intrinsic pathway through the release of platelet factor 3.

The last component of the hemostatic system consists of the blood coagulation proteins, commonly referred to as the coagulation factors of the intrinsic and extrinsic pathways to coagulation.

Intrinsic Pathway

In the normal state, the blood coagulation factors circulate in the blood in an inactive state. After an initiating stimulus, changes in the coagulation factors take place immediately. The changes that occur bear the relationship of enzyme (organic catalyst) to substrate (specific substance on which an enzyme acts). The initiation of change causes molecular alteration in any coagulation factor, converting it to an active form. The inactive coagulation factor, known as a proenzyme, is converted to an active state and becomes an active enzyme. The product of this enzymatic reaction activates the next coagulation factor. Thus, one coagulation factor will activate the next coagulation factor in a chain-like reaction, leading to final clot formation. Coagulation factors are designated by Roman numerals. They are numbered according to the order in which they were first identified by researchers. When the factors are in active form, they are designated by a lower-case "a" (eg, factor XIIa). Table 43–1 lists the factors by Roman numeral and common name.

As mentioned, disruption of the endothelial membrane lining blood vessels attracts platelets, which in turn release platelet factor 3. This platelet factor initiates the activation of the intrinsic pathway by activating factor XII (Hageman factor), and it is a necessary component for complex reactions at factor V and factor VIII levels. The exposed collagen, phospholipids from injured erythrocytes and granulocytes, antigen–antibody complexes, and endotoxins are thought to be other activators of factor XII.

These activators convert inactive factor XII to the active enzymatic form, XIIa. The enzyme XIIa acts on the

TABLE 43–1
Coagulation Factors

I. Fibrinogen
II. Prothrombin–thrombin in active form
III. Thromboplastin
IV. Calcium
V. Proaccelerin
VI. Unassigned
VII. Proconvertin
VIII. Antihemophiliac factor A
IX. Antihemophiliac factor B
X. Stuart–Prower factor
XI. Antihemophiliac factor C
XII. Hagman factor
XIII. Fibrin-stabilizing factor

next clotting proenzyme, inactive factor XI, converting it to the active enzyme XIa. Active XIa is responsible for the activation of factor IX, and requires calcium ions. The activation of the next factor, factor X, requires factor VII and platelet factor 3. The conversion of prothrombin (factor II) to thrombin (factor IIa) requires factor V, platelet factor 3, and calcium ions. Thrombin acts on fibrinogen, converting it to fibrin. This initial soluble fibrin clot is stabilized by factor XIII in the presence of calcium.

A self-perpetuating effect in the intrinsic pathway occurs as the result of the ongoing cycle of activation of factor X through the effect of thrombin on factor VIII. Thrombin enhances the activity of factor VIII so that it interacts more rapidly with factor IXa and thus catalyzes the activation of factor X. Also, thrombin interacts with platelets, resulting in the release of platelet factor 3, which activates factor XII.

Extrinsic Pathway

The triggering event initiating the extrinsic pathway is injury to tissues and blood vessels, resulting in the release of factor III, tissue thromboplastin, into the circulation. As in the intrinsic pathway, a chain of events occurs that leads to clot formation. Tissue thromboplastin catalyzed by factor VII activates factor X. In the presence of calcium ions, factor V, and platelet factor 3, active factor X catalyzes the conversion of prothrombin to thrombin and fibrinogen to fibrin clot.

The result of the interaction of the blood vessels, platelets, and blood coagulation factors is the formation of factor Xa, which converts prothrombin to thrombin and results in fibrin formation. Thus, it can be seen that at factor Xa, the intrinsic and extrinsic pathways merge into a final common pathway to clot formation. Figure 43–1 depicts diagrammatically the sequence of clot formation. Notice that the activation of factor VIII by thrombin creates the activation of factor X, resulting in the self-perpetuating effect. As noted in the figure, calcium plays an important role in several steps along the clotting cascade. Many coagulation factors carry two negative charges. Calcium, with its two positive changes, creates a strong affinity for the factors to bind at the site of clotting.

Unchecked activation of the blood clotting factors would cause clots to form on top of the platelet plug, releasing thrombin in the process of clotting, further attracting platelets to the clot site and causing additional clots to form at the local site of vessel leak. The result of this activation would be total vessel occlusion (Fig. 43–2) if there were no mechanisms operating to maintain the blood in a fluid state and prevent uncontrolled clotting.

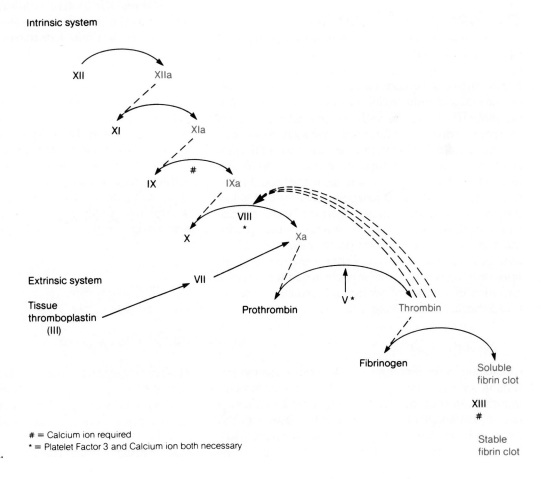

FIGURE 43–1
Sequence of coagulation.

\# = Calcium ion required
* = Platelet Factor 3 and Calcium ion both necessary

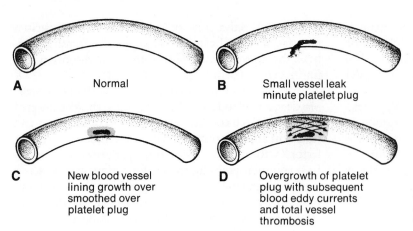

A Normal

B Small vessel leak minute platelet plug

C New blood vessel lining growth over smoothed over platelet plug

D Overgrowth of platelet plug with subsequent blood eddy currents and total vessel thrombosis

FIGURE 43–2
Sequence of thrombus formation in blood vessels.

Coagulation Inhibitors

There is a well-controlled balance between clotting and lysis in humans. Through the action of physiological coagulation inhibitors, the blood is maintained in its fluid state and vessels remain patent. These inhibitors work by limiting reactions that promote clotting and by breaking down any clots that do form, preventing total occlusion of the vessels. Coagulation inhibitors include the reticuloendothelial system, antithrombin III, adequate blood flow, mast cells, and the fibrinolytic system.

Reticuloendothelial System

The reticuloendothelial system inhibits coagulation by clearing activated factors from the blood, and the maintenance of an adequate blood flow acts to dilute activated clotting factors and quickly deliver them to the liver, where they are cleared from circulation. The liberation of antithrombin III in response to thrombin inactivates the circulating thrombin, as well as neutralizing activated factors XII, XI, IX, and X. This retards the conversion of fibrinogen to fibrin, thus stopping sequential activation of clotting factors. Mast cells located in most body tissues produce heparin, with an anticoagulant activity that is low compared to that of commercial heparin. Finally, the system antagonist, the fibrinolytic system, interferes with thrombin at its site of action on fibrinogen. In a way analogous to that of the coagulation mechanisms, the fibrinolytic system also involves a chain reaction whereby activation of a series of proenzymes produces lytic enzymes capable of dissolving clots.

Fibrinolytic System

Circulating in the blood is the proenzyme plasminogen, waiting for activation. It is believed that the endothelial cells that constitute the endothelial lining of blood vessels release plasminogen activator, converting plasminogen to plasmin. In addition, activated factor XII, thrombin, kallikrein, and substances in the tissues are thought to be involved in the conversion of plasminogen to plasmin. Plasmin is the dissolving or lytic enzyme that acts to lyse fibrin and attacks factors V, VIII, IX, and fibrinogen. Plasminogen activator levels are found to be transiently elevated in response to exercise, stress, anoxia, and pyrogens.

The lysis of fibrinogen and fibrin results in the liberation of degradation products. These products, known as fibrin degradation products (FDPs), inhibit platelet aggregation, exhibit an antithrombin effect, and interfere with formation of the fibrin clot.

Fibrinolytic System Inhibitors

Similar to the coagulation system inhibitors, there are inhibitors of the fibrinolytic system to prevent inappropriate lysis of needed clot formation. The reticuloendothelial system clears the FDPs from the circulation. Antiplasmin, a protein circulating in the blood, binds with plasmin and renders it inactive. The level of circulating antiplasmin far outweighs plasmin concentration, and plasmin is neutralized rapidly. Figure 43–3 depicts fibrinolytic activation.

It is evident that the systems of hemostasis and fibrinolysis in conjunction with their system inhibitors function within a narrow margin to ensure the liquidity of the blood and patency of the vasculature. An upset in these systems may result in clinical evidence of thrombosis, hemorrhage, or the catastrophic event of DIC.

Disseminated Intravascular Coagulation

Pathophysiological Principles

This syndrome of transient coagulation causes transformation of fibrinogen to fibrin clot and often is associated with acute hemorrhage. Paradoxically, DIC is a bleeding disorder resulting from an increased tendency to clot. The syndrome is triggered by a host of diverse states of physiological disequilibrium resulting in systemic activation of

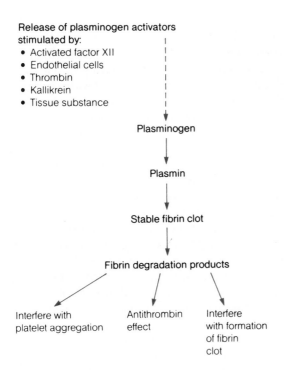

Release of plasminogen activators
stimulated by:
• Activated factor XII
• Endothelial cells
• Thrombin
• Kallikrein
• Tissue substance

Plasminogen

↓

Plasmin

↓

Stable fibrin clot

↓

Fibrin degradation products

Interfere with platelet aggregation · Antithrombin effect · Interfere with formation of fibrin clot

FIGURE 43–3
Sequential fibrinolytic activation.

coagulation and fibrinolysis. States of physiological disequilibrium that act as precipitating factors in DIC include crush syndrome, abruptio placentae, septic abortion, leukemia, carcinoma, incompatible blood transfusion, and endotoxic shock.

In all of these states, the presence of injured or lysed cells cause the release of tissue phospholipid into the bloodstream, which can trigger the intrinsic pathway. Prolonged low cardiac output states such as seen with prolonged cardiopulmonary bypass or hemorrhagic shock result in injury to the vascular endothelial lining, which also can trigger the intrinsic pathway. Abnormalities of vascular endothelium secondary to such conditions as burns, vasculitis, sepsis, and major surgical interventions also can trigger DIC.

Regardless of the precipitating event in DIC, the triggering stimulus initiates systemic coagulation activity, resulting in diffuse intravascular fibrin formation and deposition of fibrin in the microcirculation. The ultimate result is the accumulation of clot in the body's capillaries, the total length of which exceeds 100,000 miles in the average adult. The amount of blood clot sequestration in the capillaries due to DIC is enormous. Because of the rapidity of intravascular thrombin formation, clotting factors effectively are used up in the capillary clotting process at a rate exceeding factor replenishment. Circulating thrombin persists in the extravascular space waiting for its substrate, fibrinogen, to arrive. The availability of the inhibitor, antithrombin III, is greatly reduced by the excessive thrombin formation.

The activation of the coagulation mechanisms also

activates the fibrinolytic system. Recall that activated factor XII, thrombin, endothelial cells, and tissue substances stimulate the release of plasminogen activators. The breakdown of fibrin and fibrinogen results in FDPs that interfere with platelet function and the formation of the fibrin clot. Thus, the patient has a simultaneous, self-perpetuating combination of thrombotic and bleeding activity occurring in response to the precipitating event.

Almost uniformly, there is arterial hypotension, often associated with activation of the kallikrein and complement systems. Kallikrein perpetuates the activation of factor XII to XIIa, further enhancing clotting activity. In addition, kallikrein releases kinins that increase vascular permeability and vasodilation, increasing hypotension. The activation of the complement system results in an increased vascular permeability and lysis of erythrocytes, granulocytes, and platelets. This activity produces phospholipids, which provide fuel for accelerating clotting activity by activating factor XII.

Arteriole vasoconstriction and capillary dilation ensue as the result of activation of the kallikrein and complement systems. Blood is then shunted to the venous side, bypassing dilated capillaries owing to the opening of arteriovenous (AV) shunts. The dilated capillaries now contain stagnant blood, in which metabolic by-products accumulate that render the blood acidotic. There now are three concomitant procoagulating conditions present in the capillary blood: acidosis, blood stagnation, and the presence of coagulation-promoting substances. Figure 43–4 depicts the effect of AV shunting.

The DIC patient bleeds not only because of increased clotting, which results in consumption of clotting factors,

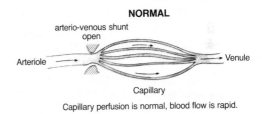

NORMAL

Capillary perfusion is normal, blood flow is rapid.

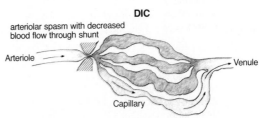

DIC

Capillary perfusion is impaired, blood flow is slow, intracapillary thrombosis occurs with blood stagnation and acidosis. Cells nourished by capillaries die of ischemia due to blood clotting.

FIGURE 43–4
Arteriole–capillary–venule relationship in normal circulation as opposed to the DIC patient. The diagram shows the effect of AV shunting in DIC.

but also because of increased fibrinolysis and diminished antithrombin III. As mentioned, the thrombin concentration is regulated by antithrombin III, and in DIC antithrombin III cannot keep up with the excessive generation of thrombin. This circulating thrombin continues to activate the conversion of plasminogen to plasmin, which compounds the bleeding diathesis. Figure 43–5 depicts the self-perpetuating cycle of thrombosis and bleeding in DIC.

Assessment

All critically ill patients are at risk for development of DIC because many are in the state of physiological disequilibrium characterized by hypovolemia, hypotension, hypoxia, and acidosis, all of which have procoagulant effects. Increased awareness of DIC as a potentially catastrophic complication in the critically ill patient has resulted in earlier recognition and intervention. The critical care nurse who is armed with a knowledge of physiological norms and who uses a systematic approach to assessment may be the first person to identify the early signs of coagulation dysfunction and its probable trigger.

Clinical Manifestations

Patients with DIC exhibit a varied constellation of problems and have the potential for development of more. The critical care nurse will be confronted with a patient bleeding from the nose, gums, and injection sites; a patient covered with purpura, petechiae, and ecchymosis; a patient immobilized by a variety of drainage tubes, intravenous lines, and hemodynamic monitoring equipment and attached to a mechanical ventilator; a frightened patient at risk for renewed bleeding; a family feeling frightened by their loved one's appearance and lacking understanding of this catastrophic event.

Assessment of the patient with possible DIC centers around several priorities. First, the patient will have a history of a possible triggering event such as a crush injury coupled with bleeding. Bleeding often is observed as oozing from venipuncture sites, development of petechiae, bleeding from mucous membranes, or occult blood present in gastric contents or stool.

Hypovolemic shock may develop in patients who are bleeding, and they must be monitored closely for signs and symptoms of its onset. Nurses also should be vigilant in preventing severe anemia. All organs can become dysfunc-

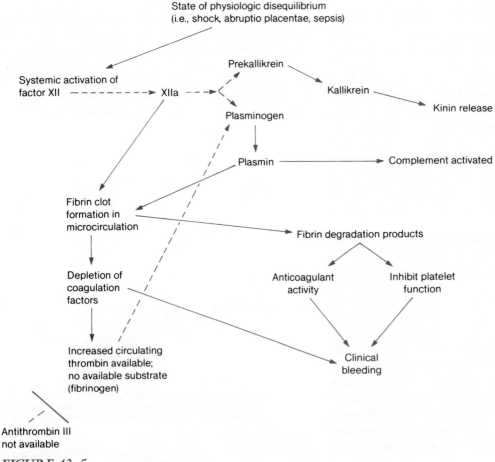

FIGURE 43–5
Self-perpetuating cycle of thrombosis and bleeding in DIC.

tional because of bleeding into tissue spaces or because of ischemia caused by thrombosis. Ongoing assessment of cerebral, pulmonary, renal, and hepatic function is vitally important.

Diagnostic Studies

A second important component of assessment is the evaluation of key laboratory data that typically are found to be abnormal with DIC. Table 43–2 outlines studies that are abnormal in DIC.

Management

Eliminate Cause

The backbone of therapy for DIC is elimination of the cause. If one's basement is flooded by a broken pipe, the problem will not be solved by mopping alone. The water supply to the broken pipe must be turned off. In DIC, the factor that activates the clotting factors must be "turned off." If the initiating state of physiological disequilibrium is septic shock, volume must be restored and antibiotic therapy initiated to eliminate the precipitating event.

Minimize Further Bleeding

A second management priority is to minimize the risk of further bleeding by protecting the patient from trauma or traumatic procedures, if possible. The third management priority will be to correct the clotting deficiencies by administering component therapy.

Attention also should be directed to correction of hypovolemia, hypotension, hypoxia, and acidosis, all of which have procoagulant effects. Correction of these imbalances must be the focus of the treatment of bleeding patients with DIC. Additionally, correction of hemostatic deficiencies that compromise the clotting mechanisms is necessary.

Replace Depleted Factor

Continued bleeding despite treatment of the underlying cause may indicate depletion of the coagulation factors. Some advocate administration of depleted factors only *after* heparin therapy is initiated so that the infused fibrinogen present in whole blood or fresh frozen plasma does not add "fuel to the fire" of circulating thrombin waiting for its substrate. Others do not support this rationale, and advocate the administration of depleted factors as the patient's condition dictates.

Heparin Therapy

Systemic heparinization was the accepted treatment for DIC in the 1970s and 1980s. Newer research has left many clinicians skeptical as to the value of heparin therapy. If the underlying cause of DIC cannot be eliminated, it can be controlled by stopping the cycle of thrombosis–hemorrhage with heparin administration. Heparin helps prevent further thrombus formation, but it does not alter clots that already have formed. Heparin also slows coagulation and permits restoration of coagulation proteins. It does this by combining with antithrombin III, and, in the presence of thrombin, forms a reversible combination in which thrombin is inactivated. In addition, this combination of heparin and antithrombin III neutralizes activated factors XII, XI, IX, and X, thus blocking the progression of the sequential activation of coagulation factors. Furthermore, heparin inhibits thrombin-mediated platelet aggregation by neutralizing the effects of thrombin. The administration of heparin therefore inhibits thrombin generation, thrombin–fibrinogen interactions, and platelet aggregation.

The dose of heparin required to treat DIC must agree with the clinical status and individual needs of the patient. There are advocates for both the subcutaneous and the intravenous routes of administration. Those who advocate intravenous administration favor continuous infusion of doses ranging up to 20,000 to 30,000 U in 24 hours. Proponents of subcutaneous heparin favor low doses that

TABLE 43–2
Laboratory Findings in Acute Disseminated Intravascular Coagulation (DIC)

Test	Normal Value	Value in DIC
Prothrombin time	11–15 seconds	Prolonged
Partial thromboplastin time	39–48 seconds	Prolonged
Thrombin time	10–13 seconds	Usually prolonged
Fibrinogen level	200–400 mg/100 ml	Decreased
Antithrombin III levels	89%–120%	Decreased
Platelet count	150,000–400,000/mm^3	Decreased
Fibrin degradation products	<10	Increased
Plasminogen levels		Decreased

range from 2,500 to 5,000 U every 4 to 8 hours. Sequential coagulation studies must be conducted to regulate the heparin dose and to determine the patient response to the heparin. Heparin should be continued until the primary precipitating cause has been removed and the clinical and the laboratory data suggest that the patient is on the way to recovery.

Antithrombin III Concentrate

Clinicians are awaiting the results of the use of investigational antithrombin III concentrate in DIC patients. Thus far, the studies have been favorable, and perhaps in the future there will be antithrombin III concentrate available to replenish the depleted stores in the patient with DIC.

Complications

A patient with DIC is vulnerable to a wide variety of complications, all of which are related either to bleeding or thrombosis.

Related to Bleeding

A serious bleeding-related complication is intracranial hemorrhage, which may manifest as headache, loss of motor or sensory function, altered level of consciousness, and changes in pupil reactions. Gastrointestinal hemorrhage may become evident in the patient who complains of abdominal pain and has distention, vomiting, signs of hypovolemia, and the presence of occult or frank blood in stool or emesis. Bleeding into the skin will manifest as petechiae and ecchymoses.

Related to Thrombosis

Thrombus formation in the microcirculation can cause problems related to ischemia. Cerebral vascular ischemia most likely will be manifested by changes in the level of consciousness, sensory abnormalities, visual disturbances, or motor weakness. Ischemia in the gastrointestinal tract can cause necrosis, resulting in severe abdominal pain, absent bowel sounds, and vomiting. Microthrombus in the renal vascular bed impairs normal renal function and could result in renal failure when prolonged hypotension or shock are present. Another danger is the formation of deep venous thromboses, which could embolize to the lungs. Pulmonary embolus is a catastrophic event that presents with hyperventilation, hemoptysis, chest pain, hypoxia, cyanosis, hypotension, and extreme apprehension in the patient.

CASE STUDY

Robert Pace is a 62-year-old man being cared for in the ICU after an abdominal aortic aneurysm repair. His aneurysm was located above the superceliac artery, and aortic cross-clamp was required for 62 minutes. Currently, he is 1 day postoperative. He is being mechanically ventilated. His abdomen is distended, tender to touch, and he has no bowel sounds. His temperature is 40°C. Dopamine hydrochloride, at a dose of 10 μg/kg/minute is being used to support his blood pressure. He has had several hypotensive episodes that have responded to fluid boluses with normal saline. The nurse caring for Mr. Pace notices that slow but constant bleeding has developed from his abdominal wound and from his central venous line insertion site. His blood is cultured for possible pathogens and screening for suspected DIC is obtained. His laboratory values are as follows:

Packed cell volume: 36%

Platelet count: 95,000/mm³

Prothrombin time: 36 seconds

Partial thromboplastin time: 57 seconds

Fibrinogen level: 100 mg/dl

His hemodynamic status continues to deteriorate and his abdomen continues to enlarge, and is increasingly tender. Peripheral perfusion is poor and petechiae are starting to develop. A repeat platelet count shows platelets to be decreased to 80,000/mm³. A repeat fibrinogen gives a value of 78 g/dl. His oxygenation has deteriorated, probably related to microthrombus in the pulmonary vascular bed. Currently, his PaO₂ has fallen to 70 mm Hg on 80% oxygen.

The studies indicate consumption of coagulation factors, fibrinogen, and platelets. The trigger for this process seems to be a portion of the bowel that became ischemic after a prolonged aortic cross-clamp during resection of his aneurysm.

The patient is treated with antibiotics because the possibility of a bowel perforation is not totally ruled out. He also is given platelets, cryoprecipitate, and fresh frozen plasma. After administration of these blood components, his laboratory studies improve as follows:

Platelet count: 110,000

Prothrombin time: 25 seconds

Partial thromboplastin time: 54 seconds

Fibrinogen level: 170 mg/dl

A decision is made to proceed with an emergency exploratory laparotomy. The patient is discovered to have a 4- to 5-inch segment of his colon that is necrotic, with evidence of a small perforation. This segment is removed along with adjoining ischemic tissue. The remainder of the bowel appears to be healthy.

Mr. Pace required treatment with antibiotics for 6 days and coagulation factor replacement for 2 days after the bowel resection. After removal of the trigger for the DIC, his coagulation status gradually normalized. His pulmonary function also improved and he was extubated on the 5th postoperative day. Although his ischemic bowel and subsequent DIC were life threatening, he made a gradual, successful recovery.

Nursing Care Plan

A detailed nursing care plan (Nursing Care Plan 43–1) follows. The problem of DIC presents the ultimate chal-
(*Text continues on page 958*)

NURSING CARE PLAN 43–1:
The Patient With Disseminated Intravascular Coagulation

NURSING DIAGNOSIS	OUTCOME CRITERIA/ PATIENT GOALS	NURSING INTERVENTIONS
Fluid volume deficit: related to hemorrhage, oozing of blood through puncture sites, tissue congestion, and slowed circulating blood volume.	• Maintain adequate hemodynamic state.	1. Assess vital signs q1h and prn. 2. Assess hemodynamic parameters (PAP, PCWP, CVP) q2h and prn. 3. Assess cardiac monitor for heart rate and rhythm. 4. Evaluate hourly urine output (amount and specific gravity). 5. Assess breath sounds q4h. 6. Assess quality and presence of peripheral pulses q4h. 7. Maintain accurate input and output. 8. Give IV fluids, as ordered. 9. Give plasma expanders and blood products, as ordered. 10. Evaluate laboratory values: Hgb, Hct, Na, K, Cl, PT, PTT, platelet count, fibrin split products, fibrinogen, and clotting times. 11. Maintain bed rest.
Decreased cardiac output: related to loss of coagulation factors resulting in hemorrhage, dysrhythmias, lactic acidosis, and intravascular thrombi.	• Maintain hemodynamic stability.	1. Minimize cardiac workload by maintaining bed rest. 2. Assess vital signs q1h until stable, and then q2h. 3. Assess hemodynamic parameters (PAP, PCWP, CVP) q2h and prn. 4. Assess cardiac monitor for heart rate, rhythm, and dysrhythmias. 5. Evaluate urine hourly for amount and specific gravity. 6. Verify acid–base status with ABGs. 7. Maintain O$_2$, as ordered. 8. Maintain IV access with large-bore needle that is adequate for blood replacement products. 9. Maintain accurate input and output. 10. Report abnormal findings to the physician.

(continued)

NURSING CARE PLAN 43–1: (Continued)
The Patient With Disseminated Intravascular Coagulation

NURSING DIAGNOSIS	OUTCOME CRITERIA/ PATIENT GOALS	NURSING INTERVENTIONS
Altered tissue perfusion: related to intravascular volume deficit, intravascular thrombosis and hemorrhage.	• Maintain adequate systemic circulation.	1. Assess for changes in mentation q1h and prn.
		2. Assess skin color, cyanosis, temperature, and diaphoresis q2h.
		3. Assess urine output and specific gravity q1h.
		4. Assess the quality and presence of peripheral pulses q2h.
		5. Assess bowel sounds q4h; place NG tube if vomiting blood or ileus appears.
		6. Evaluate laboratory values for Hgb, Hct, electrolytes, and coagulation studies.
		7. Position for relief of discomfort of pressure on dependent areas.
		8. Maintain O_2, as ordered.
		9. Evaluate all subjective symptomatic complaints.
		10. Consider the potential for multiple organ failure, and report all abnormal findings to the physician.
		11. Assess skin for presence of petechiae, ecchymosis, or oozing from puncture sites.
		12. Apply pressure to all puncture sites for 3–5 min, apply pressure dressings to all puncture sites.
		13. Maintain IV access.
Impaired gas exchange: related to intravascular volume deficit, reduced cardiac output, pulmonary hypertension, pulmonary hemorrhage, and intravascular thrombosis.	• Maintenance of adequate oxygenation and acid–base status (per ABG samples), with supplemental O_2.	1. Assess work of breathing (rate, rhythm, and depth) q2h.
		2. Assess breath sounds q2h and prn.
		3. Assess cyanosis, mottled skin, and diaphoresis, if present.
		4. Provide supplemental O_2, as ordered.
		5. Monitor O_2 saturation with a noninvasive device such as oximetry.
		6. Check ABGs, or ordered, and prn.

(continued)

NURSING CARE PLAN 43–1: (Continued)
The Patient With Disseminated Intravascular Coagulation

NURSING DIAGNOSIS	OUTCOME CRITERIA/ PATIENT GOALS	NURSING INTERVENTIONS
		7. Minimize O_2 consumption by maintaining bed rest.
		8. Correct acid–base balance with $NaHCO_3$ and fluid replacement.
		9. Review reports of chest radiographs.
		10. Administer bronchodilators, as ordered.
		11. Prevent atelectasis by TC and DB q2h.
		12. Position the patient to facilitate gas exchange (elevate the head of the bed, as tolerated).
High risk for impaired skin integrity: related to shock state, hemorrhage, tissue congestion, and decreased tissue perfusion.	• Skin will remain intact, without areas of maceration or breakdown.	1. Assess all skin surfaces q4h.
		2. Remove, examine, and replace all occlusive dressings q4–8h, as tolerated.
		3. Rotate the patient's position q2h.
		4. Evaluate all subjective complaints.
		5. Check WBC count for potential of infection.
		6. Medicate, as ordered, for comfort.
		7. Avoid excessive punctures for laboratory values, use arterial line or great vessel IV access for blood draws.
		8. Use padded soft restraints, if needed.
		9. Provide for safety by assisting with all transfer out of bed.
		10. Provide oral hygiene q4h.
		11. Assess all orifices for presence of hemorrhage or bruising.
High risk for injury: related to altered coagulation state, resulting in hemorrhage or thrombosis.	• Absence of trauma to skin and mucous membranes.	1. Assess environment for safety.
		2. Instruct patient to use call light and seek assistance before getting out of bed.
		3. If decreased level of consciousness, apply padded soft restraints, pad side rails, and observe closely.

(continued)

NURSING CARE PLAN 43–1: (Continued)
The Patient With Disseminated Intravascular Coagulation

NURSING DIAGNOSIS	OUTCOME CRITERIA/ PATIENT GOALS	NURSING INTERVENTIONS
		4. Evaluate all subjective complaints of limb, abdominal, or torso pain.
		5. Provide oral hygiene q4h.
		6. Avoid coughing, sneezing, or Valsalva maneuvers.
		7. Give simple instructions that elicit cooperation from the patient.
High risk for anxiety: related to critical illness, fear of death or disfigurement, role changes within social setting, or permanent disability.	• Patient will express anxieties to appropriate resource person.	1. Provide environment that encourages open discussion of emotional issues.
		2. Mobilize patient's support system and involve these resources as appropriate.
		3. Allow time for patient to express self.
		4. Identify possible hospital resources for patient/family support.
		5. Encourage open family-to-nurse communications regarding emotional issues.
		6. Validate patient and family knowledge base regarding the critical illness.
		7. Involve religious support systems as appropriate.

lenge to the critical care nurse—the use of the intellect for assessment and the integration of psychomotor skills for interventions—blended with the compassion required to care for the critically ill.

Summary

Disseminated intravascular coagulation is a situation in which localization of clotting and clot lysis has failed. Successful management of DIC requires that the inciting cause be recognized and treated. Treatment of the cause is the mainstay of therapy. Once this is accomplished, the whole bleeding process will begin to correct. If the precipitating factor cannot be corrected, patient survival is unlikely. Until total correction is achieved, a second major focus of management will be protection of the patient

from further bleeding and the replacement of consumed clotting factors, so that fibrin can be produced and clotting returned to a more physiologic state.

BIBLIOGRAPHY

Fischbach F: A Manual of Laboratory and Diagnostic Tests, 4th ed. Philadelphia, JB Lippincott, 1992
Guyton AC: Textbook of Medical Physiology, 8th ed. Philadelphia, WB Saunders, 1991
Kjeldsberg C, Beutler E, Bell C, Hougie C, et al: Practical Diagnosis of Hematologic Disorders. Chicago, American Society of Clinical Pathologists, 1989
Porth CM: Pathophysiology: Concepts of Altered Health States. Philadelphia, JB Lippincott, 1990
Suddarth DS: Lippincott Manual of Nursing Practice, 5th ed. Philadelphia, JB Lippincott, 1991

STUDY QUESTIONS

1. Normal inhibitors of coagulation include all but the following

   a. adequate cardiac output, which dilutes activated factors
   b. antithrombin III, which inactivates thrombin
   c. tissue thromboplastin, which interferes with fibrin formation
   d. plasminogen converting to plasmin

2. An early indication of a DIC process is bleeding associated with

   a. a decreased platelet count
   b. a decreased prothrombin time
   c. decreased levels of FDPs
   d. increased fibrinogen

3. Patients with DIC, a hypercoagulable syndrome, bleed because of all of the following except

   a. depleted clotting factors
   b. increased levels of fibrin degradation products
   c. diffuse microthrombosis
   d. decreased plasminogen levels

CHAPTER 44

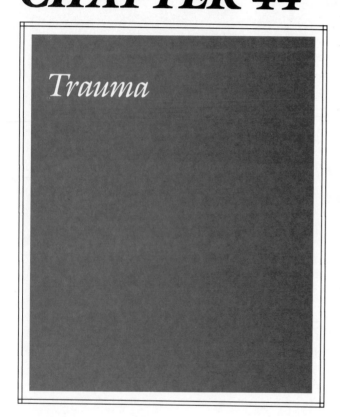

Trauma

BEHAVIORAL OBJECTIVES

Based on the content in this chapter, the reader should be able to:

1. Outline the four phases of initial assessment and care of the trauma patient.
2. Discuss the treatment of and nursing actions associated with trauma to the chest and heart.

Hudak: Critical Care Nursing:
A Holistic Approach, 6th ed. © 1994
J. B. Lippincott Company.

3. Contrast the response of solid and hollow abdominal organs to trauma.
4. Describe management of and nursing actions related to abdominal trauma.
5. Identify two serious complications of pelvic trauma.
6. Describe the nursing responsibilities associated with trauma to the extremities.
7. List the disorders involved in multiple organ failure.

Description

Trauma is the leading cause of death in people between the ages of 1 and 44 years. In older age groups, it is surpassed only by cancer and cardiovascular disease. The cost of trauma in terms of potential lost years of productive life, however, exceeds that of both cancer and cardiovascular disease.[1] As a major cause of death and disability, trauma has become a significant health and social problem.

Major advances in the care of traumatized patients have been made in the last few decades. The development of trauma centers has decreased mortality and morbidity among accident victims. Improved prehospital care and transportation have resulted in an increasing number of critically injured people reaching hospitals alive. Consequently, traumatized patients arriving in today's critical care units tend to have serious injuries involving multiple organs, and they often require extensive and complex nursing care.

Initial Assessment and Management

The severely injured person must be assessed quickly and efficiently. Criteria and protocols to facilitate initial assessment, intervention, and triage of the trauma victim have been developed by the American College of Surgeons, Committee on Trauma.[2]

Prehospital

Initial management often determines the final outcome. This phase begins at the accident scene with the rapid assessment of life-threatening injuries. After an airway is established, breathing and circulation are evaluated and supported. Initial circulatory resuscitation includes control of external hemorrhage, initiation of intravenous fluid therapy, and occasionally the application of a pneumatic antishock garment (PASG). Potential fractures also are immobilized before transport.

Hospital

Assessment and care performed on arrival at the hospital can be divided into four phases: primary evaluation, resuscitation, secondary assessment, and definitive care.

Primary Evaluation

Similar to prehospital assessment, the primary evaluation detects airway, breathing, and circulation problems, and determines threats to life and limb. Information about the mechanism of injury and the accident scene (ie, bent steering wheel) can provide clues about possible serious injuries. A brief neurologic examination also is performed.

Resuscitation

Resuscitation frequently begins during the primary evaluation and involves the treatment of life-threatening conditions. The patient may require endotracheal intubation, administration of oxygen, intravenous fluid therapy, and control of hemorrhage. Life-threatening conditions, such as tension or open pneumothorax, massive hemothorax, and cardiac tamponade, are treated quickly.[3] Unless contraindicated, a urinary catheter and nasogastric tube are inserted.

Secondary Assessment

Once the patient's condition has been stabilized, a complete history, including information on the mechanism of injury, must be obtained and a thorough physical examination performed. The examination may include an electrocardiogram (ECG), various laboratory tests, and radiologic studies (Table 44–1). If abdominal injuries are suspected, a diagnostic peritoneal lavage (DPL) also may be necessary (Table 44–2).

Patterns of Injury

Information on the pattern or mechanism of injury often is helpful in the diagnosis of potential disorders. Blunt trauma occurs in motor vehicle accidents (MVA) and falls, whereas penetrating trauma often is the result of gunshot or stab wounds. Generally, the greater the speed involved in the accident, the greater the injury (eg, high-speed MVA, high-velocity bullet, fall from a great height).

Blunt Trauma. In an automobile accident, the vehicle offers some protection and absorbs energy from the collision. The unrestrained driver or passenger, however, can be ejected from the car and receive additional injuries on impact. Motorcyclists have minimal protection and frequently sustain severe injuries when thrown.

Rapid deceleration during an MVA or fall can cause shearing forces that tear certain structures. Mobile organs such as the heart can tear away from adjacent anchoring great vessels. Likewise, abdominal organs (spleen, kidneys, intestines) may tear away from the mesentery.

A second type of blunt trauma involves compression caused by severe crushing forces. In such cases, the heart can be compressed between the sternum and spine. The liver, spleen, and pancreas also often are compressed against the spine. Crush injuries frequently cause internal damage with few external signs of trauma.

The type of damage to the vehicle often provides clues to specific injuries sustained in an MVA. A bent or broken steering wheel increases suspicion of possible injuries to the chest, ribs, heart, trachea, spine, or abdomen. Head and facial trauma, cervical spine injuries, and tracheal injuries often are associated with a damaged windshield or dashboard. A lateral impact can cause broken ribs, penetrating chest wounds from door or window handles, spleen or liver injuries, and a fractured pelvis.

Penetrating Trauma. Gunshot wounds are associated with a higher degree of damage than stab wounds.[4] Bullets may cause cavitation of surrounding tissue and can fragment or change direction inside the body, resulting in increased injury. Internal bleeding, organ perforation, and fractures all can be caused by penetrating injuries.

TABLE 44–1
Radiologic Procedures Indicated in Trauma

Procedure	Suspected Injury
Radiograph	
Chest	Pneumothorax
	Hemothorax
	Fractured ribs
	Pulmonary contusion
	Tracheobronchial injury
	Great vessel injury
Pelvis	Fracture
Extremities	Fracture
Angiogram	Great vessel injury
	Renal injury
	Vascular injury of the pelvis
	Vascular injury of the extremities
Computed tomography	Abdominal injury
	Retroperitoneal injury
	Renal injury
	Pelvic fracture
Gastrografin upper GI series	Duodenal hematoma or laceration
Radionuclide liver/spleen scan	Splenic injury
	Hepatic injury
Intravenous pyelogram	Renal injury
Retrograde urethrogram	Urethral injury
Retrograde cystogram	Bladder injury

GI, gastrointestinal.

TABLE 44–2
Diagnostic Peritoneal Lavage (DPL)

Purpose: To Detect Intraperitoneal Bleeding
Indications

- Blunt abdominal injury with:
  Altered pain response
    Decreased: head or spinal cord injury; presence of alcohol or drugs
    Increased: pelvic, lumbar spine or lower rib fractures
  Unexplained hypovolemia in multiple trauma victim
- Penetrating abdominal trauma (if exploration not indicated)

Contraindications

- History of multiple abdominal operations
- Immediate laparotomy needed

Procedure

1. Insert lavage catheter into peritoneal cavity through 1–2 cm incision.
2. Attempt to aspirate peritoneal fluid.
3. Infuse normal saline or Ringer's lactate by gravity.
4. Turn patient from side to side (unless contraindicated).
5. Allow fluid to run back into bag by gravity.
6. Send specimens to laboratory.

Positive Results

- 10–20 ml gross blood on initial aspirate
- Greater than 100,000 RBCs/mm^3
- Greater than 500 WBCs/mm^3
- Presence of bile, bacteria, or fecal matter

Using astute assessment skills and an awareness of the mechanism of injury, the critical care nurse can assist in identifying injuries that are not diagnosed in the emergency department.

Definitive Care

Although definitive care may begin in the emergency department or operating room, it consists mostly of the care provided in the intensive care unit, and, later, the surgical ward. Constant monitoring and evaluation are essential in facilitating the management of existing problems. Other important elements of definitive care include the evaluation of new signs and symptoms, the management of preexisting medical conditions, and the identification of injuries missed during treatment of life-threatening problems.

Assessment and Management

Thoracic Trauma

Approximately 25% of trauma death is due to thoracic injury.[4] Many potentially life-threatening injuries to the thorax, such as tension or open pneumothorax, massive hemothorax, flail chest, and cardiac tamponade, can be managed quickly and easily, often without major surgery. Untreated, they can be life-threatening.

Injuries to the Lungs and Rib Cage

Pneumothorax and Hemothorax

Blunt and penetrating trauma can cause pneumothorax or hemothorax (Fig. 44–1). Frequently, the only treatment needed is the placement of a chest tube. A massive hemothorax (>1,500 ml initially or >100–200 ml/hour) may require a thoracotomy, whereas chest tube reexpansion of the lung often is sufficient to tamponade most smaller sources of bleeding. Surgical intervention also may be necessary in the case of an open pneumothorax (sucking chest wound) or uncontrolled air leak.[5]

In addition to providing routine postoperative care (spirometry, coughing, and deep-breathing exercises), the critical care nurse should assess respiratory and hemodynamic function carefully. The patient with lung injuries has an increased risk for development of pulmonary complications such as atelectasis, pneumonia, and empyema. Chest tubes must be assessed for patency and function and the physician notified if drainage is excessive. For large blood loss from chest tubes, autotransfusion may be initiated (see Chapter 13).[6]

Flail Chest

A flail chest occurs when blunt trauma causes multiple rib fractures, leading to instability of the chest wall. Flail chest can be associated with pneumothorax, hemothorax, pulmonary contusion, or myocardial contusion (see p. 488).

The main goal in treatment of flail chest is promotion of adequate ventilation. If the respiratory status is compromised or surgery for an associated injury is necessary, intubation and mechanical ventilation are indicated.[4] Positive end-expiratory pressure (PEEP) may also be used. In rare instances, operative stabilization with wires or staples may be performed. Rib fractures are never taped because this only further decreases pulmonary function.

Rib fractures often are associated with severe pain. Adequate pain control promotes lung expansion without the need for lengthy mechanical ventilation. Parenteral, intramuscular, or patient-controlled analgesia often is ordered. Systemic analgesics, however, may not be potent enough to relieve the pain of a flail chest, necessitating other methods of pain relief such as intercostal blocks or epidural analgesia.[7]

Nursing care of the patient with a flail chest is aimed at pain assessment and control, along with the promotion of adequate oxygenation and gas exchange. Hypoventilation due to pain increases the risk for respiratory complications, including atelectasis and pneumonia. Various interventions to improve respiratory function may be indicated, including coughing and deep breathing, spirometry, postural drainage and chapping, mucolytics, bronchodilators, intermittent positive pressure breathing (IPPB), endotracheal or nasotracheal suctioning, and therapeutic bronchoscopy.

Serial pulmonary assessments, including chest x-rays, arterial blood gases, physical examinations, and occasionally oximetric monitoring are essential.

Pulmonary Contusion

A pulmonary contusion is a bruising of the lung parenchyma, often due to blunt trauma. This disorder may not

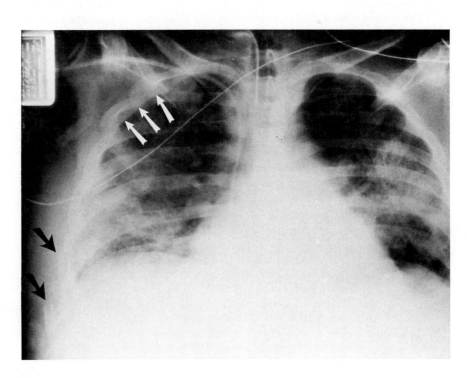

FIGURE 44–1
Chest radiograph of a 31-year-old man injured in an industrial explosion. Note rib fractures (*black arrows*) and right hemothorax (*white arrows*). Peripheral pulmonary infiltrates are the result of ARDS. (Courtesy of Winfield M. Craven, MD, Fort Collins Radiologic Associates, Fort Collins, CO)

TABLE 44–3
Differences Between Pulmonary Contusion and ARDS

Pulmonary Contusion	ARDS
Gradual onset of respiratory failure	Sudden onset of respiratory failure
Radiograph changes can be immediate	Radiograph changes frequently delayed 2–3 days after symptoms appear
Focal infiltrates	Diffuse infiltrates
Can lead to cavitation and lung abscess	Can lead to chronic pulmonary fibrosis

ARDS, adult respiratory distress syndrome.

be diagnosed on the initial chest x-ray; however, the presence of rib fractures or a flail chest should lead the to the suspicion of a possible pulmonary contusion.[5]

Pulmonary contusion occurs when rapid deceleration ruptures capillary cell walls, causing hemorrhage and extravasation of plasma and protein into alveolar and interstitial spaces. This results in atelectasis and consolidation, leading to intrapulmonary shunting and hypoxemia. Presenting signs and symptoms include dyspnea, rales, hemoptysis, and tachypnea. Severe contusions also will result in increasing peak airway pressures, hypoxemia, and respiratory acidosis. Pulmonary contusion may mimic adult respiratory distress syndrome (ARDS); both are poorly responsive to high inspired oxygen fractions (FIO_2). Table 44–3 lists the differences between ARDS and pulmonary contusion.

The patient with a mild contusion requires close observation. Frequent arterial blood gas (ABG) measurements or pulse oximetry often are necessary. Additional nursing interventions include frequent respiratory assessment, pulmonary care, and pain control. Chest physiotherapy and continuous epidural analgesia also may be beneficial. Severe pulmonary contusion may require ventilatory support with PEEP. An oximetric pulmonary artery catheter (oximetric Swan–Ganz) and arterial line usually are placed to facilitate monitoring of ABGs, hemodynamics, and respiratory parameters (oxygen delivery, oxygen consumption, intrapulmonary shunt). Although alveolar ventilation improves as PEEP is added, blood flow to alveoli may diminish, leading to an increased intrapulmonary shunt. To optimize tissue perfusion and oxygenation, each change in PEEP requires assessment of the status of the shunt, oxygen delivery, and other indicators of tissue perfusion (cardiac output, blood pressure, urine output). In severe cases of respiratory compromise, increased sedation or paralysis may be indicated to decrease energy expenditure and oxygen requirements. A rotation bed, such as the Roto-Rest (Kinetic Concepts, Inc., San Antonio, TX) also should be considered. The use of high-frequency jet ventilation for this type of injury still is controversial.[8] Severe unilateral contusions may be managed with simultaneous independent lung ventilation and positioning the patient with the injured side up.[9]

Fluid management also is important. Intake and output, daily weights, central venous pressure, and pulmonary capillary wedge pressure should be monitored. Concentration of medications may be needed to diminish excess intake, and diuretics may be required periodically. Severe fluid restriction is not indicated. Instead, fluid balance should be maintained at a near-normal level to support optimal cardiac output and oxygen delivery. Because a wet, contused lung has a decreased ability to clear bacteria, prophylactic antibiotics may be ordered. Prophylactic steroid and protein administration continues to be controversial.[8] Pneumonia and superimposed ARDS are common complications.

Clinical Research

Fink, MP, Helsmoortel CM, et al: The efficacy of an oscillating bed in the prevention of lower respiratory tract infection in critically ill victims of blunt trauma. Chest 97:132–137, 1990

The purpose of this study was to determine whether the use of continuous postural oscillation would reduce the incidence of lower respiratory tract infection (LRTI) and pneumonia. Blunt trauma victims admitted to the surgical intensive care unit (SICU) were randomly assigned to either a conventional bed or a Roto-Rest treatment table (Kinetic Concepts, Inc., San Antonio, TX). Patients in the SICU less than 24 hours were excluded from the study. The remaining subjects were monitored daily for development of LRTI or pneumonia. Twenty-eight patients in the control group (n = 48) met the criteria for LRTI, and pneumonia developed in 19. Of the 51 patients in the experimental group, 13 met the criteria for LRTI, and pneumonia developed in 7. The incidences of LRTI and pneumonia between the two groups were both statistically significant ($P = 0.0011$, $P = 0.0056$).

Tracheobronchial Injury

Injuries to the trachea or bronchi can be due to blunt or penetrating trauma and frequently are accompanied by esophageal and vascular damage. Ruptured bronchi often are present in association with upper rib fractures or pneumothorax. Severe tracheobronchial injury has a high mortality rate; however, with recent improvements in prehospital care and transport, more of these patients are surviving.[6]

Airway injuries often are subtle. Presenting signs include dyspnea (occasionally the only sign), hemoptysis, cough, and subcutaneous emphysema. A chest x-ray can alert the physician to a possible injury; however, diagnosis usually is made with a bronchoscopy or during surgery. Surgical repair with postoperative mechanical ventilation by an endotracheal tube or tracheostomy may be necessary.

Nursing care involves the assessment of oxygenation and gas exchange, along with appropriate pulmonary care. During the first few days, the physician may perform a bronchoscopy to visualize the repair site and to provide more effective suctioning. Pneumonia is a potential short-term complication, whereas tracheal stenosis may occur later.

Injuries to the Heart

Myocardial Contusion

Bruising of the myocardium is caused most often by the impact of the chest against the steering column or dashboard during an MVA. Rapid deceleration causes the mobile heart to strike the anterior chest wall. The right ventricle, due to its anterior location, is affected most commonly. A contusion also can result as the heart is compressed between the sternum and spine.

Symptoms of cardiac contusion vary from none (common) to severe congestive heart failure and cardiogenic shock. After trauma, complaints of chest pain must be evaluated carefully. Nonspecific ECG changes are seen frequently and can include any type of dysrhythmia. Sinus tachycardia, premature atrial or ventricular beats, paroxysmal supraventricular tachycardia, right bundle branch block, or ST and T wave changes are most common.[5]

Histologically, cardiac contusion is similar to myocardial infarction. Diagnosis can be difficult. Serial ECGs and serial levels of creatine kinase myocardial isoenzymes are obtained; however, these tests are not 100% sensitive. Some physicians will order a two-dimensional echocardiogram to check for complications and degree of injury once a contusion has been confirmed.

Close monitoring is necessary until cardiac contusion has been ruled out. Much more common than a confirmed myocardial contusion is a reversible "concussion" type of injury. Temporary signs and symptoms (eg, tachycardia, premature beats) will be present without changes in isoenzymes. As long as the diagnosis is uncertain, oxygenation, hemodynamics, and activity tolerance should be monitored carefully. If a tachycardia develops, alternative causes such as pain or volume depletion should be considered. Once a contusion is confirmed, treatment is similar to that for an acute myocardial infarction.

Penetrating Injury

A penetrating injury to the heart results in prehospital death of the victim in about 60% to 90% of cases.[10] In the remainder, hemorrhage and shock are common presenting signs. Small stab wounds to the ventricles occasionally seal themselves owing to the thick ventricular musculature. In the presence of ongoing hemorrhage, lost volume is replaced, and surgical repair is necessary. In severe cases, a thoracotomy in the emergency department may be required as a lifesaving measure.[11]

After surgical repair, a pulmonary artery catheter (Swan–Ganz) and arterial line are placed to facilitate careful hemodynamic monitoring. Vasopressors or inotropic agents may be necessary to maintain adequate blood pressure and cardiac output. Fluid and electrolyte balance, along with cardiac rhythm, must be monitored closely. Heart sounds should be assessed for murmurs, indicating valvular or septal defects, and for signs of congestive heart failure. Chest and mediastinal tube drainage is recorded frequently. Fresh frozen plasma and platelets are administered, as indicated, to correct coagulopathies. Complications include continued hemorrhage and postcardiotomy syndrome. In the event of multiple blood transfusions, the risk of ARDS and disseminated intravascular coagulation (DIC) is heightened (Table 44–4). An extended period of hypotension increases the possibility of renal failure.

Tamponade

Cardiac tamponade can result from both penetrating and blunt trauma. Blood fills the pericardium and compresses the heart, causing decreased cardiac filling, which leads to reduced cardiac output and eventually shock. Only a small amount of pericardial blood is necessary to produce shock.

TABLE 44–4
Complications Related to Multiple Blood Transfusions

ARDS
Coagulopathy
DIC
Hypokalemia or hyperkalemia
Hypocalcemia
Metabolic acidosis
Hypothermia
Volume overload
Transfusion reaction
Transmission of infection

ARDS, adult respiratory distress syndrome; DIC, disseminated intravascular coagulation.

Initial signs may include decreased blood pressure, increased central venous pressure as manifested by distended neck veins, and muffled heart sounds. A pericardiocentesis may be both diagnostic and therapeutic; however, surgery often is necessary for definitive treatment.[12] Postoperative nursing care is similar to that for a penetrating cardiac injury; however, surgical repair is not always needed.

Injury to the Great Vessels

Most patients with a transection or tear of the aorta exsanguinate before reaching a hospital.[13] Rapid deceleration causes shearing forces between the aortic arch and the tethered descending aorta. The most common site of injury is near the ligamentum arteriosum. Distal to this point, the aorta is closely applied to the thoracic spine, whereas proximal to this point, it is freely movable. Immediate death is prevented if the hemorrhage is contained within the aortic adventitia. This "false aneurysm" can rupture at any time, however, and thus requires prompt diagnosis and treatment.

Suspicion of an aortic or other great vessel injury is increased with fractures of the first and second ribs or a massive left hemothorax. A widened mediastinum on an upright chest x-ray frequently is indicative of aortic injury, necessitating an aortogram for diagnosis (Fig. 44–2). Additional diagnostic signs, although not always present, include hypertensive upper extremities with reduced lower extremity pulses. Injuries to the subclavian or innominate arteries may cause decreased pulses in the upper extremities.

A positive aortogram indicates the need for surgical repair. The torn aorta requires end-to-end anastomosis or, more commonly, the placement of a synthetic graft.[14] Cardiopulmonary bypass may be necessary for repair of the ascending aorta or the aortic arch. Autotransfusion also may be used. To prevent leakage from the repair site, postoperative vasodilators may be administered to reduce afterload. A vasopressor may be added to prevent hypotension. Nursing care focuses on hemodynamic monitoring with a Swan–Ganz catheter and titrating medications to maintain optimal blood pressure. Serious complications include renal failure due to ischemia, along with ARDS and DIC due to multiple transfusions. Rarely, repair or cross-clamping of the descending thoracic aorta can cause ischemia of the spinal cord, resulting in permanent paralysis of the lower extremities.

Abdominal Trauma

The abdominal cavity contains both solid and hollow organs. Blunt trauma is likely to cause serious damage to solid organs, and penetrating trauma most often injures the hollow organs. The compression and deceleration of blunt trauma leads to fractures of solid organ capsules and parenchyma, whereas the hollow organ can collapse and

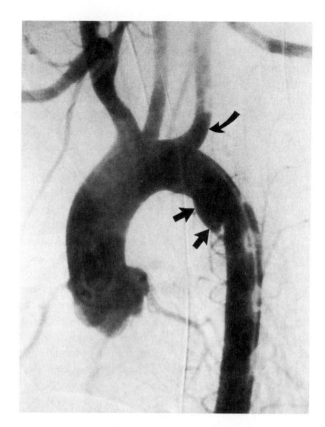

FIGURE 44–2
Arch aortogram demonstrates laceration of descending aorta (*straight arrows*) just distal to origin of left subclavian artery (*curved arrow*). Extravasated contrast material is contained by aortic adventitia. (Courtesy of Michael Mestek, MD, Denver General Hospital, Denver, CO)

absorb the force. The bowel, however, which occupies most of the abdominal cavity, is prone to injury by penetrating trauma. In general, solid organs respond to trauma with bleeding. Hollow organs rupture and release their contents into the peritoneal cavity, causing inflammation and infection.

Early diagnosis is important in abdominal trauma. Patients presenting with an abdominal injury penetrating the peritoneal deep fascia, hemodynamic instability, or signs and symptoms of an acute abdomen are surgically explored.[3] In most other cases of abdominal trauma, diagnostic peritoneal lavage (DPL) is performed. A positive DPL also necessitates surgical exploration.

Neither a DPL or a computed tomography (CT) scan is 100% diagnostic; therefore, trauma patients with negative results should be observed. Serial hematocrits and amylase levels are obtained. Pain medication may be withheld so as not to cloud potential signs and symptoms. Oral intake also is withheld in case surgery is required. The patient is assessed for the clues of an acute abdomen: distention, rigidity, guarding, and rebound tenderness. Surgical exploration becomes necessary with the onset of any signs or symptoms indicating injury. The use of abdominal CT has gained in popularity and often is used in place of, or in addition to, the DPL. Retroperitoneal injuries, frequently missed with a DPL and even exploratory surgery, often can be identified on a CT scan. The CT scan, however, may not be as reliable in detecting injury to hollow organs.[4]

Injuries to the Stomach and Small Bowel

Significant gastric injury is rare; however, the small bowel is more commonly injured. Although frequently damaged by penetrating trauma, blunt trauma also can cause the small bowel to burst. The multiple convolutions occasionally form a closed loop that is subject to rupture with increased pressure from impact with a steering wheel or seat belt. The bowel's mobility around fixed points (such as the ligament of Treitz) predisposes it to shearing injuries with deceleration.

Blunt small bowel or gastric injury can present with blood in the nasogastric aspirate or hematemesis. Physical signs often are absent, however, and diagnosis is not made until peritonitis develops.[4] Penetrating injuries usually cause a positive DPL. Although a mild bowel contusion can be managed conservatively (gastric decompression and withholding oral intake), surgery usually is necessary to repair penetrating wounds.

Postoperative decompression, either with a nasogastric or gastric tube, is maintained until bowel function returns. In most cases a feeding jejunostomy tube is placed distal to the repair site. Tube feedings can be initiated early in the postoperative course. As the concentration and rate of feedings are advanced slowly, frequent assessment for signs of intolerance (distention, vomiting) is essential. Because the stomach and small bowel contain an insignificant amount of bacteria, the risk of sepsis is small; however, prophylactic antibiotics are given any time a bowel perforation is present. On the other hand, the acidic gastric juice is irritating to the peritoneum and may cause peritonitis. Other potential complications include postoperative bleeding, hypovolemia due to "third spacing," and the development of a fistula or obstruction. Some of these conditions may necessitate additional surgical procedures. Malabsorption syndrome is rare unless over 200 cm of bowel has been removed.[4]

Injuries to the Duodenum and Pancreas

The pancreas and duodenum will be discussed together because they both are retroperitoneal organs and are closely related anatomically and physiologically. A great deal of force is necessary to injure these organs, because they are well protected, deep in the abdomen. Injuries to adjacent organs almost are always present. The retroperitoneal location makes these injuries difficult to diagnose because the DPL frequently is negative; therefore, an abdominal CT scan is very useful in this instance. Signs and symp-

toms may include an acute abdomen, increased serum amylase levels, epigastric pain radiating to the back, nausea, and vomiting.

A minor laceration or contusion may require only the placement of drains, whereas larger wounds need surgical repair. Most pancreatic injuries will require postoperative drains to prevent fistula formation. A distal pancreatectomy or Roux-en-Y anastomosis are two procedures commonly performed for injuries to the body and tail of the pancreas. Occasionally, the spleen also must be removed owing to its multiple vascular attachments. Damage to the head of the pancreas is associated with duodenal injury and severe hemorrhage because of the close proximity of vascular structures. Surgical procedures used in these cases include pancreaticoduodenectomy, Roux-en-Y anastomosis, and, on rare occasions, total pancreatectomy.

Postoperative nursing assessment and care are similar for the various procedures. Patency of drains must be maintained and the patient monitored for the development of fistulas. Skin protection is important if a fistula does develop, because of the high enzyme content of pancreatic fluid. Assessment of fluid and electrolyte balance is important because a pancreatic fistula results in fluid loss, along with potassium and bicarbonate. Pancreatic stimulation can be decreased by administering parenteral hyperalimentation or jejunal feedings instead of an oral diet. The onset of diabetes mellitus is rare unless a total pancreatectomy is performed. Other complications include bleeding from a fistula eroding into vessels, peritonitis, intra-abdominal or systemic sepsis, pancreatitis, and mechanical bowel obstruction.

Injury to the duodenum alone can be repaired by a primary anastomosis or Billroth II. A duodenostomy tube may be placed for decompression and a jejunostomy tube for feeding. Blunt trauma to the duodenum also can cause an intramural hematoma, which may lead to duodenal obstruction. The diagnosis is made with a diatrizoate (Gastrografin) upper gastrointestinal study. A complete obstruction generally requires surgical drainage of the hematoma.

Injuries to the Colon

Colon injury usually is due to penetrating trauma. The nature of the injury most often dictates immediate surgical exploration. Primary repair is the treatment of choice for lacerations of the colon. In some situations, however, an exteriorized repair or colostomy is required. A cecostomy tube may be placed for decompression. The subcutaneous tissue and skin of the incision site may be left open to decrease the chance of wound infection. The colon has a high bacterial count; spillage of the contents will predispose to intra-abdominal sepsis and abscess formation.

Postoperative nursing care focuses on the prevention of infection. Dressing changes are necessary for the open incision and prophylactic antibiotics usually are used. In the case of an exteriorized colon repair, an end-to-end anastomosis is performed and the repair site exteriorized to facilitate identification of a leak. The exteriorized colon must be kept moist and covered with a nonadhering dressing or bag to protect the integrity of the sutures. Because sepsis is the major complication of colon injuries, a series of radiographic and surgical procedures may be required to locate and drain abscesses.

Injuries to the Liver

After the spleen, the liver is the most commonly injured abdominal organ.[15] Both blunt and penetrating trauma can cause injuries (Fig. 44–3). A small percentage of patients may be managed nonoperatively with serial CT scans. In most cases, however, either the nature of the injury or a positive DPL or CT scan combined with the patient's clinical condition will dictate the need for surgery. Hepatic trauma can cause a large blood loss into the peritoneum, but bleeding may stop spontaneously. Small lacerations are repaired, whereas larger injuries may require segmental resection or debridement.[16] In the case of uncontrollable hemorrhage, the liver is packed. After packing, the abdomen may be closed or simply covered with mesh.[17] An additional surgical procedure is required within the next few days to remove the packing and repair the laceration. Large liver injuries also need postoperative drainage of bile and blood via drains (Penrose, Davol, or Jackson–Pratt).[18]

After surgery, hypovolemic shock and coagulopathies may be present. Incomplete hemostasis also is possible and must be differentiated from coagulopathy-induced bleeding. Severe bleeding due to incomplete hemostasis requires a return to the operating room for clot removal, packing, and additional repair. With a coagulopathy, bleeding arises from numerous sites, whereas with incomplete hemostasis the bleeding is mainly from the surgical site. Nursing care includes the replacement of blood products while monitoring the hematocrit and coagulation studies. Assessment of the type and amount of tube drain-

age, along with fluid balance, also is essential. Potential complications of liver injury include hepatic or perihepatic abscess, biliary obstruction or leak, sepsis, ARDS, and DIC.

Injuries to the Spleen

The spleen is the most commonly injured abdominal organ, more often as a result of blunt trauma. The presence of left lower rib fractures should increase suspicion of a splenic injury. Presenting signs and symptoms include left upper quadrant (LUQ) pain radiating to the left shoulder, hypovolemic shock, and the nonspecific finding of an increased white blood cell count. The DPL, abdominal CT scan, or radionuclide study usually are necessary for diagnosis.

Adults with minor injuries and most children are treated nonoperatively, with observation (serial abdominal examinations, serial hematocrits), and nasogastric decompression. Because the spleen and stomach are both in the LUQ, decompression of the stomach reduces pressure on the injured spleen. Surgical treatment consists of splenorrhaphy or splenectomy. Splenic autotransplantation, a fairly new and still controversial procedure, consists of implanting splenic fragments into pockets of omentum.[4]

Early complications include recurrent bleeding, subphrenic abscess, and pancreatitis due to surgical trauma. Late complications consist of thrombocytosis and overwhelming postsplenectomy sepsis (OPSS). Because the spleen plays an important role in the body's response to infection, a splenectomy predisposes to an increased risk for infection. This risk is especially high among children and highest in those under 2 years of age. *Pneumococcus*, an encapsulated microorganism resistant to phagocytosis, commonly infects patients after splenectomy. Therefore, pneumococcal pneumonia frequently is the initial presentation of OPSS, often resulting in a fulminant sepsis. Complications include adrenal insufficiency and DIC. This syndrome has a high incidence and mortality rate, especially within the first year after surgery.[4] Teaching

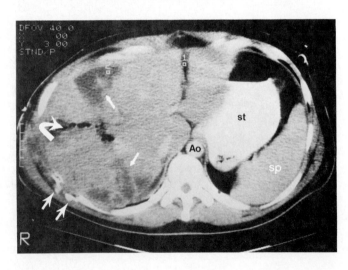

FIGURE 44–3
Cross-section from abdominal CT scan shows multiple liver lacerations that contain blood (*small straight arrows*) and air (*large curved arrow*). Rib fractures are present posteriorly on the right (*large straight arrows*). Note normal aorta (*Ao*) and spleen (*sp*). Stomach (*st*) contains oral contrast material. (Courtesy of Winfield M. Craven, MD, Fort Collins Radiologic Associates, Fort Collins, CO)

should focus on detection of signs and symptoms of infection. Splenic autotransplantation may prove beneficial in decreasing the incidence of OPSS.

Injuries to the Kidneys

Vascular Injury

Penetrating injury may lead to either a "free" hemorrhage, contained hematoma, or the development of an intraluminal thrombus. A sudden deceleration injury can cause avulsion of smaller vessels or tear the renal artery intima, which also may lead to thrombosis of the vessel. Signs and symptoms, when present, consist of hematuria, pain, and a flank mass. Because the bleeding is retroperitoneal, it will be more difficult to detect. A CT scan, intravenous pyelogram, or angiogram usually provide the diagnosis. Smaller lacerations are repaired, whereas larger injuries may necessitate a nephrectomy.

Postoperative assessment and support of renal function is imperative. Low-dose dopamine may be ordered, and optimal fluid balance must be maintained to ensure renal perfusion. The major complications consist of arterial or venous thrombosis and acute renal failure.

Parenchymal Injury

Blunt or penetrating trauma can cause a laceration or contusion of the renal parenchyma or rupture of the collecting system. Lower rib fractures should raise suspicion of an associated renal injury. Diagnosis is similar to that of renal vascular injuries. A minor injury can be managed conservatively, with observation and bed rest until gross hematuria resolves. Surgery is required for larger injuries. As with vascular injury, decreased renal function is a potential consequence. Other complications include bleeding, sepsis (especially with extravasation of infected urine), the development of a urinary fistula, and late onset of hypertension.

Pelvic Trauma

Injuries to the Bladder

The bladder can be lacerated or ruptured, most often as the consequence of blunt trauma. Bladder injuries frequently are associated with pelvic fractures. The presence of hematuria (gross or microscopic), low abdominal pain, or the inability to void require examination for urethral injuries with a retrograde urethrogram before the insertion of a urinary catheter.

A bladder injury can cause intraperitoneal or extraperitoneal urine extravasation. Extraperitoneal extravasation often can be managed with urinary catheter drainage. Intraperitoneal extravasation, however, requires surgery. A suprapubic cystostomy tube may be placed. Complications are infrequent, but infection due to the urinary catheter or sepsis from extravasation of infected urine can occur.

Pelvic Fracture

Complex pelvic fractures are associated with a high mortality. Secondary hemorrhage is the most frequent cause of early death, whereas sepsis causes most of the delayed mortality. Radiographs and a CT scan can confirm the presence and define the extent of pelvic fractures. A pelvic fracture often causes the laceration of small vessels that bleed into soft tissue in the retroperitoneal space. This area extends from the diaphragm to mid-thigh and will accommodate several liters of blood before tamponade occurs. An angiogram often is necessary to localize and embolize the source of bleeding.

Hemorrhage control is of primary concern. The PASG may be applied in the prehospital phase or in the emergency department, but is used infrequently in the intensive care unit. It serves to splint the pelvis and tamponade the hemorrhage. Because the PASG decreases tidal volume, ventilatory support may be necessary. Internal or external fixation is more effective in stabilizing the fracture as well as controlling the bleeding.[4] In addition, early fixation reduces pain and facilitates earlier ambulation. Surgical packing also may be necessary to control the hemorrhage.

The critical care nurse's primary concern is to prevent hemorrhagic shock. Multiple transfusions and hemodynamic monitoring are necessary in the case of a significant hemorrhage. A pelvic hematoma can be a source of sepsis and may require percutaneous or surgical drainage.[4] Other major complications of pelvic fractures include pelvic nerve involvement and pulmonary emboli. Prolonged physical therapy and rehabilitation frequently are necessary.

Trauma to the Extremities

Fractures

Fractures occur often in blunt trauma, less frequently in penetrating trauma. Once a radiograph confirms the fracture, stabilization or repair is undertaken. Because orthopedic procedures can be time consuming, other life-threatening injuries often take precedence, and surgical repair may be postponed until a later date. Internal fixation of fractures often allows earlier ambulation in patients with multiple injuries in whom complications of prolonged bed rest (decubitus ulcers, pulmonary embolus, muscle wasting) otherwise may develop. Fracture management also may be accomplished with external fixation or skeletal traction. Open fractures may require surgical debridement.

Nursing responsibilities include assessment of neurovascular status, along with wound and pin care. Open fractures have an increased risk of infection. Other potential complications are fat emboli from long bone fractures, and compartment syndrome. Nursing care must be directed toward the prevention and early detection of these problems. The nurse also must work closely with the physical therapist to promote strengthening and early mobilization.

Vascular Injuries

Vascular injuries frequently result in bleeding or thrombosis of a vessel. They usually are due to penetrating trauma, and less often are the consequence of fractures. Doppler ultrasonography often is used to diagnose peripheral vascular injury. An angiogram also may be performed to locate the site of injury and identify arteriovenous fistulas, pseudoaneurysms, and intimal flaps. Primary surgical repair or vascular grafting is then undertaken.

In the immediate postoperative period, there is a risk for continued bleeding or thrombotic occlusion of the vessel. Both require a return to the operating room. The nurse must assess distal pulses, color, sensation, movement, and temperature of the involved extremity. Ankle–brachial indexes (ABIs) often are helpful in detecting the development of an occlusion after lower extremity trauma. To calculate an ABI, the systolic blood pressure of the ankle is divided by the systolic blood pressure of the arm. Decreasing ABIs indicate increasing pressure gradient across a vessel. This method provides more objective data than simply palpating pulses. The nurse also must watch for the development of compartment syndrome.

Complications of Multiple Trauma

Early Cause of Death (Within 72 Hours)

Hemorrhage and Head Injury

Hemorrhage and head injuries (see Chapter 30) are the greatest causes of early death after multiple trauma. To prevent exsanguination, bleeding must be controlled. This can be accomplished by surgical ligation or packing, and embolization by angiography. Continued hemorrhage requires multiple transfusions, thus increasing the likelihood of development of ARDS and DIC. Prolonged hemorrhage leads to hypovolemic shock and eventual decrease in organ perfusion (Table 44–5). Various organs respond differently to the decreased perfusion caused by hypovolemic shock (Table 44–6).

TABLE 44–5
Mechanisms Leading to
Decreased Tissue Perfusion

Causative factor (eg, decreased volume, release of toxins)
↓
Decreased venous return
↓
Decreased stroke volume
↓
Decreased cardiac output
↓
Nonuniform decrease in tissue perfusion

Late Causes of Death (After 3 Days)

Sepsis

Sepsis is a frequent complication of multiple trauma. The release of toxins causes dilation of vessels, leading to venous pooling that results in a decrease in venous return. Initially, cardiac output rises to compensate for decreased systemic vascular resistance. Eventually, the compensatory mechanisms are overcome and cardiac output falls along with blood pressure and organ perfusion (ie, septic shock).

The infective source must be found and eradicated. Antibiotics are prescribed, cultures obtained, radiologic studies begun, and exploratory surgery frequently is performed. Intra-abdominal abscess is a frequent cause of sepsis. Some abscesses can be drained percutaneously, whereas others require surgery. After the surgical drainage of an abdominal abscess, the incision is left open, with drains in place, to allow healing and prevent recurrence. Other sources of infection to consider are invasive lines, urinary tract, and lungs. It is thought that early nutritional support decreases the development of sepsis and multiple organ failure.[4]

Multiple Organ Failure

The onset of sepsis often coincides with the onset of multiple organ failure (MOF), which occurs in 7% to 12% of critically injured patients. Infection and a history of hypovolemic shock are thought to increase the potential for development of MOF. Characterized by the failure of two or more organs, MOF is associated with a mortality rate of 25% to 95%.[4] The lungs and liver tend to fail first, followed by the kidneys, gastrointestinal tract, and heart.

Pulmonary failure in the form of ARDS usually develops 5 to 7 days postinjury. It is characterized by hypoxemia with shunting, decreased lung compliance, tachypnea, dyspnea, and the appearance of diffuse bilateral pulmonary infiltrates. The syndrome requires intensive ventilatory support. Causative factors include major pul-

TABLE 44–6
The Effects of Hypovolemic Shock on Different Systems

Cardiac System

Tachycardia
Decreased systolic blood pressure
Narrowing of pulse pressure
Eventual cardiac failure

Skin

Cool, clammy
Pale, cyanotic

Central Nervous System

Anxiety, restlessness
Confusion, altered sensorium
Decreased level of consciousness

Renal System

Decreased urine output
Decreased glomerular filtration (increased BUN, serum
  creatinine)
Acute or chronic renal failure

Pulmonary System

Tachypnea
Increased pulmonary capillary permeability (ARDS)

Hepatic System

Decreased manufacture of clotting factors
Impaired drug metabolism
Decreased synthesis of plasma proteins (decreased serum
  albumin)
Reduced serum glucose levels
Decreased elimination of ammonia (increased BUN)
Decreased phagocytosis

Gastrointestinal System

Adynamic ileus
Ulceration
Decreased absorption of nutrients
Increase in toxins passing from lumen into bloodstream

Vascular System

DIC

Cellular System

Anaerobic metabolism (lactic acidosis)

BUN, blood urea nitrogen; ARDS, adult respiratory distress
syndrome; DIC, disseminated intravascular coagulation.

monary trauma, multiple blood transfusions, sepsis, and
shock (see Chapter 21).

Liver failure can result from initial damage, vascular
compromise, shock, and sepsis. Jaundice is a common
indicator of deteriorating liver function, although other
causes such as post-traumatic biliary obstruction must be
ruled out. Liver function tests are diagnostic. Liver failure
can lead to a decrease in the level of consciousness, abnormal clotting studies, and hypoglycemia (see Chapter 37).

Renal failure can be precipitated by a renal injury,
ischemia, radiographic contrast material, hypovolemia
(due to hemorrhage, third spacing), or sepsis. Initial signs
include a rising blood urea nitrogen and serum creatinine.
Renal failure may be polyuric or oliguric. Dialysis often is
necessary (see Chapter 25).

Gastrointestinal failure manifests with stress bleeds
requiring blood transfusion. Prophylactic neutralization
of gastric acid can minimize the risk of bleeding (see
Chapter 36).

TABLE 44–7
Delayed Sequelae of Multiple Trauma

Hematologic

Hemorrhage
Coagulopathy
DIC

Cardiac

Dysrhythmia
Heart failure
Ventricular aneurysm

Pulmonary

Atelectasis
Pneumonia
Emboli (fat or thrombotic)
ARDS

Gastrointestinal

Peritonitis
Adynamic ileus
Mechanical bowel obstruction
Anastomotic leak
Fistula
Bleeding

Hepatic

Liver abscess
Liver failure

Renal

Hypertension
Renal failure

Skin

Wound infection
Dehiscence
Skin breakdown

Systemic

Sepsis

DIC, disseminated intravascular coagulation; ARDS, adult
respiratory distress syndrome.

Heart failure usually is a late complication; however, the presence of a preexisting cardiac condition can predispose the multiple trauma victim to early-onset heart failure. Hypotension, decreased cardiac output, and decreased ejection fraction may be present (see Chapter 14).

Disseminated intravascular coagulation and central nervous system changes, ranging from confusion to obtundation, also may be evident in MOF (see Chapter 43).

Complications associated with multiple trauma are numerous (Table 44–7). Because most trauma patients are in the intensive care unit when these complications develop, the critical care nurse plays an essential role in detecting and preventing these sequelae.

The unexpected nature of trauma tends to amplify fear and anxiety. Therefore, nursing care also must provide psychosocial support for the seriously injured and their families through a multidisciplinary approach that recognizes concerns and offers frequent explanations.

CASE STUDY

A 31-year-old heavy equipment operator sustained blunt trauma when an industrial tire exploded and threw him 10 feet. He arrived unconscious in the emergency department with a blood pressure of 80/palpable and heart rate of 135 beats/minute. Multiple radiologic studies, a DPL, and exploratory surgery were performed. The following injuries were identified: epidural hematoma, multiple bilateral rib fractures (flail chest), right hemothorax, left pneumothorax, severe liver lacerations, bilateral forearm fractures, and an open fracture of the left tibia and fibula. Bilateral chest tubes were placed and the patient underwent surgery for evacuation of the epidural hematoma, packing of liver lacerations, and debridement of the open fracture. All fractures were externally stabilized.

After surgery, he was maintained on a mechanical ventilator with an FIO_2 of 0.40 to 0.45 and PEEP of 5 cm. Mechanical ventilation with PEEP promoted adequate lung expansion and stabilization of the flail chest. Parenteral nutritional support was initiated. Repeated blood transfusions were administered; however, the hematocrit and systolic blood pressure remained low (Hct = 20%–25%; SBP = 90 mm Hg). Continued internal bleeding necessitated a return to the operating room for debridement and repacking of the liver. By the next day, the bleeding had resolved. The packing was then removed, liver lacerations repaired, and drains placed.

The next day, signs and symptoms of sepsis developed in the patient, including elevated temperature and white blood cell count, tachycardia, tachypnea, increased cardiac output, decreased systemic vascular resistance, and decreased level of consciousness. Cultures were obtained and antibiotics begun. Adult respiratory distress syndrome and acute renal failure then developed, requiring increased ventilatory support and hemodialysis.

Intensive nursing care was necessary to manage the existing disorders and prevent further complications (see Nursing Care Plan 44–1). Psychosocial support for the patient and his family also was provided.

After a third surgical procedure to debride necrotic tissue and drain a perihepatic abscess, the patient finally began to improve. Several weeks later, dialysis and ventilatory support were discontinued. Two months after admission, the patient was transferred out of the intensive care unit, and 3 weeks later discharged home.

Nursing Care Plan

The nursing care plan that follows (Nursing Care Plan 44–1) must be individualized to meet the needs of each multiple-trauma patient.

NURSING CARE PLAN 44–1:
The Patient With Trauma

NURSING DIAGNOSIS	OUTCOME CRITERIA/ PATIENT GOALS	NURSING INTERVENTIONS
Fluid volume deficit: related to hemorrhage, third spacing.	• Maintain optimal fluid balance.	1. Replace volume, as ordered: crystalloids or colloids.
		2. Maintain patent IV line: central line preferred.
		3. Monitor BP, HR every hour or as indicated.
		4. Monitor urine output hourly.
		5. Assess hemodynamic parameters: PCWP, CVP, cardiac output.
		6. Weigh patient daily.

(continued)

NURSING CARE PLAN 44–1: (Continued)
The Patient With Trauma

NURSING DIAGNOSIS	OUTCOME CRITERIA/ PATIENT GOALS	NURSING INTERVENTIONS
		7. Administer oxygen as needed.
		8. Monitor electrolytes, CBC, coagulation factors.
		9. Assess type and amount of drainage: mark dressings if indicated.
		10. If indicated, prepare and ensure function of autotransfusion equipment.
		11. Prepare for surgery, as necessary.
Impaired gas exchange: related to pulmonary trauma, respiratory complications (eg, ARDS), pain.	• Maintain adequate oxygenation and normal acid–base balance.	1. Assess lung sounds, respirations, temperature, sensorium, CVP, arterial and mixed venous blood gases, compliance, airway pressures, WBC.
		2. Provide oxygen as needed.
		3. Turn, cough, deep breathe if patient is not mechanically ventilated.
		4. Consider rotation bed.
		5. Maintain mechanical ventilation, as ordered.
		6. Suction, tracheal lavage as necessary.
		7. Assist with chest radiograph, bronchoscopy as needed.
		8. Obtain cultures, as ordered.
		9. Administer mucolytics, bronchodilators, as ordered.
		10. Provide chest physiotherapy, postural drainage if not contraindicated.
		11. Promote pain control: assess effectiveness.
		12. Assist with intercostal block or epidural analgesia.
		13. Sedate, as ordered, to minimize oxygen requirements.
		14. Maintain and assist with placement of chest tubes.
		15. Prepare for tracheostomy if required for long-term ventilation.

(continued)

NURSING CARE PLAN 44–1: (Continued)
The Patient With Trauma

NURSING DIAGNOSIS	OUTCOME CRITERIA/ PATIENT GOALS	NURSING INTERVENTIONS
Impaired tissue integrity: related to trauma, surgery, invasive procedures, immobility.	• Existing wounds will heal and no new skin or tissue breakdown will occur.	1. Assess wound healing, skin, tissue integrity. 2. Turn, change position q2h. 3. Consider air bed. 4. Change dressings, as ordered. 5. Protect skin from irritating drainage. 6. Monitor gastric aspirate for acidity or bleeding. 7. Administer antacids, histamine antagonists, as ordered. 8. Promote adequate nutrition.
High risk for altered tissue perfusion: related to decreased cardiac output, decreased oxygenation, decreased gas exchange.	• Maintain adequate organ function.	1. Assess organ functioning: vital signs, urine output, sensorium, cardiac output, cardiac index. 2. Monitor arterial and mixed venous blood gases, oxygen delivery, oxygen consumption, shunting. 3. Monitor BUN, creatinine, bilirubin, and liver function tests. 4. Assess for jaundice. 5. Prepare for dialysis if necessary. 6. Administer inotropic agents as ordered. 7. Maintain optimal fluid balance. 8. Sedate patient, as ordered, to decrease metabolic requirements.
High risk for infection: related to trauma, invasive procedures.	• Patient will show no signs or symptoms of infection.	1. Assess vital signs, temperature, wounds, IV sites, drain sites. 2. Monitor WBCs. 3. Obtain cultures, as ordered. 4. Administer antibiotics, as ordered. 5. Change dressings, as ordered or per protocols. 6. Assist with IV line changes. 7. Maintain patency of drains. 8. Assess amount and type of drainage. 9. Monitor hemodynamics for signs of septic shock: BP, cardiac output, systemic vascular resistance.

(continued)

NURSING CARE PLAN 44–1: *(Continued)*
The Patient With Trauma

NURSING DIAGNOSIS	OUTCOME CRITERIA/ PATIENT GOALS	NURSING INTERVENTIONS
		10. Maintain adequate fluid balance, urine output, nutrition.
		11. Prepare for diagnostic studies, surgery as needed.
High risk for anxiety: related to critical illness, fear of death or disfigurement, role changes within social setting, or permanent disability.	• Patient will express anxieties to appropriate resource person.	1. Provide environment that encourages open discussion of emotional issues.
		2. Mobilize patient's support system and involve these resources as appropriate.
		3. Allow time for patient to express self.
		4. Identify possible hospital resources for patient/family support.
		5. Encourage open family-to-nurse communications regarding emotional issues.
		6. Validate patient and family knowledge base regarding the critical illness.
		7. Involve religious support systems as appropriate.

Summary

Caring for the multiply injured person is extremely challenging. Many trauma patients have injuries to more than one body system and most present with a unique combination of injuries. The critical care nurse must be able to integrate knowledge of organ systems and consider how they interrelate. Aggressive and knowledgeable nursing care plays a crucial role in decreasing mortality and morbidity in seriously injured patients.

REFERENCES

1. Rice D, MacKenzie E, et al: Cost of injury in the United States: A Report to Congress 1989. San Francisco, Institute For Health and Aging—University of California and Injury Prevention Center—Johns Hopkins University, 1989
2. PHTLS Committee of the National Association of Emergency Medical Technicians in cooperation with the Committee on Trauma of the American College of Surgeons: Pre-Hospital Trauma Life Support. Akron, OH, Emergency Training, 1990
3. Pons P: Multiple trauma. In Hamilton G, Sanders A, et al (eds): Emergency Medicine: An Approach to Clinical Problem-Solving, pp 60–79. Philadelphia, WB Saunders, 1991
4. Moore E, Mattox K, Feliciano D (eds): Trauma. Norwalk, CT, Appleton & Lange, 1991
5. Mancini M, Klein J (eds.): Decision Making in Trauma Management: A Multidisciplinary Approach. Philadelphia, BC Decker, 1991
6. Cilley J Jr, Mure A: Chest wall and pulmonary injuries. Topics in Emergency Medicine 12:45–52, 1990
7. Martinez R, Pepe P, et al: Blunt chest trauma: Early management. Patient Care 25:24–63, 1991
8. Luchtefeld W: Pulmonary contusion. Focus on Critical Care 17:482–488, 1990
9. Ruth-Sahd L: Pulmonary contusion: The hidden danger in blunt chest trauma. Critical Care Nurse 11:46–57, 1991
10. Lewis F Jr, Krupski W: Management of the injured patient. In Way L (ed): Current Surgical Diagnosis and Treatment, pp 212–234. Norwalk, CT, Appleton & Lange, 1991
11. DelRossi A, Talucci R: Penetrating cardiac injuries. Topics in Emergency Medicine 12:17–24, 1990

12. O'Malley K, Spence R: Emergency department initial evaluation and resuscitation in chest trauma. Topics in Emergency Medicine 12:7–15, 1990
13. Alexander J, Camishion R: Thoracic vascular trauma. Topics in Emergency Medicine 12:33–34, 1990
14. Nunn D: Thoracic great vessel injuries. Trauma Quarterly 7:53–61, 1991
15. McGarvey N, Indeck M: Epidemiology of liver trauma. Trauma Quarterly 7:22–26, 1991
16. Norkus G, Samin A, et al: Diagnosis, resuscitation, classification, and decision making. Trauma Quarterly 7:27–37, 1991
17. Gannon M: Packing for control of hemorrhage in severe liver injuries. Trauma Quarterly 7:48–56, 1991
18. Ives W, Indeck M: Drainage of liver injuries. Trauma Quarterly 7:57–63, 1991

BIBLIOGRAPHY

DelRossi A, Cernaianu A: Blunt cardiac trauma. Topics in Emergency Medicine 12:25–31, 1990
Dennis J: Diagnosis of vascular injuries: A clinician's perspective. Trauma Quarterly 7:23–28, 1991
Feliciano D: Missed extremity vascular injuries: Implications and consequences. Trauma Quarterly 7:37–41, 1991
Fink M, Helsmoortel C, et al: The efficacy of an oscillating bed in the prevention of lower respiratory tract infection in critically ill victims of blunt trauma. Chest 97:132–137, 1990
Frykberg E: The role of arteriography in penetrating proximity extremity trauma: Experience at the University of Florida. Trauma Quarterly 7:29–36, 1991
Hammond S: Chest injuries in the trauma patient. Nursing Clinics of North America 25:35–43, 1990
Hayes PG, Fallon W Jr: Evaluation priorities in the multiply injured patient with potential vascular injury. Trauma Quarterly 7:6–10, 1991
Ross S, Cernaianu A: Epidemiology of thoracic injuries: Mechanisms of injury and pathophysiology. Topics in Emergency Medicine 12:1–6, 1990
Rutledge R, Sheldon G: Abdominal trauma. In Nora P (ed): Operative Surgery: Principles and Techniques, pp 476–486. Philadelphia, WB Saunders, 1990
Satiani B: Extracavitary vascular trauma. Journal of Vascular Nursing 9(3):8–11, 1991
Vonfrolio L, Bacon K: Abdominal trauma. RN 54(6):30–34, 1991
Wilf LH, Vines F: Imaging techniques for vascular trauma. Trauma Quarterly 7:11–22, 1991

STUDY QUESTIONS

1. A 31-year-old man arrives in the emergency department with multiple injuries, including a massive right hemothorax. During which phase of care should chest tubes be inserted to treat the hemothorax?

   a. primary evaluation
   b. resuscitation
   c. secondary assessment
   d. definitive care

2. Nursing care of the patient with a flail chest may include all of the following actions *except*

   a. assisting the patient to cough and deep breathe
   b. administering pain medication
   c. taping rib fractures
   d. assessing oxygenation and gas exchange

3. Hemorrhage is most likely to occur after injury to

   a. the liver
   b. the small bowel
   c. the colon
   d. the stomach

4. Abdominal injuries can be diagnosed with

   a. an abdominal CT scan
   b. exploratory surgery
   c. a diagnostic peritoneal lavage
   d. all of the above

5. A multiple-trauma patient is in the critical care unit after repair of severe liver lacerations. The nurse should monitor the patient for

   a. incomplete hemostasis
   b. development of sepsis
   c. signs and symptoms of DIC
   d. all of the above

6. The two most serious complications associated with pelvic fractures are

   a. hemorrhage and sepsis
   b. fat emboli and hemorrhage
   c. decubitus ulcers and pelvic nerve damage
   d. muscle wasting and decubitus ulcers

7. Nursing responsibilities when caring for the multiple-trauma patient with a fracture may include

   a. maintaining skeletal traction
   b. wound and pin care
   c. assessment for signs and symptoms of compartment syndrome
   d. all of the above

8. The first manifestation of multiple organ failure usually is

   a. congestive heart failure
   b. ARDS
   c. DIC
   d. gastrointestinal bleeding

CHAPTER 45

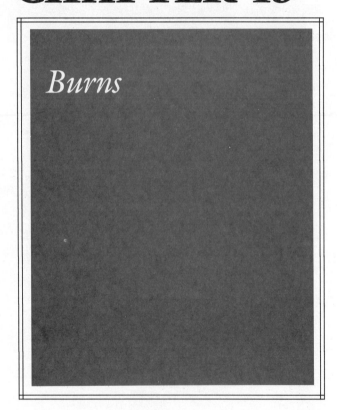

Burns

Hudak: Critical Care Nursing:
A Holistic Approach, 6th ed. © 1994
J. B. Lippincott Company.

BEHAVIORAL OBJECTIVES

Based on the content in this chapter, the reader should be able to:

1. Use a burn classification system.
2. Describe the major pathophysiological changes associated with burn injury.
3. Describe the major psychosocial changes associated with burn injury.
4. Define the phases of recovery after burn injury.
5. Identify the major clinical problems in each phase of recovery after burn injury.
6. State the rationale for specific management of major clinical problems in each phase of recovery after burn injury.
7. Develop a nursing care plan for the patient in each phase of recovery after burn injury.

Description

Burn injury is a serious problem in the United States. The United States ranks first in per capita fire deaths and property loss among the major industrialized nations, and has a rate nearly double that of second-ranked Canada.

People who suffer burn injury present one of the most challenging health care crises. A person who at one moment is well rapidly can become extensively burned. Concomitant with the dramatic physiological alterations is the emotional impact of burn injury, which affects both the burn victim and the family. Major advances have occurred in burn therapy since the early 1960s. The prognosis has changed from *expecting death* to *expecting life*.

Comprehensive nursing care given once burn injury occurs is vital to the prevention of death and disability. It is essential that the nurse have a clear understanding of the interrelated changes in all body systems after burn injury as well as an appreciation of the emotional impact of the injury on the burn victim and family. Only with such a comprehensive knowledge base can the nurse provide the therapeutic interventions necessary in all stages of recovery.

Pathophysiology

Burn injury affects all organ systems. The magnitude of this pathophysiological response is proportional to the extent of burn injury, and reaches a plateau when approximately 60% of the total body surface is burned.[1] Cardiovascular dynamics are affected significantly by burn injury, which can result in hypovolemic shock.

Hypovolemic Shock

The person sustaining major burn injury experiences a form of hypovolemic shock known as burn shock (Fig. 45–1). Immediately after thermal injury, a marked in-

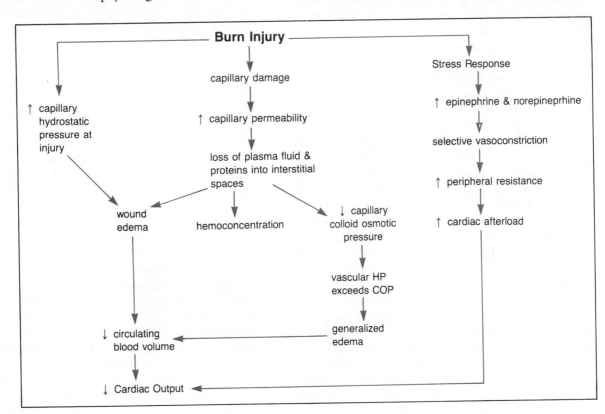

FIGURE 45–1
Fluid shifts in burn shock.

crease in capillary hydrostatic pressure occurs in the injured tissue, accompanied by an increase in capillary permeability. This results in a rapid shift of plasma fluid from the intravascular compartment across heat-damaged capillaries, into interstitial areas (resulting in edema) and to the burn wound itself. The loss of plasma fluid and proteins results in a decreased colloid osmotic pressure in the vascular compartment; hence, leakage of fluid and electrolytes from the vascular compartment continues and results in additional edema formation in the burned tissue and throughout the body.

This "leak," which consists of sodium, water, and plasma proteins, is followed by a decrease in cardiac output, hemoconcentration of red blood cells, diminished perfusion to major organs, and generalized body edema. The pathophysiological response after burn injury is biphasic. In the early postinjury phase, generalized organ hypofunction (ebb phase) develops as a consequence of decreased cardiac output. Peripheral vascular resistance increases as a result of the neurohumoral stress response after trauma. This increases cardiac afterload, resulting in a further decrease in cardiac output. The increase in peripheral vascular resistance (selective vasoconstriction), as well as the hemoconcentration resulting from plasma fluid loss, may cause the blood pressure to appear normal at first; however, if fluid replacement is inadequate, and plasma protein loss continues, hypovolemic shock soon occurs.[1-3]

In patients receiving adequate fluid resuscitation, the cardiac output usually returns to normal in the later part of the first 24 hours after burn injury. As plasma volume is replenished during the second 24 hours, the cardiac output increases to hypermetabolic levels (hyperfunction phase), and slowly returns to more normal levels as the burn wounds are closed.

In some instances, with burns exceeding 60% total body surface area (TBSA), depressed cardiac output does not respond to aggressive volume resuscitation. Some investigators have attributed this depressed cardiac performance to a circulating myocardial depressant factor; however, this factor has not been isolated, and the concept has been challenged.[1]

The response of the pulmonary vasculature is like that of the peripheral circulation; however, pulmonary vascular resistance is greater and lasts longer. Immediately after burn injury, the patient may experience a mild, transient pulmonary hypertension. A decrease in oxygen tension and lung compliance also may be evident.

The loss of fluid throughout the body's intravascular space results in a thickened, sluggish flow of the remaining circulatory blood volume. The effects reach all body systems. This slowing of circulation permits bacteria and cellular material to settle in the lower portions of blood vessels, especially in the capillaries, resulting in sludging. The antigen–antibody reaction to burned tissue adds to the circulatory congestion by the clumping or aggluti-

nation of cells. Coagulation problems occur as a result of the release of thromboplastin by the injury itself and the release of fibrinogen from injured platelets. If thrombi occur, they may cause ischemia of the affected part and lead to necrosis. The increased coagulation process may develop into disseminated intravascular coagulation. Because this is a widespread occurrence, any organ in the body may be involved, and organ failure may occur.

Classification of Burn Injury

Burn injuries are described by depth, causative agent, and severity. The nurse must have an understanding of the basic structure and functions of the skin to appreciate the classification of the various degrees of burn injury (Fig. 45–2). The skin is the largest organ of the body, and it performs several complex functions. It is the body's first line of defense against invasion by microorganisms and environmental radiation. It prevents loss of body fluids, controls body temperature, functions as an excretory and sensory organ, produces vitamin D, and influences body image.

Burn Depth

Damage to the skin frequently is described according to the depth of injury and is defined in terms of partial-thickness and full-thickness injuries, which correspond to the various layers of the skin (Table 45–1).

Partial-Thickness Burns

Partial-thickness burns are differentiated into superficial and deep partial-thickness burns. *Superficial partial-thickness burns* (ie, first-degree burns) damage the epidermis, which is the thin layer of epithelial cells that continuously is being replaced. This keratinized layer provides a protective wall between the host and the environment. A sunburn is a familiar example of a superficial partial-thickness injury. It feels painful at first and later itches due to the stimulation of sensory receptors. Because the epithelial cells of the epidermis continuously are being replaced, this type of injury will heal spontaneously without scarring.

Deep partial-thickness injuries (ie, a second-degree burns) involve varying degrees of the dermal layer. The dermis contains structures essential to normal skin function: sweat and sebaceous glands, sensory and motor nerves, capillaries, and hair follicles. A deep partial-thickness burn will be pinkish-red and painful, and it will form blisters and subcutaneous edema. Depending on the depth, these wounds will heal spontaneously in 3 to 35 days as the epidermal elements germinate and migrate until the epidermal surface is restored. If the wound be-

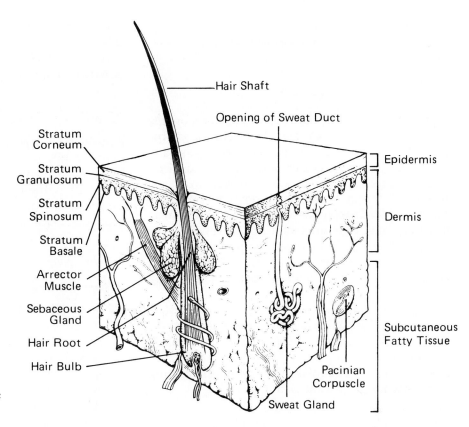

FIGURE 45–2
A three-dimensional view of the skin.

TABLE 45–1
Characteristics of Burns of Various Depths

Depth	Tissues Involved	Usual Cause	Characteristics	Pain	Healing
Superficial partial-thickness (first degree)	Minimal epithelial damage	Sun	Dry No blisters Pinkish red Blanches with pressure	Painful	About 5 days
Superficial partial-thickness (second degree)	Epidermis, minimal dermis	Flash Hot liquids	Moist Pinkish or mottled red Blisters Some blanching	Pain Hyperesthetic	About 21 days, minimal scarring
Deep dermal partial-thickness (second degree)	Entire epidermis, part of dermis, epidermal-lined hair and sweat glands intact	Above plus hot solids, flame, and intense radiant injury	Dry, pale, waxy No blanching	Sensitive to pressure	Prolonged; late hypertrophic scarring; marked contracture formation
Full-thickness (third degree)	All of above, and portion of subcutaneous fat; may involve connective tissue, muscle, bone	Sustained flame, electrical, chemical, and steam	Leathery, cracked avascular, pale yellow to brown to charred	Little pain	Cannot self-regenerate; needs grafting

From Burgess C: Initial management of a patient with extensive burn injury. *Critical Care Nursing Clinics of North America* 3(2):167, 1991.

comes infected or traumatized or if the blood supply is compromised, these burns will develop into full-thickness burns.

Full-Thickness Burns

Full-thickness burns (ie, third-degree burns) expose the fat layer, which is composed of poorly vascularized adipose tissue. This layer contains the roots of the sweat glands and hair follicles. All epidermal elements are destroyed. These burns may appear white, red, brown, or black. Reddened areas do not blanch in response to pressure because the underlying blood supply has been interrupted. Brownish streaks are evidence of thrombosed blood vessels.

These burns are completely anesthetic because the sensory receptors have been totally destroyed. In addition, they may appear sunken because of the loss of underlying fat and muscle.

The small wound (<4 cm) may be allowed to heal by granulation and migration of healthy epithelium from the wound margins. Extensive, open full-thickness wounds leave the patient highly susceptible to overwhelming infection and malnutrition. Wound closure by skin grafting restores the integrity of the skin.

Causative Agent

Burns also may be classified according to the agent causing the injury:

- Thermal (scald, contact, and flame injuries)
- Electrical
- Chemical
- Radiation

The extent and depth of burn injury are related to the intensity and duration of exposure to the causative agent.

Severity of Burn

A burn injury may range from a small blister to massive third-degree burns. Recognizing the need for a clear description of terms, the American Burn Association developed the Injury Severity Grading System, which is used to determine the magnitude of the burn injury and to provide optimal criteria for hospital resources for patient care. Burn injury has been categorized into minor, moderate, and major burns.

Minor Burn Injury

A *minor* burn injury is a partial-thickness injury of less than 15% TBSA in adults or 10% TBSA in children, or a full-thickness injury of less than 2% TBSA that is not associated with any complications. Patients with these

injuries may be treated in a hospital emergency room and followed on an outpatient basis, but they must be seen every 48 hours until the risk of infection decreases, and wound healing is underway.

Moderate Uncomplicated Burn Injury

A *moderate uncomplicated* burn injury is a partial-thickness injury of 15% to 25% TBSA in adults or 10% to 20% TBSA in children, or a full-thickness injury of less than 10% TBSA that is not associated with complications. These patients can be treated in an average hospital with appropriate facilities and personnel.

Major Burn Injury

A *major* burn injury is any of the following:

- A partial-thickness injury of more than 25% TBSA in adults or 20% in children
- A full-thickness injury of 10% or greater TBSA
- A burn involving the hands, face, eyes, ears, feet, and perineum
- An inhalation injury
- An electrical injury
- A burn associated with extenuating problems, such as a soft tissue injury, fractures, other trauma, or preexisting health problems

Patients with these injuries should be cared for in a burn unit or a burn center.

Assessment

Assessing the Burn Injury

The extent and depth of the burn as well as the time and circumstances surrounding the burn injury are vital data that must be communicated to the burn facility before transfer.

To assess the severity of the burn, several factors must be considered:

- The percentage of body surface area (BSA) burned
- The depth of the burn
- The anatomic location of the burn
- Inhalation injury
- The age of the person
- Medical history
- Concomitant injury

Burn Area Size

Several rules are available for estimating the extent of a burn in percentages of the total body surface. The "rule of nines" divides the body parts into multiples of 9% (Fig.

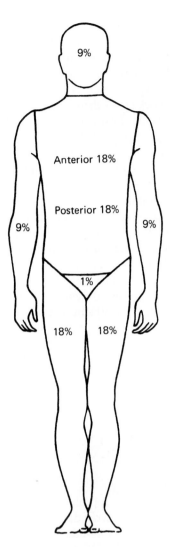

FIGURE 45-3
The "rule of nines" method for determining percentage of body area with burn injury.

45-3). The head is considered to account for 9% of TBSA, each arm for 9%, each leg 18%, the anterior trunk for 18%, the posterior trunk for 18%, and the perineum for 1%, making a total of 100%. It is important to remember that burns may either be circumferential or involve only one surface of a body part. A circumferential burn of an arm is 9%, whereas if only the anterior surface were burned, the value would be 4.5%.

Although the rule of nines is the most common method used for estimating burn area size, Berkow's method is more accurate, particularly for infants and children, because it accounts for proportionate growth. The extent of small scattered burns can be estimated by comparing the size of the nurse's hand to the patient's hand. Allowing for differences, the comparison will indicate that the palmar surface of an adult's hand equals approximately 1% of an adult's TBSA.

Burn Depth

Burn classifications are based on the tissues involved (as discussed previously) or classified as first-, second- (superficial or deep), and third-degree burns (see Table 45-1).

Anatomic Location

The location of the burn is important to healing and general rehabilitation. Burns of the face, head, neck, hands, feet, and genitalia create particular problems. Although they may be limited in surface area, these burns usually require hospitalization of the injured person and special care because they are important areas where rapid, uninfected healing with minimal scarring is desired. Facial burns may involve edema and present problems with airway management. Burns of the head that involve the external ear and burns of the hands that involve the distal phalanges are particularly difficult to heal because these structures are primarily composed of cartilage, which lacks a good blood supply. Perineal burns are difficult, if not impossible, to keep from becoming infected. Edema also can be a problem, and the patients need to be catheterized as soon as possible.

If burns in any of these special areas do not heal well, serious psychosocial and economic problems related to appearance, self-concept, manual dexterity, and locomotion can occur.

Inhalation Injury

Location of the burn also can alert staff to possible inhalation injury. The nurse should assess for these findings:

- Singed nasal hairs
- Burns of the oral or pharyngeal mucous membranes
- Burns in the perioral area or neck
- Coughing up of soot or change in voice
- History of being burned in a confined area

Patient's Age

Although burns occur in all age groups, the incidence is higher at both ends of the age continuum. People younger than age 2 and older than age 60 have a higher mortality than other age groups with burns of similar severity. A child younger than age 2 is more susceptible to infection because of the immature immune response. The older person may have degenerative processes that complicate recovery and that may be aggravated by the stress of the burn. As a general rule, children with burns of 10% or more and all adults whose injuries account for 12% to 15% or more of TBSA will require hospitalization.

Medical History

It is important to determine whether the patient has a disease that compromises the ability to manage fluid shifts and resist infection (eg, diabetes mellitus, congestive heart failure, cirrhosis) or if renal, respiratory, or gastrointestinal problems are present. Some problems, such as diabetes and renal failure, may become acute during the burn process. If inhalation injury has occurred in the presence of cardiopulmonary disease (eg, congestive heart failure, emphysema), the respiratory status is compromised tremendously.

Concomitant Injuries

It is important to obtain a brief history from the patient and check for concurrent injuries. Burn patients usually are awake and alert, so any changes in neurologic status usually indicate other injury, such as anoxia, head injury, drug use or intoxication, hypoglycemia, or myocardial infarction. Burn wounds do not bleed; therefore, any external bleeding indicates lacerations of deeper structures. Extremities should be assessed for fractures.

Clinical Manifestations and Diagnostic Findings

Inhalation Injury

When the burn is caused by a flame, or the person was burned in a confined area, or both, look for signs of carbon monoxide poisoning, smoke inhalation, and the accompanying signs of respiratory distress and pulmonary injury.

Carbon Monoxide Poisoning

Often, the burn patient has been trapped in a burning building and has inhaled significant amounts of carbon monoxide. Characteristic physical signs usually are not present, and the hallmark cherry red skin color almost is never observed in burn patients. Central nervous system manifestations of carbon monoxide poisoning may range from headache to coma to death (see Table 46–5).

The diagnosis is made by direct determination of carboxyhemaglobin levels by spectrophotometry. Carboxyhemoglobin concentrations should be measured in all fire victims. Before central nervous system abnormalities are attributed to carbon monoxide poisoning, other potentially fatal diseases sometimes present in thermally injured people must be investigated. Conditions clinically similar to carbon monoxide poisoning in thermally injured people include acute drug overdose, uncontrolled diabetes, acute alcohol intoxication, acute head injury, acute psychotic reaction, insulin overdose, and hypovolemic or septic shock.

Respiratory Distress

A decreased arterial oxygenation often is seen after burn injury. Although the exact mechanism is unknown, restoration of cardiac output improves oxygenation. Hence, this decreased oxygenation may be related to poor tissue perfusion and shock rather than airway obstruction. Therefore, a falling arterial PO_2 may indicate either an airway obstruction or declining left heart output.

The immediate cause of respiratory distress often is laryngeal edema or spasm and the accumulation of mucus. Because actual signs of obstruction may not become apparent for several hours, it is necessary to monitor the patient continuously for hoarseness, drooling, or inability to handle secretions. Hoarseness indicates a significant decrease in the diameter of the airway. The edema may continue to develop for 72 hours, and endotracheal intubation or tracheostomy may be indicated. Because airway obstruction due to laryngeal edema subsides within 3 to 5 days, endotracheal or nasotracheal intubation is preferable to a tracheostomy.

Signs of Respiratory Distress

- Hoarseness
- Drooling
- Inability to handle secretions

Pulmonary Injury

Inhalation injury usually appears within the first 24 to 48 hours postburn and is secondary to the inhalation of combustible products; it is not the result of thermal injury because most heat is dissipated at the level of the distal trachea. Most commonly, especially in closed-space injuries, inhalation of the products of incomplete combustion results in a chemical pneumonitis. Inflammatory changes occur during the first 24 hours postburn. The pulmonary tree becomes irritated and edematous; however, changes may not become apparent until the second 24 hours. Pulmonary edema is a possibility any time from the first few hours to 7 days after the injury. The patient may be irrational or even unconscious, depending on the degree of hypoxia.

Signs of Inhalation Injury

- Rapid or labored breathing
- Crackles
- Stridor
- Hacking cough

Serial arterial blood gases will show a falling PO_2. Usually, the admission chest film will appear normal because changes are not reflected until 24 to 48 hours post-burn. A sputum specimen should be obtained for culture and sensitivity studies. Laryngoscopy and bronchoscopy may be of value in determining the presence of extra-mucosal carbonaceous material (the most reliable sign of inhalation injury) and the state of the mucosa (blistering, edema, erythema), which may have an effect on bronchospasm, atelectasis, hypoxemia, and pulmonary edema.

More specific confirmation of inhalation injury is achieved with the use of fiberoptic bronchoscopy, which permits direct examination of the proximal airway, and xenon-133 scintigraphy. Xenon-133 ventilation–perfusion scanning is helpful in establishing a diagnosis of injury to small airways and lung parenchyma.[1]

Pulmonary damage, primarily as a result of inhalation, accounts for 20% to 84% of burn mortality. The three stages of injury that have been described are:

1. Acute pulmonary insufficiency—may occur during the first 36 hours
2. Pulmonary edema—occurs in 5% to 30% of burn patients between 6 and 72 hours after burn
3. Bronchopneumonia—appears in 15% to 60% of burn patients 3 to 10 days after burn

Hematologic Manifestations

The hematologic signs associated with major thermal injury are varied. Initially, the hematocrit increases secondary to capillary leak and loss of circulating plasma volume. The hematocrit usually reaches 50% to 70% and remains elevated until plasma volume is restored.

During the initial burn period, 8% to 19% of the circulating red blood cells are hemolyzed by the effects of heat as they pass through the burned area at the time of injury. The survival time of other red cells is shortened by the burn injury, resulting in an additional 10% to 25% loss of circulating red blood cells. Still other red cells are trapped in engorged capillaries and are unavailable to the general circulation. Some small amount of blood loss occurs initially at the burn site; additional blood loss is slow and constant as debridements proceed. A unit of blood is lost every 3 to 4 days in adults with over 40% TBSA burns. The burn-injured patient therefore needs frequent transfusions to maintain blood volume, correct anemia, and maintain hematocrit between 35% and 40%.

The leukocyte count may be high initially, due to hemoconcentration. If leukocytosis persists after a week, it usually indicates infection by a gram-positive organism, often *Staphylococcus aureus*.

During the resuscitative phase, platelet destruction is accelerated, resulting in a progressive thrombocytopenia. After the fifth day postburn, platelet levels return to normal or elevated levels.

As a result of increased platelet adhesiveness, increased blood viscosity, and the release of thromboplastin and

Findings:
- ↑ Hematocrit
- ↓ RBCs
- ↑ Leukocytes
- ↓ Thrombocytes

fibrinogen, clotting factors V and VIII are elevated, and thrombin times are prolonged.

Electrolytes

Electrolyte concentrations are altered not only from the leaking process but also from direct injury to burned cells. Chemical changes are due to shifts in the composition of various fluids as they move from one body compartment to another. Electrolyte studies at first show an increase in serum potassium because of intracellular potassium release secondary to cell injury. The intracellular potassium is replaced by sodium, and therefore normal cellular function is impaired.

After approximately 48 hours, the capillary walls have healed sufficiently to stop the fluid shift from the vascular tree. Fluid is then drawn back into the blood vessels, edema subsides, the plasma volume expands, and diuresis begins. At this time, large amounts of potassium are lost, and replacement may be necessary. In severe burns, the alterations in potassium levels must be monitored carefully to avoid cardiac failure.

The plasma level of both sodium and chloride is normal or slightly elevated at first but increases rapidly as excessive interstitial fluid is reabsorbed. The blood urea nitrogen may be elevated if excessive protein catabolism occurred. Blood glucose levels may be increased temporarily as a result of the action of epinephrine, which is released in reaction to the stress of the burn injury. The epinephrine acts on amino acids to produce glucose (gluconeogenesis), which the patient requires to meet the body's demands during stress.

Findings:
- ↓ K
- ↑ Na, chloride
- ↑ BUN

Renal

Urinary output decreases due to hypotension, decreased renal blood flow, and secretion of antidiuretic hormone and aldosterone. Unless fluid resuscitation measures are taken promptly and appropriately, poor tissue perfusion can result in renal shutdown. As erythrocytes are damaged by thermal injury, they release free hemoglobin; damaged muscle tissue releases myoglobin. As the free hemoglobin and myoglobin pass through the kidney, they are excreted into the urine. If these substances block the nephrons, renal failure may develop.

Findings:

• ↑ Urinary output
• Myoglobinuria

Specialized protocols for treatment of myoglobinuria have been developed. The common features of these formulas are maintenance of a high urine output and alkalinization of the urine to avoid precipitation of myoglobin or hemochromogens and subsequent acute renal failure. Myoglobinuria in the thermally injured patient cannot be treated in isolation. Overall volume deficits must be corrected and renal perfusion optimized before osmotic or loop diuretics are given.

Metabolic

The stress response elicited by burn injury (or trauma of any kind) promotes a set of physiological responses characterized by increased energy expenditure and elevated nutritional requirements. Hypermetabolism, increased glucose flow, and severe protein and fat wasting are characteristic responses to trauma and infection. In no other disease state is this response as severe as it is after thermal injury (see Chapter 35). The metabolic rate of people with burns covering more than 40% TBSA often is twice normal. This hypermetabolic state peaks between days 7 and 17 postburn. Increased oxygen consumption, metabolic rate, urinary excretion, fat breakdown, and steady erosion of body mass are related directly to burn size and return to normal as the burn wound heals or is covered.

Patients with greater than 40% TBSA burns, who have been treated vigorously with oral alimentation, have been shown to lose 25% of their preadmission weight by 3 weeks postinjury. This rapid weight loss alone can be fatal. Only recently, with the use of enteral and parenteral hy-

---

Findings:

• Hypermetabolism
• Weight loss

---

peralimentation, has it been possible to deliver sufficient exogenous energy to prevent postburn weight loss.

Management

The Resuscitative Phase

Initial Care at the Scene

The first priority at the scene of injury is to stop the burning process and to prevent self-injury. Flames should be extinguished with water or smothered with a blanket, or the victim should be rolled on the ground. Smoldering clothing, constricting clothing, belts, and jewelry should be removed before swelling begins. Clothing and jewelry retain heat and may cause burns to progress into deeper tissues.

In a chemical injury, all clothing should be removed and the wound should be flushed with copious amounts of water. In the event of an electrical injury, the victim should be removed from the current with a nonconducting object to ensure safety of the rescuer.[2]

Care in the Emergency Department

If intravenous cannulation was not initiated in the field, a large-bore cannula should be inserted in a peripheral vein or a central line should be started. All patients with burns greater than 20% to 30% TBSA should have an indwelling catheter inserted for accurate urinary output measurements. A nasogastric tube should be inserted in all patients at risk for paralytic ileus (burns greater than 25% TBSA). If inhalation injury or carbon monoxide poisoning are suspected, humidified 100% oxygen should be administered.

A tetanus toxoid booster should be administered if the patient has been immunized previously but has not received tetanus toxoid within the past 5 years. If a tetanus immunization history is unknown, the patient should receive 250 units of human tetanus-immune globulin and the first of a series of active immunizations with tetanus toxoid.

The patient should be covered with a nonadherent, nonfuzzy cover. Additional blankets can be added as needed to provide warmth and to prevent hypothermia. Burn patients chill easily because they have lost their skin's protection against temperature changes. Covers also guard the wound against contamination and ease the pain caused by air currents. Cool, sterile water or saline may be applied to the burn to ease the pain; however, it is important to guard against hypothermia and tissue damage. Ice or ice water should not be used because extreme cold can cause further tissue damage.

Nursing responsibilities include monitoring for inhalation injury, monitoring fluid resuscitation, assessing the burn wound, monitoring vital signs, obtaining an accurate history, and carrying out emergency measures.

Care in the Critical Care Unit

The critical care nurse plays an essential role in caring for the burn patient and family (see Nursing Care Plan 45–1).

Fluid Resuscitation

Fluid resuscitation is the primary intervention in this phase. Figure 45–4 shows a decision tree for the initial fluid management.

The goals for this phase of care are to:

- Correct fluid, electrolyte, and protein deficits
- Replace continuing losses and maintain fluid balance
- Prevent excessive edema formation
- Maintain a urine output in adults of 30 to 70 ml/ hour

Formulas for Fluid Administration. Numerous formulas have been developed for fluid resuscitation, each with advantages and disadvantages. They differ primarily in terms of recommended volume administration and salt content (Table 45–2). In general, rigorous replacement of lost crystalloid and colloid solutions must be made. Free water, given as 5% dextrose/water (D5W) with or without added electrolytes, is regulated so that insensible fluid loss is covered. Ringer's lactate is used as the crystalloid solu-

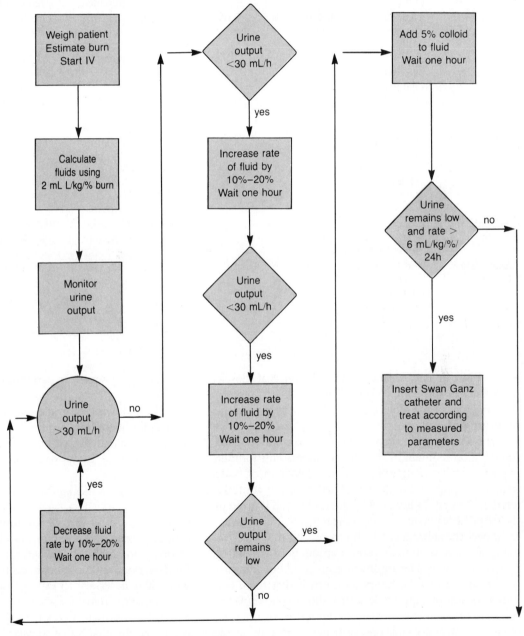

FIGURE 45–4
Initial 24-hour fluid management. (From Rue LW, Cioffi WG: Resuscitation of thermally injured patients. Critical Care Nursing Clinics of North America 3(2):186, 1991)

TABLE 45–2
Formulas for Fluid Replacement/Resuscitation

	First 24 Hours			Second 24 Hours		
	Electrolyte	Colloid	Glucose in Water	Electrolyte	Colloid	Glucose in Water
Burn budget of F.D. Moore	1,000–4,000 ml lactated Ringer's and 1,200 ml 0.5N saline	7.5% of body weight	1,500–5,000 ml	1,000–4,000 ml lactated Ringer's and 1200 ml 0.5N saline	2.5% of body weight	1,500–5,000 ml
Evans	Normal saline, 1 ml/kg/% burn	1.0 ml/kg/% burn	2,000 ml	One-half of first–24-hr requirement	One-half of first-hour requirement	2,000 ml
Brooke	Lactated Ringer's, 1.5 ml/kg/% burn	0.5 ml/kg/% burn	2,000 ml	One-half to three-quarters of first–24-hr requirement	One-half of three-quarters of first–24-hr requirement	2,000 ml
Parkland	Lactated Ringer's 4 ml/kg/% burn				20%–60% of calculated plasma volume	
Hypertonic sodium solution	Volume to maintain urine output at 30 ml/hr (fluid contains 250 mEq Na/liter)			One-third of salt solution orally, up to 3,500 ml limit		
Modified Brooke	Lactated Ringer's 2 ml/kg/% burn				0.3–0.5 ml/kg/% burn	Goal: maintain adequate urinary output
Burnett Burn Center	Isotonic or hypertonic alkaline sodium solution/% burn/kg			$n_{51/4}$ NS maintenance	Colloid 0.5 ml/% burn/kg	D_5W (% burn) (TBSAm^2)

tion because it is a balanced salt solution that closely approximates the composition of extracellular fluid. In addition, it has large molecules, which serve to expand the circulating plasma volume.

The Parkland formula is the most commonly used resuscitation regimen in the United States. This formula requires 4 ml of Ringer's lactate per kilogram of body weight per percent TBSA burn. This amount is administered in the first 24 hours postinjury. One half is given in the first 8 hours postinjury, and the remainder is administered over the subsequent 16 hours postburn. Other formulas advocated contain various amounts of colloid or hypertonic saline. The argument against colloid administration in the first 12 hours postburn is that there is a diffuse postburn capillary leak that allows colloids to extravasate through endothelial junctions, thereby not producing any demonstrable oncotic benefit over administration of a crystalloid. Hypertonic saline resuscitation lowers the amount of fluid that need be given to selected patients, but can cause severe hypernatremia and must be used cautiously.

The following example may help illustrate the very large amounts of fluid required. The Baxter, or Parkland, formula for a patient weighting 75 kg who received burns over 50% of the body would be stated as follows:

$$4 \text{ ml} \times 75 \text{ kg} \times 50\% = 15,000 \text{ ml}$$

Of this, 7,500 ml is to be administered during the first 8-hour period, and 3,750 ml is to be administered in the second and third 8-hour periods. Hence, avoidance of fluid overload and pulmonary edema is extremely difficult when it is necessary to infuse fluids so rapidly. Consequently, digoxin may be given to severely burned patients to induce maximal function of the left ventricle and to minimize the chances of transient increases in left atrial pressure. Isoproterenol infusions may be used for symptoms of decreased cardiac output.

The time postinjury at which capillary integrity is restored varies among individuals, but usually is between 12 and 14 hours. Many physicians administer colloids at this point to restore albumin levels to 2.0 to 3.0 mg/dl. Controversy exists over the type of colloid to be administered, with some centers using salt-poor albumin and others fresh frozen plasma.

Nonprotein collagens may be used in burn shock resuscitation. Dextran and hetastarch are high-molecular-weight solutions that generate colloid osmotic pressure when given intravascularly. Allergic responses have been reported with dextran, but the risk virtually is eliminated by pretreatment with Promit, a very-low-molecular-weight dextran.[3]

After the first 24 hours postinjury, replacing the massive evaporative water loss is a major consideration in fluid management. The primary solution given at this time is D5W, with the goal of keeping the patient's sodium concentration at 140 mEq/L.

Monitoring Fluid Replacement. Resuscitation formulas are considered approximations, and the patient's urine output and blood pressure must be monitored hourly to evaluate response to treatment. Urine output is the single best indicator of fluid resuscitation in patients with previously normal renal function. Central lines and Swan–Ganz catheters are not inserted routinely owing to the danger of sepsis; however, they are used in selected instances (see Figure 45–4).

Adequacy of fluid replacement is judged clinically for adults by a urinary output of 30 to 70 ml/hour, pulse rate below 120, blood pressure in normal to high ranges, central venous pressure readings less than 12 cm H_2O or a pulmonary capillary wedge pressure reading below 18 mm Hg, clear sensorium and clear lung sounds, and the absence of intestinal symptoms such as nausea and paralytic ileus. Patients usually are weighed daily. A gain of 15% of admission weight may be expected. Intake and output must be monitored meticulously.

The onset of spontaneous diuresis is a hallmark indicating the end of the resuscitative phase. Infusion rates can

be decreased by 25% for 1 hour if the urine output is satisfactory and can be maintained for 2 hours; the reduction then can be repeated. It is essential that urinary outputs be maintained in normal limits (50–70 ml/hour).

Patients who sustain deep muscle injury (ie, second- or third-degree burns) are at risk for development of acute renal insufficiency. This renal dysfunction may be the result of inadequate fluid resuscitation or it may be the consequence of the liberation of the myoglobin and hemoglobin from damaged cells. These compounds, sometimes referred to as hemochromogens, may precipitate in renal tubules, resulting in acute tubular necrosis. Hemochromogens produce a clear reddish-brown color in the urine. Should hemochromogens appear in the urine, acidosis should be corrected promptly and intravenous fluids increased to maintain a brisk urine output until the urine returns to its normal clear yellow color.

Inhalation Injury

The goals in treating inhalation injury are to:

- Improve oxygenation
- Decrease interstitial edema and airway occlusion

The conventional treatment of inhalation injury is largely supportive. Humidified oxygen is administered to prevent drying and sloughing of the mucosa. Upper airway edema peaks at 24 to 48 hours after injury. If the injury is mild or moderately severe, administration of aerosolized racemic epinephrine along with high Fowler's position may be sufficient to limit further edema formation. Severe upper airway obstruction may require endotracheal intubation to protect the airway until the edema subsides.

In patients with mild tracheobronchial injury, atelectasis may be prevented by frequent pulmonary toilet, including a high Fowler's position, coughing and deep breathing, chest physiotherapy, repositioning, frequent tracheal suctioning, and incentive spirometry. More severe inhalation injury requires more frequent suctioning and possible bronchoscopic removal of debris. These patients usually require endotracheal intubation and mechanical ventilatory support. Patients with bronchospasm should be treated with aerosolized or intravenously administered bronchodilators. Respiratory parameters should be monitored closely and extreme attention paid to breath sounds and vital signs so that fluid overload can be detected as early as possible.

Bronchopneumonia may be superimposed on other respiratory problems at any time, and it may be hematogenous or airborne. Airborne bronchopneumonia is most common, with an onset occurring soon after injury. It often is associated with a lower airway injury or aspiration. Hematogenous, or miliary, pneumonia begins as a bacterial abscess secondary to another septic source, usually the burn wound. The time of onset usually is 2 weeks after injury.

Clinical Manifestations of Adequate Fluid Replacement

Blood pressure	Normal to high ranges
Pulse rate	<120
CVP	<12 cm H_2O
PCWP	<18 mm Hg
Urinary output	30–70 ml/hr
Lungs	Clear
Sensorium	Clear
GI tract	Absence of nausea and paralytic ileus

Prophylactic antibiotics and steroids have not been demonstrated to prevent the common complications of infection encountered in patients with inhalation injury. New avenues of investigation, designed to decrease the incidence of nosocomial pneumonia in critically ill patients, include the selective decontamination of the oro-digestive tract and the use of sucralfate for stress ulcer prophylaxis.

Tissue Perfusion

Another area of concern during the resuscitative phase is tissue perfusion. With tissue injury, vessels are damaged and thrombosed. Adjacent intact vessels soon dilate, and platelets and leukocytes adhere to the vascular endothelium, resulting in eschar formation. The underlying tissues swell, but the area of a circumferential full-thickness burn is inelastic and remains contracted. The area acts like a tourniquet. An unyielding eschar contributes to a compromised vascular state with ischemic necrosis, which may eventually necessitate amputation. It is vital, therefore, that the nurse monitor tissue perfusion hourly by checking for capillary refill, neurologic changes, temperature and color of the skin, and the presence of peripheral pulses. An ultrasonic flowmeter often is useful in assessing for peripheral pulses. Pulse oximetry may be used to monitor the vascular status of extremities to identify the need for escharotomy.[3] Extremities should be elevated and put through passive range of motion at least 5 minutes per hour to prevent edema and mobilize that which does accumulate.

Escharotomy. Although elevation decreases the edema, escharotomy often is necessary. An escharotomy is an incision through the entire thickness of the eschar that allows underlying viable edematous tissues to expand, thereby restoring adequate tissue perfusion. An escharotomy is made in the midlateral or midmedial line of the involved extremity (Fig. 45–5). The procedure is performed at the bedside, and does not require local anesthesia. The escharotomy site is covered with a topical agent because viable tissue is exposed, and a light dressing may be applied.

Only rarely are fasciotomies necessary to restore peripheral perfusion. Usually, this procedure is necessary only in the setting of high-voltage electrical current or concomitant crush injury. Fasciotomies would be undertaken in the operating room under general anesthesia.

Gastrointestinal Symptoms

Because of the risk of paralytic ileus and gastric distention, the patient should receive no oral fluid or nutrition. If a nasogastric tube is not already in place, one should be inserted if distention or nausea occur. Gastric drainage initially may contain some blood. Therefore, observe the amount and type of drainage to ensure that the quantity of blood subsides.

The formation of gastroduodenal ulcers, also known as Curling's ulcers, used to be a major complication in

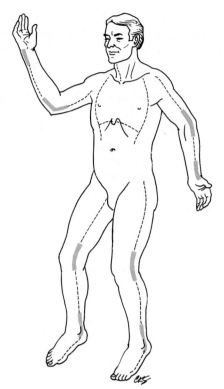

FIGURE 45–5
Preferred sites of escharotomy incisions.

burn patients. This complication now is preventable with the prophylactic administration of H2 histamine receptor antagonists and antacids. H2 histamine receptor antagonists (eg, cimetidine) are given orally or intravenously every 4 hours. Antacids are administered every 2 hours to titrate the gastric pH above 5.

Immobility

Because the burn victim is particularly susceptible to the hazards of immobility, proper body alignment and pressure relief are essential. Decubitus ulcers may develop quickly. Therefore, the patient may be placed on a pressure-relief mattress or in a special pressure-relief bed. Endotracheal and nasogastric tubes should be secured midline in the nares to prevent erosion of the nasal septum or alae. Range-of-motion exercises should be performed for 5 minutes every hour to prevent contractures and reduce edema.

Wound Care

Once hemodynamic and pulmonary stability have been achieved, attention is directed toward initial care of the burn wound. The wound should be cleaned with a surgical detergent disinfectant, gently debrided, and body hair shaved form the wound and around the wound periphery. The wound should then be covered with a topical antimicrobial agent. Owing to alterations in the immune system, protective isolation measures should be instituted.

Pain

Burn injuries are one of the most painful forms of trauma a person can experience, and pain management is a major challenge for the critical care nurse. The degree of pain experienced by patients in both the resuscitative and acute phases of care is influenced by the depth of the injury, the patient's anxiety level, and the number of invasive monitoring and wound care procedures required.

As the protective layers of the epidermis are damaged, nerve endings of pain fibers are exposed first to the atmosphere, and later to fluid exudate. Air currents moving across exposed nerve endings cause extreme discomfort. Covering wounds with a clean sheet during transfer thus will decrease pain.

As exudate accumulates in the injured area, potassium, prostanoids, and substance P serve to irritate exposed nerve endings, contributing even greater pain sensations.[4] During the resuscitative phase, pain control may be achieved by frequent administration of small doses of intravenous morphine sulfate (3–5 mg for adults) or meperidine (30–50 mg). Continuous intravenous infusion also may be used, with dosage titrated to the patient's response. Intramuscular and subcutaneous injections should be avoided. Because hypovolemia impairs soft tissue circulation, these agents will be sequestered with virtually no therapeutic effect until the patient becomes hemodynamically stable. As circulation is restored, intramuscular and subcutaneous medications would be reabsorbed, with the total circulatory dose unknown. When patients are hemodynamically stable (ie, acute phase),

medications can be administered safely intravenously, intramuscularly, or orally.

The pain experience is a complex phenomenon, involving physiological, psychological, and cognitive processes. Physiological pain (ie, burn injury) can be influenced by anxiety, fear, cultural background, and life history patterns. Various theories of pain are discussed in Chapter 27.

Because so many factors influence pain perception, a variety of techniques, other than narcotics, may be useful in alleviating pain. These methods include relaxation therapy, guided imagery techniques, biofeedback, hypnosis, patient-controlled analgesia, anxiolytic or antidepressant drug therapy, anesthesia, and transcutaneous electronic nerve stimulation. Because the pain experience is unique to each individual, the nurse must be resourceful and flexible in determining the best pain control approach for each individual patient.

Patient and Family Support

Providing psychological support for the newly admitted burn patient and the family is not the least of the many tasks facing the critical care nurse. The patient most often is awake and alert, although anxious and overwhelmed by the suddenness and magnitude of injuries. The overriding concern at this time is whether the patient will live or die. This should be handled as gently, tactfully, and honestly as possible. This often is the all-important basis for establishing a trusting relationship for the long months of rehabilitation ahead.

Burn patients are under severe, long-term stress, and

Clinical Research

Choiniere M, Melzack R, et al: Comparisons between patients' and nurses' assessment of pain and medication efficacy in severe burn injuries. Pain 40(2):143–152, 1990

To provide burn patients with adequate pain relief, the nurse must be able accurately to evaluate the patients' pain levels and to assess whether sufficient analgesia is achieved. This study examined the issue by comparing the pain ratings in 42 patients hospitalized for burn injuries, and 42 nurses. The patient and the attending nurse were asked to rate, independently of each other, the intensity of the pain felt by the patient during a therapeutic procedure and at rest. When analgesic medication was given before the procedure, both the patients and the nurses were asked to estimate the degree of pain relief. All ratings were obtained using visual analogue and verbal scales. The results revealed significant but small correlations between the nurses' and patients' ratings. Frequently, the nurses underestimated or overestimated the patients' pain. Discrepancies also were observed in the evaluation of pain medication efficacy, with the nurses showing a tendency to overestimate the degree of pain relief. The accuracy of the nurses' perceptions did not vary as a function of the patients' age, socioeconomic status, or burn severity. The number of years of experience in burn nursing, however, had a significant influence on the nurses' estimation of the patients' pain during therapeutic procedures. Theoretical and clinical implications of these results are discussed, with a particular emphasis on the need to implement systematic procedures to assess pain and the success of analgesia. Additional recommendations to optimize pain management in burn patients also are made.

they nearly always manifest personality variants. Four of the most common are

- depression
- regression
- paranoia
- schizophrenia

Often, burn patients become depressed and withdrawn, asking to be left alone and not to be made uncomfortable. The nurse should respond by making certain *expectations* clear—expecting the patient to feed himself or herself, go to the bathroom, or do as much as the physical condition permits, communicating to the patient that the condition is not hopeless, and recovery is expected.

The best way to handle regression in a burn patient is to acknowledge it. First, the nurse must accept the fact that the patient may be unable to cope on an adult level, and that the patient may be unstable emotionally as well as physically. Second, the nurse must devise ways to help the patient cope on an appropriate level. Interventions that usually help include following a regular schedule so that the patient knows what is expected, rewarding the patient for adult behavior, and permitting the patient as much control and choice as possible.

It is not uncommon for severely burned patients to transfer their fears to a specific caregiver (physician, nurse, therapist) and to complain that they are being treated unjustly or unkindly. Working with a psychiatric liaison nurse may help the burn victim recognize and deal with his or her fears more effectively, and also help the caregiver support the patient and respond therapeutically.

Hallucinations, confusion, and combativeness are common in severely burned patients for physical as well as mental reasons. Exhaustion, pain, and medications may distort reality and produce schizophrenic behavior.

All four of the listed personality variants are temporary. The schizophrenia and paranoia almost always disappear by the time the patient is discharged from the hospital. The regression and depression may continue into the rehabilitation period.

Family Needs. The resuscitative phase is a traumatic time for the family as well. With high anxiety levels and lack of knowledge of burn care, the family approaches the burn unit with fear, hesitancy, and sometimes hysteria. The physical appearance of the patient and the high-technology atmosphere of the burn unit are indeed frightening. Preparing the family for the initial visit by explaining what to expect and escorting them to the bedside is extremely important. Visitors often are overwhelmed on the first visit and stand silently with feelings of anxiety and helplessness growing. It may be helpful for the nurse to suggest that the family members leave and return when they feel stronger.

Although the patient tends to concentrate on the present, the family members look to the future and want to know what to expect. Information about the patient's condition and treatments should be shared with them. The trusting relationship that was established initially provides a strong base for patient and family teaching and rehabilitation in the months to follow.

The Acute Phase: Managing the Burn Wound

Once the patient's general condition has stabilized, attention can be directed toward the burn itself. The goals of topical burn care are to promote healing, to control infection, and to help alleviate pain. Care is outlined in Nursing Care Plan 45–2.

Sepsis

The most significant complication in the acute phase of injury is sepsis. It may arise from the burn wound, pneumonia, suppurative thrombophlebitis, urinary tract infection or infection elsewhere in the body, invasive procedures, and invasive monitoring devices. The burn wound is the most frequent source of infection, which may be caused by a variety of organisms. Early after the injury, the organisms tend to be gram positive; after the first week, the organisms tend to be gram negative.

Septic shock, seen most often in patients with extensive full-thickness burns, is caused by invading bacteria from the wound entering the bloodstream. Clinically, the symptoms listed in Display Box 45–1 are expected.

A major function of viable skin is to prevent infection. Thus, when skin integrity is impaired, the patient is susceptible to infection from a variety of organisms. The nonviable and frequently necrotic burn wound eschar and granulating surfaces present a constant potential reservoir for contamination. Burn wound surfaces provide a warm, moist, protein-laden growth medium for microorganisms. There is general consensus that it is unrealistic to maintain the burn wound sterile; however, control of the microbial flora is realistic and achievable. Systemic antibiotics are of little value in controlling this bacterial popula-

---

DISPLAY BOX 45–1
Symptoms of Septic Shock

Temperature (varies)
Pulse (140–170—sinus tachycardia)
Decreased blood pressure
Paralytic ileus
Petechiae
Frank bleeding from wounds
Disorientation

tion because they are unable to reach the injured tissue owing to impaired circulation. The best method of limiting bacterial proliferation in the burn eschar is the use of topical antimicrobial agents.[5]

Wound Care

Management of wound healing entails:

- Daily hydrotherapy and debridement techniques
- Maintaining adequate nutrition
- Preventing hypothermia
- Controlling pain
- Maintaining joint mobility
- Adhering to infection control procedures
- Astute wound assessment and monitoring

All burned areas should be cleaned once or twice a day with an antimicrobial liquid detergent (eg, chlorhexidine), and initial debridement begun. After daily hydrotherapy, the burn wound is covered with a topical antimicrobial agent.

Hydrotherapy

Some centers immerse patients in a Hubbard tank to loosen exudates, clean and assess the wound, and provide range-of-motion exercises. Bath solutions vary, and may contain salt, povidone–iodine solutions, and bleaches. Because the baths usually are painful, patients should receive an analgesic 20 to 30 minutes before tubbing. In addition, the patient should receive a complete explanation of and assistance with pain-controlling techniques (eg, imagery).

Care must be taken to avoid cross-contamination of wounds during bathing procedures. For this reason, many centers no longer immerse patients in Hubbard tanks. Clean or healing wounds should be cleaned separately from contaminated ones.

Topical Antimicrobial Agents

Antimicrobial agents used from time of admission to a burn unit include 0.5% silver nitrate, mafenide acetate (Sulfamylon), nitrofurazone, povidone–iodine, silver sulfadiazine, gentamycin, and nystatin. It is important to realize that no single agent is totally effective against all burn wound infections. Treatment is guided by *in vitro* testing or *in vivo* results. Biopsies of eschar and granulating wound surfaces may be done three times weekly to identify contaminating organisms and to determine antibiotic sensitivity.

Silver sulfadiazine is the primary topical agent of choice on admission. The most common adverse reaction is leukopenia; therefore, serial complete blood counts must be monitored. If the white blood count falls below 3,000, the physician probably will change to another topical agent. When the leukocyte count returns to normal (4,000–5,000), silver sulfadiazone may be reinstituted.

If the colony counts increase, the topical agent of choice usually is mafenide acetate cream (Sulfamylon), a very effective broad-spectrum bacteriostatic agent. Mafenide acetate diffuses through third-degree eschar to the burn wound margin within 3 hours after application. It causes metabolic acidosis as it enters the blood. This acidosis initially is compensated for by hyperventilation. Oral administration of Bicitra or intravenous sodium bicarbonate usually corrects this acid–base imbalance.

The application of topical antimicrobial agents inhibits the rate of wound epithelialization and may increase the metabolic rate. Electrolyte imbalances (eg, sodium leaching by silver nitrate) and acid–base abnormalities may occur. The best topical agents are water soluble because they will not hold in heat and macerate the wound. The nurse may apply the topical agent as indicated in Table 45–3.

Debridement of the Burn Wound

The eschar will cover the burn wound until it is excised or has separated spontaneously. In theory, burn wound management is simple. It calls for debridement of the eschar and skin graft closure before the eschar becomes infected. The sometimes serious systemic complications of burn injury, such as hypovolemia and sepsis, however, may delay this course of action significantly.

Mechanical Debridement. Mechanical debridement may be accomplished using forceps and scissors to lift gently and trim loose necrotic tissue. Another form of mechanical debridement is dressing the wound with coarse gauze in the form of wet-to-dry or wet-to-wet dressings.

Wet-to-dry dressings consist of layers of moistened coarse mesh gauze. As the inner layer dries, it adheres to the wound, entrapping exudate and wound debris. The dressing should be removed at a 90° angle, and every effort should be made to avoid damaging fragile, newly granulating tissue.

As the wound forms increasing amounts of granulation tissue, wet-to-wet dressings may be used to prevent desiccation and trauma. These dressings remain moist until the next dressing change. The dressing should be removed by first gently lifting from the edges toward the center of the wound, and then removed it at a 180° angle. This procedure prevents detachment of newly formed epithelial tissue.

Enzymatic Debridement. Enzymatic debridement involves the application of a proteolytic substance to burn wounds to shorten the time of eschar separation. Travase and Elase are the most commonly used agents. The wound is first cleaned and debrided of any loose necrotic material, and the agent is applied directly to the wound bed and covered with a layer of fine mesh gauze. A topical antimicrobial agent is then applied, and the entire area is covered with saline-soaked gauze. The dressing is changed two to four times per day.

Enzymatic debridement has the advantage of eliminating the need for surgical excision; however, there are

TABLE 45–3
Topical Antimicrobial Agents for Burn Wound Management

Agent	Indications	Nursing Considerations
Mafenide acetate (Sulfamylon)	Active agent against most gram-positive and gram-negative wound pathogens; drug of choice for electrical and ear burns	Apply once or twice daily with sterile glove; do not use dressings that reduce effectiveness and cause maceration; monitor respiratory rate, electrolyte values, and arterial pH for evidence of metabolic acidosis; painful on application to partial-thickness burns for about 30 min
Silver nitrate	Effective against wide spectrum of common wound pathogens and candidal infections; used in patients with sulfa allergy or toxic epidermal necrolysis. Poor penetration of eschar	Apply 0.5% solution wet dressings twice or three times a day; ensure that dressings remain moist by wetting every 2 hours; preserve solution in a light-resistant container; protect walls, floors, etc., with plastic to prevent staining; monitor for hyponatremia and hypochloremia
Silver sulfadiazine	Active against a wide spectrum of microbial pathogens; use with caution in patients with impaired renal or hepatic function	Apply once or twice daily with a sterile gloved hand; leave wounds exposed or wrap lightly with gauze dressings; painless

From Duncan DJ, Driscoll DM: Burn wound management. Critical Care Nursing Clinics of North America 3(2):205, 1991.

complications that must be considered. Hypovolemia may occur as a result of excessive fluid loss through the wound. Hence, no more than 20% TBSA should be treated in this manner. Cellulitis and maceration of normal skin may occur around the wound periphery, and patients often complain of a burning sensation lasting 30 to 60 minutes after enzyme application.

Surgical Excision. In surgical excision, the wound is excised to viable bleeding points while minimizing the loss of viable tissue. Early excision has contributed significantly to the survival of major burn victims. The open burn causes hypermetabolism and a stress response that will not be corrected until wound closure occurs. Surgical excision should be done as soon as the patient is hemodynamically stable, usually within 72 hours.

After excision is completed, hemostasis must be achieved. This may be accomplished by topical thrombin sprayed on the wound, or application sponges soaked in a 1:10,000 epinephrine solution.

After removal of necrotic tissue, the exposed underlying structures must be dressed with a temporary or permanent covering to provide protection and prevent infection.

Grafting

The ideal substitute for lost skin is an autograft of similar color, texture, and thickness from a close location on the body. Sheets of the patient's epidermis and a partial layer of the dermis are harvested from unburned locations using a dermatome. These grafts are referred to as split thickness and can be applied to the wound as a sheet or in a meshed form.

A *sheet graft* is one in which harvested skin is placed on the recipient in sheets. The graft must be inspected frequently for collections of fluid under the graft. Fluid accumulation is prevented by rolling the graft with a cotton-tipped applicator. *Mesh grafts* are those in which the harvested skin is slit to allow it to expand and then placed on the burn site. This allows for greater coverage and drainage and is draped more easily over uneven surfaces. Over exposed areas, such as the face and hands, sheet grafts give a more natural appearance than do mesh grafts.

Mesh grafts frequently have to be expanded to get maximum coverage from each piece of autograft. An expansion rate of 1:3 or 1:4 often is practical. Sometimes ratios such as 1:6 or 1:7 are used to cover large burns. With these larger ratios, the expanded autograft is covered with either cadaver skin allografts or synthetic skin (Biobrane; Winthrop Pharmaceuticals). In addition to physically stabilizing the fragile mesh, the cover decreases evaporation, heat loss, and bacterial contamination.

A new technique that involves the growth and subsequent graft placement of cultured epithelial autographs has become an important adjunct to permanent coverage of extensive burn wounds. Biopsies are taken from unburned skin and cells are cultured in the laboratory. Sheets of cultured epithelial cells are attached to petroleum jelly gauze and applied to the wound. After 7 to 10 days, the petroleum jelly gauze is removed and a nonadherent dressing applied to prevent mechanical trauma.[5]

Biologic Dressings. Biologic dressings used in the management of burn wounds includes homograft skin (allograft) or heterograph skin (xenograft). Homograft skin is obtained from living or deceased human donors, usually the latter. Amniotic membranes have been used in the past, but are not used commonly at present. It is possible to transmit disease through the use of homograft skin, and thus it is important to test donor skin for human immunodeficiency virus, hepatitis B, and syphilis before use.

Because the demand for homograft skin exceeds the supply, heterografts have been used to achieve temporary wound closure. Porcine skin is the most commonly used substance.

Synthetic Dressings. Synthetic dressings are being developed in an attempt to overcome the pitfalls of biologic dressings, namely disease transmission, storage problems, and limited supply.

Biobrane is a collagen-based substance that adheres to the wound surface within 48 hours after application. The membrane forms an occlusive barrier to protect against bacterial infection and fluid losses while permitting drainage of exudate and penetration of topical antimicrobial agents. The membrane is translucent, permitting direct visualization of the wound bed. Other synthetic substitutes used in small, clean, temporary wound closures are polyurethane films.

Hypothermia

Hypothermia is a potential problem for the extensively burned patient, especially during hydrotherapy and immediately after surgery. Heat is lost through the open burn wounds by means of radiation and evaporation. Body temperature should be maintained at 99°F to 101°F by maintaining environmental temperatures at 82°F to 91°F with heat lamps or shields, foil blankets, and temperature-controlled air beds, if used, and by limiting body surface areas exposed at any one time.

Nutrition

The precise energy requirements needed to achieve weight and nitrogen balance and energy equilibrium depend on variables such as burn size, patient age, and other coexisting medical conditions. This requirement has been found to be approximately 25 kcal/kg plus 40 kcal/percent TBSA burn/24 hours. In some cases, this caloric load can exceed 5,000 kcal/day. Approximately 50 g of nitrogen a day are needed in addition to some polyunsaturated fats to prevent essential fatty acid deficiency. The precise protein requirements for each person are modified based on nitrogen balance studies and serum urea nitrogen values.[6] Mul-

tivitamins and increased amounts of vitamin C, potassium, zinc, and magnesium also are required.

A burn patient's appetite seldom exceeds preburn levels, and voluntary eating rarely meets protein, fat, and caloric requirements in patients with large burns. High caloric supplements between meals may be sufficient in patients with moderate burns, but those with large burns require constant interval feedings through feeding tubes. With around-the-clock administration, caloric loads of 5,000 kcal/day can be tolerated. Diarrhea may occur and can be treated with kaolin–pectin, Metamucil (Procter and Gamble, Cincinnati, OH), or bran.

In some instances (ie, prolonged paralytic ileus, malnutrition before injury, failure to gain weight), parenteral hyperalimentation may be required. When peripheral or central parenteral hyperalimentation is required, absolute aseptic technique for line insertion and alteration of intravenous sites every 3 days is essential to prevent septic thrombophlebitis. Insulin supplementation may be necessary; frequent serum and urine glucose determinations as well as serial liver function tests are required for patients on parenteral hyperalimentation.

Failure to reach the large caloric loads required for weight maintenance, nitrogen balance, and energy equilibrium results in delayed and abnormal wound healing.

The Rehabilitative Phase

Patients who have sustained extensive burns obviously will require many months for recovery and rehabilitation. Physical and psychological rehabilitation measures are begun in the critical care unit and continued through the entire recovery period.

Physical Rehabilitation

Two very important physical measures are nutrition and prevention of scarring and contractures, as discussed in Nursing Care Plan 45–3.

Promoting Nutrition
The diet should remain high in protein until all wounds have healed. As healing takes place, the diet should be tapered to meet normal caloric requirements. Burn patients may become accustomed to eating frequently and in large amounts. After healing is complete, metabolism returns to normal, and weight will be gained if eating habits are not controlled properly.

Preventing Scarring and Contractures
Once regarded as inevitable, hypertrophic scarring and joint contractures now largely are preventable. Preventive measures start when the person is admitted to the hospital (*Text continues on page 998*)

NURSING CARE PLAN 45–1:
The Patient With Burns: Resuscitative Phase

NURSING DIAGNOSIS	OUTCOME CRITERIA/ PATIENT GOALS	NURSING INTERVENTIONS
Fluid volume deficit: related to increased capillary permeability, increased capillary hydrostatic pressure, decreased capillary colloid osmotic pressure, increase evaporative loss.	• Patient will maintain fluid balance and hydration.	1. Intake and output q1h. Evaluate trends. 2. Titrate IV fluids to maintain urine output. 3. Daily weight VS q1h. 4. Report urine output < 30 or > 70 ml/h. 5. Monitor Hct, BUN, electrolytes q12h, as ordered. 6. Obtain urine specimens and monitor as ordered for hemachromagens, sugar, or acetone. 7. Monitor sensorium q1h.
Impaired gas exchange: related to carbon monoxide poisoning and/or inhalation injury.	• Patient will maintain adequate oxygenation.	1. Assess and document breath sounds q4h. 2. Administer humidified O_2 as ordered. 3. Monitor O_2 saturation with oximetry. 4. Elevate HOB. 5. Monitor carboxyhemoglobin levels as ordered.
	• Patient will be able to mobilize pulmonary secretions.	1. Turn q2h. 2. Cough, deep breath, and incentive spirometry q1h. 3. Suction q1–2h. 4. Assess and document pulmonary secretions. 5. Monitor O_2 saturation with oximetry. Evaluate ABGs prn. 6. Assess for inhalation injury: singed nasal hairs, burns around mouth or neck, coughing up soot, burn in a confined area. 7. Monitor for indications of impending airway obstruction: stridor, wheezing, rales, hoarseness, O_2 desaturation. 8. Prepare for endotracheal intubation and mechanical ventilation, as ordered.
Pain: related to burn trauma, tissue damage.	• Patient experiences a manageable level of discomfort.	1. Explain procedures before and during intervention. 2. Assess need for sedative agents.

(continued)

NURSING CARE PLAN 45–1: (Continued)
The Patient With Burns: Resuscitative Phase

NURSING DIAGNOSIS	OUTCOME CRITERIA/ PATIENT GOALS	NURSING INTERVENTIONS
		3. Assess need for analgesia: verbalization, changes in VS, agitation.
		4. Teach patient alterative methods of pain control (ie, imagery, music therapy, relaxation therapy).
		5. Administer IV analgesia as ordered, before painful procedures, and per assessment.
		6. Monitor and document response to medications.
High risk for injury: related to impaired tissue perfusion, stress response, immobility, and loss of skin integrity.	• Patient will have adequate arterial perfusion to all extremities with circumferential burns.	1. Remove constricting clothing and jewelry.
		2. Monitor extremities hourly for signs and symptoms of decreased blood flow: pulse oximeter, ultrasonic flow detector hourly, color and temperature, capillary refill, presence of peripheral pulses.
		3. Elevate burned extremities above the level of the heart.
		4. Encourage exercise of extremities for 5 minutes every hour
		5. Prepare for escharotomy or transfer to OR for fasciotomy.
	• Patient will have an absence of gastrointestinal bleeding.	1. Measure and hematest NG drainage.
		2. Measure NG drainage pH every 2 hours.
		3. Assess gastric pH q shift.
		4. Report gastric pH < 5.
		5. Administer antacids and H2 histamine receptor antagonists per MD order.
	• Patient's uninjured skin or tissues will remain intact.	1. Pad footboard and side rails.
		2. Pad pressure areas.
		3. Protect ears and nasal septum from pressure exerted by facial ties on ET and NG tubes.
		4. Provide active and passive ROM hourly.
		5. Apply positioning splints as needed.
		6. Apply eye-lubricating ointment q2h.

(continued)

NURSING CARE PLAN 45–1: (Continued)
The Patient With Burns: Resuscitative Phase

NURSING DIAGNOSIS	OUTCOME CRITERIA/ PATIENT GOALS	NURSING INTERVENTIONS
High risk for infection: related to burn injury, impaired immune response, invasive procedures, immobility.	• Patient will be free of burn wound infection.	1. Cover wounds with sterile sheets during patient transfer. 2. Clean wound according to protocol: gently debride, shave hair from areas in close proximity to wounds. 3. Cover wound with topical antimicrobials, as ordered. 4. Administer tetanus toxoid prophylaxis, as ordered. 5. Use heat lamps to maintain body temperature. 6. Assess invasive line insertion sites bid. 7. Obtain specimens as ordered for culture and sensitivity, and monitor results. 8. Report temperature spikes (> 101°F, rectal) or increased WBC (> 10,000).
High risk for ineffective individual/family coping: related to pain, fear, anxiety, and lack of information.	• Patient and family demonstrate effective coping mechanisms.	1. Offer explanations in a warm, confident manner. 2. Provide honest answers to questions. 3. Encourage appropriate coping measures: follow a regular schedule, reward positive behaviors, permit the patient as much control as possible. 4. Prepare family for initial visit and escort them to bedside. 5. Provide emotional support during visiting times. 6. Provide family with daily updates on patient's condition. 7. Refer family to available support services.

and continue for at least 12 months or until the scar is fully mature.

These preventive measures, positioning the body and helping the patient perform range-of-motion exercises, are not new to the nurse. Positioning the body with extremities extended is extremely important. Although tightly flexed positions are preferred by patients for comfort, they will result in severe contractures. The range-of-motion exercises should be carried out with each dressing change, or more often if indicated. Special splints are used to maintain arms, legs, and hands in extended yet functional positions. Later, when the wounds have healed sufficiently, the person is custom-fitted for a special pressure garment. The garment, by applying continuous uniform pressure

NURSING CARE PLAN 45–2:
The Patient With Burns: Acute Phase

NURSING DIAGNOSIS	OUTCOME CRITERIA/ PATIENT GOALS	NURSING INTERVENTIONS
High risk for injury: related to burn wound and immobility.	• Wounds will heal in a reasonable time frame.	1. Clean wounds with antimicrobial soap at least once per day. 2. Assess and document at least once per shift: burn wound and donor sites, skin grafts.
	• Skin in uninjured areas will remain intact.	1. Prevent pressure injury by padding bony prominences. 2. Protect wound and uninjured skin from secretions and excretions. 3. Assess need for pressure relief with airflow bed. 4. Immobilize graft sites to prevent trauma. 5. Moisten mesh grafts or roll-sheet grafts to promote adherence. 6. Protect grafted areas: bed cradle, dressings, splints, do not apply external devices (eg, BP cuff). 7. Promote healing of donor sites by using heat lamps and dressings as indicated.
	• Absence of contractures. • Adequate tissue perfusion.	1. Passive ROM for 5 min qh. 2. Maintain proper body alignment. 3. Elevate extremities to prevent edema. 4. Remove all constricting bands (eg, BP cuffs) when not in use. 5. Maintain environmental temperature to prevent vasoconstriction. 6. Check circulation distal to restraints q1h. 7. Check circulation of digits in splints q1h.
High risk for infection: related to impaired skin integrity, altered immune response, and invasive procedures.	• Wound and catheter sites free from infection.	1. Maintain protective isolation procedures. 2. Use strict aseptic technique for all procedures. 3. Follow protocol for care of invasive lines.

(continued)

NURSING CARE PLAN 45–2: (Continued)
The Patient With Burns: Acute Phase

NURSING DIAGNOSIS	OUTCOME CRITERIA/ PATIENT GOALS	NURSING INTERVENTIONS
		4. Assess wound and catheter sites at least once per shift for signs of infection.
		5. Perform routine wound cultures and biopsies.
		6. Instruct all visitors to maintain protective isolation.
		7. Keep wound covered with topical antimicrobials and temporary wound coverings, as ordered.
	• Negative urine, blood, sputum cultures.	8. Obtain specimens as ordered.
		9. Assess and record temperature and vital signs.
		10. Monitor for clinical signs of sepsis: tachycardia, decreased BP, increased respirations, decreased bowel sounds, altered sensorium, petechiae, bleeding.
Altered nutrition, less than body requirements: related to intake less than body requirements (hypermetabolism).	• Ingests 80%–90% of desired nutritional intake.	1. Provide high-protein, high-carbohydrate diet.
		2. Consult with dietician.
		3. Provide oral care q shift and prn.
		4. Provide adequate time to eat.
		5. Offer supplements.
		6. Monitor intake and output.
	• Tolerates tube feeding, maintaining 80% of preburn weight.	1. Assess for: abdominal distention, NG output <600 ml/24 h, abdominal cramps, diarrhea.
		2. Daily weight.
		3. Monitor intake and output.
	• Tolerates parenteral nutrition.	1. Assist with insertion of central line.
		2. Chest radiograph to verify position.
		3. Change infusion equipment q24h.
		4. Monitor VS q2h. Obtain blood, urine, sputum cultures during febrile episodes.
		5. Assess insertion site daily.
		6. Monitor infusion rate.

(continued)

NURSING CARE PLAN 45–2: (Continued)
The Patient With Burns: Acute Phase

NURSING DIAGNOSIS	OUTCOME CRITERIA/ PATIENT GOALS	NURSING INTERVENTIONS
		7. Maintain constant rate of infusion intake and output q8h.
		8. Urine glucose q2h. Serum electrolytes, chemistries, and CBC daily, as ordered.
Ineffective thermoregulation: related to impaired skin integrity.	• Body temperature 99°F–101°F.	1. Monitor and document body temperature q1h.
		2. If body temperature < 98°F (hypothermia): apply heat lamps or heat shields, cover patient with a foil blanket, apply warm moist dressings, limit exposure of body surface areas.
		3. If body temperature > 102.5°F (hyperthermia): limit physical activity, obtain blood, urine, sputum cultures, administer antipyretic agents as ordered, use cooling measures according to institutional protocol.
Knowledge deficit: related to care of burn wound.	• Patient will apply principles of burn wound management.	1. Provide information.
		2. Have patient explain rationale for wound care during procedure.
		3. Have patient perform as much self-care as possible daily.

over the entire area of the burn, prevents hypertrophic scarring and must be worn 24 hours a day for approximately 1 year. The smooth elastic garment forms a shield that permits the person to wear normal clothing and resume ordinary activities much sooner.

Psychological Rehabilitation

Psychological care of the burn patient is extremely difficult; the patient may, in the course of therapy, run the full gamut of behavioral responses. Initially, the combination of physical pain and emotional disturbance may lead to abnormal behavior, as discussed. Guilt may be particularly severe if the patient feels that his or her carelessness was the cause of injuries to others, especially if others died as a result of the accident.

If burns involve the face, eyes, or hands, additional emotional support will be needed because damage to these structures will have a long-term effect on the patient's life and livelihood.

A consistent, truthful team approach that includes the patient and family is necessary. Several supportive measures will allow the patient time to assimilate what has happened and to grow in the ability to cope.

- Staff should be stabilized as much as possible so that they become familiar with the patient's needs and so that a sense of identification between patient and nurse is established.
- Family members can be very helpful if incorporated into the overall plan of care and instructed in selected procedures.
- Diversional therapy (ie, reading, watching television, listening to music) should be encouraged as soon as possible.
- Occupational therapy should be started as soon as the patient is able to participate.

NURSING CARE PLAN 45-3:
The Patient With Burns: Rehabilitation

NURSING DIAGNOSIS	OUTCOME CRITERIA/ PATIENT GOALS	NURSING INTERVENTIONS
Altered nutrition, potential for more than body requirements: related to burn injury.	• Caloric intake will be adjusted and no unnecessary weight gain will result.	1. Teach patient about a well-balanced diet high in protein and vitamin C to meet caloric needs. 2. Explain rationale for adjusting intake.
	• Return to preburn weight.	3. Monitor intake and weight. 4. Consult with dietician.
Self–esteem disturbance: related to sequelae of burn injury.	• Patient will integrate changed body image and develop a realistic self-image.	1. Assess body image and anxiety about returning to home and job. 2. Refer to self-help groups and community resources. 3. Note signs of maladaptation and refer to counseling if necessary.
Pain: related to burn injury and pruritus.	• Pain and pruritus will be controlled.	1. Assess and document type and occurrence of pain. 2. Plan pain management techniques. 3. If pruritus occurs: maintain cool, dry environment; apply lotion as needed; use mild soap for bathing; and recommend cotton underwear. 4. Medicate with analgesics, as ordered.
Impaired skin integrity: related to burn injury.	• Wound will heal.	1. Continue to assess and monitor skin integrity. 2. Instruct patient and family about wound care, susceptibility to skin breakdown, sunburn, and skin cancer.
High risk for ineffective individual coping: related to alteration in body image, critical illness, and possible life-style changes.	• Patient will demonstrate positive coping behaviors.	1. Assess current coping skills and obtain coping history; compare. 2. Teach about home care. 3. Include family in care. 4. Consult with occupational therapist. 5. Make expectations clear. 6. Use positive reinforcement. 7. Note signs of maladaptation (depression, withdrawal, isolation, regression) and refer for counseling.
	• Scarring and contractures will be minimized.	1. Maintain proper alignment of body parts. 2. Instruct patient on ROM exercises. 3. Instruct patient about splints or special pressure garments.

In addition to the emotional support of the patient, support for the nursing staff is advisable. Faced with long and arduous care of these patients, where progress is slow and setbacks are common, staff quickly develop "burnout" unless some of their emotional reactions and problems can be aired and solved (see Chapter 10).

Summary

The skin serves multiple physiological functions that render it indispensable to life. When a large area of skin surface is destroyed, severe systemic reactions occur.

The burn victim goes through phases of recovery, each with its own special problems. The resuscitative phase begins with the burn injury and lasts until diuresis occurs (1–5 days). The major problems for the patient at this time are maintenance of an airway and adequate tissue perfusion. After diuresis, the patient enters the acute phase, during which the major problem is sepsis. Burn wound management is essential during this phase. Rehabilitation focuses on adequate nutrition and prevention of scarring and contractures. Psychological support is essential throughout the entire experience. A firm, compassionate team approach is essential throughout recovery.

REFERENCES

1. Rue LW, Cloffl WG: Resuscitation of thermally injured patients. Critical Care Nursing Clinics of North America 3:181–189, 1991
2. Burgess M: Initial management of the patient with extensive burn injury. Critical Care Nursing Clinics of North America 3:165–179, 1991
3. Robins EV: Burn shock. Critical Care Nursing Clinics of North America 2:299–307, 1990
4. Smith D, Rennie MJ: Management of burn injuries: Rationale for the use of synthetic substitutes? Professional Nurse 6:571–574, 1991
5. Duncan DJ, Driscoll DM: Burn management. Critical Care Nursing Clinics of North America 3:199–220, 1991
6. Carlson DE, Jordan BS: Implementing nutritional therapy in the thermally injured patient. Critical Care Nursing Clinics of North America 3:221–235, 1991

BIBLIOGRAPHY

Andrews I: A unique specialty . . . varied roles of the burns nurse specialist. Nursing Standard 5(26):52, 1992

Bayley EW, Carrougher GJ, et al: Research priorities for burn nursing: Patient, nurse, and burn prevention education. J Burn Care Rehabil 12:377–383, 1991

Carrougher GJ, Marvin JA, et al: Research priorities of burn nursing: Report of the wound care and infection control group. J Burn Care Rehabil 12:272–277, 1991

Casey N: Care of the burns patient. Nursing Standard 5(19): 53–55, 1991

Cioffi WG, Rue LW: Diagnosis and treatment of inhalation injuries. Critical Care Nursing Clinics of North America 3:191–198, 1991

Dyer C, Roberts D: Thermal trauma. Nursing Clinics of North America 25:85–117, 1990

Holmes P: Caring for burns. Nursing Times 87(6):18–19, 1991

Jarlsberg CR: Action STAT! neck and chest burns. Nursing 20(1):33, 1990

Lee JJ, Marvin, JA, et al: Infection control in a burn center. J Burn Care Rehabil 11:575–580, 1990

Locke G, Gazzard A: Receiving and caring for a burned patient. Nursing Standard 5(21):48–50, 1991

McSweeney P: Psychosocial effects of burns. Nursing 4(7): 15–18, 1990

Waymack JP, Pruitt BA: burn wound care. Adv Surg 23:261, 1990

STUDY QUESTIONS

1. Mr. John Frye is a victim of a house fire. He sustains burns that damage the epidermis, dermis, and subcutaneous tissue. Which of the following classifications of burns best describes his injuries?

   a. second-degree burns
   b. third-degree burns
   c. superficial burns
   d. partial-thickness burns

2. Which of the following statements best describe the development of burn shock?

   a. increased capillary permeability causes an increase in vascular colloid osmotic pressure and a decrease in hydrostatic pressure
   b. release of epinephrine produces increased heart rate, but it is ineffective, and cardiogenic shock occurs

   c. increased capillary permeability results in decreased vascular colloid osmotic pressure and increased hydrostatic pressure

   d. the stress response (epinephrine and norepinephrine) causes selective vasoconstriction, resulting in shock

3. Mr. Frye complains of headache, nausea, and vertigo. What might these symptoms indicate?

   a. smoke inhalation
   b. carbon monoxide poisoning
   c. cerebral edema
   d. overhydration

4. Mr. Frye has sustained burns to his entire right arm and his anterior trunk. Using the "rule of nines" method, what is the percentage of his burn injury?

   a. 48%
   b. 27%
   c. 18%
   d. 9%

5. During the resuscitative phase, an elevated serum potassium may occur. This is primarily the result of

   a. cellular injury
   b. fluid volume loss
   c. increased capillary permeability
   d. interstitial edema

6. The primary nursing diagnosis during the resuscitative phase is

   a. altered nutrition (less than body requirements), related to hypermetabolism
   b. impaired skin integrity, related to burn injury
   c. fluid volume deficit, related to increased capillary permeability
   d. ineffective thermoregulation, related to impaired skin integrity

7. Intramuscular injection of analgesics during the resuscitative phase is not recommended because

   a. narcotics can severely depress the respiratory system
   b. narcotics can further decrease the blood pressure
   c. inadequate peripheral perfusion results in uneven absorption of the medication
   d. tolerance to pain medication develops easily

8. Silver sulfadiazine is the topical antimicrobial agent selected for Mr. Frye. Which of the following nursing actions is appropriate when using this drug?

   a. premedicate Mr. Frye for pain before application
   b. monitor acid–base balance
   c. monitor white blood cell count
   d. observe for signs of hepatotoxicity

9. On-site first aid for thermal injuries should include

   a. application of ice
   b. covering with butter or petroleum jelly

c. flushing with cool water

d. covering with clean flannel blanket

10. Nursing care during the acute phase is directed primarily toward

a. fluid volume resuscitation

b. burn wound management

c. detection of smoke inhalation injury

d. maintenance of body temperature

CHAPTER 46

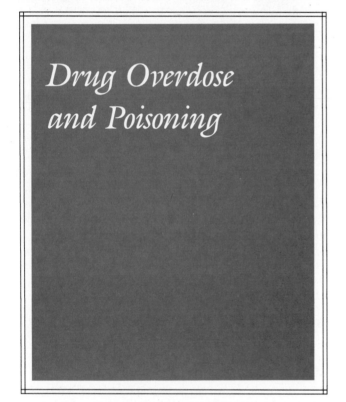

Drug Overdose and Poisoning

BEHAVIORAL OBJECTIVES

Based on the content in this chapter, the reader should be able to:

1. Discuss the initial assessment and management for acutely poisoned patients.
2. Describe the different methods to prevent absorption and enhance elimination in the management of the acutely poisoned patient.
3. Describe the groups of symptoms or toxidromes that may assist in identifying the drug(s) or toxin(s) to which the patient may have been exposed.
4. Develop a care plan for the poisoned patient.

Hudak: Critical Care Nursing:
A Holistic Approach, 6th ed. © 1994
J. B. Lippincott Company.

Description

The 1991 annual report of the American Association of Poison Control Centers National Data Collection System reported over 1.8 million poison exposures.[1] These exposures included accidental childhood ingestions, intentional overdoses, use and abuse of recreational drugs, and chronic exposures. Although all age groups are affected, children account for 59% of accidental poisonings. The remaining 41% includes adolescents and adults. Other studies have shown that up to 70% of all cases of poisoning are not reported,[2] and many deaths due to drug overdoses are not reflected in the national data base.

Therapy for the many different types of poisoning is changing rapidly as a result of new information and experience. Most nurses find it difficult to keep abreast of the latest treatment. Nurses nevertheless can impress on parents of small children the importance of poison-proofing the home.

Although most poison center cases involve children, adults attempting suicide will be seen and cared for most often in a critical care environment. The intent of this chapter is to present general guidelines for assessment and management of the acutely poisoned patient. A review of the current concepts in the initial management of ingestions of toxic substances is followed by a chart of commonly observed poisonings, their basic clinical course, and their general management. Nursing Care Plan 46–1 describes the case of the patient with cocaine toxicity.

Assessment

The evaluation and treatment plan for the poisoned patient include the following:

1. Stabilization
2. General history
3. Identification/presence of a toxic syndrome

Stabilization

Treatment of the poisoned patient is directed at the stabilization of immediate life-threatening problems of airway,

breathing, and circulation. Stabilization care includes the following steps:

1. Assess, establish, and manage the airway. Intubate the patient if necessary. Frequent suctioning may be necessary.
2. Assess and control bleeding. Prevent and treat shock with blood products if necessary. To prevent fluid overload, fluids are given cautiously and only to hydrate the person.
3. Assess for any associated injuries or other disease processes.
4. Assess, establish, and manage acid–base and electrolyte status.
5. Assess cardiac status. Cardiac monitoring is essential in a comatose patient. Many overdoses predispose the patient to cardiac irregularities and dysrhythmias.

The vital signs, including blood pressure, pulse, respirations, temperature, and level of consciousness are measured often and recorded. Once the patient is stable, specific decontamination procedures can be initiated. In certain cases, health care providers may need to protect themselves against contamination by toxic substances while the patient is being stabilized. Cases of this nature include poisonings with insecticides and cyanide. If the patient has any compromise of ABCs (airway, breathing, and circulation) or sensorium, an intravenous line should be started and supplemental oxygen should be administered. Thiamine also should be given to all alcoholic patients with altered mental status.

All unconscious patients and patients who are convulsing should receive dextrose, naloxone, and oxygen. The initial dose of naloxone in an unconscious adult patient is 2 mg.[3] In some cases, more than 2 mg of naloxone may be required to reverse the effects of drugs such as propoxyphene.[4]

History Taking

Once the patient has been stabilized, efforts can be made to obtain a history of the exposure. The history should be obtained from the patient, family members, friends, rescuers, or bystanders. Important points are the identity of toxic substance(s), amount and time of exposure, the presence of allergies or underlying diseases, and whether any first aid treatment has been administered. Family, friends, or the police may need to search the home. Clothing and personal effects should be examined for ingestants.

Identification of Toxic Syndrome (Toxidromes)

The presence of a toxic syndrome may help establish a differential diagnosis by suggesting the class of poison(s)

Evaluate Severity

Is life in

- immediate danger?
- potential danger?
- no immediate danger?

to which the patient may have been exposed. Table 46–1 lists five common toxic syndromes and their most common causes.

Management

The process of managing an overdose or poisoning may be approached at two levels: (1) general management, and (2) advanced general management.

General management includes the first aid treatment given to prevent absorption of the agent and, if indicated, to eliminate continued exposure or reexposure. Advanced general management refers to specific treatment modalities, which may include further steps of prevention of absorption, enhanced elimination of the drug(s) or toxin(s), patient monitoring (eg, acid–base status, hemodynamics), antidote, antitoxin, or antivenin administration, and symptomatic and supportive care. The purpose of this section is to discuss general management and advanced general management procedures for managing an overdose or poisoning.

General Management

Preventing Absorption

Initial first aid treatment is directed at preventing absorption of the drug(s) or toxin(s). Physiochemical properties of the drug or toxin, amount (eg, quantity ingested), route (eg, ingestion or inhalation), and the time of expo-

sure help determine the type and extent of decontamination. The following outlines the first-line decontamination of four common routes of exposure to toxic agents: ocular, dermal, inhalation, and ingestion.

Ocular Exposure

In the case of an ocular exposure, decontamination is achieved by a lukewarm water or normal saline irrigation immediately on exposure. Using a large glass or a low-pressure shower, the eye may be flooded continuously for 15 to 30 minutes while it is blinked open and closed. The length of the irrigation may be dictated by the pH of the toxin. In cases of exposure to alkaline substances, 30 minutes of irrigation is indicated. Determination of the pH of the tears after irrigation also may afford a parameter for the length of the flush. If symptoms of ocular irritation or visual disturbances persist after irrigation, an eye examination is warranted.

Dermal Exposure

After removal of contaminated clothing, skin decontamination is accomplished by flooding the skin with lukewarm water for 15 to 30 minutes and then proceeding gently to wash the contaminated area with soap and water, rinsing thoroughly. Certain toxins may require further skin decontamination. For example, such dermally absorbed pesticides as the organophosphates (eg, Malathion or diazinon) warrant three separate washings or showers with soap and water.

In cases of dermally absorbed toxins, the health care provider may be at risk for toxicity if dermal contamination occurs while assisting the victim to decontaminate.

TABLE 46–1
Toxic Syndromes

Syndrome	Symptoms	Common Causes
Cholinergic	Decreased vital signs, excessive salivation, lacrimation, urination, emesis and diaphoresis, central nervous system depression, muscle fasiculations, pulmonary edema, miosis, bradycardia, and seizures	Organophosphate and carbamate insecticides, physostigmine, some mushrooms
Opiate/sedative hypnotic	Decreased vital signs, coma, respiratory depression, miosis, hypotension, bradycardia, decreased bowel sounds, pulmonary edema (propoxyphene may cause seizures)	Narcotics, benzodiazepines, barbiturates, ethanol, clonidine, methaqualone
Anticholinergic	Delirium, dry, flushed skin, dilated pupils, elevated temperature, urinary retention, decreased bowel sounds, tachycardia, seizures	Antihistamines, atropine, antidepressant agents, some plants and mushrooms
Sympathomimetic	Delusions, paranoia, tachycardia, hypertension, mydriasis, seizures	Cocaine, theophyllin, caffeine, LSD, amphetamines, phenylpropanolamine
Withdrawal	Diarrhea, mydriasis, tachycardia, hallucinations, cramps	Alcohol, barbiturates, narcotics, benzodiazepines

Contamination may occur while handling contaminated clothing or body fluids, or during the decontamination of the patient's skin.

Neutralization of an acid or base on the skin is not recommended. Neutralization is the reaction between an acid and a base, in which the H^+ of the acid and the OH^- of the base react to produce H_2O (water). This exothermic reaction may result in a thermal burn.

Inhalation Exposure

The first step in inhalation exposures is to move the victim to fresh air while ensuring that the responder or health care provider is not exposed to the airborne toxin. A patent airway must be established and respiratory status assessed. Artificial breathing may be necessary if the victim does not breathe spontaneously. If symptoms of respiratory tract irritation or failure persist after exposure to fresh air, further medical evaluation is required.

Ingestions

Dilution with milk or water is indicated for ingested irritants or caustics. Ingestions in adults may be diluted with one glass of milk or water, whereas children may be given 2 to 8 ounces of fluids, based on their size. Evidence of mucosal irritation or burns after dilution indicates that further medical evaluation may be necessary. In exposures complicated by seizures, depressed mental status, or loss of gag reflex, dilution is not advised owing to the risk for aspiration.

As with dermal exposures, neutralization of an acid or base generates heat. The exothermic reaction may lead to further injury of the gastrointestinal tract, and neutralization therefore is not advised.

Advanced General Management

The second level of managing an overdose or poisoning, advanced general management, incorporates gastrointestinal decontamination, enhanced elimination of the drug(s) or toxin(s), patient monitoring, specific antidote, antitoxin, or antivenin administration, and support of the patient's vital functions throughout the toxic event.

Gut Decontamination

Gastrointestinal decontamination with the use of emetics, gastric lavage, or the administration of adsorbents and cathartics may be useful to prevent absorption and forestall toxicity resulting from ingestion of nearly all drugs and a variety of other toxins, ranging from long-acting anticoagulant rodenticides to poisonous mushrooms.

Emetics

Retrieving the ingested drug or toxin by inducing emesis with an emetic is one method of gut decontamination.

Syrup of ipecac (SOI) is a commonly used emetic that will partially empty the stomach when given immediately after ingestion of the drug or toxin. This over-the-counter medication may be of benefit for home use in minor pediatric overdoses under the supervision of a physician or poison control center. Its value, however, is limited for two reasons: (1) it may empty the stomach completely, and (2) the vomiting may delay activated charcoal administration (see Adsorbents section, later).[5]

Syrup of ipecac may be given to adults and children aged 6 months and older, but its administration to children ages 6 to 12 months best is done under the guidance of a health care provider to avoid aspiration of vomitus.[6] The SOI is to be administered as soon as possible after the ingestion (within 30 minutes) and followed with water and increased patient physical activity. If the initial dose fails to produce results in 20 to 30 minutes, one repeat dose may be given. Once the emesis is clear, withhold food and fluids for 1 to 2 hours to settle the stomach. Adverse effects of SOI include protracted vomiting, lethargy, and diarrhea.[7] Rare complications of SOI-induced emesis include Mallory–Weiss syndrome,[8] pneumomediastinum, and retropneumoperitoneum.[9]

To avoid the aspiration of vomitus, gastric emptying by emesis is contraindicated in situations of (1) depressed mental status, (2) absent gag reflex, (3) seizures, and (4) ingestion of an agent that may produce rapid onset of central nervous system (CNS) depression. Gastric emptying by emesis also is contraindicated when caustic agents have been ingested. This is to prevent the reexposure and possible new injury to the gastrointestinal tract by the caustic agent.

Other emetics such as apomorphine, cupric sulfate, and salt have been suggested but are not advisable. Apomorphine may cause CNS depression.[10] Salt water used as an emetic has produced fatal hypernatremia.[11–13] Death from toxicity has been reported with use of cupric sulfate as an emetic.[14]

Gastric Lavage

Gastric lavage is a common alternative method of gastric emptying, in which fluid such as normal saline is introduced into the stomach through a large-bore orogastric or nasogastric tube and then removed in an attempt to reclaim part of the ingested agent before it is absorbed. During lavage, gastric contents can be collected for toxin or drug identification. Gastric lavage is suggested for patients with a depressed mental status or absent gag reflex, or for those in whom SOI has failed to produce emesis.

To evacuate particulate matter effectively, including whole capsules or tablets, a large, preferably orogastric, tube should be used. The orogastric tube size in an adult or adolescent is 36 to 40 Fr, and in children, 16 to 28 Fr. Standard nasogastric tubes are not preferred because of their small size. Large nasogastric tubes may be used, but may cause mucosal trauma and epistaxis.[15]

The patient is positioned in the left lateral decubitus position, with the head lower than the feet, for the lavage. The procedure entails attaching a funnel (or a catheter-tip syringe) to the end of the orogastric tube and instilling 150 to 200 ml of water or saline solution (50–100 ml in children) into the stomach. Lowering the funnel and tube below the patient will allow the fluid to return by gravity.[15] This procedure is repeated until clear fluid returns or a minimum of 2 L of fluid has been used.[16] Nasotracheal or endotracheal intubation may be necessary to protect the airway.

Complications of gastric lavage include esophageal perforation,[17] pulmonary aspiration, electrolyte imbalance, tension pneumothorax, and hypothermia in small children when cold lavage solutions are used.[16]

Lavage is contraindicated in the ingestion of caustics owing to the risk of esophageal perforation, and in uncontrolled seizures because of risk of trauma and aspiration.[18]

Adsorbents

An adsorbent is a solid substance that has the ability to attract and hold to its surface ("to adsorb") another substance.[19] Activated charcoal (AC) is an effective nonspecific adsorbent of many drugs[6] and toxins. Activated charcoal adsorbs or traps the drug or toxin to its large surface area and prevents absorption from the gastrointestinal tract. Caustics, hydrocarbons, iron, and lithium are not adsorbed effectively by AC. Table 46–2 lists drugs or toxins that are adsorbed effectively by AC, and Table 46–3 identifies drugs or toxins that are not adsorbed effectively by AC.

Activated charcoal is a fine, black powder that is given as slurry with water, either orally or by nasogastric or orogastric tube, as soon as possible after the ingestion. Commercially available AC products may be mixed with 70% sorbitol to decrease grittiness, increase palatability, and serve as a cathartic.

Activated charcoal must be used cautiously in patients with diminished bowel sounds, and it is contraindicated in patients with bowel obstruction. Serial doses of AC may be useful in the treatment of many drug overdoses, including phenobarbital, phenytoin, and theophylline. This use is discussed in greater detail in the section on Enhanced Elimination.

TABLE 46–2
Charcoal-Adsorbed Drugs and Substances

Acetaminophen	Pentobarbital
Amitriptyline	Phenol
Amphetamines	Propoxyphene
Codeine	Salicylates
Morphine	Strychnine
N-acetylcysteine	Theophylline

TABLE 46–3
Substances Not Well Adsorbed by Charcoal

Acids	Ferrous sulfate
Alkalis	Lithium
Ethanol	Potassium chloride

Cathartics

It generally is accepted that cathartics decrease absorption of drugs and toxins by speeding their passage through the gastrointestinal tract, thereby limiting their contact with mucosal surfaces. Although scientific evidence is lacking, their routine use in poisonings and overdose continues.[20] The cathartic is administered concomitantly with the first dose of AC. Commonly used preparations include magnesium citrate, magnesium sulfate, sodium sulfate, and sorbitol 70%.

Cathartics are given orally or by nasogastric or orogastric tube in all overdoses or poisonings in which activated charcoal is indicated, except in small children. In children younger than 1 year of age, the cathartic is omitted to avoid dehydration. The safety of more than one dose of cathartic has not been established. Hypermagnesemia has been reported after repeated doses of magnesium-containing cathartics in overdose patients.[21,22]

Enhancement of Elimination

The pharmacologic characteristics of a drug or toxin greatly influence the severity and length of the clinical course in the acutely poisoned patient. These properties—absorption rate, body distribution, and elimination rate—must be considered in choosing ways to eliminate the drug or toxin from the body. This review focuses on seven methods of enhanced elimination:

1. Multidose activated charcoal
2. Whole-bowel irrigation
3. Alteration of urine pH
4. Hemodialysis
5. Hemoperfusion
6. Hyperbaric oxygenation therapy
7. Exchange transfusion

Multidose Activated Charcoal

Administration of multidose AC may result in greater adsorption of many drugs or toxins than with a single dose of AC, owing to the poor binding characteristics of the drug, interference by food with binding, or the drug being a sustained-release pharmaceutical.[23] Systemic clearance of drugs also may be enhanced by adsorption of drugs that enter the gastrointestinal tract through routes other than ingestion, such as passive diffusion, active secretion, facilitated transport, or biliary excretion.[24]

Levy suggested that drugs diffuse from the systemic

circulation into the gastrointestinal lumen because of the large surface area of the intestine and the concentration gradient that some membrane-permeable drugs create.[25] The AC reduces the concentration of drug in the lumen and inhibits back-diffusion of the drug into the systemic circulation. The process is maintained by administration of repeated doses of AC that "propel" the drug through the intestine and allow the drug to be excreted in the feces.

Biliary secretion, also termed "enterohepatic circulation," occurs when some drugs or their active metabolites are excreted with bile into the intestine, where they can be reabsorbed into the systemic circulation. Systemic drug clearance may be enhanced when AC prevents reabsorption of the drug or its active metabolites.

Levy described this process of drug clearance by AC in the gut as "gastrointestinal dialysis," and likened it to drug clearance by hemodialysis.[25]

Multidose AC given orally or per nasogastric or orogastric tube every 2 to 6 hours is of benefit in the clearance of theophylline, phenytoin, and phenobarbital. Complications of multidose AC include bowel obstruction[26,27] and aspiration.[28]

Whole-Bowel Irrigation

Whole-bowel irrigation is the rapid enteral administration of large volumes of a balanced electrolyte solution to flush the bowel mechanically without creating electrolyte disturbances.[29] Already routinely used as a bowel preparation for colonoscopy, its successful use as a gastrointestinal decontamination procedure has been reported in overdoses of specific drugs such as zinc sulfate,[30] in cocaine body packer,[31] and also with the ingestion of modified-release pharmaceuticals.[32,33]

Commercially available products for use in whole-bowel irrigation include Golytely and Colyte. Both products are dispensed as a powder and require addition of water for administration. The solution is given orally or via nasogastric or orogastric tube. Whole-bowel irrigation is contraindicated in the patient with bowel obstruction or perforation.

Alteration of Urine pH

Drugs or toxins may be weak acids or bases that become ionized in solution. Urine alkalinization uses this property to enhance excretion of the drug by altering the urine pH and subsequently increasing the amount of ionized drug in the urine. This form of enhanced elimination, also termed "ion-trapping," usually is accomplished with intravenous fluid therapy (eg, continuous infusion of an intravenous fluid with 1 to 3 ampules of sodium bicarbonate). Urine alkalinization is used in salicylate and phenobarbital overdoses. Urine acidification has been suggested for phencyclidine (ie, "angel dust") and amphetamine poisonings; however, it no longer is considered appropriate in any situation because of potential complications and low drug clearance.[15]

Complications have been observed with both of these therapies. Cerebral edema, pulmonary edema, and electrolyte imbalances may develop with urine alkalinization. Urine acidification may complicate a preexisting metabolic acidosis, and, in the patient with myoglobinuria, may predispose to renal injury.[34]

Hemodialysis

Hemodialysis is the process of altering the solute composition of the blood by diffusion across a semipermeable membrane between blood and a salt solution.[35] It is used in moderate to severe intoxications to remove a drug or toxin rapidly when more conservative methods (ie, gastric emptying, AC, antidotes) have failed. Low molecular weight, low protein binding, and water solubility are factors that make a toxin or drug suitable for hemodialysis. Toxins that may be removed by hemodialysis include methanol, ethylene glycol, theophylline, and salicylates.

Hemoperfusion

Hemoperfusion is a method of removing drugs and toxins from the blood by pumping the blood through a cartridge of adsorbent material such as AC. An advantage of hemoperfusion over hemodialysis is that the total surface area of the dialyzing membrane is much greater with the hemoperfusion cartridges.[36] As in hemodialysis, drugs with large volumes of distribution or significant tissue-binding characteristics are not good candidates for hemoperfusion because little drug is available in the blood.

Although not a commonly used procedure, hemoperfusion has been used successfully in theophylline overdose.

Hyperbaric Oxygenation Therapy

Hyperbaric oxygenation therapy (HBO) is the process of administering oxygen to a patient in an enclosed chamber at a pressure greater than the pressure at sea level (ie, 1 atmosphere absolute—1 ATA). Its primary mechanisms are to reduce the volume of gas-filled spaces (eg, arterial gas embolism) and to hyperoxygenate perfused tissue beds.[37] It is used in methylene chloride[38] and in carbon monoxide poisonings. Methylene chloride is metabolized to CO in the body after it is absorbed through inhalation.

Hyperbaric oxygenation therapy is an important therapy in reducing the half-life ($t_{1/2}$) of CO, thereby enhancing elimination. For example, the $t_{1/2}$ of CO in room air is 5 to 6 hours, but in 100% oxygen is 90 minutes. The $t_{1/2}$ is reduced further to 20 minutes with HBO.[18] Some reports support that HBO initiated soon after exposure may decrease delayed neurologic sequelae.[37] The small number of HBO chambers limits the wide use of this therapy.

Complications of HBO include pressure-related otalgia, sinus pain, tooth pain, and tympanic membrane rupture.[39] Confinement anxiety, convulsion,[40] and tension pneumothorax[41] also have been observed in patients receiving HBO.

Exchange Transfusion

Exchange transfusion is an infrequently used technique of removing a portion of the patient's blood and replacing it with whole fresh blood. In the toxicologic literature, its effective use has been reported in an iatrogenic caffeine overdose in a newborn,[42] in an accidental analine poisoning of a 4.5-year old girl in whom persistent methemoglobinemia developed,[43] and in a preterm infant with iatrogenic theophylline poisoning. In the latter case, exchange transfusion was implemented because hemodialysis or hemoperfusion were considered impractical owing to the infant's size and hemodynamic status.[44]

Antagonists

Myth of the Universal Antidote

"The universal antidote" has been the touted treatment for poisonings; however, it has no clinical significance. It consists of the following:

2 parts burnt toast = activated charcoal

1 part milk of magnesium = cathartic

1 part strong tea = tannic acid

The antidote is not effective in part because burnt toast is not activated charcoal. Furthermore, tannic acid is potentially hepatotoxic.

Although it commonly is believed that there is an antidote for every toxin, the opposite is closer to the truth. There are, in fact, very few antidotes. Antidotes for specific intoxications are listed in Table 46–4.

TABLE 46–4
Antidotes

Toxin	Antidote
Opiates	Naloxone
Methanol, ethylene glycol	Ethanol
Anticholinergics	Physostigmine
Organophosphates or carbamate insecticides	Atropine
	Pyridoxine
β-Blockers	Glucagon
Digitalis, glycosides	Digoxin-specific antibody fragments
Benzodiazepines	Flumazenil
Carbon monoxide	Oxygen
Nitrites	Methylene blue
Acetaminophen	N-acetylcysteine (Mucomyst)
Cyanide	Amyl nitrite
	Sodium nitrite
	Sodium thiosulfate
Calcium channel blockers	Calcium gluconate

Antivenin

Antivenins are antitoxins that neutralize the venom of the offending snake or spider. Antivenin (*Crotalidae*) Polyvalent (Equine) is active against snake venoms of members of the family *Crotalidae*, native to North, Central, and South America.[6] Antivenin (*Latrodectus mactans*) (Equine) is available for black widow spider bites and Antivenin (*Micrurus fulvius*) (Equine) is available for envenomations by the eastern coral snake and the Texas coral snake.[6]

Antitoxin

Antitoxins neutralize a toxin such as that of botulism. Botulism Antitoxin Trivalent (Equine) is available through the Centers for Disease Control and Prevention, Atlanta, GA.

Patient Monitoring

Seriously poisoned or overdosed patients may require continued monitoring for hours or days after exposure. Diagnostic tools and clinical signs and symptoms will provide information about the patient's progress and direct medical and nursing management.

Monitoring Parameters Useful in Toxicology

1. *Electrocardiography.* Electrocardiography may provide evidence of drugs causing dysrhythmias or conduction delays (eg, tricyclic antidepressants).
2. *Radiology.* Many substances are radiopaque (eg, heavy metals, button batteries, enteric coated tablets). Chest x-rays also will provide evidence of aspiration and pulmonary edema.
3. *Electrolytes, arterial blood gases, and other laboratory tests.* Acute poisoning can cause an imbalance in electrolyte levels, including sodium, potassium, chloride, CO_2 content, magnesium, and calcium. Signs of inadequate oxygenation include cyanosis, tachycardia, hypoventilation, intercostal retractions, and altered mental status. Any signs of inadequate ventilation or oxygenation should be evaluated further by arterial blood gas (ABG) measurements. Seriously poisoned patients require routine screening of electrolytes, creatinine, and glucose, complete blood count, urinalysis, ABGs, and chest x-ray.
4. *Anion gap.* The anion gap (AG) is a simple, cost-effective tool that uses commonly measured serum components (eg, sodium, chloride, bicarbonate) to assist in evaluating the poisoned patient for certain toxins. The normal value for the AG is approximately 8 to 16 mEq/L.[45] An AG that exceeds the upper normal value may indicate metabolic acidosis. Toxins that can cause an elevated AG include methanol (eg, windshield washer fluids), alcohol, ethylene glycol (eg, automobile antifreeze), and salicylates (eg, aspirin). Newer re-

search suggests that the anion gap is not sensitive in the diagnosis of toxic metabolic acidosis, and that a normal AG does not preclude a toxic ingestion.[46]

5. *Osmolality*. The osmolal gap (OG) is the difference between the measured osmolality (by the freezing point depression method) and the calculated osmolality determined by using the major osmotically active substances in the serum (ie, sodium, glucose, blood urea nitrogen).[16] Like the AG, it is a simple, cost-effective tool for evaluating the poisoned patient for certain toxins. An OG that exceeds 10 mOsm is abnormal. Toxins that can cause an OG include ethylene glycol and methanol.

6. *Toxicology screen*. Toxicology screen may be helpful in the diagnosis of the poisoned patient. A negative screen does not necessarily mean that a toxin is not present, but only that none of the toxins screened for is present. It is important for the nurse to know what toxins his or her laboratory routinely screens for to use a toxicology screen effectively.

Summary

Because there are so few antidotes, the care of the poisoned patient usually is directed at maintaining the ABCs. This may entail the use of intravenous fluids, vasopressors, ventilators, antiarrhythmics, and other measures specific to the abnormalities, such as external cooling. In light of

Commonly Observed Poisonings Described in Table 46-5

Benzodiazepines
Propoxyphene
Iron
Amphetamines
Hydrocarbons
LSD
Barbituates
Carbon monoxide
Cyclic antidepressants
Marijuana
Opioids
Ethylene glycol
Acetaminophen
Organophosphates
Salicylates
Methanol

the massive number of toxins patients encounter, and the limited number of antidotes, symptomatic and supportive care most likely will continue to be the mainstay in poisonings and overdoses.

The nursing assessments, diagnostic tests, interventions, and comments related to commonly observed poisonings follow in Table 46-5. Figure 46-1 shows a nomogram for acetaminophen poisoning.

(*Text continues on page 1023*)

TABLE 46-5
Commonly Observed Poisonings

Substance/Examples	Nursing Assessment	Diagnostic	Intervention	Comments
Benzodiazepines				
Diazepam (Valium) Chlordiazepoxide (Librium) Flurazepam (Dalmane) Clorazepate (Tranxene) Oxazepam (Serax)	Vital signs: hypotension, tachycardia, respiratory depression Neurologic: ataxia, lethargy, slurred speech	Plasma levels not usually clinically useful	Supportive care: 1. airway 2. breathing 3. circulation Prevention of absorption: 1. lavage 2. activated charcoal 3. cathartic Fluids for hypotension Antidotes: Flumazenil has reversed coma and respiratory depression in severely poisoned patients, contraindicated in tricyclic antidepressant overdose	Benzodiazepines cause CNS depression effects. Because of their long half-life, these drugs may cause prolonged drowsiness in the overdose situation. Fatalities are unlikely from the ingestion of these agents alone, but frequently they are involved in the multiple overdose, most notably with alcohol. Ingestions of 500–1,500 mg have occurred with only minor toxicity. Physical dependence can

(continued)

TABLE 46–5
Commonly Observed Poisonings (Continued)

Substance/Examples	Nursing Assessment	Diagnostic	Intervention	Comments
				occur with chronic ingestion; therefore, withdrawal may be anticipated if a person arrives with an acute oral benzodiazepine overdose.
Propoxyphene				
Darvon Darvon compound Darvocet N-100	Vital signs: hypotension, respiratory depression CV: cardiac dysrhythmias Neurologic: CNS depression, drowsiness progressing to coma, convulsions, pinpoint pupils	Arterial blood gases Propoxyphene levels are not clinically useful	Supportive care: 1. airway 2. breathing 3. circulation Prevention of absorption: 1. lavage 2. activated charcoal 3. cathartic Cardiac monitoring Seizure precaution Antidote: naloxone	Propoxyphene is a synthetic narcotic found in a variety of preparations, and acts directly on the CNS. Its rapid action allows for observable symptoms within 30 min of ingestion, and effects may be exhibited for 8–12 hr. A diagnostic clue to propoxyphene overdose is that the person will present with seizures and pinpoint pupils. The propensity toward seizures makes lavage preferable to ipecac. Large amounts of naloxone have been required for reversal of the effects of propoxyphene overdose. Most deaths occur within first 2 hr of ingestion, many within 15 min.
Iron				

Multivitamin with iron
Ferrous gluconate
Intron
Fergon
Ferrous sulfate
Mol-iron
Feosol
Fer-In-Sol
Ferous fumarate
	Iron toxicity is best described in four distinct phases:
	1. Phase I (30 min–2 hr)
	GI:
	hemorrhagic gastritis, vomiting, diarrhea
	CNS:
	lethargy, coma
	2. Phase II (up to 12 hr after exposure)
	Deceptive period of improvement and stabilization; stage may be brief
	3. Phase III (12–48 hr)
	GI:
	hematemesis, melena, GI perforation
		Serum iron total iron binding capacity
		Abdominal radiograph
		Electrolytes
		White blood cell count
		Blood glucose
		Type and cross-matching for blood
			Supportive care:
			1. airway
			2. breathing
			3. circulation (check for hypovolemia)
			Prevention of absorption:
			1. ipecac/lavage
			2. charcoal
			3. cathartic (unless pt already has diarrhea)
			Antidotes/chelation
			Deferoxamine
			Indications:
			1. Peak serum iron levels above 350 µg/dl
			2. symptomatic patients
			  a. hypotension
			  b. bleeding
			  c. protracted vomiting
				Iron is found in a number of preparations, including multivitamins with iron and prenatal vitamins. Iron has a direct effect on the gastrointestinal mucosa. In less than 2 hr, there can be severe hemorrhagic necrosis with large losses of blood and fluid. The plasma iron concentration and total iron-binding capacity may vary and are regulated by hemoglobin synthesis. Careful calculations must be made as to the amount of elemental iron ingested.
				
				(continued)

TABLE 46–5
Commonly Observed Poisonings (*Continued*)

Substance/Examples	Nursing Assessment	Diagnostic	Intervention	Comments
	CNS: lethargy, coma, seizures CV: vascular collapse, cyanosis, pulmonary edema Metabolic: acidosis, hypoglycemia Liver/kidney: coagulation defects, hepatorenal failure 4. Phase 4 (2–4 days) possible hepatic necrosis		Replace fluid loss aggressively	
Amphetamines: Diet pills Illicit drugs (MDA, MMDA, "Ice") Methyl phenidate (Cylert)	Vital signs: hypothermia, hyperventilation, hypertension, tachycardia CV: myocardial stimulation, dysrhythmias Neurologic: hyperactivity, restlessness, seizures GI: nausea, vomiting, diarrhea, anorexia Fluid–electrolyte: hypokalemia, hyperkalemia, dehydration Psychiatric: aggressive behavior, delusions	Urine drug screen for amphetamine	Supportive care: 1. airway 2. breathing 3. circulation Prevention of absorption: 1. lavage 2. activated charcoal 3. cathartic Cardiac monitoring Seizure precautions Nitroprusside for severe hypertension External cooling for hyperthermia Calm environment	Used to treat narcolepsy and attention deficit disorder and hyperkinetic syndrome in children, amphetamines also play a role as street drugs. "Ice" is a new form of methamphetamine that is gaining popularity in Hawaii and the West Coast of the United States.

Hydrocarbons	Vital signs:
	respiratory distress cyanosis, tachypnea
	Neurologic:
	the volatile aromatic hydrocarbons induce higher degrees of CNS toxicity, and their effects may include lethargy, irritability, dizziness, stupor, and coma
	GI:
	irritations of the mouth, burning sensation in the mucous membranes of mouth and esophagus, nausea and vomiting
	CV:
	dysrhythmia
	Dermal:
	skin irritation
		Baseline chest radiograph
		Arterial blood gases
			Supportive care:
			1. airway
			2. breathing
			3. circulation
			Prevention of absorption:
			1. ipecac is recommended in the alert patient with ingestion of:
			  a. large amounts of petroleum distillates
			  b. petroleum distillates with seriously toxic additives (heavy metals, insecticides)
			  c. halogenated aromatic hydrocarbons
			  d. do not induce emesis for min-
				The most serious toxic effect after ingestion is aspiration pneumonitis. Ingestion of low-viscosity hydrocarbons poses the greatest risk of aspiration and toxicity. Intentional inhalation may result in cardiac dysrhthmias, respiratory arrest, and CNS toxicity. Gastric emptying is not indicated unless there is a history of large ingestion (intentional poisoning) or ingestion of hydrocarbons that may produce renal, liver CNS, or pulmonary toxicity (halogenated hydrocarbons or

(*continued*)

TABLE 46–5
Commonly Observed Poisonings (*Continued*)

Substance/Examples	Nursing Assessment	Diagnostic	Intervention	Comments
	Ocular: corneal burns		eral seal oil, signal oil, or furniture polish 2. lavage in patients who require decontamination but are too obtunded to take ipecac 3. charcoal 4. saline cathartics Cardiac monitor in symptomatic patients Positive end-expiratory pressure may be necessary to maintain adequate oxygenation Decontamination eye exposure: irrigate 15 min with tepid water Dermal-wash area with soap and water Steroids are not useful Antibiotics are to be used only if indicated	petroleum distillates with additives).
LSD				
Morning glory seeds	HEENT: mydriasis and impaired color preception CV: hypertension, hypotension, tachycardia Neurologic: acute anxiety, hallucination, fluctuations in mood, paranoia, psychotic reactions, flashbacks GI: vomiting diarrhea Temperature regulation: hyperthermia	Urine drug screen	Supportive care 1. airway 2. breathing 3. circulation Prevention of absorption: 1. activated charcoal 2. cathartic Acute anxiety: 1. IV or PO diazepam Psychological and supportive care	LSD is available on the street in the form of tablets, capsules, sugar cubes, or solution on blotting paper ("blotter acid" or "postage stamps"). Street name includes "California sunshine." A quite, nonthreatening environment may be helpful in "talking down" patients. Trauma as result of altered behavior may be noted.
Barbiturates				
Short acting: 1. Pentobarbital 2. Butalbital Long acting: 1. Phenobarbital 2. Primidone	Neurologic: CNS depression, including coma CV: hypotension, cardiovascular collapse Respiratory: respiratory arrest Temperature regulation: hypothermia Dermal: hemorrhagic blisters—"barb burns"	Plasma levels (serial)	Supportive care: 1. airway 2. breathing 3. circulation Prevention of absorption: 1. lavage 2. activated charcoal (serial) 3. cathartic Specific therapy for phenobarbital: 1. urine alkalinization Symptomatic and supportive care	Barbiturates are used as anticonvulsants and sedatives. Drug withdrawal may occur.

(*continued*)

TABLE 46–5
Commonly Observed Poisonings (Continued)

Substance/Examples	Nursing Assessment	Diagnostic	Intervention	Comments
Carbon Monoxide				
Incomplete combustion of carbon-containing fuels Sources: 1. Exhaust from automobiles or any gas engines 2. Faulty wood/coal stoves 3. Fire 4. Methylene chloride found in paint and varnish remover converts to carbon monoxide	Vital signs: hypotension CV: myocardial depression, conduction defects Neurologic: headache, lethargy, agitation, confusion, coma, seizures, cerebral edema GI: nausea gastroenteritis Metabolic: acidosis	Carboxyhemoglobin level LDH, CPK, SGOT Arterial blood gases CT scan if indicated Cardiac monitor Chest radiograph	Supportive care: 1. airway 2. breathing 3. circulation 100% oxygen through a tight-fitting mask or endotracheal tube if patient lacks adequate ventilation Hyperbaric oxygen therapy for symptomatic patients Correct acidosis	Carbon monoxide (CO) is the leading cause of poisoning deaths in the United States. CO combines with hemoglobin with an affinity over 200 times greater than that of oxygen. Toxicity results from impaired oxygen delivery and affects primarily the organs most susceptible to hypoxia (heart, brain).
Cyclic Antidepressants				
Amitriptyline Imipramine Desipramine Nortriptyline Trimipramine Doxepin Amoxapine Protriptyline Tetracyclics	Vital signs: tachycardia, hypertension followed by hypotension, respiratory depression CV: ventricular dysrhythmias and conduction block Neurologic: lethargy, coma, seizures, myoclonus GI: decreased bowel sounds, dry mouth, urinary retention	Urine/blood for tricyclics Electrolytes Arterial blood gases Serial 12-lead ECG	Supportive care: 1. airway 2. breathing 3. circulation Prevention of absorption: 1. lavage 2. activated charcoal 3. cathartic Hypotension: fluids, and, if necessary, norepinephrine is the vasopressor of choice Cardiac monitor Seizure precautions Correct acidosis with sodium bicarbonate or hyperventilation on ventilator Correct conduction disturbances with serum alkalinization to a pH of 7.45–7.55 Monitor bowel sounds	Cyclic antidepressants are used in the treatment of endogenous depression. CNS and CV toxicity are the major complications of this overdose. Certain newer compounds such as amoxapine appear to have more CNS than CV affects.
Marijuana	Vital signs: tachycardia, postural hypotension Neurologic: alteration in mood, cognition, motor coordination and heightened sensory awareness, lethargy, euphoria GI: stimulation of appetite, dry mouth, nausea	Urine/plasma screen	Supportive care: 1. airway 2. breathing 3. circulation Prevention of absorption: 1. ipecac 2. charcoal 3. cathartic Benzodiazepines for sedation Calm environment IV fluids and Trendelenburg position for hypotension	The individual response to recreational use of marijuana depends on the dose, the personality and expectations of the user, and the setting. Initial effects range from euphoria and relaxation to paranoia and manic psychosis. Adults usually require only supportive care after overdose. Accidental ingestion by children may require preven-

(continued)

TABLE 46-5
Commonly Observed Poisonings (*Continued*)

Substance/Examples	Nursing Assessment	Diagnostic	Intervention	Comments
				tion of absorption if seen within 3 hr of exposure.
Opioids	Vital signs: hypotension, bradycardia, decreased respirations, hypothermia CV: bradycardia Neurologic: pinpoint pupils, coma, respiratory depression, seizures	Urine/plasma screen Arterial blood gases	Supportive care: 1. airway 2. breathing 3. circulation Prevention of absorption: 1. lavage 2. charcoal 3. cathartic Cardiac monitor Management of withdrawal Antidote: Naloxone Evaluation for pulmonary edema	An attempt should be made to get a complete history of the overdose, including route of exposure, quantities, and type of drug used, and history of addiction. Monitor in an intensive care facility.
Ethylene Glycol				
Antifreeze	Neurologic: ataxia, lethargy, coma, seizures GU: calcium oxaluria, hematuria, proteinuria, renal insufficiency Respiratory: pulmonary edema CV: cardiomegaly	Serum ethylene glycol level Electrolytes Arterial blood gases Renal function tests Urinalysis Osmolar gap (use plasma osmolaity measured with freezing point depression method)	Supportive care: 1. airway 2. breathing 3. circulation Prevention of absorption: 1. ipecac 2. lavage 3. activated charcoal 4. cathartic Correction of acidosis with IV sodium bicarbonate Ethanol drip: 1. monitor glucose 2. monitor blood alcohol level Hemodialysis (may be indicated for levels > 50 mg/dl, renal failure, or uncorrected acid–base or electrolyte abnormalities) Evaluation of renal function	Ethylene glycol toxicity may result in CNS effects similar to those seen with ethanol toxicity. Anion gap metabolic acidosis may result from the production of toxic metabolites. Oxalic acid formation may contribute to renal injury. Supplying ethanol competitively inhibits alcohol dehydrogenase, subsequently impairing the metabolism of ethylene glycol to its toxic metabolic. If IV ethanol is not available, oral ethanol may be given until the IV form is available.
Acetaminophen				
Acetaminophen-containing commercial products: Excedrin Extra Strength Tablet Liquiprin Tablet Tempura Chewable Table Tylenol PM	Phase 1 (up to 24 hr postingestion): anorexia, nausea, vomiting, diaphoresis, malaise Phase 2 (after 24 hr): RUQ pain, increased liver function tests and total bilirubin Phase 3 (3–5 days): characterized by se-	Acetaminophen level at 4 or more hr postingestion Daily monitoring of SGOT, total bilirubin, blood urea nitrogen, creatinine, and prothrombin time.	Supportive care: 1. airway 2. breathing 3. circulation Prevention of absorption: 1. ipecac 2. activated charcoal 3. cathartic Determination of 4 hr postingestion	Acetaminophen is an antipyretic and analgesic over-the-counter preparation. It also is a component of many combination products. Indication for n-acetylcysteine (NAC) therapy is determined by plotting the serum level on the Rumack–

(continued)

TABLE 46–5
Commonly Observed Poisonings (*Continued*)

Substance/Examples	Nursing Assessment	Diagnostic	Intervention	Comments
	quelae of hepatic necrosis: coagulation defects, jaundice, renal failure, hepatic encephalopathy Phase 4: recovery		acetaminophen level (plotted on Rumack–Matthew nomogram) Antidote: N-acetylcysteine (NAC, Mucomyst) 1. loading dose: 140 mg/kg po of 20% solution × 1 dose 2. Maintenance dose: 70 mg/kg of 20% solution × 17 doses q4h 3. Dilute doses 3:1 with soft drink or juice Repeat dose if patient vomits within 1 hr of dose; for persisting vomiting, consider an antiemetic or administration of undiluted drug via nasogastric or duodenal tube	Matthew nomogram (Fig. 46–1). NAC is most effective if administered within 8 hr postingestion. Oral NAC is the only approved drug treatment of acetaminophen poisoning in the U.S. Intravenous NAC is investigational in the U.S. Activated charcoal will interfere with NAC; therefore, do not adminster the drugs concurrently.
Organophosphates Chlorphyrifos Dursban Malathion Ortho Malathion 50 Insect Spray Parathion	1. Muscarinic effects: a. Increased salivation b. increased lacrimination c. sweating d. vomiting e. diarrhea 2. Nicotinic effects: a. muscle weakness b. respiratory paralysis c. fasiculations	Plasma pseduocholinesterase and/or red cell acetylcholinesterase	Supportive care: 1. airway 2. breathing 3. circulation Prevention of absorption: 1. ipecac 2. activated charcoal 3. cathartic Dermal decontamination: 1. Repeated washings with soap and water 2. discard leather products 3. protect health care provider from dermal exposure Assessment of oral secretions (suction prn) Pulmonary status monitoring: 1. breath sounds 2. chest radiograph Antidotes: 1. atropine 2. pralidoxime	Organophosphates are widely used in agriculture and for home/garden pest control. Rapid-acting organophosphates such as Tabun, Sarin, and Soman have been developed as nerve gases for chemical warfare. Well absorbed via oral, dermal, or inhalation routes, these agents exhibit their main effects by preventing the breakdown of the neurotransmitter acetylcholine. The acetylcholine accumulates at the synapses and myoneural junctions, leading to a cholinergic crisis. The efficient dermal absorption requires a rigorous skin decontamination. Leather products are difficult to decontaminate; therefore, the patient's leather shoes, watchband, and belt must be discarded. Atropine blocks the effects

(*continued*)

TABLE 46–5
Commonly Observed Poisonings (*Continued*)

Substance/Examples	Nursing Assessment	Diagnostic	Intervention	Comments
				of excessive acetylcholine if it persists in high enough concentrations. The administration of over 2,000 mg of atropine has been reported to reverse effects of severe poisoning.[3]
Salicylates Aspirin AlkaSeltzer Aspergum Pepto Bismol Sunscreens Liniments Methyl salicylate (oil of wintergreen)	Respiratory: tachypnea, pulmonary edema, respiratory alkalosis GI: nausea, vomiting, hemorrhage Metabolic: fluid and electrolyte disturbances, metabolic acidosis, hyperthermia, hypokalemia, dehydration, fever Neurologic: tinnitus, confusion, lethargy, coma, seizures Hematologic: hypothrombinemia, platelet dysfunction CV: tachycardia	Serial salicylate levels Arterial blood gases Electrolytes Complete blood count, prothrombin time, partial thromboplastin time Platelet count Chest radiograph	Supportive care: 1. airway 2. breathing 3. circulation Prevention of absorption: 1. ipecac 2. lavage 3. activated charcoal (serial doses) 4. cathartic Enhancement of excretion: 1. urine alkalinization to pH 7.5–8.0 Monitor respiratory status Hemodialysis may be indicated	Salicylates are used as antipyretic, analgesic, antiinflammatory medications. Absorption may be erratic. Large doses may form concretions in stomach and delay absorption and toxicity. At least two salicylate levels are needed to ensure levels are declining and absorption is not continuing. Urine alkalinization may be difficult without adequate serum potassium.
Methanol Antifreeze Windshield washer solvent Varnish Sterno Wood alcohol	Vital signs: monitor for apnea Neurologic: headache, vertigo, lethargy confusion; coma and seizures may occur in severe cases Ocular: blurred vision, decreased visual acuity, photophobia GI: nausea, vomiting, abdominal pain	Blood methanol Arterial blood gases Electrolytes Anion gap Glucose, blood alcohol while on ethanol drip	Supportive care: 1. airway 2. breathing 3. circulation Prevention of absorption: 1. ipecac/lavage 2. charcoal/cathartic ineffective Antidotes: 1. ethanol drip for blood methanol level greater than 20 mg/dl 2. Folic acid to enhance the metabolism of formic acid Correct acidosis with sodium bicarbonate Monitor electrolytes, creatinine, calcium, blood urea nitrogen and serum methanol and ethanol levels	Methanol is an alcohol commonly found in antifreeze, windshield washer fluid, and Sterno. Methanol is metabolized to formaldehyde and formic acid, both of which are much more toxic than methanol itself. These two end products produce severe acidosis and blindness, with the onset of symptoms in several hours to several days. The administration of intravenous alcohol is the treatment of choice. Alcohol competes with methanol at the enzyme site in the liver, blocking the formation of toxic metabolites and

(*continued*)

TABLE 46–5
Commonly Observed Poisonings (*Continued*)

Substance/Examples	Nursing Assessment	Diagnostic	Intervention	Comments

			Enhancement of elimination:
			1. Hemodialysis indications:
			  a. Methanol level over 50 mg/dl
			  b. Metabolic acidosis not immediately correctable with bicarbonate therapy
			  c. Visual impairment
			  d. Renal failure
				allowing methanol to be excreted unchanged. The drip must be continued until the blood methanol level is less than 20 mg/dl and acidosis is corrected.

CNS, central nervous system; CV, cardiovascular; GI, gastrointestinal; HEENT, head, eyes, ear, nose, throat; LDH, lactate dehydrogenase; CPK, creatinine phosphokinase; SGOT, serum glutamic oxaloacetic transaminase; CT, computed tomography; ECG, electrocardiogram; GU, genitourinary; IV, intravenous.

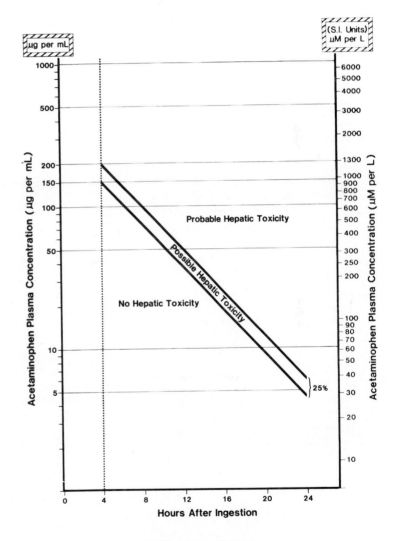

RUMACK – MATTHEW NOMOGRAM
FOR ACETAMINOPHEN POISONING

FIGURE 46–1
Semilogarithmic plot of plasma acetaminophen levels versus time. (With permission, from Rumack BH, Matthew HJ: Acetaminophen poisoning and toxicity. Pediatrics 55:871–876, 1975)

CAUTIONS FOR USE OF THIS CHART:
1) The time coordinates refer to time of ingestion.
2) Serum levels drawn before 4 hours may not represent peak levels.
3) The graph should be used only in relation to a single acute ingestion.
4) The lower solid line 25% below the standard nomogram is included to allow for possible errors in acetaminophen plasma assays and estimated time from ingestion of an overdose.

1022 Multisystem Organ Failure Conditions

NURSING CARE PLAN 46–1:
The Patient With Cocaine Toxicity

NURSING DIAGNOSIS	OUTCOME CRITERIA/ PATIENT GOALS	NURSING INTERVENTIONS
High risk for altered cardiac tissue perfusion: related to dysrhythmias and increased myocardial oxygen demand.	• Vital signs will return to or remain within normal limits.	1. Assess vital signs q15min initially and prn. 2. Note changes in blood pressure, heart rate, and rhythm. 3. Maintain bed rest. 4. Auscultate heart sounds q2h and prn. 5. Administer oxygen and medications, as ordered. 6. Monitor pulse oximetry or arterial blood gases, as ordered.
Hyperthermia: related to drug toxicity.	• Normal body temperature will be maintained.	1. Monitor temperature q15min initially and prn. 2. Place patient in cool room. 3. Minimize physical activity. 4. Sponge patient with tepid water. 5. Institute external cooling therapies as ordered (eg, cooling blanket).
High risk for injury: related to seizures, restlessness, and agitation.	• Patient will remain free of physical injury.	1. Monitor for seizure activity. 2. Pad side rails. 3. Place oral airway at bedside. 4. Suction equipment available at bedside. 5. Place bed in lower position, all side rails elevated. 6. Administer anticonvulsants, as ordered. 7. Administer sedation, as ordered. 8. Use soft restraints for agitation (not for seizure control).
Anxiety: related to use of a stimulant fear of the unknown, or fear of legal repercussions.	• Patient will demonstrate effective coping skills.	1. Decrease environmental stimuli. 2. Acknowledge and support effective coping mechanisms used by patient. 3. Identify major support systems or people. 4. Enlist patient's cooperation and allow him or her to participate in care when possible. 5. Explain all procedures in simple terms.

(continued)

NURSING CARE PLAN 46–1: *(Continued)*
The Patient With Cocaine Toxicity

NURSING DIAGNOSIS	OUTCOME CRITERIA/ PATIENT GOALS	NURSING INTERVENTIONS
Knowledge deficit: related to cocaine abuse.	• Patient will verbalize understanding of the physical manifestations of cocaine abuse.	1. Assess patient's and family's understanding of cocaine toxicity and treatment. 2. Assess learning ability and readiness to learn. 3. Provide information about the physical effects of cocaine abuse. 4. Clarify misconceptions.

REFERENCES

1. Litovitz T, Holm K: 1991 Annual report of the American Association of Poison Control Centers national data collection system. Am J Emerg Med 10:5, 1992
2. Caravati EM, McElwee NE: Use of clinical toxicology resources by emergency physicians and its impact on poison control centers. Ann Emerg Med 20:147–150, 1991
3. Rumack BH (ed): POISINDEX Information System, vol. 74. Denver, Micromedex, 1993, edition expires 11/30/92 (updated yearly)
4. Ford M, Hoffman RS, Goldfrank LR: Opioids and designer drugs. Emerg Med Clin North Am 8:495–511, 1990
5. Kornberg A, Dolgin J: Pediatric ingestions: Charcoal alone versus ipecac and charcoal. Ann Emerg Med 20:648–651, 1991
6. McEvoy G: AHFS Drug Information 92. Bethesda, MD, American Society of Hospital Pharmacists, 1992
7. Chafee-Bahamon C, Lacouture P, Lovejoy F: Risk assessment of ipecac in the home. Pediatrics 75:1106, 1985
8. Timberlake G: Ipecac as a cause of the Mallory–Weiss syndrome. South Med J 77:804–805, 1984
9. Wolowodiuk O, McMicken D, O'Brien P: Pneumomediastinum and retropneumoperitoneum: An unusual complication of syrup-of-ipecac-induced emesis. Ann Emerg Med 13:1148–1151, 1984
10. Olin B: Facts and Comparisons. St. Louis, JB Lippincott, 1992
11. Robertson W: A further warning on the use of salt as an emetic agent. J Pediatr 79:877, 1971
12. Streat S: Fatal salt poisoning in a child. New Zealand Medical Journal 706(95):285–286, 1982
13. Gresham G, Mashru M: Fatal poisoning with sodium chloride. Forensic Sci Int 20:87–88, 1982
14. Stein R, Jenkins D, Korns M: Death after use of cupric sulfate as emetic. JAMA 235:801, 1976
15. Goldfrank L, Flomenbaum N, Lewin N, Weisman R, Howland M (eds): Goldfrank Toxicologic Emergencies. Norwalk, CT, Appleton & Lange, 1990
16. Ellenhorn M, Bareloux D: Medical Toxicology: Diagnosis and Treatment of Human Poisonings. New York, Elsevier Science Publishing, 1988
17. Askenasi R, Abramowicz M, Jeanmart J, Ansay J, Degaute J: Esophageal perforation: An unusual complication of gastric lavage. Ann Emerg Med 13:146, 1984
18. Rakel R: Conn's Current Therapy. Philadelphia, WB Saunders, 1991
19. Hensyl W: Stedman's Medical Dictionary. Baltimore, Williams & Wilkins, 1990
20. DiPiro J: Pharmacotherapy: A Physiologic Approach. New York, Elsevier Science Publishing, 1989
21. Smilkstein M, Smolinske S, Kulig K, Rumack B: Severe hypermagnesemia due to multiple-dose cathartic therapy. West J Med 148:208–211, 1988
22. Weber C, Santiago R: Hypermagnesemia, a potential complication during treatment of theophylline intoxication with oral activated charcoal and magnesium-containing cathartics. Chest 95:56–59, 1989
23. McLuckie A, Forbes A, Ilett K: Role of repeated doses of oral activated charcoal in the treatment of acute intoxications. Anaesth Intensive Care 18:375–384, 1990
24. Young LY, Koda-Kimble M (eds): Applied Therapeutics: The Clinical Use of Drugs. Vancouver, WA, Applied Therapeutics, 1992
25. Levy G: Gastrointestinal clearance of drugs with activated charcoal. N Engl J Med 307:677, 1982
26. Watson C, Cremer K, Chapman J: Gastrointestinal obstruction associated with multiple-dose activated charcoal. J Emerg Med 4:401–407, 1986
27. Ray M, Padin D, Condie J, Halls J: Charcoal bezoar, small-bowel obstruction secondary to amitryptyline overdose therapy. Dig Dis Sci 33:106–107, 1988
28. Harsch H: Aspiration of activated charcoal. N Engl J Med 314:318, 1986
29. Rosenberg P, Livingston D, McLellan B: Effect of whole-

bowel irrigation on the antidotal efficacy of oral activated charcoal. Ann Emerg Med 17:681, 1988
30. Burkhart K, Kulig K, Rumack B: Whole-bowel irrigation as treatment for zinc sulfate overdose. Ann Emerg Med 19: 1167–1170, 1990
31. Hoffman R, Smilkstein M, Goldfrank L: Whole bowel irrigation and the cocaine body-packer: A new approach to a common problem. Am J Emerg Med 8:523–527, 1990
32. Kirshenbaum L, Mathews S, Sitar D, Tenenbein M: Whole-bowel irrigation versus activated charcoal in sorbitol for the ingestion of modified-released pharmaceuticals. Clin Pharmacol Ther 46:264–271, 1989
33. Smith S, Ling L, Halstenson C: Whole-bowel irrigation as a treatment for acute lithium overdose. Ann Emerg Med 20:536–539, 1991
34. Haddad L, Winchester J (eds): Clinical Management of Poisoning and Drug Overdose. Philadelphia, WB Saunders, 1990
35. Jameson M, Wiegmann T: Principles, uses, and complications of hemodialysis. Med Clin North Am 74:946, 1990
36. Garella S: Extra corporeal techniques in the treatment of exogenous intoxication. Kidney Int 33:737–738, 1988
37. Thom S: Hyperbaric oxygen therapy. J Intensive Care Med 4:58–59, 1989
38. Rioux J, Myers R: Hyperbaric oxygen for methylene chloride poisoning: Report on two cases. Ann Emerg Med 18:691–695, 1989
39. Sloan E, Murphy D, Hart R, Cooper M, Turnbull T, Barecca R, Ellerson R: Complications and protocol considerations in carbon-monoxide poisoned patients who require hyperbaric oxygen therapy: Report from a ten-year experience. Ann Emerg Med 18:629–634, 1989
40. Davis J: Hyperbaric oxygen therapy. J Intensive Care Med 4:57, 1989
41. Murphy D, Sloan E, Hart R, Narasimhan K, Barreca R: Tension pneumothorax associated with hyperbaric oxygen therapy. Am J Emerg Med 9:176–179, 1991
42. Perrin C, Debruyne D, Lacolte J, Laloum D, Bonte J, Moulin M: Treatment of caffeine intoxication by exchange transfusion in a newborn. Acta Paediatr Scand 76:679–681, 1987
43. Mier RJ: Treatment of aniline poisoning with exchange transfusion. Clinical Toxicology 26(5–6):357–364, 1988
44. Shannon M, Wernovsky G, Morris C: Exchange transfusion in the treatment of severe theophylline poisoning. Pediatrics 89:145–147, 1992
45. Smilkenstein MJ, Bronstein AC, Pickett HM, Rumack BH: Hyperbaric oxygen therapy for severe hydrogen sulfide poisoning. J Emerg Med 3(1):27–30, 1985
46. Brent J, Wang J, Foley M, Kulig K: Anion gap is not sensitive in the diagnosis of toxic metabolic acidosis. Ann Emerg Med 20:475, 1991

BIBLIOGRAPHY

Brogden R, Goa K: Flumazenil: A reappraisal of its pharmacological properties and therapeutic efficacy as a benzodiazepine antagonist. Drugs 42:1061–1089, 1991
Caravati E, Bossart P: Demographic and electrocardiographic factors associated with severe tricyclic antidepressant toxicity. Clinical Toxicology 29(1):31–43, 1991
DeSilva H, Wijewickrema R, Senanayake N: Does pralidoxime affect outcome of management in acute organophosphorous poisoning? Lancet 339:1136–38, 1992
Graziano J, Lolacono N, Moulton T, Mitchell M, Slavkovich V, Zarate C: Controlled study of meso-2, 3-dimercaptosuccinic acid for the management of childhood lead intoxication. J Pediatr 120:133–139, 1992
Hall A: Ethylene glycol and methanol: Poisons with toxic metabolic activation. Emergency Medicine Reports 12:29–38, 1992
Hall A: Gastrointestinal decontaminations: Sifting through supportive therapeutic options. Emergency Medicine Reports 12:171–178, 1991
Kuhn M: Drug overdoes: Salicylates. Crit Care Nurse 12(1):16, 25, 27, 1992
Litovits T, Manoguerra A: Comparison of pediatric poisoning hazards: An analysis of 3.8 million exposure incidents. Pediatrics 89:999–1006, 1992
Mayer A, Sitar D, Tenenbein M: Multiple-dose charcoal and whole-bowel irrigation do not increase clearance of absorbed salicylate. Arch Intern Med 152:393–396, 1992
Rottman S: Carbon monoxide screening in the ED. Am J Emerg Med 9:204–205, 1991
Schubert C, Wason S: Cocaine toxicity in an infant following intranasal instillation of a four percent cocaine solution. Pediatr Emerg Care 8:82–83, 1992
Shapiro B, Cane R: Blood gas monitoring: Yesterday, today and tomorrow. Crit Care Med 17:573–581, 1989
Tenebein M: Multiple doses of activated charcoal: Time for reappraisal? Ann Emerg Med 20:529–531, 1991
Woolf A, Wenger T, Smith T, Lovejoy F: The use of digoxin-specific fragments for severe digitalis intoxication in children. N Engl J Med 326:1739–1744, 1992

STUDY QUESTIONS

1. All of the following are examples of gut decontamination except

   a. syrup of ipecac
   b. activated charcoal
   c. gastric lavage
   d. exchange transfusion

2. Activated charcoal is not an effective adsorbent of the following

   a. cyclic antidepressants
   b. salicylates

    c. lithium carbonate

    d. acetaminophen

3. Urine alkalinization may increase renal clearance of

    a. all drugs

    b. salicylates

    c. cyclic antidepressants

    d. acetaminophen

4. A patient presents to the emergency room with tinnitus, nausea, vomiting, hypo-kalemia, and mild pulmonary edema. The clinical findings may be related to

    a. an anticholinergic drug

    b. salicylate toxicity

    c. cyclic antidepressant toxicity

    d. organophosphate poisoning

5. Tricyclic antidepressant overdose may cause all of the following except

    a. cardiac dysrhythmias

    b. seizures

    c. anticholinergic effects

    d. alkalosis

6. Symptoms of cholinergic syndrome include

    a. decreased vital signs

    b. excessive secretions

    c. muscle fasciculations

    d. all of the above

CHAPTER 47

Immune System-Compromising Conditions

BEHAVIORAL OBJECTIVES

Based on the content in this chapter, the reader should be able to:

1. Describe the physiology of adaptive immune responses.

Hudak: Critical Care Nursing:
A Holistic Approach, 6th ed. © 1994
J. B. Lippincott Company.

2. Discuss the etiologies of impaired host defenses and resistance.
3. Outline appropriate nursing assessment parameters related to immunocompetence of the critically ill patient.
4. Describe the etiology, immunopathology, and medical and nursing interventions associated with acquired immunodeficiency syndrome.
5. Discuss the incidence and development of nosocomial infections in the critically ill patient.
6. Explain universal precautions and their implementation in the critical care unit.

Description

Virtually all patients cared for in a critical care unit probably have some degree of immune system dysfunction related to disruptions caused by their underlying disease processes or alterations in their physical, chemical, and inflammatory responses associated with diagnostic, therapeutic, and supportive medical interventions. Bringing renewed attention to this problem is the patient with acquired immunodeficiency syndrome (AIDS)/human immunodeficiency virus (HIV) infection. Therefore, as the knowledge base in immunology grows, critical care nurses must incorporate this knowledge into their practice to care competently for the critically ill patient.

This chapter presents an overview of the immune system, its anatomy and physiology, etiologies of dysfunction in host defenses, guidelines for assessment of immunocompetence, and considerations for patients with AIDS and nosocomial infections.

Physiological Principles

Immune Responses

Under normal circumstances, the human body is equipped with numerous mechanisms that enable it to resist almost all types of organisms and toxins that damage tissues and organs. Usually, infections in most people are short in duration and leave little or no damage to the immune system. The body's protective mechanisms can be divided into two major groups: *innate* and *adaptive*. A healthy immune system consists of all the components of these two groups of defense mechanisms, and performs three major functions:

1. Protection of the body from destruction by foreign agents and microbial pathogens
2. Degradation and removal of damaged and dead cells
3. Surveillance and destruction of malignant cells

Innate Immunity

Innate immunities are present in all normal people and form the first line of defense against illness. A previous exposure to an organism or toxin is not required. These mechanisms are general and do not distinguish between microorganisms of different species, and do not alter in intensity on reexposure. Innate immunities include physical, chemical, and mechanical barriers, biologic defenses, phagocytes, inflammatory processes, interferons, and natural killer cells.

Physical, Chemical, and Mechanical Barriers
Physical barriers, such as skin, prevent harmful organisms and other substances from gaining entrance into the body or body cavities. Chemical defense factors include antibacterial agents, antibodies, and acid solutions that create an environment hostile to many pathogens. Other mechanisms, such as normal intestinal peristalsis, function through mechanical actions to help rid the body of potentially harmful substances. Additional examples of these types of barriers are listed below.

Biologic Defenses
Under normal conditions, large areas of the human body are colonized with microorganisms. The skin and mucous membranes of the oropharynx, nasopharynx, intestinal tract, and parts of the genital tract each have their own microflora, referred to as normal flora. These microorganisms influence patterns of colonization by competing with more harmful organisms for essential nutrients, as well as by producing substances that inhibit the growth of other microorganisms.

Nonspecific Physical, Chemical, and Mechanical Barriers

Physical

Skin
Mucous membranes
Epiglottis
Respiratory tract cilia
Sphincters

Chemical

Tears (lysozyme)
Vaginal secretions (lactic acid)
Gastric acidity (hydrochloric acid)

Mechanical

Lacrimation
Intestinal peristalsis
Urinary flow

Phagocytes and Phagocytosis

Phagocytosis is a nonspecific response in which injured cells and foreign invaders are ingested by certain white blood cells (leukocytes). The two main phagocytic leukocytes are the polymorphonuclear neutrophils and the mononuclear monocytes. Both cells originate from stem cells in the bone marrow, and, although structurally different, both approach phagocytosis in a similar manner. Surface receptors on their cell membranes allow them to attach to foreign substances and then to engulf, internalize, and destroy these substances using enzymatic mechanisms present within their cellular interior.

Neutrophils constitute approximately 60% of the white blood cells of the peripheral blood, are produced in the bone marrow at the rate of approximately 80 million per minute, and generally survive for only 2 to 3 days. Neutrophils provide the "first-wave" cellular attack on invading organisms during acute inflammatory processes.

Monocytes comprise 2% to 12% of the white blood cells found in peripheral blood and are mobile, phagocytic cells that spend only a short time in the bloodstream before escaping through the capillary membranes into the tissue. Once in the tissue, they swell to much larger sizes to become tissue macrophages. Monocytes will either attach to certain tissues and destroy bacteria, or wander through the tissue phagocytizing foreign matter. These tissue macrophages form the basis of the reticuloendothelial system, and can be found strategically placed throughout the body tissues where they can exist for months and even years to function as a first line of defense against invading microorganisms. Macrophages in different tissues differ in appearance because of environmental variations, and are known by different names.

Inflammatory Responses

Inflammation is an acute, nonspecific physiological response of the body to tissue injury caused by factors such as chemicals, heat, trauma, or microbial invasion. It is the primary process through which the body repairs tissue damage and defends itself against infection. Inflammation may be initiated by either immune or nonspecific pathways. The major events of the inflammatory process, which

are mediated by chemical substances released from injured cells, include:

1. Increased blood flow and increased vessel permeability at the site of injury
2. The movement of leukocytes from surrounding blood vessels into the tissues
3. The formation of a fibrin clot that walls off the injured area to delay or limit spread of toxic products or bacteria

The single most important result of this process is accumulation of large numbers of polymorphonuclear neutrophil and macrophage phagocytes at the injury site, which act to inactivate or destroy invaders, remove debris, and begin the initial tissue repair. The neutrophils react quickly and are the initial "attack troops," whereas the macrophages, the "big eaters," finish the job by acting as the clean-up troops.

Interferons and Natural Killer Cells

When infected by viruses, certain types of cells respond by secreting glycoproteins called interferons. Interferons provide some protection to the body against invasion by viruses until more slowly reacting specific immune responses can take over.

In addition, interferons appear to be involved in protecting the body against some forms of cancer. These substances have been demonstrated to interfere with cellular division and proliferation of abnormal cells. They also enhance the activity of a specialized group of lymphoid cells called natural killer cells. Natural killer cells are a population of lymphocytes that do not carry markers for either T or B lymphocytes. These cells act directly, without prior sensitization, to lyse a variety of malignant cells and also play a significant role in cancer immunity.

Adaptive Immune Responses

When a foreign agent gains entrance to the body, innate defenses will attempt to destroy it. If the agent persists, the body's second line of defense, activation of the acquired or adaptive immune system, is initiated. These adaptive immune responses generally require previous exposure to a foreign agent or organism to be most effective. In contrast to innate defense mechanisms, the cellular components of these types of responses are capable of distinguishing between microorganisms and can alter their intensity and response time significantly on reexposure to foreign agents. Adaptive immune responses are not always beneficial, however, and they sometimes are responsible for hypersensitivity reactions (allergies) and other harmful reactions such as autoimmune diseases.

Two major arms of the adaptive immune response have been identified: cell-mediated immunity and humoral immunity. Certain mononuclear leukocytes known as lymphocytes are central to both these types of immunity. Lymphocytes referred to as B lymphocytes belong to

---

Macrophages Localized in Various Tissues

Kupffer's cells	Liver
Tissue macrophages	Lymph nodes
	Spleen
	Bone marrow
Alveolar macrophages	Lung
Histiocytes	Skin
	Subcutaneous tissue
Microglia	Brain

the humoral response and are the source of the protein substances known as antibodies, which bind to foreign substances and aid in their removal or destruction. Cells known as T lymphocytes are the mediators of cell-mediated immune response. This second type of acquired immunity is achieved through the formation of large numbers of activated T lymphocytes that are designed specifically to destroy the foreign agent. Most foreign substances stimulate both cellular and humoral immune responses, which results in an overlapping of their reactions and maximum protection against damage from these invaders. Macrophages, another cellular component essential to these responses, function to present foreign agents to both T and B cells and initiate their subsequent reactions.

Any foreign substance capable of eliciting a specific immune response is referred to as an antigen. Antigens most often are composed of proteins, but polysaccharides, complex lipids, and nucleic acids sometimes may act as antigenic materials.

Lymphoid System
Acquired immunity is the result of all the cells, tissues, and organs that participate in adaptive immune responses and are collectively referred to as the lymphoid system. This system consists of primary and secondary lymphoid organs and tissues.

The B and T lymphocytes originate from stem cells produced in the bone marrow. During fetal development and shortly after birth, primary lymphoid organs are the site where these cells differentiate and mature into the competent cells responsible for humoral and cellular immune responses. For T lymphocytes, this preprocessing occurs in the thymus gland, and for B lymphocytes it is believed to occur in the bone marrow and possibly the fetal liver. As they develop, both B and T lymphocytes acquire specific receptors for antigens that commit them to a single antigenic specificity for their lifetime. Subsequently, each of these "preprogrammed" T or B lymphocytes (on activation by its specific antigen) is capable of producing tremendous numbers of clones or duplicate lymphocytes.

The thymus gland, in addition to providing the site for T cell differentiation, also produces factors known as thymic hormones. These factors not only influence thymic T cell maturation, but also circulate throughout the body, inducing competent T and B lymphocyte function throughout life.

After preprocessing in the primary lymphoid organs, B and T lymphocytes migrate to secondary lymphoid tissues where the interaction with antigens and immune responses actually occurs. Secondary lymphatic tissue is located extensively in the lymph nodes. It also is found in special lymphoid tissue such as that of the spleen, tonsils, adenoids, appendix, bone marrow, and gastrointestinal tract. This lymphoid tissue is placed advantageously throughout the body to intercept invading organisms or

toxins before they can enter the bloodstream and disseminate too widely.

Cell-Mediated Immune Responses
Cell-mediated immune responses are important in providing adaptive immune resistance to viruses, fungi, parasites, and intracellular bacteria. They also play a major role in rejection or acceptance of certain tissue grafts, in the stimulation and regulation of antibody production, and in the defense against various cancers. In fact, T lymphocytes are the primary cells of cell-mediated immunity and are involved in almost all adaptive immune reactions—either by acting as effector cells while directly attacking antigens and malignant cells, or by acting as regulators of both the humoral and cellular immune response.

The cell-mediated response is begun by antigenic stimulation of T lymphocytes found in the lymphoid tissues. This step of the response is mediated by macrophages that bind to the antigen, facilitating recognition of the antigen. The macrophages then produce a chemical substance known as interleukin-1 that serves to activate antigen-specific T lymphocytes. Once activated, these cells clone themselves, giving rise to a large number of subpopulations of T cells that subsequently carry out the functions attributed to the cell-mediated immune response.

The different types of T cells produced are categorized according to their functions, and include: (1) cytotoxic T cells; (2) helper–inducer T cells; (3) delayed hypersensitivity T cells; (4) suppressor T cells; and (5) memory T cells. The T cells also may be classified structurally by the surface antigens present on their cell membrane. Once mature, T cells either display the T4 antigen or the T8 antigen. The T4 subset consists mainly of helper–inducer cells; the T8 subset contains predominantly cytotoxic–suppressor cells.

Cytotoxic T cells (T8) are direct-attack cells capable of killing many microorganisms, and are the predominant effector cell of cell-mediated immune responses. Virus-infected cells, cancer cells, and transplanted cells appear to be particularly susceptible to the deadly effects of the cytotoxic T cells.

Helper–inducer T cells (T4) are the most numerous and also the most important of all the subpopulations of T lymphocytes. These T lymphocytes play a pivotal role in the overall regulation of the immune response and often are referred to as the "master conductor" of the specific immune system. On activation by antigen-infected macrophages, helper–inducer T cells secrete substances known as lymphokines that modulate and enhance the activity of all other lymphoid cells, including macrophages, antibody-producing B lymphocytes, cytotoxic and suppressor T cells, and natural killer cells. Given the central role of the helper T4 cell, reduction in the normal number of these cells, as occurs in AIDS, can seriously impair the overall immune response and the level of host resistance.

Suppressor T cells (T8) act as negative feedback controllers of the helper–inducer T4 cells, causing cessation of the immune response when it no longer is needed and thus preventing excessive reactions that might severely damage the body. It is speculated that these cells also limit the ability of the immune system to attack body tissues, creating what is called "immune tolerance."

Delayed-type hypersensitivity cells mediate inflammation and activate macrophages in delayed-type hypersensitivity (allergic) reactions. *Memory T lymphocytes* are the subpopulation sensitized to antigens during specific immune responses that remain stored in the body and are capable of initiating a far more rapid response by the T cells on reexposure to the same antigen.

Humoral Immunity

Humoral immune responses, involving B lymphocytes, are important in providing specific immune resistance to most bacteria, bacterial toxins, and the extracellular phase of viral infections. On stimulation (within the blood or lymphoid tissues by an antigen and in conjunction with signals from macrophages and T4 helper–inducer lymphocytes), antigen-specific B lymphocytes multiply, differentiate, and mature into plasma cells and memory cells. The plasma cells produce antibodies that bind to antigens to form antigen–antibody complexes that neutralize or destroy the antigen. After the antigen is eliminated, the plasma cells disappear, but the memory B cells remain in circulation and in the lymphoid tissue to mature into plasma cells if the antigen is encountered again.

Complement System

Complement is a collective term used to describe a system of about 20 different proteins that, when activated, play a major role in immune defense responses, primarily by:

1. Directly causing destruction of antigens by cellular membrane lysis
2. Facilitating interaction of antigens and antibodies
3. Enhancing all aspects of the inflammatory process, especially with respect to increasing vascular permeability and phagocytosis

The main components of this system are 11 proteins that normally reside among the plasma proteins of the blood in an inactive form. Activation of these complement proteins involves a cascade type of sequence, and may be accomplished by one of two pathways. The classic pathway is activated by antibody–antigen complexes. The alternative pathway can activate complement in response to certain microbial products in the absence of antibody–antigen complexes.

Combined Immune Responses

The adaptive immune response is complex and involves the interaction of macrophages, complement proteins, and the cellular components of both the cellular and humoral systems. Macrophages initially function to recognize, process, and present the antigen to antigen-specific

T lymphocytes within the lymphoid tissues. Helper–inducer T4 cells subsequently are activated with the help of a chemical factor (interleukin-1) released by the presenting macrophage. The T4 cells proliferate and produce their own chemical substances, known as lymphokines, which in turn stimulate the activation and proliferation of antibody-producing B lymphocytes, cytotoxic T cells, suppressor T cells, and phagocytic macrophages. The production of antibodies leads to the activation of complement proteins. All of these components work together to destroy the antigen, either through complex processes involving direct attack or through modulation by chemical processes. Suppressor T cells provide feedback to the T4 helper cells to halt these defense reactions when they are no longer needed, and memory cells serve to reactivate them on reexposure to the antigen. Figure 47–1 is a schematic representation of these processes.

Impaired Host Resistance

As the previous section has demonstrated, the various components of the immune system provide an exquisitely complex network of mechanisms that, when intact, function to defend the body against foreign microorganisms and malignant cells. In some situations, however, components of either the nonspecific or specific immune responses can fail, resulting in host defense impairment. A number of conditions that can affect various aspects of the immune system are presented in Table 47–1. People who acquire an infection because of a deficiency in any of their multifaceted host defenses are referred to as compromised hosts. People with major defects related to specific immune responses are referred to as immunosuppressed hosts. These two terms often are used interchangeably, although in theory they do have different connotations.

The exact effects and symptoms related to defects in host defenses will vary according to the part of the immune system affected. General features associated with compromised host defects, however, include recurrent infections, infections caused by usually harmless agents (opportunistic organisms), chronic infections, skin rashes, diarrhea, growth impairment, and increased susceptibility to certain cancers.

Assessment

The ability of the human body to protect itself against disease is described by the term immunocompetence. Immunocompetence can be assessed by the critical care nurse through seven major areas—history, nutritional status, skin integrity, chronic disease, immunosuppressed states, medications and treatment, and diagnostic studies (Fig. 47–2).

It is essential that assessment of immunocompetence be performed on the critically ill patient at frequent, regular

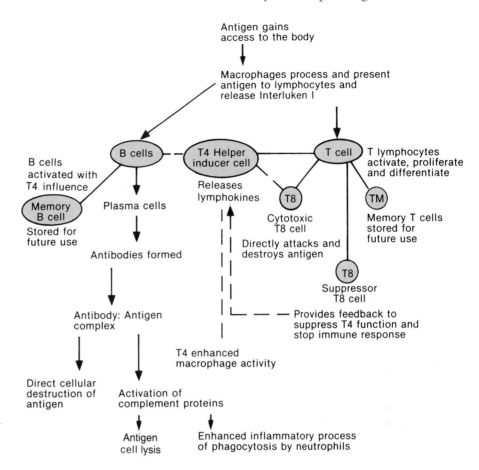

FIGURE 47–1
A schematic representation of the combined immune responses.

intervals. During assessment, the nurse should be extremely attentive to possible sites of infection, changes in body temperature, and laboratory findings that may provide an early indication of compromise in immune functioning.

History

A careful history to identify susceptibility to infection is of major importance in assessing a patient's immunocompetence. The type of infection often provides the first clue as to the nature of the immune defect. For example, patients with defects in humoral immunity may have recurrent or chronic bacterial infections such as meningitis or bacteremia. Repeated viral or fungal infections indicate a defect in cell-mediated immunity.

The patient's chronologic age also influences immunocompetence. Immune response may be depressed in the very young owing to the underdevelopment of the thymus gland. In elderly people, atrophy of the thymus gland may increase susceptibility to infection.

Nutritional Status

The patient's nutritional status has a major impact on immune function. Inadequate protein and calories can alter immune responses and resistance to infection by decreasing lymphocyte and antibody production. A team approach using a nutritionist can assist the nurse in assessing dietary intake and nutritional requirements for the critically ill immunocompromised person.

Skin Integrity

The integumentary system, including skin and mucous membranes, has been identified as a physical barrier to infection. Surgical or traumatic wounds, burn injuries, or pressure sores breach these physical defenses and predispose the critically ill patient to infection. In a critical care setting, in which intravenous and intra-arterial catheters, urethral catheters, or endotracheal tubes are used, multiple portals of entry for pathogens can provide simultaneous sites for potential infection. All wounds and portals of entry should be assessed for signs and symptoms of infection.

Chronic Disease

Many chronic diseases are associated with compromised immune functioning. Diabetes, cancer, and aplastic anemia are just a few examples of diseases during the course of which immune deficiencies occur (see Table 47–1). Be-

TABLE 47–1
Factors Predisposing to Specific Aspects of Compromised Host Defenses

Host Defect	Diseases, Therapies and Other Conditions Associated With Host Defects
Impaired phagocyte functioning	Radiation therapy
	Nutritional deficiencies
	Diabetes mellitus
	Acute leukemias
	Corticosteroids
	Cytotoxic chemotherapeutic drugs
	Aplastic anemia
	Congenital hematologic disorders
	Alcoholism
Complement system deficiencies	Liver disease
	Systemic lupus erythematosus
	Sickle cell anemia
	Splenectomy
	Congenital deficiencies
Impaired cell-mediated (T lymphocyte) immune response	Radiation therapy
	Nutritional deficiencies
	Aging
	Thymic aplasia
	AIDS
	Hodgkin's disease/lymphomas
	Corticosteroids
	Antilymphocyte globulin
	Congenital thymic dysfunctions
Impaired humoral (antibody) immunity	Chronic lymphocytic leukemia
	Multiple myeloma
	Congenital hypogammaglobulinemia
	Protein-liosing enteropathies (inflammatory bowel disease)
Interruption of physical/mechanical/chemical barriers	Traumatic injury
	Decubitus ulcers/skin defect
	Invasive medical procedures
	Vascular disease
	Skin diseases
	Nutritional impairments
	Burns
	Respiratory intubation
	Mechanical obstruction of body drainage systems such as lacrimal and urinary systems
	Decreased level of consciousness
Impaired reticuloendothelial system	Liver disease
	Splenectomy

From Larson E: Infection control issues in critical care: An update. Heart Lung 14:149–155.

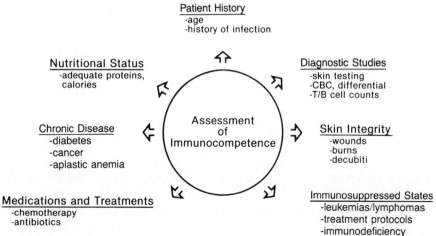

FIGURE 47–2
Assessment of immunocompetence in the critically ill patient should cover seven major areas.

cause many critically ill patients have underlying chronic disease, the existence of such diseases should be considered contributing factors when the immunocompetence of these patients is assessed.

Immunosuppressed States

In addition to cancer, leukemias and lymphomas can severely compromise cell-mediated immunity by decreasing functional T cells. Chemotherapy and radiation therapy commonly used to treat these disorders also decrease normal T cells in the body and further compromise immune functioning.

Congenital and acquired immunodeficiency states also result in the suppression of the body's immune response. Primary immunodeficiencies may be either congenital or acquired and involve defects in either the development or differentiation of T and B cells. Secondary immunodeficiencies result from underlying disease, malnutrition, cytotoxic drugs, and infectious agents. A prime example of a secondary immunodeficiency is AIDS, which may follow infection with HIV.

Medications and Treatments

Treatment protocols for increasing numbers of cancer patients being cared for in the critical care unit can lead to life-threatening complications such as infection and sepsis. Chemotherapeutic agents primarily affect the bone marrow's ability to produce stem cells, which are the precursors for the white blood cells in the body.

Antibiotics such as tetracycline and chloramphenicol inhibit cellular immunity. Steroids display many immunologic effects, including decreased lymphocyte and antibody concentration. Patients placed on treatment regimes with these agents should be monitored for compromise in immune functioning as part of their total response to the therapy.

It is clear that the immune response of the critically ill patient can be affected by underlying disease, therapeutic protocols, and environmental influences. Accurate and timely assessment of these factors can assist the critical care nurse in providing individualized care to patients with compromised immune functioning.

Diagnostic Studies

Laboratory tests to assess immunocompetence include intradermal skin testing, complete blood count with differential, and circulating T and B cell counts. Additional data may be obtained for specific infections through radiography and culture specimens.

AIDS: Acquired Immunodeficiency Syndrome

Description

Acquired immunodeficiency syndrome was first recognized in 1981 as a severe disease characterized by impaired cellular immunity caused by a previously unknown retrovirus, known as HIV. In 1982 AIDS was defined by the Centers for Disease Control and Prevention (CDC). Today, AIDS remains a uniformly fatal disease, with most patients requiring sophisticated medical and nursing care during the course of the illness.

Epidemiology

People at greatest risk for AIDS–HIV infection in the United States include homosexual–bisexual men who are sexually active outside a monogamous relationship, intravenous drug users who share needles or syringes with an infected person, hemophiliacs and people with coagulation disorders, sexual partners of any of the above, and babies of mothers with HIV–AIDS infections who may become infected *in utero* (Table 47–2).[1] People who have had blood transfusions since 1977 are at small risk for the infection. Of all the statistics, perhaps the most alarming is the growing number of adolescents who have become infected from heterosexual intercourse.[2]

Pathophysiology

Etiology and Transmission

The cause of the immune defects in AIDS is a viral agent called HIV from the group of viruses known as retroviruses. Retroviruses are transmitted by blood and intimate contact (sexual), and have a strong affinity for T lymphocytes.

In the retrovirus, the genetic information is transmitted as a single strand of RNA. For the RNA to replicate, this information is transferred into a double strand of DNA in the host cell nucleus. This backward or "retro" flow of information from RNA to DNA is made possible by the enzyme reverse transcriptase that exists in the retrovirus particle. A model of the HIV retrovirus is presented in Figure 47–3.

Transmission of HIV follows a pattern similar to that of hepatitis B, having enteric, parenteral, and sexual routes of transmission. Thus, precautions in the critical care setting against contact with blood and bodily fluids should be used when a patient is hospitalized with AIDS (see Display Box 47–1).

Transmission in the workplace can be related to the following areas (see Display Box 47–2):

1. Needle stick or parenteral exposures, including punctures, lacerations, and superficial cuts.

TABLE 47–2
Overview of the Epidemiology of AIDS

Occurrence	Worldwide and increasing everywhere. Highest in persons with identified risk factors: homosexual and bisexual males, heterosexual contact with persons with AIDS, intravenous drug abuse, transfusion recipients, hemophilia or coagulation disorder, infant born of HIV-positive mother.
Etiologic agent	Human immunodeficiency virus (HIV); two types of HIV virus have been identified: HIV-1 (prevalent in the United States) and HIV-2 (prevalent in West Africa and countries with epidemiologic links to West Africa).
Reservoir	Humans.
Transmission	The virus is present in blood and serum-derived body fluids; transmitted person to person through anal or vaginal intercourse, transplacentally, and by breastfeeding; transmitted indirectly by transfusion of contaminated blood or blood products, use of contaminated needles or syringes, or direct contact with infected blood or body fluids on mucous membranes or open wounds; theoretically possible to transmit by oral/genital contact and deep French kissing. There are no reports of transmission from saliva, tears, urine, bronchial secretions, biting insects or any type of casual contact.
Incubation period	Variable. The time from exposure to seroconversion is 4 weeks to 6 months. The time to symptomatic immune suppression and to AIDS diagnosis can be up to 20 years.
Period of communicability	Lifelong; from presence of HIV in sera until death. The degree of contagiousness may vary during the course of HIV infection.
Susceptibility and resistance	Unknown; presumed to be general. Antibody response is not protective.
Report to local health authority	AIDS case report required. Report of HIV positive status varies by state.

Data from Benensen A (ed): Control of Communicable Diseases in Man, 15th ed. Washington, DC, The American Public Health Association, 1990.
Reproduced by permission from Grimes E: Infectious Diseases. St. Louis, Mosby Year Book, 1991.

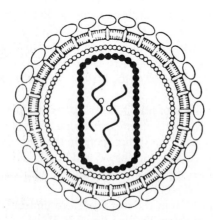

FIGURE 47–3
Model of the retrovirus HIV, the causative agent of AIDS.

DISPLAY BOX 47–1
Safety Practices in the Workplace

Three essentials for safe workplace practices are:

1. Knowledge of the disease and its transmission
2. Strict adherence to universal precautions
3. Use of the following engineering controls:
   - Prohibit needle capping without the use of a mechanical device
   - Placement of needle containers of rigid construction at site of use
   - Convenient placement of soap and running water for handwashing

---

2. Mucosal exposures, including splashes to the eyes, mouth and nose.
3. Large-volume exposure to intact skin surfaces.

In some hospitals and other health care providerships, AZT (zidovudine; formerly azidothymidine) therapy has been adopted as a means of treatment and prevention for the exposed health care worker. The worker, however, must begin the treatment within 4 hours of the exposure for optimum coverage, and not later than 24 hours for the treatment to have effect. Display Box 47–3 illustrates the course of AIDS–HIV infection.[3]

Immune Defects

Immunologically, AIDS patients exhibit impaired activation of both cellular and humoral immunity. The AIDS virus, HIV, primarily infects the T4 helper cell of the immune system. As previously described, the T4 helper cell plays a major role in the overall immune response. Infection of the T4 helper cell with HIV results in profound lymphopenia with decreased functional abilities, including decreased response to antigens and loss of stimulus for T and B cell activation. In addition, the cytotoxic activity of the T8 killer cell is impaired. The functional abilities of macrophages also are affected, with decreased phagocytosis and diminished chemotaxis. In humoral immunity, there is diminished antibody response to antigens, along with deregulation of antibody production. In essence, serum antibodies are increased, but their functional abilities are decreased. The total effect of these immune defects is increased susceptibility to opportunistic infections and neoplasms. A summary of the immune defects associated with AIDS is presented in Figure 47–4.

Assessment

Clinical Manifestations

The clinical course of AIDS is characterized by a progressive decline in immunocompetence and by repeated episodes of severe opportunistic infections. The entire spectrum of clinical findings ranges from asymptomatic infection with HIV to a variety of infections and symptoms of decreasing immunocompetence with AIDS-related complex, to full-blown AIDS with the diagnosis of opportunistic infection as defined by the CDC (Table 47–3).[4] The AIDS patient typically gives a history that may include weight loss, fever, night sweats, lymphadenopathy, diarrhea, and a persistent nonproductive cough.

Although patients with AIDS are seriously ill and frequently hospitalized, their need for critical care is limited. The critical care nurse more often encounters patients with AIDS when they have life-threatening opportunistic infections. The most common of the opportunistic infections is *Pneumocystis carinii* pneumonia (PCP), an interstitial pneumonia caused by a protozoan. This pneumonia is accompanied by dyspnea, tachypnea, cyanosis, a nonproductive cough, and initial respiratory alkalosis. The major indication for critical care of AIDS patients is impending or actual respiratory failure due to PCP. Symptoms of respiratory compromise often are more severe than diagnostic studies such as chest x-rays and blood gas values indicate. Therefore, early aggressive therapy with intravenous trimethoprim and sulfamethoxazole (Bactrim,

Clinical Research

McNabb K, Keller M: Nurses' risk taking regarding HIV transmission in the workplace. Western Journal of Nursing Research 13:732–745, 1991

Over 300 nurses answered a questionnaire designed to explore their knowledge regarding transmission of HIV in the workplace and to determine if this knowledge influenced their risk-taking behavior on the job. Although the results of the study indicate that the nurses possessed accurate knowledge about HIV causes and transmission and preventive measures, they still took risks when acceptable protective materials were not available. Specifically, the nurses admitted to starting an IV without protection either because of being in a hurry or due to the difficulty of starting an IV with gloves on. Because starting an IV is a common procedure for critical care nurses, having gloves of acceptable quality becomes a significant issue in reducing risk-taking behavior in the critical care unit.

Septra) or with pentamidine is the treatment of choice for the person with diagnosed or suspected PCP. Even with urgent, aggressive treatment, many patients require mechanical ventilation for progressive alveolar hypoventilation.

Other opportunistic infections associated with AIDS include meningitis, candidiasis, cytomegalovirus, and atypical mycobacteria. Patients may present with esophagitis caused by candidiasis, leading to dysphagia and malnutrition. It is important to note that although single infections may develop in critically ill patients with AIDS, they often have multiple infections occurring simultaneously and requiring a variety of treatment strategies.

Opportunistic infections may strike the central nervous system (CNS). These infections may cause intracranial abscesses, meningitis, or encephalopathy. Minor symptoms of CNS involvement include headache, fever, malaise, and weight loss. More severe symptoms include seizures, hemiparesis, cognitive and sensory defects, or coma. Patients with CNS involvement in AIDS may arrive at the hospital requiring critical care, or signs and symptoms may develop in them, necessitating transfer to an intensive care unit during the course of their hospitalization.

A disseminated form of the neoplasm known as Kaposi's sarcoma strikes homosexual and bisexual patients

DISPLAY BOX 47–3
Phases of HIV Infection and AIDS

Phase	Length of Phase	Antibodies Detectable	Symptoms	Can be Transmitted
1. Window period	4 wks to 6 mos after infection	No	None	Yes
2. Acute primary HIV infection	1–2 wks	Possible	Flu-like illness	Yes
3. Asymptomatic infection	1–15 or more yrs	Yes	None	Yes
4. Symptomomatic immune suppression	Up to 3 yrs	Yes	Fever, night sweats, weight loss, diarrhea, neuropathy, fatigue, rashes, lymphadenopathy, cognitive slowing, oral lesions	Yes
5. AIDS	Variable: 1–5 yrs from first AIDS-defining condition	Yes	Severe opportunistic infections and tumors in any body system; neurologic manifestations	Yes

From Grimes E: Infectious Diseases. St. Louis, Mosby Year Book, 1991.

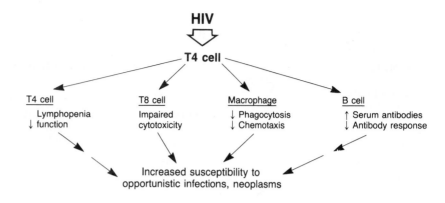

FIGURE 47-4
Summary of immune defects in AIDS.

TABLE 47-3
1993 Revision of Case Definition for AIDS for Surveillance Purposes

Conditions Included in the 1993 AIDS Surveillance Case Definition

- Candidiasis of bronchi, trachea, or lungs
- Candidiasis, esophageal
- Cervical cancer, invasive*
- Coccidioidomycosis, disseminated or extrapulmonary
- Cryptococcosis, extrapulmonary
- Cryptosporidiosis, chronic intestinal (>1 month's duration)
- Cytomegalovirus disease (other than liver, spleen, or nodes)
- Cytomegalovirus retinitis (with loss of vision)
- Encephalopathy, HIV-related
- Herpes simplex: chronic ulcer(s) (>1 month's duration); or bronchitis, pneumonitis, or esophagitis
- Histoplasmosis, disseminated or extrapulmonary
- Isosporiasis, chronic intestinal (>1 month's duration)
- Kaposi's sarcoma
- Lymphoma, Burkitt's (or equivalent term)
- Lymphoma, immunoblastic (or equivalent term)
- Lymphoma, primary, of brain
- *Mycobacterium avium* complex or *M. kansasii*, disseminated or extrapulmonary
- *Mycobacterium tuberculosis*, any site (pulmonary* or extrapulmonary)
- *Mycobacterium*, other species or unidentified species, disseminated or extrapulmonary
- *Pneumocystis carinii* pneumonia
- Pneumonia, recurrent*
- Progressive multifocal leukoencephalopathy
- *Salmonella* septicemia, recurrent
- Toxoplasmosis of brain
- Wasting syndrome due to HIV
- Also included as an AIDS indicator is a CD4 count of 200 or less cells/μL.

*Added in the 1993 expansion of the AIDS surveillance case definition.
From Centers for Disease Control: 1993 Revised Classification System for HIV Infection and Expanded Surveillance Case Definition for AIDS Among Adolescents and Adults. MMWR 41, No. RR-17, December 18, 1992.

with AIDS more often than any other group. This tumor can disseminate through the viscera, causing airway obstruction, gastrointestinal bleeding, and malnutrition. Chemotherapy and radiation therapy have been effective in its treatment (Table 47–4).

Management

Management of the patient with AIDS is a problem involving a complex, multisystem disease process, multiple hospitalizations, invasive diagnostic testing, and an extremely high mortality rate. The prognosis is related to the nature of the secondary disease that develops and the degree of immunocompromisation. Patients with multiple opportunistic infections tend to be more seriously immunosuppressed and have a poorer prognosis.

Control Opportunistic Infection

The primary goal of management for the critically ill AIDS patient is the absence, control, or resolution of opportunistic infection, nosocomial infection, or sepsis. Management of the opportunistic infection(s) is aimed at support of the involved system(s). Specific pharmacologic agents for identified organisms as well as experimental agents for uncommon organisms are used. In the critical care setting, additional isolation procedures such as neutropenic precautions may be necessary to prevent health care workers from transmitting common environmental organisms to patients with AIDS. Staphylococcal infection is of major concern in the critical care setting. Patients with AIDS infected with this bacteria may become septic, as evidenced by fever, hypotension, and tachycardia. Safe infection control measures to prevent bacterial contamination and complications resulting in sepsis must be maintained for the AIDS patient in the critical care setting.

TABLE 47–4
Clinical Manifestations of AIDS

Possible Causes	Possible Effects
Oral Manifestations	
Lesions due to: *Candida*, herpes simplex, Kaposi's sarcoma; papillomavirus oral warts; HIV gingivitis or peridontits; oral leukoplakia	Oral pain leading to difficulty in chewing and swallowing, decreased fluid and nutritional intake, dehydration, weight loss and fatigue, disfigurement
Neurologic Manifestations	
AIDS dementia complex due to: direct attack of HIV in nerve cells	Personality changes; impaired cognition, concentration, and judgment; impaired motor ability; weakness; needs assistance with ADL or unable to perform ADL; unable to talk or comprehend; paresis and/or plegia; incontinence; caregiver burden; inability to comply with medical regimen; inability to work; social isolation
Acute encephalopathy due to: therapeutic drug reactions; drug overdose; hypoxia; hypoglycemia from drug-induced pancreatitis; electrolyte imbalance; meningitis or encephalitis resulting from *Cryptococcus*, herpes simplex virus, cytomegalovirus, *Mycobacterium tuberculosis*, syphilis, *Candida*, *Toxoplasma gondii*; lymphoma; **Cerebral infarction** resulting from: vasculitis, meningovascular syphilis, systemic hypotension, and marantic endocarditis	Headache, malaise, fever; full or partial paralysis; loss of cognitive ability, memory, judgment, orientation or appropriate affect; sensory distortion; seizures, coma, death
Neuropathy due to: inflammatory demyelination resulting from direct HIV attack; drug reactions; Kaposi's sarcoma lesions	Loss of motor control; ataxia; peripheral numbness, tingling, burning sensation; depressed reflexes; inability to work; caregiver burden; social isolation
Gastrointestinal Manifestations	
Diarrhea due to: *Cryptosporidum, Isopora belli, Microsporidium, Strongyloides stercoides*, cytomegalovirus, herpes simplex, enterovirusus, adenovirus, *Mycobacterium avium intracellulare, Salmonella, Shigella, Campylobacter, Vibrio parahaemolyticus, Candida, Histoplasma capsulatum, Giardia, Entamoeba histolytica*, normal flora overgrowth, lymphoma, and Kaposi's sarcoma	Weight loss, anorexia, fever; dehydration, malabsorption; malaise, weakness and fatigue; loss of ability to perform social functions due to inability to leave house; incontinence and caregiver burden
Hepatitis due to: *Mycobacterium avium intracellulare, Cryptococcus*, cytomegalovirus, *Histoplasma, Coccidiomycosis, Microsporidium*, Epstein–Barr virus, hepatitis A, B, C, D (delta agent) and E viruses, lymphoma, Kaposi's sarcoma, illegal drug use, alcohol abuse, and prescribed drug use (particularly sulfa drugs)	Anorexia, nausea, vomiting, abdominal pain, jaundice; fever, malaise, rash, joint pain, fatigue; hepatomegaly, hepatic failure, death
Biliary dysfunction due to: Cholangitis from cytomegalovirus and *Cryptosporidum;* lymphoma and Kaposi's sarcoma	Abdominal pain, anorexia, nausea, vomiting and jaundice
Anorectal disease due to: perirectal abscesses and fistulas, perianal ulcers and inflammation resulting from infections with *Chlamydia, Lymphogranulum venereum*, gonorrhea, syphilis, *Shigella, Campylobacter, M. tuberculosis*, herpes simplex, cytomegalovirus, *Candida ablicans* obstruction from lymphoma; Kaposi's sarcoma and papillomovirus warts	Difficult and painful elimination; rectal pain, itching, diarrhea
Respiratory Manifestations	
Infection due to: *Pneumocystis carinii, M. avium intracellulare, M. tuberculosis, Candida, Chlamydia, Histoplasma capsulatum, Toxoplasma gondii, Coccidioides immitis, Cryptococcus neoforms*, cytomegalovirus, influenza viruses, *Pneumococcus, Strongyloides*	Shortness of breath, cough, pain; hypoxia, activity intolerance, fatigue; respiratory failure and death
Lymphoma and Kaposi's sarcoma	Same as above
Dermatologic Manifestations	
Staphylococcal skin lesions (bullous impetigo, ecthyma, folliculitis); herpes simplex virus lesions (oral, facial, anal; vulvovaginal); herpes zoster; chronic mycobacterial lesions	Pain, itching, burning, secondary infection and sepsis; disfigurement and altered self-image

(continued)

TABLE 47–4
Clinical Manifestations of AIDS (*Continued*)

Possible Causes	Possible Effects
appearing over lymph nodes or as ulcerations or hemorrhagic macules; other lesions related to infection with *Pseudomonas aeruginosa*, *Molluscum contagiosum*, *Candida albicans*, ringworm, *Cryptococcus*, *Sporotrichosis*; xerosis-induced dermatitis, seborrheic dermatitis; drug reactions (particularly from sulfa-based drugs); lesions from parasites such as scabies or lice; Kaposi's sarcoma; decubiti and impairment in the integrity of the skin resulting from prolonged pressure and incontinence	
Sensory System	
Vision: Kaposi's sarcoma on conjunctiva or eyelid; cytomegalovirus retinitis	Blindness
Hearing: Acute external otitis and otitis media; hearing loss related to myelopathy, meningitis, cytomegalovirus, and drug reactions	Pain and hearing loss

ADL, activities of daily living.
Reproduced by permission from Grimes, Deanna E.: Infectious Diseases, St. Louis, 1991, Mosby-Year Book, Inc.

AZT Therapy

In 1987, use of the antiviral drug AZT was approved by the Federal Drug Administration; it remains the only antiviral therapy effective against AIDS. The drug inhibits viral replication of HIV by inhibiting the enzyme reverse transcriptase. Previously, AZT was available to AIDS patients who had an episode of PCP or who had a T4 cell count of less than 200 mm³. AZT is now available to HIV-positive patients who are asymptomatic and have T cell counts greater than 500 mm³.

New Antiviral Therapy

Several new antiviral treatment protocols have been introduced for the patient with HIV infection–AIDS that boost the activity of the immune system by either inhibiting the replication of the virus or breaking the reproductive sequences at specific links in the process. These new drugs are:

- Didanosine (dideoxyinosine)
- Ribavirin
- Dideoxycytidine
- Recombinant soluble CD4

Vaccines and Immune Reconstruction

Other therapeutic challenges for the treatment of AIDS remain. Since the causative agent in HIV infection and AIDS was isolated, vaccine development has been researched actively. Attempts at immune reconstruction also are being studied with such agents as interferon. Future research no doubt will develop additional drugs and protocols for the treatment of this disease.

As progress toward a cure for AIDS continues, critical care nurses are challenged to use their expertise in assessment, nursing diagnosis, and research to contribute to the understanding and success of future therapies and management strategies to combat AIDS.

CASE STUDY

Arthur Jacobs is a 33-year-old man with HIV disease. His social history involves both homosexuality and intravenous drug abuse (IVDA) risk factors. He converted HIV positive in 1989 and was diagnosed with AIDS in 1990. He remains homosexual with a steady partner and denies IVDA since 1991. He has been involved in various HIV treatment protocols with both AZT and dideoxyinosine, and is on AZT currently.

Mr. Jacobs presented to the Emergency Department with complaints of increasing shortness of breath, fevers, and pain. He is emaciated (50 kg) and has Kaposi's sarcoma to his face, arms, and trunk. Chest radiography revealed dense infiltrates in all lobes. Arterial blood gases (ABGs) were pH 7.6, PO₂ 45 mm Hg, PCO₂ 50 mm Hg, HCO₃ 25 meq. He was placed on humidified oxygen via nonrebreather mask and admitted to the medical ICU with the diagnosis R/O *Pneumocystis carinii* pneumonia. He was started on pentamidine, 200 mg daily (due to a Bactrim/Sulfa allergy), and was closely monitored with aggressive respiratory therapy.

After 12 hours in the ICU, Mr. Jacobs' condition deteriorated. His ABGs revealed worsening gas exchange with a PO₂ of 40 mm Hg and a PCO₂ of 60 mm Hg. Mr. Jacobs had decided previously on no CPR or resuscitation in the event of a cardiac arrest, but had stated that he would like to have his pulmonary status aggressively managed until it seemed evident that this episode would not resolve. He did not want to be "lingering on a respirator." The medical team intubated Mr. Jacobs and he was placed on a ventilator. His postintubation ABGs showed pH 7.33, PO₂ 60 mm Hg, PCO₂ 36 mm Hg, and HCO₃ 18; chest radiography showed the endotracheal tube in good position.

Mr. Jacobs required suctioning every 1 to 2 hours, frequent positioning for postural drainage, and aggressive respiratory therapy. He was receiving 200 mg intravenous pentamidine every day. During his pentamidine therapy, his blood pressure remained stable; however, his blood sugar frequently fell and usually was treated with D_{50} when symptomatic. The nurses placed Mr. Jacobs on a specialty bed to enhance his respiratory function and maintain his skin integrity. He was medicated with morphine sulfate for pain (secondary to his Kaposi's sarcoma). His family and significant other (SO) visited often and were appropriately concerned, yet remained optimistic. Mr. Jacobs was able to communicate by writing, but as he became weaker, this was more difficult.

On hospital day 6, Mr. Jacobs was showing no improvement. His respiratory status is unchanged and his WBC count dropped to 700 (secondary to the pentamidine/AZT therapy). The nurses moved Mr. Jacobs to a private room and instituted neutropenic precautions as a protective measure. Mr. Jacobs' electrolytes were abnormal, and he required frequent potassium boluses to maintain a therapeutic potassium level. Mr. Jacobs' mental status fluctuated between obtunded and confused and he was no longer able to communicate coherently with his family and SO.

His clinical picture deteriorated further on hospital day 7 when he began showing signs of sepsis and septic shock. His COR status was readdressed with his family and SO, and everyone agreed that in light of this clinical development (septic shock) it would be unlikely that Mr. Jacobs would survive this hospitalization. His COR status was readdressed and decisions were made to limit his care to supportive and comfort measures. He remained ventilated and received morphine, and within 6 hours he suffered a cardiac arrest and died without medical resuscitation efforts.

Nursing Care Plan

Nursing Care Plan 47–1 details the nursing care for the patient with AIDS.

Nosocomial Infections

Description

The CDC defines a nosocomial infection as any infection acquired during hospitalization that was neither present nor incubating at the time of admission and was not related to a previous hospitalization.

Epidemiology

Given that all critical care patients most likely have some degree of altered host defenses, they are conceivably at great risk for development of nosocomial infections. This notion has been supported by various investigations that have revealed hospital-acquired infection rates of 25% to 30% among critical care patients, compared to 5% to 10% among all hospitalized patients. The impact of nosocomial infections on critical care patients is significantly greater than on hospitalized patients in general, and is associated with a higher incidence of morbidity and mortality. It is essential, therefore, that critical care nurses understand the causes of nosocomial infections and implement protocols to decrease the risk of infection for their patients.

Pathophysiology

Etiology and Transmission

The specific nosocomial infections that most frequently arise in critical care patients include respiratory tract infections, urinary tract infections, surgical wound infections, and bacteremias often associated with invasive devices. The sources of microorganisms causing these infections fall into two categories: endogenous sources (derived from the flora of the patient's own body) and exogenous sources (originating from the hospital environment, such as from the hands of health care workers). Infections caused by both sources can have equally serious consequences for the compromised patient. Nosocomial infections caused by exogenous sources are the more preventable by adherence to appropriate infection control procedures. The most common type of microorganisms isolated as causative agents of hospital-acquired infections in the critical care patient include a disproportionate fraction of *Staphylococcus aureus*, gram-negative bacilli, and yeast organisms with gram-negative bacilli.

Within critical care units, the spread of exogenous hospital-acquired infections appears to take place primarily through hand transmission by hospital personnel, followed by contaminated drugs, fluids, or equipment, and last through the use of invasive devices that bypass normal defensive mechanisms. Previously suspected mechanisms of transmission such as airborne routes and environmental contamination appear to be a less significant cause of infection.

Management

Controlling Nosocomial Infections

One of the most important mechanisms for control of nosocomial infections has been shown to be *handwashing*. Numerous studies, however, have demonstrated that critical care staff frequently overlook the importance of this procedure. Readily accessible sinks equipped with antiseptic solutions are essential for all critical care units. But most important, the staff providing care to patients in these units must use this equipment conscientiously to practice adequate and timely handwashing procedures.

Other interventions that can decrease the incidence of the spread of microorganisms among critical care patients include those outlined in Display Box 47–4.

NURSING CARE PLAN 47–1:
The Patient With AIDS

NURSING DIAGNOSIS	OUTCOME CRITERIA/ PATIENT GOALS	NURSING INTERVENTIONS
High risk for infection: related to HIV immunodeficiency and malnutrition.	• Patient will be free from nosocomial infections.	1. Use universal precautions. 2. Assess baseline immunologic studies: T cell count, WBC, differential. 3. Stress proper handwashing techniques by all caregivers. 4. Monitor visitors/caregivers to protect compromised host. 5. Monitor for signs and symptoms of sepsis: fever, hypotension, positive blood cultures. 6. Assist patient and family in learning about preventing infection.
High risk for impaired gas exchange: related to alveolar–capillary membrane changes with PCP infection.	• Patient will maintain adequate oxygenation.	1. Monitor for signs and symptoms of respiratory compromise: tachypnea, cyanosis, changes in mentation, fatigue. 2. Review pertinent laboratory data: CBC, chest radiograph, ABG. 3. Assess activity tolerance. 4. Administer oxygen. 5. Monitor therapeutic and adverse effects of antibiotic therapy. 6. Monitor oxygen saturation with oximetry.
High risk for fluid volume deficit: related to diarrhea, dysphagia.	• Patient will maintain fluid and electrolyte balance.	1. Assess risk factors: fever, diarrhea, dysphagia. 2. Monitor weight and intake and output. 3. Assess vital sign changes: hypotension, tachycardia, fever. 4. Encourage increased oral intake of fluids. 5. Provide supplemental fluids, as ordered: IV, tube feeding. 6. Administer medications, as ordered (antidiarrheals, antipyretics). 7. Assess lab data, as ordered.
High risk for altered thought processes: related to HIV or opportunistic infection of CNS.	• Patient will maintain or improve level of consciousness.	1. Assess neurologic status q4h. 2. Assess for changes in behavior, slowing and slurring of speech. 3. Maintain safe environment.

(continued)

NURSING CARE PLAN 47–1: (Continued)
The Patient With AIDS

NURSING DIAGNOSIS	OUTCOME CRITERIA/ PATIENT GOALS	NURSING INTERVENTIONS
High risk for knowledge deficit: related to illness and impact on patient's future.	• Patient will verbalize understanding of AIDS and treatment.	1. Initiate nurse–patient relationship to encourage learning. 2. Include family in teaching. 3. Provide discharge teaching that emphasizes avoidance of exposure to infection, safe sex practices, diet, and maintaining high level of wellness. 4. Assist patient in identifying community support groups and resources available.
High risk for anxiety: related to critical illness, fear of death.	• Patient will begin to identify source of anxiety.	1. Provide environment that encourages open discussion of emotional issues. 2. Mobilize patient's support system and involve these resources as appropriate. 3. Allow time for patient to express self. 4. Identify possible hospital resources for patient and family support. 5. Encourage open family-to-nurse communications regarding emotional issues. 6. Validate patient and family knowledge base regarding the critical illness. 7. Involve religious support systems as appropriate.
High risk for infection transmission: related to AIDS.	• Patient will not contaminate health care team, other patients, or family.	1. Use universal precautions with every patient. 2. Instruct patient to handwash after handling own secretions. 3. Use extra care with disposal of body secretions, needles. 4. Use "needleless" IV system for IVPB meds, etc. 5. Observe all health team members' technique for universal precautions, and give feedback.

DISPLAY BOX 47-4
Interventions to Decrease Nosocomial Infections

- Handwashing between patients
- Limit visitors and employees that may be infected
- Proper insertion and maintenance of invasive devices such as Foley catheters, intravenous lines, and pressure-monitoring devices
- The appropriate use of sterile equipment and aseptic technique, such as during surgical dressing changes and respiratory suctioning
- Attention to proper skin care and respiratory hygiene
- Provisions for sufficient nutrition and hydration
- Programs of decontamination, sterilization, and maintenance of respiratory therapy devices
- The use of appropriate body substance barrier precautions
- Adequate staffing patterns
- The ongoing surveillance of all critical care nosocomial infections to monitor trends and possible problem areas

ocomial infections. The reader is referred to these publications, readily available from either organization, for more specific recommendations for the prevention of hospital-acquired infections.

REFERENCES

1. Bennensen A (ed): Control of Communicable Disease in Man, 15th ed. Washington, DC, American Public Health Association, 1990
2. Centers for Disease Control and Prevention: Update: Universal precautions for the prevention of transmission of human immunodeficiency virus, hepatitis B virus, and other bloodborne pathogens in the health care setting. MMWR 37(24):377–388, 1988
3. Grimes DE, Grimes RM, Hamelink M: Infectious Disease. St. Louis, Mosby's Clinical Nursing Series, 1991
4. Centers for Disease Control and Prevention: 1993 Revised Classification System for HIV Infection and Expanded Surveillance Case Definition for AIDS Among Adolescents and Adults. MMWR 41, No. RR-17, December 18, 1992, pp 1–19

BIBLIOGRAPHY

Ganong WF: Review of Medical Physiology, 15th ed. Norwalk, CT, Appleton & Lange, 1991
Guyton AC: Textbook of Medical Physiology, 8th ed. Philadelphia, WB Saunders, 1991
Hole JW Jr: Essentials of Human Anatomy and Physiology, 4th ed. Dubuque, IA, WC Brown, 1992
Porth CM: Pathophysiology: Concepts of Altered Health States. Philadelphia, JB Lippincott, 1990

Standards for Preventing Nosocomial Infections

Agencies and organizations such as the CDC and the American Nurses' Association have published extensive standards and guidelines related to the prevention of nos-

---

STUDY QUESTIONS

1. All of the following are functions of the immune system *except*

   a. degradation and removal of damaged and dead cells
   b. protection of the body from destruction by foreign agents
   c. surveillance and destruction of malignant cells
   d. none of the above

2. The average time from exposure to HIV and conversion to seropositivity is

   a. 2 to 6 weeks
   b. 6 weeks to 6 months
   c. 6 months to 12 months
   d. 8 months to 18 months

3. The use of protective gloves is warranted for

   1. phlebotomy and placement of IV lines
   2. contact with specimens and changing simple dressings

3. lumbar punctures and oral procedures
4. removing IV lines and lumbar punctures

    a. 1 and 2
    b. 2 and 3
    c. 1, 2, and 4
    d. 1, 3, and 4

4. Wearing gloves, masks, and protective eyewear is sufficient for all of the following procedures *except*

    a. placement of arterial catheters
    b. intubation
    c. oral procedures
    d. airway manipulation

5. Nursing measures effective in reducing the incidence of nosocomial infections include all of the following *except*

    a. appropriate handwashing techniques
    b. proper care of invasive devices
    c. eliminating airborne routes of transmission
    d. proper skin care and respiratory hygiene

Behavioral Objectives

Description

Assessment and Management

Potential Problems in the Postanesthesia Patient
    Hypoxemia
    Hypoventilation
    Hypotension
    Hypertension
    Cardiac Dysrhythmias
    Hypothermia
    Hyperthermia
    Malignant Hyperthermia
    Nausea and Vomiting
    Pain

Nursing Care Plan: Recovery From Anesthesia

Study Questions

BEHAVIORAL OBJECTIVES

Based on the content in this chapter, the reader should be able to:

1. Identify four anesthetic options that could be used during surgery.
2. Differentiate between anesthetic agents appropriate for the conscious patient and those appropriate for the unconscious patient.
3. List five potential problems encountered in the immediate postanesthetic period and state a nursing diagnosis and nursing intervention for each problem.

APPENDIX 1

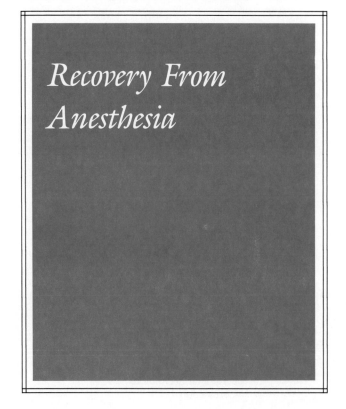

Recovery From Anesthesia

Hudak: Critical Care Nursing:
A Holistic Approach, 6th ed. © 1994
J. B. Lippincott Company.

Description

The time immediately after surgery, when the patient is taken to the postanesthesia care unit (PACU) or the intensive care unit, is the most crucial period in the patient's recovery from anesthesia. Most patients are taken to the PACU for close observation and care by a qualified PCU nurse; others are taken directly to the ICU, where it is important that nurses be trained in postanesthesia nursing care. The critical care nurse must have a basic understanding of anesthetic options available for use during the intraoperative phase. After examining the patient before surgery, the anesthesiologist decides which option and technique to use based on the patient's condition, age, previous surgical and anesthetic experiences, ongoing disease processes, operation to be performed, the surgeon's experience, and the position required for the surgical procedure. The anesthesiologist's options range from maintaining a conscious state with the use of minimal, regional, or intravenous agents to inducing an unconscious state with the use of intravenous or inhalation agents (Tables 1 and 2).

What happens in the operating room may affect the patient's immediate postoperative care as well as the overall recovery. To convey what has occurred in the operating suite, the anesthesiologist is expected to give a detailed and complete report to the nurse assuming postoperative care of the anesthetized patient (Table 3).

While receiving report from the anesthesiologist, the nurse simultaneously must assess the patient's condition

TABLE 1
Anesthetic Options

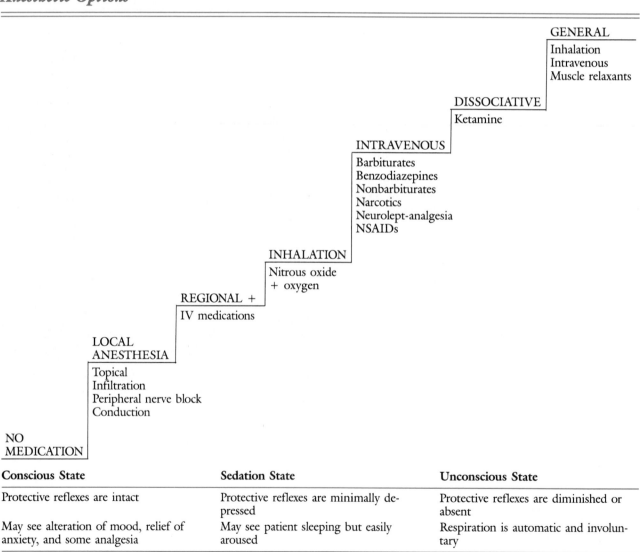

Conscious State	Sedation State	Unconscious State
Protective reflexes are intact	Protective reflexes are minimally depressed	Protective reflexes are diminished or absent
May see alteration of mood, relief of anxiety, and some analgesia	May see patient sleeping but easily aroused	Respiration is automatic and involuntary

NSAIDs, nonsteroidal anti-inflammatory drugs; IV, intravenous.

and individualize the nursing care plan. Initial assessment factors reported to the anesthesiologist are the patient's vital signs (blood pressure, pulse, respiration, and temperature), pulse oximetry, and level of consciousness. Cardiac monitoring, pressure readings, and urine output monitoring also may be indicated. Vital signs are monitored every 15 minutes, or more often if the patient's condition warrants. The American Society of Post Anesthesia Nurses, as endorsed by the American Society of Anesthesiologists, recommends all assessment data be collected and documented on the patient's postoperative record.[1]

Some of the major problems that can occur in the immediate postoperative period, and their causes and interventions, will be the focus of this section. A detailed nursing care plan for the patient recovering from anesthesia (Nursing Care Plan 1) will be found at the end of Appendix I.

Assessment and Management

Potential Problems in the Postanesthesia Patient

Hypoxemia

Hypoxemia is a common occurrence in the immediate postoperative period. Severe hypoxemia is characterized by a PaO_2 less than 50 mm Hg and is life threatening.

TABLE 2
Medication Choices for Anesthetic Options

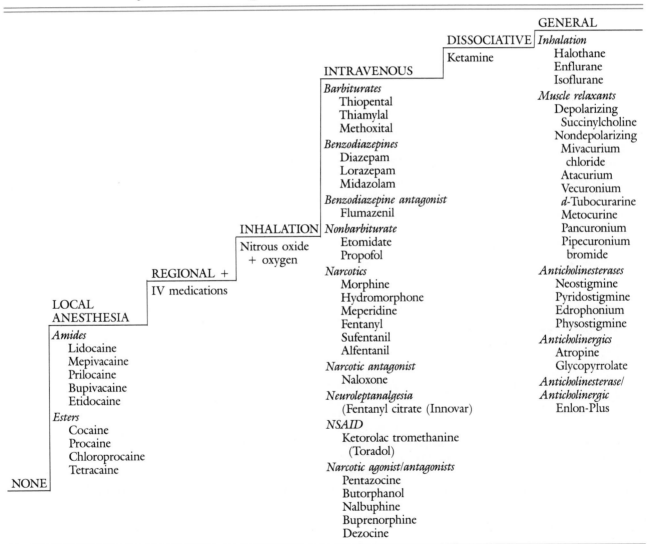

NSAID, nonsteroidal anti-inflammatory drugs.

TABLE 3
Anesthesiologist-to-Nurse Report:
Information to Convey

Name of patient
Surgical procedure
Anesthetic options (agents and reversal agents used)
Estimated blood loss/fluid loss
Fluid/blood replacement
Vital signs—significant problems
Complications encountered (anesthetic or surgical)
Preoperative condition (diabetes, hypertension, allergies, etc.)
Considerations for immediate postoperative period (pain
  management, reversals, vent settings)
Language barrier

Ideally, the anesthesiologist should not leave the patient until the nurse is satisfied with the patient's airway and immediate condition.

Hypoventilation leads to hypoxia, which is difficult to diagnose because of its multiple presentations. Clinical manifestations of hypoxia can include hypotension or hypertension, tachycardia or bradycardia, cardiac dysrhythmias, dyspnea, tachypnea, hypoventilation, disorientation with agitation, decreased PCO_2, and cyanosis.

When investigating the etiology of hypoxemia related to anesthetic agents, the nurse should consider the effects of a prolonged block that traveled too high, narcotic use, deep sedation, use of inhalation agents such as enflurane (Ethrane), isoflurane (Forane), halothane, and nitrous oxide, and the use of neuromuscular blockers, particularly if they have not been reversed adequately. Diffusion hypoxia may occur when nitrous oxide is used, but administering 100% oxygen for 3 to 4 minutes after the nitrous oxide is terminated can prevent this complication.

All patients who received a general anesthetic or sedation should receive supplemental oxygen in the immediate postoperative period. The oxygen can be weaned subsequently using pulse oximetry readings. Because pulse oximetry offers a noninvasive method of continuously monitoring oxygen saturation, increasing numbers of patients are receiving supplemental oxygen for 24 hours after surgery.

In addition to being aware of hypoxia, the nurse should use a "stir-up" regimen for every patient in the postoperative period. This regimen involves encouraging the patient to deep breathe, cough, and move about in bed. An integral part of recovery from anesthesia, this routine should be encouraged every time vital signs are checked.

Reversal agents may be required while the patient is still under the effects of muscle relaxants, benzodiazepines, and narcotics. Close monitoring always is indicated when reversal agents are administered. The effects of muscle relaxants, benzodiazepines, and narcotics may last longer than the reversal medication, resulting in hypoventilation and hypoxia at some point after the reversal medication is given. Knowledge of the onset and duration of action of reversal agents are important data for the nurse.

Hypoventilation

Hypoventilation leading to hypercarbia may result from:

- Inadequate respiratory drive secondary to the effects of residual anesthesia (ie, narcotics and inhalation agents).
- Inadequate functioning of the respiratory muscles. The lungs may be unable to move an adequate tidal volume owing to pain or inadequate reversal of neuromuscular blockade.
- Intrinsic lung disease, which often requires postoperative ventilatory support of the patient.

Clinical Research

Berels D, Marz MS: SaO₂ monitoring in the postanesthesia care unit. Journal of Post Anesthesia Nursing 6:394–401, 1991

A 3-month pilot study conducted in a Michigan hospital compared a discharge scoring system with the SaO_2 readings of patients in a postanesthesia care unit. The purposes of the study were determining the need for respiratory support; assessing the relationship between patients temperature and SaO_2 readings; and providing baseline data to set policy for pulse oximetry use and supplemental oxygen administration. The study showed that warming shivering patients decreased oxygen demand and improved oxygen saturation. The length of stay in the PACU was inversely related to the SaO_2 value on room air. Patients with a pulse oximetry reading of 90% or less were potential candidates for hypoxemia and required supplemental oxygen postoperatively. Pulse oximetry has become a required measurement for all patients and a standard of care for the PACU.

Chronic obstructive pulmonary disease is a classic example.

In the immediate postoperative phase, it is important to institute the stir-up routine to stimulate the patient, especially if narcotics and muscle relaxants were used during surgery. Also, consider the length of time since reversal agents were administered to antagonize neuromuscular blockade (Tables 4 and 5). The patient may reparalyze because the effects of the reversal agent were shorter acting than the effects of the muscle relaxant.

Because hypothermia prolongs nondepolarizing blocks, it is important to monitor the patient's temperature. The nurse also must consider other conditions that might potentiate the effect of neuromuscular blocking agents (Display Box 1).

Hypotension

Hypotension is probably the most common cardiovascular complication seen in the postoperative period, and is caused most often by a decreased circulating blood volume.[4] The term refers to a 25% to 30% decrease in systolic blood pressure from resting baseline values. Intervention is indicated if the pressure falls more than 30% (Table 6).

Anesthetic agents can affect the blood pressure in various ways. Regional anesthetics such as lidocaine and procaine may decrease blood pressure by sympathetic blockade, vasodilation, and myocardial depression. Intravenous agents, including narcotics, cause vasodilation and histamine release, resulting in lowered blood pressure. Tranquilizers, especially droperidol and chlorpromazine hydrochloride, produce sympathetic blockade and subsequent decreased blood pressure. Barbiturates cause myocardial depression, as do inhalation agents such as Forane, Ethrane, and halothane. Muscle relaxants can cause hypotension by ganglionic blockade and histamine release.

Because decreased venous return is seen with hypovolemia and myocardial depression, the nurse should consider the adequacy of fluid and blood replacement, bleeding, third spacing, or excessive diuresis. Orthostatic hypotension should be checked for by taking vital signs with the patient supine and after raising the head of the bed 60° (if not contraindicated by the surgical procedure). Cardiac dysrhythmias can produce hypotension, espe-

---

TABLE 4
Neuromuscular Blocking Agents

Muscle Relaxants

- Neuromuscular blockers pharmacologically paralyze patients and provide no sedation or analgesia.
- Neuromuscular agents are used to facilitate endotracheal intubation, relax muscles for surgical procedures, terminate laryngospasm, eliminate chest wall rigidity, and for mechanical ventilation if indicated.
- There are two groups of muscle relaxants: depolarizing and nondepolarizing neuroblockers that work at the myoneural junction, affecting the chemical transmitter, acetylcholine.[2,3]

Depolarizing Agents (Sucostrin, Anectine)

- These drugs combine with acetylcholine receptors at the myoneural junction and mimic the action of acetylcholine.
- Onset of action is 1–2 min and duration of action is 4–6 min.
- The enzyme pseudocholinesterase removes succinylcholine from plasma, so in conditions involving a decrease in pseudocholinesterase, the length of action of succinylcholine increases, keeping patients paralyzed for longer periods.
- Increased pseudocholinesterase enzyme may be seen in pregnancy, liver disease, malnutrition states, severe anemia, cancer, and with other pharmacologic agents such as quinidine, phospholine eye drops, and propranolol.

Nondepolarizing Agents

- Nondepolarizing agents (atacurium, mivacurium chloride, pipecuronium bromide, vecuronium, *d*-tubocurarine, metocurine, pancuronium) compete with acetylcholine at the myoneural junction for muscle membrane receptors.
- Onset of action is within 2–3 min.
- Duration of action ranges from 20 min to 2 hr, depending on the medication and dosage.
- May be reversed pharmacologically with anticholinesterase drugs (neostigmine, pyridostigmine, edrophonium). Duration of action of anticholinesterase is brief, so there is a chance the patient may have continued muscle weakness or respiratory depression. Anticholinesterases may induce muscarinic side effects, including bradycardia, increased salivary, and bronchial secretions. These side effects are counteracted with the routine administration of anticholinergic drugs (atropine, glycopyrrolate) in conjunction with the anticholinesterase.

TABLE 5
Muscle Relaxant Comparison

	Succinylcholine	Mivacurium Chloride	Atacurium	Vecuronium	d-Tubocurarine	Metocurine	Pancuronium	Pipecuronium Bromide
Onset of action Duration of action	Within 1–2 min 4–6 min	2–2.5 min 10–15 min	Within 2min 30–45 min	Within 3 min 30–40 min	Within 3 min 45–60 min	Within 4 min > 60 min	Within 4 min 1–1½ hr	5 min 1–2 hr
Dose	1 mg/kg	0.10–0.25 mg/kg	0.4–0.5 mg/kg	0.75–1 mg/kg	up to 0.6 mg/kg	0.2 mg/kg	0.04–0.1 mg/kg	0.07–0.85 mg/kg
Metabolism elimination	Enzyme pseudo-cholinesterase	Plasmacholines-terase Renal and biliary path	Hoffman elimination and ester hydrolysis	Hepatic and renal function	Kidney and liver	Kidney and liver	Kidney and liver	Eliminated by kidneys
Histamine release	Possible	Yes	Mild	Very mild	Yes, causing hypotension and bradycardia	Yes, causing hypotension	Isolated cases	Yes
Side effects	↓ Pulse fasciculation Cardiac dysrhythmias Hyperkalemia ↑ICP ↑Intraocular pressure	Flushing, hypotension, dysrhythmia, rash, bronchospasm, muscle spasms			Histamine-like reactions	↓ BP	Avoid with myasthenia gravis, true renal disease, hypersensitivity to bromide	Hypertension, atrial fibrillation, CVA, hypoglycemia, hyperkalemia, CNS depressant, respiratory depressant
Advantages		Use with continuous drip; no refrigeration	Little or no cardiovascular effect Easily reversed Block not prolonged	Little or no cardiovascular effect Easily reversed		Useful if cardiovascular disease and hypertension present		Does not cause increased heart rate
	Short acting	Short acting	Intermediate acting	Intermediate acting	Long acting		Long acting	

Short acting   Intermediate acting   Long acting

ICP, intracranial pressure; CVA, cerebro vascular accident; CNS, central nervous system.

TABLE 6
Hypotension Etiologies

Anesthetic Agents

Regional agents
Narcotics
Tranquilizers
Barbiturates
Muscle relaxants
Inhalation agents

Decreased Venous Return

Hypovolemia
 Inadequate replacement
 Continued blood loss
Hypothermia
Myocardial depression
Third spacing
Sepsis
Transfusion reaction
Tight abdominal dressing
Increased intrathoracic pressure

Cardiac

Dysrhythmias
 Supraventricular tachycardia
Myocardial infarction
Congestive heart failure

Pulmonary

Hypoxia
Acidosis
Pulmonary embolism
Pneumothorax

Vasovagal Reactions

Bradycardia
Pain
Bladder/abdominal distention

Technical Problems

Blood pressure cuff size and position
Transducer balance and calibration
Stethoscope position

DISPLAY BOX 1
Conditions and Medications That Increase the Effects of Nondepolarizing Muscle Relaxants

Local anesthetics
General anesthetics
Antibiotics: aminoglycosides, polypeptides, Polymyxin
Antiarrhythmics: quinidine, procainamide
Furosemide
Acid–base status: respiratory acidosis, metabolic alkalosis
Electrolyte imbalance: hypokalemia, hypocalcemia, dehydration, magnesium administration
Hypothermia

---

lated. Anesthetic drugs may require reversal, including muscle relaxant reversal, with anticholinesterase and anticholinergic agents, narcotic reversal with naloxone, or vasopressor drugs to increase blood pressure. Intravenous fluids including blood, plasma expanders, and crystalloids should be administered as ordered and dressings and surgical sites inspected frequently for hemorrhage. Elevation of the legs or the Trendelenburg position may be indicated to increase blood pressure.

An important consideration when assessing and treating hypotension is the possibility of technical rather than physiological problems. Is the blood pressure cuff the correct size and positioned correctly? Is the stethoscope positioned correctly? Is the patient's position a factor? If an arterial line is present, is the patient peripherally constricted, or does peripheral vascular disease exist? Is the transducer balanced and correctly calibrated?

Hypertension

Hypertension is classified according to its degree of severity, ranging from mild with a diastolic pressure between 90 and 104 mm Hg, severe with the diastolic pressure above 115 mm Hg, to malignant with the diastolic pressure greater than 120 mm Hg.

The two most common causes of postoperative hypertension are a prior history of hypertension and pain. It can be associated with peripheral vasoconstriction and shivering. Inhalation and intravenous anesthetic agents may produce hypoxia and hypercarbia with a resultant increase in catecholamine release and blood pressure elevation. Ketalar, a dissociative drug used for surgery patients, stimulates the sympathetic nervous system and can cause tachycardia and hypertension. Also, if given too rapidly, naloxone may precipitate hypertension, which in turn may precipitate pulmonary edema or cerebral hemorrhage.

cially when cardiac output is decreased, as it is with supraventricular tachycardia. Other causes of early postoperative hypotension include sepsis, pulmonary embolism, transfusion reaction, and pain.

Deliberate, controlled hypotensive techniques are used during specific procedures such as head and neck or neurosurgical procedures and some cancer operations. The advantage of this technique is that it minimizes blood loss and the need for transfusion, decreases oozing, and requires minimal anesthesia.

Treatment of hypotension is directed to the underlying cause. This complication illustrates the need for the nurse to receive a complete report from the anesthesiologist, including the techniques used during surgery and any untoward events that occurred.

The patient must be adequately oxygenated and venti-

TABLE 7
Cardiac Dysrhythmias Associated With Anesthetic Options

Anesthetic Option	Dysrhythmia
Local anesthesia with epinephrine	Tachycardia
Spinal and epidural	Bradycardia 2° vagal response; PACs, PVCs, supraventricular tachycardia, atrial fibrillation 2° sympathetic stimulation; wandering pacemaker and heart block 2° increased vagal tone.
Barbiturates	
Pentothal	Bradycardia, AV dissociation, occasional PVC
Nonbarbiturate etomidate	Sinus tachycardia
Narcotics	
Morphine sulfate	Transient bradycardia
Meperidine hydrochloride	Transient tachycardia
Fentanyl	Bradycardia
Narcotic antagonist	PVCs, ventricular tachycardia, occasional ventricular fibrillation
Neuroleptanalgesia (droperidol component)	Tachycardia
Dissociative agent	Myocardial depression, ventricular ectopy, tachycardia
Inhalation agents	
Halothane	AV dissociation, ventricular dysrhythmias if hypercarbia occurs
Halothane plus aminophylline, cocaine, lidocaine	Bradycardia
Halothane plus pancuronium	PACs and PVCs
Isoflurane	Tachycardia
Enflurane	AV dissociation
Muscle relaxants	
Succinylcholine	Sinus bradycardia, junctional rhythms, PVCs. Patients with burns, trauma, paraplegia or quadriplegia prone to ST depression, peaked T waves, widening QRS leading to ventricular tachycardia, ventricular fibrillation, or asystole
Pipecuronium bromide	Atrial fibrillation, ventricular extrasystole
Pancuronium	Tachycardia and nodal rhythms
d-Tubocurarine	Tachycardia
Anticholinesterases	Bradycardia, slowed AV conduction, PVC
Anticholinergics	Tachycardia

PAC, premature atrial contraction; PVC, premature ventricular contraction; AV, atrioventricular.

Other causes of hypertension include hyperthermia, anxiety, urinary bladder distention, fluid overload, pain, a too-narrow blood pressure cuff, and withholding of antihypertensive therapy before surgery.

Transient hypertension may occur during induction, intubation, positioning, making the surgical incision, or on awakening from anesthesia.

Treatment of hypertension is directed first to the cause, if known. Unless contraindicated, patients should be instructed to continue their hypertensive medication up to the time of the surgical procedure. The nurse must be alert to administering analgesics if the patient is in pain, starting oxygen if hypoxemia is suspected, and stimulating the patient to deep breathe if hypoventilation occurs. Changing blood pressure cuffs if the wrong size is in use as well as checking the function of all equipment should be an integral part of the nurse's problem solving.

Antihypertensive medications may be ordered if the severity of hypertension indicates. Short-acting peripheral vasodilators such as hydralazine and nifedipine may be used. The adrenergic inhibitor, labetalol, also might be prescribed. Continuous vasodilator drips of sodium nitroprusside or nitroglycerine sometimes are needed to bring the blood pressure within safe limits. When hypertension accompanies emergence delirium, narcotics or physostigmine, an anticholinesterase, may be required. If the patient is hypertensive due to anxiety, and verbal reassurance is ineffective, tranquilizers such as diazepam, midazolam, or droperidol may be indicated.

Urinary catheterization and aggressive treatment with diuretics such as furosemide may be indicated if the patient was fluid overloaded during surgery.

The pregnant, preeclamptic patient who presents with high blood pressure (which sometimes takes 48 hours after delivery to subside) may require magnesium sulfate to control seizure activity and intravenous hydralazine to lower blood pressure. Hydralazine also increases uterine blood flow.

Hypothermia, with its associated vasoconstriction and initial increase in blood pressure, requires special attention in the postoperative phase. Care must be taken in rewarming because too rapid rewarming of the patient can result in an acute drop in blood pressure, as well as other significant problems. The hypertensive patient definitely requires reassurance, close observation, and aggressive postoperative treatment.

Cardiac Dysrhythmias

Discussion of dysrhythmias will be limited to those induced by anesthetic agents and complications frequently seen in the immediate postoperative period (Table 7). Refer to Chapters 12 and 13 for detailed information on identifying and treating specific cardiac dysrhythmias. There are many causes of cardiac dysrhythmias in the immediate postoperative period. Some of the most common are anesthetic agents, reversal anticholinesterase drugs, hypoxemia, hypoventilation, hypovolemia, fluid overload, and pain (Display Box 2).

Hypothermia

Hypothermia is present when the body temperature is less than 35°C or 95°F. Heat loss during surgery occurs secondary to reduced basal metabolism and the vasodilation caused by inhalation anesthetic agents; to vasodilation related to sympathetic blockade with inhibition of motor and sensory nerve fibers when spinal and regional techniques are used; and to the inability of the patient to shiver when muscle relaxants are given. Other intraoperative causes include prolonged exposure of body surface, lying under saturated drapes (especially in long procedures), use of antiseptic prepping solutions, use of cold irrigation or intravenous solutions, and the actual temperature of the operating suite. In other words, heat is lost through radiation, exposure, convection, and conduction. Elderly, debilitated patients and infants are more intolerant of temperature changes and thus more prone to hypothermia.

> **DISPLAY BOX 2**
> **Conditions That Precipitate Dysrhythmias**
>
> **Hypoxemia**
> Sinus bradycardia, sinus tachycardia, PVCs, supraventricular tachycardia
>
> **Hypoventilation**
> Sinus tachycardia, PVCs, sinus bradycardia
>
> **Hypovolemia**
> Sinus tachycardia
>
> **Fluid overload**
> PVCs, supraventricular tachycardia, PACs, atrial fibrillation/flutter
>
> **Hyperthermia**
> Sinus tachycardia, PVCs
>
> **Pain**
> Sinus tachycardia, PVCs

For specific management of the hypothermic patient, see Nursing Care Plan Appendix I–1.

Hyperthermia

Hyperthermia is a body temperature greater than 39°C or 102.2°F. Elevated temperature can occur in the anesthetized patient secondary to thermal insulation from the operating drapes, and to the administration of inhalation anesthetics and anticholinergic drugs that can induce a pharmacologic loss of thermoregulatory capacity. Most patients with elevated temperature either arrive in the surgical suite with fever or have a pyrogenic response from septicemia. Other causes of postoperative hyperthermia might include allergic reactions to blood or drugs, central nervous system disorders, or infection.

For specific interventions for the hyperthermic patient, see Nursing Care Plan Appendix I–1.

Malignant Hyperthermia

One of the most catastrophic events that can occur in the immediate postoperative period is malignant hyperthermia. Malignant hyperthermia is a hypermetabolic syndrome that may be triggered by depolarizing neuromuscular blockers, halogenated inhalation agents, and postoperative pain.

This syndrome is a rare, inherited disorder of skeletal muscle and is more prevalent in those with muscular abnormalities such as ptosis, strabismus, and kyphoscoliosis.

Clinical manifestations include an increase in temperature of 0.5°C or more since the induction of anesthesia, muscle rigidity, unexplained tachycardia, sweating, unstable blood pressure, and very hot skin. Masseter muscle rigidity after the administration of succinylcholine is the earliest warning sign of malignant hyperthermia.[5] If the patient's temperature rises rapidly and the anesthetic is not discontinued, death may occur.

Malignant hyperthermia is treated vigorously with dantrolene sodium, cooling measures, oxygen administration, and correction of acid–base imbalances. Most institutions that administer anesthesia have a malignant hyperthermia kit that is readily available in the operating suite (Display Box 3).

Nausea and Vomiting

Nausea and vomiting occur frequently in the immediate postoperative period and can be the result of any of the anesthetic options. Other frequent causes include use of preoperative and intraoperative narcotics, increased gastric secretions, anesthesia techniques, particularly spinal anesthesia, and surgical procedures involving manipulation of eye muscles, abdominal muscles, and genitourinary muscles.

The critical care nurse must be cognizant of the potential for regurgitation or aspiration in all patients who have been anesthetized. Vomiting is an active process, whereas regurgitation is a passive one. *Adequate positioning of the unconscious patient is essential*, and the ideal position is on the side with the head and neck extended. If the surgical procedure precludes turning the patient on the side, then the patient must not be left unattended until consciousness is regained.

Antiemetics frequently are ordered in the immediate postoperative period. The critical care nurse should recognize that many antiemetics potentiate the effect of other medications, particularly narcotics. Therefore, decreased doses of narcotic for pain relief may be indicated.

DISPLAY BOX 3
Contents of Malignant Hyperthermia Kit

Arterial blood gas sets	Methylprednisolone
Blood specimen tubes	Procainamide
Dantrolene sodium	Sodium bicarbonate
Furosemide	Sterile water
Dextrose (50%)	Nasogastric tubes
Insulin	Foley catheter tray
Mannitol	

DISPLAY BOX 4
Factors Influencing Pain

Surgical procedure: Site and nature of the operation
Anxiety level: Fear of surgery, disfigurement, death, loss of control
Patient expectations: Effectiveness of preoperative teaching, adequately prepared for outcome
Pain tolerance: Prior use of medications including analgesics, individual differences
Anesthesia technique: Analgesics used during the intraoperative period, use of naloxone

---

Often, nausea and vomiting can be relieved by identifying the causative factor (gastric distention, hypotension, administration of narcotics) and making the appropriate intervention.

Pain

Patients normally expect to feel pain when their surgical procedure is over. The incidence of pain and its severity depend on the person. All pain assessment in the immediate postoperative period must be individualized. A number of factors will affect the severity of pain, including the site of the operation, the psychological state of the patient, and the anesthetic technique used.

If the anesthetic option chosen was use of inhalation agents without the use of narcotics or local agents, the patient may have more pain than one who received some form of analgesia during surgery. Patients who have been given analgesic medication during the procedure and who then receive naloxone at the end also may experience severe pain because naloxone will reverse the analgesic effects of any prior medication. Because these patients may renarcotize, the nurse must wait 15 to 45 minutes after the naloxone was given before medicating the patient with an analgesic. Display Box 4 outlines some of the factors that can influence the patient's response to pain.

Intravenous titration of narcotics in the immediate postoperative period offers the quickest and most effective method of pain relief. Because the patient's basal metabolic rate is decreased during surgery, the uptake of intramuscular medication is difficult to predict.

One intramuscular medication, ketorolac tromethamine, (Toradol; Syntex Laboratories, Inc., Palo Alto, CA), administered during surgery, has proven very effective in the management of postoperative pain. Ketorolac tromethamine is a nonsteroidal anti-inflammatory drug that exhibits analgesic, anti-inflammatory, and antipyretic activity. Intramuscular doses are recommended on a regular schedule rather than intermittently. An intramuscular loading dose administered in the operating room by the anesthesiologist is followed by half the loading dose every 6 hours.[6]

Newer trends in pain control include use of patient controlled analgesia (PCA) devices and epidural analgesia. The use of PCA pumps has increased significantly over recent years, and it is believed that patients maintain autonomy when they control administration of narcotics for their pain relief.

Epidural analgesia has proven successful in treating acute pain due to trauma or surgery and for chronic pain as in cancer. Patients receiving epidural narcotics are less sedated and therefore ambulate earlier and have improved respiratory function. Medications given epidurally may be administered as a bolus injection or by a continuous infusion.

When administering continuous infusions an infusion pump should be used. Safeguards to be taken include using preservative-free medications in the epidural infusion; using infusion sets that have *no* injection ports; and labeling infusing pump, infusion bag, and infusion tubing with the word *epidural*. The reason for such safeguards is that accidental infusion of vasodilators, chemotherapy medications, antibiotics, and medications with any type of preservative could permanently destroy nerve tissue, and paralyze or even kill the patient.

Preservative-free medications frequently used epidurally include morphine, hydromorphone, meperidine, and fentanyl. The duration of sensory analgesia varies with the narcotic administered. Covino and Scott identified that the more lipid-soluble agents penetrate the dura mater more rapidly, resulting in a more rapid diffusion away from the spinal cord and subarachnoid space, and hence a shorter duration of action.[7] The most frequently used narcotics for epidural administration for which average duration times have been identified are morphine, with a duration that varies from 2 to 24 hours; hydromorphone, with an average duration of 10 to 14 hours; meperidine, with an average duration of 6 to 8 hours; and fentanyl, with an average duration of 4 to 6 hours.

Dilute local anesthetic solutions are used either in conjunction with the above narcotics or used alone. Local anesthetics used alone and in conjunction with narcotics are lidocaine, mepivacaine, prilocaine, bupivacaine, and etidocaine. The combination of local anesthetics and narcotics has been used to obtain both a rapid onset and prolonged duration of analgesia. The local agents work more rapidly and the narcotics have a more prolonged action. Side effects may occur with the use of narcotics and anesthetic solutions in the epidural space. Nurses have the primary responsibility for recognizing and preventing side effects when caring for patients receiving epidural analgesia (Table 8). Adequate pain relief during the postopera-

TABLE 8
Management of Side Effects From Epidural Analgesia

Specific protocols for epidural management are essential for each individual hospital

Urinary retention
Catheterization may be needed

Postural hypotension
Fluid (volume) replacement
Ephedrine 5 mg IV

Pruritus (itching of face, head, and neck)
Treat with benadryl 25 mg PO, IM, IV
Treat with naloxone 01. mg IV

Nausea and vomiting
Metoclopramide 10 mg IV
Droperidol 0.25 mg IV
Scopolamine patch

Respiratory depression (risk increases with age)
First signs may be change in level of consciousness
May occur up to 24 hr after narcotic injection with naloxone 0.1 mg up to a maximum of 0.4 mg IV
Continuous observation is imperative because naloxone's duration is 30 min

Naloxone and ephedrine should be available at the bedside of patients who have received epidural narcotics or anesthetics.

PO, orally; IM, intramuscularly; IV, intravenously.

tive period allows the patient to cough, deep breathe, and ambulate sooner, thus preventing complications.

Other techniques investigated as alternatives in pain management include intrathecal methods, interpleural methods, transdermal patches, and transmucosal–nasal aerosol. Intrathecal analgesia occurs when the anesthesiologist injects, usually as a one-time dose, medication directly into the cerebrospinal fluid of the subarachnoid space.[8] Interpleural techniques involve administration of local anesthetics into the interpleural space. The catheter is placed during the perioperative period, but occasionally may be placed in the ICU. Continuous infusions as well as bolus injections may be given. Transdermal patches of fentanyl are being studied, as are transmucosal–nasal aerosol delivery systems.[4,8–10]

Nursing Care Plan

Acute and challenging situations arise in the early postoperative period as the patient recovers from anesthesia. An understanding of the anesthetic options and anticipated responses enables the critical care nurse to assist the patient to a safe, uncomplicated, postoperative recovery. Nursing Care Plan Appendix I–1 details the nursing care of the patient recovering from anesthesia.

(*Text continues on page 1062*)

NURSING CARE PLAN APPENDIX 1–1:
Recovery From Anesthesia

NURSING DIAGNOSIS	OUTCOME CRITERIA/ PATIENT GOALS	NURSING INTERVENTIONS
High risk for ineffective breathing pattern: related to anesthetic agents.	• Effective breathing pattern will be evidenced by normal rate and rhythm, depth, and blood gases WNL.	1. Check breathing pattern q15m and prn. 2. Assess and record rate, depth of breath sounds, use of accessory muscles. 3. Monitor oxygen saturation and $ETCO_2$ if intubated. 4. Monitor ABGs. 5. Reposition q2h and prn. 6. Consult physician if ineffective breathing pattern is sustained or impaired gas exchange signs and symptoms present (confusion, restlessness, cyanosis, irritability, abnormal ABG ($\uparrow PCO_2$ and $\downarrow PO_2$).
High risk for ineffective airway clearance: related to depressant anesthetic medications (narcotics and muscle relaxants).	• Maintain patent, clear airway.	1. Maintain airway by jaw thrust, hyperextended neck or repositioning the patient. 2. Insert artificial airway (oral and nasal), if indicated. 3. Differentiate between adult and child airway management. 4. Stir up regimen: cough, deep breathe, turn. 5. Assess for equal breath sounds and bilateral, symmetrical chest excursion. 6. Administer reversal agents, as ordered. 7. Suction prn. Monitor for signs that indicate need for suctioning (dyspnea, increased secretions, excessive coughing, peak pressure alarms if on ventilator). 8. Implement measures to liquefy tenacious secretions.
High risk for impaired gas exchange: related to anesthetic agents.	• Maintain adequate oxygenation and ventilation.	1. Assess respiratory status frequently. Note: • $\uparrow$ rate—compensatory mechanism for hypoxia • Work of breathing—intercostal retraction and nasal flaring reflect increased respiratory effort

(continued)

NURSING CARE PLAN APPENDIX 1–1: (*Continued*)
Recovery From Anesthesia

NURSING DIAGNOSIS	OUTCOME CRITERIA/ PATIENT GOALS	NURSING INTERVENTIONS
		• Presence of adventitious sounds
		• Chest excursion
		• Presence of cyanosis
		2. Monitor cardiac rhythm.
		3. Monitor intake and output.
		4. Administer IV fluids, as indicated.
		5. Assess mechanical ventilator if used.
High risk for altered tissue perfusion: related to the surgical procedures or anesthetic agents.	• Preoperative health status will be restored with controlled vital signs and cardiac rhythm.	1. Accept report from anesthesiologist and assume patient care.
		2. Assess vital signs q15m and prn.
		3. Assess for patent airway.
		4. Assess breath sounds.
		5. Administer oxygen and monitor oxygen saturations with oximeter.
		6. Assess cardiovascular status.
		7. Monitor and analyze rhythm strip on admission and prn.
		8. Note skin condition.
		9. Assess level of consciousness.
		10. Assess regional level when used as anesthetic option.
		11. Assess fluid status.
		12. Monitor intake and output.
		13. Administer IV fluids, as indicated.
		14. Check surgical site.
		15. Monitor laboratory values.
		16. Initiate physician's orders.
High risk for altered tissue perfusion: related to hypotension, decreased cardiac output.	• Maintain systolic blood pressure within 10–20 mm Hg of preoperative status.	1. Notify anesthesiologist/surgeon of decreased blood pressure.
		2. Elevate legs/Trendelenburg if not contraindicated.
		3. Increase IV solutions if not contraindicated.
		4. Check surgical site for bleeding.

(*continued*)

NURSING CARE PLAN APPENDIX 1–1: (Continued)
Recovery From Anesthesia

NURSING DIAGNOSIS	OUTCOME CRITERIA/ PATIENT GOALS	NURSING INTERVENTIONS
		5. Administer medications as ordered.
		6. Monitor cardiac rhythm.
		7. Check for accurate functioning of equipment.
High risk for altered tissue perfusion: related to hypertension.	• Maintain blood pressure within 10–20 mm Hg of preoperative status.	1. Notify anesthesiologist/surgeon of increased blood pressure.
		2. Elevate head of bed if not contraindicated.
		3. Evaluate for cause of hypertension: preop status, fluid status, pain, bladder distention, gastric distention, technical problems (cuff size, transducer, patient's position).
		4. Administer medications, as ordered.
High risk for altered tissue perfusion: related to dysrhythmias.	• Maintain stable cardiac rhythm.	1. Monitor lead II or V_5 to detect ischemia on admission and prn. MCL I may be used for monitoring for bundle branch block.
		2. Notify anesthesiologist/surgeon of dysrhythmia.
		3. Administer drugs, as ordered.
		4. Administer oxygen.
		5. Assess airway for patency.
		6. Offer support and reassurance.
		7. Obtain 12-lead ECG if ordered.
High risk for fluid volume deficit: related to surgical procedure and anesthetic technique.	• Fluid–electrolyte balance will be evidenced by stable blood pressure and adequate intake and output.	1. Monitor for signs and symptoms of fluid volume deficit—assess for: skin turgor, dry mucous membranes, thirst, orthostatic pressure changes, weak thready pulse, urine specific gravity.
		2. Hyponatremia—assess for nausea and vomiting, abdominal cramps, weakness, confusion.
		3. Hypokalemia—assess for irregular pulse, muscle weakness, cramping, nausea and vomiting, drowsiness, dysrhythmias.
		4. Hypochloremia—assess for depressed respiration, twitching, tetanus, dizziness, nervousness, tingling fingers, toes and muscle twitching.

(continued)

NURSING CARE PLAN APPENDIX 1–1: (*Continued*)
Recovery From Anesthesia

NURSING DIAGNOSIS	OUTCOME CRITERIA/ PATIENT GOALS	NURSING INTERVENTIONS
		5. Implement measures to prevent and treat fluid and electrolyte imbalance.
		6. Assess status of fluid intake and output from anesthesia record.
		7. Perform actions to prevent nausea and vomiting and consult physician if signs and symptoms persist.
		8. Administer and maintain IV solutions as indicated.
		9. Administer and note effect of fluid challenges and volume expanding solutions if ordered.
		10. Note presence and types of all drainage systems, the amount and character of drainage, and maintain patency of all tubes.
	• Nausea and vomiting will be minimized.	11. Administer oxygen if indicated.
		12. Suction prn.
		13. Reposition on side for comfort and safety.
		14. Assess and monitor fluid status.
		15. Administer medications, as ordered.
		16. Provide reassurance and support.
		17. Offer oral solutions if appropriate.
High risk for fluid volume excess: related to heart failure, kidney failure, fluids given during surgery.	• Fluid–electrolyte balance will be evidenced by stable BP and heart rate and adequate intake and output.	1. Monitor for signs and symptoms of fluid volume excess: hypertension, change in mental status, crackles, diminished or absent breath sounds, low serum sodium and osmolality, decreased Hct, decreased specific gravity, peripheral edema, distended neck veins.
High risk for altered body temperature: related to hypothermia (body temperature less than 35.0°C [95°F]).	• Maintenance of body temperature within normal limits.	1. Monitor temperature on arrival and every hour if not normothermic.
		2. Monitor patient's ability to shiver—shivering increases oxygen consumption up to 400%.
		3. Apply warm blankets.

(*continued*)

NURSING CARE PLAN APPENDIX 1–1: (Continued)
Recovery From Anesthesia

NURSING DIAGNOSIS	OUTCOME CRITERIA/ PATIENT GOALS	NURSING INTERVENTIONS
		4. Use heat lamps to warm.
		5. Use warm/room-temperature IV solutions.
		6. Use hyperthermic blanket to warm patient.
		7. Cover head with warm blanket.
		8. Administer oxygen, use warm humidified oxygen.
		9. Monitor oxygen saturations and ABGs.
		10. Monitor cardiac rhythm.
		11. Assess level of consciousness.
		12. Administer Demerol, of ordered for shivering.
High risk for altered body temperature: related to hyperthermia (body temperature greater than 39.0°C [102.2°F]).	• Maintain body temperature within normal limits.	1. Apply hypothermia blanket to decrease temperature.
		2. Infuse cool solutions.
		3. Cool sponge baths.
		4. Ice to axilla and groin.
		5. Administer oxygen.
		6. Monitor oxygen saturations with oximeter.
		7. Monitor cardiac rhythm.
		8. Assess level of consciousness.
High risk for altered body temperature: related to malignant hyperthermia.	• Body temperature will be restored to within normal limits.	1. Procure malignant hyperthermia kit and crash cart.
		2. Reconstitute dantrolene.
		3. Administer dantrolene sodium, as ordered.
		4. Cool patient: submerge in ice if child; infuse iced solutions; lavage with cold saline.
		5. Hyperventilate if intubated.
		6. Monitor cardiac rhythm.
		7. Treat dysrhythmia with procainamide.
		8. Monitor ABGs frequently.
		9. Correct acidosis.
		10. Insert Foley catheter.
		11. Administer Lasix and mannitol, as ordered.
		12. Administer other medications, as ordered.

(continued)

NURSING CARE PLAN APPENDIX 1–1: (*Continued*)
Recovery From Anesthesia

NURSING DIAGNOSIS	OUTCOME CRITERIA/ PATIENT GOALS	NURSING INTERVENTIONS
		13. Have monitoring lines available for insertion of CVP, A-line, thermodilution catheter.
		14. Provide emotional support and appropriate explanations to the patient and family.
		15. Encourage follow-up test for patient and other blood relatives.
High risk for altered comfort: related to pain associated with surgical procedure or positioning of patient.	• Pain will be relieved or controlled.	1. Assess vital signs (BP, PR, RR, temp) on admission and q15m.
		2. Assess description, location, and severity of pain.
		3. Administer IV narcotics prn for effect, as ordered.
		4. Discuss availability of pain medications with patient.
		5. Assess and record effectiveness of medications for pain relief.
		6. Position and reposition prn to facilitate comfort.
		7. Observe for minimum of 20 min after narcotic before discharge from PACU.
		8. Offer reassurance and support during immediate postoperative recovery from surgery.
		9. Encourage patient to verbalize discomfort.
		10. Administer oxygen if indicated.
		11. Check circulation if surgery on extremity; check peripheral pulse; check color and temperature; check sensation.
		12. Check for level of regional anesthetic and reassure patient sensation and movement will return.
		13. If spinal/epidural: motor and sensory must return before discharge from unit—must be able to lift hips off bed.
		14. Promote safe environment with adequate functioning equipment; side rails up.

(*continued*)

NURSING CARE PLAN APPENDIX 1–1: (Continued)
Recovery From Anesthesia

NURSING DIAGNOSIS	OUTCOME CRITERIA/ PATIENT GOALS	NURSING INTERVENTIONS
High risk for anxiety: related to critical illness, fear of death or disfigurement, role changes within social setting, or permanent disability.	• Patient will begin to identify source of anxiety.	1. Provide environment that encourages open discussion of emotional issues. 2. Mobilize patient's support system and involve these resources as appropriate. 3. Allow time for patient to express self. 4. Identify possible hospital resources for patient/family support. 5. Encourage open family-to-nurse communications regarding emotional issues. 6. Validate patient and family knowledge base regarding the critical illness. 7. Involve religious support systems as appropriate.

REFERENCES

1. American Society of Post Anesthesia Nurses: Standards of Post Anesthesia Nursing Practice. Philadelphia, WB Saunders, 1992
2. Davidson J: Neuromuscular blockers. Focus on Critical Care 18:512–520, 1991
3. Dripps RD, Eckenhoff JE, Vandam RD: Introduction to Anesthesia: The Principles of Safe Practice, 7th ed. Philadelphia, WB Saunders, 1988
4. Breslow M, Miller C, Rogers M: Perioperative Management. St. Louis, CV Mosby, 1990
5. Rosenberg H: The hotline. The Communicator IX(3):2, 1991
6. Syntex Laboratories, Inc.: Toradol. Palo Alto, CA, Syntex Laboratories, Inc., 1991
7. Covino BG, Scott DB: Handbook of Epidural Anaesthesia and Analgesia. Orlando FL, Grune & Stratton, Inc., 1985
8. Bragg C: Interpleural analgesia. Heart Lung 20:30–38, 1991
9. Gilbert H: Pain relief methods in the PACU. Journal of Post Anesthesia Nursing 5:(1):6–15, 1990
10. Vender J, Spiess BD: Post Anesthesia Care. Philadelphia, WB Saunders, 1992

BIBLIOGRAPHY

Chien B, Burke R, Hunter D: An extensive experience with postoperative pain relief using postoperative fentanyl infusion. Arch Surg 126:692–695, 1991
Karch AK: Handbook of Drugs and the Nursing Process. Philadelphia, JB Lippincott, 1992
Shevde K, Panagopoulos G: A survery of 800 patients' knowledge, attitudes, and concerns regarding anesthesia. Anesth Analg 73:190–198, 1991
Suddarth DS: The Lippincott Manual of Nursing Practice. Philadelphia, JB Lippincott, 1991
Wild L, Coyne C: Epidural analgesia: The basics and beyond. Am J Nurs 92(4):26–34, 1992

**STUDY
QUESTIONS**

1. Which of the following medications should be kept at the bedside of the patient who has received epidural narcotics?

   a. naloxone and morphine
   b. naloxone and ephedrine
   c. dopamine and nitroglycerine
   d. benadryl and droperidol

2. One of the earliest warming signs for malignant hyperthermia after the administration of succinylcholine is

   a. elevated temperature
   b. cyanosis
   c. diaphoresis
   d. masseter muscle rigidity

3. Nondepolarizing muscle relaxants may be reversed with

   a. anticholinesterase medications
   b. narcotics
   c. depolarizing muscle relaxants
   d. acetylcholine

APPENDIX 2

Answer Key to Study Questions

Chapter 1 Integrating Nursing Process and Nursing Diagnosis Within a Holistic Framework

1. d
2. d
3. d

Chapter 2 Psychosocial Concepts and the Patient's Experience With Critical Illness

1. d
2. b
3. d
4. d
5. d
6. a
7. a

Chapter 3 Caring for the Patient's Family

1. c
2. a
3. d
4. d
5. c
6. c

Chapter 4 Psychosocial Impact of the Critical Care Environment

1. b
2. c
3. a
4. d
5. c

Chapter 5 The Dynamics of Touch in Patient Care

1. c
2. d
3. b
4. d

Chapter 6 Patient and Family Teaching

1. a
2. d
3. b
4. d
5. c

Chapter 7 The Critically Ill Elderly Patient

1. a
2. c
3. b
4. d
5. c
6. b

Chapter 8 Bioethical Issues in Critical Care

1. d
2. d
3. b
4. a
5. b

Chapter 9 Applied Legal Principles

1. a
2. c
3. c
4. a

Chapter 10 Effects of the Critical Care Unit on the Nurse

1. c
2. b
3. a
4. d

Chapter 11 Anatomy and Physiology of the Cardiovascular System

1. c
2. a
3. d
4. b

Hudak: Critical Care Nursing:
A Holistic Approach, 6th ed. © 1994
J. B. Lippincott Company.

Chapter 12 Assessment: Cardiovascular System
Auscultation of the Heart

1. d   *3.* c
2. d

Cardiac Enzyme Studies

1. c   *2.* a

Cardiovascular Diagnostic Techniques

1. c   *3.* d
2. b

Electrocardiographic Monitoring

1. b   *3.* a
2. c

Dysrhythmias and Conduction Disturbances

1. c   *3.* a
2. d   *4.* b

Effects of Serum Electrolytes on the ECG

1. c   *2.* b

Hemodynamic Monitoring

1. b   *4.* c
2. d   *5.* d
3. b   *6.* b

Chapter 13 Management Modalities: Cardiovascular System
Cardiac Pacing

1. c   *3.* c
2. c

Commonly Used Antiarrhythmic Agents and Cardioversion

1. c   *3.* b
2. a   *4.* d

PTCA and PBV

1. c   *3.* b
2. a   *4.* d

IABP and Other Ventricular Assist Devices

1. b   *3.* c
2. c

Autologous Blood Transfusion

1. c, d   *3.* a
2. a, b, c, d   *4.* b

Cardiopulmonary Resuscitation

1. c   *3.* c
2. d

Chapter 14 Heart Failure

1. b   *3.* a
2. c   *4.* a

Chapter 15 Acute Myocardial Infarction

1. d   *4.* b
2. b   *5.* c
3. c

Chapter 16 Cardiac Surgery and Heart Transplantation

1. c   *4.* d
2. b   *5.* a
3. d   *6.* c

Chapter 17 Anatomy and Physiology of the Respiratory System

1. a   *3.* b
2. c   *4.* d

Chapter 18 Assessment: Respiratory System

1. c   *4.* b
2. a   *5.* a
3. d   *6.* b

Chapter 19 Management Modalities: Respiratory System
Bronchial Hygiene

1. c   *3.* a
2. a & d

Artificial Airways

1. d   *2.* c

Chest Tubes

1. c   *3.* b
2. d

Pharmacologic Agents

1. b   *2.* c

Ventilatory Support

1. d   *4.* c
2. c   *5.* d
3. d

Chapter 20 Common Pulmonary Disorders

1. c   *3.* b
2. a   *4.* d

Chapter 21 Adult Respiratory Distress Syndrome

1. a   *3.* b
2. c   *4.* c

Chapter 22 Anatomy and Physiology of the Renal System

1. b   *3.* b
2. c   *4.* a

Chapter 23 Assessment: Renal System

1. c   *3.* b
2. a   *4.* a

Chapter 24 Management Modalities: Renal System

1. b   6. d
2. c   7. b
3. c   8. a
4. d   9. c
5. a   10. b

Chapter 25 Acute Renal Failure

1. d   5. b
2. c   6. d
3. a   7. b
4. d

Chapter 26 Renal Transplantation

1. d   4. c
2. d   5. a
3. a   6. c

Chapter 27 Anatomy and Physiology of the Nervous System

1. b   4. a
2. d   5. c
3. c   6. d

Chapter 28 Assessment: Nervous System

1. d   4. d
2. a   5. b
3. c   6. c

Chapter 29 Management Modalities: Nervous System Intracranial Pressure Monitoring

1. b   5. c
2. d   6. a
3. b   7. c
4. a   8. a

Hypothermia

1. d   3. d
2. d

Chapter 30 Head Injury

1. d   4. c
2. a   5. c
3. b

Chapter 31 Common Neurologic Disorders

1. b   4. b
2. c   5. a
3. c   6. d

Chapter 32 Spinal Cord Injury

1. b   5. c
2. a   6. d
3. c   7. b
4. d

Chapter 33 Anatomy and Physiology of the Gastrointestinal System

1. a   3. b
2. c   4. b

Chapter 34 Assessment: Gastrointestinal System

1. b   3. b
2. a   4. d

Chapter 35 Management Modalities: Gastrointestinal System

1. d   3. c
2. a   4. c

Chapter 36 Acute Gastrointestinal Bleeding

1. c   3. b
2. c

Chapter 37 Hepatic Disorders

1. c   3. c
2. a   4. d

Chapter 38 Acute Pancreatitis

1. b   4. c
2. d   5. d
3. c

Chapter 39 Anatomy and Physiology of the Endocrine System

1. d   4. a
2. c   5. a
3. b

Chapter 40 Diabetic Emergencies

1. b   6. d
2. c   7. c
3. b   8. d
4. a   9. a
5. a

Chapter 41 Common Endocrine Emergencies

1. a   3. d
2. b

Chapter 42 Septic Shock

1. d   4. a
2. c   5. c
3. b   6. b

Chapter 43 Disseminated Intravascular Coagulation

1. c   3. d
2. a

Chapter 44 Trauma

1. b   5. d
2. c   6. a
3. a   7. d
4. d   8. b

Chapter 45 Burns

1.	b	*6.*	c
2.	c	*7.*	c
3.	b	*8.*	c
4.	b	*9.*	c
5.	a	*10.*	b

Chapter 46 Drug Overdose and Poisoning

1.	d	*4.*	b
2.	c	*5.*	d
3.	b	*6.*	d

Chapter 47 Immune System-Compromising Conditions

1.	d	*4.*	a
2.	b	*5.*	c
3.	c		

Appendix I Recovery From Anesthesia

1.	b	*3.*	a
2.	d		

APPENDIX 3

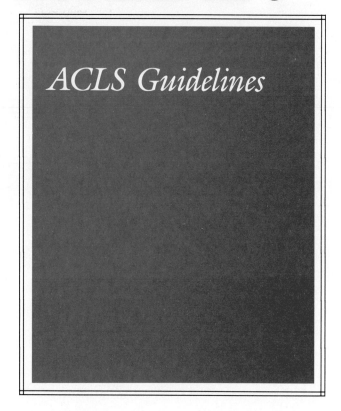

ACLS Guidelines

Hudak: Critical Care Nursing:
A Holistic Approach, 6th ed. © 1994
J. B. Lippincott Company.

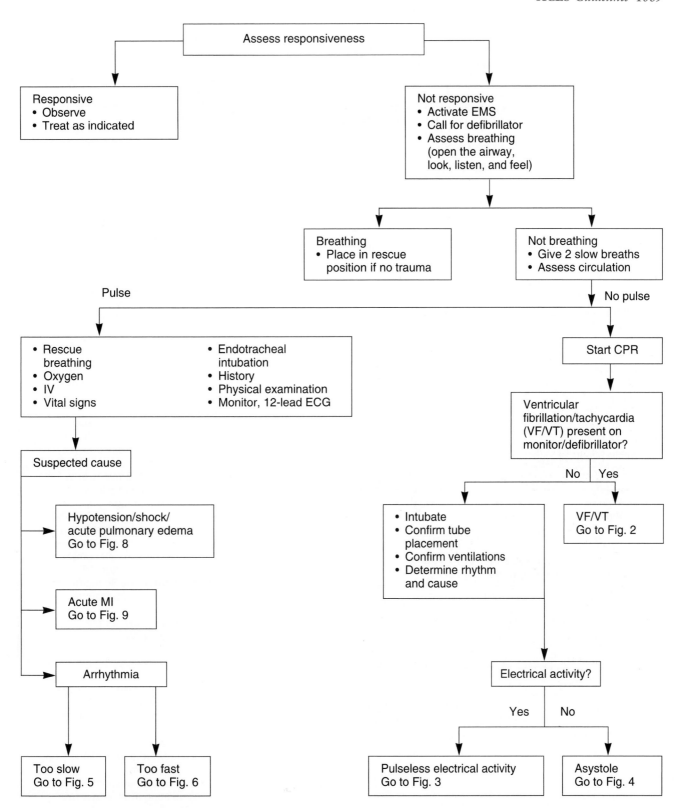

Fig. 1.—Universal algorithm for adult emergency cardiac care (ECC). (JAMA 286[16]:2216.)

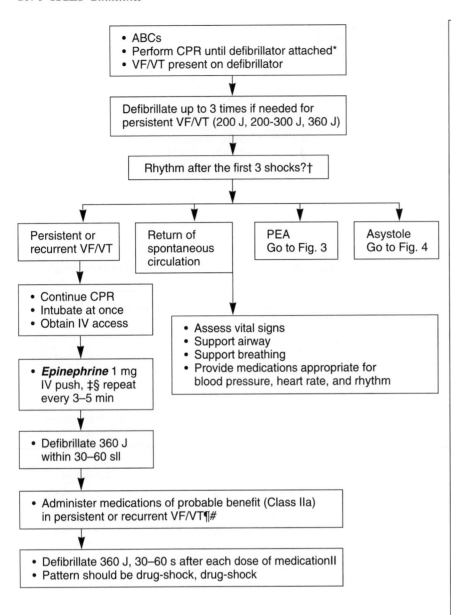

- ABCs
- Perform CPR until defibrillator attached*
- VF/VT present on defibrillator

↓

Defibrillate up to 3 times if needed for persistent VF/VT (200 J, 200-300 J, 360 J)

↓

Rhythm after the first 3 shocks?†

| Persistent or recurrent VF/VT | Return of spontaneous circulation | PEA Go to Fig. 3 | Asystole Go to Fig. 4 |

Persistent or recurrent VF/VT:

- Continue CPR
- Intubate at once
- Obtain IV access

↓

- *Epinephrine* 1 mg IV push, ‡§ repeat every 3–5 min

↓

- Defibrillate 360 J within 30–60 s‖

↓

- Administer medications of probable benefit (Class IIa) in persistent or recurrent VF/VT¶#

↓

- Defibrillate 360 J, 30–60 s after each dose of medication‖
- Pattern should be drug-shock, drug-shock

Return of spontaneous circulation:

- Assess vital signs
- Support airway
- Support breathing
- Provide medications appropriate for blood pressure, heart rate, and rhythm

Class I: definitely helpful
Class IIa: acceptable, probably helpful
Class IIb: acceptable, possibly helpful
Class III: not indicated, may be harmful

* Precordial thump is a Class IIb action in witnessed arrest, no pulse, and no defibrillator immediately available.

† Hypothermic cardiac arrest is treated differently after this point. See section on hypothermia.

‡ The recommended dose of *epinephrine* is 1 mg IV push every 3–5 min. If this approach fails, several Class IIb dosing regimens can be considered:
- Intermediate: *epinephrine* 2–5 mg IV push, every 3–5 min
- Escalating: *epinephrine* 1 mg–3 mg–5 mg IV push (3 min apart)
- High: *epinephrine* 0.1mg/kg IV push, every 3–5 min

§ *Sodium bicarbonate* (1 mEq/kg) is Class I if patient has known preexisting hyperkalemia.

‖ Multiple sequenced shocks (200 J, 200–300 J, 360 J) are acceptable here (Class I), especially when medications are delayed.

¶ • *Lidocaine* 1.5 mg/kg IV push. Repeat in 3–5 min to total loading dose of 3 mg/kg; then use
- *Bretylium* 5 mg/kg IV push. Repeat in 5 min at 10 mg/kg
- *Magnesium sulfate* 1–2 g IV in torsades de pointes or suspected hypomagnesemic state or severe refractory VF
- *Procainamide* 30 mg/min in refractory VF (maximum total 17 mg/kg)

• *Sodium bicarbonate* (1 mEq/kg IV):
Class IIa
- if known preexisting bicarbonate-responsive acidosis
- if overdose with tricyclic antidepressants
- to alkalinize the urine in drug overdoses
Class IIb
- if intubated and continued long arrest interval
- upon return of spontaneous circulation after long arrest interval
Class III
- hypoxic lactic acidosis

Fig. 2.—Algorithm for ventricular fibrillation and pulseless ventricular tachycardia (VF/VT). (JAMA 268[16]:2217.)

PEA includes
- Electromechanical dissociation (EMD)
- Pseudo-EMD
- Idioventricular rhythms
- Ventricular escape rhythms
- Bradyasystolic rhythms
- Postdefibrillation idioventricular rhythms

- Continue CPR
- Intubate at once
- Obtain IV access
- Assess blood flow using Doppler ultrasound

Consider possible causes
(Parentheses=possible therapies and treatments)
- Hypovolemia (volume infusion)
- Hypoxia (ventilation)
- Cardiac tamponade (pericardiocentesis)
- Tension pneumothorax (needle decompression)
- Hypothermia (see hypothermia algorithm, Section IV)
- Massive pulmonary embolism (surgery, **thrombolytics**)
- Drug overdoses such as tricyclics, digitalis, ß-blockers, calcium channel blockers
- Hyperkalemia*
- Acidosis†
- Massive acute myocardial infarction (go to Fig. 9)

- **Epinephrine** 1 mg IV push, *‡repeat every 3–5 min

- If absolute bradycardia (<60 beats/min) or relative bradycardia, give **atropine** 1 mg IV
- Repeat every 3–5 min up to a total of 0.04 mg/kg§

Class I: definitely helpful
Class IIa: acceptable, probably helpful
Class IIb: acceptable, possibly helpful
Class III: not indicated, may be harmful
***Sodium bicarbonate** 1 mEq/kg is Class I if patient has known preexisting hyperkalemia.
†**Sodium bicarbonate** 1 mEq/kg:
 Class IIa
 • if known preexisting bicarbonate-responsive acidosis
 • if overdose with tricyclic antidepressants
 • to alkalinize the urine in drug overdoses
 Class IIb
 • if intubated and long arrest interval
 • upon return of spontaneous circulation after long arrest interval
 Class III
 • hypoxic lactic acidosis
‡The recommended dose of **epinephrine** is 1 mg IV push every 3–5 min.
 If this approach fails, several Class IIb dosing regimens can be considered.
 • Intermediate: **epinephrine** 2–5 mg IV push, every 3–5 min
 • Escalating: **epinephrine** 1 mg–3 mg–5 mg IV push (3 min apart)
 • High: **epinephrine** 0.1 mg/kg IV push, every 3–5 min
§Shorter **atropine** dosing intervals are possibly helpful in cardiac arrest (Class IIb).

Fig. 3.—Algorithm for pulseless electrical activity (PEA) (electromechanical dissociation [EMD]). (JAMA 268[16]:2219.)

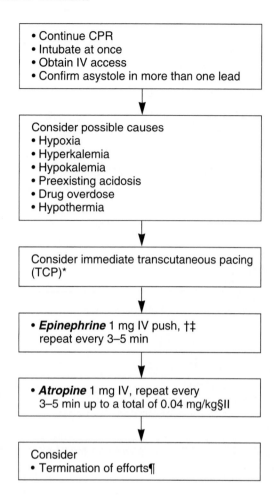

- Continue CPR
- Intubate at once
- Obtain IV access
- Confirm asystole in more than one lead

Consider possible causes
- Hypoxia
- Hyperkalemia
- Hypokalemia
- Preexisting acidosis
- Drug overdose
- Hypothermia

Consider immediate transcutaneous pacing (TCP)*

- *Epinephrine* 1 mg IV push, †‡ repeat every 3–5 min

- *Atropine* 1 mg IV, repeat every 3–5 min up to a total of 0.04 mg/kg§II

Consider
- Termination of efforts¶

Class I: definitely helpful
Class IIa: acceptable, probably helpful
Class IIb: acceptable, possibly helpful
Class III: not indicated, may be harmful
* TCP is a Class IIb intervention. Lack of success may be due to delays in pacing. To be effective TCP must be performed early, simultaneously with drugs. Evidence does not support routine use of TCP for asystole.
†The recommended dose of *epinephrine* is 1 mg IV push every 3–5 min. If this approach fails, several Class IIb dosing regimens can be considered:
- Intermediate: *epinephrine* 2–5 mg IV push, every 3–5 min
- Escalating: *epinephrine* 1 mg–3 mg–5 mg IV push (3 min apart)
- High: *epinephrine* 0.1 mg/kg IV push, every 3–5 min
‡ *Sodium bicarbonate* 1 mEq/kg is Class I if patient has known preexisting hyperkalemia.
§Shorter *atropine* dosing intervals are Class IIb in asystolic arrest.
II *Sodium bicarbonate* 1 mEq/kg:
Class IIa
- if known preexisting bicarbonate-responsive acidosis
- if overdose with tricyclic antidepressants
- to alkalinize the urine in drug overdoses
Class IIb
- if intubated and continued long arrest interval
- upon return of spontaneous circulation after long arrest interval
Class III
¶ If patient remains in asystole or other agonal rhythms after successful intubation and initial medications and no reversible causes are identified, consider termination of resuscitative efforts by a physician. Consider interval since arrest.

Fig. 4.—Asystole treatment algorithm. (JAMA 286[16]:2220.)

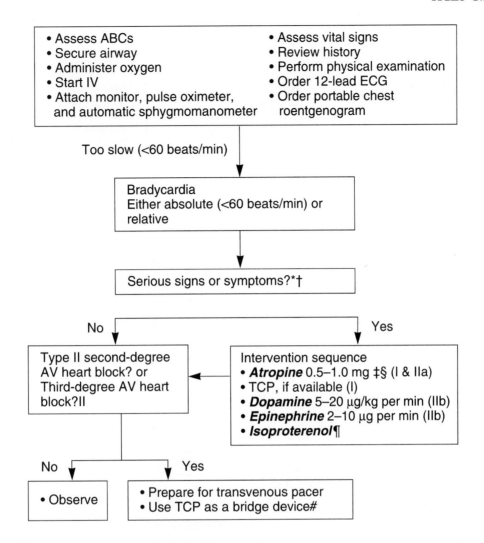

* Assess ABCs
* Secure airway
* Administer oxygen
* Start IV
* Attach monitor, pulse oximeter, and automatic sphygmomanometer

* Assess vital signs
* Review history
* Perform physical examination
* Order 12-lead ECG
* Order portable chest roentgenogram

Too slow (<60 beats/min)

Bradycardia
Either absolute (<60 beats/min) or relative

Serious signs or symptoms?*†

No

Type II second-degree AV heart block? or Third-degree AV heart block?||

Yes

Intervention sequence
* *Atropine* 0.5–1.0 mg ‡§ (I & IIa)
* TCP, if available (I)
* *Dopamine* 5–20 µg/kg per min (IIb)
* *Epinephrine* 2–10 µg per min (IIb)
* *Isoproterenol*¶

No

* Observe

Yes

* Prepare for transvenous pacer
* Use TCP as a bridge device#

* Serious signs or symptoms must be related to the slow rate. Clinical manifestations include:
  symptoms (chest pain, shortness of breath, decreased level of consciousness) and
  signs (low BP, shock, pulmonary congestion, CHF, acute MI).
†Do not delay TCP while awaiting IV access or for *atropine* to take effect if patient is symptomatic.
‡Denervated transplanted hearts will not respond to *atropine*. Go at once to pacing, *catecholamine* infusion, or both.
§*Atropine* should be given in repeat doses in 3–5 min up to total of 0.04 mg/kg. Consider shorter dosing intervals in severe clinical conditions. It has been suggested that atropine should be used with caution in atrioventricular (AV) block at the His-Purkinje level (type II AV block and new third-degree block with wide QRS complexes) (Class IIb).
||Never treat third-degree heart block plus ventricular escape beats with *lidocaine*.
¶*Isoproterenol* should be used, if at all, with extreme caution. At low doses it is Class IIb (possibly helpful); at higher doses it is Class III (harmful).
#Verify patient tolerance and mechanical capture. Use analgesia and sedation as needed.

Fig. 5.—Bradycardia algorithm (with the patient not in cardiac arrest). (JAMA 268[16]:2221.)

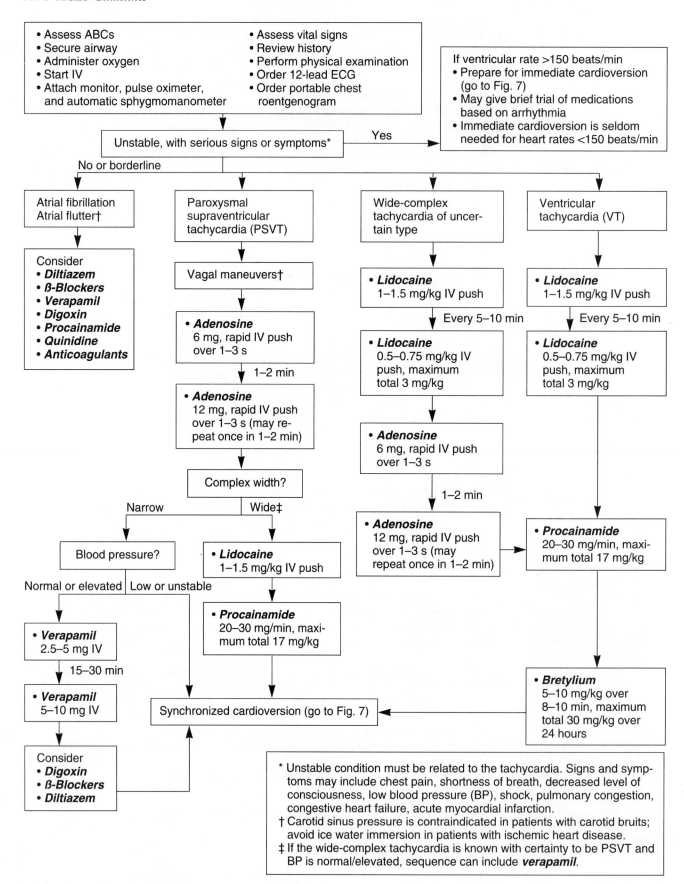

Fig. 6.—Tachycardia algorithm. (JAMA 268[16]:2223.)

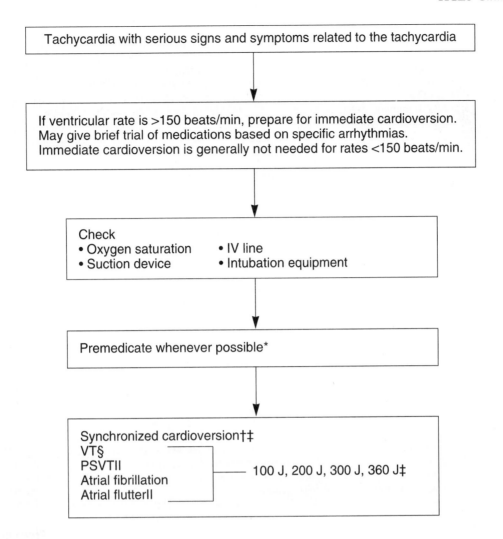

* Effective regimens have included a sedative (eg, *diazepam, midazolam, barbiturates, etomidate, keta-mine, methohexital*) with or without an analgesic agent (eg, *fentanyl, morphine, meperidine*).
  Many experts recommend anesthesia if service is readily available.
†Note possible need to resynchronize after each cardioversion.
‡If delays in synchronization occur and clinical conditions are critical, go to immediate unsynchronized shocks.
§Treat polymorphic VT (irregular form and rate) like VF: 200 J, 200–300 J, 360 J.
IIPSVT and atrial flutter often respond to lower energy levels (start with 50 J).

Fig. 7.—Electrical cardioversion algorithm (with the patient not in cardiac arrest). (JAMA 268[16]:2224.)

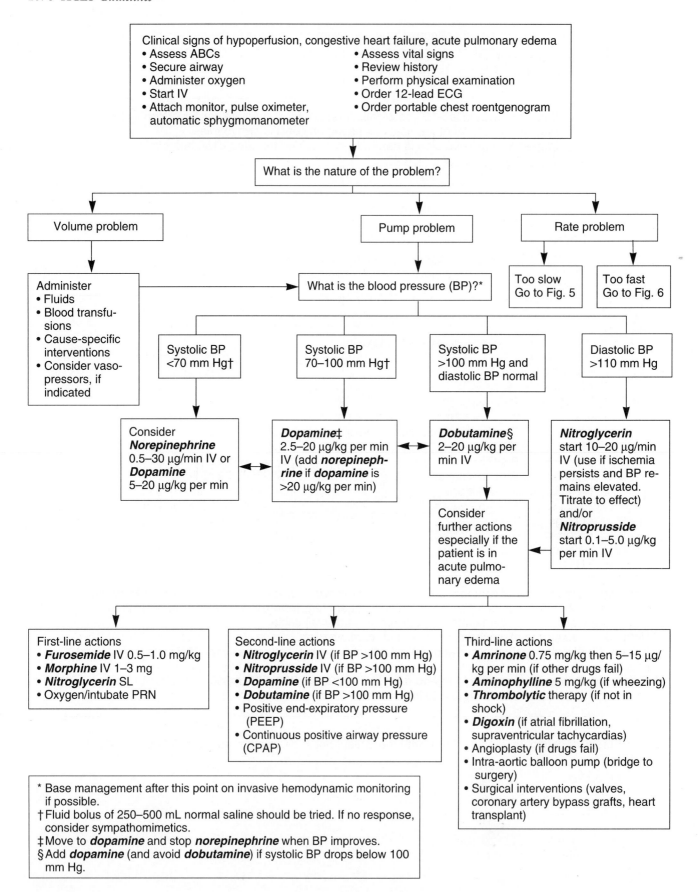

Fig. 8.—Algorithm for hypotension, shock, and acute pulmonary edema. (JAMA 268[16]:2227.)

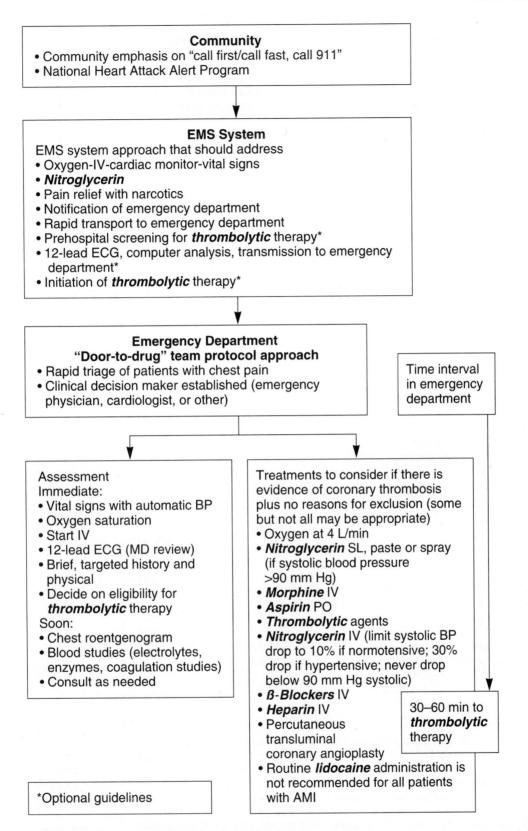

Community
- Community emphasis on "call first/call fast, call 911"
- National Heart Attack Alert Program

EMS System
EMS system approach that should address
- Oxygen-IV-cardiac monitor-vital signs
- *Nitroglycerin*
- Pain relief with narcotics
- Notification of emergency department
- Rapid transport to emergency department
- Prehospital screening for *thrombolytic* therapy*
- 12-lead ECG, computer analysis, transmission to emergency department*
- Initiation of *thrombolytic* therapy*

**Emergency Department
"Door-to-drug" team protocol approach**
- Rapid triage of patients with chest pain
- Clinical decision maker established (emergency physician, cardiologist, or other)

Time interval in emergency department

Assessment
Immediate:
- Vital signs with automatic BP
- Oxygen saturation
- Start IV
- 12-lead ECG (MD review)
- Brief, targeted history and physical
- Decide on eligibility for *thrombolytic* therapy
Soon:
- Chest roentgenogram
- Blood studies (electrolytes, enzymes, coagulation studies)
- Consult as needed

Treatments to consider if there is evidence of coronary thrombosis plus no reasons for exclusion (some but not all may be appropriate)
- Oxygen at 4 L/min
- *Nitroglycerin* SL, paste or spray (if systolic blood pressure >90 mm Hg)
- *Morphine* IV
- *Aspirin* PO
- *Thrombolytic* agents
- *Nitroglycerin* IV (limit systolic BP drop to 10% if normotensive; 30% drop if hypertensive; never drop below 90 mm Hg systolic)
- *ß-Blockers* IV
- *Heparin* IV
- Percutaneous transluminal coronary angioplasty
- Routine *lidocaine* administration is not recommended for all patients with AMI

30–60 min to *thrombolytic* therapy

*Optional guidelines

Fig. 9.—Acute myocardial infarction (AMI) algorithm. Recommendations for early treatment of patients with chest pain and possible AMI. (JAMA 268[16]:2230.)

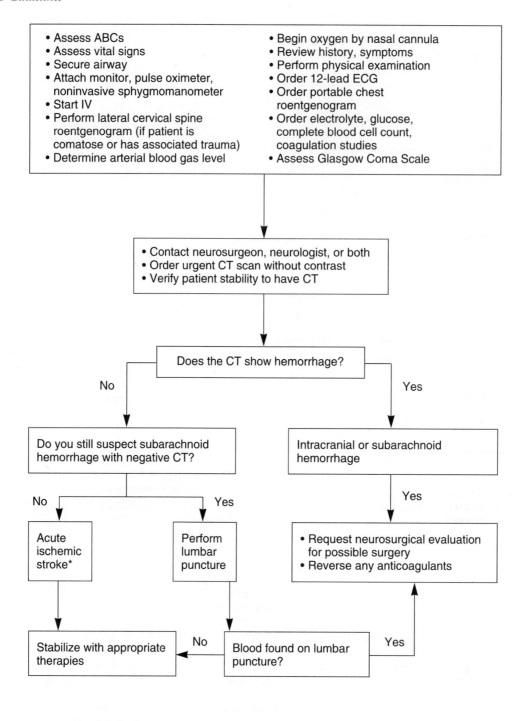

Fig. 10.—Algorithm for initial evaluation of suspected stroke. (JAMA 268[16]:2243.)

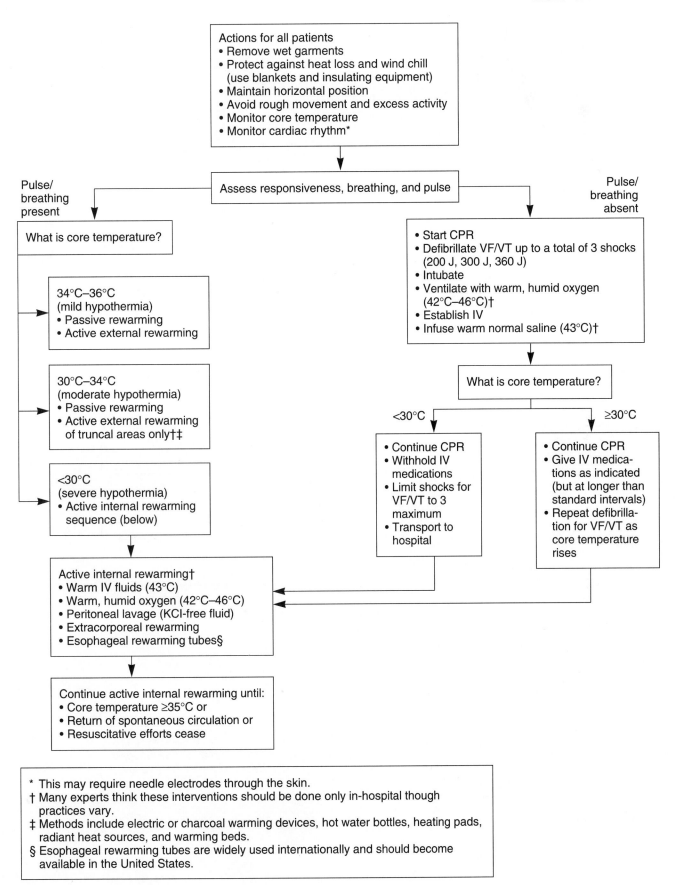

Actions for all patients
• Remove wet garments
• Protect against heat loss and wind chill
  (use blankets and insulating equipment)
• Maintain horizontal position
• Avoid rough movement and excess activity
• Monitor core temperature
• Monitor cardiac rhythm*

Assess responsiveness, breathing, and pulse

Pulse/
breathing
present

What is core temperature?

34°C–36°C
(mild hypothermia)
• Passive rewarming
• Active external rewarming

30°C–34°C
(moderate hypothermia)
• Passive rewarming
• Active external rewarming
  of truncal areas only†‡

<30°C
(severe hypothermia)
• Active internal rewarming
  sequence (below)

Pulse/
breathing
absent

• Start CPR
• Defibrillate VF/VT up to a total of 3 shocks
  (200 J, 300 J, 360 J)
• Intubate
• Ventilate with warm, humid oxygen
  (42°C–46°C)†
• Establish IV
• Infuse warm normal saline (43°C)†

What is core temperature?

<30°C

• Continue CPR
• Withhold IV
  medications
• Limit shocks for
  VF/VT to 3
  maximum
• Transport to
  hospital

≥30°C

• Continue CPR
• Give IV medica-
  tions as indicated
  (but at longer than
  standard intervals)
• Repeat defibrilla-
  tion for VF/VT as
  core temperature
  rises

Active internal rewarming†
• Warm IV fluids (43°C)
• Warm, humid oxygen (42°C–46°C)
• Peritoneal lavage (KCI-free fluid)
• Extracorporeal rewarming
• Esophageal rewarming tubes§

Continue active internal rewarming until:
• Core temperature ≥35°C or
• Return of spontaneous circulation or
• Resuscitative efforts cease

* This may require needle electrodes through the skin.
† Many experts think these interventions should be done only in-hospital though
  practices vary.
‡ Methods include electric or charcoal warming devices, hot water bottles, heating pads,
  radiant heat sources, and warming beds.
§ Esophageal rewarming tubes are widely used internationally and should become
  available in the United States.

Fig. 11.—Algorithm for treatment of hypothermia. (JAMA 268[16]:2245.)

Index